Rheumatoid Arthritis

Rheumatoid Arthritis

EDITORS

E. William St. Clair, MD
Professor of Medicine and Immunology
Departments of Medicine and Immunology
Division of Rheumatology and Immunology
Duke University Medical Center
Durham, North Carolina

David S. Pisetsky, MD, PHD
Professor of Medicine and Immunology
Departments of Medicine and Immunology
Division of Rheumatology and Immunology
Chief of Rheumatology and Immunology
Duke University Medical Center
Durham VA Medical Center
Durham, North Carolina

Barton F. Haynes, MD
Frederic M. Hanes Professor of Medicine
Professor of Immunology
Departments of Medicine and Immunology
Duke University School of Medicine
Director
Human Vaccine Institute
Duke University Medical Center
Durham, North Carolina

WITH CONTRIBUTING AUTHORS

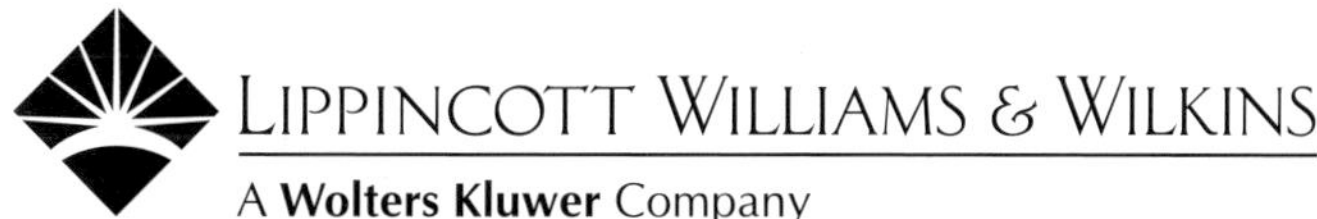

Philadelphia • Baltimore • New York • London
Buenos Aires • Hong Kong • Sydney • Tokyo

Acquisitions Editor: Danette Somers
Developmental Editor: Lisa Consoli
Supervising Editor: Mary Ann McLaughlin
Production Editor: Kate Sallwasser, Silverchair Science + Communications
Manufacturing Manager: Colin Warnock
Cover Designer: Brian Crede
Compositor: Silverchair Science + Communications
Printer: Quebecor World-Kingsport

530 Walnut Street
Philadelphia, PA 19106 USA
LWW.com

Printed in the USA

Library of Congress Cataloging-in-Publication Data

Rheumatoid arthritis / edited by E. William St. Clair, David S. Pisetsky, Barton F. Haynes ; with contributing authors.
p. ; cm.
Includes bibliographical references.
ISBN 0-7817-4149-1
1. Rheumatoid arthritis. I. St. Clair, E. William. II. Pisetsky, David S. III. Haynes, Barton F.
[DNLM: 1. Arthritis, Rheumatoid. WE 346 R469 2004]
RC933.R39 2004
616.7'227--dc22
2004006104

---

10 9 8 7 6 5 4 3 2 1

To my lovely wife, Barbara, and my daughters, Becky and Sarah
—E.W.S

To my wife, Ingrid, and my children, Michael and Emily
—D.S.P.

To my partner and wife, Caroline, and my children, Charlotte, Ben, and Laura
—B.F.H.

Contents

Contributing Authors

Steven B. Abramson, MD
Professor of Medicine and Pathology
Department of Medicine
Division of Rheumatology
New York University School of Medicine
New York, New York

Graciela S. Alarcón, MD, MPH
Jane Knight Lowe Chair of Medicine in Rheumatology
Department of Medicine
Division of Clinical Immunology and Rheumatology
University of Alabama School of Medicine
Birmingham, Alabama

Ronald J. Anderson, MD
Associate Professor
Department of Medicine
Division of Rheumatology, Immunology, and Allergy
Harvard Medical School
Brigham and Women's Hospital
Boston, Massachusetts

Evangelos T. H. Andreakos, BSc, DIC, PhD
Senior Research Fellow
Kennedy Institute of Rheumatology Division
Imperial College London Faculty of Medicine
London, United Kingdom

William P. Arend, MD
Scoville Professor of Rheumatology
Department of Medicine
University of Colorado School of Medicine
Denver, Colorado

John Patterson Atkinson, MD
Samuel B. Grant Professor of Medicine, Professor of Molecular Biology
Department of Medicine
Division of Rheumatology
Washington University School of Medicine
St. Louis, Missouri

Catherine L. Backman, PhD, OT(C)
Associate Professor
School of Rehabilitation Sciences
University of British Columbia Faculty of Medicine
Research Scientist
Arthritis Research Centre of Canada
Vancouver, British Columbia, Canada

Philip E. Blazar, MD
Assistant Professor of Orthopaedic Surgery
Department of Orthopaedics
Harvard Medical School
Brigham and Women's Hospital
Boston, Massachusetts

Ferdinand C. Breedveld, MD
Professor
Department of Rheumatology
Leiden University Medical Center
Leiden, The Netherlands

Fionula M. Brennan, BSc, PhD
Professor of Cytokine Immunopathology
Kennedy Institute of Rheumatology Division
Imperial College London Faculty of Medicine
London, United Kingdom

S. Louis Bridges, Jr., MD, PhD
Associate Professor
Departments of Medicine and Microbiology
University of Alabama School of Medicine
Birmingham, Alabama

Nathalie D. Burg, MD
Postdoctoral Fellow
Laboratory of Blood and Vascular Biology
The Rockefeller University
New York, New York

Lisa C. Campbell, PhD
Department of Psychiatry and Behavioral Sciences
Duke University Medical Center
Durham, North Carolina

Grant W. Cannon, MD
Professor of Medicine
Division of Rheumatology
University of Utah School of Medicine
Associate Chief of Staff for Academic Affiliations
VA Salt Lake City Health Care System
Salt Lake City, Utah

Wayne K. Cheng, MD
Instructor
Department of Orthopaedics
Loma Linda University Medical Center
Loma Linda, California

Philip G. Conaghan, MB, MS, FRACP
Senior Lecturer
Department of Musculoskeletal Disease
University of Leeds School of Medicine
Honorary Consultant
Leeds General Infirmary
Leeds, United Kingdom

R. Lee Cothran, Jr., MD
Clinical Associate
Department of Radiology
Duke University School of Medicine
Duke University Medical Center
Durham, North Carolina

Leslie J. Crofford, MD
Associate Professor
Department of Internal Medicine
University of Michigan Medical School
Ann Arbor, Michigan

Anne Davidson, MBBS
Professor
Departments of Medicine and Microbiology and Immunology
Albert Einstein College of Medicine of Yeshiva University
Bronx, New York

Paola de Pablo, MD, MPH
Postdoctoral Fellow
Department of Rheumatology, Immunology, and Allergy
Harvard Medical School
Brigham and Women's Hospital
Boston, Massachusetts

Mark E. Easley, MD
Assistant Professor of Surgery
Department of Orthopaedic Surgery
Duke University Medical Center
Durham, North Carolina

Paul Emery, MA, MD, FRCP
ARC Professor of Rheumatology
Head of Academic Unit of Musculoskeletal Disease
Department of Musculoskeletal Disease
University of Leeds Medical School
Clinical Director
Leeds Teaching Hospitals Trust
Leeds, United Kingdom

Angela Fairleigh, OT (Reg) BC
Department of Occupational Therapy
Mary Pack Arthritis Centre
Vancouver General Hospital
Vancouver, British Columbia, Canada

Marc Feldmann, MBBS, BSc, PhD, FRCP, FRCPath
Professor of Immunology
Kennedy Institute of Rheumatology Division
Imperial College London Faculty of Medicine
London, United Kingdom

Beverley F. Fermor, PhD
Assistant Professor
Department of Surgery
Duke University Medical Center
Durham, North Carolina

Brian M. J. Foxwell, BSc, PhD
Professor of Immune Cell Signaling
Department of Cytokine Biology and Cellular Immunology
Imperial College London Faculty of Medicine
London, United Kingdom

Daniel E. Furst, AB, MD
Carl M. Pearson Professor of Rheumatology
Department of Rheumatology
University of California, Los Angeles, David Geffen School of Medicine at UCLA
Los Angeles, California

Cem Gabay, MD
Associate Professor of Medicine
Departments of Internal Medicine and Pathology/Immunology
Division of Rheumatology
University Hospital of Geneva
Geneva, Switzerland

Sherine E. Gabriel, MD, MSc
Professor of Medicine (Rheumatology) and Epidemiology
Department of Health Sciences Research

Mayo Clinic
Rochester, Minnesota

Renate E. Gay, MD
Professor of Experimental Rheumatology
Department of Rheumatology
University of Zurich
University Hospital
Zurich, Switzerland

Steffen Gay, MD
Professor of Experimental Rheumatology
Department of Rheumatology
University of Zurich
University Hospital
Zurich, Switzerland

Mary B. Goldring, PhD
Division of Rheumatology
Beth Israel Deaconess Medical Center
New England Baptist Bone & Joint Institute
Boston, Massachusetts

Steven R. Goldring, MD
Division of Rheumatology
Beth Israel Deaconess Medical Center
New England Baptist Bone & Joint Institute
Boston, Massachusetts

Jörg J. Goronzy, MD, PhD
Professor of Medicine
Lowance Center for Human Immunology
Emory University School of Medicine
Atlanta, Georgia

Peter K. Gregersen, MD
Professor of Medicine and Pathology
Robert S. Boas Center for Genomics and Human Genetics
New York University School of Medicine
New York, New York
North Shore LIJ Research Institute
Manhasset, New York

Farshid Guilak, PhD
Associate Professor
Department of Surgery
Duke University Medical Center
Durham, North Carolina

Boulos Haraoui, MD, FRCPC
Clinical Associate Professor of Medicine
Department of Medicine
Université de Montréal, Faculty of Medicine
CHUM, Hôpital Notre-Dome
Montréal, Quebec, Canada

Barton F. Haynes, MD
Frederic M. Hanes Professor of Medicine
Professor of Immunology
Departments of Medicine and Immunology
Duke University School of Medicine
Director
Human Vaccine Institute
Duke University Medical Center
Durham, North Carolina

Glenn J. Jaffe, MD
Professor of Ophthalmology
Department of Ophthalmology
Duke University School of Medicine
Duke University Medical Center
Durham, North Carolina

Marcela Juárez, MD
Research Fellow in Rheumatology
Department of Medicine
Division of Clinical Immunology and Rheumatology
University of Alabama School of Medicine
Birmingham, Alabama

Jeffrey N. Katz, MD, MSc
Associate Professor of Medicine
Division of Rheumatology, Immunology, and Allergy
Harvard Medical School
Brigham and Women's Hospital
Boston, Massachusetts

Francis J. Keefe, PhD
Professor
Department of Medical Psychiatry
Duke University Medical Center
Durham, North Carolina

Peter D. Kent, MD
Instructor of Medicine
Department of Rheumatology
Mayo Clinic
Rochester, Minnesota

Edward C. Keystone, MD, FRCP(C)
Professor of Medicine
Department of Rheumatology
Mount Sinai Hospital
Toronto, Ontario, Canada

Dinesh Khanna, MD
Clinical Instructor
Department of Medicine
Division of Rheumatology
University of California, Los Angeles, David Geffen School of Medicine at UCLA
UCLA Medical Center
Los Angeles, California

Alice V. Klinkhoff, MD, FRCP
Associate Professor
Department of Medicine
University of British Columbia Faculty of Medicine
Mary Pack Arthritis Centre
Vancouver General Hospital
Vancouver, British Columbia, Canada

Alisa E. Koch, MD
William D. Robinson and Frederick Huetwell Endowed Professor
Department of Internal Medicine
Division of Rheumatology
University of Michigan Medical School
Ann Arbor, Michigan

Gay Kuchta, OT (Reg) BC
Department of Occupational Therapy
Mary Pack Arthritis Centre
Vancouver General Hospital
Vancouver, British Columbia, Canada

Nancy E. Lane, MD
Associate Professor
Department of Medicine
University of California, San Francisco, School of Medicine
San Francisco General Hospital
San Francisco, California

David M. Lee, MD, PhD
Instructor
Department of Medicine
Division of Rheumatology, Immunology, and Allergy
Harvard Medical School
Brigham and Women's Hospital
Boston, Massachusetts

Robert E. Lins, MD
Total Spine Specialists
Charlotte, North Carolina

Peter E. Lipsky, MD
Scientific Director
National Institute of Arthritis and Musculoskeletal and Skin Diseases
National Institutes of Health, NIAMS
Bethesda, Maryland

Hilal Maradit Kremers, MD, MSc
Assistant Professor of Epidemiology
Department of Health Science Research
Mayo Clinic
Rochester, Minnesota

Salutario Martinez, MD
Professor of Radiology
Department of Radiology
Duke University Medical Center
Durham, North Carolina

Eric L. Matteson, MD, MPH
Professor of Medicine
Department of Internal Medicine
Division of Rheumatology
Mayo Clinic
Rochester, Minnesota

Rex M. McCallum, MD
Clinical Professor of Medicine
Department of Medicine
Division of Rheumatology
Duke University School of Medicine
Duke University Hospital
Durham, North Carolina

J. Lee Nelson, MD
Professor
Department of Rheumatology
University of Washington School of Medicine
Member
Division of Clinical Research
Fred Hutchinson Cancer Research Center
Seattle, Washington

James A. Nunley, MD
Professor and Chief
Department of Orthopaedics
Duke University School of Medicine
Durham, North Carolina

James R. O'Dell, MD
Professor
Department of Internal Medicine
University of Nebraska College of Medicine
Nebraska Medical Center
Omaha, Nebraska

Monika E. Østensen, MD, PhD
Professor of Medicine
Department of Rheumatology
University Hospital of Berne
Berne, Switzerland

Thomas Pap, MD
Division of Experimental Rheumatology
Otto-von-Guericke University Magdeburg
University Hospital
Magdeburg, Germany

Peter D. Pardubsky, MD
Orthopaedic and Rheumatology Associates
Moline, Illinois

Jerry C. Parker, PhD
Clinical Professor of Physical Medicine and Rehabilitation
University of Missouri—Columbia School of Medicine
Associate Chief of Staff for Research and Development
Harry S. Truman Memorial Veteran's Hospital
Columbia, Missouri

Harold E. Paulus, MD
Professor
Department of Medicine
Division of Rheumatology
University of California, Los Angeles, David Geffen School of Medicine at UCLA
UCLA Medical Center
Los Angeles, California

Michael H. Pillinger, MD
Assistant Professor of Medicine and Pharmacology
Department of Medicine
Division of Rheumatology
New York University School of Medicine
Hospital for Joint Diseases
New York, New York

David S. Pisetsky, MD, PhD
Professor of Medicine and Immunology
Departments of Medicine and Immunology
Division of Rheumatology and Immunology
Chief of Rheumatology and Immunology
Duke University Medical Center
Durham VA Medical Center
Durham, North Carolina

Qaiser Rehman, MD, FACA
South Central Kansas Bone and Joint Center
Pratt, Kansas

Christopher Glen Richardson, MD, FRCSC
Department of Orthopaedics
Dalhousie University Faculty of Medicine
Nova Scotia, Canada
Saint John Regional Hospital
Saint John, New Brunswick, Canada

William James Richardson, MD
Associate Professor
Department of Orthopaedic Surgery
Duke University School of Medicine
Durham, North Carolina

Allen D. Sawitzke, MD
Associate Professor
Department of Medicine
University of Utah School of Medicine
Salt Lake City, Utah

Hendrik Schulze-Koops, MD, PhD
Clinical Research Group III
Nikolaus Fiebiger Center for Molecular Medicine
Department of Internal Medicine III
University of Erlangen-Nuremberg
Erlangen, Germany

David L. Scott, BSc, MD, FRCP
Professor
Department of Rheumatology
King's College Hospital
Denmark Hill, London, United Kingdom

Barry P. Simmons, MD
Associate Professor of Orthopaedic Surgery
Harvard Medical School
Chief, Hand and Upper Extremity Service
Department of Orthopaedic Surgery
Brigham and Women's Hospital
Boston, Massachusetts

James R. Slaughter, MD
Clinical Associate Professor
Departments of Psychiatry, Neurology, and Family and Community Medicine
University of Missouri—Columbia School of Medicine
Columbia, Missouri

Josef S. Smolen, MD
Professor of Medicine
Department of Rheumatology–Internal Medicine
Medical University of Vienna
Vienna General Hospital
Vienna, Austria

E. William St. Clair, MD
Professor of Medicine and Immunology
Departments of Medicine and Immunology
Division of Rheumatology and Immunology
Duke University Medical Center
Durham, North Carolina

Christina H. Stenström, PhD, RPT
Associate Professor
Neurotec Department
Division of Physical Therapy
Karolinska Institutet
Huddinge, Sweden

John S. Sundy, MD, PhD
Assistant Professor
Department of Medicine
Duke University School of Medicine
Durham, North Carolina

Zoltán Szekanecz, MD, PhD
Associate Professor of Medicine, Rheumatology, and Immunology
Department of Medicine
Division of Rheumatology
University of Debrecen Medical and Health Science Center
Debrecen, Hungary

Thomas Parker Vail, MD
Associate Professor of Orthopaedic Surgery
Director of Adult Reconstructive Surgery
Department of Surgery
Duke University Medical Center
Durham, North Carolina

Wim B. van den Berg, PhD
Professor of Experimental Rheumatology
Department of Rheumatology Research and Advanced Therapeutics
University Medical Center Nymegen
Nymegen, The Netherlands

Désirée M. F. M. van der Heijde, MD, PhD
Professor of Rheumatology
Department of Internal Medicine
Division of Rheumatology
University Hospital Maastricht
Maastricht, The Netherlands

Richard J. Wakefield, MRCP
Senior Lecturer
Department of Musculoskeletal Disease
University of Leeds Faculty of Medicine
Honorary Consultant
Leeds General Infirmary
Leeds, United Kingdom

Michael M. Ward, MD, MPH
Investigator
Intramural Research Program
National Institute of Arthritis and Musculoskeletal and Skin Disease
National Institutes of Health
U.S. Department of Health and Human Services
Bethesda, Maryland

Sandra J. Waters, PhD
Department of Medical Psychiatry
Duke University Medical Center
Durham, North Carolina

J. Brice Weinberg, MD
Professor of Medicine and Immunology
Department of Medicine
Duke University Medical Center
Durham VA Medical Center
Durham, North Carolina

Michael E. Weinblatt, MD
Professor of Medicine
Department of Rheumatology
Harvard Medical School
Brigham and Women's Hospital
Boston, Massachusetts

Mark H. Wener, MD
Associate Professor
Department of Laboratory Medicine
University of Washington School of Medicine
Seattle, Washington

Cornelia M. Weyand, MD, PhD
Professor of Medicine
Lowance Center for Human Immunology
Emory University School of Medicine
Atlanta, Georgia

Frederick Wolfe, MD
Clinical Professor of Internal Medicine and Family and Community Medicine
National Data Bank for Rheumatic Diseases
Wichita, Kansas

David E. Yocum, MD
Professor
Department of Medicine
Chief of Rheumatology
University of Arizona College of Medicine
Tucson, Arizona

Foreword

Advances in scientific knowledge, new medicines, changing demography, socioeconomic progress, and the empowerment of patients are among the forces that are shaping contemporary medical practice. Rheumatoid arthritis can be viewed as a prime example of a common disabling chronic disease that has provided a crucible for this revolution. This book, *Rheumatoid Arthritis*, provides a solid foundation in what is known, how we got there, and where we are heading. For the practitioner, *Rheumatoid Arthritis* provides a practical handbook. For the scholarly reader and researcher, it should stimulate the formulation of unanswered questions and future solutions.

The initial part of *Rheumatoid Arthritis* sets the scene with chapters on epidemiology, description of classical features, outcome, and clinical investigation. It will be evident that we have come a long way in refining clinical methods of measurement, laboratory tests, and imaging technologies in the past decade. The level of sophistication is a tribute to generations of leaders in the field devoted to the study of a disease entity described only 150 years ago.

The generally similar prevalence of rheumatoid arthritis worldwide raises interesting epidemiologic questions about selection pressures impacting genetic imprints, with a few striking exceptions—for example, overrepresentation in certain Native American tribes and scarcity in West Africans—challenging thinking regarding disease etiology. Other questions concern the incidence of rheumatoid arthritis and its clinical pattern in Western countries. For example, is the clinical pattern of extraarticular disease changing? Is the polyarthritis associated with rheumatoid factor or antibodies to citrullinated peptides different from polyarthritis occurring in association with other, diagnostically specific autoantibodies to nuclear and cytoplasmic antigens in connective tissue diseases? Do the differences define discrete pathogenic mechanisms or simply reflect the response of a diverse human genome to the same initiating cause? Does knowledge of the immunotaxonomy of rheumatic disease make any difference to strategies of management and future discoveries of better treatments?

These and many other questions are considered in the first two sections of this book. The contribution of genes in the major histocompatibility complex, encoding the shared epitope to susceptibility and severity of disease, is an elegant example of progress in molecular medicine that is proving valuable in unraveling the etiology of rheumatoid arthritis. The trend of applying pharmacogenomics to clinical medicine is evolving and will, no doubt, contribute in the future to tailoring therapies for individual patients and deselecting patients who might react adversely to specific targeted drugs.

Whether the functional importance of the major histocompatability complex and susceptibility to disease lies in antigen presentation and activation of T cells and their cooperation with B cells has been difficult to prove in rheumatoid disease. The analysis of disease tissue and cells from rheumatoid joints in the following chapters of this book should provide a fascinating insight into the biology, immunopathology, and pathogenesis of cell recruitment, survival, apoptosis, and cell-to-cell interactions that are engaging the interest of scientists. It is safe to conclude that cytokines, chemokines, and growth factors (also described) play a key role in integrating cellular responses of the innate and adaptive immune system that result in inflammation, tissue destruction, and repair. Because at least 40 cell types and perhaps thousands of gene products—some defined and some yet to be discovered—are involved in pathogenesis, the picture that emerges is bound to be complex and incomplete.

Many of the hypotheses that emerge from such studies require validation in physiologic systems in which the gain or loss of function of molecules by gene manipulation and targeted therapies can now be investigated in a unique fashion in animal models. The scientific basis of pathogenesis should make the reader more appreciative of the fact that much of the empiricism of clinical practice is beginning to yield to rational thought. More important, for the first time, scientific knowledge is leading to the development of targeted therapies. The advent of anti–tumor necrosis factor biologics as "blockbuster" drugs for the treatment of rheumatoid arthritis illustrates the new paradigm.

The next section of *Rheumatoid Arthritis,* on management, provides a comprehensive and informative perspective on drugs used in the treatment of rheumatoid arthritis. Reflecting the variety of medicines used to treat rheumatoid arthritis, the following chapters examine in detail the expanding class of nonsteroidal antiinflammatory and analgesic drugs, corticosteroids, and disease-modifying antirheumatic drugs, including methotrexate, azathioprine, sulfasalazine, gold compounds, hydroxychloroquine, minocycline, leflunomide, and, last, but not least, the biologics. The debate regarding whether there is a hierarchy of efficacy among these agents and a rational algorithm on how best to use them is thoughtfully considered in these and subsequent chapters. Other therapies are not forgotten and include behavioral, physical, and occupational therapies, which underpin the holistic approach and teamwork that go into the best care of patients.

Evidence is accumulating that remission of disease can be achieved in at least a proportion of patients in the short term. Apparently, best results are obtained by vigorous treatment soon after the onset of disease—a time when the disease activity of most patients can be subdued. Thus, there is little doubt that, at least in the 5- to 10-year timeframe, the quality of life in terms of physical function and psychosocial health, employment, and family life of the majority of patients can be restored and maintained. Attention to these issues and surgical treatment play an important part in the life of patients. In addition, surgery is becoming safer and more effective. It is gratifying that the book contains additional chapters on various aspects of medical and surgical treatment to provide a complete picture of the available therapeutic armamentarium.

The editors of *Rheumatoid Arthritis* have put together an exciting vision that is philosophically and intellectually coherent. The publication of this book is timely, bringing together, as it does, the foremost exponents of the science and art of medicine that underpin the specialty. *Rheumatoid Arthritis* deserves a wide readership and a place in the library of every student and practitioner working with rheumatoid arthritis.

Professor Sir Ravinder Maini, BA, MB, BChir, FRCP, FRCP(E), FMed Sci
Emeritus Professor of Rheumatology
The Kennedy Institute of Rheumatology Division
Imperial College London
London, United Kingdom

Preface

Of all diseases in clinical medicine, rheumatoid arthritis (RA) has undergone probably the greatest transformation with respect to its conceptualization and the approach to its treatment. Until the last decade or so, RA was viewed as a chronic disease that progressed inexorably to disability, with its symptoms of pain and inflammation resistant to medical therapy. Few drugs were available for treatment, with those capable of slowing progression characterized by either limited efficacy or unacceptable toxicity. Not surprisingly, surgery to correct deformity was a mainstay of management. Indeed, most textbooks in rheumatology were filled with pictures or x-rays of joints before and after surgery, showing destroyed joints realigned or replaced by metal or plastic.

Because of rapid advances in basic research, as well as the introduction of new and highly effective drugs into the armamentarium, the whole landscape of RA treatment has changed. RA, rather than being considered a chronic disorder, is now viewed as an acute or subacute disease that is amenable to early intervention. Progression is now viewed as the consequence of events occurring early in disease that can and must be stopped. Expectant therapy has given way to early aggressive management. The need for surgery, once the only hope to reduce symptoms, has become much less common, reflecting the success of early aggressive therapy in retarding or preventing joint damage.

The field of rheumatology remains in rapid flux. Like other immune-mediated diseases, RA is at the center of exciting clinical and basic research that is allowing investigators in the field to seriously contemplate the possibility of inducing remission or even permanently curing this disease. Not since the development of corticosteroids has the specialty of rheumatology been so energized and excited by the tangible improvements in the efficacy of new drugs. Fortunately, unlike corticosteroids, agents such as the tumor necrosis factor blockers appear relatively free of serious, long-term side effects, promising sustained benefits for patients who previously could often expect a life of unrelenting pain and disability.

At this key juncture in the history of rheumatology, the time appears right for a new textbook, focusing exclusively on RA, that attempts to capture the revolutionary change that has occurred in our understanding of this disease and its treatment. We have, therefore, endeavored to develop a new type of book that has, at its core, both cutting-edge science and an evidence-based approach. Fortunately, rheumatology has long been at the forefront of evidence-based research, pioneering quantitative measures of disease outcomes relevant to the patient, as well as to the investigator. At their best, these measures translate laboratory tests and x-ray images into indices of quality of life, the ultimate goal of all therapy. Although these measures were developed at a time when therapy for RA was primitive by current standards, they have enormously facilitated the testing of new drugs and the implementation of early, aggressive therapy.

Rheumatoid Arthritis has been designed as a definitive work on the most prevalent of all inflammatory arthritides. In the development of this book, we have enlisted some of the most distinguished basic and clinical investigators in the field of arthritis research to provide a comprehensive picture of RA, to describe the modern science that underpins ongoing research, and to lay out the evidence on new treatment. The approach can be termed *bench to bedside*, although the advances in treatment have kept patients out of the hospital and made the bedside a rare place for the physician and other providers to encounter RA.

Although the assembly of information is always gratifying, as editors, we want *Rheumatoid Arthritis* to be more than a compendium. We want this text to be a guidebook and a map providing the reader with the options in current therapy and a means for making informed choices. At present, there are hundreds, if not thousands, of different and effective ways to treat RA. This abundance reflects the availability of a host of effective medications, used alone or in combination, in conjunction with nonmedical approaches, such as physical and occupational therapy. Thus, *Rheumatoid Arthritis* covers the full gamut of such treatments, with key chapters describing their application in a comprehensive and integrated approach.

In designing *Rheumatoid Arthritis*, we have endeavored to be as current as possible, but the field is moving rapidly. Just as ideas on pathogenesis will evolve, our assessment of treatments will change. As we become more confident in the ability of drugs to alter disease course, the inclination to treat early disease aggressively will grow, making assessment of diagnosis and prognosis in early disease a major challenge for the future. As editors and investigators in the field, we cannot accurately predict this future. We have provided, however, a full and complete picture of the past and present to glimpse, at least, the outlines of the future.

As an evidence-based text, *Rheumatoid Arthritis* is about populations, not individuals, and trends, not narratives. As rheumatologists who have participated in the revolution in the care of RA patients, we can attest to the reality of recent advances embodied in impersonal numbers, with the sure knowledge that statistics do not lie and that the course of patients with RA is much better now than it was in the past. It has been a great thrill for us as physicians to witness the extraordinary improvements in the lives of our patients. Unlike doctors, patients feel comfortable in using the word "miracle" to describe how new treatments have renewed their lives. In *Rheumatoid Arthritis*, miracles are described. We are fortunate that our patients have experienced such miracles and hope that our book will allow many more to occur.

E. William St. Clair, MD
David S. Pisetsky, MD, PhD
Barton F. Haynes, MD
The Editors

Acknowledgments

The editors wish to acknowledge their colleagues at Lippincott Williams & Wilkins for their invaluable advice and help in bringing *Rheumatoid Arthritis* to fruition: Richard Winters, for his vision to develop a new textbook to capture the excitement in the field of rheumatology and amalgamate state-of-the-art science with current clinical practice; Danette Somers, for her strong editorial guidance in producing an accessible, authoritative, and attractive textbook to match Richard Winters' vision; and Lisa Consoli, for her diligence and fortitude in helping us meet schedules and her consummate skill in overseeing the myriad details that go into assembling a new book.

The editors also wish to acknowledge the authors of this book for their outstanding scholarship and commitment to contribute their expertise generously, despite busy and hectic lives, in a way that will advance both inquiry into rheumatoid arthritis and the care of patients with this disease.

E.W.S.
D.S.P.
B.F.H.

CHAPTER 1

Epidemiology

Hilal Maradit Kremers and Sherine E. Gabriel

ROLE OF EPIDEMIOLOGY IN IMPROVING OUR UNDERSTANDING OF RHEUMATOID ARTHRITIS

Epidemiology is the study of the distribution and determinants of disease in human populations (1). This definition is based on two fundamental assumptions. First, that human disease does not occur at random and second, that human disease has causal and preventive factors that can be identified through systematic investigation of different populations or subgroups of individuals within a population in different places or at different times. Thus, epidemiologic studies include simple descriptions of the manner in which disease appears in a population (i.e., levels of disease frequency—incidence and prevalence, mortality, trends over time, geographic distributions, and clinical characteristics) and studies that describe the role of putative risk factors for disease occurrence. Incidence studies include all new cases of a specified condition arising in a defined population over a specified time period, whereas prevalence studies include all cases with the condition who are present in a population at a particular point in time. As shown in Figure 1.1, prevalence cohorts exclude cases who died or left the population soon after their incidence date, and they include cases arising in different populations who moved into the cohort after their incidence date. Because of this, there is a greater potential for bias to be introduced in prevalence as compared to incidence cohorts. Thus, population-based incidence cohorts are superior to prevalence cohorts for descriptive epidemiologic studies.

Epidemiologic studies of risk factors fall into three major categories: prospective cohort studies, retrospective cohort studies, and case control studies. The relationship between these is illustrated in Figure 1.2. In a prospective cohort study, a study population is assembled, none of whom has experienced the outcome of interest, and followed into the future. People in the cohort are classified according to those characteristics that might be related to outcome—that is, putative risk factors. These people are then observed over time to determine which of them experience the outcome. The analysis addresses the question of whether people who are exposed to the risk factor are more likely to develop the outcome compared to those who are not exposed. In a retrospective cohort study, the cohort of individuals is identified from past records and followed up to the present. Data regarding historic exposure to the putative risk factor are collected retrospectively, typically by examination of medical records. As with prospective cohort studies, retrospective cohort studies also compare the frequency of the outcome in exposed compared to unexposed individuals. In a case control study, two cohorts are assembled: one that has the outcome of interest and another that is free of the outcome of interest. Data regarding exposure to the putative risk factor in both groups are collected retrospectively to determine whether cases with the outcome of interest were more likely to have had a history of the exposure of interest, compared to controls who were free of the outcome of interest. Of these three study designs, prospective cohort studies are susceptible to fewer potential biases than the other two. However, prospective cohort studies are frequently not feasible because they typically require extended follow-up, often 5 to 10 years or more into the future. Detailed comparison of the potential biases involved in retrospective cohort studies and case control studies is beyond the scope of this chapter (1–3). In this chapter, we will review data on the descriptive epidemiology (incidence, prevalence, comorbidity, and survival) and risk factors (genetics, infections, estrogens, smoking, coffee consumption, and formal education) associated with rheumatoid arthritis (RA). We will also briefly summarize the economics of RA.

DESCRIPTIVE EPIDEMIOLOGY OF RHEUMATOID ARTHRITIS

Incidence

The most reliable estimates of incidence, prevalence, and mortality in RA are those derived from population-based studies. Several of these have been conducted in a variety of geographically and ethnically diverse populations. The Norfolk Arthritis Register (NOAR) is a prospective population-based database that was established to study new cases of inflammatory arthritis as they occur in the community and to follow them prospectively to investigate the natural history of the condition. This data resource is the first primary care–based register of incidence cases of RA ever assembled (4). One hundred four newly diagnosed cases of RA who fulfilled the 1987 American College of Rheumatology (ACR) criteria (5) for RA at the time of presentation between 1990 and 1991 were identified. The age- and sex-adjusted annual incidence rate per 100,000 population was 35.9 for women and 14.3 for men (Table 1.1). RA was rare in men

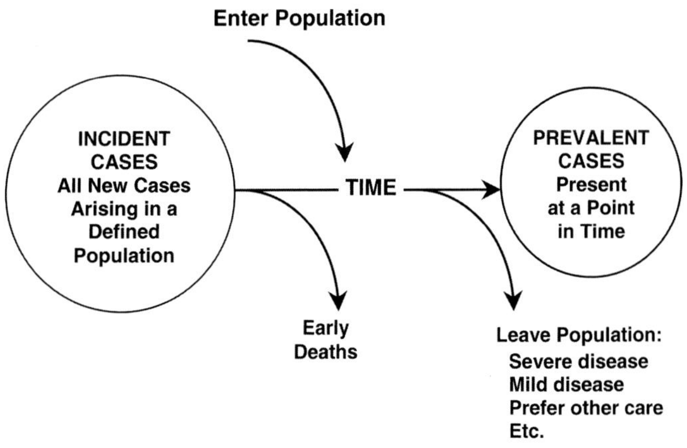

Enter Population

INCIDENT CASES
All New Cases Arising in a Defined Population

TIME

PREVALENT CASES
Present at a Point in Time

Early Deaths

Leave Population:
Severe disease
Mild disease
Prefer other care
Etc.

Figure 1.1. The difference in cases for incidence and prevalence studies. (Adapted from Fletcher RH, Fletcher SW, Wagner EH, eds. *Clinical epidemiology—the essentials*, vol. 2. Baltimore: Williams & Wilkins, 1988:87.)

younger than 45 years of age. The incidence of RA in men rose steeply with age, whereas in women, the incidence increased to age 45 and plateaued until 75 years, after which it declined (4). In a subsequent report, the same investigators explored the estimation of the incidence of RA in 1990 by allowing each criterion to "carry forward" once it had been satisfied on a single occasion (6). They showed that, if up to 5 years elapsed between symptom onset and the time the criteria were applied cumulatively, the incidence estimates rose by 75% and 93% for women and men, respectively, reaching 54.0 per 100,000 for women and 24.5 per 100,000 for men. These estimates more accurately reflect the true incidence of RA. These findings emphasize the importance of long-term follow-up of patients with undifferentiated polyarthritis and of applying the ACR criteria cumulatively to accurately estimate the incidence of RA.

Numerous studies have been undertaken in Finland describing the epidemiology of RA. Estimates of the incidence and prevalence have been derived from several surveys based on computerized data registers covering the entire Finnish population (7–11). The incidence of clinically significant RA in these surveys was approximately 29 to 35.5 per 100,000 adult population over the study years (1975, 1980, 1985, 1990, and 1995) (Table 1.1). Trends in RA incidence between 1975 and 1995 were also examined (8,11). Among the 1,321 incident cases identified between 1975 and 1990, the authors noted a rise in the mean age at onset (increasing from 50.2 to 57.8 years) and a simultaneous decline in the age-specific incidence rates in the younger individuals (11). A further rise to 59.0 years was reported in 1995, and these figures correspond to a mean increase of 8.8 years in age at onset from 1975 to 1995 (8). The same authors studied the incidence of rheumatoid factor (RF)–positive RA and RF-negative polyarthritis (10). In that study, the investigators demonstrated a decline of approximately 40% in the number of RF-negative RA cases in 1990 compared with the earlier years. This declining trend was statistically significant ($p = .008$). In fact, the decline in incidence of approximately 15% compared with previous study years was noted to affect, nearly exclusively, RF-negative disease.

Gabriel and colleagues (12,13) assembled an inception cohort of Rochester, Minn, residents who were 18 years of age or older and had RA, as defined by the 1987 ACR criteria for RA, first diagnosed between January 1, 1955, and December 31, 1994. The overall age- and sex-adjusted annual incidence of RA among Rochester, Minn, residents 18 years of age or older (1955–1994) was 44.6 per 100,000 [95% confidence interval (CI): 41.0–48.2]. The incidence was approximately double in women compared with that in men and increased steadily with age until age 85, after which the incidence decreased. Incidence peaked earlier in women than in men. The incidence rate fell progressively during the 4 decades of study, from 61.2 per 100,000 in 1955 through 1964, to 32.7 per 100,000 in 1985 through 1994 (Fig. 1.3). Birth cohort analysis showed diminishing incidence rates through successive cohorts after a peak in the 1880 to 1890 cohorts (13).

Incidence cases of RA were identified among a population-based cohort of Pima Indians in Arizona during the period 1965 to 1990 (14). Among 2,894 subjects, 78 incidence cases of RA were identified. The total age- and sex-adjusted incidence rate per 100,000 population was 890 (95% CI: 590–1,190) in 1966 to 1973,

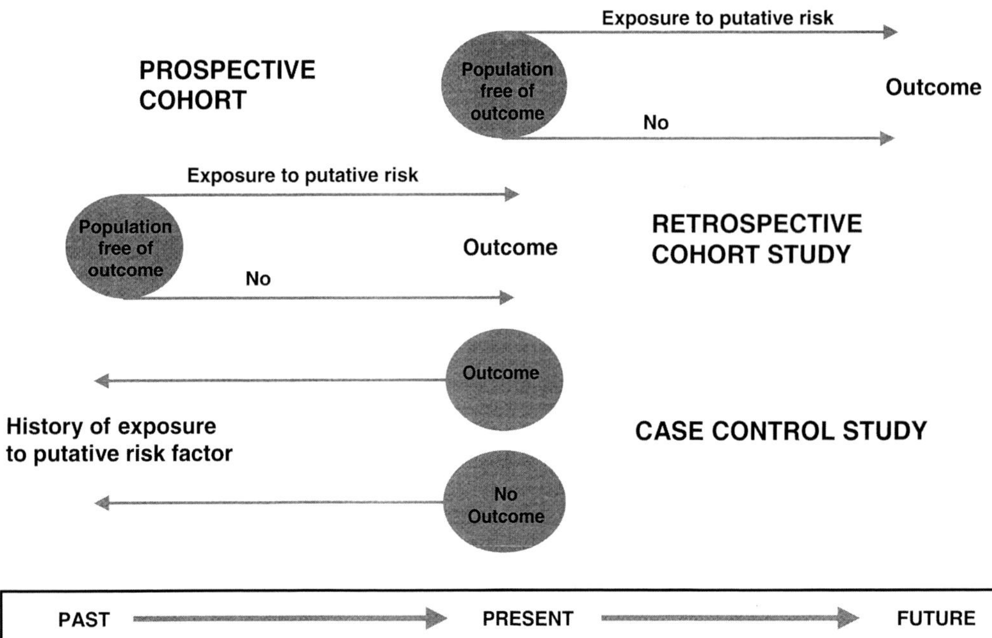

Figure 1.2. Epidemiologic studies of risk factors.

TABLE 1.1. Incidence of Rheumatoid Arthritis

Author, Yr (Reference)	County/Region	Yrs of Study	Age Range	Sample Size	Annual Incidence Rate per 100,000
Dugowson, 1991 (16)	Seattle, Wash, USA	1987–1989	18–64	81[a]	F: 23.9 (95% CI: 18.5–29.3)
Chan, 1993 (215)	Massachusetts, USA	1987–1990	18–70+	81	O: 42 (95% CI: 23–60) F: 60 (95% CI: 46–75) M: 22 (95% CI: 13–32)
Symmons, 1994 (4)	Manchester, UK	1990–1991	15–85+	104[a]	F: 35.9 (95% CI: 26.9–43.1) M: 14.3 (95% CI: 8.2–18.7)
Jacobsson, 1994 (14)	Pima Indians, Arizona, USA	1965–1990	25–65+	78	1966–1973: 890 (95% CI: 590–1,190) 1974–1982: 620 (95% CI: 380–860) 1983–1990: 380 (95% CI: 170–590)
Aho, 1998, and Kaipiainen-Seppanen, 1996 and 2000 (7,8,10,11)	Finland	5 (1-yr periods): 1975, 1980, 1985, 1990, and 1995	16–85+	1,321[a] 366[a]	1975: 29.0 1980: 35.5 1985: 35.0 1990: 29.5 1995: 33.7 (O) (95% CI: 30.4–37.4) F: 43.2 (95% CI: 37.9–49.0) M: 23.5 (95% CI: 19.6–28.1)
Drosos, 1997 (15)	Northwest Greece (Ioannina)	1987–1995	16–75+	428[a]	O: 24 (95% CI: 15–33) F: 36 (95% CI: 21–51) M: 12 (95% CI: 4–20)
Uhlig, 1998 (216)	Oslo, Norway	1988–1993	20–79	550[a]	O: 25.7 (95% CI: 23.6–28.0) F: 36.7 (95% CI: 33.4–40.6) M: 13.8 (95% CI: 11.6–16.2)
Shichikawa, 1999 (217)	Wakayama, Japan	1965–1996		16	1965–1975: 39 (95% CI: 12–66) 1975–1985: 24 (95% CI: 3–46) 1985–1996: 8 (95% CI: 0–17)
Riise, 2000 (28)	Troms County, Norway	1987–1996	20+	316[a]	O: 28.7 (95% CI: 25.6–32.0) F: 34.9 (95% CI: 30.2–40.1) M: 22.2 (95% CI: 18.4–26.6)
Gabriel, 1999, and Doran, 2002 (12,13)	Olmsted County, Minn, USA	1955–1994	18–85+	609[a]	O: 44.6 (95% CI: 41.0–48.2) F: 57.8 (95% CI: 52.4–63.2) M: 30.4 (95% CI: 25.6–35.1)

CI, confidence interval; F, female; M, male; O, overall.
[a]American College of Rheumatology 1987 criteria.

620 (95% CI: 380–860) in 1974 to 1982, and 380 (95% CI: 170–590) in 1983 to 1990. The age-adjusted incidence declined by 55% in men (p trend = .225) and by 57% in women (p trend = .017) after controlling for contraceptive use, estrogen use, and pregnancy experience. Drosos and colleagues (15) investigated the records of patients at rheumatology clinics of universities, general hospitals, and private clinics in Ioannina, Greece. Cases were identified according to the 1987 ACR criteria for RA, and population data were based on the 1991 national census. A total of 428 cases of RA were identified during the study period, with annual incidence rates fluctuating between 12 and 36 per 100,000 population.

A review of the incidence rates from the ten major population-based epidemiologic studies (Table 1.1) reveals substantial variation in incidence rates across the different studies and across time periods within the studies. These data emphasize the dynamic nature of the epidemiology of RA. A substantial decline in RA incidence over time with a shift toward a more elderly age of onset was a consistent finding across various studies (10,11,13,14,16–18). The etiologic role of various environmental, infectious, and hormonal factors in the decline in RA incidence is being investigated.

Prevalence

Several studies in the literature provide estimates of the number of people with current disease (prevalence) in a defined population (Table 1.2). Although these studies suffer from a number of methodologic limitations (19), the remarkable finding across these studies is the uniformity of prevalence figures in developed populations, generally between 0.5% and 1% of the adult population (7,12,14,15,20–29). Our own data demonstrated an overall prevalence of RA on January 1, 1985, of 1.07% (95% CI:

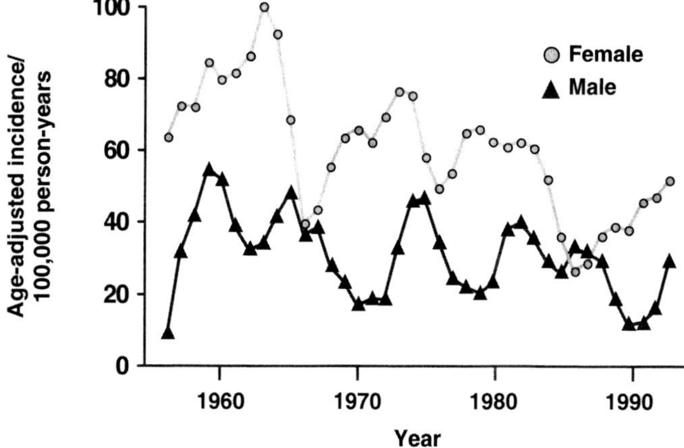

Figure 1.3. Annual incidence of rheumatoid arthritis in Rochester, Minn: annual incidence rate per 100,000 population by gender, 1955 to 1995. Each rate was calculated as a 3-year centered moving average. [From Doran MF, Pond GR, Crowson CS, et al. Trends in incidence and mortality in rheumatoid arthritis in Rochester, Minnesota, over a forty-year period. *Arthritis Rheum* 2002;46(3):625–631, with permission.]

TABLE 1.2. Prevalence of Rheumatoid Arthritis

Author	County/Region	Prevalence Rate (%)
Jacobsson, 1994 (14)	Pima Indians, Arizona, USA	0.15–1.00
Kvien, 1997 (23)	Oslo, Norway	0.437
Drosos, 1997 (15)	Northwest Greece	0.21–0.48
Stojanovic, 1998 (22)	Belgrade, Yugoslavia	0.69
Cimmino, 1998 (21)	Genova, Italy	0.33
Boyer, 1998 (20)	Anchorage, Alaska, USA	0.62–1.78
Aho, 1998 (7)	Finland	0.80
Power, 1999 (24)	Dublin, Ireland	0.50
Saraux, 1999 (25)	Brittany, France	0.62
Simonsson, 1999 (26)	Halland, Sweden	0.51
Gabriel, 1999 (12)	Olmsted County, Minn, USA	1.07
Carmona, 2002 (27)	Spain	0.50
Riise, 2000 (28)	Troms, Norway	0.39–0.47
Symmons, 2002 (29)	Norfolk, UK	0.81

0.94–1.20). The prevalence among women was approximately double that in men. Women had a prevalence of RA of 1.37%, compared to 0.74% in men (12).

Comorbidity

Several studies have reported that RA patients have a higher chronic disease burden compared to age- and gender-matched peers in the general population (30–42). The major comorbidities in RA include cardiovascular disease, infections, malignancies, gastrointestinal disease, and osteoporosis leading to fractures (40–42). Pincus and Callahan considered arthritis as a risk factor for other comorbid conditions, such as hypertension, cardiovascular disease, chronic pulmonary disease, or upper gastrointestinal disease (33–35,37–39). Gabriel and colleagues (40) reported that the presence of RA is highly predictive of the development of future comorbidities (Table 1.3). Some of the observed excess morbidity was attributable to the use of nonsteroidal antiinflammatory drugs (NSAIDs) (e.g., peptic ulcer disease and renal disease) or disease-modifying antirheumatic drugs (e.g., liver disease). However, RA patients also had a higher likelihood of developing several other comorbidities (e.g., congestive heart failure, myocardial infarction, peripheral vascular disease, chronic pulmonary disease). Moreover, the level of comorbidity increased significantly over time, even after controlling for the effects of age, gender, and baseline comorbidity (40).

TABLE 1.3. Relative Risk for the Development of Selected Comorbidities among 450 Prevalence Cases of Rheumatoid Arthritis (RA) and Matched Community Controls

Comorbidity	Relative Risk (95% CI),[a] RA vs. RA Controls
Myocardial infarction	1.35 (0.92–1.97)
Congestive heart failure	1.60 (1.12–2.27)
Peripheral vascular disease	1.51 (0.99–2.30)
Cerebrovascular disease	0.90 (0.61–1.32)
Dementia	1.53 (1.03–2.29)
Chronic pulmonary disease	2.33 (1.44–3.77)
Peptic ulcer disease	1.92 (1.12–3.28)
Liver disease	1.84 (0.77–4.41)
Diabetes	1.24 (0.73–2.12)
Hemiplegia or paraplegia	0.64 (0.25–1.65)
Renal disease	1.31 (0.74–2.32)
Any malignancy	0.99 (0.68–1.43)

[a]From the Cox Proportional Hazards Models adjusting for age, sex, and baseline comorbidity.
From Gabriel SE, Crowson CS, O'Fallon WM. Comorbidity in arthritis. *J Rheumatol* 1999;26(11):2475–2479, with permission.

TABLE 1.4. Results of Rheumatoid Arthritis (RA) Mortality Studies

Author, Publication Yr (Reference)	No. of RA Cases	Standardized Mortality Ratio
Cobb, 1953 (45)	583	1.29
van Dam, 1961 (60)	231	1.66
Duthie, 1964 (61)	307	1.66
Uddin, 1970 (75)	475	1.29
Isomaki, 1975 (53)	1,000	1.77
Monson, 1976 (49)[a]	1,035	1.86
Linos, 1980 (64)[a]	521	1.16
Lewis, 1980 (63)	311	1.40
Allebeck, 1981 (56)[a]	293	1.32
Allebeck, 1982 (57)	1,165	2.48
Prior, 1984 (58)	489	2.98
Pincus, 1984 (55)	75	1.31
Vandenbroucke, 1984 (54)	209	1.14
Mutru, 1985 (65)	1,000	1.64
Mitchell, 1986 (66)	805	1.51
Reilly, 1990 (62)	100	1.40
Jacobsson, 1993 (59)[a]	2,979	1.28
Wolfe, 1994 (46)	3,501	2.26
Myllykangas-Luosujarvi, 1995 (52)[a]	1,666	1.37
Callahan, 1996 (76)	1,384	1.54
Wallberg-Jonsson, 1997 (67)	606	1.57
Symmons, 1998 (69)	448	2.70
Lindqvist, 1999 (218)	183	0.87
Sokka, 1999 (68)	135	1.28
Kvalvik, 2000 (70)	149	1.49
Cheheta, 2001 (71)	309	1.65
Krause, 2000 (72)	271	2.60
Martinez, 2001 (73)	182	1.85
Riise, 2001 (74)	187	2.00
Gabriel, 1999 (51)[a]	425	1.38
Doran, 2002 (13)[a]	609	1.27

[a]Population-based studies.

Doran and colleagues (43) reported that RA patients are at almost twice the risk of developing an infection compared with age- and sex-matched individuals in the same community who do not have RA (hazard ratio, 1.70; 95% CI: 1.42–2.03). The most common infection sites were the bone, joints, skin, and soft tissues. The same investigators reported that various RA severity markers (e.g., RF positivity, rheumatoid nodules, extraarticular manifestations), as well as coexisting medical conditions, are strong predictors of infections (44).

Survival

The first mortality study of RA was published by Cobb (45). In that study, 583 RA patients admitted to the Massachusetts General Hospital were followed for a mean of 9.6 years. The mortality rates among the RA patients were higher than non-RA controls (24.4 deaths per 1,000 patients per year compared with an expected number of 18.9). There have been numerous subsequent studies examining mortality in RA (13,14,45–76). These studies have consistently demonstrated an increased mortality in patients with RA when compared to expected rates in the general population (Table 1.4). The standardized mortality ratios in these studies varied from 1.28 to 2.98. Two studies have examined specifically trends in mortality over time using a population-based design. Both concluded that the excess mortality associated with RA remained unchanged during the past 2 to 3 decades (48,51). Although some studies have reported an apparent improvement in survival, a recent critical review indicates that these observations are likely due to referral selection bias (77). These findings suggest that the introduction and widespread use of effective disease-modifying antirheumatic drugs have had little impact to date on RA mortality in the community. However, the effect of these new agents on RA mortality may not be readily apparent for another 5 to 10 years. Clearly, there is a need for additional research examining the impact of new treatments on RA mortality.

A number of investigators have examined the underlying causes for the observed excess mortality in RA (40,48,58,63,65–67,78,79). These reports suggest increased risk from cardiovascular, infectious, hematologic, gastrointestinal, and respiratory diseases among RA patients compared to controls. Various disease severity and disease activity markers in RA (e.g., extraarticular manifestations, erythrocyte sedimentation rate seropositivity, higher joint count, functional status) have been shown to be associated with increased mortality (80–85).

Cardiovascular diseases are responsible for almost one-half of all deaths in patients with RA (67,83,86–88). Studies are ongoing to clarify predictors of excess cardiovascular morbidity and mortality in RA and whether the excess is due to an increased prevalence of traditional coronary heart disease risk factors, or is independent of these (78,80,83,89–93). There is also growing interest in the potential preventive role of pharmacotherapies, including biologics, methotrexate, NSAIDs, and cyclooxygenase-2 inhibitors in improving outcomes (94–96).

In summary, RA not only takes its toll on functional status and quality of life, but also significantly reduces life expectancy. The mechanisms underlying this reduction in mortality are not fully understood.

RISK FACTORS ASSOCIATED WITH RHEUMATOID ARTHRITIS

A number of risk factors have been suggested as important contributors to the development or progression of RA. Of these, the best studied have been genetics, infectious agents, oral contraceptives, smoking, coffee consumption, and formal education.

Genetics

The familiality of RA has long been recognized (97,98), suggesting that genetic risk factors are important in the etiology of this disease. Until recently, genetic studies of RA have focused primarily on the role of the major histocompatibility complex locus in RA in various distinct populations. Several investigators have demonstrated important associations between specific HLA alleles (i.e., HLA-DR4 and HLA-DR1) and susceptibility to RA (99–107). There is still controversy, however, regarding the mode of inheritance (i.e., recessive vs. dominant) (108–112) and the characteristics of the association (i.e., are there specific disease susceptibility loci, or do they simply affect disease severity?) (108,113–118).

Irrespective of the mode of inheritance and the role of HLA-associated susceptibility gene(s), the relationship between HLA-DR alleles and RA is insufficient to explain the familiality of the disease (119–121). The observations of high RA incidence rates, more severe clinical disease, and familial aggregation among certain North American Indian populations (14,98,122–126), combined with the unusually low incidence of RA in other populations (15), all lend support to the hypothesis of a genetic predisposition to RA.

The magnitude of the genetic contribution of RA has been estimated using twin studies and first-degree relatives of affected individuals. The concordance rate in monozygotic twins is approximately 15% (127–129), which is four to five times greater than the rates observed among dizygotic twins and siblings of RA probands (119,130). The heritability of RA is estimated at 65% (95% CI: 50–77) (131), suggesting that genetic factors account for a substantial portion of the disease risk. A genealogic study from Iceland demonstrated that the familial component of RA extends beyond the nuclear family into second- and third-degree relatives (132).

Various studies have examined other important variables associated with susceptibility and disease severity in first-degree relatives of probands (126,133–135). Gender and age at onset in the proband are identified as important risk factors, with relatives of male probands having the greatest cumulative risk of RA (126). Complex segregation analyses have indicated that a small proportion of all cases of RA may be attributed to a highly penetrant recessive gene. Under this model, the largest proportion of genetic cases of RA would be expected to occur in men affected before the age of 40 years. Significant heterogeneity in the inheritance of RA and in the distribution of risk for RA among first-degree relatives was demonstrated. In another study from the Netherlands, the prevalence of familial RA was 9.8%, and familial aggregation of RA occurred preferentially in large sibships (133). Probands with familial RA were more often RF positive and had a longer follow-up period. Male gender and history of joint replacements were associated with higher concordance for RA.

Efforts to identify both HLA- and non–HLA-linked genes are now strengthened by the genome-wide scans (136–139). These scans have identified various predisposing genes both within and outside the HLA region, and studies are ongoing on the relative contribution of these candidate genes and gene–gene interactions, not only to disease susceptibility and severity, but also response to therapy (139–144).

Infectious Agents

One feature of RA disease occurrence that might point to an environmental component is evidence of secular trends or disease clusters in time or space. Data from the population-based incidence studies in Olmsted County, Minn, demonstrate secular trends in the incidence of RA (Fig. 1.3) (12,13). Using NOAR, based in the east Anglian region of the United Kingdom, Silman and colleagues conducted time trend and spatial clustering analyses on 687 incident cases of inflammatory joint disease identified between January 1, 1990, and December 31, 1994. These results demonstrated no evidence of a consistent seasonal variation in the onset of disease; in other words, there was no suggestion of any localized "epidemic" in time. Modest evidence for spatial clustering was demonstrated with nonrandom distribution observed in one geographic area. There was also no evidence of time or seasonal clustering of these incident cases. However, these investigators did demonstrate some evidence of time-independent spatial clustering within the northwest part of the study area. Unfortunately, the small sample size precluded any definitive conclusions. Further investigation into local factors, which might explain this finding, is under way (145,146).

The possibility of a host–environment interaction has been discussed in detail in a number of review articles (147–150). Human parvovirus infection has been linked to the occurrence of inflammatory polyarthritis, but its role in the development of RA is less clear. Data from NOAR, which has the benefit of ascertaining cases close in time to disease onset, showed that only 2.7% of patients with polyarthritis had evidence of recent human parvovirus B19 infection, suggesting that such infection does not explain more than a very small proportion of RA cases (151).

Estrogens

The possibility that oral contraceptives protect against the development of RA has been proposed by numerous investigators.

Brennan and colleagues (152) reviewed 17 studies investigating this association and noted that 11 showed a protective effect and six did not. Brennan et al. also provided their own results, based on 115 incident cases of inflammatory polyarthritis, showing that current oral contraceptive use does protect against the development of RA [adjusted odds ratio (OR), 0.22; 95% CI: 0.06–0.85].

There have been a smaller number of studies, including three case control and two cohort studies, on the association between postmenopausal estrogen use and RA, again yielding conflicting results. One case control study by Carette and colleagues (153) found no effect, while another by Vandenbroucke (154) found a sevenfold reduction in risk among current users. These studies have been criticized for inconsistent inclusion criteria for RA cases, potential recall bias, incomplete evaluation of postmenopausal use of estrogen, and responder bias. The first cohort study by Hernandez-Avila and colleagues (155) included too few women using estrogen replacement therapy (ERT) to provide a reliable estimate of its effect. A later cohort study (156) found a relative risk (RR) of 1.62 (95% CI: 0.56–4.74), which reduced toward unity (RR, 1.08; 95% CI: 0.30–6.75) after adjustment for potential confounders. A number of limitations exist within this study, including that of protopathic bias (i.e., that self-selection occurs for estrogen therapy at the menopause of those with undiagnosed joint symptoms). Other biases may exist in the ERT cohort in this study, as they were selected from a menopause clinic. This study also had extremely low power (20%) to be able to detect a large (50%) reduction in risk, as too few individuals in the study were ever on ERT.

Doran and colleagues observed an inverse association between use of oral contraceptives and the risk of RA, which persisted after adjusting for potential confounders (OR, 0.56; 95% CI: 0.34–0.92). Exposure to oral contraceptives in earlier years, when higher doses of estrogen and progestins were used in the formulations, was associated with a further lowering of risk, such that women who received oral contraceptives before 1970 had only one-fourth the risk of unexposed women. There was no evidence of an association of ERT with RA risk (OR, 1.11; 95% CI: 0.69–1.78) (157).

Thus, the bulk of the evidence points to a protective role for estrogens in the etiology of RA. Additional research is needed to elucidate the mechanism underlying this association.

Smoking

Several studies assessed the relationship between smoking and the development and severity of RA (158). Uhlig and colleagues identified a significant association for the development of RA among male cigarette smokers compared to nonsmokers (OR, 2.38; 95% CI: 1.45–3.92). Although the risk in women was also elevated, it was not statistically significant (OR, 1.14; 95% CI: 0.80–1.62). The effect in men was stronger for seropositive RA where the odds ratio was 4.77 (95% CI: 2.09–10.9) (159). More recently, Karlson and colleagues (160) studied the association of cigarette smoking with risk of RA among 377,481 female health professionals in the Women's Health Cohort Study. After adjusting for potential confounders, duration (but not intensity) of smoking was associated with a significantly increased risk of RA (p <.01). Wolfe and colleagues (161) reported that the RF concentration was linearly related to the number of years spent smoking. Smoking was related to rheumatoid nodule formation and radiographic abnormalities, even controlling for RF, but had no effect on disease process variables such as erythrocyte sedimentation rate, pain, joint count, global severity, or functional ability. These findings add to the growing body of evidence suggesting that smoking is an independent risk factor in the development of RA (162,163). The increased risk of RA associated with smoking is speculated to be mediated through antiestrogenic effects of smoking.

Coffee Consumption

Due to the observed association between RA and smoking, two studies examined the association between coffee consumption and the development of RA (164,165). In a cross-sectional survey of almost 7,000 people, the number of cups of coffee drunk daily was directly proportional to the prevalence of RF positivity (164). The same authors also prospectively followed up nearly 20,000 people for the development of RA and reported that people who consume more than four cups of coffee per day were more than twice as likely to develop seropositive RA compared with those drinking less (RR, 2.2; 95% CI: 1.13–4.27) (164). Mikuls and colleagues (165) examined the types of coffee consumed and reported that decaffeinated coffee intake is positively associated with RA onset (RR, 3.1; 95% CI: 1.75–5.48), whereas tea consumption was protective (RR, 0.24; 95% CI: 0.06–0.98).

Formal Education

The risk of self-reported arthritis, as well as several other chronic diseases, has been found to be inversely related to the level of formal education (166). Low levels of formal education also have been associated with increased mortality (167), as well as poor clinical status (33,167,168) in patients with RA. No relationship was found between the onset of RA and indicators of socioeconomic deprivation using employment categories as indicators for social class (169). Thus, although some evidence points to low formal education as a risk factor for RA, there is no apparent association with socioeconomic deprivation. Moreover, the mechanism for this possible excess risk is unknown.

ECONOMICS OF RHEUMATOID ARTHRITIS

Studies examining the medical and economic burden of RA are referred to as *cost-of-illness* studies. These studies estimate the total societal cost of caring for RA patients compared with people without the illness. Such studies consider costs in three categories. *Direct costs* refer to either costs associated with the provision of health care (e.g., physician and hospital costs, medications) or costs incurred due to the disease or the need to seek medical care (e.g., transportation). *Indirect costs* (or productivity costs) typically refer to wage losses resulting from the morbidity or mortality associated with the disease. Finally, *intangible costs* are defined as the costs associated with disability, pain, and suffering and mainly represent deterioration in quality of life of patients and their families.

Musculoskeletal diseases in general, and RA in particular, have considerable social and economic impact due to their chronic nature, associated morbidity, and long-term disability. Average per capita medical expenditure in 1996 for people with musculoskeletal diseases was $3,578, and this amount translated into a national total of $193 billion, equivalent to 2.5% of the gross domestic product (170). Some investigators recently summarized published estimates of economic impact of RA and concluded that there is substantial variation in the estimates (171–173).

Indirect costs of RA are usually two to three times higher than direct costs, which results in a total of $26 to $32 billion of RA-related costs in the United States alone (172). Direct costs of RA are also substantial, and they rise considerably with increasing age and disease duration. Hospitalization costs are the biggest component of direct costs, whereas costs of medications currently represent only a small proportion. According to a recent review, the published direct costs estimates (in 1996 U.S. dollars) ranged from $2,299 per person per year in Canada to $13,549 in the United States (174). With the availability and widespread use of biological therapy, pharmacologic treatment of RA will constitute a larger proportion of direct cost in the future.

Indirect costs are, in general, proportional to the prevalence of work disability. Gabriel and colleagues (175) reported that more than five times as many community-based residents with arthritis incurred some indirect and nonmedical expenditures compared to nonarthritic residents, and these expenditures were nearly 2.5-fold greater among arthritics compared to nonarthritics. The same group also simulated the lifetime incremental costs of RA using a mathematical model with data inputs from cross-sectional population-based prevalence cohorts (176). The results indicate that the median incremental costs over 25 years of disease vary from $61,000 to $122,000. Incremental costs were higher for younger individuals, and there was no systematic relationship between the incremental costs of women versus men (176).

In addition to cost-of-illness studies, there are several published cost-effectiveness evaluations of RA. These studies typically evaluate costs and consequences of various alternatives (i.e., medical intervention or therapeutic agent). The bulk were published after 1995 and conducted mainly in the United States, United Kingdom, and Canada. Various investigators reviewed the methodologic quality and major findings of these evaluations (177–181). Although most of the evaluations were found to be of high quality according to published methodologic guidelines, there was considerable heterogeneity in their methodology, and it was almost impossible to compare across studies. The most common intervention studied was prevention of NSAID-induced upper gastrointestinal ulcers (182–190). Also, a number of evaluations assessed the value of preventive or primary care–based interventions (191–197), traditional NSAIDs in comparison to cyclooxygenase-2 inhibitors (198–203), and the cost-effectiveness of newer disease-modifying antirheumatic drugs (204–209).

Economic evaluations in RA will become increasingly important in the future because cost-effectiveness findings are now an integral part of registration of new pharmaceuticals (210–213). Also, with disability and lost productivity being the major determinants of costs in RA patients, all future therapies will be expected to show economic advantage by delaying onset of disability. Efforts are currently under way to develop methodologic standards for economic evaluations in rheumatology. The OMERACT (Outcome Measures in Arthritis Clinical Trials) Task Force on economic evaluation recently published the consensus-based reference case for economic evaluations in RA (214).

SUMMARY

Epidemiologic research is an essential contributor to our understanding of RA. Studies of the descriptive epidemiology of RA indicate a population prevalence of 0.5% to 1.0% and highly variable annual incidence rates (from 8 to 900 per 100,000), depending on gender, race or ethnicity, and calendar year time period. Secular trends in RA incidence over time have been shown in several studies, supporting the hypothesis of a host–environment interaction. People with RA have a significantly increased risk of death compared to age- and sex-matched non-RA controls from the same community. The determinants of this excess mortality remain, although reports suggest increased risk of cardiovascular, infectious, gastrointestinal, respiratory, and hematologic diseases. Despite extensive epidemiologic research, the etiology of RA is unknown. Several risk factors have been suggested as important in the development or progression of RA. These include genetics, infectious agents, oral contraceptives, smoking, coffee consumption, and formal education. The economic impact of RA is substantial, mainly due to associated morbidity and long-term disability. Lifetime incremental cost of RA is estimated to be approximately $61,000 to $122,000.

ACKNOWLEDGMENTS

This chapter has been reprinted from Gabriel S. The epidemiology of rheumatic arthritis. *Rheum Dis Clin North Am* 2001;27(2):269–281, with permission from Elsevier Science. The authors wish to acknowledge Ms. Deborah Fogarty for her assistance in the preparation of this manuscript, and Michele Doran, M.D., for her contribution to the section *Risk Factors Associated with Rheumatoid Arthritis: Estrogens.*

REFERENCES

1. Fletcher R, Fletcher S, Wagner E. *Clinical epidemiology—the essentials,* 3rd ed. Baltimore: Williams & Wilkins, 1996.
2. Sackett D, Haynes R, Tugwell P. *Clinical epidemiology: a basic science for clinical medicine,* 2nd ed. Boston: Little, Brown and Company, 1991.
3. Hennekens C, Buring J. *Epidemiology in medicine.* Boston: Little, Brown and Company, 1987.
4. Symmons DPM, Barrett EM, Bankhead CR, et al. The incidence of rheumatoid arthritis in the United Kingdom: results from the Norfolk Arthritis Register. *Br J Rheumatol* 1994;33:735–739.
5. Arnett FC, Edworthy SM, Bloch DA, et al. The American Rheumatism Association 1987 revised criteria for the classification of rheumatoid arthritis. *Arthritis Rheum* 1988;31:315–324.
6. Wiles N, Symmons DP, Harrison B, et al. Estimating the incidence of rheumatoid arthritis: trying to hit a moving target? *Arthritis Rheum* 1999;42:1339–1346.
7. Aho K, Kaipiainen-Seppanen O, Heliovaara M, et al. Epidemiology of rheumatoid arthritis in Finland. *Semin Arthritis Rheum* 1998;27:325–334.
8. Kaipiainen-Seppanen O, Aho K. Incidence of chronic inflammatory joint diseases in Finland in 1995. *J Rheumatol* 2000;27:94–100.
9. Kaipiainen-Seppanen O, Aho K, Nikkarinen M. Regional differences in the incidence of rheumatoid arthritis in Finland in 1995. *Ann Rheum Dis* 2001; 60:128–132.
10. Kaipiainen-Seppanen O, Aho K, Isomaki H, et al. Incidence of rheumatoid arthritis in Finland during 1980–1990. *Ann Rheum Dis* 1996;55:608–611.
11. Kaipiainen-Seppanen O, Aho K, Laakso M. Shift in the incidence of rheumatoid arthritis toward elderly patients in Finland during 1975–1990. *Clin Exp Rheumatol* 1996;14:537–542.
12. Gabriel SE, Crowson CS, O'Fallon WM. The epidemiology of rheumatoid arthritis in Rochester, Minnesota, 1955–1985. *Arthritis Rheum* 1999;42:415–420.
13. Doran MF, Pond GR, Crowson CS, et al. Trends in incidence and mortality in rheumatoid arthritis in Rochester, Minnesota, over a forty-year period. *Arthritis Rheum* 2002;46:625–631.
14. Jacobsson LTH, Hanson RL, Knowler WC, et al. Decreasing incidence and prevalence of rheumatoid arthritis in Pima Indians over a twenty-five-year period. *Arthritis Rheum* 1994;37:1158–1165.
15. Drosos AA, Alamanos I, Voulgari PV, et al. Epidemiology of adult rheumatoid arthritis in northwest Greece 1987–1995. *J Rheumatol* 1997;24:2129–2133.
16. Dugowson CE, Koepsell TD, Voigt LF, et al. Rheumatoid arthritis in women. Incidence rates in Group Health Cooperative, Seattle, Washington, 1987–1989. *Arthritis Rheum* 1991;34:1502–1507.
17. Hochberg MC. Changes in the incidence and prevalence of rheumatoid arthritis in England and Wales, 1970–1982. *Semin Arthritis Rheum* 1990;19: 294–302.
18. Imanaka T, Shichikawa K, Inoue K, et al. Increase in age at onset of rheumatoid arthritis in Japan over a 30 year period. *Ann Rheum Dis* 1997;56:313–336.
19. MacGregor AJ, Silman AJ. A reappraisal of the measurement of disease occurrence in rheumatoid arthritis. *J Rheumatol* 1992;19:1163–1165.
20. Boyer GS, Benevolenskaya LI, Templin DW, et al. Prevalence of rheumatoid arthritis in circumpolar native populations. *J Rheumatol* 1998;25:23–29.
21. Cimmino MA. Prevalence of rheumatoid arthritis in Italy: the Chiavari study. *Ann Rheum Dis* 1998;57:315–318.
22. Stojanovic R, Vlajinac H, Palic-Obradovic D, et al. Prevalence of rheumatoid arthritis in Belgrade, Yugoslavia. *Br J Rheumatol* 1998;37:729–732.
23. Kvien TK, Glennas A, Knudsrod OG, et al. The prevalence and severity of rheumatoid arthritis in Oslo. Results from a county register and a population survey. *Scand J Rheumatol* 1997;26:412–418.
24. Power D, Codd M, Ivers L, et al. Prevalence of rheumatoid arthritis in Dublin, Ireland: a population based survey. *Ir J Med Sci* 1999;168:197–200.
25. Saraux A, Guedes C, Allain J, et al. Prevalence of rheumatoid arthritis and spondyloarthropathy in Brittany, France. Societe de Rhumatologie de l'Ouest. *J Rheumatol* 1999;26:2622–2627.
26. Simonsson M, Bergman S, Jacobsson LT, et al. The prevalence of rheumatoid arthritis in Sweden. *Scand J Rheumatol* 1999;28:340–343.
27. Carmona L, Villaverde V, Hernandez-Garcia C, et al. The prevalence of rheumatoid arthritis in the general population of Spain. *Rheumatology (Oxford)* 2002;41:88–95.

28. Riise T, Jacobsen BK, Gran JT. Incidence and prevalence of rheumatoid arthritis in the county of Troms, northern Norway. *J Rheumatol* 2000;27:1386–1389.
29. Symmons D, Turner G, Webb R, et al. The prevalence of rheumatoid arthritis in the United Kingdom: new estimates for a new century. *Rheumatology (Oxford)*; 2002;41:793–800.
30. Lawrence JS. Hypertension in relation to musculoskeletal disorders. *Ann Rheum Dis* 1975;34:451–456.
31. Holbrook TL, Wingard DL, Barrett-Connor E. Self-reported arthritis among men and women in an adult community. *J Community Health* 1990;15:195–208.
32. Scott JC, Hochberg MC, Stevens MB, et al. Arthritis in Maryland: prevalence and health care utilization. *Clin Res* 1986;34:872A.
33. Pincus T, Callahan LF. Taking mortality in rheumatoid arthritis seriously—predictive markers, socioeconomic status and comorbidity. *J Rheumatol* 1986;13:841–845.
34. Pincus T, Callahan LF, Vaughn WK. Questionnaire, walking time and button test measures of functional capacity as predictive markers for mortality in rheumatoid arthritis. *J Rheumatol* 1987;14:240–251.
35. Pincus T. Baseline information can help predict who is at risk. Is mortality increased in rheumatoid arthritis? *J Musculoskelet Med* 1988;5:27–46.
36. Berkanovic E, Hurwicz ML. Rheumatoid arthritis and comorbidity. *J Rheumatol* 1990;17:888–892.
37. Pincus T. New concepts in prognosis of rheumatic diseases for the 1990s. In: Bellamy N, ed. *Prognosis in the rheumatic diseases*. Dordrecht: Kluwer Academic, 1991:451–492.
38. Pincus T, Callahan LF. Quantitative measures to assess, monitor and predict morbidity and mortality in rheumatoid arthritis. *Baillieres Best Pract Res Clin Rheumatol* 1992;6:161–191.
39. Pincus T, Callahan LF. Remodeling the pyramid or remodeling the paradigms concerning rheumatoid arthritis—lessons from Hodgkin's disease and coronary artery disease. *J Rheumatol* 1990;17:1582–1585.
40. Gabriel SE, Crowson CS, O'Fallon WM. Comorbidity in arthritis. *J Rheumatol* 1999;26:2475–2479.
41. Kroot EJ, Van Gestel AM, Swinkels HL, et al. Chronic comorbidity in patients with early rheumatoid arthritis: a descriptive study. *J Rheumatol* 2001;28:1511–1517.
42. Mikuls TR, Saag KG. Comorbidity in rheumatoid arthritis. *Rheum Dis Clin North Am* 2001;27:283–303.
43. Doran M, Crowson C, Pond G, et al. Frequency of infection in patients with rheumatoid arthritis compared with controls: a population-based study. *Arthritis Rheum* 2002;46:2287–2293.
44. Doran M, Crowson C, Pond G, et al. Predictors of infection in rheumatoid arthritis. *Arthritis Rheum* 2002;46:2294–2300.
45. Cobb S, Anderson F, Bauer W. Length of life and cause of death in rheumatoid arthritis. *N Engl J Med* 1953;249:553–556.
46. Wolfe F, Mitchell DM, Sibley JT, et al. The mortality of rheumatoid arthritis. *Arthritis Rheum* 1994;37:481–494.
47. Pincus T, Brooks RH, Callahan LF. Prediction of long-term mortality in patients with rheumatoid arthritis according to simple questionnaire and joint count measures. *Ann Intern Med* 1994;120:26–34.
48. Coste J, Jougla E. Mortality from rheumatoid arthritis in France, 1970–1990. *Int J Epidemiol* 1994;23:545–552.
49. Monson RR, Hall AP. Mortality among arthritics. *J Chron Dis* 1976;29:459–467.
50. Myllykangas-Luosujarvi RA, Aho K, Isomaki HA. Mortality in rheumatoid arthritis. *Semin Arthritis Rheum* 1995;25:193–202.
51. Gabriel SE, Crowson CS, O'Fallon WM. Mortality in rheumatoid arthritis: have we made an impact in 4 decades? *J Rheumatol* 1999;26:2529–2533.
52. Myllykangas-Luosujarvi R, Aho K, Kautiainen H, et al. Shortening of life span and causes of excess mortality in a population-based series of subjects with rheumatoid arthritis. *Clin Exp Rheumatol* 1995;13:149–153.
53. Isomaki HA, Mutru O, Koota K. Death rate and causes of death in patients with rheumatoid arthritis. *Scand J Rheumatol* 1975;4:205–208.
54. Vandenbroucke JP, Hazevoet HM, Cats A. Survival and cause of death in rheumatoid arthritis: a 25-year prospective followup. *J Rheumatol* 1984;11:158–161.
55. Pincus T, Callahan LF, Sale WG, et al. Severe functional declines, work disability, and increased mortality in seventy-five rheumatoid arthritis patients studied over nine years. *Arthritis Rheum* 1984;27:864–872.
56. Allebeck P, Ahlbom A, Allander E. Increased mortality among persons with rheumatoid arthritis, but where RA does not appear on death certificate. Eleven-year follow-up of an epidemiological study. *Scand J Rheumatol* 1981;10:301–306.
57. Allebeck P. Increased mortality in rheumatoid arthritis. *Scand J Rheumatol* 1982;11:81–86.
58. Prior P, Symmons DPM, Scott DL, et al. Cause of death in rheumatoid arthritis. *Br J Rheumatol* 1984;23:92–99.
59. Jacobsson LTH, Knowler WC, Pillemer S, et al. Rheumatoid arthritis and mortality: a longitudinal study in Pima Indians. *Arthritis Rheum* 1993;36:1045–1053.
60. van Dam G, Lezwign A, Bos JG. Death rate in patients with rheumatoid arthritis. *Minerva Med* 1961;1:161–164.
61. Duthie JJR, Brown PE, Truelove LH, et al. Course and prognosis in rheumatoid arthritis. A further report. *Ann Rheum Dis* 1964;23:193–204.
62. Reilly PA, Cosh JA, Maddison PJ, et al. Mortality and survival in rheumatoid arthritis: a 25 year prospective study of 100 patients. *Ann Rheum Dis* 1990; 49:363–369.
63. Lewis P, Hazleman BL, Hanka R, et al. Cause of death in patients with rheumatoid arthritis with particular reference to azathioprine. *Ann Rheum Dis* 1980;39:457–461.
64. Linos A, Worthington JW, O'Fallon WM, et al. The epidemiology of rheumatoid arthritis in Rochester, Minnesota: a study of incidence, prevalence, and mortality. *Am J Epidemiol* 1980;111:87–98.
65. Mutru O, Laakso M, Isomaki H, et al. Ten year mortality and causes of death in patients with rheumatoid arthritis. *BMJ* 1985;290:1797–1799.
66. Mitchell DM, Spitz PW, Young DY, et al. Survival, prognosis, and causes of death in rheumatoid arthritis. *Arthritis Rheum* 1986;29:706–714.
67. Wallberg-Jonsson S, Ohman ML, Dahlqvist SR. Cardiovascular morbidity and mortality in patients with seropositive rheumatoid arthritis in Northern Sweden. *J Rheumatol* 1997;24:445–451.
68. Sokka T, Mottonen T, Hannonen P. Mortality in early "sawtooth" treated rheumatoid arthritis patients during the first 8–14 years. *Scand J Rheumatol* 1999;28:282–287.
69. Symmons DP, Jones MA, Scott DL, Prior P. Longterm mortality outcome in patients with rheumatoid arthritis: early presenters continue to do well. *J Rheumatol* 1998;25:1072–1077.
70. Kvalvik AG, Jones MA, Symmons DP. Mortality in a cohort of Norwegian patients with rheumatoid arthritis followed from 1977 to 1992. *Scand J Rheumatol* 2000;29:29–37.
71. Chehata JC, Hassell AB, Clarke SA, et al. Mortality in rheumatoid arthritis: relationship to single and composite measures of disease activity. *Rheumatology (Oxford)* 2001;40:447–452.
72. Krause D, Schleusser B, Herborn G, et al. Response to methotrexate treatment is associated with reduced mortality in patients with severe rheumatoid arthritis. *Arthritis Rheum* 2000;43:14–21.
73. Martinez MS, Garcia-Monforte A, Rivera J. Survival study of rheumatoid arthritis patients in Madrid (Spain). A 9-year prospective follow-up. *Scand J Rheumatol* 2001;30:195–198.
74. Riise T, Jacobsen BK, Gran JT, et al. Total mortality is increased in rheumatoid arthritis. A 17-year prospective study. *Clin Rheumatol* 2001;20:123–127.
75. Uddin J, Kraus AS, Kelly HG. Survivorship and death in rheumatoid arthritis. *Arthritis Rheum* 1970;13:125–130.
76. Callahan LF, Cordray DS, Wells G, et al. Formal education and five-year mortality in rheumatoid arthritis: mediation by helplessness scale score. *Arthritis Care Research* 1996;9:463–472.
77. Ward MM. Recent improvements in survival in patients with rheumatoid arthritis: better outcomes or different study designs? *Arthritis Rheum* 2001; 44:1467–1469.
78. Goodson NJ, Wiles NJ, Lunt M, et al. Mortality in early inflammatory polyarthritis: cardiovascular mortality is increased in seropositive patients. *Arthritis Rheum* 2002;46:2010–2019.
79. Mutru O, Laakso M, Isomaki H, et al. Ten year mortality and causes of death in patients with rheumatoid arthritis. *BMJ (Clin Res Ed)* 1985;290: 1797–1799.
80. Gabriel SE, Crowson CS, Maradit Kremers H, et al. Survival in rheumatoid arthritis: a population-based analysis of trends over 40 years. *Arthritis Rheum* 2003;48:54–58.
81. Soderlin MK, Nieminen P, Hakala M. Functional status predicts mortality in a community based rheumatoid arthritis population. *J Rheumatol* 1998; 25:1895–1899.
82. Erhardt CC, Mumford PA, Venables PJ, et al. Factors predicting a poor life prognosis in rheumatoid arthritis: an eight year prospective study. *Ann Rheum Dis* 1989;48:7–13.
83. Wallberg-Jonsson S, Johansson H, Ohman ML, et al. Extent of inflammation predicts cardiovascular disease and overall mortality in seropositive rheumatoid arthritis. A retrospective cohort study from disease onset. *J Rheumatol* 1999;26:2562–2571.
84. Leigh JP, Fries JF. Mortality predictors among 263 patients with rheumatoid arthritis. *J Rheumatol* 1991;18:1307–1312.
85. Turesson C, O'Fallon WM, Crowson CS, et al. Occurrence of extraarticular disease manifestations is associated with excess mortality in a community based cohort of patients with rheumatoid arthritis. *J Rheumatol* 2002;29:62–67.
86. Mutru O, Laakso M, Isomaki H, et al. Cardiovascular mortality in patients with rheumatoid arthritis. *Cardiology* 1989;76:71–77.
87. Jacobsson LT, Knowler WC, Pillemer S, et al. Rheumatoid arthritis and mortality. A longitudinal study in Pima Indians. *Arthritis Rheum* 1993;36:1045–1053.
88. Myllykangas-Luosujarvi R, Aho K, Kautiainen H, et al. Cardiovascular mortality in women with rheumatoid arthritis. *J Rheumatol* 1995;22:1065–1067.
89. Asanuma Y, Kawai S, Aoshima H, et al. Serum lipoprotein(a) and apolipoprotein(a) phenotypes in patients with rheumatoid arthritis [see comments]. *Arthritis Rheum* 1999;42:443–447.
90. Wallberg-Jonsson S, Cederfelt M, Dahlqvist SR. Hemostatic factors and cardiovascular disease in active rheumatoid arthritis: an 8 year followup study. *J Rheumatol* 2000;27:71–75.
91. del Rincon ID. High incidence of cardiovascular events in a rheumatoid arthritis cohort not explained by traditional cardiac risk factors. *Arthritis Rheum* 2001;44:2737–2745.
92. Jacobsson LT, Turesson C, Hanson RL, et al. Joint swelling as a predictor of death from cardiovascular disease in a population study of Pima Indians. *Arthritis Rheum* 2001;44:1170–1176.
93. Hurt-Camejo E, Paredes S, Masana L, et al. Elevated levels of small, low-density lipoprotein with high affinity for arterial matrix components in patients with rheumatoid arthritis. *Arthritis Rheum* 2001;44:2761–2767.
94. Choi HK, Hernán MA, Seeger JD, et al. Methotrexate and mortality in patients with rheumatoid arthritis: a prospective study. *Lancet* 2002;359: 1173–1177.

95. Ray WA, Stein CM, Hall K, et al. Non-steroidal anti-inflammatory drugs and risk of serious coronary heart disease: an observational cohort study. *Lancet* 2002;359:118–123.
96. Dalen J. Selective COX-2 inhibitors, NSAIDs, aspirin, and myocardial infarction. *Arch Intern Med* 2002;162:1091–1092.
97. Hochberg MC. Adult and juvenile rheumatoid arthritis: current epidemiologic concepts. *Epidemiol Rev* 1981;3:27–44.
98. Deighton CM, Walker DJ. The familial nature of rheumatoid arthritis. *Ann Rheum Dis* 1991;50:62–65.
99. Stastny P. Association of the B-cell alloantigen DRw4 with rheumatoid arthritis. *N Engl J Med* 1978;298:869–871.
100. Gregerson P, Silver J, Winchester R. The shared epitope hypothesis: an approach to understanding the molecular genetics of susceptibility to rheumatoid arthritis. *Arthritis Rheum* 1987;30:1205–1213.
101. Nepom GT, Hansen JA, Nepom BS. The molecular basis for HLA class II associations with rheumatoid arthritis. *J Clin Immunol* 1987;7:1–7.
102. Willkens RF, Nepom GT, Marks CR, et al. Association of HLA-Dw16 with rheumatoid arthritis in Yakima Indians. Further evidence for the "shared epitope" hypothesis. *Arthritis Rheum* 1991;34:43–47.
103. del Rincon I, Escalante A. HLA-DRB1 alleles associated with susceptibility or resistance to rheumatoid arthritis, articular deformities, and disability in Mexican Americans. *Arthritis Rheum* 1999;42:1329–1338.
104. Pascual M, Nieto A, Lopez-Nevot MA, et al. Rheumatoid arthritis in southern Spain: toward elucidation of a unifying role of the HLA class II region in disease predisposition. *Arthritis Rheum* 2001;44:307–314.
105. Tuokko J, Nejentsev S, Luukkainen R. HLA haplotype analysis in Finnish patients with rheumatoid arthritis. *Arthritis Rheum* 2001;44:315–322.
106. Gonzalez-Gay MA, Garcia-Porrua C, Hajeer AH. Influence of human leukocyte antigen-DRB1 on the susceptibility and severity of rheumatoid arthritis. *Semin Arthritis Rheum* 2002;31:355–360.
107. Ioannidis JP, Tarassi K, Papadopoulos IA, et al. Shared epitopes and rheumatoid arthritis: disease associations in Greece and meta-analysis of Mediterranean European populations. *Semin Arthritis Rheum* 2002;31:361–370.
108. Deighton CM, Cavanagh G, Rigby AS, et al. Both inherited HLA-haplotypes are important in the predisposition to rheumatoid arthritis. *Br J Rheumatol* 1993;32:893–898.
109. Yamashita TS, Khan MA, Kushner I. Genetic analysis of families with multiple cases of rheumatoid arthritis. *Dis Markers* 1986;4:113–119.
110. Hasstedt S, Cartwright P. PAP: pedigree analysis package. Salt Lake City: University of Utah Medical Center, Tech report 13, rev. 2.
111. Rigby AS, Voelm L, Silman AJ. Epistatic modeling in rheumatoid arthritis: an application of the Risch theory. *Genet Epidemiol* 1993;10[Suppl]:311–320.
112. Genin E, Babron MC, McDermott MF, et al. Modelling the major histocompatibility complex susceptibility to RA using the MASC method. *Genet Epidemiol* 1998;15[Suppl]:419–430.
113. Weyand CM, Hicok KC, Conn DL, et al. The influence of HLA-DRB1 genes on disease severity in rheumatoid arthritis. *Ann Intern Med* 1992;117:801–806.
114. Harrison B, Thomson W, Symmons D, et al. The influence of HLA-DRB1 alleles and rheumatoid factor on disease outcome in an inception cohort of patients with early inflammatory arthritis. *Arthritis Rheum* 1999;42:2174–2183.
115. Reveille JD. The genetic contribution to the pathogenesis of rheumatoid arthritis. *Curr Opin Rheumatol* 1998;10:187–200.
116. Criswell LA, Mu H, Such CL, et al. Inheritance of the shared epitope and long-term outcomes of rheumatoid arthritis among community-based Caucasian females. *Genet Epidemiol* 1998;15[Suppl]:61–72.
117. Moxley G, Cohen HJ. Genetic studies, clinical heterogeneity, and disease outcome studies in rheumatoid arthritis. *Rheum Dis Clin North Am* 2002;28:39–58.
118. Gorman JD, Criswell LA. The shared epitope and severity of rheumatoid arthritis. *Rheum Dis Clin North Am* 2002;28:59–78.
119. Hasstedt SJ, Clegg DO, Ingles L, et al. HLA-linked rheumatoid arthritis. *Am J Hum Genet* 1994;55:738–746.
120. Rigby AS, Silman AJ, Voelm L, et al. Investigating the HLA component in rheumatoid arthritis: an additive (dominant) mode of inheritance is rejected, a recessive mode is preferred. *Genet Epidemiol* 1991;8:153–175.
121. Rigby AS, MacGregor AJ, Thomson G. HLA haplotype sharing in rheumatoid arthritis sibships: risk estimates subdivided by proband genotype. *Genet Epidemiol* 1998;15[Suppl 4]:403–418.
122. Del Puente A, Knowler WC, Pettitt DJ, et al. High incidence and prevalence of rheumatoid arthritis in Pima Indians. *Am J Epidemiol* 1989;129:1170–1178.
123. Oen K, Postl B, Chalmers IM, et al. Rheumatic diseases in an Inuit population. *Arthritis Rheum* 1986;29:65–74.
124. Hirsch R, Lin JP, Scott WW Jr., et al. Rheumatoid arthritis in the Pima Indians: the intersection of epidemiologic, demographic, and genealogic data. *Arthritis Rheum* 1998;41:1464–1469.
125. Silman AJ. The genetic epidemiology of rheumatoid arthritis. *Clin Exp Rheumatol* 1992;10:309–312.
126. Lynn AH, Kwoh CK, Venglish CM, et al. Genetic epidemiology of rheumatoid arthritis. *Am J Hum Genet* 1995;57:150–159.
127. Aho K, Koskenvuo M, Tuominen J, et al. Occurrence of rheumatoid arthritis in a nationwide series of twins. *J Rheumatol* 1986;13:899–902.
128. Silman AJ, MacGregor AJ, Thomson W, et al. Twin concordance rates for rheumatoid arthritis: results from a nationwide study. *Br J Rheumatol* 1993;32:903–907.
129. Jarvinen P, Aho K. Twin studies in rheumatic diseases. *Semin Arthritis Rheum* 1994;24:19–28.
130. Wolfe F, Kleinheksel SM, Khan MA. Familial vs sporadic rheumatoid arthritis: a comparison of the demographic and clinical characteristics of 956 patients. *J Rheumatol* 1988;15:400–404.
131. MacGregor AJ, Snieder H, Rigby AS, et al. Characterizing the quantitative genetic contribution to rheumatoid arthritis using data from twins. *Arthritis Rheum* 2000;43:30–37.
132. Grant SF, Thorleifsson G, Frigge ML, et al. The inheritance of rheumatoid arthritis in Iceland. *Arthritis Rheum* 2001;44:2247–2254.
133. Barrera P, Radstake TR, Albers JM, et al. Familial aggregation of rheumatoid arthritis in The Netherlands: a cross-sectional hospital-based survey. European Consortium on Rheumatoid Arthritis Families (ECRAF). *Rheumatology (Oxford)* 1999;38:415–422.
134. Radstake TR, Barrera P, Albers JM, et al. Familial vs sporadic rheumatoid arthritis (RA). A prospective study in an early RA inception cohort. *Rheumatology* 2000;39:267–273.
135. Laivoranta-Nyman S, Mottonen T, Luukkainen R, et al. Immunogenetic differences between patients with familial and non-familial rheumatoid arthritis. *Ann Rheum Dis* 2000;59:173–177.
136. Cornelis F, Faure S, Martinez M, et al. New susceptibility locus for rheumatoid arthritis suggested by a genome-wide linkage study. *Proc Natl Acad Sci U S A* 1998;95:10746–10750.
137. Shiozawa S, Hayashi S, Tsukamoto Y, et al. Identification of the gene loci that predispose to rheumatoid arthritis. *Int Immunol* 1998;10:1891–1895.
138. MacKay K, Eyre S, Myerscough A, et al. Whole-genome linkage analysis of rheumatoid arthritis susceptibility loci in 252 affected sibling pairs in the United Kingdom. *Arthritis Rheum* 2002;46:632–639.
139. Jawaheer D, Seldin MF, Amos CI, et al. A genomewide screen in multiplex rheumatoid arthritis families suggests genetic overlap with other autoimmune diseases. *Am J Hum Genet* 2001;68:927–936.
140. Mattey DL, Hassell AB, Dawes PT, et al. Interaction between tumor necrosis factor microsatellite polymorphisms and the HLA-DRB1 shared epitope in rheumatoid arthritis: influence on disease outcome. *Arthritis Rheum* 1999; 42:2698–2704.
141. Martinez A, Fernandez-Arquero M, Pascual-Salcedo D, et al. Primary association of tumor necrosis factor-region genetic markers with susceptibility to rheumatoid arthritis. *Arthritis Rheum* 2000;43:1366–1370.
142. Barton A, John S, Ollier WE, et al. Association between rheumatoid arthritis and polymorphism of tumor necrosis factor receptor II, but not tumor necrosis factor receptor I, in Caucasians. *Arthritis Rheum* 2001;44:61–65.
143. Bridges SL Jr., Jenq G, Moran M, et al. Single-nucleotide polymorphisms in tumor necrosis factor receptor genes: definition of novel haplotypes and racial/ethnic differences. *Arthritis Rheum* 2002;46:2045–2050.
144. Lard LR, Boers M, Verhoeven A, et al. Early and aggressive treatment of rheumatoid arthritis patients affects the association of HLA class II antigens with progression of joint damage. *Arthritis Rheum* 2002;46:899–905.
145. Silman A, Bankhead C, Rowlingson B, et al. Do new cases of rheumatoid arthritis cluster in time or in space? *Int J Epidemiol* 1997;26:628–634.
146. Silman A, Harrison B, Barrett E, et al. The existence of geographical clusters of cases of inflammatory polyarthritis in a primary care based register. *Ann Rheum Dis* 2000;59:152–154.
147. Silman AJ. Trends in the incidence and severity of rheumatoid arthritis. *J Rheumatol* 1992[Suppl 32]19:71–73.
148. Silman AJ. Are there secular trends in the occurrence and severity of rheumatoid arthritis? *Scand J Rheumatol* 1989[Suppl 79]:25–30.
149. Silman AJ. Epidemiology of rheumatoid arthritis [Review]. *APMIS* 1994; 102:721–728.
150. Hochberg MC, Spector TD. Epidemiology of rheumatoid arthritis: update. *Epidemiol Rev* 1990;12:247–252.
151. Harrison B, Silman A, Barrett E, et al. Low frequency of recent parvovirus infection in a population-based cohort of patients with early inflammatory polyarthritis. *Ann Rheum Dis* 1998;57:375–377.
152. Brennan P, Bankhead C, Silman A, et al. Oral contraceptives and rheumatoid arthritis: results from a primary care-based incident case-control study. *Semin Arthritis Rheum* 1997;26:817–823.
153. Carette S, Marcoux S, Gingras S. Postmenopausal hormones and the incidence of rheumatoid arthritis. *J Rheumatol* 1989;16:911–913.
154. Vandenbroucke JP, Witteman JC, Valkenburg HA, et al. Noncontraceptive hormones and rheumatoid arthritis in perimenopausal and postmenopausal women. *JAMA* 1986;255:1299–1303.
155. Hernandez-Avila M, Liang MH, Willett WC, et al. Oral contraceptives, replacement oestrogens and the risk of rheumatoid arthritis. *Br J Rheumatol* 1989;28[Suppl 1]:31; discussion, 42–45.
156. Spector TD, Brennan P, Harris P, et al. Does estrogen replacement therapy protect against rheumatoid arthritis? *J Rheumatol* 1991;18:1473–1476.
157. Doran M. The effect of oral contraceptives and estrogen replacement therapy on the risk of rheumatoid arthritis: a population-based study. *J Rheumotol* 2004;31.
158. Harrison BJ. Influence of cigarette smoking on disease outcome in rheumatoid arthritis. *Curr Opin Rheumatol* 2002;14:93–97.
159. Uhlig T, Hagen KB, Kvien TK. Current tobacco smoking, formal education, and the risk of rheumatoid arthritis. *J Rheumatol* 1999;26:47–54.
160. Karlson EW, Lee IM, Cook NR, et al. A retrospective cohort study of cigarette smoking and risk of rheumatoid arthritis in female health professionals. *Arthritis Rheum* 1999;42:910–917.
161. Wolfe F. The effect of smoking on clinical, laboratory, and radiographic status in rheumatoid arthritis. *J Rheumatol* 2000;27:630–637.

162. Silman AJ, Newman J, MacGregor AJ. Cigarette smoking increases the risk of rheumatoid arthritis. Results from a nationwide study of disease-discordant twins. *Arthritis Rheum* 1996;39:732–735.
163. Heliovaara M, Aho K, Aromaa A, et al. Smoking and risk of rheumatoid arthritis. *J Rheumatol* 1993;20:1830–1835.
164. Heliovaara M, Aho K, Knekt P, et al. Coffee consumption, rheumatoid factor, and the risk of rheumatoid arthritis. *Ann Rheum Dis* 2000;59:631–635.
165. Mikuls TR, Cerhan JR, Criswell LA, et al. Coffee, tea, and caffeine consumption and risk of rheumatoid arthritis: results from the Iowa Women's Health Study. *Arthritis Rheum* 2002;46:83–91.
166. Pincus T, Callahan LF, Burkhauser RV. Most chronic diseases are reported more frequently by individuals with fewer than 12 years of formal education in the age 18–64 United States population. *J Chron Dis* 1987;40:865–874.
167. Pincus T, Callahan LF. Formal education as a marker for increased mortality and morbidity in rheumatoid arthritis. *J Chron Dis* 1985;38:973–984.
168. Callahan LF, Pincus T. Formal education level as a significant marker of clinical status in rheumatoid arthritis. *Arthritis Rheum* 1988;31:1346–1357.
169. Bankhead C, Silman A, Barrett B, et al. Incidence of rheumatoid arthritis is not related to indicators of socioeconomic deprivation. *J Rheumatol* 1996;23:2039–2042.
170. Yelin E, Herrndorf A, Trupin L, et al. A national study of medical care expenditures for musculoskeletal conditions: the impact of health insurance and managed care. *Arthritis Rheum* 2001;44:1160–1169.
171. Hunsche E, Chancellor JV, Bruce N. The burden of arthritis and nonsteroidal anti-inflammatory treatment. A European literature review. *Pharmacoeconomics* 2001;19[Suppl 1]:1–15.
172. Pugner KM, Scott DI, Holmes JW, et al. The costs of rheumatoid arthritis: an international long-term view. *Semin Arthritis Rheum* 2000;29:305–320.
173. Cooper N. Economic burden of rheumatoid arthritis: a systemic review. *Rheumatology* 2000;39:28–33.
174. Lubeck DP. A review of the direct costs of rheumatoid arthritis: managed care versus fee-for-service settings. *Pharmacoeconomics* 2001;19:811–818.
175. Gabriel SE, Crowson CS, Campion ME, et al. Indirect and nonmedical costs among people with rheumatoid arthritis and osteoarthritis compared with nonarthritic controls. *J Rheumatol* 1997;24:43–48.
176. Gabriel SE, Crowson CS, Luthra HS, et al. Modeling the lifetime costs of rheumatoid arthritis. *J Rheumatol* 1999;26:1269–1274.
177. Ferraz MB, Maetzel A, Bombardier C. A summary of economic evaluations published in the field of rheumatology and related disciplines. *Arthritis Rheum* 1997;40:1587–1593.
178. Maetzel A, Ferraz MB, Bombardier C. A review of cost-effectiveness analyses in rheumatology and related disciplines. *Curr Opin Rheumatol* 1998;10 :136–140.
179. Rothfuss J, Mau W, Zeidler H, et al. Socioeconomic evaluation of rheumatoid arthritis and osteoarthritis: a literature review. *Semin Arthritis Rheum* 1997; 26:771–779.
180. Ruchlin HS, Elkin EB, Paget SA. Assessing cost-effectiveness analyses in rheumatoid arthritis and osteoarthritis. *Arthritis Care Research* 1997;10:413–421.
181. Maradit Kremers H, Gabriel SE, Drummond D. Principles of health economic and application to rheumatic diseases. In: Hochberg MC, Silman A, Smolen JS, Weinblatt ME, Weisman MH, eds. *Rheumatology*, 3rd ed. Philadelphia: Elsevier Science, 2004:45–54.
182. Al MJ, Michel BC, Rutten FFH. The cost effectiveness of diclofenac plus misoprostol compared with diclofenac monotherapy in patients with rheumatoid arthritis. *Pharmacoeconomics* 1996;10:141–151.
183. Gabriel SE, Campion ME, O'Fallon WM. A cost-utility analysis of misoprostol prophylaxis for rheumatoid arthritis patients receiving nonsteroidal anti-inflammatory drugs. *Arthritis Rheum* 1994;37:333–341.
184. Schwarz B. Die Kosten-Effektivitat der Misoprostoltherapie in der Pravention NSAR-induzierter Magenulzera. *Wien Klin Wochenschr* 1995;107:366–372.
185. Goldstein JL, Larson LR, Yamashita BD, et al. Management of NSAID-induced gastropathy: an economic decision analysis. *Clin Ther* 1997;19:1496–1509; discussion, 24–25.
186. Maetzel A, Ferraz MB, Bombardier C. The cost-effectiveness of misoprostol in preventing serious gastrointestinal events associated with the use of nonsteroidal antiinflammatory drugs. *Arthritis Rheum* 1998;41:16–25.
187. McCabe CJ, Akehurst RL, Kirsch J, et al. Choice of NSAID and management strategy in rheumatoid arthritis and osteoarthritis: the impact on costs and outcomes in the UK. *Pharmacoeconomics* 1998;14:191–199.
188. Walan A, Wahlqvist P. Pharmacoeconomic aspects of non-steroidal anti-inflammatory drug gastropathy. *Ital J Gastroenterol Hepatol* 1999;31[Suppl 1]:S79–88.
189. Kristiansen IS, Kvien TK, Nord E. Cost effectiveness of replacing diclofenac with a fixed combination of misoprostol and diclofenac in patients with rheumatoid arthritis. *Arthritis Rheum* 1999;42:2293–2302.
190. Davey PJ, Meyer E. The cost effectiveness of misoprostol prophylaxis alongside long term nonsteroidal anti-inflammatory drugs: implications of the MUCOSA trial. *Pharmacoeconomics* 2000;17:295–304.
191. Anderson RB, Needleman RD, Gatter RA, et al. Patient outcome following inpatient vs outpatient treatment of rheumatoid arthritis. *J Rheumatol* 1988; 15:556–560.
192. Helewa A, Bombardier C, Goldsmith CH, et al. Cost-effectiveness of inpatient and intensive outpatient treatment of rheumatoid arthritis. A randomized, controlled trial. *Arthritis Rheum* 1989;32:1505–1514.
193. Lorig KR, Mazonson PD, Holman HR. Evidence suggesting that health education for self-management in patients with chronic arthritis has sustained health benefits while reducing health care costs. *Arthritis Rheum* 1993;36:439–446.
194. Nordstrom DC, Konttinen YT, Solovieva S, et al. In- and out-patient rehabilitation in rheumatoid arthritis. A controlled, open, longitudinal, cost-effectiveness study. *Scand J Rheumatol* 1996;25:200–206.
195. Kruger JM, Helmick CG, Callahan LF, et al. Cost-effectiveness of the arthritis self-help course. *Arch Intern Med* 1998;158:1245–1249.
196. Lambert CM, Hurst NP, Forbes JF, et al. Is day care equivalent to inpatient care for active rheumatoid arthritis? Randomised controlled clinical and economic evaluation. *BMJ* 1998;316:965–969.
197. Lambert CM, Hurst NP, Lochhead A, et al. A pilot study of the economic cost and clinical outcome of day patient vs inpatient management of active rheumatoid arthritis. *Br J Rheumatol* 1994;33:383–388.
198. Motheral BR, Bataoel JR, Armstrong EP. A strategy for evaluating the novel COX-2 inhibitors versus NSAIDs for arthritis. *Hosp Formul* 1999;34:855–863.
199. Svarvar P, Aly A. Use of the ACCES model to predict the health economic impact of celecoxib in patients with osteoarthritis or rheumatoid arthritis in Norway. *Rheumatology (Oxford)* 2000;39[Suppl 2]:43–50.
200. Haglund U, Svarvar P. The Swedish ACCES model: predicting the health economic impact of celecoxib in patients with osteoarthritis or rheumatoid arthritis. *Rheumatology (Oxford)* 2000;39[Suppl 2]:51–56.
201. Zabinski RA, Burke TA, Johnson J, et al. An economic model for determining the costs and consequences of using various treatment alternatives for the management of arthritis in Canada. *Pharmacoeconomics* 2001;19[Suppl 1]:49–58.
202. Chancellor JV, Hunsche E, de Cruz E, et al. Economic evaluation of celecoxib, a new cyclo-oxygenase 2 specific inhibitor, in Switzerland. *Pharmacoeconomics* 2001;19[Suppl 1]:59–75.
203. Marshall JK, Pellissier JM, Attard CL, et al. Incremental cost-effectiveness analysis comparing rofecoxib with nonselective NSAIDs in osteoarthritis: Ontario Ministry of Health perspective. *Pharmacoeconomics* 2001;19:1039–1049.
204. Choi HK, Seeger JD, Kuntz KM. A cost-effectiveness analysis of treatment options for patients with methotrexate-resistant rheumatoid arthritis. *Arthritis Rheum* 2000;43:2316–2327.
205. Choi HK, Seeger JD, Kuntz KM. A cost effectiveness analysis of treatment options for methotrexate-naive rheumatoid arthritis. *J Rheumatol* 2002;29: 1156–1165.
206. Kavanaugh A, Heudebert G, Cush J, et al. Cost evaluation of novel therapeutics in rheumatoid arthritis (CENTRA): a decision analysis model. *Semin Arthritis Rheum* 1996;25:297–307.
207. Maetzel A, Strand V, Tugwell P, et al. Economic comparison of leflunomide and methotrexate in patients with rheumatoid arthritis: an evaluation based on a 1-year randomised controlled trial. *Pharmacoeconomics* 2002;20:61–70.
208. Suarez-Almazor M, Connor-Spady B. Rating of arthritis health states by patients, physicians, and the general public. Implications for cost-utility analyses. *J Rheumatol* 2001;28:648–656.
209. Slothuus U, Brooks RG. Willingness to pay in arthritis: a Danish contribution. *Rheumatology (Oxford)* 2000;39:791–799.
210. Nuijten MJ, Starzewski J. Applications of modelling studies. *Pharmacoeconomics* 1998;13:289–291.
211. Bloor K, Maynard A, Freemantle N. Lessons from international experience in controlling pharmaceutical expenditure. III: Regulating industry. *BMJ* 1996; 313:33–35.
212. Jacobs P, Bachynsky J, Baladi JF. A comparative review of pharmacoeconomic guidelines. *Pharmacoeconomics* 1995;8:182–189.
213. Henry D. Economic analysis as an aid to subsidisation decisions: the development of Australian guidelines for pharmaceuticals. *Pharmacoeconomics* 1992;1:54–67.
214. Gabriel SE, Drummond M, Maetzel A, et al. OMERACT 6 Economics working group report: a proposal for a reference case for economic evaluation in rheumatoid arthritis. *J Rheumatol* 2003;30:886–890.
215. Chan K-WA, Felson DT, Yood RA, et al. Incidence of rheumatoid arthritis in central Massachusetts. *Arthritis Rheum* 1993;36:1691–1696.
216. Uhlig T, Kvien TK, Glennas A, et al. The incidence and severity of rheumatoid arthritis, results from a county register in Oslo, Norway. *J Rheumatol* 1998;25:1078–1084.
217. Shichikawa K, Inoue K, Hirota S, et al. Changes in the incidence and prevalence of rheumatoid arthritis in Kamitonda, Wakayama, Japan, 1965–1996. *Ann Rheum Dis* 1999;58:751–756.
218. Lindqvist E, Eberhardt K. Mortality in rheumatoid arthritis patients with disease onset in the 1980s. *Ann Rheum Dis* 1999;58:11–14.

CHAPTER 2

Clinical Features and Differential Diagnosis

Peter D. Kent and Eric L. Matteson

Rheumatoid arthritis (RA) is a chronic, usually progressive, systemic inflammatory condition of unknown cause. It is characterized by synovial proliferation and a symmetric, erosive arthritis of peripheral joints, but it may also cause systemic manifestations.

CLINICAL FEATURES

The diagnosis of RA is made using the patient's history and examination results in conjunction with laboratory and radiographic data. Patient characteristics, including age, gender, and ethnicity, are important, as they are related to disease risk and severity. Approximately 75% of patients with RA are women. RA with involvement limited to the hands and feet—sparing the more proximal joints, such as the shoulders, hips, and cervical spine—is more common in women than in men (1). In contrast, there is a higher rate of large-joint involvement in men. Erosive disease is found in long-term follow-up in up to 73% of men and 55% of women (1). Although a higher percentage of men have erosive disease, women undergo almost twice as many orthopedic surgeries as men, principally hand and foot joint procedures. This difference may be a consequence of increased small-joint involvement in women, but other factors may also contribute. The presence of a positive rheumatoid factor (RF) and of rheumatoid nodules are also risk factors for joint surgery (2).

Of the extraarticular manifestations, nodules, as well as lung and pericardial involvement, are more common in men, whereas the sicca syndrome occurs more frequently in women (1). Native Americans are at a higher risk for developing RA than Northern Europeans and often have early-onset seropositive disease with extraarticular manifestations (3). The incidence of disease-related complications increases with disease duration, and patients with longer disease duration may not respond as well to treatment as those with early disease (4,5). There are no specific laboratory findings in RA, although the RF is positive in approximately 60% of patients at diagnosis and 80% to 90% of patients with established disease (6).

Patients with RA usually report joint pain at rest and with motion, in addition to joint swelling and stiffness. Morning stiffness secondary to an inflammatory arthritis such as RA usually lasts longer than 45 minutes if not modified by treatment, and mornings are typically the worst time of day for function. Stiffness can be difficult to define but may best be described as slowness or difficulty moving joints when getting out of bed or after remaining stationary for a period. Stiffness improves with movement.

To distinguish RA from other forms of arthritis, classification criteria were developed by the American Rheumatism Association (Table 2.1) (7). These criteria are useful when evaluating patients with potential RA and provide a 91% to 94% sensitivity and an 89% specificity for the diagnosis of RA (7). In very early RA, however, nodules and erosive changes may not be present. The pattern of joint involvement, especially in early disease, may not satisfy the criteria, and, as a result, they are less sensitive for classifying patients with early disease. The diminished sensitivity of the criteria in early disease helps to illustrate an important point: The criteria are intended to ensure standardization of patient groups for clinical studies and not specifically for making a diagnosis or as the basis of medical decision making.

A complete history includes asking about the symptoms of extraarticular RA (ExRA) and recording joint surgeries and past serious infections, including tuberculosis, fungal infections, and hepatitis B and C. A complete review of systems is essential, as RA can affect almost any organ system. Detection of organ involvement frequently influences therapeutic decisions. Patients not uncommonly report or even present with constitutional symptoms such as lethargy, weight loss, malaise, or fever. A positive family history of RA should increase suspicion for RA in a patient presenting with articular complaints.

PHYSICAL EXAMINATION

Physical examination of patients with arthritis includes a standardized assessment of joint swelling, tenderness, and limitation of motion, as well as a thorough general medical examination.

Joint tenderness is assessed by palpation with a standard amount of compression, usually just enough to cause blanching of the examiner's nail bed. Squeezing the metacarpal and metatarsal rows is a sensitive test for synovitis in these areas, and individual joint examination can then follow. Although swelling and tenderness may not correlate with radiographic evidence of erosions, the number of deformed joints [as defined by malalignment or impaired range of motion (ROM)] corresponds very well with the extent of radiographic joint damage (8,9). Clinically, joint damage and deformity may be noted as reduced ROM, malalignment, subluxation, crepitus, and collateral ligament instability. A joint may be considered "active" if it is swollen, tender to palpation, or painful with passive motion.

TABLE 2.1. 1987 Revised American Rheumatism Association Criteria for the Classification of Rheumatoid Arthritis[a]

Criterion	Definition
1. Morning stiffness	Morning stiffness in and around the joints, lasting at least 1 h.
2. Arthritis in three or more joint areas	At least three joint areas simultaneously have had soft tissue swelling or fluid (not bony overgrowth alone) observed by a physician. The 14 possible areas are right or left PIP, MCP, wrist, elbow, knee, ankle, and MTP joints.
3. Arthritis of hand joints	At least one area swollen (as defined above) in a wrist, MCP, or PIP joint.
4. Symmetric arthritis	Simultaneous involvement of the same joint areas (as defined in Criterion 2) on both sides of the body (bilateral involvement of PIPs, MCPs, or MTPs is acceptable without absolute symmetry).
5. Rheumatoid nodules	Subcutaneous nodules over bony prominences or extensor surfaces or juxtaarticular regions observed by a physician.
6. Serum rheumatoid factor	Demonstration of abnormal amounts of serum rheumatoid factor by any method for which the result has been positive in <5% of normal control subjects.
7. Radiographic changes	Radiographic changes typical of rheumatoid arthritis on the posteroanterior hand and wrist radiographs, which must include erosions or unequivocal decalcification localized in, or most marked adjacent to, the involved joints (osteoarthritis changes alone do not qualify).

MCP, metacarpophalangeal; MTP, metatarsophalangeal; PIP, proximal interphalangeal.

[a]For classification purposes, a patient shall be said to have rheumatoid arthritis if he or she has satisfied at least four of these seven criteria. Criteria 1 through 4 must have been present for at least 6 weeks. Patients with two clinical diagnoses are not excluded. Designation as classic, definite, or probable rheumatoid arthritis is *not* to be made.

From Arnett FC, Edworthy SM, Bloch DA, et al. The American Rheumatism Association 1987 revised criteria for the classification of rheumatoid arthritis. *Arthritis Rheum* 1988;31(3):315–324.

Other intraarticular pathology and periarticular disease, such as chondromalacia, meniscal tears, and tendonitis, may also cause painful passive joint motion. The presence of both joint tenderness and swelling correlates better with C-reactive protein levels than either variable alone (10). A high median erythrocyte sedimentation rate and elevated median joint count in active RA are predictive of later erosive disease and the need for subsequent joint surgery (11).

The assessment of joints begins with inspection for signs of swelling, erythema, and deformity. It is instructive for the patient to move each joint through active ROM, observing for pain and limitation of joint function before attempting palpation or passive ROM. This strategy enables the examiner to immediately assess pain and discomfort, and avoids causing the patient unnecessary pain. The extremes of ROM may be observed and recorded with ease. The assessment of all joints may be completed in minutes and includes assessment of temporomandibular joints, spinal mobility, and gait, and is then followed by a more exacting evaluation of abnormal joints.

Joint ROM in the hands is first assessed actively by having the patient flex the distal interphalangeal (DIP) and proximal interphalangeal (PIP) joints with the metacarpophalangeal (MCP) joints in the neutral position. Normally, the pads of the fingers can touch the palm distal to the distal palmar crease. Finger flexion limitation points to pathology in the PIP or DIP joints. With normal hand function, the patient can make complete fists with good grip strength, which can be roughly quantified using a sphygmomanometer or exactly quantified with a dynamometer. Thumb ROM is assessed in all planes. The patient is then asked to position the hands in the "praying" position, permitting assessment of extension limitations of the finger and wrist joints. The dorsum of the hands can then be placed together (similar to a Phalen's test) to assess wrist flexion. The presence of a joint effusion in smaller joints may be assessed using the four-finger technique: The examiner squeezes a joint in one plane between his or her thumb and second finger while feeling for the hydraulic effect of displaced fluid in a perpendicular plane with the thumb and second finger of his or her other hand (12).

Elbow motion can be measured by asking the patient to bend and straighten his or her elbows maximally. A simple screen for shoulder motion involves complete abduction, followed by having the patient place both hands behind his or her neck (external rotation) and then both hands on his or her lower back (internal rotation). Hip motion can be easily assessed even in a seated position by internal and external rotation. Knee mobility is measured by having the patient maximally flex and extend the joint. Ankle motion is measured with active dorsiflexion, plantar flexion, inversion, and eversion. Examination of the feet should first be done with the patient in the standing position, as deformities often become more apparent with weightbearing and their effect on gait can be assessed. Pressure points seen at the base of the feet and toes should be noted as a risk for future ulceration and infection.

The complete physical examination also reveals the presence of extraarticular features such as scleritis, nodules, pericardial rub, pleural effusions, splenomegaly, and lower extremity skin ulcers.

CLINICAL SYNDROMES OF EARLY RHEUMATOID ARTHRITIS

The majority of patients with RA have a slow onset of disease over several weeks to months. Uncommonly, patients present with acute onset of symptoms over days. The onset is polyarticular (more than six joints) in 75% of cases. The joints initially involved in RA are commonly the MCPs, PIPs, metatarsophalangeals (MTPs), ankles, and wrists in a symmetric distribution (13). However, in up to 25% of cases, the initial presentation is asymmetric or mono- or oligoarticular, or involves large joints such as the knees (initial joint involved in 50% of such cases), hips, and shoulders.

A unique, although unusual, presentation of early RA is palindromic rheumatism (PR). This condition is characterized by multiple recurring episodes of arthritis or periarthritis, or both, lasting from hours to days and then resolving completely. Attacks are usually monarticular; the small joints of the hands, as well as the shoulders and knees, are commonly involved. Most patients with PR are eventually diagnosed with a chronic form of inflammatory arthritis. Patients with PR and a positive RF have a 33% to 50% chance of developing RA (14). Early involvement of the wrist and PIP joints is associated with an increased risk for developing RA or a connective tissue disease. Other diseases, such as crystalline arthropathies and connective tissue diseases that cause intermittent inflammatory arthritis, should be excluded before diagnosing PR.

SPECIFIC JOINTS

Overview

Although an attempt has been made to provide up-to-date information, long-term (10- to 15-year follow-up) studies involving new therapies, such as tumor necrosis factor inhibitors, are not yet available. It appears likely that current therapeutic strategies will significantly modify the disease course of RA. Therefore, some of the long-term studies presented below, which reflect the "pre-biologic era" (and even inadequate application of available disease-modifying antirheumatic treatments) may over-represent the erosive and functional burden a patient with newly diagnosed RA can expect.

The descriptions of joint involvement in RA will begin with the hands and cover the upper extremity joints, followed by the feet and lower extremity joints, and, finally, describe the spine and other axial joints.

Upper Extremity

WRIST AND HAND

The three major compartments of the wrist are the radiocarpal, midcarpal, and radioulnar. These compartments, as well as the overlying dorsal and volar tendon sheaths, are lined by synovium and can be involved in RA. As with other joints, chronic synovitis in the wrist and hand eventually results in laxity of joint capsules and ligaments, allowing the tendons crossing the wrist to deform it. This eventually leads to ulnar and volar shifting of the carpus on the radius, dislocation of the radioulnar joint, radial deviation of the metacarpals at the wrist, and ulnar shift of the fingers at the MCP joints (15) (Fig. 2.1). The forces involved with hand grip also pull the fingers in an ulnar direction and potentiate hand deformities in RA (12).

PIP and MCP joint involvement are common in RA, resulting in pain, swelling, and loss of finger motion. As the capsule of the MCP joints is weakened, volar migration of the fingers relative to the metacarpal bones occurs.

Swan-neck deformities are characterized by PIP joint hyperextension with concurrent flexion of the DIP joint. This deformity results from laxity of the joint capsule, volar plate, and collateral ligaments, with concurrent tightening of the dorsally displaced lateral bands and central extensor tendon. MCP joint hyperextension, PIP joint flexion, and DIP joint hyperextension characterize the boutonnière deformity. This deformity results from stretching of the extensor mechanism, attenuation of the central slip over the PIP joint, and secondary contraction of the volarly displaced lateral bands (15).

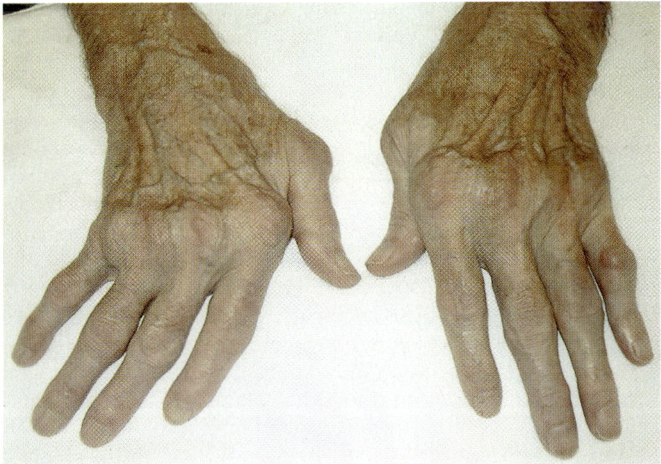

Figure 2.1. Hands of a patient demonstrating ulnar deviation of the fingers, greater on the dominant (right) side; synovial thickening at proximal interphalangeal, metacarpophalangeal, and wrist joints; interosseous atrophy; and a rheumatoid nodule over the left fifth proximal interphalangeal joint.

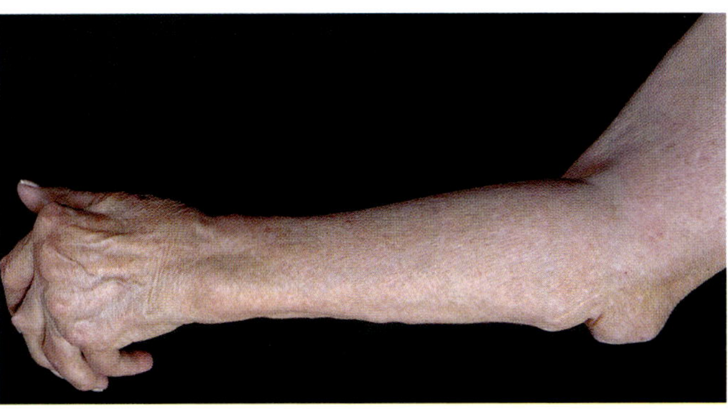

Figure 2.2. Olecranon nodule and bursitis in a patient with destructive nodular rheumatoid changes of the hand.

Disease of the thumb can lead to a flail interphalangeal (IP) joint, the boutonnière deformity, or a "duckbill thumb" (12). The flail IP joint results from synovitis of the IP joint and secondary laxity, causing patients to pinch with the proximal phalanx of the thumb. The duckbill thumb is due to dislocation of the first carpometacarpal joint and secondary adduction of the first metacarpal.

Tenosynovitis of the volar or dorsal tendon sheaths may be painless but can result in swelling, triggering, tendon rupture, or carpal tunnel syndrome. A clue that tenosynovitis is present is when passive flexion is greater than active flexion (12). Extensor tendon rupture may result from wear against exposed jagged bone, usually over the distal ulna. Ulnar subluxation of the extensor tendons may cause them to slip between the metacarpal heads during flexion, causing a painful catching while attempting finger extension.

Swelling in the region of the ulnar styloid and loss of wrist extension are early signs of RA. Later in the disease, rotation and subluxation of the wrist prevent the normal function of the extensor carpi ulnaris as a wrist extensor (12).

ELBOW

The elbow is composed of the humeroradial, humeroulnar, and radioulnar articulations. Erosive involvement of the elbow has been observed in up to 61% of patients with RA after 15 years of disease (16). Clinically, elbow effusions are noted as a palpable fullness between the lateral epicondyle and the olecranon, and should be distinguished from olecranon bursitis. Although bursitis does not significantly limit elbow mobility, significant elbow joint involvement or effusion can lead to lack of full extension and, eventually, to flexion contracture. Olecranon bursitis is more frequent in patients with a positive RF (Fig. 2.2). The white blood cell count of the bursal fluid is usually lower than that of actively inflamed joints. As with inflamed joints, olecranon bursitis from RA must be distinguished from septic bursitis and crystalline disease.

SHOULDER

Shoulder involvement in RA is common, presenting with pain and limitation of motion secondary to tendonitis, bursitis, or distention of the joint capsule by synovial fluid or hypertrophic synovitis. To minimize discomfort, the patient may hold his or her shoulder in slight flexion and internal rotation, maximizing joint volume but also predisposing to frozen shoulder. Fifteen years after onset of RA, 55% and 68% of patients have erosive involvement of the glenohumeral (17) and acromioclavicular joints, respectively (18). Subdeltoid, subacromial, and scapulothoracic bursitis can occur. Tears of the supraspinatus tendon can result from adjacent bursal synovitis, chronic impingement, or exposure of the tendon to glenohumeral synovitis at its insertion on the greater tuberosity. Rotator cuff tears often limit external rotation and abduction, are associated with glenohumeral arthritis, and are a cause of significant morbidity.

Lower Extremity

ANKLE AND FOOT

Initial involvement with RA occurs as often in the feet as in the hands. The most frequently affected foot joints are the MTP, talonavicular, and ankle joints (19). Weightbearing results in greater dysfunction and pain in lower extremity joints, particularly the feet and ankles (19). Synovitis at the MTP joints causes laxity of the capsules and ligaments. In the presence of active forefoot synovitis, dorsiflexion of the toes during walking results in dorsal subluxation of the phalanges and plantar subluxation of the metatarsal heads (20). This condition may lead to painful callus formation under the metatarsal heads. Chronic cutaneous fistulas can develop from ulceration of the bursae under the metatarsal heads (12).

The imbalance of foot intrinsic and extrinsic muscles caused by dislocation of the MTP joints combined with the fixed length of the toe flexor tendons eventually results in hammer toe deformities (MTP extension and PIP and DIP flexion) (20). Hallux valgus often occurs when the lateral support for the first toe is lost as the lesser metatarsals are displaced in a plantar direction and the extensor hallucis longus tendon begins to act more as an adductor than an extensor.

The midfoot consists of the navicular, the cuboid, and the cuneiform bones with their intertarsal and tarsometatarsal articulations. Forefoot deformities correlate with destruction of the midfoot joints, particularly the cuneonavicular and cuneometatarsal joints (21).

The hindfoot consists of the talus and calcaneus and three articulations—the talonavicular, the talocalcaneal, and the calcaneocuboid. Of these, the talonavicular is most commonly affected in RA (22). The ankle is made up of the tibia, fibula, and talus with three articulations—the tibiotalar, the distal tibiofibular, and the fibulotalar. Hindfoot involvement and deformity become more prevalent after 5 years of disease duration, and ankle joint deformity probably results from the stress of talocalcaneal (subtalar) joint malalignment (23). Patients often are found to have pes planus with hindfoot valgus deformity (Fig. 2.3). Whether this is due to hindfoot joint synovitis, posterior tibial tendon dysfunction, laxity of supporting ligaments, or a combination of these factors is controversial (24). Patients with RA may also develop Achilles tendonitis, retrocalcaneal bursitis, or ankle joint effusions.

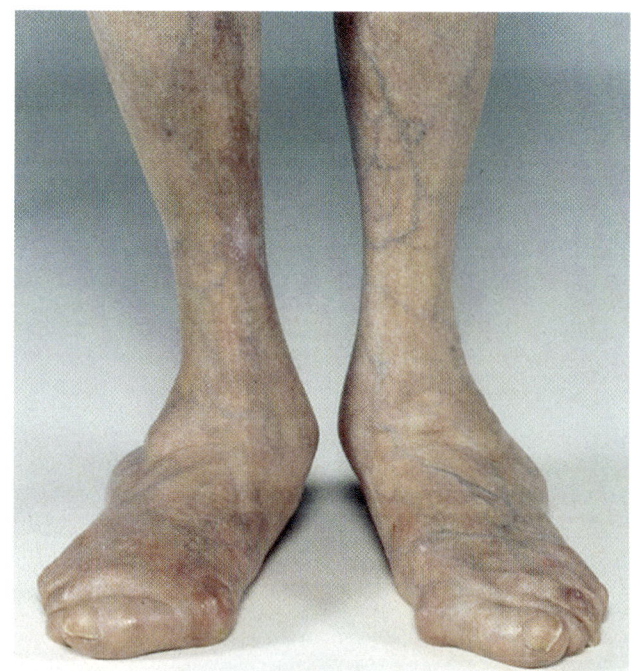

Figure 2.3. Severe pes planus, hindfoot valgus, and hallux valgus deformities with bunions.

KNEE

Bilateral knee involvement is common in patients with RA. The presence of fluid in the knee may be confirmed by eliciting a bulge sign or by ballottement of the patella. The presence of fluid or synovitis limits knee flexion and may prevent full extension. Activation of nociceptors around the knee secondary to effusions and synovitis leads to quadriceps inhibition and secondary atrophy. Popliteal cysts are often present and best detected by observing the patient in the standing position from behind. Eventually, a valgus deformity with or without flexion contracture can develop, and these are often accompanied by pes planovalgus deformity of the feet.

HIP

Signs and symptoms of hip involvement are abnormal gait, groin discomfort, and limitation of motion and pain during internal and external rotation. In a group of patients with seropositive erosive RA, 31% had severe radiographic changes 15 years after disease onset (25). A high number of peripheral joint erosions, impaired function as noted by health assessment questionnaire responses, the presence of HLA-B27 antigen, and elevated acute phase markers are all associated with an increased risk for hip joint destruction in RA.

Spine and Axial Joints

SPINE

Involvement of the cervical spine with RA has been reported in 17% to 86% of patients and correlates with longer duration of disease, multiple joint involvement, extent of peripheral erosions, seropositivity, rheumatoid nodules, steroid use, and vasculitis (26). Spinal cord compression can result from atlantoaxial subluxation, basilar invagination, or subaxial subluxation. *Atlantoaxial subluxation* is defined as greater than 3 mm of space between the odontoid process of second cervical vertebra (C-2) and the anterior arch of the atlas (C-1) (12). Subluxation greater than 10 mm greatly increases the risk of cervical myelopathy (Fig. 2.4).

Up to 50% of patients with cervical spine involvement from RA do not have neck or occipital pain or any symptoms of neurologic impairment (27). Pain is the earliest and most common clinical manifestation, often experienced in the occipital or posterior neck areas. Suboccipital headaches may be due to synovitis at C1-2, bony disease, or compression of the greater occipital nerve. Degenerative disc disease, facet arthropathy, and subaxial subluxation can cause neck pain. Neurologic deficits have been reported in 11% of patients during an average follow-up of 10 years (27). Compression of the posterior aspect of the spinal cord and vertebrobasilar arteries may result in symptoms of tinnitus, vertigo, diplopia, or posterior column impingement with loss of proprioception. Rarely, rheumatoid pannus or reactive osteophyte formation of the cervical spine can compress the esophagus, causing dysphagia. Disc disease and cervical radiculopathy can occur at any level. Symptoms of cervical myelopathy can include weakness, numbness, clumsiness, and even

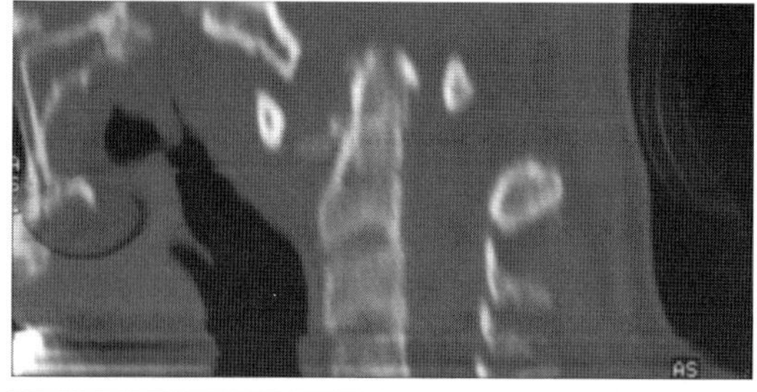
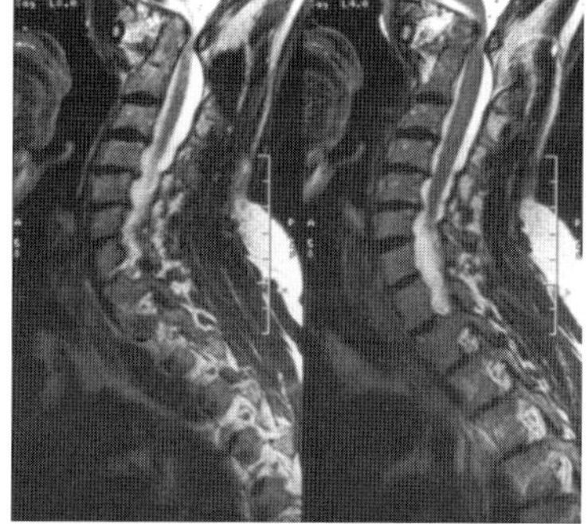
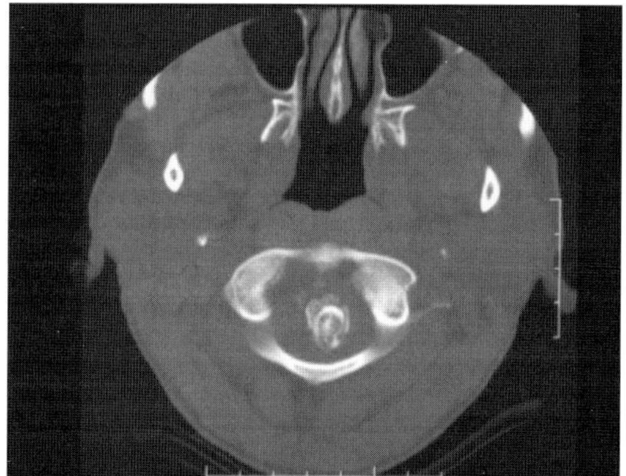
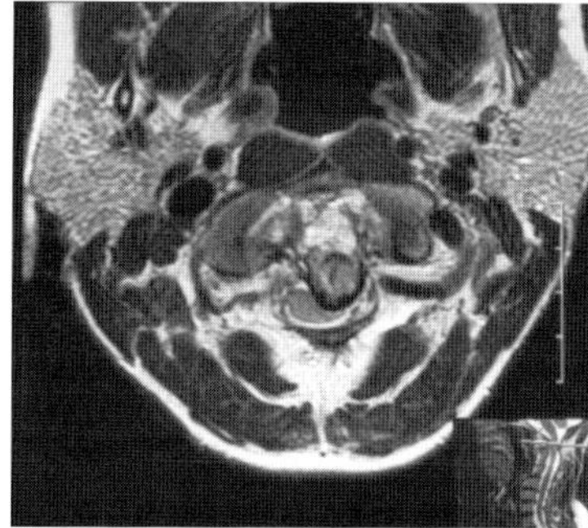

A,B

Figure 2.4. A: Atlantoaxial subluxation (AAS) of 14 mm seen on computed tomographic sagittal reconstruction (*top*). There are erosive changes at the dens and associated dystrophic calcification. The bottom portion shows an axial computed tomographic scan through the atlas (C-1) of the same patient, with posterior displacement of the dens and a space of only 4 mm for the spinal cord. **B:** Corresponding T2-weighted sagittal magnetic resonance image showing AAS, pannus anterior to the dens, and compression of the spinal cord between the posterior aspect of the dens and the posterior arch of C-1 (*top*). The bottom portion shows T2-weighted axial magnetic resonance image at the C-1 level with compression and displacement of the cervical spinal cord by the dens.

respiratory embarrassment. Spasticity, sensory deficits, hyperreflexia, and upper motor neuron signs such as Babinski or Hoffmann may be present on physical examination (26).

The thoracic and lumbar portions of the spine are not commonly involved in RA, although pain and radiculopathy may result from pannus formation, especially at the zygapophyseal joints. Compression fractures from disease- and corticosteroid-related osteoporosis are frequent.

TEMPOROMANDIBULAR JOINT

There is a wide range of clinical and radiologic involvement of the temporomandibular joints (TMJs) in RA. In one study, 31% of patients with RA described pain or locking of the jaw at some point, whereas only 4% of a control group described such symptoms (28). Patients with RA more commonly report pain on palpation of and clicking of the TMJs than controls. Severe arthritic involvement of the TMJ has been associated with a higher incidence of upper-airway obstruction (29).

CRICOARYTENOID JOINT

Although laryngoscopy and computed tomography (CT) may show cricoarytenoid abnormalities in up to 75% of patients with RA, clinically significant disease is much less common (30). Cricoarytenoid arthritis tends to affect patients with longstanding seropositive erosive disease. Signs and symptoms include sore throat, respiratory difficulty during inspiration, tenderness over the larynx, dysphagia, hoarseness, cough, dyspnea, and stridor (31). CT of the larynx and indirect laryngoscopy are often abnormal, especially in the setting of dysphagia and dyspnea, but may be abnormal in the absence of symptoms. Acute laryngeal obstruction is rare but potentially fatal.

MIDDLE EAR

The incudomalleolar and incudostapedial joints are synovial joints and may be involved in RA. Abnormal middle-ear mechanics have been detected with multiple-frequency tympanometry in 40% of patients with RA, usually due to stiffness of the tympano-ossicular system (32). However, most middle-ear involvement is asymptomatic, and there is no difference in hearing acuity among patients with RA compared to control subjects.

STERNOCLAVICULAR AND STERNOMANUBRIAL JOINTS

Approximately one-third of RA patients have clinical manifestations of sternoclavicular involvement, as evidenced by asymmetry, swelling, crepitus, tenderness, hypertrophy, pain, or limitation of motion (33), and a similar percentage have erosions on tomography (34).

Synovitis of the sternomanubrial joint is also common, but, because of the relative immobility of this amphiarthrodial joint, symptoms are uncommon (35). Sternomanubrial joint arthritis should be considered in the differential diagnosis of chest pain in a patient with RA. Subluxation of the sternomanubrial joint is present in 2.5% of patients with RA (35). These patients tend to have severe erosive disease with cervical spine involvement.

EXTRAARTICULAR COMPLICATIONS OF RHEUMATOID ARTHRITIS

Extraarticular manifestations of RA occur in approximately 40% of patients and are associated with an overall mortality risk ratio of three times that of patients without these manifestations (Fig. 2.5) (5,36,37). Often present are constitutional symptoms such as fatigue, low-grade fevers, and weight loss. Rheumatoid nodules, in addition to positive antinuclear antibodies and high-titer RFs, predict the occurrence of other extraarticular manifestations (38).

Extraarticular manifestations in a community-based cohort of patients incident between 1955 and 1995 and followed to 2000 were more frequent in each successive decade (39). This increasing incidence of extraarticular manifestations is mainly due to an increase in the number of patients found to have nodules, which may reflect either detection bias or the increased use of nodule-inducing methotrexate therapy. The incidence of other ExRA in aggregate was stable. These data likely do not fully reflect more aggressive treatments for RA in

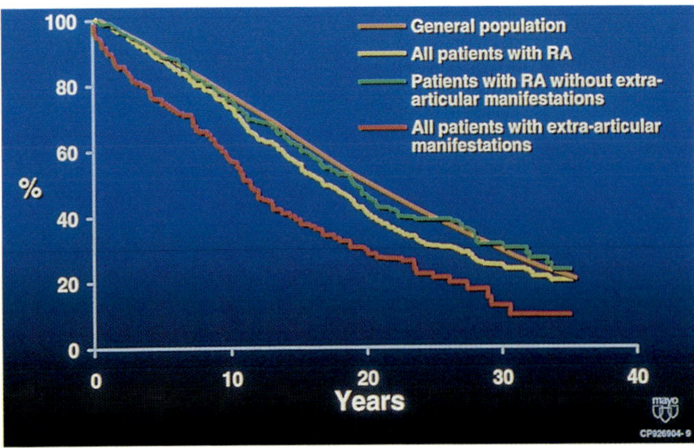

Figure 2.5. Survival curves for patients with rheumatoid arthritis (RA) with and without extraarticular manifestations compared to those of the general population.

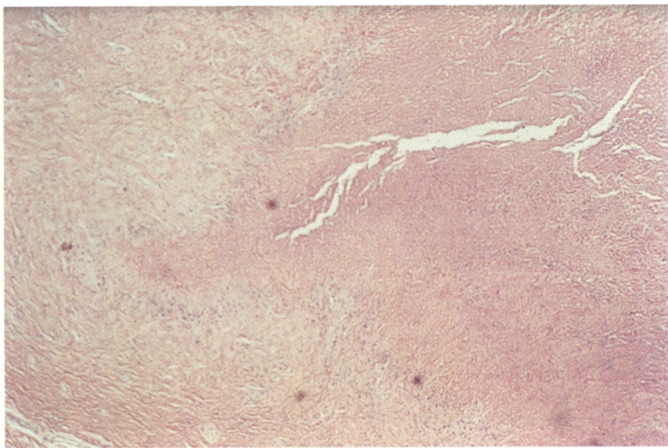

Figure 2.6. Histopathology of a rheumatoid nodule with central fibrinoid necrosis surrounded by a rim of palisading histiocytes and an outer zone of fibrosing connective tissue with fibroblasts, plasma cells, and lymphocytes (magnification, 15×).

recent years, including the recent introduction of potent biologic therapies such as tumor necrosis factor blockers and interleukin-1 receptor antagonists. It is possible that these therapeutic approaches have decreased the incidence of extraarticular complications in recent years, but this remains unstudied.

Skin

Nailfold infarcts and rheumatoid nodules are common findings in extraarticular RA, and both are suggestive of more severe disease. Rheumatoid neutrophilic dermatitis is a rare, nonvasculitic eruption of red-purple plaques and papules, sometimes with pustules or vesicles, occurring on extensor surfaces (40). Treatment-related skin pigmentation from drugs, such as minocycline, hydroxychloroquine, and gold (chrysiasis), can also occur.

Oral

There is an association between increased disease activity and decreased saliva production, and oral sicca symptoms have been reported in up to 50% of patients with RA (41). Secondary Sjögren's syndrome with reduced salivary flow can lead to difficulty swallowing, difficulty speaking, oral burning, oral candidiasis, difficulty with dentures, and increased caries. Periodontal disease, including loss of alveolar bone and teeth, occurs with an increased frequency in patients with longstanding RA.

Nodules

Rheumatoid nodules occur in approximately 30% of patients and are associated with seropositive, erosive, and more severe disease (5). Rheumatoid nodules should be distinguished from other types of nodules, including xanthomas and gouty tophi.

A very small subset of patients with multiple nodules, bone cysts without erosions on radiographs, elevated RF, and little active arthritis or synovitis are said to constitute a relatively benign variant of rheumatoid disease called *rheumatoid nodulosis* (42).

Patients tend to develop nodules in areas of increased friction or pressure, such as the extensor aspects of the elbow, olecranon bursae, finger joints, and Achilles tendons. In bedridden patients, the ischial, sacral, and occipital prominences can develop nodules (43). Nodules can occur not only in the skin and subcutaneous tissue, but also have been reported in the larynx, pericardium, heart valves, pleura, lung, peritoneum, eye, bridge of the nose, pinna of the ear, kidney, and meninges. Accelerated nodulosis can occur after the institution of methotrexate or antitumor necrosis factor alpha therapy (44,45).

Histologic examination of the nodules reveals a central necrotic core surrounded by a corona of palisading mononuclear cells and an outer zone of fibroblasts, plasma cells, and lymphocytes (43) (Fig. 2.6). Rheumatoid nodules may result from small-vessel vasculitis and complement activation. They may develop central necrosis and become sites for local ulceration and infection.

Hematologic Abnormalities

Anemia is among the most common extraarticular manifestations of RA (46). The prevalence of anemia among patients with RA depends on the group sampled. In outpatients with RA, anemia has been found in up to 27%, and the average hemoglobin in that subset was 10.0 g per dL (46). Anemia of chronic disease is the most common type of anemia in RA, followed by iron deficiency and, less commonly, pure red cell aplasia and autoimmune hemolytic anemia. More than one type of anemia may be present simultaneously. Interpretation of the ferritin level in RA can be confusing, as the level may be elevated because of the acute phase response despite absent bone marrow iron stores. However, a ferritin of less than 50 ng per mL in patients with RA is always associated with iron deficiency (47).

Abnormalities of leukocyte counts in RA are likely to be related to medications. Corticosteroids cause a neutrophilic leukocytosis, whereas disease-modifying agents such as methotrexate and sulfasalazine can cause leukopenia. Leukopenia is also seen in Felty's syndrome (FS). Eosinophilia is common in severe seropositive RA but may also be related to drug therapy with methotrexate, gold, or penicillamine.

Thrombocytosis often accompanies active RA and correlates well with other laboratory parameters of disease activity, such as erythrocyte sedimentation rate, C-reactive protein, and plasma fibrinogen. Elevation of the platelet count may represent the response of the bone marrow to stress or overcompensation by the marrow for shortened platelet survival time. Thrombocytopenia is usually secondary to drugs, FS, or splenomegaly.

The increase in plasma proteins, fibrinogen, and immunoglobulins that occurs in RA results in an increased plasma viscosity that parallels increases in the sedimentation rate (48). Hyperviscosity syndrome, characterized by an insidious onset of headache, retinal vein dilation, somnolence, and bleeding diathesis, has rarely been described in RA (49).

Lymphadenopathy has been reported to occur in 19% to 96% of patients with RA, particularly those with active disease (50). The lymph nodes are usually small, mobile, nontender, and generally occur in the axillary, inguinal, and epitrochlear areas. The adenopathy resolves or decreases with improved disease control. Histologic examination usually reveals follicular hyperplasia (51). Even in the absence of FS, splenomegaly is clinically detectable in 5% to 10% of patients with RA (52).

Other causes of lymphadenopathy in RA may be more ominous. Granulomatous infection with lymphadenopathy may occur in patients on immunosuppressive medications such as methotrexate, etanercept, and infliximab. Lymphoma is more common in patients with RA and may occur in the setting of secondary Sjögren's syndrome or with use of immunosuppressive drugs such as methotrexate (53). Rarely, intrathoracic lymphadenopathy can occur in the setting of interstitial lung disease with RA. Necrotizing lymphadenitis in the form of Kikuchi's syndrome is an unusual complication of RA and other collagen vascular diseases. Lymphadenopathy has also rarely been related to drugs such as gold, to a granulomatous reaction to silastic prostheses used in hand joint reconstruction, or to a condition known as *proteinaceous lymphadenopathy* (which can be confused with amyloidosis).

Lymphedema

Lymphedema is an uncommon extraarticular feature of RA, presenting with gradual onset of uncomfortable swelling of a limb. Lymphoscintigraphy usually shows lymphatic obstruction not related to lymphadenopathy (54).

Amyloidosis

Clinically significant amyloidosis, of the AA type, is uncommon and has had a declining incidence in RA since the 1950s, which has been ascribed to more effective medical treatment (55). Serum amyloid-A protein levels are elevated by the increased cytokine production associated with active RA. Parenchymal organ amyloidosis occurs at a mean of 15 to 17 years of disease duration, presenting most commonly with proteinuria, diarrhea, or organomegaly. Amyloid is detected on tissue biopsy (usually fat aspirate) by Congo red stain and polarized microscopy. The prognosis for reactive AA amyloidosis is better than AL amyloidosis, although the 4-year survival rate is only 58% for the former (56).

Felty's Syndrome

The triad of RA, leukopenia, and splenomegaly is termed *FS* (Fig. 2.7). It is a rare extraarticular manifestation of RA, occurring in less than 1% of patients (57). Its pathogenesis is incompletely understood and likely multifactorial. The majority of cases are women, aged 55 to 65 years, with a disease duration of 10 to 15 years. Usually, these patients have had significantly worse articular disease than controls, although, at the time they develop FS, little or no active synovitis may be present. The degree of neutropenia in FS is not related to the severity of splenomegaly. Patients with FS usually have high titers of RF and an increased incidence of other extraarticular features (58). The major complication and cause of mortality with FS is infection, which appears to be directly related to the degree of neutropenia. Infections are most common in patients with less than 0.1×10^9 per L circulating polymorphonuclear cells (59). Hepatomegaly, abnormal liver function tests, and refractory leg ulcers are other manifestations of FS.

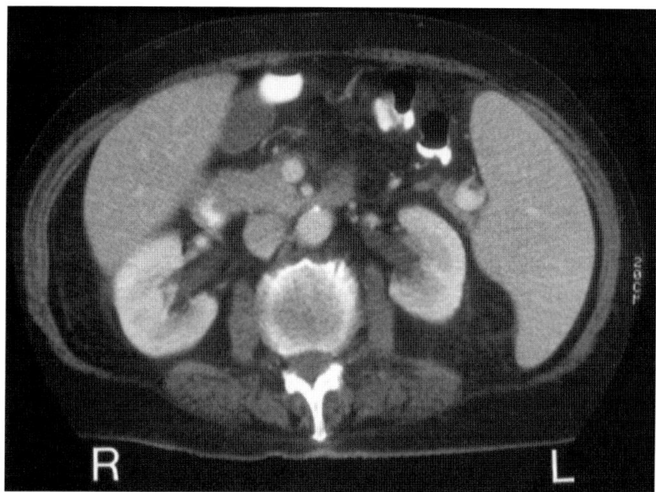

Figure 2.7. Splenomegaly in a patient with Felty's syndrome seen on computed tomography of the abdomen.

Pseudo-Felty's Syndrome

Pseudo-Felty's syndrome is a chronic lymphoproliferative disorder of large granular lymphocytes associated with neutropenia, splenomegaly, and recurrent pyogenic infections. It may be distinguished from FS by its onset earlier in the course of RA, paucity of erosive disease and other extraarticular features, lymphocytosis with lack of leukopenia, and T-cell gene rearrangement studies showing a clonally expanded population of large granular lymphocyte cells (57). Despite the fact that this is a clonal disorder, survival appears good, with 90% of patients alive after nearly 4 years of follow-up (60).

Ocular

Dry eyes occur in as many as 38% of patients with RA (41), but most authors have cited a prevalence of approximately 15% to 25%. Keratoconjunctivitis sicca is, thus, the most common ophthalmic manifestation of RA. Symptoms include dryness, burning, and sensation of a foreign body in the eyes. Severe dryness results in devitalization of corneal epithelial cells and punctate epithelial erosions, which are apparent with 1% rose-bengal staining. Decreased tear production may be detected by an abnormal Schirmer test (less than 5 mm of wetting of a filter paper strip after 5 minutes).

Inflammatory eye disease is much less common than keratoconjunctivitis sicca. Episcleritis does not affect visual acuity and usually correlates with the activity of RA and subsides spontaneously. It appears acutely as a red eye with mild, if any, associated discomfort. Necrotizing nodular scleritis is painful and associated with longstanding arthritis, active joint disease, and visceral vasculitis and can lead to scleromalacia perforans and blindness (Fig. 2.8A).

Retinal vasculitis is a rare complication in RA. Corticosteroid treatment places RA patients at higher risk of cataracts. Hydroxychloroquine treatment can uncommonly result in retinopathy.

Peripheral ulcerative keratitis is a severe form of keratitis that develops as an extension of scleritis and may lead to corneal thinning and perforation (corneal melt) (Fig. 2.8B). Both

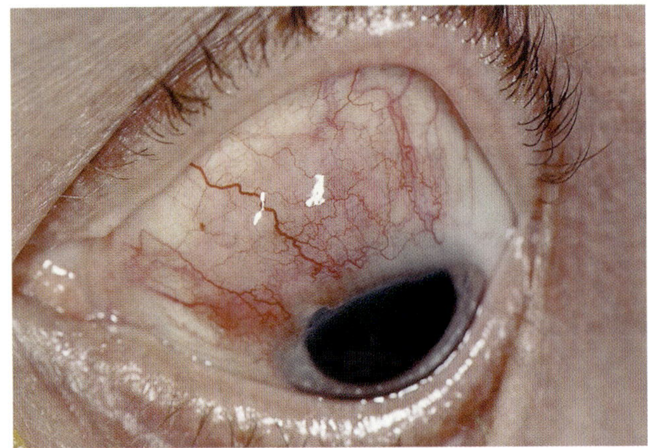

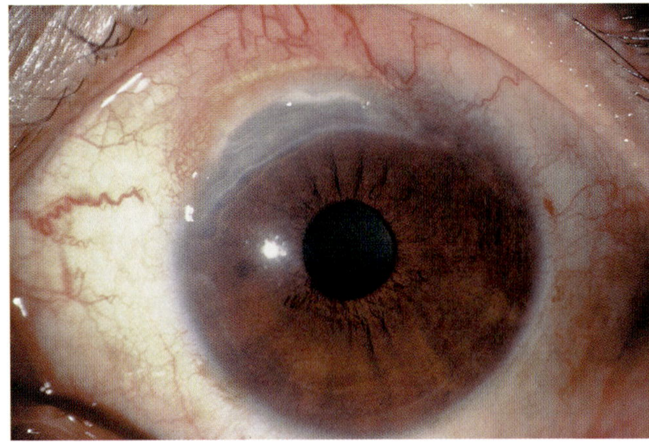

Figure 2.8. **A:** Raised nodular scleritis. **B:** Corneal melt at the superior limbus. (Courtesy of Thomas P. Link and Jay A. Rostvold, Department of Ophthalmology, Mayo Clinic, Rochester, Minn.)

necrotizing scleritis and peripheral ulcerative keratitis portend a high mortality in the absence of treatment, likely because of their association with underlying systemic vasculitis (61). Anterior uveitis commonly accompanies episcleritis or scleritis in RA patients, but seldom occurs in isolation (62).

Neurologic

Neurologic complications of RA include nerve compression from synovial proliferation, vasculitis, and sensory or sensorimotor neuropathies. Atlantoaxial subluxation, vertical subluxation with basilar invagination, and subaxial subluxation can result in spinal cord impingement or radiculopathy. Uncommonly, rheumatoid pannus formation from synovial facet joints in the spine can cause nerve root compression or cauda equina syndrome. Vasculitis of the central nervous system (CNS) is rare in RA and occurs in the setting of diffuse systemic vasculitis. As in other forms of CNS vasculitis, stroke, seizure, intracranial hemorrhage, and leptomeningitis can occur. Rheumatoid nodules rarely develop in the dura or choroid plexus and can impinge on the CNS, causing neurologic symptoms (63).

Some type of neuropathy affects up to one-third of RA patients (64). Carpal tunnel syndrome is the most common compressive neuropathy in RA, resulting from tenosynovitis of the flexor tendons of the fingers with pressure on the median nerve within the carpal tunnel. Patients may have numbness and tingling in the radial four fingers accompanied by a positive Tinel's, Phalen's, or carpal tunnel compression test. Less common is tarsal tunnel syndrome, which results from posterior tibial nerve compression by adjacent tenosynovitis of the posterior tibial tendon as both structures pass through the tarsal tunnel (formed by the medial malleolus and the flexor retinaculum) (63). Clinically, tarsal tunnel syndrome may be asymptomatic, but it may cause pain, paresthesia, and burning in the toes and plantar aspect of the foot. Other compressive neuropathies are very rare, but include the anterior interosseous branch of the median nerve, the ulnar nerve at the wrist or elbow (cubital tunnel syndrome), the posterior interosseous branch of the radial nerve, and the common peroneal or tibial nerves (63). Very rarely, iliopsoas bursitis may cause unilateral femoral nerve palsy. Nerve conduction studies and electromyography can assist in the diagnosis of a compressive neuropathy. Treatment is usually aimed at controlling the responsible tenosynovial proliferation with medications, corticosteroid injections, or splinting, but, occasionally, decompressive surgery is needed.

Distal sensory neuropathy and combined sensorimotor neuropathy are more common than the compressive neuropathies in patients with RA (63,64). Distal sensory neuropathy has an insidious onset with symptoms of numbness, paresthesia, and burning in the feet. Often, this form of neuropathy remains stable over time or may even improve. In contrast, combined sensorimotor neuropathy can present acutely and has a poorer outcome. Mononeuritis multiplex is a form of combined sensorimotor neuropathy caused by vasculitis of epineural arteries and can present with acute foot or wrist drop. Such patients usually have severe longstanding RA with other extraarticular features. Pathologically, both sensory and sensorimotor neuropathy in RA are caused by epineural or perineural vasculitis, or both (65), resulting in axonal degeneration. The presence of multifocal neuropathy, low C-4 complement levels, and concomitant cutaneous vasculitis are associated with decreased survivorship (65).

Muscular

Myopathy in RA is usually due to disuse atrophy, corticosteroid therapy, or both. Hip and knee flexor and extensor strength are significantly reduced in RA patients compared with controls (66). Both hydroxychloroquine and penicillamine therapy may rarely cause a myopathy. Clinically significant disease-related myositis is very rare. Denervation atrophy from peripheral neuropathy is another cause of muscle weakness.

Pulmonary Disease

Pleural disease is found in up to 73% of RA patients at autopsy (67). It is more common in men and may be clinically silent or cause pleurisy or dyspnea. Nodules may develop in the pleura. Pleural effusions are usually unilateral and small to moderate in size (67). Rheumatoid pleural effusions can be transudates but are usually exudative with an increase in mononuclear cells, a high lactate dehydrogenase, high protein, and low glucose and pH (67). The low glucose is probably caused by impaired glucose transport into the pleural space (68). RF may be present in the fluid, and hemolytic complement levels may be low. Pleural effusions usually resolve over months with treatment of the underlying disease, but therapeutic and diagnostic aspiration may be required to confirm the fluid's relation to RA or to investigate the possibilities of infection, malignancy, or congestive heart failure.

Pulmonary rheumatoid nodules are usually asymptomatic and typically occur in seropositive patients who have subcutaneous nodules (69). The pulmonary nodules can be single or multiple but tend to be peripheral and upper lobe in location. Spontaneous pneumothorax can occur from rupture of a necrobiotic nodule into the pleural space and may cause secondary sterile empyema. Nodules can cavitate, erode into bronchi, and cause bronchopleural fistulas. Excisional biopsy may be required to exclude the possibility of neoplastic disease and granulomatous infection. Caplan's syndrome is, classically, the presence of multiple pulmonary nodules in coal workers with RA and pneumonoconiosis from extensive exposure to coal dust but can be associated with exposure to other substances, such as silica (70).

The most common pulmonary manifestation of RA is interstitial lung disease (ILD) (67) (Fig. 2.9). Male gender, high RF, more severe articular disease, and smoking are risk factors for this complication. In the majority of patients with ILD, joint involvement precedes lung involvement. ILD usually develops within 5 years of onset of joint disease (69). Bi-basilar interstitial infiltrates that may have honeycombing are seen on chest radiography or CT. CT has ten times the sensitivity of plain radiography for detecting ILD, and ILD may be found in as many as 47% of patients on high-resolution CT scanning (71). Clinically, findings are indistinguishable from idiopathic pulmonary fibrosis, although patients with RA are less likely to have digital clubbing (72). Bronchoalveolar lavage usually demonstrates a neutrophilic alveolitis, which carries a worse prognosis than lymphocytic alveolitis (73).

Since the advent of high resolution CT scanning, bronchiectasis is detected in as many as 30% of patients with RA. The pathogenesis of bronchiectasis in RA is unknown but may relate to recurrent infections, underlying obstructive airway disease, or genetic susceptibility (67).

Bronchiolitis obliterans (BO) organizing pneumonia is another entity that can be idiopathic but may affect patients with RA. Its presenting symptoms include fever, cough, and dyspnea. Consolidative infiltrates are found on CT scan. The diagnosis usually requires lung biopsy, and prognosis is favorable with corticosteroid treatment (69).

BO is less common than BO organizing pneumonia. Patients with BO tend to be women with longstanding seropositive disease. On occasion, BO may be related to medications such as penicillamine. Patients present with nonproductive cough and dyspnea but are usually afebrile. Chest radiographs are usually normal or show air trapping. Histopathologically, the disease results from peribronchial and submucosal fibrosis, which causes narrowing of the bronchiolar lumens with little active inflammation (74). There is an obstructive pattern on pulmonary function tests. Lung biopsy is often required for the diagnosis.

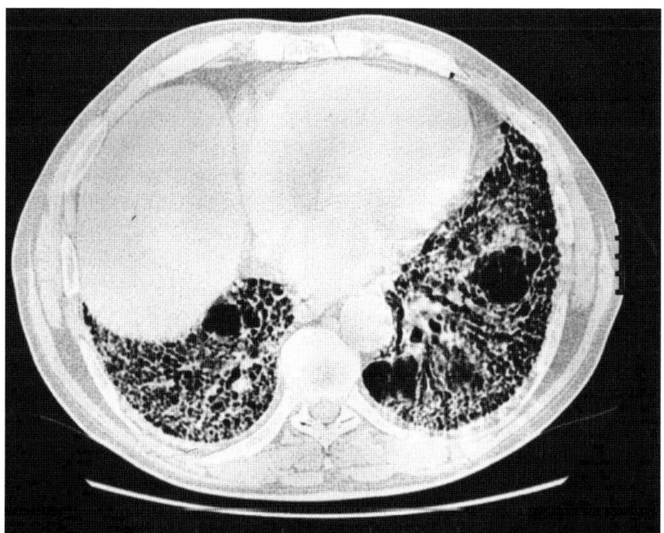

Figure 2.9. Advanced changes of interstitial lung disease with honeycombing seen on computed tomography of the chest.

Primary pulmonary vasculitis in RA is extremely rare, as is primary pulmonary hypertension. Secondary pulmonary hypertension may result from underlying ILD (67).

Drugs such as gold, penicillamine, and methotrexate can rarely be the cause of lung problems in patients with RA. Pulmonary toxicity from methotrexate usually presents subacutely with interstitial pneumonitis, fever, cough, dyspnea, and eosinophilia (75). Prompt recognition of this syndrome and discontinuation of methotrexate may be life-saving.

Cardiac

Coronary artery disease and accelerated atherosclerosis are now recognized as perhaps the most common extraarticular manifestations of RA (76). Compared to patients with osteoarthritis (OA), those with RA have an increased prevalence of myocardial infarction, congestive heart failure, and stroke (77). There is an increased incidence of cardiovascular events in RA patients independent of traditional risk factors (78).

Inflammation plays a role in atherogenesis, as evidenced by the presence of inflammatory cells in atherosclerotic plaques. Certain T-cell populations ($CD4^{+}CD28^{null}$) are expanded in the blood of patients with RA (79). These same cells are found in ruptured coronary plaques of patients with unstable angina (80). At their first coronary angiogram, rheumatoid patients have an increased coronary atherosclerotic burden compared to control patients who required coronary angiography (81). Furthermore, elevated C-reactive protein levels, often detected in patients with RA, have been shown to carry an increased risk for coronary heart disease and portend a worse prognosis in patients with angina (82).

Although pericardial inflammation or effusion as detected by echocardiography and at autopsy is common, clinical signs and symptoms of pericarditis are not (83,84) (Fig. 2.10). Symptomatic pericarditis usually occurs in patients who have a positive RF and nodules and can result in pericardial tamponade or chronic constriction (85). In a review of 41 episodes, the median duration of RA among patients with pericarditis was 9 years. Typically, symptomatic patients present with dyspnea, orthopnea, and positional or pleuritic chest pain. On examination, tachycardia and tachypnea are common (85). Approximately two-thirds of patients will have a pericardial friction rub, jugular venous distention, or rales, whereas pulsus paradoxus, Kussmaul's sign, and pericardial knock are uncommon (85). Like pleural fluid, pericardial fluid in RA tends to have an elevated leukocyte count, high protein and lactate dehydrogenase, low glucose and complement, and positive RF. The diagnosis of constrictive pericarditis should be entertained in patients with RA who develop unexplained right heart failure. Pericardial aspiration, intrapericardial corticosteroid therapy, or pericardiectomy may be required for successful management of pericardial disease.

Myocarditis, when present, is usually asymptomatic and diagnosed at autopsy (83). If rheumatoid nodules and inflammation occur near the atrioventricular node, complete heart block can result (86). Nonspecific endocardial inflammation is not infrequently noted at autopsy, and valvular thickening can

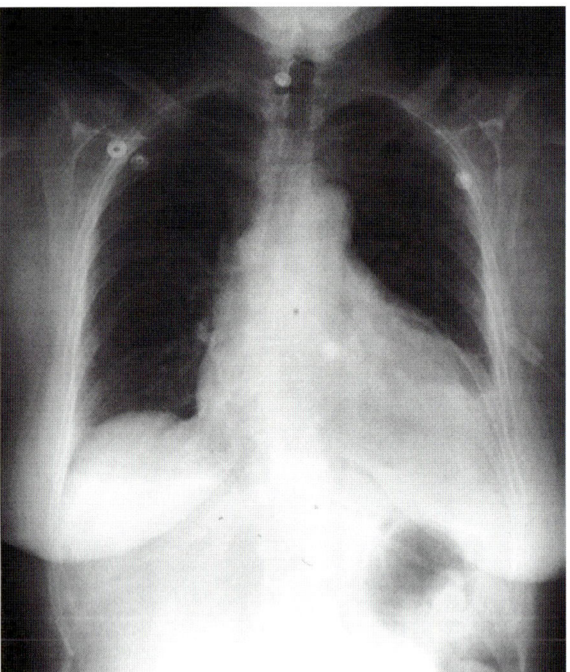

Figure 2.10. Posterior-anterior chest radiograph showing enlarged cardiac silhouette of a patient with rheumatoid pericarditis and pericardial effusion. A left pleural effusion is also present.

be seen on echocardiography. These are usually asymptomatic (84). Rheumatoid nodule formation within valve leaflets or extruding from the endocardium can rarely lead to valvular incompetence or mimic atrial myxoma (87,88). Coronary arteritis has been rarely described as the cause of myocardial infarction (89). Similarly, aortitis from RA is uncommon, can be fatal, and is seldom diagnosed before autopsy (90).

Rheumatoid Vasculitis

Isolated nailfold infarctions are not associated with a worse prognosis in patients with RA and, in isolation, are not an indication for intensification of therapy directed against vasculitis. However, the presence of these lesions should prompt a search for other dermatologic and systemic manifestations of rheumatoid vasculitis (91).

Clinically significant rheumatoid vasculitis most commonly presents with mononeuritis multiplex and skin involvement (ulcers, digital tip gangrene, purpura, petechia) (92). The ischemic ulcers tend to affect the legs (Fig. 2.11). Although leg ulcers are initiated by vasculitis, they are often potentiated by comorbid factors such as chronic venous insufficiency, occlusive arterial disease, peripheral edema, trauma, and friable skin from corticosteroid use.

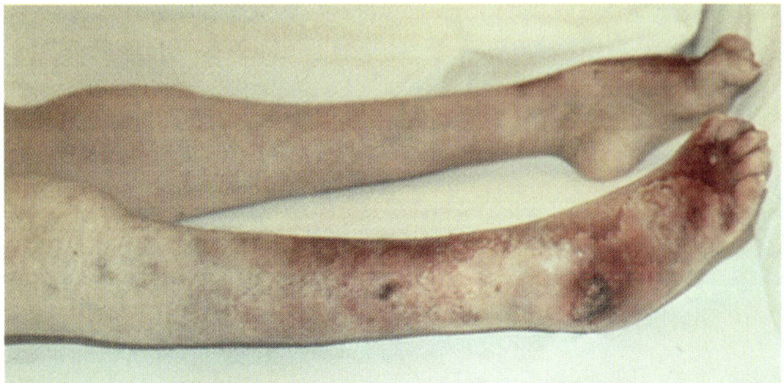

Figure 2.11. Rheumatoid vasculitis with several punched out ulcers on the lower extremities.

Rheumatoid vasculitis may be associated with scleritis. Vasculitis occurs in up to 10% of patients with FS (93). Other organ system involvement with vasculitis is uncommon, but the process may involve the mesenteric, cerebral, and coronary arteries.

Men who are seropositive and have nodular erosive disease of long duration are at greatest risk for developing rheumatoid vasculitis. Patients may have systemic constitutional symptoms and weight loss. Joint inflammation may be quiescent in these patients (91).

Patients with rheumatoid vasculitis typically have a high sedimentation rate, anemia of chronic disease, reactive thrombocytosis, hypoalbuminemia, high-titer RF and may have low C-3 and C-4 complement levels (94). Circulating immune complexes and activation of complement are believed to play a pathogenic role. Cryoglobulins may be present in one-third of patients (95). Angiography or biopsy of skin or nerve may be required to confirm the diagnosis. Leukocytoclastic vasculitis is the most common abnormality on skin biopsy (91).

Despite therapy, mortality rates are high with rheumatoid vasculitis, which is due mainly to infection and target organ involvement.

Hepatic

Clinically significant liver disease related to RA is uncommon. Serum transaminases are usually normal, but alkaline phosphatase is not uncommonly elevated in active disease; in approximately two-thirds of cases, this is of hepatic origin (96).

Histologically, liver biopsies obtained before starting methotrexate in RA patients reveal that 28% have mild portal triad inflammation and 38% have mild fatty infiltration (97). The liver is frequently involved in amyloidosis. Patients with FS may develop nodular regenerative hyperplasia, portal fibrosis, portal hypertension, and bleeding esophageal varices (98). Hepatotoxicity is a known complication of many disease-modifying antirheumatic drugs and nonsteroidal antiinflammatory agents.

Renal Disease

Although RA is not typically thought to cause renal disease, 17% of patients were found to have microscopic hematuria, elevated serum creatinine, or significant proteinuria in one prospective study (99). Serum creatinine may be normal in the setting of decreased glomerular filtration rate because of muscle atrophy in RA patients.

Generally, renal disease in patients with RA is either secondary to drugs or related to RA and its complications. A raised serum creatinine or proteinuria is likely to be drug related, whereas isolated hematuria is associated with active rheumatoid disease (99). Numerous drugs used in the treatment of RA can cause renal disease, including nonsteroidal antiinflammatory agents, gold, penicillamine, and cyclosporine. Clinically significant amyloidosis of the AA type, if it occurs in RA, almost invariably affects the kidneys, causing progressive proteinuria and decline in renal function. Renal involvement can occur in the setting of rheumatoid vasculitis, and membranous, membranoproliferative, and proliferative glomerulonephritis have been described in autopsy series (100). It is unclear whether the renal diseases associated with primary Sjögren's syndrome, such as interstitial nephritis and distal renal tubular acidosis, are seen with increased frequency in RA patients with secondary Sjögren's.

Infection

Infections are clearly increased in RA patients. Corticosteroid use, leukopenia, the presence of extraarticular features, and comorbid conditions such as diabetes, alcoholism, and chronic lung disease are all strong predictors of serious infection in this disease (101).

Malignancy

There are conflicting data regarding the overall risk of cancer in RA patients compared to the general population. Certainly, RA patients do have an increased risk of lymphoproliferative malignancies, and the risk is further increased by immunosuppressive medications used in treatment, including methotrexate, azathioprine, cyclosporine, and cyclophosphamide (102,103). A confounding factor in the assessment of this risk is the higher incidence of Sjögren's syndrome among patients with RA, which itself is a risk factor for lymphoma. Many lymphomas in patients treated with methotrexate are Epstein-Barr virus related, similar to those seen in patients with human immunodeficiency virus infection or in organ transplant patients.

DIFFERENTIAL DIAGNOSIS

The diagnosis of the patient with symmetric polyarthritis, nodules, positive RF, and typical erosions is straightforward. However, early RA may be subtle or atypical in presentation. The RF may be negative. The hallmarks of RA are those of an inflammatory arthritis—namely, morning stiffness, pain, and joint warmth and swelling. The history and physical examination are the keys to the proper diagnosis of an inflammatory arthritis.

The differential diagnosis for a patient with arthritis that may mimic RA is broad (104). Many diseases encountered in clinical practice may be confused with RA (Table 2.2).

Crystalline Arthritis

Acute gouty arthritis is usually easily diagnosed, but the patient with tophaceous gout may present to the physician with a chronic, symmetric inflammatory polyarthritis, even with subcutaneous nodules. Even the radiologic changes of gout can mimic RA, but typically with gout there is a lack of periarticular osteoporosis and the erosions may be displaced from the joint and often have a sclerotic margin. Although patients with RA may rarely develop gout, the correct diagnosis of the polyarthritis can usually be resolved by aspiration of an affected joint and examination of the fluid for monosodium urate crystals under polarized light microscopy.

TABLE 2.2. Differential Diagnosis of Rheumatoid Arthritis

Crystalline arthropathy (gout, pseudogout, or chronic pyrophosphate arthropathy)
Infectious arthritis (rubella, parvovirus, hepatitis B and C, human immunodeficiency virus, disseminated gonococcal infection, Lyme disease, Whipple's disease, bacterial endocarditis, septic arthritis)
Rheumatic fever
Spondyloarthropathy
Arthritis related to connective tissue disease or systemic vasculitis
Behçet's disease
Adult Still's disease
Palindromic rheumatism
Polymyalgia rheumatica
Remitting seronegative synovitis with pitting edema
Malignancy-related arthritis
Hypertrophic osteoarthropathy
Osteoarthritis
Fibromyalgia
Infiltrative disorders (amyloidosis, sarcoidosis)
Hemochromatosis
Endocrinopathies (hypothyroidism, hyperthyroidism, hyperparathyroidism)
Hemophilic arthropathy
Pigmented villonodular synovitis

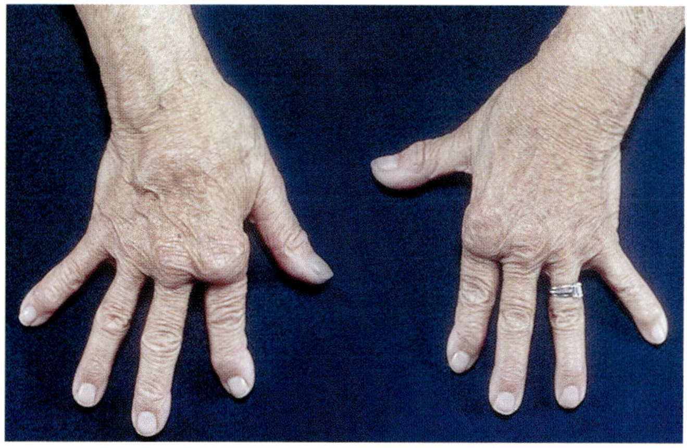

Figure 2.12. Calcium pyrophosphate dihydrate crystalline arthropathy with a "pseudo-rheumatoid" appearance of the hands. There is bony hypertrophy of the second and third metacarpophalangeal (MCP) joints and volar subluxation of the second and third fingers at the MCP joints. There is also cystic swelling of the dorsal aspect of the right hand.

In 2% to 6% of patients with clinically manifest calcium pyrophosphate dihydrate (CPPD) crystal deposition disease, the arthritis simulates RA (sometimes called *pseudorheumatoid arthritis*) (105) (Fig. 2.12). More commonly, however, it simulates and coexists with OA. The acute inflammatory arthritis of CPPD is usually mono- or oligoarticular, involving the knee, wrist, ankle, MCP, hip, or shoulder joints. The presence of chondrocalcinosis on joint radiographs can be helpful, but it is not always present. Radiographic findings of OA at the MCP joints should suggest CPPD disease. Aspiration of an affected joint and the finding of intracellular positively birefringent rhomboid-shaped crystals under polarized microscopy is diagnostic.

Infectious Arthritis

Rubella is a childhood disease characterized by rash, adenopathy, and constitutional symptoms. Rubella infection or immunization in young women is not infrequently followed by arthralgias or frank polyarthritis (106). The involved joints may include small joints of the hands, knees, wrists, elbows, ankles, hips, and toes. The arthritis typically resolves within 1 month of onset, but a minority of patients can develop chronic arthritis.

Parvovirus B19 most frequently affects children who present with erythema infectiosum (107). Like rubella, the arthropathy of parvovirus usually affects young women as a symmetric polyarthritis of acute onset with pain, swelling, and morning stiffness. The hands are usually affected. In most patients, the arthropathy resolves over several weeks, but it can be chronic or recurrent. Occasionally, cases may meet the classification criteria for RA. However, these patients usually lack RF, and erosive changes are absent. The diagnosis of parvovirus is confirmed with the finding of immunoglobulin M antibodies to the virus. It has been suggested that an antecedent viral infection, with parvovirus, for example, may be associated with some cases of subsequent RA.

Hepatitis B can present with an inflammatory polyarthritis in the absence of other clinical manifestations, but the arthritis is usually of short duration (108). Liver transaminases are usually elevated at presentation of the arthritis. Similarly, arthritis can be a manifestation of *hepatitis* C. Patients with mixed cryoglobulinemia from hepatitis C frequently have a positive RF and may develop a symmetric arthritis that can be confused with RA (109). However, like other forms of viral arthritis, these patients lack subcutaneous nodules and erosive radiographic findings.

Patients with early *human immunodeficiency virus* infection may develop clinical entities resembling RA or one of the spondyloarthropathies.

Disseminated gonococcal infection typically presents in young, sexually active adults with asymmetric polyarthralgia, which may be migratory and cause a rash. It is often accompanied by isolated tenosynovitis. The pustular, necrotic, or vesicular lesions that can be seen with disseminated gonococcal infection are not features of RA.

Lyme disease, after months of untreated infection, may produce mono- or oligoarticular arthritis usually involving large joints, especially the knee (110). The attacks tend to be intermittent, and usually, the arthritis resolves after months or years. Usually, patients will have had erythema migrans, and the RF is typically negative.

Whipple's disease, due to chronic infection with *Tropheryma whippelii*, can cause diarrhea, weight loss, and arthritis. Classically, the arthritis takes the form of a chronic seronegative oligo- or polyarthritis with a relapsing course, typically involving the knee(s) (111). In most cases, the arthritis precedes the onset of gastrointestinal symptoms, making it difficult to distinguish from other forms of inflammatory arthritis. The diagnosis can be confirmed by small bowel biopsy. Periodic acid-Schiff staining reveals inclusions within the macrophages, corresponding to bacterial structures. Polymerase chain reaction for the bacterium on joint fluid, synovial tissue, or gastrointestinal biopsy specimens can also confirm the diagnosis of Whipple's disease.

Bacterial endocarditis frequently causes musculoskeletal symptoms, including arthralgia, back pain, and frank arthritis (usually in large proximal joints). Synovial fluid cultures are usually negative. The RF is transiently positive in one-third of patients, which can be a source of confusion (112).

Nongonococcal septic arthritis usually causes a monoarticular and profoundly inflammatory arthritis. Synovial fluid cultures are positive in 90% of patients (112). RA and immunosuppression are risk factors for polyarticular septic arthritis. During acute "flares" of RA, whether mono-, oligo-, or polyarticular, it is always important to consider infection.

Rheumatic fever often causes a migratory large-joint inflammatory arthritis. Like RA, acute rheumatic fever (ARF) can cause subcutaneous nodules. However, the nodules in ARF appear in crops, are smaller than rheumatoid nodules, and are only present for several weeks (113). Unlike ARF, RA is not associated with antecedent streptococcal pharyngitis, chorea, erythema marginatum, or pancarditis. Jaccoud's arthropathy is a rare deforming arthritis associated with ARF that can resemble the chronic hand changes seen in RA but is not erosive (113).

The *spondyloarthropathies* include ankylosing spondylitis, reactive arthritis, psoriatic arthritis (PA), inflammatory bowel disease–associated arthritis, and undifferentiated spondyloarthropathy. Postinfectious inflammatory joint disease from organisms such as *Shigella*, *Salmonella*, *Yersinia*, *Campylobacter*, and *Chlamydia* tends to affect young adults and causes an additive, asymmetric arthritis that has a predilection for the lower extremities and sacroiliac joints (104). The urethritis, conjunctivitis, and iritis that may accompany reactive arthritis typically do not occur in RA. The HLA-B27 antigen is present in the majority of patients with Reiter's syndrome.

The peripheral arthritis that develops in 50% of patients with ankylosing spondylitis may be indistinguishable from RA, but the presence of back pain and sacroiliitis aids in arriving at the correct diagnosis. PA can cause a symmetric inflammatory arthritis identical to RA. Separating the diseases is the presence of psoriasis, the occurrence of DIP involvement with PA, and the usual lack of RF in PA. There are also patients with RA who have psoriasis. Distinguishing characteristics of RA in this setting include positive RF, presence of nodules, the typical pattern of rheumatoid joint erosions on radiography, and lack of DIP involvement.

The diagnosis of inflammatory bowel disease–associated arthritis is only confusing if it precedes the overt bowel involvement. The peripheral arthritis tends to be more asymmetric than in RA, involves the large joints of the lower extremities, and may parallel the activity of the bowel disease (104). Principal distinguishing factors of all the spondyloarthropathies from RA are the findings of enthesopathy (inflammatory changes in which ligaments attach to bone) and dactylitis presenting as "sausage digits."

Polyarthritis may occur in *connective tissue diseases*. Systemic lupus erythematosus (SLE) not uncommonly causes a symmetric peripheral-joint arthritis. A history of photosensitivity, oral ulcerations, typical malar or discoid rash, and/or renal disease can be helpful in differentiating SLE from RA. Jaccoud's arthropathy can occur in lupus and is characterized by deformation of the hands with ulnar deviation, swan-neck deformities, "Z" deformity of thumb, subluxations, absence of erosions, and paucity of synovitis. It is distinguished from the chronic findings of the rheumatoid hand because all the deformities are reducible. Patients with lupus may develop subcutaneous nodules, but these are generally transient. The antinuclear antibody test is almost always positive, and the RF should be negative. *Rhupus syndrome* was a term coined to describe patients with a mixture of features of SLE and RA (114). Mixed connective tissue disease can cause edema and synovitis of the hands, but is distinguished from RA by the presence of U1-RNP antibodies, Raynaud's phenomenon, and acrosclerosis. However, Raynaud's phenomenon may occur in up to 17% of patients with RA (115).

Systemic vasculitides, such as polyarteritis nodosa and Wegener's granulomatosis, can cause arthritis, but, usually, other findings, such as skin lesions, renal disease, neuropathy, and the lack of erosive disease, distinguish these entities from RA.

Behçet's disease, marked by oral and genital ulcers, iritis, and a myriad of other symptoms and signs, may also cause an asymmetric inflammatory polyarthritis.

Adult Still's disease can cause arthralgia, oligoarthritis, or polyarthritis. Joint involvement is often symmetric and affects knees, wrists, ankles, and MCP joints. The high fever, sore throat, typical rash, lymphadenopathy, pleuropericarditis, organomegaly, leukocytosis, absent RF, and high levels of serum ferritin help to distinguish adult Still's from RA. RF and antinuclear antibodies are negative in adult Still's disease, and these patients lack subcutaneous nodules.

PR has been described earlier in the chapter as a possible presenting syndrome of RA as well as a separate disease entity. Patients with PR who have a positive RF are likely to develop RA.

Polymyalgia rheumatica (PMR) presents with stiffness and pain in the neck, shoulder girdles, and pelvic girdles. Small-joint involvement is unusual, and the arthritis is nonerosive. Patients with PMR are at least 50 years old and usually have elevated acute phase markers. Patients with seronegative RA can also present with symptoms of shoulder and hip pain with stiffness. Coexistent symptoms of giant cell arteritis and the exquisite response of PMR to relatively low doses of corticosteroids can help clarify the diagnosis.

RS3PE, or remitting seronegative symmetric synovitis with pitting edema, is a syndrome in elderly patients of acute onset of symmetric synovitis with pitting edema in the hands, feet, and legs. Patients with RS3PE do not develop bony erosions, lack RF, and the predominant inflammatory involvement is of the tenosynovial sheaths rather than of the joints. Most patients with RS3PE, unlike patients with RA, go into complete remission. RS3PE may be associated with PMR.

Malignancies, including solid tumors and hematologic cancers, can cause musculoskeletal symptoms and even symmetric polyarthritis but are usually RF negative and nonerosive (104). *Hypertrophic osteoarthropathy* (HOA) may be associated with pulmonary malignancy. Other lung conditions and chronic hypoxemic states, such as cyanotic heart disease, may also cause HOA. However, HOA is usually distinguished from RA because the pain is along the bones, as a result of subperiosteal new bone formation rather than from joint-centered synovitis. Clubbing is often a feature of HOA, whereas the erosive disease and RF typical of RA are absent.

OA typically affects the DIP, PIP, and first carpometacarpal (CMC) joints. It can cause stiffness, pain, loss of motion, and even deformities. Osteophyte formation leads to bony enlargement of the joints in OA, whereas the typical synovial proliferation of RA results in a "boggy" feeling when palpating the joints.

A subset of patients, usually middle-aged women, can develop erosive OA characterized by red, warm PIP joints, but almost no synovial proliferation is present, and RF and nodules are absent (116). However, joint destruction and ankylosis of the affected joints can occur in erosive OA, which, in the terminal stages, is radiographically indistinguishable from RA.

Fibromyalgia, although a painful musculoskeletal syndrome and often accompanied by arthralgias, lacks the cardinal features of RA—synovial inflammation and proliferation. The tender points of fibromyalgia are separated from the joints themselves.

Amyloidosis of the AL type is rarely confused with RA but can result in periarticular deposition and pseudoarthritis. The "shoulder pad sign" can occur from amyloid deposition in the soft tissue surrounding the shoulders. Patients can develop joint effusions that contain particulate material, staining positive with Congo red (117).

Sarcoidosis can cause migratory polyarthralgia, often of the large joints of the lower extremities (104). Löfgren's syndrome consists of hilar adenopathy, erythema nodosum, and periarticular ankle inflammation. RF is positive in 10% to 30% of patients with sarcoidosis, but the typical erosive changes of RA are absent.

Hemochromatosis might be confused with RA because it can cause bony enlargement and even low-grade inflammation of the second and third MCP joints. Cystic degenerative changes with osteophytes, and, occasionally, chondrocalcinosis are characteristic radiologic features (118).

Patients with *hypothyroidism* can present with stiffness, arthralgias, and carpal tunnel syndrome. Deposition of hyaluronic acid at various soft tissue sites may be responsible for these symptoms (104). Large-joint effusions can occur, and the fluid is noninflammatory. Hypothyroidism may also lead to chondrocalcinosis, CPPD arthropathy, and pseudogout. Similarly, *primary hyperparathyroidism* can cause arthralgias and myalgias and predisposes to CPPD crystal deposition. *Hyperthyroidism*, usually in the setting of exophthalmos and pretibial myxedema, can cause thyroid acropachy (119). This syndrome presents with insidious onset of hand swelling, clubbing, and periosteal reaction.

Hemophilic arthropathy can result from recurrent hemorrhage into a joint. The hemorrhage appears to occur most frequently in the knees and ankles and can provoke proliferative synovitis and joint destruction. The patient and family history usually helps to distinguish this disorder from RA.

Pigmented villonodular synovitis is a proliferative disease of synovium that usually affects a single joint, most often the knee. Magnetic resonance imaging findings are characteristic.

CONCLUSION

Armed with knowledge of the clinical features, examination findings, and differential diagnosis, the clinician is equipped to make an accurate and timely diagnosis of RA. Patients with RA then benefit from early introduction of effective therapies that lower the incidence and prevalence of many of the joint-specific and extraarticular disease complications described in this chapter.

REFERENCES

1. Weyand CM, Schmidt D, Wagner U, et al. The influence of sex on the phenotype of rheumatoid arthritis. *Arthritis Rheum* 1998;41(5):817–822.
2. Massardo L, Gabriel SE, Crowson CS, et al. A population based assessment of the use of orthopedic surgery in patients with rheumatoid arthritis. *J Rheumatol* 2002;29(1):52–56.
3. Peschken CA, Esdaile JM. Rheumatic diseases in North America's indigenous peoples. *Semin Arthritis Rheum* 1999;28(6):368–391.
4. Anderson JJ, Wells G, Verhoeven AC, et al. Factors predicting response to treatment in rheumatoid arthritis: the importance of disease duration. *Arthritis Rheum* 2000;43(1):22–29.
5. Turesson C, O'Fallon WM, Crowson CS, et al. Incidence of extraarticular disease manifestations in a population based cohort of patients with rheumatoid arthritis. *Arthritis Rheum* 2000;43(9S):S152.
6. Hakala M, Sajanti E, Ikaheimo I, et al. High prevalence of rheumatoid factor in community-based series of patients with rheumatoid arthritis meeting the new (1987) ARA criteria: RF-negative non-erosive rheumatoid arthritis is very rare. *Scand J Rheumatol* 1998;27(5):368–372.
7. Arnett FC, Edworthy SM, Bloch DA, et al. The American Rheumatism Association 1987 revised criteria for the classification of rheumatoid arthritis. *Arthritis Rheum* 1988;31(3):315–324.
8. Kirwan JR. The relationship between synovitis and erosions in rheumatoid arthritis. *Br J Rheumatol* 1997;36(2):225–228.
9. Orces CH, Del Rincon I, Abel MP, et al. The number of deformed joints as a surrogate measure of damage in rheumatoid arthritis. *Arthritis Rheum* 2002;47(1):67–72.
10. Thompson PW, Silman AJ, Kirwan JR, et al. Articular indices of joint inflammation in rheumatoid arthritis. Correlation with the acute-phase response. *Arthritis Rheum* 1987;30(6):618–623.
11. Eberhardt K, Fex E, Johnsson K, et al. Hip involvement in early rheumatoid arthritis. *Ann Rheum Dis* 1995;54(1):458.
12. Gordon DA, Hastings DE. Clinical features of early, progressive and late disease. In: Klippel JH, Dieppe PA, eds. *Rheumatology*, 2nd ed. Barcelona: Mosby, 1998:1–13
13. Fleming A, Benn RT, Corbett M, et al. Early rheumatoid disease. II. Patterns of joint involvement. *Ann Rheum Dis* 1976;35(4):361–364.
14. Schumacher HR. Palindromic onset of rheumatoid arthritis. Clinical, synovial fluid, and biopsy studies. *Arthritis Rheum* 1982;25(4):361–369.
15. Rosen A, Weiland AJ. Rheumatoid arthritis of the wrist and hand. *Rheum Dis Clin North Am* 1998;24(1):101–128.
16. Lehtinen JT, Kaarela K, Ikavalko M, et al. Incidence of elbow involvement in rheumatoid arthritis. A 15 year endpoint study. *J Rheumatol* 2001;28(1):70–74.
17. Lehtinen JT, Kaarela K, Belt EA, et al. Incidence of glenohumeral joint involvement in seropositive rheumatoid arthritis. A 15 year endpoint study. *J Rheumatol* 2000;27(2):347–350.
18. Lehtinen JT, Kaarela K, Belt EA, et al. Incidence of acromioclavicular joint involvement in rheumatoid arthritis: a 15 year endpoint study. *J Rheumatol* 1999;26(6):1239–1241.
19. Anderson RJ. Rheumatoid arthritis: clinical and laboratory features. In: Klippel JH, ed. *Primer on the rheumatic diseases*, 12th ed. Atlanta: Arthritis Foundation, 2001:221.
20. Burra G, Katchis SD. Rheumatoid arthritis of the forefoot. *Rheum Dis Clin North Am* 1998;24(1):173–180.
21. Mizumura T, Momohara S, Tomatsu T, et al. Radiological evaluation of foot deformities in rheumatoid arthritis. *Ryumachi* 2000;40(6):891–897.
22. Ritchie GW, Keim HA. Major foot deformities: their classification and x-ray analysis. *J Can Assoc Radiol* 1968;19(3):155–166.
23. Spiegel TM, Spiegel JS. Rheumatoid arthritis in the foot and ankle—diagnosis, pathology, and treatment. The relationship between foot and ankle deformity and disease duration in 50 patients. *Foot Ankle Int* 1982;2(6):318–324.
24. Michelson J, Easley M, Wigley FM, et al. Posterior tibial tendon dysfunction in rheumatoid arthritis. *Foot Ankle Int* 1995;16(3):156–161.

25. Lehtimaki MY, Kautiainen H, Hamalainen MM, et al. Hip involvement in seropositive rheumatoid arthritis. Survivorship analysis with a 15-year follow-up. *Scand J Rheumatol* 1998;27(6):406–409.
26. Rawlins BA, Girardi FP, Boachie-Adjei O. Rheumatoid arthritis of the cervical spine. *Rheum Dis Clin North Am* 1998;24(1):55–65.
27. Fujiwara K, Owaki H, Fujimoto M, et al. A long-term follow-up study of cervical lesions in rheumatoid arthritis. *J Spinal Disord* 2000;13(6):519–526.
28. Goupille P, Fouquet B, Goga D, et al. The temporomandibular joint in rheumatoid arthritis: correlations between clinical and tomographic features. *J Dent* 1993;21(3):141–146.
29. Redlund-Johnell I. Upper airway obstruction in patients with rheumatoid arthritis and temporomandibular joint destruction. *Scand J Rheumatol* 1988;17(4):273–279.
30. Geterud A, Ejnell H, Mansson I, et al. Severe airway obstruction caused by laryngeal rheumatoid arthritis. *J Rheumatol* 1986;13(5):948–951.
31. Lawry GV, Finerman ML, Hanafee WN, et al. Laryngeal involvement in rheumatoid arthritis. A clinical, laryngoscopic, and computerized tomographic study. *Arthritis Rheum* 1984;27(8):873–882.
32. Colletti V, Fiorino FG, Bruni L, et al. Middle ear mechanics in subjects with rheumatoid arthritis. *Audiology* 1997;36(3):136–146.
33. Yood RA, Goldenberg DL. Sternoclavicular joint arthritis. *Arthritis Rheum* 1980;23(2):232–239.
34. Kalliomaki JL, Viitanen SM, Virtama P. Radiological findings of sternoclavicular joints in rheumatoid arthritis. *Acta Rheumatol Scand* 1968;14(3):233–240.
35. Khong TK, Rooney PJ. Manubriosternal joint subluxation in rheumatoid arthritis. *J Rheumatol* 1982;9(5):712–715.
36. Turesson C, O'Fallon WM, Crowson CS, et al. Occurrence of extraarticular disease manifestations is associated with excess mortality in a community based cohort of patients with rheumatoid arthritis. *J Rheumatol* 2002;29(1):62–67.
37. Turesson C, Jacobsson L, Bergstrom U. Extraarticular rheumatoid arthritis: prevalence and mortality. *Rheumatology (Oxford)* 1999;38(7):668–674.
38. Turesson C, Jacobsson L, Bergstrom U, et al. Predictors of extraarticular manifestations in rheumatoid arthritis. *Scand J Rheumatol* 2000;29(6):358–364.
39. Turesson C, O'Fallon WM, Crowson CS, et al. No decrease over time in the incidence of extraarticular disease manifestations in rheumatoid arthritis—results from a community based study of patients diagnosed during a 40-year period. *Arthritis Rheum* 2002;46(9):S247.
40. Ichikawa MM, Murata Y, Higaki Y, et al. Rheumatoid neutrophilic dermatitis. *Eur J Dermatol* 1998;8(5):347–349.
41. Uhlig T, Kvien TK, Jensen JL, et al. Sicca symptoms, saliva and tear production, and disease variables in 636 patients with rheumatoid arthritis. *Ann Rheum Dis* 1999;58(7):415–422.
42. Wisnieski JJ, Askari AD. Rheumatoid nodulosis: a relatively benign rheumatoid variant. *Arch Intern Med* 1981;141(5):615–619.
43. Palmer DG. The anatomy of the rheumatoid lesion. *Br Med Bull* 1995;51 (2):286–295.
44. Segal R, Caspi D, Tishler M, et al. Accelerated nodulosis and vasculitis during methotrexate therapy for rheumatoid arthritis. *Arthritis Rheum* 1988;31(9):1182–1185.
45. Cunnane G, Warnock M, Rehman Q, et al. Accelerated nodulosis and vasculitis following etanercept therapy for rheumatoid arthritis. *Arthritis Rheum* 2001;44(9):S373.
46. Baer AN, Dessypris EN, Krantz SB. The pathogenesis of anemia in rheumatoid arthritis: a clinical and laboratory analysis. *Semin Arthritis Rheum* 1990;19(4):209–223.
47. Bentley DP, Williams P. Serum ferritin concentration as an index of storage iron in rheumatoid arthritis. *J Clin Pathol* 1974;27(10):786–788.
48. Harreby M, Danneskiold-Samsoe B, Kjer J, et al. Viscosity of plasma in patients with rheumatoid arthritis. *Ann Rheum Dis* 1987;46(8):601–604.
49. Bach LA, Buchanan RR, Scarlett JD, et al. Hyperviscosity syndrome secondary to rheumatoid arthritis. *Aust N Z J Med* 1989;19(6):710–712.
50. Kelly CA, Malcolm AJ, Griffiths I. Lymphadenopathy in rheumatic patients. *Ann Rheum Dis* 1987;46(3):224–227.
51. Kondratowicz GM, Symmons DP, Bacon PA, et al. Rheumatoid lymphadenopathy: a morphological and immunohistochemical study. *J Clin Pathol* 1990;43(2):106–113.
52. Isomaki H, Koivisto O, Kiviniitty K. Splenomegaly in rheumatoid arthritis. *Acta Rheumatol Scand* 1971;17(1):23–26.
53. Georgescu L, Quinn GC, Schwartzman S, et al. Lymphoma in patients with rheumatoid arthritis: association with the disease state or methotrexate treatment. *Semin Arthritis Rheum* 1997;26(6):794–804.
54. Sant SM, Tormey VJ, Freyne P, et al. Lymphatic obstruction in rheumatoid arthritis. *Clin Rheumatol* 1995;14(4):445–450.
55. Husby G. Amyloidosis and rheumatoid arthritis. *Clin Exp Rheumatol* 1985;3(2):173–180.
56. Okuda Y, Takasugi K, Oyama T, et al. Amyloidosis in rheumatoid arthritis—clinical study of 124 histologically proven cases. *Ryumachi* 1994;34(6):939–946.
57. Rosenstein ED, Kramer N. Felty's and pseudo-Felty's syndromes. *Semin Arthritis Rheum* 1991;21(3):129–142.
58. Goldberg J, Pinals RS. Felty syndrome. *Semin Arthritis Rheum* 1980;10(1):52–65.
59. Breedveld FC, Fibbe WE, Cats A. Neutropenia and infections in Felty's syndrome. *Br J Rheumatol* 1988;27(3):191–197.
60. Dhodapkar MV, Li CY, Lust JA, et al. Clinical spectrum of clonal proliferations of T-large granular lymphocytes: a T-cell clonopathy of undetermined significance? *Blood* 1994;84(5):1620–1627.
61. Foster CS, Forstot SL, Wilson LA. Mortality rate in rheumatoid arthritis patients developing necrotizing scleritis or peripheral ulcerative keratitis: effects of systemic immunosuppression. *Ophthalmology* 1984;91(10):1253–1263.
62. Reddy SC, Rao UR. Ocular complications of adult rheumatoid arthritis. *Rheumatol Int* 1996;16(2):49–52.
63. Chang DJ, Paget SA. Neurologic complications of rheumatoid arthritis. *Rheum Dis Clin North Am* 1993;19(4):955–973.
64. Nadkar MY, Agarwal R, Samant RS, et al. Neuropathy in rheumatoid arthritis. *J Assoc Physicians India* 2001;49:217–220.
65. Puechal X, Said G, Hilliquin P, et al. Peripheral neuropathy with necrotizing vasculitis in rheumatoid arthritis: a clinicopathologic and prognostic study of thirty-two patients. *Arthritis Rheum* 1995;38(11):1618–1629.
66. Ekdahl C, Broman G. Muscle strength, endurance, and aerobic capacity in rheumatoid arthritis: a comparative study with healthy subjects. *Ann Rheum Dis* 1992;51(1):35–40.
67. Tanoue LT. Pulmonary manifestations of rheumatoid arthritis. *Clin Chest Med* 1998;19(4):667–685.
68. Bywaters EG. The mechanism of low glucose concentration in rheumatoid pleural effusions: a primary transport defect? *J Rheumatol* 1981;8(1):175–176.
69. Anaya JM, Diethelm L, Ortiz LA, et al. Pulmonary involvement in rheumatoid arthritis. *Semin Arthritis Rheum* 1995;24(4):242–254.
70. Caplan A. Certain unusual radiologic appearances in the chest of coal miners suffering from rheumatoid arthritis. *Thorax* 1953;8:29–36.
71. Fujii M, Adachi S, Shimizu T, et al. Interstitial lung disease in rheumatoid arthritis: assessment with high-resolution computed tomography. *J Thorac Imaging* 1993;8(1):54–62.
72. Rajasekaran BA, Shovlin D, Lord P, et al. Interstitial lung disease in patients with rheumatoid arthritis: a comparison with cryptogenic fibrosing alveolitis. *Rheumatology (Oxford)* 2001;40(9):1022–1025.
73. Haslam PL, Turton CW, Heard B, et al. Bronchoalveolar lavage in pulmonary fibrosis: comparison of cells obtained with lung biopsy and clinical features. *Thorax* 1980;35(1):9–18.
74. Muller NL, Miller RR. Diseases of the bronchioles: CT and histopathologic findings. *Radiology* 1995;196(1):3–12.
75. Kremer JM, Alarcon GS, Weinblatt ME, et al. Clinical, laboratory, radiographic, and histopathologic features of methotrexate-associated lung injury in patients with rheumatoid arthritis: a multicenter study with literature review. *Arthritis Rheum* 1997;40(10):1829–1837.
76. Van Doornum S, McColl G, Wicks IP. Accelerated atherosclerosis: an extraarticular feature of rheumatoid arthritis? *Arthritis Rheum* 2002;46(4):862–873.
77. Wolfe F, Straus WL. Increased prevalence of cardiovascular and cerebrovascular disease in rheumatoid arthritis compared with osteoarthritis. *Arthritis Rheum* 2000;43:S133.
78. del Rincon ID, Williams K, Stern MP, et al. High incidence of cardiovascular events in a rheumatoid arthritis cohort not explained by traditional cardiac risk factors. *Arthritis Rheum* 2001;44(12):2737–2745.
79. Warrington KJ, Takemura S, Goronzy JJ, et al. CD4+,CD28-T cells in rheumatoid arthritis patients combine features of the innate and adaptive immune systems. *Arthritis Rheum* 2001;44(1):13–20.
80. Liuzzo G, Goronzy JJ, Yang H, et al. Monoclonal T-cell proliferation and plaque instability in acute coronary syndromes. *Circulation* 2000;101(25):2883–2888.
81. Warrington KJ, Kent P, Nakajima T, et al. Rheumatoid arthritis is an independent risk factor for accelerated coronary artery disease. *Arthritis Rheum* 2001;44:S378.
82. Haverkate F, Thompson SG, Pyke SD, et al. Production of C-reactive protein and risk of coronary events in stable and unstable angina. European Concerted Action on Thrombosis and Disabilities Angina Pectoris Study Group. *Lancet* 1997;349(9050):462–466.
83. Bonfiglio T, Atwater EC. Heart disease in patients with seropositive rheumatoid arthritis; a controlled autopsy study and review. *Arch Intern Med* 1969;124(6):714–719.
84. Bacon PA, Gibson DG. Cardiac involvement in rheumatoid arthritis. An echocardiographic study. *Ann Rheum Dis* 1974;33(1):20–24.
85. Hara KS, Ballard DJ, Ilstrup DM, et al. Rheumatoid pericarditis: clinical features and survival. *Medicine (Baltimore)* 1990;69(2):81–91.
86. Ahern M, Lever JV, Cosh J. Complete heart block in rheumatoid arthritis. *Ann Rheum Dis* 1983;42(4):389–397.
87. Chand EM, Freant LJ, Rubin JW. Aortic valve rheumatoid nodules producing clinical aortic regurgitation and a review of the literature. *Cardiovasc Pathol* 1999;8(6):333–338.
88. Webber MD, Selsky EJ, Roper PA. Identification of a mobile intracardiac rheumatoid nodule mimicking an atrial myxoma. *J Am Soc Echocardiogr* 1995;8(6):961–964.
89. Voyles WF, Searles RP, Bankhurst AD. Myocardial infarction caused by rheumatoid vasculitis. *Arthritis Rheum* 1980;23(7):860–863.
90. Gravallese EM, Corson JM, Coblyn JS, et al. Rheumatoid aortitis: a rarely recognized but clinically significant entity. *Medicine (Baltimore)* 1989;68(2):95–106.
91. Scott DG, Bacon PA, Tribe CR. Systemic rheumatoid vasculitis: a clinical and laboratory study of 50 cases. *Medicine (Baltimore)* 1981;60(4):288–297.
92. Vollertsen RS, Conn DL. Vasculitis associated with rheumatoid arthritis. *Rheum Dis Clin North Am* 1990;16(2):445–461.
93. Vollertsen RS, Conn DL, Ballard DJ, et al. Rheumatoid vasculitis: survival and associated risk factors. *Medicine (Baltimore)* 1986;65(6):365–375.

94. Mongan ES, Cass RM, Jacox RF, et al. A study of the relation of seronegative and seropositive rheumatoid arthritis to each other and to necrotizing vasculitis. *Am J Med* 1969;47(1):23–35.
95. Weisman M, Zvaifler N. Cryoimmunoglobulinemia in rheumatoid arthritis. Significance in serum of patients with rheumatoid vasculitis. *J Clin Invest* 1975;56(3):725–739.
96. Sullivan S, Hamilton EB, Williams R. Rheumatoid arthritis and liver involvement. *J R Coll Physicians Lond* 1978;12(5):416–422.
97. Brick JE, Moreland LW, Al-Kawas F, et al. Prospective analysis of liver biopsies before and after methotrexate therapy in rheumatoid patients. *Semin Arthritis Rheum* 1989;19(1):31–44.
98. Thorne C, Urowitz MB, Wanless I, et al. Liver disease in Felty's syndrome. *Am J Med* 1982;73(1):35–40.
99. Koseki Y, Terai C, Moriguchi M, et al. A prospective study of renal disease in patients with early rheumatoid arthritis. *Ann Rheum Dis* 2001;60(4):327–331.
100. Boers M, Croonen AM, Dijkmans BA, et al. Renal findings in rheumatoid arthritis: clinical aspects of 132 necropsies. *Ann Rheum Dis* 1987;46(9):658–663.
101. Doran MF, Crowson CS, Pond GR, et al. Predictors of infection in rheumatoid arthritis. *Arthritis Rheum* 2002;46(9):2294–2300.
102. Mikuls TR, Saag KG. Comorbidity in rheumatoid arthritis. *Rheum Dis Clin North Am* 2001;27(2):283–303.
103. Matteson EL, Hickey AR, Maguire L, et al. Occurrence of neoplasia in patients with rheumatoid arthritis enrolled in a DMARD Registry. Rheumatoid Arthritis Azathioprine Registry Steering Committee. *J Rheumatol* 1991;18(6):809–814.
104. Hoffman GS. Polyarthritis: the differential diagnosis of rheumatoid arthritis. *Semin Arthritis Rheum* 1978;8(2):115–141.
105. Steinbach LS, Resnick D. Calcium pyrophosphate dihydrate crystal deposition disease revisited. *Radiology* 1996;200(1):1–9.
106. Smith CA, Petty RE, Tingle AJ. Rubella virus and arthritis. *Rheum Dis Clin North Am* 1987;13(2):265–274.
107. Smith CA, Woolf AD, Lenci M. Parvoviruses: infections and arthropathies. *Rheum Dis Clin North Am* 1987;13(2):249–263.
108. Pease C, Keat A. Arthritis as the main or only symptom of hepatitis B infection. *Postgrad Med J* 1985;61(716):545–547.
109. Zuckerman E, Keren D, Rozenbaum M, et al. Hepatitis C virus-related arthritis: characteristics and response to therapy with interferon alpha. *Clin Exp Rheumatol* 2000;18(5):579–584.
110. Steere AC. Diagnosis and treatment of Lyme arthritis. *Med Clin North Am* 1997;81(1):179–194.
111. Puechal X. Whipple disease and arthritis. *Curr Opin Rheumatol* 2001;13(1):74–79.
112. Pinals RS. Polyarthritis and fever. *N Engl J Med* 1994;330(11):769–774.
113. Amigo MC, Martinez-Lavin M, Reyes PA. Acute rheumatic fever. *Rheum Dis Clin North Am* 1993;19(2):333–350.
114. Panush RS, Edwards NL, Longley S, et al. "Rhupus" syndrome. *Arch Intern Med* 1988;148(7):1633–1636.
115. Saraux A, Allain J, Guedes C, et al. Raynaud's phenomenon in rheumatoid arthritis. *Br J Rheumatol* 1996;35(8):752–754.
116. Ehrlich GE. Erosive osteoarthritis: presentation, clinical pearls, and therapy. *Curr Rheumatol Rep* 2001;3(6):484–488.
117. Hannon RC, Limas C, Cigtay OS, et al. Bone and joint involvement in primary amyloidosis. *J Can Assoc Radiol* 1975;26(2):112–115.
118. Ines LS, da Silva JA, Malcata AB, et al. Arthropathy of genetic hemochromatosis: a major and distinctive manifestation of the disease. *Clin Exp Rheumatol* 2001;19(1):98–102.
119. Vanhoenacker FM, Pelckmans MC, De Beuckeleer LH, et al. Thyroid acropachy: correlation of imaging and pathology. *Eur Radiol* 2001;11(6):1058–1062.

CHAPTER 3

Prognosis and Clinical Course

David L. Scott

BACKGROUND

When patients develop rheumatoid arthritis (RA), they want to have a realistic assessment of what is likely to happen to them and some appreciation of the ability of their clinician to give an accurate prediction. These related concepts form the basis of defining the clinical course and prognosis of RA. Unfortunately, an accurate prediction of an individual patient's clinical course is virtually impossible. The best that can be achieved is an approximate estimation of future patterns of disease in the overall group of RA patients seen in the setting of specialist clinics. There are many reasons for clinicians' inability to accurately predict the clinical course of a patient with RA. Chance events, the unknown impact of new treatments, changes in the pattern of disease with time, and the complex effects of lifestyle factors and comorbidity all have an impact on prognosis and increase the difficulty of giving an individual patient a precise assessment of future events.

When a patient presents with RA, there are many potential disease courses. Some patients will enter complete and permanent remission. Others will enter a temporary remission. Many will have persisting synovitis, increasing joint damage, and disability. A few will have a rapidly progressive and destructive course. Patients with RA have an increased mortality in comparison with the general population and are more likely to have one of a large range of comorbidities. Treatment reduces the overall burden of disease and reduces the chance of joint damage, disability, and death. Improved treatments should dramatically reduce the chance of a poor end result. However, estimating the overall outcome is complex because the way in which patients are selected to enter observational studies of the natural history of treated RA has a major impact on the likely results, and patients from community-based studies of all cases of polyarthritis will show far better overall outcomes than patients selected from tertiary referral centers. It is also likely that all observational studies give selective representations, as the very act of studying patients is relatively unusual, and most patients are not studied in this way, making those cases that are studied an unusual and probably unrepresentative group. Comparing different observational studies of disease course and outcome is therefore fraught with difficulties and uncertainties. Changes in outcomes, which are usually in the direction of improvement, may reflect genuine improvements but could also be partially or completely explained by variations in case selection and differences between units and investigators.

Describing the Course and Outcome of Rheumatoid Arthritis

The conventional view is that synovitis results in joint damage and that this damage, in turn, leads to disability and handicap. This scenario is shown in Figure 3.1. There is no doubt that persisting synovitis is associated with increasing erosive damage in patients with RA and that, in many ways, such a conventional view is a realistic summary of the course of the disease. However, it is also too simplistic because, for example, synovitis itself is often an immediate cause of disability, and, as a result, it causes a reduced quality of life. Despite such limitations in methods of assessment, it is reasonable to make the reduction of synovitis the principal aim of treatment because reaching this goal should reduce disability directly and also have the indirect benefit of reducing erosive damage, thereby limiting a secondary cause of disability.

Other consequences of RA, including increased mortality, comorbidity, drug side effects, and social factors, such as work disability, lie outside the axis defined by synovitis, damage, and disability. Although patients with the most severe RA have the greatest synovitis and are most likely to have an increased mortality and greater comorbidities, it is best to describe these events separately.

Prognostic Markers

Prognosis means forecast or prediction and in clinical practice refers to "the possible outcomes of a disease and the frequency with which they can be expected to occur" (1). Prognostic factors fall into several classes, including demographic factors such as age, disease-specific factors such as the presence of autoantibodies, and comorbidities. Prognostic factors do not necessarily cause specific outcomes, but are associated with them strongly enough to predict their development. Prognostic factors must be distinguished from risk factors, which are those characteristics associated with the development of disease.

ASSESSING DISEASE COURSE

Synovitis

There is agreement on a core data set to assess disease activity, including synovitis, in RA. This core data set comprises swollen joint counts, tender joint counts, pain assessment, patient's glo-

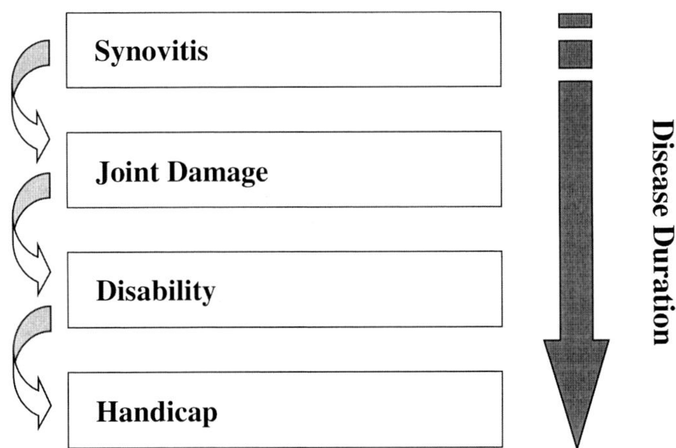

Figure 3.1. Conventional view of the relationships among synovitis, damage, and disability in rheumatoid arthritis.

bal assessment, and an acute phase marker such as the erythrocyte sedimentation rate (ESR) (2). Combined or overall indices are often used, and, in Europe, the Disease Activity Score (DAS) dominates. This score combines data on swollen and tender joints, ESR, and global health, with 28-joint counts preferred over counting all joints (3). Another widely used combined assessment measure is the American College of Rheumatology (ACR) response criteria (4). The ACR response criteria are principally designed for clinical trials. They show comparable changes to DAS scores (5).

Disability and Quality of Life

Quality of life, health status, handicap, and disability are overlapping concepts that can be used to define the course of RA. Their subjective, multidimensional nature means they are usually assessed using validated questionnaires that are completed by patients. Assessments by health care professionals are often considered inappropriate, because patients' views on quality of life may diverge from those of their physicians. A wide range of instruments has been developed to measure quality of life, and these are divided into global, generic, and disease-specific instruments.

UTILITY MEASURES

Single index measures of health status, such as the EuroQuol, provide a unitary value of health status, primarily for use in cost-utility analyses. The EuroQuol assesses perceived health in five dimensions (mobility, self-care, usual activities, pain/discomfort, and anxiety/depression) with an overall assessment of health status. It is available in English and many other European languages, and the patient completes it. The content of the EuroQuol is restricted, and it has been criticized as being skewed and relatively unresponsive—it seems rather insensitive to the clinical changes in RA.

GENERIC HEALTH PROFILES

Health profiles provide a measure of the impact of disease on a number of areas of patients' lives, each area being scored and presented separately. Commonly used health profiles include the Nottingham Health Profile (NHP) and questionnaires from the Rand Health Insurance Study Batteries Experiment, particularly the Medical Outcomes Study 36-Item Short Form (SF-36).

Nottingham Health Profile. This self-completed questionnaire comprises 38 statements that are answered yes or no. They measure subjective health status in six dimensions: physical mobility, pain, sleep, emotional reaction, social isolation, and energy. The results are presented as total scores in each category to give a profile; scores range from zero, indicating no problems, to 100, indicating all problems were present.

Medical Outcomes Study 36-Item Short Form. The SF-36 is the most widely used general health status measure. It has three levels: 36 individual items, eight scales that each aggregate two to ten items, and two summary measures that aggregate scales. The eight scales form two clusters—physical and mental health. The SF-36 is suitable for self-administration, computerized administration, or administration by a trained interviewer in person or by telephone. Its scaling is the inverse of many other questionnaires, in that zero is normal and 100 represents maximal difficulty.

CLASSIFICATION SYSTEMS FOR DISABILITY

The oldest, simplest measure is the Steinbrocker functional class (6), revised by Hochberg and colleagues in 1992 (7). It classifies patients with RA in four classes from normal (I) to completely disabled (IV). It is useful for broad comparisons between groups of patients but is less useful for monitoring changes in individual patients. It is now rarely used in clinical practice or research.

DISABILITY QUESTIONNAIRES

Although a number of instruments are available to measure disability in RA, only two have achieved widespread use—the Health Assessment Questionnaire (HAQ) and the Arthritis Impact Measurement Scales (AIMS) and its revision (AIMS-2).

Health Assessment Questionnaire. The HAQ is a self-completed questionnaire. Its complete form includes assessments of mortality, disability, discomfort and symptom levels, drug side effects, and economic impact. However, in practice, studies only use the physical disability scale. This scale assesses upper and lower limb function in relation to the degree of difficulty encountered in performing daily living tasks. These tasks include walking, dressing, bathing, and shopping. The HAQ features 20 items distributed across eight components. HAQ scores range from zero (without any difficulty) to three (unable to do). The highest score on any item within one component represents the component score. The respondent also indicates whether he or she uses devices or help from other people. Scores for each section are corrected for the use of aids or devices, summed, and transformed to give an overall disability score of zero to three. The range of HAQ scores is shown in Table 3.1. A score of zero represents no disability and three very severe, high-dependency disability.

Arthritis Impact Measurement Scales. AIMS was developed by Meenan and colleagues by adapting preexisting instruments, such as the activity of daily living, the Rand Health Insurance Study Scales, and the Quality of Well-Being Scale (6). It assesses physical, social, and emotional well-being in nine

TABLE 3.1. Ranges of Health Assessment Questionnaire (HAQ) Scores

HAQ Score	Disability	Functional Class
0	None	I
0–1	Mild	II
1–2	Moderate	III
2–3	Severe	IV

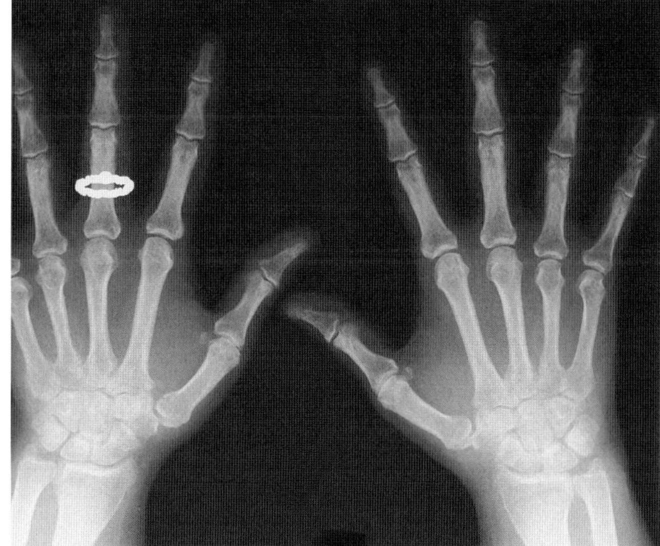

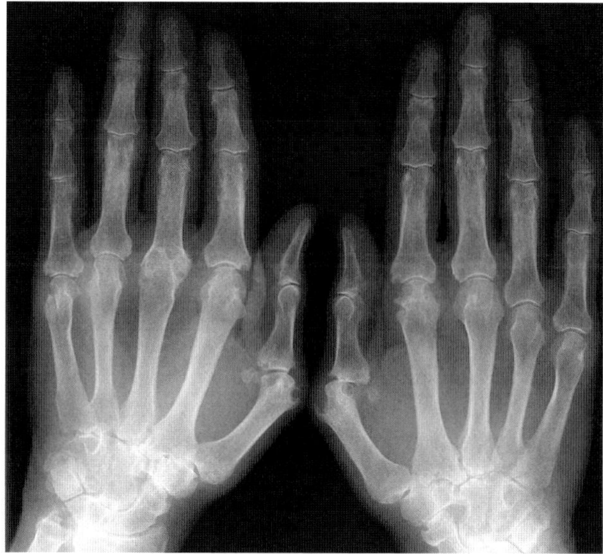

Figure 3.2. A,B: The progression of joint damage in rheumatoid arthritis. X-rays of the hands show illustrations of early- and intermediate-stage RA, with joint space loss and erosions being prominent changes.

dimensions: mobility, physical activity, activities of daily living, dexterity, household activities, pain, social activity, depression, and anxiety. An additional 19 items define general health, health perceptions, and demographic details. Scale scores are adjusted to fall within a range of zero to ten. The original AIMS takes 15 to 20 minutes to complete (8). Shorter and longer versions have been developed that have comparable sensitivity to change, including AIMS-2 (9).

Anderson et al. (10) found that improvements in AIMS parallel changes in traditional clinical outcome, such as tender joint count, morning stiffness, and ESR. The content of the AIMS overlaps with that of the full HAQ by approximately 65%, and both instruments measure three major dimensions of health status: physical disability, psychologic disability, and pain.

Joint Damage

Assessing x-ray progression in RA provides an objective measure of the extent of anatomic joint damage. Once the cascade of radiologic damage starts, there is relatively rapid progression in the early years (11). An example of x-ray damage is shown in Figure 3.2. New techniques such as MRI and ultrasound can visualize the earliest stages, although these techniques are still being developed. Currently, plain x-rays remain the most appropriate approach to evaluate the progression of damage in established RA. Serial measurements of radiologic progression are better than a single reading for evaluating increasing damage. Rapid x-ray progression suggests that patients need aggressive treatment. X-ray damage increases throughout the course of RA (12,13).

Many systems score x-ray damage in RA. Dominant methods include those of Sharp, modified by van der Heijde (14), and those of Larsen, modified by Scott et al. (15) and by Rau et al. (16). Current opinion favors the Sharp/van der Heijde system to detect meaningful clinical change (17,18). However, there remains considerable debate about the best method of scoring x-rays (19). Conventional x-ray films are still used, but, during the next few years, these will be replaced by digital images (20,21).

Mortality and Comorbidity

Causes of death should be defined from a register of cases. These data are used to calculate the standardized mortality ratio (SMR), which is the ratio of observed to expected number of deaths. Knowledge of the number of expected deaths in the observed population is obtained from age-, sex-, and year-specific mortality rates in the general population.

Comorbidity is difficult to define. There is no exact definition of "chronic coexisting diseases," and deciding whether a specific symptom is attributable to an extraarticular manifestation of RA, a drug side effect, or a completely unrelated illness is problematic. It is conventionally decided by the clinical judgment of experienced medical staff. Chronic coexisting disease should last more than 6 weeks. At present, there are only descriptive studies of coexisting diseases and extraarticular features of RA.

DISEASE ACTIVITY, DISABILITY, AND QUALITY OF LIFE

Disease Activity

Patients with RA have persistent synovitis throughout their disease. This synovitis results in continuing joint swelling, pain, and an elevated ESR. The belief that RA will "burn out" with time is based on the relatively small numbers of patients with long-duration RA who have no disease activity. The available evidence suggests the converse is the case with RA patients having active synovitis for most of their disease. Wolfe and Pincus (22) showed this persistence using serial data on 1,897 patients with RA seen in one unit from 1974 to 2000. During this period, there were 26,442 clinic visits. They found that the ESR, which reflects synovitis, had a value of 34 mm per hour in these cases. There was a small decrease (4 mm per hour) during the first ten years of disease. The ESR then stabilized for the next 25 years. Patients with recent onset of RA, stratified in quartiles of ESR, maintained their position over time. Experience from the author's unit confirms the stability of both ESR and pain measures throughout the course of RA, with little reduction during 25 years of RA. This result is shown for 725 patients in Figure 3.3.

The persistence of active synovitis has also been illustrated clearly in a 9-year observational study of 378 patients with early RA from Nijmegen in the Netherlands. This study

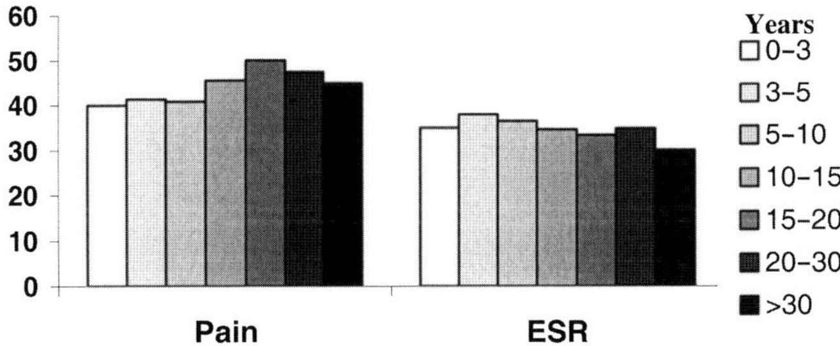

Figure 3.3. Pain and erythrocyte sedimentation rate (ESR) and disease duration in rheumatoid arthritis. Mean scores are shown from a cross-sectional study of 725 cases.

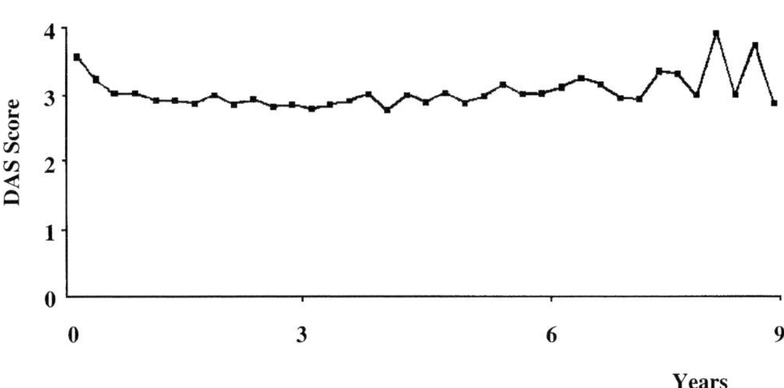

Figure 3.4. Mean Disease Activity scores (DASs) during the first 9 years of rheumatoid arthritis. (Adapted from Welsing PM, van Gestel AM, Swinkels HL, et al. The relationship between disease activity, joint destruction, and functional capacity over the course of rheumatoid arthritis. *Arthritis Rheum* 2001;44:2009–2017.)

followed DAS during conventional antirheumatic drug therapy (23). There was a small initial reduction in the extent of disease activity, but, thereafter, mean DAS remained more or less stable during the course of the disease. DAS levels were between three and four, as shown in Figure 3.4.

Functional Class

Studies before 1980 used Steinbrocker's functional classes to assess disability. The results of these reports are summarized in Table 3.2. Ragan and Farrington (24) studied 500 cases: 15% of patients who had RA for less than 5 years were class III/IV and 48% of patients with RA for more than 15 years. Duthie and colleagues (25) studied 307 cases: 25% of patients who had RA for less than 5 years were class III/IV and 38% of patients with RA for more than 15 years. Rasker and Cosh (26) studied 100 patients: 5% of patients who had RA for less than 5 years were class III/IV and 33%of patients with RA for more than 15 years. Other reports were by Short et al. (27), Scott et al. (28), Pincus et al. (29), Sherrer et al. (30), and Isacson et al. (31). The average results were 15% in class III/IV before 5 years and 40% after 15 years.

Although treatment effects are largely outside the scope of this chapter, this chapter presents evidence that aggressive treatment with antirheumatic drugs improves RA outcomes and reduces the number of cases ending up in functional classes III and IV. Möttönen et al. (32) reported a prospective study of 142 patients with early RA treated actively with slow-acting antirheumatic drugs and followed up for an average of 6 years; only 24% of cases deteriorated and entered functional class III or IV. This suggested that such a "sawtooth" treatment strategy might improve outcome in early RA. Under the "sawtooth" strategy, disease-modifying drugs are used soon after the onset of RA, and they are continued throughout the course of the disease with the aim of maintaining patients' levels of disability as close to normal levels as possible (33).

Health Assessment Questionnaire

HEALTH ASSESSMENT QUESTIONNAIRE AND DISEASE DURATION

Since 1980, outcome studies have predominantly assessed disability using HAQ scores. The range of available HAQ scores is from zero to three. Mean HAQ scores invariably increase with disease duration. Consequently, there are correlations between disease duration and HAQ scores. Studies by Pincus et al. (34) and Houssien et al. (35) evaluated 200 to 259 cases with wide ranges in disease duration and found correlations of approximately 0.3. An alternative approach to showing the progression of disability, suggested by Lassere et al. (36), is to construct percentile curve reference charts from HAQ scores. Such centile charts can be derived for most RA populations and an illustrative example (Fig. 3.5) is shown for 715 RA outpatients attending four European units. Finally, Wolfe and colleagues (37) showed that, in 400 current clinic attenders, mean baseline disease duration was 7.5 years in those with HAQ scores ≤1 and 14.2 years in those with HAQ scores ≥2.

PROGRESSION OF HEALTH ASSESSMENT QUESTIONNAIRE

As HAQ scores have only been widely used for 2 decades, there is little long-term longitudinal data. Cross-sectional data can be used to show time trends with the HAQ. The results from four cross-sectional studies are shown in Figure 3.6 (30,36,38,39). These studies show changes in mean HAQ scores in groups of 264 to 725 patients with disease durations from 1 to 25 years. At

TABLE 3.2. Long-Term Studies Reporting Functional Class in Rheumatoid Arthritis (RA) Patients

Study, Reference	Yr	Cases	Follow-Up (Yr)	Source	Functional Class III/IV at Onset (%)	Functional Class III/IV at End (%)
Short et al. (27)	1957	239	14	Inpatients	20	63
Ragan and Farrington (24)	1962	500	13	Outpatients	18	50
Duthie et al. (25)	1964	307	9	Inpatients	65	39
Rasker et al. (26)	1984	100	15	Early RA	5	51
Scott et al. (28)	1987	112	20	Inpatients	77	82
Pincus et al. (29)	1984	75	9	Outpatients	12	42
Sherrer et al. (30)	1986	1,043	12	Regional clinic	12	35
Isacson et al. (31)	1987	127	17	Population	9	22

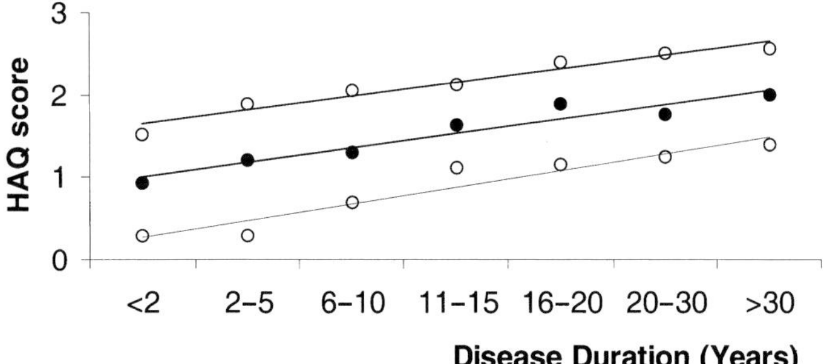

Figure 3.5. The progression of functional disability in rheumatoid arthritis. Median Health Assessment Questionnaire (HAQ) scores and 25% and 75% centiles constructed from a cross-sectional study of 725 cases.

7 years, the average HAQ score was approximately 1.00, at 12 years, it was 1.25, and at 18 years, 1.50.

Data from one study in Finland are shown after 20 years (Fig. 3.7). There was a wide range in end-point HAQ scores in the 81 patients in whom data were available. Sixteen percent showed poor outcomes (HAQ scores 2 to 3), and 60% had good outcomes, with HAQ scores of 1 or less (40).

ANNUAL PROGRESSION OF HEALTH ASSESSMENT QUESTIONNAIRE

An alternative approach to assessing the progression of disability is to calculate the average annual increase in HAQ scores. This increase has been reported in several prospective studies, following the concept of Leigh et al. (41). This study found an average annual increase in HAQ scores of 0.018 in 209 patients followed between 1981 and 1989. Patients who were maximally disabled showed average annual increases of 0.045. Data from a variety of cross-sectional and longitudinal studies can be transformed and expressed as such average annual increases in HAQ scores, as shown in Figure 3.8 (30,38,39,42–48), including two unpublished data sets (Truro, Cornwall, U.K. and Whipps Cross Hospital, London, U.K.). Two studies showed no change during 2 to 5 years, but the average increases in HAQ scores were 0.031 per year (approximately 1% of possible maximum disability). This finding means that, over 25 years, the average HAQ score would increase by less than one.

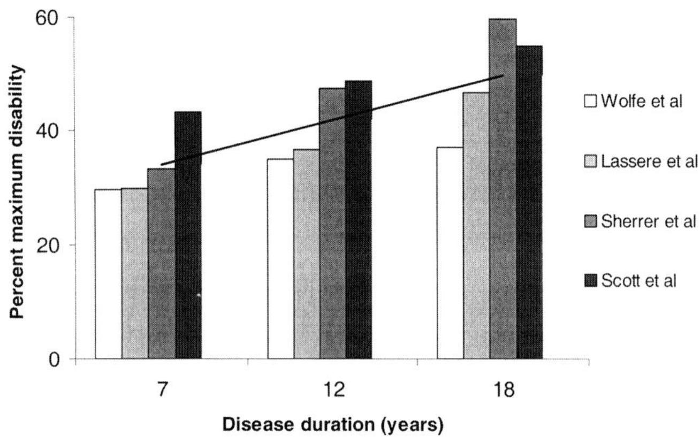

Figure 3.6. The increase in disability shown by combining results from four studies using the Health Assessment Questionnaire to assess disability. The average increase in disability, shown by the trend line, was an annual increase of 1.4% of possible maximum disability. (Data from Wolfe F, Hawley DJ, Cathey MA. Clinical and health status measures over time: prognosis and outcome assessment in rheumatoid arthritis. *J Rheumatol* 1991;18:190–197; Lassere M, Wells G, Tugwell P, et al. Percentile curve reference charts of physical function: rheumatoid arthritis population. *J Rheumatol* 1995;22:1241–1246; Sherrer YS, Bloch DA, Mitchell DM, et al. The development of disability in rheumatoid arthritis. *Arthritis Rheum* 1986;29:494–500; and Greenwood M, Scott DL, Carr AJ, et al. Pain and disability in rheumatoid arthritis. *Ann Rheum Dis* 1999;58[Suppl]:110.)

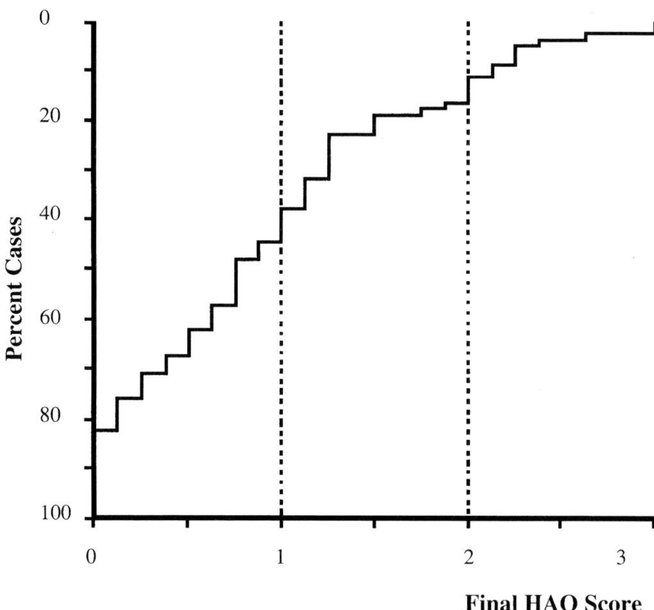

Figure 3.7. Health Assessment Questionnaire (HAQ) scores after 20 years in a cohort of six patients with rheumatoid arthritis from Finland (40). (Modified from Jantti JK, Kaarela K, Belt EA, et al. Incidence of severe outcome in rheumatoid arthritis during 20 years. *J Rheumatol* 2002;29:688–692.)

EARLY RHEUMATOID ARTHRITIS

The Norfolk Arthritis Register (NOAR) enrolls all patients with inflammatory polyarthritis from a community near Norwich in the United Kingdom. The NOAR cohort shows that, during the first 3 years of RA, disability scores were highest at baseline, with an improvement at 12 months (49). By 3 years, the average HAQ score was 0.63 in the whole NOAR group and 0.88 in patients classified as having RA. The Nijmegen study (23) reported a similar initial decline in HAQ scores, followed by an annual increase of 0.02 units per year, and, by 9 years, mean HAQ scores were 0.64 (Fig. 3.9).

INDIVIDUAL VARIATION

HAQ is usually applied to groups of RA patients and mean values used. However, when individual cases are followed over time, a

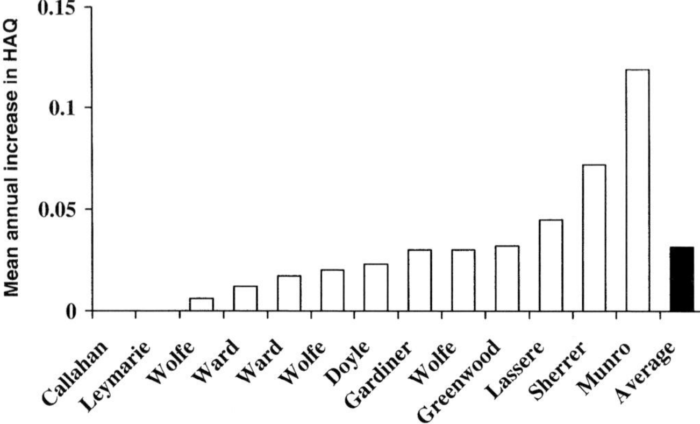

Figure 3.8. Annual increases in Health Assessment Questionnaire (HAQ) scores. Based on prospective observational studies (30,39–48).

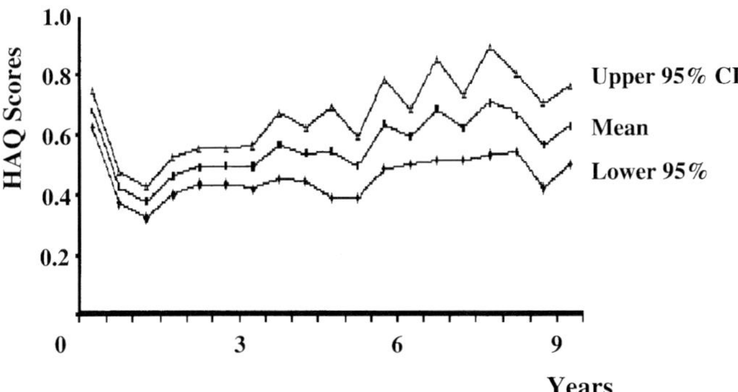

Figure 3.9. Mean Health Assessment Questionnaire (HAQ) scores at 95% confidence intervals (CI) during 9 years in prospective series. (Data from Welsing PM, van Gestel AM, Swinkels HL, et al. The relationship between disease activity, joint destruction, and functional capacity over the course of rheumatoid arthritis. *Arthritis Rheum* 2001;44:2009–2017.)

different pattern emerges. The extent of individual variations was shown by Eberhardt and Fex (50) in a 5-year prospective study of 63 patients with early RA. Median HAQ scores were stable and at 5 years were 0.7 for men and 1.1 for women with a median change over 5 years of 0.1 (annual average increase of 0.020). However, individual variation was considerable, with maximum changes varying from –1 to +1.

Similar variations were reported by Wiles and colleagues (51) in the 433 early RA patients in NOAR. Instead of following the centile lines as proposed by Lassere et al. (52), most cases showed marked volatility. Over 5 years, only 19% of cases remained in the same quartile. By the fifth year, the numbers of cases remaining in the same quartile increased, with 65% staying in one quartile for the year. This finding implies that the levels of disability may begin to stabilize after 4 to 5 years. An example of these individual changes in HAQ scores is shown for 25 patients followed in a single unit (Whipps Cross Hospital, London, U.K.) during a 4-year period (Fig. 3.10).

EuroQuol

An initial study by Hurst et al. (53) in 233 RA patients gave a favorable view of the EuroQuol, reporting that it had high correlations with measures of impairment and disability. Regression models showed that 70% of the variation in EuroQuol utility values were explained by pain, disability, disease activity, and mood. The reliability of the EuroQuol seemed as good as other instruments, except the HAQ.

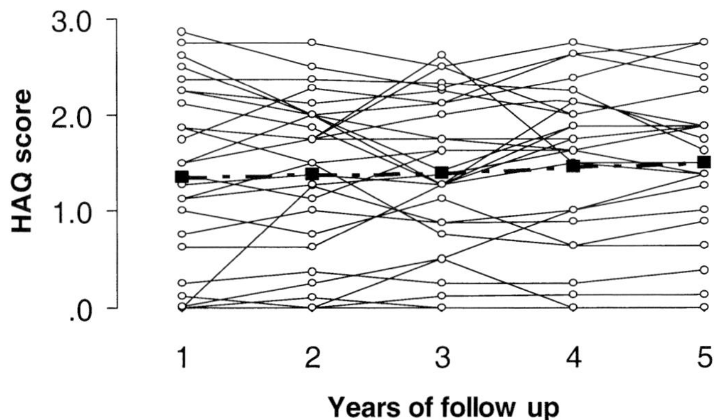

Figure 3.10. Changes in individual Health Assessment Questionnaire (HAQ) scores in 25 patients followed for 4 years. The bold line shows mean scores.

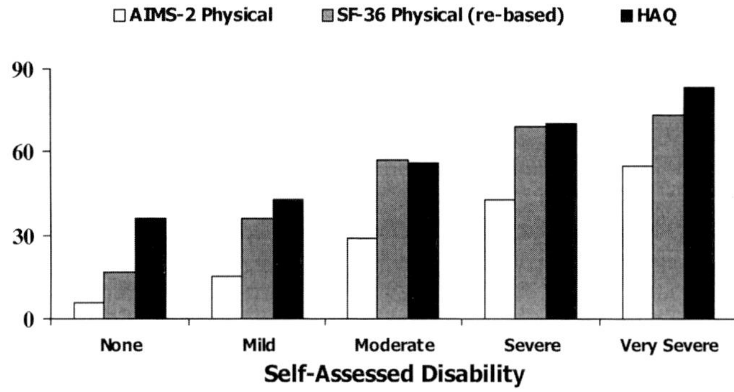

Figure 3.11. Comparison of Medical Outcomes Study 36-Item Short Form (SF-36), Arthritis Impact Measurement Scales Revision (AIMS-2), and Health Assessment Questionnaire (HAQ) physical function scores in 1,030 Norwegian patients with rheumatoid arthritis. (Modified from Kvien TK, Kaasa S, Smedstad LM. Performance of the Norwegian SF-36 Health Survey in patients with rheumatoid arthritis. II. A comparison of the SF-36 with disease-specific measures. *J Clin Epidemiol* 1998;51:1077–1086.)

A subsequent report by Wolfe and Hawley (54) on 537 patients with RA was less certain about the value of EuroQuol scores. These scores were lower than visual analog scale health state scores and arthritis-related global severity scores. The distribution of EuroQuol scores had many gaps and was not continuous. Thus, EuroQuol confirms the significant disability of RA but seems unhelpful in capturing the individual impact of the disease in a meaningful manner.

Nottingham Health Profile

An initial evaluation of the NHP in 56 RA patients followed for 6 months (55) showed that it reflected disease severity. A subsequent cross-sectional study of 200 RA patients (56) showed significant associations between NHP scores and DAS scores. There is evidence that NHP scores reflect changes in clinical and laboratory indicators of disease activity during methotrexate therapy (57). A multinational pilot study (58) that examined how different quality-of-life measures reflect changes due to methotrexate therapy found NHP gave large percentage improvements (22%) and a high standardized response mean (0.54), suggesting that it is sensitive to treatment effects. Despite these advantages, the NHP has not been used extensively in the evaluation of outcomes in RA.

Medical Outcomes Study 36-Item Short Form

The SF-36 has measurement properties similar to the NHP. In a study of 233 RA patients, Ruta et al. (59) showed the SF-36 scales were reliable with intraclass correlation coefficients of 0.76 to 0.93. They correlated with clinical and laboratory disease activity measures and were responsive to improvements in health (standardized response means, 0.27 to 0.9). A comparable Norwegian study of 1,030 RA patients (60) showed the SF-36 physical functioning scale had strong correlations with the HAQ and AIMS-2 physical scales (r = –0.69 and –0.73, respectively). The SF-36 performed well in RA, and although the physical function subscale did not capture all aspects of physical health, it may be more sensitive than disease-specific measures at low levels of physical disability. These results are illustrated in Figure 3.11.

The SF-36 was included in a hypothetical model to explore the factors causing disability in RA (61). The model explained 59% of overall disability, defined by the physical function scale of the SF-36 and HAQ. The main disease-disability pathway—articular signs and symptoms—explained 33% of disability. External modifiers and contextual variables, such as age, sex, and psychologic status, explained 26% of disability.

An SF-36 Arthritis-Specific Health Index (ASHI) has been constructed to improve its responsiveness using arthritis-specific scoring algorithms. Longitudinal data from 835 RA patients participating in placebo-controlled trials (62) showed that short-term (2-week) changes were assessed better using the ASHI rather than the generic SF-36 summary measures and the most valid SF-36 scale (bodily pain) as well. The ASHI was 5% to 19% better than the best SF-36 scale. Further analysis of this data set suggests that ASHI predominantly assesses pain severity (63).

Ethgen et al. (64) used the SF-36 and other measures of quality of life to evaluate direct costs and other components of future health care resource utilization in 642 patients with RA. There were significant associations between health care costs and the poor quality of life, including low scores in the SF-36. Poor quality-of-life scores on the summary scales of the SF-36 were associated with a 45% increase in visits to patients' family doctors.

PROGRESSION OF DAMAGE

Rate of Progression with Disease Duration

Joint damage increases with disease duration. Almost any population of RA patients currently attending a specialist clinic shows this increase. For example, a sample of 134 patients attending rheumatology outpatient clinics at the author's unit showed a highly significant relationship between disease duration and Larsen score, with a correlation of 0.47. There is some doubt whether disease duration influences the rate of progression. Larsen and Thoen (65) followed 200 RA patients for 12 months and found the rate of increase in the Larsen score fell in late RA. However, this fall may reflect how the rate of progression is calculated (66). A detailed study of 256 RA patients by Wolfe and Sharp (67) found constant progression over 19 years.

Prospective Cohort Studies Reporting Sequential Changes in Larsen Score

Three published studies report longitudinal changes in Larsen scores (68–70). These studies evaluated between 103 and 142 patients who were initially seen with a disease duration of less than 3 years and were followed prospectively for up to 20 years. Initially, average Larsen scores were less than 4% of possible maximum damage. By 9 years, they were 23% of possible maximum damage, and, after 15 years, they exceeded 50% of possible maximum damage in the one study in which data were available. The overall average annual increase in Larsen score was approximately 2% maximal possible damage.

Prospective Cohort Studies Reporting Sequential Changes in Sharp Score

Another three published studies reported longitudinal changes in the Sharp score. These studies evaluated between 123 and 378 patients seen within 2 years of disease onset and followed for up to 19 years (23,71,72). Initially, average Sharp scores were less than 4% of possible maximum damage. By 9 years, they were 20% of possible maximum damage, and, after 15 years, they exceeded 28% of possible maximum damage in the one study in which data were available. The overall average annual increase in Larsen score was approximately 1.8% of maximal possible damage.

Combining Longitudinal Studies Using Larsen and Sharp Scores

The results of these six studies are amalgamated in Figure 3.12. Initially, there was less than 3% of maximum possible damage. This percentage rose to 11% of maximal damage by 5 years and to more than 40% by 20 years. The rate of progression changed from an initial rate of 1.6% maximal progression annually to a later rate of 2.0% annually.

Patterns of Progression

Plant et al. (73) described four patterns of damage in 114 patients with early RA followed for 8 years. These patterns of damage are linear progression, which occurred in 51 cases; a lag pattern that was seen in 13 cases; a plateau pattern in 19 cases; and a nonerosive RA in 29 cases. Graudal et al. (74) studied 109 patients who were followed for up to 30 years and identified five patterns of progression. These patterns comprised no progression at all (under 1%), slow onset with a later exponential increase (39%), fast onset with a later stable rate of progression (11%), fast onset with a later slow rate of progression (30%), and slow onset with acceleration and then deceleration in progression (20%).

Kuper and colleagues (75) suggested a ceiling effect, with many patients reaching maximum scores for erosions. In a follow-up study of 87 patients with RA followed for 6 years, they found that 50% of patients had maximum scores in one joint and 20% had maximum scores in more than ten joints.

Developing New Erosions

Five prospective studies of hospital-based cases (73–79) reported between 1977 and 1998, which included 40 to 147 patients seen within 12 months of the onset of their RA, described results after 3 to 8 years of prospective follow-up. In these studies, 60% to 73% of patients developed one or more erosions in the hands and wrists. However, the situation is complex. Many patients have erosions when first seen in the clinic. For example, Jansen et al. (80) described 130 patients with early RA followed for 12 months, by which time 86% were erosive. However, when first seen, many patients already had erosions, and the extent of joint damage was related to the duration of symptoms before patients were initially seen.

There is evidence that the development of erosions is influenced by ceiling effects. Hulsmans et al. (81) described radiologic outcome at 6 years in a longitudinal study of 502 patients with recent-onset RA who were seen with disease duration of less than 1 year. There was a pronounced ceiling effect in the percentage of patients who developed more than one erosion. This means that, by setting a low level for assessing the amount of damage, its progression is underestimated. After 6 years, 95% of the patients had already developed more than one erosive joint. Finally, case selection is very important

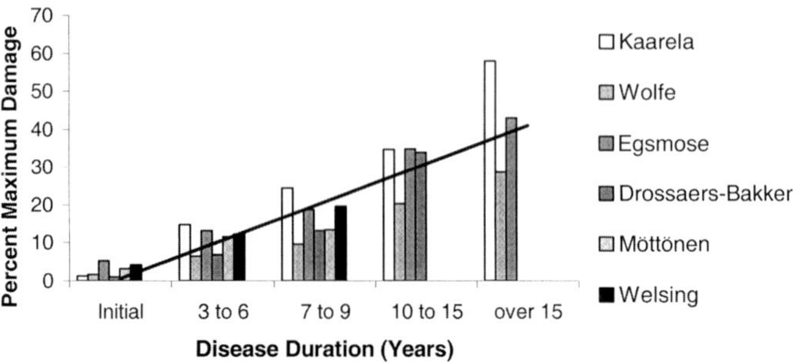

Figure 3.12. Progression of joint damage in long-term observational studies. Data are shown from six studies: three used Larsen scores (Egsmose, Möttönen, Kaarela), and three used Sharp scores (Welsing, Wolfe, Drossaers-Bakker). The results are shown as percent maximum damage.

in determining whether patients will develop erosions. NOAR reported less erosive disease: 399 (80%) of the 486 patients in the NOAR study satisfied the criteria to be x-rayed, and 335 patients had available x-rays (49); only 41% developed erosions. There is evidence that the development of erosions is influenced by ceiling effects in the methods used to judge x-ray damage. This means that the apparent upper score hides greater amounts of damage because patients have reached the maximum assessable score, so they are still having further damage.

Healing of Erosions

Healing of erosive damage is rarely reported but can occur. It has been described in a number of case reports (82–84). Healing phenomena include recortication of erosions, filling in of erosions with new bone, and secondary osteoarthrosis with sclerosis and osteophytes. Menninger (85) examined radiographs of hands and forefeet for 3 years and found repair in 9% of joints compared.

Progression in Different Joints

The most comprehensive assessment of changes in different joints is the Finnish series reported in many studies by Kaarela. These reports are based on 103 patients with seropositive RA followed for 15 to 25 years. The patients were first seen within the first year of diagnosis and followed prospectively while receiving standard treatment with disease-modifying antirheumatic drugs (86).

Wrist joints had the most destruction and the greatest need for reconstructive surgery (87). At the 15-year follow-up, mean Larsen scores showed 50% of maximal damage to wrist joints. After 20 years, 18% of wrists were completely destroyed. Only 25% of wrists were nonerosive. The metatarsophalangeal (MTP) joints were also frequently damaged; after 20 years, 62% had erosions and 24% were severely damaged (88). The first MTP joints showed the least damage and the fifth MTPs the greatest destruction. Erosive changes occur early in the MTP joints.

Involvement of other joints varied in comparison to wrist, hand, and knee involvement. For example, by 15 years, 51% of elbow joints had erosive involvement, with 30 of 74 patients showing bilateral changes (89). Similarly, after 15 years, severe radiologic changes in the hips were seen in 31 (32%) cases, with acetabular protrusion in five (90), and erosive involvement was seen in 96 of 148 (65%) shoulders evaluated (91).

Joint Replacements

Joint replacement is one way to define joint destruction independently of x-rays. Wolfe and Zwillich (92) reported the likelihood of RA patients needing total joint arthroplasty in 34,040 patient visits from 1,600 consecutive RA patients observed for 23 years. Kaplan-Meier life-table estimates showed that 25% would undergo total joint arthroplasty after 22 years of RA. Massardo et al. (93) reported a retrospective medical record review of RA cases in Rochester, Minn, between 1955 and 1985. There were 424 RA cases, and 35% of patients had one or more surgical procedures involving joints during a median of 15 years' follow-up. The most frequent procedure performed was total joint arthroplasty, with an estimated cumulative incidence at 30 years of 32%. The knee was the most frequent site, which involved 68 procedures, followed by the hip, which involved 31 procedures. Metacarpophalangeal, wrist, and shoulder arthroplasties were done less often.

RELATIONSHIPS AMONG SYNOVITIS, DAMAGE, AND DISABILITY

Inevitably, in the long term, joint destruction results in disability, with persistent synovitis predating most joint damage. Kirwan (94) outlined how these variables interact (Fig. 3.13). Joint destruction is the dominant factor underlying disability late in disease, whereas inflammatory joint symptoms are the main determinant of disability in early RA.

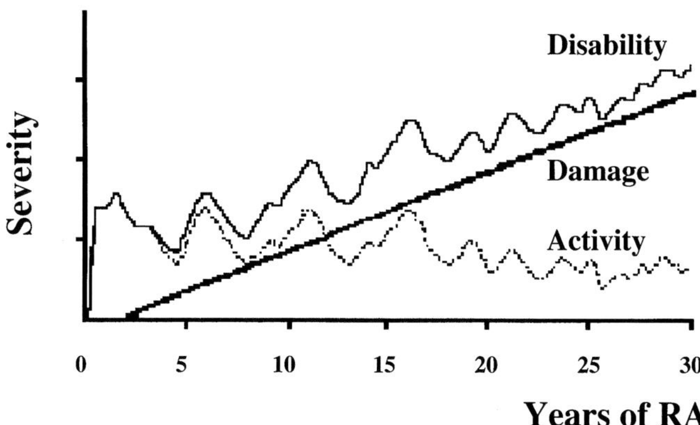

Figure 3.13. Theoretical view of the links between activity, disability, and damage in rheumatoid arthritis (RA). (Modified from Kirwan JR. Links between radiological change, disability, and pathology in rheumatoid arthritis. *J Rheumatol* 2001;28:881–886.)

Several prospective longitudinal studies report the interrelationships of function and radiologic damage in early (95,96) and established RA (97–103) (Table 3.3). Initially, patients have little radiologic damage but considerable disability as a consequence of having active arthritis. During the next 3 to 9 years, the extent of joint damage gradually increases, and a significant relationship can be seen with correlation coefficients varying from 0.3 to 0.5. After 5 years of RA, relationships between damage and disability are more pronounced. In patients with established RA, six studies showed significant correlations ranging from 0.31 to 0.68. Only Regan-Smith et al. (100) failed to show a significant relationship.

MORTALITY

Overall Mortality

It has been known for many years that RA results in excess mortality (104), though the extent of this excess is variable across different studies. Most studies suggest that patients with RA have a higher rate of all-cause mortality compared with age- and sex-matched control subjects without RA. The mortality rate is approximately twice as high in these patients compared with the general population, with calculated standardized mortality ratios (SMRs) that range from 0.87 to 3.0 (105–112). Possibly the highest mortality was seen in a series of 489 RA patients from Birmingham in the United Kingdom, reported in 1984 (113). These cases had a threefold increase in mortality overall compared with age- and sex-specific rates in the general population. The excess deaths were mainly from circulatory, respiratory, and musculoskeletal disorders. Malignant disease and digestive system disorders accounted for a small excess of borderline significance. Subsequent follow-up over 27 years (114) showed the SMR remained high at 2.7, with most excess deaths due to cardiovascular disease. SMRs from infection, renal failure, and non-Hodgkin's lymphoma rose with disease duration. Patients who presented early had less risk of premature death. There is some evidence that hospital-based cases of RA now have lower mortality rates, with one study from London reporting an SMR of only 1.3 for long-term hospital cases (115).

Gabriel and co-workers looked at population-based cohorts of all Rochester, Minn, residents older than 35 years with RA (116). They had worse mortality than expected for the general popula-

TABLE 3.3. Relationship between Radiologic Joint Damage and Functional Disability

Study, Reference	Yr	Patients	Study Type	Disease Duration	Correlation	Significance
Fex et al. (96)	1995	63	5-yr follow-up	Under 2 yr	0.27	NS
van Leeuwen et al. (95)	1994	149	3-yr follow-up	Under 1 yr	0.31	p <.001
Kaarela and Sarna (98)	1993	103	8-yr follow-up	Over 8 yr	0.68	p <.001
Larsen (99)	1988	200	Cross-sectional	Mean 15 yr	Not given	p <.01
Regan-Smith et al. (100)	1989	54	Cross-sectional	Mean 8 yr	NS	NS
Pincus et al. (97)	1989	259	Cross-sectional	Mean 12 yr	0.31	p <.001
Brühlmann et al. (101)	1994	62	Cross-sectional	—	0.39	p <.01
Hakala et al. (103)	1994	103	Cross-sectional	Mean 16 yr	0.46	p <.001
Houssein et al. (102)	1997	126	Cross-sectional	Mean 11 yr	0.38	p <.001

NS, not significant.

tion. The excess was unchanged over 4 decades, and people with RA had not shown the same improvements in survival experienced by non-RA peers. Overall, the risk of mortality in RA was 38% greater than for the general population. The risk was even greater for women, who had a 55% increased risk. Translating this into lost years shows that a 50-year-old woman with RA can expect to live 4 fewer years (30 more years instead of 34 more years) than a woman without RA.

Cardiovascular Mortality

There is considerable interest in the finding that RA is specifically associated with increased mortality from cardiovascular diseases (117). In nearly all studies, the most commonly reported cause of mortality was cardiovascular disease, accounting for more than half the deaths and up to 30% to 40% of the excess mortality associated with RA (Table 3.4). The relationship may be partly explained by RA patients having persistent inflammation and an increased likelihood of thrombosis. However, not all studies have shown increased cardiovascular deaths. A study from Norway by Riise et al. (110) found no increased cardiovascular mortality in RA patients followed up for 17 years, despite finding increased all-cause mortality in the RA group. An additional three inception cohorts studies of RA patients with disease onset in the 1980s also failed to detect any increase in cardiovascular mortality rates (118–120). However, results from NOAR (121) showed that patients who were seropositive at disease presentation had moderately increased mortality rates, and seropositive women had twice the expected mortality occurring from cardiovascular disease.

MORBIDITY

Coexisting Diseases

The most comprehensive account of coexisting diseases and comorbidity comes from Nijmegen, where a cohort of early RA patients was followed prospectively (122). The patients were enrolled between 1985 and 1990; they were assessed between 1991 and 1992 and were reviewed 3 and 6 years later. Results were available for 186 patients; 50 (27%) had one chronic coexisting disease and 28 (15%) had more than one, of whom 19 patients (10%) reported two chronic coexisting diseases, seven patients (4%) reported three, and two patients (1%) reported four. The number of cases with varying categories of coexisting diseases is shown in Table 3.5. The most common disorders were cardiovascular (29%), respiratory (18%), and dermatologic (11%).

These results reflect findings in an observational study of 288 RA patients reported by Berkanovic and Hurwicz (123). This study found 54% of cases had other chronic conditions, and, in 20%, one of these other conditions was severe. The frequency and severity of comorbidities affected scores on the AIMS. Another study by Gabriel et al. (124) evaluated selected comorbidities in a population-based prevalence cohort of 450 RA patients in Olmsted County, Minn. RA patients developed more congestive heart failure, chronic pulmonary disease, dementia, and peptic ulcer disease than expected for the general population.

There is an increased cardiovascular morbidity in RA. del Rincon et al. (125) showed this association in an evaluation of 236 RA patients assessed for the 1-year occurrence of cardiovascular-related hospitalizations, including myocardial infarction, stroke

TABLE 3.4. Deaths Attributed to Cardiovascular (CV) Disease in Patients with Rheumatoid Arthritis

Study, Reference	Cases	All Deaths	CV Disease	CV Deaths	SMR
Mutru et al. (105)	1,000	356	Ischemic heart disease	90	1.13
			Heart failure	21	5.25
			Cerebrovascular disease	29	1.16
			Other CV disease	26	2.60
Wolfe et al. (106)	3,501	922	Cerebrovascular disease	62	2.45
			Other CV disease	364	2.24
Myllykangas-Luosujärvi et al. (108)	—	1,186	Ischemic heart disease	319	1.51
			Other CV disease	274	1.14
Wållberg-Jonsson et al. (111)	606	265	Ischemic heart disease	80	1.54
			Cerebrovascular disease	21	1.10
			Total CV disease	140	1.46
Bjornadal et al. (112)	46,917	25,353	Coronary artery disease	6,991	1.79
			Cardiovascular, including stroke	12,431	1.81
Prior et al. (113)	409	199	Ischemic heart disease	40	2.14
			Cerebrovascular disease	15	1.79
			Other CV disease	23	3.85

SMR, standardized mortality ratio.

TABLE 3.5. Distribution of Chronic Coexisting Diseases in 186 Rheumatoid Arthritis Patients

Disease	Cases	% of Total Number of Coexisting Diseases
Hypertension	14	16
Angina pectoris	8	9
Other cardiovascular	4	4
Lung disease	16	18
Dermatosis	10	11
Eye disease	6	7
Kidney disease	5	6
Cancer	5	6
Gastrointestinal	5	6
Diabetes	5	6
Peripheral venous	4	4
Psychiatric	4	4
Hypothyroidism	2	2
Neurologic	1	1

Modified from Kroot EJ, van Gestel AM, Swinkels HL, et al. Chronic comorbidity in patients with early rheumatoid arthritis: a descriptive study. *J Rheumatol* 2001;28: 1511–1517.

or other arterial occlusive events, or arterial revascularization procedures, such as coronary artery surgery. The cardiovascular events in these participants were compared to the cardiovascular events occurring during an 8-year period in subjects representative of the overall population. The RA patients were observed for 252 person-years, during which 15 cardiovascular events occurred, which is an incidence of 3.4 per 100 person-years. The incidence of cardiovascular events in the control patients was 0.59 per 100 person-years This increased incidence of cardiovascular events in RA seemed independent of traditional risk factors, suggesting risks due to RA.

Extraarticular Disease

The United Kingdom–based Early Rheumatoid Arthritis Study reported its experience when 732 patients had completed 5 years of follow-up (126). A total of 270 patients (37%) developed extraarticular manifestations during this time. The main features were nodules (29%) and Sjögren's syndrome (7%); 2% of cases each had lung disease, neuropathy, Felty's syndrome, and localized and systemic vasculitis (Fig. 3.14). These findings are similar

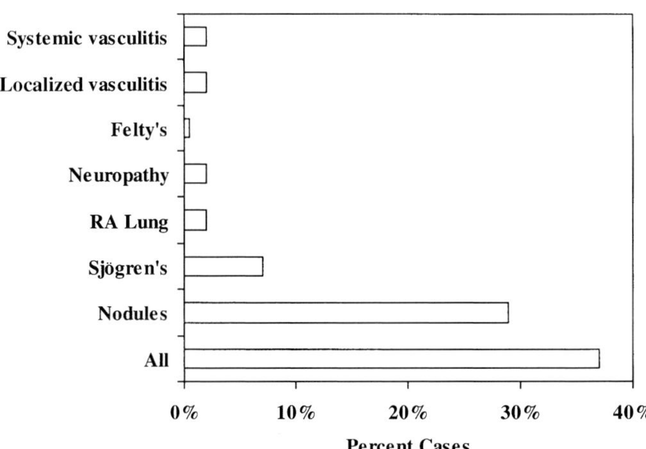

Figure 3.14. The extraarticular features of rheumatoid arthritis (RA) at 5 years. [Modified from Young A, Dixey J, Cox N, et al. How does functional disability in early rheumatoid arthritis (RA) affect patients and their lives? Results of 5 years of follow-up in 732 patients from the Early RA Study (ERAS). *Rheumatology (Oxford)* 2000;39:603–611.]

to those seen in a cross-sectional study of 587 current attenders with established RA from nine Italian rheumatology clinics (127). In this latter study, 240 (41%) patients had extraarticular features. The most common features were sicca syndrome (18%) and rheumatoid nodules (17%). Other extraarticular features included pulmonary disease in 6%, cutaneous vasculitis in 4%, and Felty's syndrome in 1%. Not all RA patients show the same extent of extraarticular disease. For example, a survey of 153 Southern Chinese patients with RA (128) found that the only extraarticular manifestations were rheumatoid nodules, which were present in 4.6%, and episcleritis (0.7%) and cutaneous vasculitis (0.7%), with a further 12% showing mild sicca symptoms.

There is a difference between the prevalence of specific extraarticular features recorded in observational studies of all such features and studies that focus on one specific feature. Such focused studies usually find a far higher frequency of extraarticular disease. A good example of this is rheumatoid lung disease. The observational studies from the Early Rheumatoid Arthritis Study and Italy reported that 2% and 6% of RA patients have lung disease. By contrast, a study by Dawson et al. (129) specifically identified interstitial lung disease using high-resolution computed tomography and found that 28 (19%) of 150 RA patients had evidence of rheumatoid lung disease. Finding higher levels of extraarticular features is an inevitable consequence of undertaking detailed clinical studies and does not indicate that most of these patients had a clinically relevant abnormality. Such focus studies usually find a far higher frequency of extraarticular disease. A good example of extraarticular problems is rheumatoid lung disease.

PROGNOSTIC FACTORS

Predicting Disability

AGE AND SEX

HAQ scores increase with age (130) and are higher in women (131). These age and sex differences were shown by Pease et al. (132) in a comparison of 214 patients whose RA started after the age of 65 years and 186 patients who developed RA before the age of 65 years. After 3 years, follow-up HAQ scores (mean, 1.81) were highest in elderly-onset cases compared with younger patients (mean, 1.13). Women with high HAQ scores at presentation had the worst functional outcomes. The effect of sex on HAQ scores may reflect women having more severe disease or differences in the relative age of onset between sexes, not to women overrating symptom severity (133).

SOCIOECONOMIC STATUS

Low socioeconomic status is associated with higher HAQ scores (134). This relationship was shown by McEntegart et al. (135), who related social deprivation to HAQ scores in 814 RA patients treated with gold or sulfasalazine. Patients from deprived areas had significantly worse HAQ scores at outset of treatment and after 5 years of therapy. This finding was not attributable to differences in disease duration in patients from the most deprived regions or compliance with treatment. The link between poor functional outcomes and deprivation is multifactorial. Likely contributory factors include comorbidities, especially other chronic diseases, smoking, and poor diets.

GENETIC FACTORS

A number of studies suggest there is a link between HAQ scores and genetic factors, in particular HLA-DR4 (136–138). However, not all studies show a strong association (139), and the issue remains open to debate.

DISEASE ACTIVITY

High HAQ scores are linked with high pain scores (140) and other features of active RA. A cross-sectional study of 259 North American RA patients (141) showed that HAQ scores correlated with joint counts, ESR, global self-assessment, and radiographic scores. Another cross-sectional study of 706 European RA patients showed that the Ritchie articular index and ESR correlated with HAQ scores (142). van der Heide and colleagues (143) followed 95 patients with recently diagnosed RA for 12 months and showed that cumulative HAQ scores were strongly related to pain scores. van Leeuwen (95) followed 149 patients with early RA for 3 years and showed that HAQ scores were determined by joint tenderness, which is closely linked to pain, with no clear relationship to joint swelling. The relationship of disability with active RA transcends cultures. When HAQ was modified for Chinese patients in an Asian setting, it still correlated with pain and physicians' assessments of disease activity (144).

OTHER VARIABLE FACTORS

Other variable factors that influence HAQ include rheumatoid factor positivity (145,146), especially immunoglobulin A rheumatoid factor (147); fatigue, which is related to pain (148); and depression, with higher HAQ scores in depressed patients (149,150).

Predicting Damage

RHEUMATOID FACTOR

Data from NOAR suggest that rheumatoid factor is the dominant predictor of erosive damage. The most recent publication from this register (151) analyzed 439 cases with inflammatory polyarthritis. Rheumatoid factor status, C-reactive protein (CRP) levels, nodules, and the number of swollen joints at baseline all predicted x-ray damage. After adjusting for baseline severity, a high titer of rheumatoid factor was an independent predictor of deterioration over 5 years. Patients with an initial high RF showed more than twice the progression in their Larsen score than did seronegative cases.

Many other studies suggest there is a strong link between x-ray damage and rheumatoid factor status. Bukhari and coworkers identified twelve such studies. These studies enrolled 1,395 patients with disease durations between 1 and 10 years. Five studies looked at a single time point (152–156) and eight looked at changes with time (73,143,157–162). The studies included assessments of new erosions, total damage, progression, the Sharp score, and the Larsen score. Rheumatoid factor when patients are first evaluated is a powerful predictor of deteriorating radiographic damage in RA patients receiving conventional therapy.

Antikeratin Antibodies and Anticyclic Citrullinated Peptide Enzyme-Linked Immunosorbent Assay Tests

Antikeratin antibodies are strongly associated with RA, but, because they can only be detected by immunofluorescence, they have little value in routine practice. Identifying filaggrin as the antigen involved led to specific tests. Using these tests, Aho et al. (163) showed that pre-illness serum antifilaggrin antibody levels are proportional to the risk of developing rheumatoid factor–positive RA.

The subsequent development of synthetic peptides containing citrulline, an amino acid present in filaggrin, enabled the introduction of an accurate enzyme-linked immunosorbent assay (ELISA). Initial reports suggested anticyclic citrullinated peptide (anti-CCP) ELISA (164) tests have high specificity for RA. Combining anti-CCP and immunoglobulin M rheumatoid factor, ELISAs gave a high positive predictive value for RA and predicted erosive disease at 2 years (165). Kroot and colleagues (166) reported that almost 70% of RA patients were positive for anti-CCP in early RA and that these cases had more radiologic damage. However, multiple regression analysis suggested that the additional predictive value of anti-CCP ELISAs was only moderate. Furthermore, van Jaarsveld et al. (167), who evaluated the clinical value of the anti-CCP ELISA in combination with rheumatoid factor status in 249 patients with early RA, concluded that the prognostic value of combining both tests lies in their ability to predict mild disease.

A further report by Visser et al. (168) looked at 524 newly referred patients with early arthritis. The combination of seven variables—symptom duration at first visit, morning stiffness over 60 minutes, arthritis in three or more joints, bilateral compression pain in the MTP joints, rheumatoid factor positivity, anti-CCP positivity, and the presence of erosions—predicted the likelihood of developing persistent erosive arthritis. For the present, the value of anti-CCP ELISA in predicting outcome and progression remains unclear, although it has much future potential.

DISEASE ACTIVITY

Because patients who have active disease are more likely to be seropositive for rheumatoid factor, it can be difficult to distinguish the effects of these different variables. Combe et al. (169) attempted to differentiate the effects of disease activity for rheumatoid factor in 191 patients with early RA prospectively followed for 3 years. Radiologic progression, seen in 71 of the 172 patients, closely correlated with the baseline ESR, CRP, and rheumatoid factor positivity.

CRP is a good surrogate measure of disease activity and, since the early work of McConkey et al. (170), it has been known to predict erosive damage. The time lag between synovial inflammation and joint damage has been shown by Matsuda et al. (171) in a study of 98 patients. This investigation showed that increases in the number of erosive joints after 12 months correlated with CRP and inflammatory markers at 6 months. Furthermore, the number of erosive joints was high in patients whose levels of CRP were high at 6 months but suppressed by 12 months and was less in patients whose levels of CRP were suppressed by 6 months.

van Leeuwen et al. (172) has established that there are individual relationships between CRP and the progression of radiologic damage. This relationship was modelled mathematically using adjustments for discontinuity in the radiographic scoring system in 149 patients with early RA followed prospectively for 3 years. Time-integrated CRP values correlated closely with radiologic progression in each patient, but there was considerable variation between individuals with similar radiographic scores. Time-integrated CRP values correlated closely with radiologic progression in each patient, but there was considerable variation between individual patients with similar radiographic scores in the elevation of their CRP. In simple terms, this means that, although there is an association between elevated CRP and x-ray damage, it is incomplete.

Subsequent research by the same group (173) provided evidence that early aggressive drug treatment to control the CRP reduces x-ray progression. Stenger and colleagues (174) undertook a prospective follow-up study with an experimental group and historical controls divided into high-risk and low-risk subgroups based on prognostic factors. Overall, they investigated 228 consecutive patients with recent-onset RA. After 2 years of follow-up, the aggressively treated cases had significantly lower radiographic progression than controls. Cumulative CRP values were also significantly lower than in the control group.

Another study by Plant et al. (175) confirmed the link between high CRP levels and joint damage. This study showed that suppressing disease activity judged by CRP levels reduced new joint involvement to a greater extent than progression in already damaged joints. This conclusion was based on a secondary analysis of

TABLE 3.6. Studies Using Multivariate Techniques to Investigate Clinical Prognostic Variables in Patients with Early Inflammatory Polyarthritis

Study Location, Reference	Cases	Initial Disease Duration	Length of Follow-Up (Yr)	Outcome	Prognostic Variables Identified	Accuracy of Prediction (%)
Memphis (177)	50	<6 mo	5	Swelling/erosions	Rheumatoid factor; articular index; female sex; white race; Raynaud's syndrome; malaise	80
Heinola (178)	200	—	8	Larsen score	Rheumatoid factor; articular index; ESR; grip strength; initial x-ray score	43
Middlesex Hospital (179)	111	<12 mo	10	Erosions	Rheumatoid factor; articular index; grip strength; function	70
Lund (180)	63	<24 mo	5	HAQ score	Rheumatoid factor; articular index; function; female sex; education	75
ERAS (181)	111	<24 mo	2.5	Steinbrocker Functional Grade	Rheumatoid factor; articular index; function; hemoglobin; platelets	90
Nijmegan (182)	149	<12 mo	3	Radiologic	Rheumatoid factor; HLA-DR2–negative; age; CRP; initial x-ray scores	43
Utrecht (183)	95	<12 mo	1	Radiologic progression	Rheumatoid factor; articular index; initial x-ray scores	82

CRP, C-reactive protein; ESR, erythrocyte sedimentation rate; HAQ, Health Assessment Questionnaire.
Adapted from Harrison B, Symmons DP. Early inflammatory polyarthritis: results from the Norfolk Arthritis Register with a review of the literature. Outcome at three years. *Rheumatology* 2000;39:939–949.

359 patients with active RA enrolled in a 5-year randomized, prospective, open-label study of disease-modifying antirheumatic drug therapy. Time-averaged CRP values correlated with increases in Larsen score, and the percentage of new joint involvement over 5 years varied markedly with time-integrated CRP. X-ray progression was 7% with low CRP values and 39% with high CRP levels, a fivefold increase.

Despite these studies, variations in CRP levels between patients with similar x-ray scores make it difficult to generalize from an initial single CRP value in individual cases. Furthermore, not all investigations show a similar relationship between CRP levels and joint damage. For example, one study from Leeds in the United Kingdom, in which 63 patients with early RA were followed up for 6 months, found that high initial CRP levels did not predict the persistence of arthritis at 6 months (176). The conventional view that high CRP levels indicate poor prognosis may not apply in very early RA.

MULTIPLE VARIABLES

Harrison et al. (49) reviewed the interactions between different prognostic variables in the NOAR study and seven other prospective studies of early RA (178–183). Overall, these studies show that the presence of rheumatoid factor and articular index are strong predictors of progressive joint damage, with other variables having less overall impact (Table 3.6). For example, one study from Lund evaluated predictive variables in 63 RA patients and focused on determination of HAQ scores. This report found that, at study end, HAQ scores could be correctly classified in 75% of the cases using three factors—baseline HAQ score, female sex, and low educational level. Another study from Utrecht (183) involved 95 cases and found that odds ratios for progression of total damage were 12 for the presence of rheumatoid factor, five for the presence of damage at baseline, and two for cumulative joint inflammation. Inevitably, these studies have looked at slightly different outcomes in slightly different patient groups and, therefore, do not give a single optimal set of prognostic markers.

Data from NOAR have also been used to develop simple algorithms (Table 3.7) that can be used easily in clinical practice. This algorithm was based on two predictors—rheumatoid factor and initial disease duration—for erosions and, following recursive partitioning to reduce the number of variables in the model from five to two, used initial HAQ scores and disease duration to predict disability. Although such simple models are helpful in a primary care setting when deciding which patients need specialist referral, they have limited value in helping define optimal care for individual cases.

TABLE 3.7. Simple Algorithms to Categorize Patients According to Risk of Developing Erosions and Risk of High Health Assessment Questionnaire (HAQ) Scores (≥1.0) after 3 Years of Rheumatoid Arthritis

Risk of Erosions	Rheumatoid Factor–Positive	Initial Disease Duration > 3 mo	Probability of Erosions
1	+	+	.79
2	+	–	.52
3	–	+	.33
4	–	–	.10
Risk of Disability	**Baseline HAQ ≥1.0**	**Initial Disease Duration >3 mo**	**Probability of HAQ ≥1.0**
1	+	+	.73
2	+	–	.45
3	–	+ or –	.19

NOAR, Norfolk Arthritis Register.
Adapted from Harrison B, Symmons DP. Early inflammatory polyarthritis: results from the Norfolk Arthritis Register with a review of the literature. Outcome at three years. *Rheumatology* 2000;39:939–949.

Predicting Death

Patients with severe RA have a higher mortality. Pincus et al. (184) reported mortality over 15 years in 75 RA patients who were followed up in a university hospital outpatient clinic. Few deaths were seen in the first 3 years, but the SMR over 15 years was 1.62. Significant predictors of mortality included age, formal education level, joint count, activities-of-daily-living questionnaire scores, disease adjustment scores, morning stiffness, comorbid cardiovascular disease, grip strength, modified walking time, and button test. Five-year survival in patients with the poorest status according to these quantitative measures was 40% to 60%, comparable to the expected survival at that time of patients with three-vessel coronary artery disease or with stage 4 Hodgkin disease. Subsequently, Callahan et al. (44) showed the predictors of death in a 5-year prospective study of 210 patients, during which 37 died. Mortality at 5 years was predicted significantly in univariable analysis by functional class, limited joint motion, HAQ scores, comorbidities, and disease duration. Multivariable regressions showed age and comorbidities; HAQ and other measures of functional status were the most effective predictors of mortality.

Extraarticular features of RA affect mortality. In a cohort of 424 cases of RA in Olmsted County, Minn (185), 169 had extraarticular features, an incidence of 3.67 per 100 person-years. Compared to the general population, survival among patients with RA was decreased. Survival among RA patients with extraarticular features was markedly reduced compared to the general population and to RA patients without these features. There was a particularly poor prognosis in 63 patients with vasculitis, pericarditis, pleuritis, or Felty's syndrome.

There is some evidence that the changing pattern of treatment for RA, especially the increased use of methotrexate, is reducing mortality rates. This reduction was shown in a cohort of 1,240 RA patients seen at the Wichita Arthritis Centre, an outpatient rheumatology setting, in which 191 individuals died during follow-up (186). Patients who began treatment with methotrexate had worse prognostic factors for mortality. After adjustment for this confounding by indication, the mortality hazard ratio for methotrexate use compared with no methotrexate use was 0.4. This finding suggests that methotrexate may provide a substantial survival benefit, and this benefit was attributed to reduced cardiovascular mortality. Set against this positive finding, other data from Minnesota (187) suggest that the survival rate in RA patients was significantly lower than the expected rate in the general population and that there has been no improvement noted over time.

CONCLUSION

This chapter describes the natural history of treated RA in terms of the course of the disease and the predictive factor for that course. The disease course can be assessed by measuring synovitis, disability, quality, and joint damage. It is also reflected by the increased comorbidity and the mortality of RA. The average patient with RA has persistent synovitis, increasing disability, and increasing joint narrowing. Treatment improves the prognosis but does not return the outcome to normal. Functional disability increases on average by 1% to 2% of maximal disability per year. The same is true of x-ray progression that increases by 1% to 2% of maximal possible damage annually. There is a relationship between the amount of inflammation and the likelihood of damage and disability. There is also an increased mortality in RA, although most recent studies suggested the excess mortality is declining as treatment potentially improves. A substantial amount of mortality is due to cardiovascular disease.

A number of prognostic factors affect the likelihood of RA being severe—it is worse in the elderly, in women, and in patients of low socioeconomic status. There is a general relationship between HLA-DR4 and poor outcomes with persisting disease activity and rheumatoid factor positivity, and, also, anti-CCP ELISA assays are more likely to show progressive disease.

The development of new biologic therapy may significantly change the relationship between conventional clinical assessments and progressive joint damage, although the evidence for this is at present incomplete.

REFERENCES

1. Laupacis A, Wells G, Richardson WS, et al. Users' guides to the medical literature. V. How to use an article about prognosis. Evidence-Based Medicine Working Group. *JAMA* 1994;272:234–237.
2. Scott DL, Houssien DA. Clinical and laboratory assessments in rheumatoid arthritis and osteoarthritis. *Br J Rheumatol* 1996 Dec;35[Suppl 3]:6–9.
3. Prevoo ML, van't Hof MA, Kuper HH, et al. Modified disease activity scores that include twenty-eight-joint counts. Development and validation in a prospective longitudinal study of patients with rheumatoid arthritis. *Arthritis Rheum* 1995;38:44–48.
4. Felson DT, Anderson JJ, Boers M, et al. American College of Rheumatology. Preliminary definition of improvement in rheumatoid arthritis. *Arthritis Rheum* 1995;38:727–735.
5. van Gestel AM, Anderson JJ, van Riel PL, et al. ACR and EULAR improvement criteria have comparable validity in rheumatoid arthritis trials. American College of Rheumatology European League of Associations for Rheumatology. *J Rheumatol* 1999;26:705–711.
6. Steinbrocker O, Traeger CH, Batterman RC. Therapeutic criteria in rheumatoid arthritis. *JAMA* 1949;140:659–662.
7. Hochberg MC, Chang RW, Dwosh I, et al. The American College of Rheumatology 1991 revised criteria for the classification of global functional status in rheumatoid arthritis. *Arthritis Rheum* 1992;35:498–502.
8. Meenan RF, Gertman PM, Mason JH. Measuring health status in arthritis. The arthritis impact measurement scales. *Arthritis Rheum* 1980;23:146–152.
9. Meenan RF, Mason JH, Anderson JJ, et al. AIMS2. The content and properties of a revised and expanded Arthritis Impact Measurement Scales Health Status Questionnaire. *Arthritis Rheum* 1992;35:1–10.
10. Anderson JJ, Firschein HE, Meenan RF. Sensitivity of a health status measure to short-term clinical changes in arthritis. *Arthritis Rheum* 1989;32:844–850.
11. Sharp JT, Wolfe F, Mitchell DM. The progression of erosion and joint space narrowing scores in rheumatoid arthritis during the first twenty-five years of disease. *Arthritis Rheum* 1991;34:660–668.
12. Sharp JT. Radiographic evaluation of the course of articular disease. *Clin Rheum Dis* 1983;9:541–557.
13. Weisman MH. Use of radiographs to measure outcome in rheumatoid arthritis. *Am J Med* 1987;83:96–100.
14. van der Heijde D. How to read radiographs according to the Sharp/van der Heijde method. *J Rheumatol* 2000;27:261–263.
15. Scott DL, Houssien DA, Laasonen L. Proposed modification to Larsen's scoring methods for hand and wrist radiographs. *Br J Rheumatol* 1995;34:56.
16. Rau R, Wassenberg S, Herborn G, et al. A new method of scoring radiographic change in rheumatoid arthritis. *J Rheumatol* 1998;25:2094–2107.
17. Bruynesteyn K, van der Heijde D, Boers M, et al. Minimal clinically important difference in radiological progression of joint damage over 1 year in rheumatoid arthritis: preliminary results of a validation study with clinical experts. *J Rheumatol* 2001;28:904–910.
18. Bruynesteyn K, van der Heijde D, Boers M, et al. Determination of the minimal clinically important difference in rheumatoid arthritis joint damage of the Sharp/van der Heijde and Larsen/Scott scoring methods by clinical experts and comparison with the smallest detectable difference. *Arthritis Rheum* 2002;46:913–920.
19. Rau R, Wassenberg S. Scoring methods. *J Rheumatol* 2002;29:653–655.
20. Jonsson A, Borg A, Hannesson P, et al. Film-screen vs. digital radiography in rheumatoid arthritis of the hand. An ROC analysis. *Acta Radiol* 1994;35:311–318.
21. Doyle AJ, Gunn ML, Gamble GD, et al. Personal computer-based PACS display system: comparison with a dedicated PACS workstation for review of computed radiographic images in rheumatoid arthritis. *Acad Radiol* 2002;9:646–653.
22. Wolfe F, Pincus T. The level of inflammation in rheumatoid arthritis is determined early and remains stable over the long-term course of the illness. *J Rheumatol* 2001;28:1817–1824.
23. Welsing PM, van Gestel AM, Swinkels HL, et al. The relationship between disease activity, joint destruction, and functional capacity over the course of rheumatoid arthritis. *Arthritis Rheum* 2001;44:2009–2017.
24. Ragan C, Farrington E. The clinical features of rheumatoid arthritis. *JAMA* 1962;181:663–667.
25. Duthie JJR, Brown PE, Truelove LH, et al. Course and prognosis in rheumatoid arthritis. A further report. *Ann Rheum Dis* 1964;23:193–202.

26. Rasker JJ, Cosh JA. The natural history of rheumatoid arthritis: a fifteen year follow up study. *Clin Rheumatol* 1984;3:11–20.
27. Short CL, Bauer W, Reynolds WE. *Rheumatoid arthritis*. Cambridge: Harvard University Press, 1957.
28. Scott DL, Symmons DP, Coulton BL, et al. Long-term outcome of treating rheumatoid arthritis: results after 20 years. *Lancet* 1987;1:1108–1111.
29. Pincus T, Callahan LF, Sale WG, et al. Severe functional declines, work disability, and increased mortality in seventy-five rheumatoid arthritis patients studied over nine years. *Arthritis Rheum* 1984;27:864–872.
30. Sherrer YS, Bloch DA, Mitchell DM, et al. The development of disability in rheumatoid arthritis. *Arthritis Rheum* 1986;29:494–500.
31. Isacson J, Allander E, Brostrom LA. 17-year follow-up of symptoms and signs in the knee joint in rheumatoid arthritis. *Scand J Rheumatol* 1988;17:325–331.
32. Möttönen T, Paimela L, Leirisalo-Repo M, et al. Only high disease activity and positive rheumatoid factor indicate poor prognosis in patients with early rheumatoid arthritis treated with "sawtooth" strategy. *Ann Rheum Dis* 1998;57:533–539.
33. Fries JF. Current treatment paradigms in rheumatoid arthritis. *Rheumatology (Oxford)* 2000;39[Suppl 1]:30–35.
34. Pincus T, Callahan LF, Brooks RH, et al. Self-report questionnaire scores in rheumatoid arthritis compared with traditional physical, radiographic and laboratory measures. *Ann Intern Med* 1989;110:259–266.
35. Houssien DA, McKenna SP, Scott DL. The Nottingham Health Profile as a measure of disease activity and outcome in rheumatoid arthritis. *Br J Rheumatol* 1997;36:69–73.
36. Lassere M, Wells G, Tugwell P, et al. Percentile curve reference charts of physical function: rheumatoid arthritis population. *J Rheumatol* 1995;22:1241–1246.
37. Wolfe F, Kleinheksel SM, Cathay MA, et al. The clinical value of the Stanford Health Assessment Questionnaire Functional Disability Index in patients with rheumatoid arthritis. *J Rheumatol* 1988;15:1480–1488.
38. Wolfe F, Hawley DJ, Cathey MA. Clinical and health status measures over time: prognosis and outcome assessment in rheumatoid arthritis. *J Rheumatol* 1991;18:190–197.
39. Greenwood M, Scott DL, Carr AJ, et al. Pain and disability in rheumatoid arthritis. *Ann Rheum Dis* 1999;58[Suppl]:110.
40. Jantti JK, Kaarela K, Belt EA, et al. Incidence of severe outcome in rheumatoid arthritis during 20 years. *J Rheumatol* 2002;29:688–692.
41. Leigh JP, Fries JF, Parikh N. Severity of disability and duration of disease in rheumatoid arthritis. *J Rheumatol* 1992;9:1906–1911.
42. Ward MM, Leigh JP, Fries JF. Progression of functional disability in patients with rheumatoid arthritis. Associations with rheumatology subspecialty care. *Arch Intern Med* 1993;153:2229–2237.
43. Gardiner PV, Sykes HR, Hassey GA, et al. An evaluation of the health assessment questionnaire in the long-term longitudinal follow-up of disability in rheumatoid arthritis. *Br J Rheumatol* 1993;32:724–728.
44. Callahan LF, Pincus T, Huston JW, et al. Measures of activity and damage in rheumatoid arthritis: depiction of changes and prediction of mortality over five years. *Arthritis Care Res* 1997;10:381–394.
45. Leymarie F, Jolly D, Sanderman R, et al. Life events and disability in rheumatoid arthritis: a European cohort. *Br J Rheumatol* 1997;36:1106–1112.
46. Ward MM, Lubeck D, Leigh JP. Longterm health outcomes of patients with rheumatoid arthritis treated in managed care and fee-for-service practice settings. *J Rheumatol* 1998;25:641–649.
47. Munro R, Hampson R, McEntegart A, et al. Improved functional outcome in patients with early rheumatoid arthritis treated with intramuscular gold: results of a five year prospective study. *Ann Rheum Dis* 1998;57:88–93.
48. Wolfe F. A reappraisal of HAQ disability in rheumatoid arthritis. *Arthritis Rheum* 2000;43:2751–2761.
49. Harrison B, Symmons DP. Early inflammatory polyarthritis: results from the Norfolk Arthritis Register with a review of the literature. Outcome at three years. *Rheumatology* 2000;39:939–949.
50. Eberhardt KB, Fex E. Functional impairment and disability in early rheumatoid arthritis. Development over 5 years. *J Rheumatol* 1995;22:1037–1042.
51. Wiles NJ, Symmons DPM, Barrett EM, et al. Is it possible to construct percentile reference charts of disability for patients with early inflammatory polyarthritis? *Br J Rheumatol* 1998;37:136.
52. Lassere M, Houssein D, Scott D, et al. Reference curves of radiographic damage in patients with RA: application of quantile regression and fractional polynomials. *J Rheumatol* 1997;24:1288–1294.
53. Hurst NP, Kind P, Ruta D, et al. Measuring health-related quality of life in rheumatoid arthritis: validity, responsiveness and reliability of EuroQol (EQ-5D). *Br J Rheumatol* 1997;36:551–559.
54. Wolfe F, Hawley DJ. Measurement of the quality of life in rheumatic disorders using the EuroQol. *Br J Rheumatol* 1997;36:786–793.
55. Fitzpatrick R, Ziebland S, Jenkinson C, et al. The social dimension of health status measures in rheumatoid arthritis. *Int Disabil Stud* 1991;13:34–37.
56. Houssein D, McKenna SP, Scott DL. The Nottingham Health Profile as a measure of disease activity and outcome in rheumatoid arthritis. *Br J Rheumatol* 1997;36:69–73.
57. Pouchot J, Guillemin F, Coste J, et al. Validation of the French version of the arthritis impact measurement scales 2 and comparison with the French version of the Nottingham Health Profile. "Quality of Life in Rheumatology" Task Force. *Rev Rhum Engl Ed* 1996;63:389–404.
58. Wells G, Boers M, Shea B, et al. Sensitivity to change of generic quality of life instruments in patients with rheumatoid arthritis: preliminary findings in the generic health OMERACT study. OMERACT/ILAR Task Force on Generic Quality of Life. Life Outcome Measures in Rheumatology. International League of Associations for Rheumatology. *J Rheumatol* 1999;26:217–221.
59. Ruta DA, Hurst NP, Kind P, et al. Measuring health status in British patients with rheumatoid arthritis: reliability, validity and responsiveness of the short form 36-item health survey (SF-36). *Br J Rheumatol* 1998;37:425–436.
60. Kvien TK, Kaasa S, Smedstad LM. Performance of the Norwegian SF-36 Health Survey in patients with rheumatoid arthritis. II. A comparison of the SF-36 with disease-specific measures. *J Clin Epidemiol* 1998;51:1077–1086.
61. Escalante A, del Rincon I. How much disability in rheumatoid arthritis is explained by rheumatoid arthritis? *Arthritis Rheum* 1999;42:1712–1721.
62. Keller SD, Ware JE Jr, Hatoum HT, et al. The SF-36 Arthritis-Specific Health Index (ASHI): II. Tests of validity in four clinical trials. *Med Care* 1999;37[Suppl 5]:MS51–60.
63. Ware JE Jr, Keller SD, Hatoum HT, et al. The SF-36 Arthritis-Specific Health Index (ASHI): I. Development and cross-validation of scoring algorithms. *Med Care* 1999;37[Suppl 5]:MS40–50.
64. Ethgen O, Kahler KH, Kong SX, et al. The effect of health related quality of life on reported use of health care resources in patients with osteoarthritis and rheumatoid arthritis: a longitudinal analysis. *J Rheumatol* 2002;29:1147–1155.
65. Larsen A, Thoen J. Hand radiography of 200 patients with rheumatoid arthritis repeated after an interval of one year. *Scand J Rheumatol* 1987;16:395–401.
66. Scott DL, Dawes PT, Fowler PD, et al. Calculating radiological progression in rheumatoid arthritis. *Clin Rheumatol* 1986;5:445–449.
67. Wolfe F, Sharp JT. Radiographic outcome of recent-onset rheumatoid arthritis. *Arthritis Rheum* 1998;41:1571–1582.
68. Egsmose C, Lund B, Borg G, et al. Patients with rheumatoid arthritis benefit from early 2nd line therapy: 5 year follow up of a prospective double blind placebo controlled study. *J Rheumatol* 1995;22:2208–2213.
69. Möttönen T, Paimela L, Ahonen J, et al. Outcome in patients with early rheumatoid arthritis treated according to the 'sawtooth' strategy. *Arthritis Rheum* 1996;39:996–1005.
70. Kaarela K, Kautiainen H. Continuous progression of radiological destruction in seropositive RA. *J Rheumatol* 1997;24:1280–1284.
71. Wolfe F, Sharp JT. Radiographic outcome of recent-onset rheumatoid arthritis. *Arthritis Rheum* 1998;41:1571–1582.
72. Drossaers-Bakker KW, Amesz E, Zwinderman AH, et al. A comparison of three radiologic scoring systems for the long-term assessment of rheumatoid arthritis: findings of an ongoing prospective inception cohort study of 132 women followed up for a median of twelve years. *Arthritis Rheum* 2001; 43:1465–1472.
73. Plant MJ, Jones PW, Sklatvala J, et al. Patterns of radiological progression in early rheumatoid arthritis—results of an 8 year prospective study. *J Rheumatol* 1998;25:417–426.
74. Graudal NA, Jurik AG, de Carvalho A, et al. Radiographic progression in rheumatoid arthritis. A long-term prospective study of 109 patients. *Arthritis Rheum* 1998;41:1470–1480.
75. Kuper IH, van Leeuwen MA, van Riel PL, et al. Influence of a ceiling effect on the assessment of radiographic progression in rheumatoid arthritis during the first 6 years of disease. *J Rheumatol* 1999;26:268–276.
76. Brook A, Corbett M. Radiographic changes in early RA. *Ann Rheum Dis* 1977;36:71–73.
77. Paimela L, Heiskanen A, Kurki P, et al. Serum hyaluronate as a predictor of radiological progression in early rheumatoid arthritis. *Arthritis Rheum* 1991;34:815–821.
78. van der Heijde DMFM, van Leeuwen MA, van Riel PLCM, et al. Biannual radiographic assessments of hands and feet in a three-year prospective follow-up of patients with early rheumatoid arthritis. *Arthritis Rheum* 1992;35:26–34.
79. Fex E, Jonsson K, Johnson U, et al. Development of radiographic damage during the first 5–6 yr of rheumatoid arthritis. A prospective follow-up study of a Swedish cohort. *Br J Rheumatol* 1996;35:1106–1115.
80. Jansen LM, van der Horst-Bruinsma IE, van Schaardenburg D, et al. Predictors of radiographic joint damage in patients with early rheumatoid arthritis. *Ann Rheum Dis* 2001;60:924–927.
81. Hulsmans HM, Jacobs JW, van der Heijde DM, et al. The course of radiologic damage during the first six years of rheumatoid arthritis. *Arthritis Rheum* 2000;43:1927–1940.
82. Sokka T, Hannonen P. Healing of erosions in rheumatoid arthritis. *Ann Rheum Dis* 2000;59:647–649.
83. Jalava S, Reunanen K. Healing of erosions in rheumatoid arthritis. *Scand J Rheumatol* 1982;11:97–100.
84. Rau R, Herborn G. Healing phenomena of erosive changes in rheumatoid arthritis patients undergoing disease-modifying antirheumatic drug therapy. *Arthritis Rheum* 1996;39:162–168.
85. Menninger H, Meixner C, Sondgen W. Progression and repair in radiographs of hands and forefeet in early rheumatoid arthritis. *J Rheumatol* 1995;22:1048–1054.
86. Kaarela K, Kautiainen H. Continuous progression of radiological destruction in seropositive rheumatoid arthritis. *J Rheumatol* 1997;24:1285–1287.
87. Belt EA, Kaarela K, Lehto MU. Destruction and reconstruction of hand joints in rheumatoid arthritis. A 20 year followup study. *J Rheumatol* 1998;25:459–461.

88. Belt EA, Kaarela K, Lehto MU. Destruction and arthroplasties of the metatarsophalangeal joints in seropositive rheumatoid arthritis. A 20-year follow-up study. *Scand J Rheumatol* 1998;27:194–196.
89. Lehtinen JT, Kaarela K, Ikavalko M, et al. Incidence of elbow involvement in rheumatoid arthritis. A 15 year endpoint study. *J Rheumatol* 2001;28:70–74.
90. Lehtimaki MY, Kautiainen H, Hamalainen MM, et al. Hip involvement in seropositive rheumatoid arthritis. Survivorship analysis with a 15-year follow-up. *Scand J Rheumatol* 1998;27:406–409.
91. Lehtinen JT, Kaarela K, Belt EA, et al. Relation of glenohumeral and acromioclavicular joint destruction in rheumatoid shoulder. A 15 year follow up study. *Ann Rheum Dis* 2000;59:158–160.
92. Wolfe F, Zwillich SH. The long-term outcomes of rheumatoid arthritis: a 23-year prospective, longitudinal study of total joint replacement and its predictors in 1,600 patients with rheumatoid arthritis. *Arthritis Rheum* 1998;41:1072–1082.
93. Massardo L, Gabriel SE, Crowson CS, et al. A population based assessment of the use of orthopedic surgery in patients with rheumatoid arthritis. *J Rheumatol* 2002;29:52–56.
94. Kirwan JR. Links between radiological change, disability, and pathology in rheumatoid arthritis. *J Rheumatol* 2001;28:881–886.
95. van Leeuwen MA, van der Heijde DM, Van Riel PL, et al. Interrelationship of outcome measures and process variables in early rheumatoid arthritis: a comparison of radiological damage, physical disability, joints counts, and acute phase reactants. *J Rheumatol* 1994;21:425–459.
96. Fex E, Jonsson K, Johnson U, et al. Development of radiographic damage during the first 5–6 years of rheumatoid arthritis. A prospective follow-up study of a Swedish cohort. *Br J Rheumatol* 1996;35:1106–1115.
97. Pincus T, Callahan LF, Fuchs HA, et al. Quantitative analysis of hand radiographs in rheumatoid arthritis: time course of radiographic changes, relation to joint examination measures and comparison of different scoring methods. *J Rheumatol* 1995;22:1983 1989.
98. Kaarela K, Sarna S. Correlations between clinical facets of outcome in rheumatoid arthritis. *Clin Exp Rheumatol* 1993;11:643–644.
99. Larsen A. The relation of radiographic changes to serum acute-phase proteins and rheumatoid factor in 200 patients with rheumatoid arthritis. *Scand J Rheumatol* 1988;17:123–129.
100. Regan-Smith MG, O'Connor GT, Kwoh CK, et al. Lack of correlation between the Steinbrocker staging of hand radiographs and the functional health status of individuals with rheumatoid arthritis. *Arthritis Rheum* 1989;32:128–133.
101. Brühlmann P, Stucki G, Michel BA. Evaluation of a German version of the physical dimensions of the Health Assessment Questionnaire in patients with rheumatoid arthritis. *J Rheumatol* 1994;21:1245–1249.
102. Houssein DA, Choy EHS, Berry H, et al. Differences between the clinical and radiological progression of rheumatoid arthritis. *Br J Rheumatol* 1996;35[Suppl 1]:199.
103. Hakala M, Nieminen P, Koivisto O. More evidence from a community based series of better outcome in rheumatoid arthritis. Data on the effect of multidisciplinary care on the retention of functional ability. *J Rheumatol* 1994;21:1432–1437.
104. Spector TD, Scott DL. What happens to patients with rheumatoid arthritis? The long-term outcome of treatment. *Clin Rheumatol* 1988;7:315–330.
105. Mutru O, Laakso M, Isomaki H, et al. Cardiovascular mortality in patients with rheumatoid arthritis. *Cardiology* 1989;76:71–77.
106. Wolfe F, Mitchell DM, Sibley JT, et al. The mortality of rheumatoid arthritis. *Arthritis Rheum* 1994;37:481–494.
107. Martinez MS, Garcia-Monforte A, Rivera J. Survival study of rheumatoid arthritis patients in Madrid (Spain). A 9-year prospective follow-up. *Scand J Rheumatol* 2001;30:195–198.
108. Myllykangas-Luosujärvi RA, Aho K, Isomaki HA. Mortality in rheumatoid arthritis. *Semin Arthritis Rheum* 1995;25:193–202.
109. Guedes C, Dumont-Fischer D, Leichter-Nakache S, et al. Mortality in rheumatoid arthritis. *Rev Rhum Engl Ed* 1999;66:492–498.
110. Riise T, Jacobsen BK, Gran JT, et al. Total mortality is increased in rheumatoid arthritis. A 17-year prospective study. *Clin Rheumatol* 2001;20:123–127.
111. Wållberg-Jonsson S, Ohman M-L, Rantapaa-Dahlqvist S. Cardiovascular morbidity and mortality in patients with seropositive rheumatoid arthritis in Northern Sweden. *J Rheumatol* 1997;24:445–451.
112. Bjornadal L, Baecklund E, Yin L, et al. Decreasing mortality in patients with rheumatoid arthritis: results from a large population based cohort in Sweden, 1964–95. *J Rheumatol* 2002;29:906–912.
113. Prior P, Symmons DP, Scott DL, et al. Cause of death in rheumatoid arthritis. *Br J Rheumatol* 1984;23:92–99.
114. Symmons DP, Jones MA, Scott DL, et al. Longterm mortality outcome in patients with rheumatoid arthritis: early presenters continue to do well. *J Rheumatol* 1998;25:1072–1077.
115. Gordon P, West J, Jones H, et al. A 10 year prospective followup of patients with rheumatoid arthritis 1986–96. *J Rheumatol* 2001;28:2409–2415.
116. Gabriel SE, Crowson CS, O'Fallon WM. Mortality in rheumatoid arthritis: have we made an impact in 4 decades? *J Rheumatol* 1999;26:2529–2533.
117. DeMaria AN. Relative risk of cardiovascular events in patients with rheumatoid arthritis. *Am J Cardiol* 2002;89:33D–38D.
118. Lindqvist E, Eberhardt K. Mortality in rheumatoid arthritis patients with disease onset in the 1980s. *Ann Rheum Dis* 1999;58:11–14.
119. Kroot EJA, van Leeuwen MA, van Rijswijk MH, et al. No increased mortality in patients with rheumatoid arthritis: up to 10 years of follow-up from disease onset. *Ann Rheum Dis* 2000;59:954–958.
120. Sokka T, Möttönen T, Hannonen P. Mortality in early "sawtooth" treated rheumatoid arthritis patients during the first 8–14 years. *Scand J Rheumatol* 1999;28:282–287.
121. Goodson NJ, Wiles NJ, Lunt M, et al. Mortality in early inflammatory polyarthritis cardiovascular mortality is increased in seropositive patients. *Arthritis Rheum* 2002;46:2010–2019.
122. Kroot EJ, van Gestel AM, Swinkels HL, et al. Chronic comorbidity in patients with early rheumatoid arthritis: a descriptive study. *J Rheumatol* 2001;28:1511–1517.
123. Berkanovic E, Hurwicz ML. Rheumatoid arthritis and comorbidity. *J Rheumatol* 1990;7:888–892.
124. Gabriel SE, Crowson CS, O'Fallon WM. Comorbidity in arthritis. *J Rheumatol* 1999;26:2475–2479.
125. del Rincon ID, Williams K, Stern MP, et al. High incidence of cardiovascular events in a rheumatoid arthritis cohort not explained by traditional cardiac risk factors. *Arthritis Rheum* 2001;44:2737–2745.
126. Young A, Dixey J, Cox N, et al. How does functional disability in early rheumatoid arthritis (RA) affect patients and their lives? Results of 5 years of follow-up in 732 patients from the Early RA Study (ERAS). *Rheumatology (Oxford)* 2000; 39:603–611.
127. Cimmino MA, Salvarani C, Macchioni P, et al. Extra-articular manifestations in 587 Italian patients with rheumatoid arthritis. *Rheumatol Int* 2000;19:213–217.
128. Cohen MG, Li EK, Ng PY, et al. Extra-articular manifestations are uncommon in southern Chinese with rheumatoid arthritis. *Br J Rheumatol* 1993;32:209–211.
129. Dawson JK, Fewins HE, Desmond J, et al. Fibrosing alveolitis in patients with rheumatoid arthritis as assessed by high resolution computed tomography, chest radiography, and pulmonary function tests. *Thorax* 2001;56:622–627.
130. Anderson KO, Keefe FJ, Bradley LA, et al. Prediction of pain behaviour and functional status of rheumatoid arthritis patients using medical status and psychological variables. *Pain* 1988;33:25–32.
131. Thompson PW, Pegley FS. A comparison of disability measured by the Stanford Health Assessment Questionnaire disability scales (HAQ) in male and female rheumatoid outpatients. *Br J Rheumatol* 1991;30:298–300.
132. Pease CT, Bhakta BB, Devlin J, et al. Does the age of onset of rheumatoid arthritis influence phenotype: a prospective study of outcome and prognostic factors. *Rheumatology (Oxford)* 1999;38:228–234.
133. Katz PP, Criswell LA. Differences in symptom reports between men and women with rheumatoid arthritis. *Arthritis Care Res* 1996;9:441–448.
134. Vliet Vlieland TP, Buitenhuis NA, van Zeben D, et al. Sociodemographic factors and the outcome of rheumatoid arthritis in young women. *Ann Rheum Dis* 1994;53:803–806.
135. McEntegart A, Morrison E, Capell HA, et al. Effect of social deprivation on disease severity and outcome in patients with rheumatoid arthritis. *Ann Rheum Dis* 1997;56:410–413.
136. Gough A, Faint J, Salmon M, et al. Genetic typing of patients with inflammatory arthritis at presentation can be used to predict outcome. *Arthritis Rheum* 1994;37:1166–1170.
137. van Zeben D, Hazes JM, Zwinderman AH, et al. Association of HLA-DR4 with a more progressive disease course in patients with rheumatoid arthritis. Results of a followup study. *Arthritis Rheum* 1991;34:822–830.
138. Moreno I, Valenzuela A, Garcia A, et al. Association of the shared epitope with radiological severity of rheumatoid arthritis. *J Rheumatol* 1996;23:6–9.
139. Eberhardt K, Fex E, Johnson U, et al. Associations of HLA-DRB and -DQB genes with two and five year outcome in rheumatoid arthritis. *Ann Rheum Dis* 1996;55:34–39.
140. Ward MM, Leigh JP. The relative importance of pain and functional disability to patients with rheumatoid arthritis. *J Rheumatol* 1993;20:1494–1499.
141. Pincus T, Callahan LF, Brooks RH, et al. Self-report questionnaire scores in rheumatoid arthritis compared with traditional physical, radiographic, and laboratory measures. *Ann Intern Med* 1989;110:259–266.
142. Smedstad LM, Moum T, Guillemin F, et al. Correlates of functional disability in early rheumatoid arthritis: a cross-sectional study of 706 patients in four European countries. *Br J Rheumatol* 1996;35:746–751.
143. van der Heide A, Remme CA, Hoffman DM, et al. Prediction of progression of radiographic damage in newly diagnosed rheumatoid arthritis. *Arthritis Rheum* 1995;38:1466–1475.
144. Koh ET, Seow A, Pong LY, et al. Cross cultural adaptation and validation of the Chinese Health Assessment Questionnaire for use in rheumatoid arthritis. *J Rheumatol* 1998;25:1705–1708.
145. Woolf AD, Hall ND, Goulding NJ, et al. Predictors of the long-term outcome of early synovitis: a 5-year follow-up study. *Br J Rheumatol* 1991;30:251–254.
146. van Zeben D, Hazes JM, Zwinderman AH, et al. Factors predicting outcome of rheumatoid arthritis: results of a follow-up study. *J Rheumatol* 1993;20:1288–1296.
147. Houssien DA, Jonsson T, Davies E, et al. Clinical significance of IgA rheumatoid factor subclasses in rheumatoid arthritis. *J Rheumatol* 1997;24:2119–2122.
148. Wolfe F, Hawley DJ, Wilson K. The prevalence and meaning of fatigue in rheumatic disease. *J Rheumatol* 1996;23:1407–1417.
149. Wolfe F, Hawley DJ. The relationship between clinical activity and depression in rheumatoid arthritis. *J Rheumatol* 1993;20:2032–2037.
150. Abdel-Nasser AM, Abd El-Azim S, Taal E, et al. Depression and depressive symptoms in rheumatoid arthritis patients: an analysis of their occurrence and determinants. *Br J Rheumatol* 1998;37:391–397.

151. Bukhari M, Lunt M, Harrison BJ, et al. Rheumatoid factor is the major predictor of increasing severity of radiographic erosions in rheumatoid arthritis: results from the Norfolk Arthritis Register Study, a large inception cohort. *Arthritis Rheum* 2002;46:906–912.
152. Kaarela K. Prognostic factors and diagnostic criteria in early rheumatoid arthritis. *Scand J Rheumatol* 1985;S57[Suppl]:5–50.
153. Van Zeben D, Hazes JMW, Zwinderman AH, et al. Clinical significance of rheumatoid factors in early rheumatoid arthritis: results of a follow-up study. *Ann Rheum Dis* 1992;51:1029–1033.
154. Feigenbaum SL, Masi AT, Kaplan SB. Prognosis in rheumatoid arthritis: a longitudinal study of newly diagnosed younger adult patients. *Am J Med* 1979;66:377–384.
155. Corbett M, Young A. The Middlesex Hospital prospective study of early rheumatoid disease. *Br J Rheumatol* 1988;27[Suppl 2]:171–172.
156. Valenzuale-Castano A, Garcia-Lopez A, Perez-Vilches D, et al. The predictive value of the HLA shared epitope for severity of radiographic joint damage in patients with rheumatoid arthritis: a 10 year observational prospective study. *J Rheumatol* 2000;27:571–574.
157. Plant MJ, Jones PW, Saklatvala J, et al. Patterns of radiographic progression in early rheumatoid arthritis: results of an 8 year prospective study. *J Rheumatol* 1998;25:417–426.
158. Van der Heijde DMFM, van Riel PLCM, van Leeuwen MA, et al. Prognostic factors for radiographic damage and physical disability in early rheumatoid arthritis: a prospective follow-up study of 147 patients. *Br J Rheumatol* 1992;31:519–525.
159. Fex E, Jonsson K, Johnson U, et al. Development of radiographic damage during the first 5–6 years of rheumatoid arthritis: a prospective follow-up study of a Swedish cohort. *Br J Rheumatol* 1996;35:1106–1115.
160. Van Leeuwen MA, Westra J, van Riel PLCM, et al. IgM, IgA and IgG rheumatoid factors in early rheumatoid arthritis: predictive of radiographic progression? *Scand J Rheumatol* 1995;24:146–153.
161. Matsuda Y, Yamanaka H, Higami K, et al. Time lag between active joint inflammation and radiographic progression in patients with early rheumatoid arthritis. *J Rheumatol* 1998;25:427–432.
162. Sjoblom KG, Saxne T, Petterson H, et al. Factors related to the progression of joint destruction in rheumatoid arthritis. *Scand J Rheumatol* 1984;13:21–27.
163. Aho K, Palosuo T, Heliovaara M, et al. Antifilaggrin antibodies within "normal" range predict rheumatoid arthritis in a linear fashion. *J Rheumatol* 2000;27:2743–2746.
164. Schellekens GA, de Jong BAW, van den Hoogen FHJ, et al. Citrulline is an essential constituent of antigenic determinants recognized by rheumatoid arthritis-specific autoantibodies. *J Clin Invest* 1998;101:273–281.
165. Schellekens GA, Visser H, de Jong BAW, et al. The diagnostic properties of rheumatoid arthritis antibodies recognizing a cyclic citrullinated peptide. *Arthritis Rheum* 2000;43:155–163.
166. Kroot E, de Jong BAW, van Leeuwen MA, et al. The prognostic value of the anti-cyclic citrullinated peptide antibody in patients with recent-onset rheumatoid arthritis. *Arthritis Rheum* 2000;43:1831–1835.
167. van Jaarsveld CH, ter Borg EJ, Jacobs JW, et al. The prognostic value of the antiperinuclear factor, anti-citrullinated peptide antibodies and rheumatoid factor in early rheumatoid arthritis. *Clin Exp Rheumatol* 1999;17:689–697.
168. Visser H, le Cessie S, Vos K, et al. How to diagnose rheumatoid arthritis early: a prediction model for persistent (erosive) arthritis. *Arthritis Rheum* 2002;46:357–365.
169. Combe B, Dougados M, Goupille P, et al. Prognostic factors for radiographic damage in early rheumatoid arthritis: a multiparameter prospective study. *Arthritis Rheum* 2001;44:1736–1743.
170. Amos RS, Constable TJ, Crockson RA, et al. Rheumatoid arthritis: relation of serum C-reactive protein and erythrocyte sedimentation rates to radiographic changes. *BMJ* 1977;1:195–197.
171. Matsuda Y, Yamanaka H, Higami K, et al. Time lag between active joint inflammation and radiological progression in patients with early rheumatoid arthritis. *J Rheumatol* 1998;25:427–432.
172. van Leeuwen MA, van Rijswijk MH, Sluiter WJ, et al. Individual relationship between progression of radiological damage and the acute phase response in early rheumatoid arthritis. Towards development of a decision support system. *J Rheumatol* 1997;24:20–27.
173. Stenger AA, Van Leeuwen MA, Houtman PM, et al. Early effective suppression of inflammation in rheumatoid arthritis reduces radiographic progression. *Br J Rheumatol* 1998;37:1157–1163.
174. Stenger AA, Van Leeuwen MA, Houtman PM, et al. Early effective suppression of inflammation in rheumatoid arthritis reduces radiographic progression. *Br J Rheumatol* 1998;37:1157–1163.
175. Plant MJ, Williams AL, O'Sullivan MM, et al. Relationship between time-integrated C-reactive protein levels and radiologic progression in patients with rheumatoid arthritis. *Arthritis Rheum* 2000;43:1473–1477.
176. Green M, Marzo-Ortega H, McGonagle D, et al. Persistence of mild, early inflammatory arthritis: the importance of disease duration, rheumatoid factor, and the shared epitope. *Arthritis Rheum* 1999;42:2184–2188.
177. Feigenbaum SL, Masi AT, Kaplan SB. Prognosis in rheumatoid arthritis. A longitudinal study of newly diagnosed younger adult patients. *Am J Med* 1979;66:377–384.
178. Kaarela K. Prognostic factors and diagnostic criteria in early rheumatoid arthritis. *Scand J Rheumatol* 1985;57[Suppl]:1–54.
179. Corbett M, Young A. The Middlesex Hospital prospective study of early rheumatoid disease. *Br J Rheumatol* 1988;27[Suppl 2]:171–172.
180. Eberhardt KB, Fex E. Functional impairment and disability in early rheumatoid arthritis—development over 5 years. *J Rheumatol* 1995;22:1037–1042.
181. Young A, Cox N, Dixie J, et al. Early rheumatoid arthritis study (ERAS). Report of first 506 patients. *Arthritis Rheum* 1991;34:S48.
182. van Leeuwen MA, Westra J, van Riel PLCM, et al. IgM, IgA and IgG rheumatoid factors in early rheumatoid arthritis. Predictive of radiological progression? *Scand J Rheumatol* 1995;24:146–153.
183. van der Heide A, Jacobs JWG, Haanen HCM, et al. Is it possible to predict the first year extent of pain and disability for patients with rheumatoid arthritis? *J Rheumatol* 1995;22:1466–1470.
184. Pincus T, Brooks RH, Callahan LF. Prediction of long-term mortality in patients with rheumatoid arthritis according to simple questionnaire and joint count measures. *Ann Intern Med* 1994;120:26–34.
185. Turesson C, O'Fallon WM, Crowson CS, et al. Occurrence of extraarticular disease manifestations is associated with excess mortality in a community based cohort of patients with rheumatoid arthritis. *J Rheumatol* 2002;29:62–67.
186. Choi HK, Hernan MA, Seeger JD, et al. Methotrexate and mortality in patients with rheumatoid arthritis: a prospective study. *Lancet* 2002;359:1173–1177.
187. Doran MF, Pond GR, Crowson CS, et al. Trends in incidence and mortality in rheumatoid arthritis in Rochester, Minnesota, over a forty-year period. *Arthritis Rheum* 2002;46:625–631.

CHAPTER 4

Self-Report Questionnaires in Clinical Care

Frederick Wolfe

The responsibility of the rheumatologist to the rheumatoid arthritis (RA) patient is to maximize the patient's quality of life in the domains that are important to the patient during the different periods of his or her lifespan. At the beginning of the twenty-first century, despite the best therapy, most patients with RA still have continuing disease activity, pain, and functional loss, and the average course of RA is downhill (1–4). Good therapy minimizes the slope of illness progression and may alter, retard, or even prevent the adverse outcomes of RA (5).

If the goal of clinical intervention is to maximize the patient's quality of life, the clinician must be able to measure (a) activity and severity of illness across physical, psychological, and social domains; (b) predict the course of illness; and (c) understand those aspects of quality of life that are most important to the patient now and will be most important in the future. Most of these goals can be met with the aid of patients' self-report questionnaires and one or two clinical observations. The key to understanding what is happening to the patient lies in asking the patient. For reference in understanding the various scales involved in self-report questionnaires, the Clinical Health Assessment Questionnaire (CLINHAQ) (6) is reprinted in Appendix E.

USE OF QUESTIONNAIRES IN THE CLINIC

The primary requirement for clinical decision making is quantitative information regarding patient status, change in status, and prognosis. In RA, *status* refers to inflammatory activity, functional ability, and emotional or affective characteristics. These areas overlap, and the often-asked question to the patient, "How are you doing?" is really an amalgamation of the three domains. Prognosis is usually thought of in terms of risk for mortality, work loss, income loss, and major arthritis surgery (7,8).

MEASUREMENT OF FUNCTION

Functional ability (or disability) is an unobserved variable that lies on the continuum from complete ability to complete inability (9). It is assessed with a surrogate, observed variable, such as the HAQ disability index (10,11), with the expectation that the surrogate measure will provide an adequate representation of the disability state. Considering the ways by which an individual may lose function and the external factors that may influence day-to-day ability, a short questionnaire is, at best, an imperfect measure. One may think of functional ability as if it is a continuum that is laid out on a 10-cm ruler. At one end of the continuum is a person who is unconscious and close to death. At the other end is a world-class athlete. Practically, such a scale needs to be shortened to make it useful in arthritis. In general, the 0 point represents ordinary activities of daily living and their extensions that the average person should be able to do. At the upper point, activities are arbitrarily selected that all but the most severe RA patient should be able to accomplish. It is expected that, at the lower end of the scale, a small number of patients who have functional limitations will not be detected because their limitations are slight (floor effect). To illustrate this range, data from the National Data Bank for Rheumatic Diseases (NDB) are used (12). Using the HAQ, for example (NDB: N = 10,398), 12.5% of RA patients have 0 scores, and 0.4% have the maximum score of 3. For the Modified HAQ (MHAQ) (13), these percentages are 26.4% and 0.1%. At the floor, there are patients who truly have no limitations and some patients who have limitations but are not detected by the questionnaire because of problems the questionnaire has in identifying patients with slight limitations.

The scores from the HAQ questionnaires increase from 0 to 3 in 0.125-unit steps. Using the 0-to-3 scales of the HAQ group of questionnaires, we would ideally expect that each step of functional loss would be reflected linearly on our functional ability/disability ruler. If this were the case, there would be just as much functional loss occurring when the scale changes from 0 to 0.5 as it does when it changes from 1.25 to 1.75. However, this is not true with current scales, as the real loss of function is much greater between 0 and 0.5 than it is between 1.25 and 1.75. The HAQ is much more linear between 0.75 and 2.00 than at levels above and below these ranges, however. Therefore, clinicians can use the HAQ as an approximate ruler within these ranges. It can be seen, however, that the practice of assuming a 20% change has the same meaning regardless of whether its beginning position on the scale is not correct.

Sometimes it has been thought that to measure disability in RA, questions must address all of the impairments that occur in this illness, in particular, hand function. This is not true. The Short Form-36 (SF-36) functional scale (14–16), for example, performs very well in RA but asks no questions about hand function. The HAQ, by contrast, has several questions that relate to hand function. Considering the 0-to-10-cm functional ruler, it is not the specific task itself that is important but the difficulty of the task and where the task lies on the continuum of disability as measured by the functional ruler. The original HAQ questionnaire classifies questions into groups (e.g., dressing and grooming, walking, and eating), but such groupings, that are familiar to clinicians, have no intrinsic meaning in the assessment of disability. If it is important to measure hand function, then a specific hand questionnaire should be used.

What do functional scales actually measure? A scale is said to be *unidimensional* when it measures only one thing (one domain); in this instance, function. Unidimensionality can sometimes be a tricky concept, as is the case when some apparent functional activities are, in fact, measuring a different domain. For example, participating in vigorous athletics may really be measuring the domain of athleticism rather than function. When rheumatologists speak of functional loss, they often mean impairment caused by structural (joint) damage, weakness, or neurologic loss. But questionnaire results do not differentiate functional loss according to cause, and cardiopulmonary disease, as well as arthritis, can influence functional scores. In addition, pain, not structural damage, is the major determinant of functional limitations among persons with RA. This is an important point: Functional status questionnaires do not differentiate functional loss caused by structural problems from those caused by pain. Because pain is such a prominent aspect of functional disability, it is not surprising to find high levels of self-reported disability at the onset of RA. Response to questionnaires is also influenced by psychosocial factors. Anxiety and depression are associated with higher levels of reported functional disability. Functional disability scores are also more abnormal in persons with less education and lower income. Women report more impaired function than do men. Functional scores may be influenced by minor illnesses, normal day-to-day variation, and the sheer randomness of the world.

How accurate is questionnaire functional assessment? Among persons reporting no difference in their health during the previous 6 months, the within-patient standard deviation of HAQ scores is 0.19 (NDB: 24,164 observations). The Bland-Altman limits of agreement test (17) indicates that the 95% limits of agreement is approximately 0.61 units within this similar group of patients. In addition, as pointed out above, the HAQ score is influenced by psychosocial factors. These observations have led some to the conclusion that the HAQ varies too much to be used in the clinic and is only suitable for research (18). This conclusion is wrong on several accounts (19). The interpretation of HAQ and HAQ scores, as with any clinical measure, is context-dependent (the who, how, where, and why of the physician–patient encounter). Of all clinical measures, including laboratory tests, the HAQ has the least variability. Clinical uncertainty exists for all tests. It is a rare clinician who has not discarded an abnormal erythrocyte sedimentation rate (ESR) or C-reactive protein (CRP) result in a patient who is otherwise doing well. The use of tests is discussed further below.

WHICH FUNCTIONAL QUESTIONNAIRE SHOULD BE USED?

A series of functional questionnaires is available, including the HAQ and its derivatives, the physical function subscale of the SF-36, and full and shortened versions of the Arthritis Impact Measurement Scales (AIMS) (20), among others (13,21–26). Practically, measurement of function in clinical trials is almost always accomplished using HAQ disability index or a shortened version, the modified MHAQ. The AIMS has not been shown to offer any advantages compared with other questionnaires, is much longer than the other questionnaires, and has had little use in rheumatology care and studies, even in its shortened version (27,28). The physical function subscale of the SF-36 is an excellent short questionnaire with very good psychometric properties. It works as well as the HAQ and is simple to score. Its major limitation is that it is not commonly used except as part of the larger SF-36, and there have been few studies of its predictive ability and sensitivity to change within RA. The SF-36 functional subscale is more sensitive than the HAQ in identifying difference in functional ability in persons with few limitations, whereas the HAQ questionnaire is more sensitive at the upper end of the impairment scale than the SF-36 functional scale. Practically, however, the differences noted above make little difference. In addition, because of its limited use, there is no clear sense of what scores mean in clinic patients. Even so, the SF-36 functional subscale is likely to work as well as the HAQ and would be a reasonable choice to use in the clinic and in RA studies.

The HAQ is a 20-item questionnaire that also inquires about the use of aides and devices, resulting in a total of 42 questions (10) (see Appendix E). It takes 2 to 4 minutes to complete and can be scored in 15 seconds. The MHAQ is a version of the HAQ that retains only 8 of the original 20 HAQ questions and does not account for aides and devices (29). It takes less than 2 minutes to complete and can be scored in seconds. The main advantage of the MHAQ is its brevity. The MHAQ, however, has a number of disadvantages (30). It has a large floor effect: 37% of RA patients score 0.125 or less on the MHAQ compared to 17% for the HAQ (NDB: N = 10,398). Considering the 0-to-10-cm functional ruler, the MHAQ is distinctly nonlinear compared with the HAQ, and it has considerably less ability to describe functional status accurately and to distinguish functional change in RA patients who have few limitations. These differences are shown in Figure 4.1. An attempt has been made to remove the floor effect from the MHAQ by adding two additional "difficult items" (MDHAQ) (31). Although successful in reducing the floor effect, the additional questions have introduced substantial additional psychometric problems, including loss of unidimensionality and differences in the meaning of scores according to age and sex (item response bias). Wolfe et al. have recently proposed a ten-item HAQ-2 questionnaire that has floor effects similar to the HAQ but that is shorter and has better linear scaling properties (32) (see Appendix F). All of the HAQ family of questionnaires have different means and medians, and scores from one HAQ questionnaire (e.g., the HAQ) cannot be converted or compared to another HAQ questionnaire (e.g., MHAQ or MDHAQ). For comparison with clinical trial and epidemiologic data, the HAQ is probably the best instrument for the clinician. However, its use comes at the cost of a two-page questionnaire compared to a one-page questionnaire and an extra minute or two in questionnaire completion. This extra time usually makes little practical difference, as it is unused time when a patient is in a waiting room, as opposed to using staff time.

MEASUREMENT OF PAIN IN THE CLINIC

Pain is a complex phenomenon that can be described in a number of ways, with separate attention to its sensory and affective components, severity, and other effects (33). The multidimensional nature of pain has led to the development of multidimensional pain scales (33–35). However, such scales are difficult to interpret clinically, and there is no evidence that they provide more useful information than simpler scales. In fact, the opposite appears to be the case. Pain may be measured in terms of current pain, pain over a given period (e.g., the last week, the last 6 months), worst pain, and average pain. In addition, pain is sometimes assessed in terms of pain relief rather than pain intensity. In general, however, pain is usually assessed in RA clinical trials and in the clinic as current pain intensity or pain intensity over the last week or month. Most often, intensity is

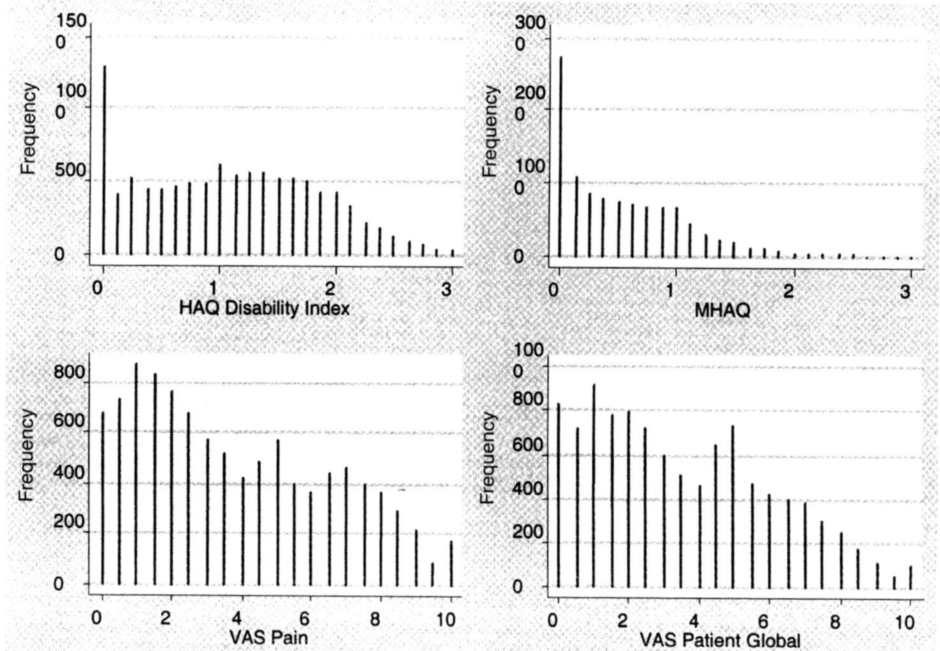

Figure 4.1. Distribution of Health Assessment Questionnaire (HAQ), Modified Health Assessment Questionnaire (MHAQ), visual analog scale (VAS) pain, and VAS patient global scores in 10,314 rheumatoid arthritis patients.

assessed as over the previous week (see Appendixes E and F). The distribution of pain scores is shown in Figure 4.1.

Pain intensity may be measured with a rating scale (none, mild, moderate, severe, very severe, and so on). Another method is to use a visual analog scale (VAS). A VAS is a single line 10 or 15 cm in length that is anchored at each end with descriptors such as "No Pain" and "Very Severe Pain." To score such a scale, a ruler is used to measure the point on the line identified by the patient. It is often possible to put marks on the line at 10 or 20 equidistant points. In contrast to measuring the line with a ruler, this method is much easier for the scorer, who then merely has to look at the line to score it rather than having to measure it. This technique is illustrated in the squares and circles of the VASs shown in Appendixes E and F. With a maximum of 10 or 20 points on the line, it is not possible to achieve the fine continuous scale of the single-line VAS. However, there is no evidence that persons completing a pain questionnaire can reliably distinguish more than 7 points. In practice, it matters little how the VAS scale is constructed. Scales can be ladder-like (vertical) or horizontal. However, there is no general agreement in clinical trials as to how scales should be oriented or drawn. There is a considerable literature on the construction and orientation of pain scales that may be consulted (36). The authors of the HAQ, MHAQ, and CLINHAQ use horizontal scales scored from 0 to 10, and such scales are recommended to rheumatologists.

MEASUREMENT OF PATIENT GLOBAL SEVERITY

Patient global severity is assessed with a rating scale or VAS scale, such as Measurement of Pain in the Clinic. A typical question to assess global severity is, "Considering all the ways that your arthritis affects you, rate how you are doing on the following scale. Place an X in the box (or a line if you are using a single line) below that best describes how you are doing on a scale of 0 to 10" (see Appendixes E and F). The distribution of patient global severity scores is shown in Figure 4.1. It is not clear whether patients can reliably distinguish between arthritis activity and arthritis severity, the latter encompassing the consequences of inflammation as well as inflammation itself. Patient global severity correlates with HAQ at r = 0.620 and with pain at r = 0.662 (NDB: N = 15,791).

MEASUREMENT OF PHYSICIAN GLOBAL SCORE(S)

Physician global scores may be differentiated into a global estimate of disease activity or a global estimate of disease severity. Disease activity and disease severity are allied concepts but have different meanings. In interpreting patient global scores in studies or in the clinic, it is important to distinguish between disease activity and severity. *Global disease activity* refers to inflammatory activity. Extraarticular manifestations of RA, such as pleural effusion, pulmonary fibrosis, or vasculitis, may occur in the absence of usual RA activity and should not be included in "global activity." A physician global disease activity scale can be a VAS scale with anchors at "no activity" and "extreme activity." Alternatively, a categorical scale can be used with the following five labeled boxes: none, mild, moderate, severe, extreme, with four unlabeled boxes in between the labeled boxes.

A "global severity" scale, on the other hand, includes extraarticular manifestations, functional ability, disease activity, and outcomes of RA—all of the manifestations and consequences of RA. The problem with a physician's estimate of global severity is that physicians cannot know all of the details of severity that the patient experiences, nor all of the consequences. It is better to rate disease activity, describe severity features, and then use the HAQ to describe function than it is to try to rate global severity. Although rheumatologists may be expected to rate disease activity similarly, disease severity has different meanings for different rheumatologists.

FATIGUE, ANXIETY, AND DEPRESSION

Clinical trials do not usually measure fatigue, anxiety, and depression, primarily because they are not sensitive to intervention-related change. However, these mental states are key features in clinical practice (37–39). In addition, they allow us to see how emotional factors can influence and be influenced by disease activity. In particular, they may allow the clinician to sort out inflammatory from noninflammatory aspects for pain and functional loss. Fatigue can be measured easily and accurately with a simple VAS anchored by "No fatigue" and "Very severe fatigue" (see Appendixes E and F). Although detailed multidimensional fatigue scales exist (40–42), there is no evidence that they perform better than simple scales. In addition, longer scales make it more difficult to assess this important component of illness by increasing patient and physician burden.

In contrast to measurement of fatigue, longer scales are better for measuring anxiety and depression or mood (practically, a combination of the two related concepts). Shorter scales do not accurately and reliably measure these complex concepts. On the other hand, standard psychological instruments are too long for use in the clinic and may be too intrusive on patients' privacy. One approach to psychological assessment is to use the five mood questions from the SF-36 (14): Have you been a very nervous person? Have you felt so down in the dumps that nothing could cheer you up? Have you felt calm and peaceful? Have you felt downhearted and blue? Have you been a happy person? We have used the ten questions from the AIMS-I (20), but an eight-question mood section is available in the AIMS-II (22). The AIMS and SF-36 questions were derived from the same sources, and are quite similar. The MDHAQ uses a single four-category question for anxiety and a four-category question for depression (31). In general, the longer the psychological question is, the more distinct categories of response can be detected accurately and the more reliably can change be detected.

PRACTICAL USE OF QUESTIONNAIRES IN THE CLINICAL SETTING

Questionnaires should be administered when the patient checks into the clinic and before he or she is seen by the physician (see reference 37). The questionnaires in Appendixes E and F are used in actual practice, and they illustrate the simplicity and ease of administration that can accompany questionnaire assessments. In administering the questionnaire, it can be helpful to provide the patient with a clipboard and pen. The process of completing the questionnaire can take 5 to 10 minutes, depending on the length and complexity of the questionnaire. There is almost always sufficient waiting room time for this task. The questionnaires should be collected just before the clinical interview. Scoring is usually quite simple. However, it is important to record the results on a flow sheet record so that changes in patient response over time can be seen. Part of the power of questionnaires is observing how they are answered over time. Flow sheets can be made with simple pen-and-ink entry. There are usually only five or six scores to be entered, a process that takes less than a minute for a staff person to do. Questionnaires can be scored by a nonmedical person to avoid using valuable medical time. Scoring instructions and questionnaires are available at http://www.arthritis-research.org.

USING INFORMATION IN THE CLINIC

The clinician should review the questionnaire results before or at the time of the patient encounter. All findings, whether they represent laboratory tests, physical examination results, or questionnaire responses, must be interpreted in the clinical context. For example, for the same degree of apparent RA severity, some patients always report a greater number of tender joints, whereas some consistently report fewer tender joints. The reporting behavior can also be true for pain scores, HAQ scores, and global severity. This pattern of responsiveness reveals something about the patient, but it also indicates that clinicians have to put the reported results into context. Physicians may have to interpret up the self-reports of the stoic patient and interpret down the reports of the more sensitive patient. Just as with any test in medicine, the usefulness and interpretation of self-report questionnaires depend on other information that clinicians have. This information may come from many years of interaction with the patient and family, knowledge of previous response to therapy, and knowledge of other problems in the life of the patient. It is this bayesian approach (use of preexisting information) to data interpretation that makes the apparently large interpersonal standard deviation of HAQ scores and scores on many measures in medicine much more reliable, in fact, than they seem when looking at the presentation of crude, noninformative scores.

The apparent subjectivity of self-report questionnaires bothers some physicians, who feel more comfortable with the apparent objectivity of swollen joint counts and ESR/CRP tests. The problems with objective data are several. Objective data do not do nearly as good a job at measuring response to therapy in the clinical trial or in clinical practice as self-report data (43). In fact, in clinical trials, the placebo effect is greatest for physician examination measures compared with laboratory and self-report results (43). In addition, the pain and function that is much more clinically relevant is the patient's pain function, not the physician's surrogate assessment through the test measure by "objective" tests. In evaluating patients in the clinic, both physician measurements and patient self-reports are important. The wise clinician disregards a patient's report when it is inaccurate, as, for example, when the number of swollen joints increases to 15 from three but the patient says he or she is doing fine. But it is usually the other way around; with laboratory tests and physical findings that seem satisfactory, yet the patient is reporting he or she is feeling worse.

INTERPRETING QUESTIONNAIRES IN THE CLINIC: STATUS

Whether it is ESR/CRP, joint count, or questionnaire data, there are no gold standards to establish the relationship between test values and categorical levels of severity. Through experience, the clinician learns to make appropriate interpretation of those interrelationships. However, clinical data may be interpreted in several ways. Score severity can be defined in terms of (a) relative severity, or how this patient's score is compared with other patients (44,45), and (b) the absolute level of severity of this patient's score. Table 4.1 presents rankings of scores for questionnaire variables in terms of the 5th, 25th, 50th, 75th, and 95th percentiles from a large RA population in the NBD. Separate sub-tables are presented for each gender. The median duration of disease in these tables is 7.6 years. A clinician can use these tables to obtain a sense of where his or her patients are with respect to other patients with RA and also a sense of the meaning of individual patient scores.

For the VASs, the median score for both genders is approximately 4, and the 25th and 75th percentiles are approximately 2 and 6. It is, therefore, relatively easy to understand how a given patient is doing using these simple markers. The median HAQ is 1.1 with 25th and 75th percentile at 0.50 and 1.75. For more detail by gender, the sub-tables should be consulted. The anxiety and depression scores are from AIMS-2 (22).

Percentiles represent an accurate measure of the distribution of scores in the RA population, and are, therefore, useful to

TABLE 4.1. Percentile (P) Scores for 10,314 Rheumatoid Arthritis Patients in the National Data Bank for Rheumatic Diseases

Variable	Mean	P5	P25	Median	P75	P95
All patients						
HAQ (0–3)	1.15	0.00	0.50	1.13	1.75	2.38
Pain (0–10)	4.24	0.50	2.00	4.00	6.50	9.00
Global severity (0–10)	4.00	0.50	2.00	4.00	5.50	8.50
Fatigue (0–10)	4.39	0.50	2.00	4.50	6.50	9.00
GI severity (0–10)	2.17	0.00	0.00	1.50	3.50	7.50
Sleep disturbance (0–10)	3.76	0.00	1.00	3.50	6.50	9.00
Anxiety (0–10)	4.12	0.99	2.64	3.96	5.61	7.59
Depression (0–10)	2.88	0.33	1.60	2.64	3.96	6.60
Women						
HAQ (0–3)	1.22	0.00	0.63	1.25	1.75	2.50
Pain (0–10)	4.33	0.50	2.00	4.00	6.50	9.00
Global severity (0–10)	4.05	0.50	2.00	4.00	5.50	8.50
Fatigue (0–10)	4.59	0.50	2.50	4.50	7.00	9.00
GI severity (0–10)	2.33	0.00	0.50	1.50	4.00	7.50
Sleep disturbance (0–10)	3.89	0.00	1.00	3.50	6.50	9.00
Anxiety (0–10)	4.26	0.99	2.64	4.29	5.61	7.59
Depression (0–10)	2.96	0.33	1.65	2.64	3.96	6.60
Men						
HAQ (0–3)	0.92	0.00	0.25	0.88	1.38	2.25
Pain (0–10)	3.98	0.50	2.00	3.50	6.00	8.50
Global severity (0–10)	3.89	0.50	2.00	4.00	5.50	8.00
Fatigue (0–10)	3.79	0.00	1.50	3.50	6.00	8.50
GI severity (0–10)	1.68	0.00	0.00	0.50	2.50	6.50
Sleep disturbance (0–10)	3.41	0.00	0.50	2.50	5.50	8.50
Anxiety (0–10)	3.70	0.33	1.98	3.63	5.20	7.26
Depression (0–10)	2.63	0.00	1.32	2.31	3.63	6.20

GI, gastrointestinal; HAQ, Health Assessment Questionnaire.

answer the question, "How is this patient doing compared to other patients?" They do not, however, address the issue of absolute severity of the measure under study. Patients in the NDB were asked to categorize their health status by indicating how satisfied they were with their health. The choices were very satisfied, somewhat satisfied, neither satisfied nor dissatisfied, somewhat dissatisfied, and very dissatisfied. Satisfaction results correlate well with long-term outcomes such as mortality and work disability. In Table 4.2, these satisfaction levels are transformed to levels of severity. Each score represents the median score at the level of severity noted in column 1. The median HAQ score for persons with very mild severity (very satisfied with health) is 0.38, whereas the median score for a patient with very severe severity is 1.88. The median "moderate" pain score is 4.5, similar to the 50th-percentile score in Table 4.1. Table 4.2 provides treating clinicians a guide to how patients see severity and how acceptable abnormalities are to them. It also provides a series of benchmarks that can serve as goals for improvement.

Clinically significant changes in the HAQ have also been addressed in several studies. Redelmeier and Lorig interviewed 103 RA patients and found that HAQ scores needed to differ by 0.23 units (95% confidence interval, 0.13, 0.23) before respondents stopped rating themselves as "about the same" (46). A

TABLE 4.2. Self-Report Scores for 10,314 Rheumatoid Arthritis Patients in the National Data Bank for Rheumatic Diseases Stratified by Severity Category

Satisfaction	HAQ	Pain	Global	Fatigue	GI Scale	Sleep	Anxiety	Depression
All patients								
Very mild	0.38	1.50	1.00	1.50	0.50	0.50	1.98	1.32
Mild	0.75	3.00	2.50	3.50	0.50	2.50	3.30	1.98
Moderate	1.25	4.50	4.50	5.00	1.50	4.50	4.29	2.64
Severe	1.38	5.50	5.00	6.00	1.50	5.25	4.62	3.30
Very severe	1.88	7.50	7.00	7.50	2.50	7.00	5.94	4.62
Women								
Very mild	0.50	1.50	1.00	2.00	0.50	1.00	2.31	1.32
Mild	0.88	3.00	2.50	3.50	1.00	2.50	3.63	1.98
Moderate	1.38	4.50	4.50	5.50	1.50	4.50	4.62	2.97
Severe	1.38	5.50	5.00	6.00	2.00	5.50	4.95	3.30
Very severe	1.88	7.50	7.00	7.50	2.50	7.00	5.94	4.62
Men								
Very mild	0.13	1.00	1.00	1.00	0.50	0.50	1.98	0.99
Mild	0.50	2.50	2.50	2.50	0.50	2.00	2.64	1.65
Moderate	1.00	4.50	4.00	4.50	0.50	3.50	3.96	2.64
Severe	1.13	5.00	5.00	5.25	1.50	4.50	4.45	2.97
Very severe	1.63	7.50	7.00	7.00	2.00	7.00	5.28	4.29

GI, gastrointestinal; HAQ, Health Assessment Questionnaire.

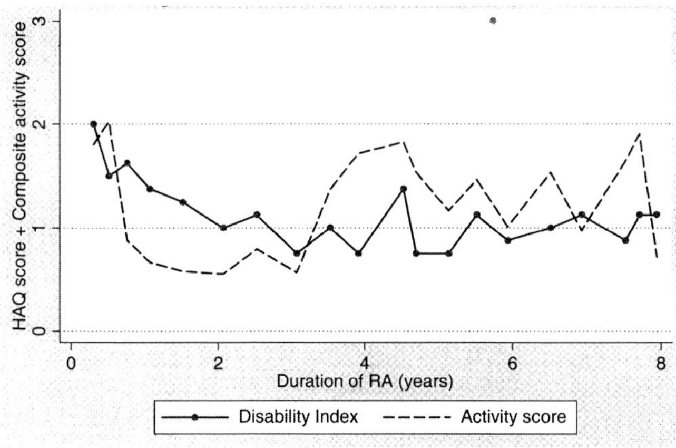

Figure 4.2. Change in Health Assessment Questionnaire (HAQ) disability and composite disease activity over time for one rheumatoid arthritis (RA) patient followed for 8 years. The composite activity score is computed from principal component analysis of erythrocyte sedimentation rate, tender joint count, visual acuity scale (VAS) pain, and VAS patient global. HAQ disability improves to its nadir at 3.5 years. Thereafter, it increases by approximately 0.1 U per year during the next 5 years.

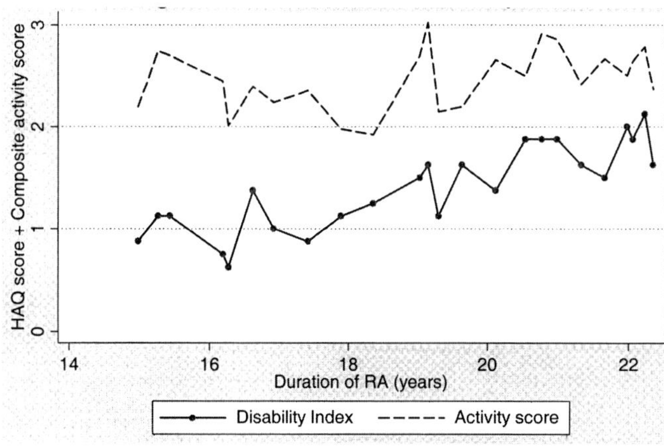

Figure 4.3. Change in Health Assessment Questionnaire (HAQ) disability and composite disease activity over time for one rheumatoid arthritis (RA) patient followed for 7 years. The composite activity score is computed from principal component analysis of erythrocyte sedimentation rate, tender joint count, visual acuity score (VAS) pain, and VAS patient global. There is a continual high level of disease activity, resulting in an approximate increase of the HAQ score of 1 U in 7 years or 0.14 U per year.

similar interpretation was made by Wells et al. in a review of data from clinical trials (47). They found the minimal clinically important difference to be 0.22 units, or approximately two steps in the HAQ score (Fig. 4.2).

INTERPRETING QUESTIONNAIRES IN THE CLINIC: CHANGE IN STATUS

Clinicians need to know whether patients are improving, remaining stable, or getting worse. Such changes must be assessed in the short term and the long term. The questions asked in the short-term assessments are

1. Has the patient changed between visits?
2. How much has he or she changed?
3. How important is the change?

Equally important is long-term change. For example, a patient may change imperceptibly between visits. Yet, at the end of 1 to 2 years, substantial change may have occurred. Verna Wright's oft-quoted comment that "Clinicians may all too easily spend years writing 'doing well' in the notes of a patient who has become progressively crippled before their eyes" is particularly apt (48).

Without patient questionnaire data, depression, functional losses, pain, and fatigue—essential matters in the patient-physician encounter—are consistently missed or underestimated. In addition, particularly in current circumstances in which physicians are allotted limited time with patients, many of these assessments are all too brief. "How are you doing?" asks the physician. "Better" (or "Not as well"), replies the patient. But without written quantitative information, possible differences between status at this patient–physician encounter and one that occurred 6 months previously are lost to the exigencies of memory and time. It is not realistic or accurate to compare patient status from one visit to another without a quantitative written record of status at an earlier time point, and the only efficient and reliable method to gather such data is through a patient questionnaire.

To see how a patient is doing over time, the clinician must observe longitudinally using quantitative data. Figures 4.2 and 4.3 demonstrate changes in disease activity over time and the effect of disease activity on HAQ progression. Even without a graph, the clinician should be able to see the changes in HAQ, provided a flow sheet is used so that all of the longitudinal data can be evaluated. Because HAQ score changes between visits are often very small, they can be missed unless longitudinal comparisons are made. In Figure 4.2, for example, the HAQ is at its nadir at 3.5 years after RA onset. However, the score can be seen to increase by approximately 0.5 U over the next 3.5 years, or 0.1 U per year. Figure 4.3 shows change in function over 7 years in which the HAQ changes by 1 U overall, or approximately 0.14 U per year. Such a change in function could not be detected clinically without serial quantitative measurement.

Self-report questionnaires also provide a way to understand and document the degree of disease activity and to measure the changes in activity. The dashed line in Figures 4.2 and 4.3 represents a computed disease activity variable that was derived from pain, patient global severity, ESR, and joint count. For illustration purposes, the composite variable is standardized to the same mean and standard deviation as the HAQ. As illustrated in Figure 4.2, the change in disease activity parallels the change in HAQ. In Figure 4.3, persistently high levels of disease activity lead to the increased HAQ score over time. Small changes in disease activity can be detected by serial observation. Figure 4.4 breaks the disease activity score into two components. The first (solid line) is a composite variable of HAQ, pain, and patient global. The dashed line represents a composite of ESR and tender joint count. As illustrated in the graph, the level of disease activity is similar in both curves, and one follows the other closely. These data indicate that self-report questionnaires and objective measure report similar information. The effects of the combined measures are seen in the dashed lines of Figures 4.2 and 4.3. Using flow sheets rather than graphs, the clinician can synthesize the results in a similar manner.

In general, changes of 20% in a single self-report measure are likely to be clinically important, provided most self-report scores are in the same direction of improvement or worsening. Wells and Tugwell suggested that clinically significant changes in pain and global severity scores occurred at a change level of 10%, a level similar to the level of clinically significant change in HAQ scores (47). Thus, on a 0-to-10 VAS scale, a 1-U change would be clinically important; on a 1-to-3 VAS scale, a 0.3-U change would be important. Sleep or fatigue scales are increasingly being used in clinical

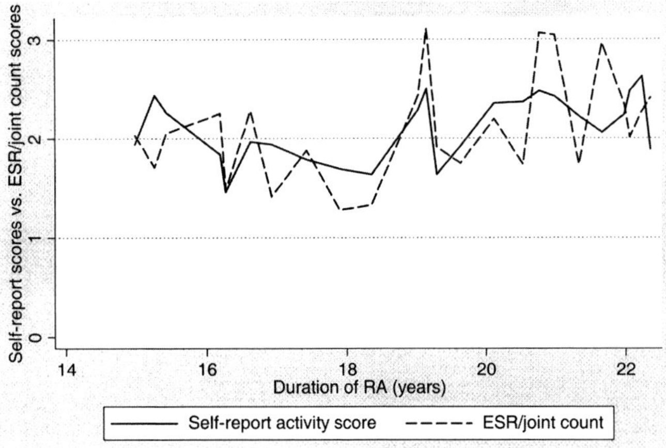

Figure 4.4. Composite scores for erythrocyte sedimentation rate (ESR)/tender joint count and Health Assessment Questionnaire (HAQ), visual acuity score (VAS) pain, and VAS patient global from principal component analyses for patient in Figure 4.3. Note that the "objective" ESR and tender joint count and the "subjective" self-report measure yield similar information.

trials and clinical care, but, as yet, no data are available on clinically significant changes for these scales. Even so, the 10% level of change suggested for pain and global scores seems likely to apply here as well. Perhaps more important than single guidelines is the trend suggested when the results of several questionnaire scales are examined together, along with standard clinical measures such as the joint examination and acute phase reactants. When considering many scales in concert, small changes in clinical activity can be detected that cannot be detected when only physician and laboratory measures are used. The 10% change that has been judged to be important to patients can only be reliably stated to be a "true" 10% when it is in agreement with most other self-report measures. If the multiple measures seem randomly "up and down," then a 10% change is not to be considered reliable. Consistency of change and clinical context impart meaning to questionnaire values and allow meaning to be extracted from them.

PREDICTIVE VALUE OF SELF-REPORT QUESTIONNAIRES

Clinical measures are sometimes categorized as being either process measures or outcome measures. A *process measure* is one that, if the inflammatory process were turned off, as with an effective treatment, the measure would return to normal. Specifically, one might expect pain, ESR, and joint count to return to normal with the removal of the inflammatory process. The component of functional disability due to structural damage, however, would not return to normal because damaged and deformed joints are permanent conditions. Nor would comorbidities, such as cardiovascular disease, remit with the resolution of inflammation. Therefore, it should come as no surprise that functional status is a much better predictor of long-term outcomes than process measures. In fact, that process measures predict long-term outcome at all is only the result of inflammation that does not remit.

RELEVANCE OF QUESTIONNAIRE DATA: RESEARCH EVIDENCE

The recommendation to use self-report measures, particularly functional measures, is supported by a vast body of research evidence. For every long-term outcome, self-report questionnaires, by far, have greater predictive ability for that outcome than do physician or laboratory measures, or both. Abnormal scores on HAQ questionnaires identify patients who are at greater risk for subsequent work disability (49–53). Functional status questionnaires are, similarly, most effective in predicting mortality (5,7,52,54–58). As shown in a recent report, pain and global severity were significantly more effective than laboratory tests to predict mortality, but HAQ is substantially better than all laboratory and self-report measures. In multivariate analyses, HAQ, depression, comorbidity, rheumatoid factors, ESR, age, and gender, but not other clinical variables, predicted mortality in 1,387 RA patients, and HAQ was the strongest predictor (59). In addition, self-report measures provide important information in regard to total joint replacement (60), response to therapy (61–63), radiographic progression (64,65), utilization of services (66,67), depression (68–72), fatigue (39,73,74), sleep disturbance (39), helplessness (75–77), and global quality of life (78,79).

In predicting outcome, clinicians know that it is not merely the degree of clinical abnormality present that is important, but also its persistence. This observation has been confirmed in long-term studies of work disability (50), joint replacement (60), and mortality (59) in which prolonged observations much better predicted outcome than single or few assessments.

Taken together, the evidence indicates that questionnaire data are useful in the clinic and in research. In fact, self-report data may afford an even more powerful tool than would otherwise be suggested by the data. Although physicians may examine some or all joints, they rarely record this information. In addition, laboratory tests are usually not available at the time of the clinical interview. Practically, questionnaire data may represent the only quantitative information available to the clinician at the visit.

Although the measurement of pain, function, and other self-report items is important in the evaluation of patients with RA, these tools can be applied to the assessment of patients with illnesses such as scleroderma (81), systemic lupus erythematosus (81), fibromyalgia (66,74,82), and other disorders (39,80). This observation is particularly important, as it suggests that questionnaires can be used for all patients to improve medical decisions. Sometimes clinicians think that they will use questionnaires just for RA patients or just for lupus patients. Under such conditions, questionnaires usually fail, because it is not easy to keep organized within the administrative aspects of the clinic which patients have which diagnosis. Soon data begin to be missed, and the process becomes haphazard and discouraging. Because the benefits of questionnaire data are great in all rheumatic illnesses and the costs of administration are low, the best path is to use questionnaires in all patients regardless of diagnosis.

REFERENCES

1. Gabriel SE, Crowson CS, O'Fallon WM. Mortality in rheumatoid arthritis: have we made an impact in 4 decades? *J Rheumatol* 1999;26:2529–2533.
2. Goodson N, Symmons D. Rheumatoid arthritis in women: still associated with an increased mortality. *Ann Rheum Dis* 2002;61:955–956.
3. Wiles NJ, Lunt M, Barrett EM, et al. Reduced disability at five years with early treatment of inflammatory polyarthritis: results from a large observational cohort, using propensity models to adjust for disease severity. *Arthritis Rheum* 2001;44:1033–1042.
4. Wolfe F. A reappraisal of HAQ disability in rheumatoid arthritis. *Arthritis Rheum* 2000;43:2751–2761.
5. Choi HK, Hernan MA, Seeger JD, et al. Methotrexate therapy and mortality in patients with rheumatoid arthritis: a prospective study. *Lancet* 2002;359:1173–1177.
6. Wolfe F. A brief health status instrument: CLINHAQ. *Arthritis Rheum* 1989; 32:S99.

7. Wolfe F. The prognosis of rheumatoid arthritis: assessment of disease activity and disease severity in the clinic. *Am J Med* 1997;103:12S–18S.
8. Wolfe F. Rheumatoid arthritis. 1991;3:37–82.
9. Wolfe F. The determination and measurement of functional disability in rheumatoid arthritis. *Arthritis Res* 2002;4[Suppl 2]:S11–S15.
10. Fries JF, Spitz PW, Kraines RG, et al. Measurement of patient outcome in arthritis. *Arthritis Rheum* 1980;23:137–145.
11. Ramey DR, Raynauld JP, Fries JF. The health assessment questionnaire 1992: status and review. *Arthritis Care Res* 1992;5:119–129.
12. Wolfe F, Flowers N, Anderson J. The National Rheumatic Disease Data Bank: case mix and severity characteristics of patients in rheumatological practice. *Arthritis Rheum* 1998;41:S132.
13. Pincus T, Summey JA, Soraci SA, et al. Assessment of patient satisfaction in activities of daily living using a modified Stanford Health Assessment Questionnaire. *Arthritis Rheum* 1983;26:1346–1353.
14. Ware JEJ, Kosinski M. The SF-36® Physical and Mental Health Summary Scales: A Manual for Users of Version 1, 2nd ed. Lincoln, RI: QualityMetric, 2001:1.
15. Ware JE, Jr. Using generic measures of functional health and well-being to increase understanding of disease burden. *Spine* 2000;25:1467.
16. Keller SD, Majkut TC, Kosinski M, et al. Monitoring health outcomes among patients with arthritis using the SF-36 Health Survey: overview. *Med Care* 1999;37[Suppl 5]:MS1–MS9.
17. Bland JM, Altman DG. Comparing methods of measurement: why plotting difference against standard method is misleading. *Lancet* 1995;346:1087.
18. Greenwood MC, Doyle DV, Ensor M. Does the Stanford Health Assessment Questionnaire have potential as a monitoring tool for subjects with rheumatoid arthritis? *Ann Rheum Dis* 2001;60:344–348.
19. Wolfe F, Pincus T, Fries JF. Usefulness of the HAQ in the clinic. *Ann Rheum Dis* 2001;60:811.
20. Meenan RF, Gertman PM, Mason JH. Measuring health status in arthritis: the arthritis impact measurement scales. *Arthritis Rheum* 1980;23:146–152.
21. Wolfe F. Data collection and utilization: a methodology for clinical practice and clinical research. 1994;22:463–514.
22. Meenan RF, Mason JH, Anderson JJ, et al. AIMS2. The content and properties of a revised and expanded Arthritis Impact Measurement Scales Health Status Questionnaire. *Arthritis Rheum* 1992;35:1–10.
23. Tugwell P, Bombardier C, Buchanan WW, Goldsmith CH, Grace E, Hanna B. The MACTAR patient preference disability questionnaire—an individualized functional priority approach for assessing improvement in physical disability in clinical trials in rheumatoid arthritis. *J Rheumatol* 1987;14:446–451.
24. Ware J Jr, Kosinski M, Keller SD. A 12-item short form health survey: construction of scales and preliminary tests of reliability and validity. *Med Care* 1996;34:220–233.
25. Bergner M, Bobbitt RA, Carter WB, et al. The Sickness Impact Profile: development and final revision of a health status measure. *Med Care* 1981;19:787–805.
26. Hunt SM, McKenna SP, McEwen J, et al. The Nottingham Health Profile: subjective health status and medical consultations. *Soc Sci Med* 1981;15A:221–229.
27. Haavardsholm EA, Kvien TK, Uhlig T, et al. Comparison of agreement and sensitivity to change between AIMS2 and a short form of AIMS2 (AIMS2-SF) in more than 1000 rheumatoid arthritis patients. *J Rheumatol* 2000;27:2810–2816.
28. Wallston KA, Brown GK, Stein MJ, et al. Comparing the short and long versions of the Arthritis Impact Measurement Scales. *J Rheumatol* 1989;16:1105–1109.
29. Pincus T, Larsen A, Brooks RH, et al. Comparison of 3 quantitative measures of hand radiographs in patients with rheumatoid arthritis: Steinbrocker stage, Kaye modified Sharp score, and Larsen score. *J Rheumatol* 1997; 24:2106–2112.
30. Wolfe F. Which HAQ is best? A comparison of the HAQ, MHAQ and RA-HAQ, a difficult 8 item HAQ (DHAQ), and a rescored 20 item HAQ (HAQ20): analyses in 2,491 rheumatoid arthritis patients following leflunomide initiation. *J Rheumatol* 2001;28:982–989.
31. Pincus T, Swearingen C, Wolfe F. Toward a multidimensional Health Assessment Questionnaire (MDHAQ)—assessment of advanced activities of daily living and psychological status in the patient-friendly health assessment questionnaire format. *Arthritis Rheum* 1999;42:2220–2230.
32. Wolfe F, Pincus T, Tennant A. HAQ-II: application of modern item response theory to the design of an improved HAQ questionnaire. *Ann Rheum Dis* 2002.
33. Melzack R. The McGill pain questionnaire: major properties and scoring methods. *Pain* 1975;1:277–299.
34. Zaza C, Reyno L, Moulin DE. The Multidimensional Pain Inventory profiles in patients with chronic cancer-related pain: an examination of generalizability. *Pain* 2000;87:75–82.
35. Kerns RD, Turk DC, Rudy TE. The West Haven-Yale multidimensional pain inventory (WHYMPI). *Pain* 1985;24:345–356.
36. Paul-Dauphin A, Guillemin F, Virion JM, et al. Bias and precision in visual analogue scales: a randomized controlled trial. *Am J Epidemiol* 1999;150:1117–1127.
37. Wolfe F, Pincus T. Current comment—listening to the patient—a practical guide to self-report questionnaires in clinical care. *Arthritis Rheum* 1999; 42:1797–1808.
38. Wolfe F. Determinants of WOMAC function, pain and stiffness scores: evidence for the role of low back pain, symptom counts, fatigue and depression in osteoarthritis, rheumatoid arthritis and fibromyalgia. *Rheumatology (Oxford)* 1999;38:355–361.
39. Wolfe F, Hawley DJ, Wilson K. The prevalence and meaning of fatigue in rheumatic disease. *J Rheumatol* 1996;23:1407–1417.
40. Taylor RR, Jason LA, Torres A. Fatigue rating scales: an empirical comparison. *Psychol Med* 2000;30:849–856.
41. Belza BL. Multidimensional assessment of fatigue (MAF) scale: users guide. 1990.
42. Krupp LB, LaRocca NG, Muir-Nash J, et al. The fatigue severity scale. Application to patients with multiple sclerosis and systemic lupus erythematosus. *Arch Neurol* 1989;46:1121–1123.
43. Pincus T, Wolfe F, Strand V, et al. Patient questionnaire data discriminate between drug versus placebo as effectively as the ACR20 in a clinical trial of patients with rheumatoid arthritis (RA). *Arthritis Rheum Suppl* 2001;43:S288.
44. Wiles NJ, Scott DG, Barrett EM, et al. Benchmarking: the five year outcome of rheumatoid arthritis assessed using a pain score, the Health Assessment Questionnaire, and the Short Form-36 (SF-36) in a community and a clinic based sample. *Ann Rheum Dis* 2001;60:956–961.
45. Wolfe F, Choi HK. Benchmarking and the percentile assessment of RA: adding a new dimension to rheumatic disease measurement. *Ann Rheum Dis* 2001;60:994–995.
46. Redelmeier DA, Lorig K. Assessing the clinical importance of symptomatic improvements—an illustration in rheumatology. *Arch Intern Med* 1993;153:1337–1342.
47. Wells GA, Tugwell P, Kraag GR, et al. Minimum important difference between patients with rheumatoid arthritis: the patient's perspective. *J Rheumatol* 1993;20:557–560.
48. Wright V. Questions on clinical trials [Editorial]. *BMJ* 1983;287:569.
49. Yelin EH. Work disability and rheumatoid arthritis. Rheumatoid arthritis: pathogenesis, assessment, outcome, 1994.
50. Wolfe F, Hawley DJ. The long-term outcomes of rheumatoid arthritis: work disability: a prospective 18 year study of 823 patients. *J Rheumatol* 1998;25:2108–2117.
51. Sokka T, Pincus T. Markers for work disability in rheumatoid arthritis. *J Rheumatol* 2001;28:1718–1722.
52. Pincus T, Callahan LF, Sale WG, et al. Severe functional declines, work disability, and increased mortality in seventy-five rheumatoid arthritis patients studied over nine years. *Arthritis Rheum* 1984;27:864–872.
53. Pincus T, Mitchell JM, Burkhauser RV. Substantial work disability and earnings losses in individuals less than age 65 with osteoarthritis: comparisons with rheumatoid arthritis. *J Clin Epidemiol* 1989;42:449–457.
54. Pincus T, Callahan LF. Taking mortality in rheumatoid arthritis seriously—predictive markers, socioeconomic status and comorbidity [Editorial]. *J Rheumatol* 1986;13:841–845.
55. Pincus T, Sokka T, Wolfe F. Premature mortality in patients with rheumatoid arthritis: evolving concepts. *Arthritis Rheum* 2001;44:1234–1236.
56. Soderlin MK, Nieminen P, Hakala M. Functional status predicts mortality in a community based rheumatoid arthritis population. *J Rheumatol* 1998;25:1895–1899.
57. Symmons DPM, Jones MA, Scott DL, et al. Longterm mortality outcome in patients with rheumatoid arthritis: early presenters continue to do well. *J Rheumatol* 1998;25:1072–1077.
58. Wolfe F, Mitchell DM, Sibley JT, et al. The mortality of rheumatoid arthritis. *Arthritis Rheum* 1994;37:481–494.
59. Wolfe F, Michaud K, Gefeller O, Choi HK. Predicting mortality in rheumatoid arthritis. *Arthritis Rheum* 2003;48:1530–1542.
60. Wolfe F, Zwillich SH. The long-term outcomes of rheumatoid arthritis: a 23-year prospective, longitudinal study of total joint replacement and its predictors in 1,600 patients with rheumatoid arthritis. *Arthritis Rheum* 1998;41: 1072–1082.
61. Wolfe F, Cathey MA. Analysis of methotrexate treatment effect in a longitudinal observational study: utility of cluster analysis. *J Rheumatol* 1991;18:672–677.
62. Fries JF, Williams CA, Singh G, et al. Response to therapy in rheumatoid arthritis is influenced by immediately prior therapy. *J Rheumatol* 1997;24: 838–844.
63. Fries JF, Williams CA, Morfeld D, et al. Reduction in long-term disability in patients with rheumatoid arthritis by disease-modifying antirheumatic drug-based treatment strategies. *Arthritis Rheum* 1996;39:616–622.
64. Summers MN, Haley WE, Reveille JD, et al. Radiographic assessment and psychologic variables as predictors of pain and functional impairment in osteoarthritis of the knee or hip. *Arthritis Rheum* 1988;31:204–209.
65. Wolfe F, Sharp JT. Radiographic outcome of recent-onset rheumatoid arthritis: a 19-year study of radiographic progression. *Arthritis Rheum* 1998;41:1571–1582.
66. Wolfe F, Anderson J, Harkness D, et al. A prospective, longitudinal, multicenter study of service utilization and costs in fibromyalgia [see comments]. *Arthritis Rheum* 1997;40:1560–1570.
67. Wolfe F, Kleinheksel SM, Spitz PW, et al. A multicenter study of hospitalization in rheumatoid arthritis: effect of health care system, severity, and regional difference. *J Rheumatol* 1986;13:277–284.
68. Wolfe F. What use are fibromyalgia control points? *J Rheumatol* 1998;25:546–550.
69. Anderson JJ, Firschein HE, Meenan RF. Sensitivity of a health status measure to short-term clinical changes in arthritis. *Arthritis Rheum* 1989;32:844–850.
70. Hawley DJ, Wolfe F. Effect of light and season on pain and depression in subjects with rheumatic disorders. *Pain* 1994;59:227–234.

71. Hawley DJ, Wolfe F. Depression is not more common in rheumatoid arthritis: a 10 year longitudinal study of 6,608 rheumatic disease patients. *J Rheumatol* 1993;20:2025–2031.
72. Hawley DJ, Wolfe F. Anxiety and depression in patients with rheumatoid arthritis: a prospective study of 400 patients. *J Rheumatol* 1988;15:932–941.
73. Wolfe F, Anderson J, Harkness D, et al. Health status and disease severity in fibromyalgia: results of a six-center longitudinal study [see comments]. *Arthritis Rheum* 1997;40:1571–1579.
74. Wolfe F. The relation between tender points and fibromyalgia symptom variables: evidence that fibromyalgia is not a discrete disorder in the clinic. *Ann Rheum Dis* 1997;56:268–271.
75. Pincus T. Eosinophilia-myalgia syndrome: patient status 2–4 years after onset. *J Rheumatol* 1996;23:19–24.
76. Callahan LF, Brooks RH, Pincus T. Further analysis of learned helplessness in rheumatoid arthritis using a "Rheumatology Attitudes Index." *J Rheumatol* 1988;15:418–426.
77. Nicassio PM, Wallston KA, Callahan LF, et al. The measurement of helplessness in rheumatoid arthritis. The development of the arthritis helplessness index. *J Rheumatol* 1985;12:462–467.
78. Wolfe F, Hawley DJ. Measurement of the quality of life in rheumatic disorders using the EuroQol. *Br J Rheumatol* 1997;36:786–793.
79. Fries JF, Ramey DR. "Arthritis specific" global health analog scales assess "generic" health related quality-of-life in patients with rheumatoid arthritis. *J Rheumatol* 1997;24:1697–1702.
80. Bellamy N. Pain assessment in osteoarthritis: experience with the WOMAC osteoarthritis index. *Semin Arthritis Rheum* 1989;18:14–17.
81. Callahan LF, Smith WJ, Pincus T. Self report questionnaires in five rheumatic diseases: comparisons of health status constructs and associations with formal education level. *Arthritis Care Res* 1989;2:122–131.
82. Callahan LF, Pincus T. A clue from a self-report questionnaire to distinguish rheumatoid arthritis from noninflammatory diffuse musculoskeletal pain. The P-VAS:D-ADL ratio. *Arthritis Rheum* 1990;33:1317–1322.

CHAPTER 5

Clinical and Laboratory Measures

Michael M. Ward

Clinical assessment serves three functions: to aid diagnosis, to permit accurate prognosis, and to evaluate the current status of patients and assess their responses to treatment (1). Measures that are useful for diagnostic purposes are those that accurately distinguish persons with the disease of interest from those who are not affected. Measures that are good prognostic guides are those that accurately predict future health outcomes. Good evaluative measures are those that accurately reflect the severity of symptoms and signs of the disease. Changes in evaluative measures tell if a patient has improved or worsened. Measures that are useful for evaluation may not be useful for diagnosis or prognosis, and vice versa. For example, the severity of joint pain is an excellent evaluative measure but a poor diagnostic and prognostic measure. In contrast, the serum rheumatoid factor (RF) concentration is a useful diagnostic measure but is a poor measure of the activity of a patient's arthritis. This chapter reviews commonly used individual evaluative measures of rheumatoid arthritis (RA), composite indexes of RA activity, and indexes of improvement.

PROPERTIES OF GOOD EVALUATIVE MEASURES

Evaluative measures are judged by their ability to detect changes in clinical status or disease activity over time. Because the goals of evaluation are different from those of diagnosis and prognosis, the methods used to assess evaluative measures also differ from those used to assess diagnostic or prognostic measures. Familiar concepts of diagnostic testing, such as sensitivity, specificity, and predictive values of tests, for example, are not applicable to the assessment of evaluative measures. The focus of evaluation is on intra-individual variation and requires serial observation of patients. The important properties of good evaluative measures are validity, reliability, and sensitivity to change (1–3).

Validity is the measurement properly concerned with whether a questionnaire, laboratory test, or other clinical assessment is a true measure of what it purports to measure. There are two main ways to determine if an evaluative measure is a valid measure of disease activity: criterion validity and construct validity (4). Criterion validity is used when a gold standard measure of disease activity exists and is tested by determining if changes in a candidate measure correlate with simultaneous changes in the gold standard. High correlation of changes in both measures over time within individual patients provides evidence that the new measure is a valid evaluative measure. However, in RA and many other diseases, there is no gold-standard measure of disease activity. In these cases, a group of measures, each reflecting some aspect of disease activity, is used to substitute for a gold standard. This group of measures is considered to represent aspects of the underlying construct of "RA activity," and high within-patient correlations between changes in a candidate measure and simultaneous changes in this group of measures provide evidence for validity of the new measure (Fig. 5.1). This type of validity, based on serial assessments of related measures, is known as *longitudinal construct validity* and is the most appropriate method to assess the validity of measures in the absence of a gold standard (1,2,4). Cross-sectional studies, in which interpatient differences in measures of RA activity are correlated, cannot assess how well these measures capture changes over time and cannot be used to establish the validity of evaluative measures.

Alternatively, validity can be established if measures predict long-term health outcomes. This is most convincingly demonstrated if serial longitudinal assessments of the measure are associated with the outcomes.

Reliability of evaluative measures commonly refers to test–retest reliability (2). Highly reliable measures are those in which repeated assessments in clinically stable patients give closely similar results (3). *Sensitivity to change*, or *responsiveness*, refers to the magnitude of change in a measure that occurs during a change in clinical status. This is most commonly tested by examining the change in a measure before and after administering a known effective treatment to a group of patients with active disease. Measures that are sensitive to change will register large changes with the resultant clinical improvement, whereas measures that are poorly responsive will not change much despite clinical improvement (1–3).

To compute estimates of sensitivity to change, the change in a measure that occurs with treatment is indexed to the variability of the measure in clinically stable patients. Several different statistics are available to compute sensitivity to change, including the effect size, the standardized response mean, and the responsiveness statistic (5–7). The effect size, for example, is computed as the change in the measure before and after treatment, divided by the standard deviation of the pretreatment scores. Larger effect sizes indicate measures that are more sensitive to change. Continuous measures, which can capture gradations of responses, are often more sensitive to change than measures that have only a few categories (e.g., excellent, good, fair, poor), and measures that are disease specific tend to be more sensitive to change than generic measures (3–8). Sensitiv-

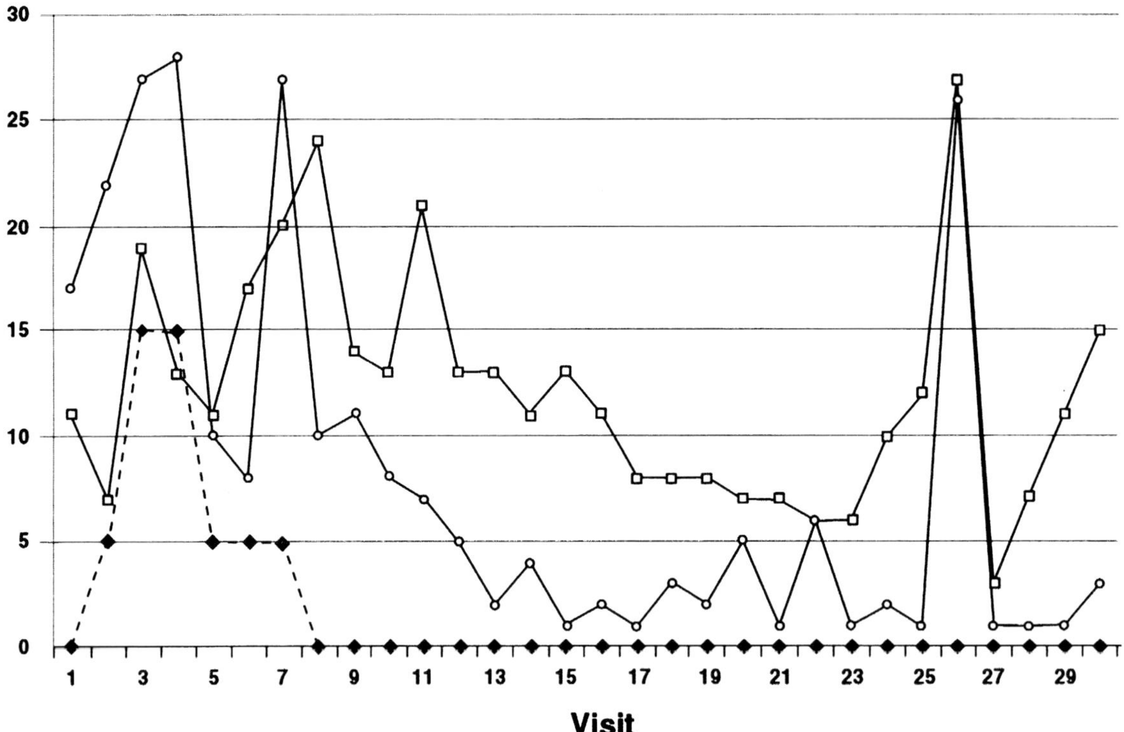

Figure 5.1. Serial measurements of the tender joint count (*squares*), patient-reported pain score (*circles*), and duration of morning stiffness (*diamonds*) in a patient with rheumatoid arthritis recorded on 30 visits made every 2 weeks for 60 weeks (see reference 25). Changes in the duration of morning stiffness do not follow those of the other measures, indicating lower longitudinal construct validity for this measure.

ity to change is best used as a relative measure, providing comparisons among different measures when the measures are assessed simultaneously in the same group of patients.

INDIVIDUAL CLINICAL MEASURES

Joint Counts

Because arthritis is the dominant clinical manifestation of RA, assessment of the extent of joint inflammation has been considered central to the evaluation of RA activity. Because of their key role in defining the disease process and predicting health outcomes, measures to assess joint tenderness and swelling have been universally recommended as core measures of RA activity by the Outcome Measures in Rheumatoid Arthritis Clinical Trials group, the American College of Rheumatology (ACR), the European League Against Rheumatism (EULAR), and the World Health Organization/International League of Associations for Rheumatology (9–12). Although informal assessments of the degree of joint inflammation are typically done in clinical practice, more formal methods are required for clinical trials and observational studies of health outcomes. Despite the fact that there is wide consensus on the importance of these measures in the assessment of RA activity, there is debate on the best ways to quantitate the degree of joint tenderness and swelling.

Several different methods to score joint tenderness and swelling have been developed (Table 5.1) (13–20). Each relies on a count of the number of involved joints, based on the premise that more widespread arthritis indicates more active RA. However, the number of joints assessed varies among measures, and recently proposed counts of 28 joints appear to measure RA activity just as well as counts of larger numbers of joints, despite the exclusion of the ankles and feet (20,21). Some joint count measures, such as the Lansbury index, Ritchie index, and Hart index, measure tender joints only, whereas others, including the American Rheumatism Association counts, the Cooperative Systemic Studies of Rheumatic Diseases counts, the Reduced Joint Survey, and the 28-joint counts, can be used to measure tender joint counts and swollen joint counts separately. The Thompson index records joints as involved only if they are both tender and swollen. The Lansbury and Thompson indexes weigh joints according to the articular surface area, so that larger joints contribute more to the total index than smaller joints. The other indexes weigh each involved joint equally. Weighting by joint size improves the cross-sectional correlations between the joint count measure and acute phase reactants, but the improvement is small in some studies (18,21). The Ritchie index, Cooperative Systemic Studies of Rheumatic Diseases index, and Reduced Joint Survey grade the degree of tenderness (0 = none, 1 = complaint, 2 = wince, 3 = withdraw) or swelling (0 = none, 1 = minimal, 2 = definite, 3 = bulging), whereas other indexes record only the presence or absence of tenderness or swelling.

The longitudinal construct validity of joint count measures for the assessment of RA activity has been demonstrated in numerous clinical trials and observational studies (22–25). In one of the few studies that compared the evaluative performance of different joint counts over time, 28-joint counts and the Reduced Joint Survey were as highly correlated with changes in patients' global assessments, Health Assessment Questionnaire (HAQ) Disability Index scores, and erythrocyte sedimentation rate (ESR) measurements as were more extensive joint counts; unweighted and ungraded counts performed as well as weighted or graded counts (26).

The reliability of joint count measures, particularly between observers, has been found to be low, with intraclass correlations

TABLE 5.1. Joint Count Measures, Including the Number and Type of Joints Included, Whether They Are Weighted or Graded for Severity, and Whether the Measure Includes Tender or Swollen Joints[a]

	Lansbury	ARA	Ritchie	Hart	CSSRD	Thompson	Reduced Joint Survey	28-Joint Count
Number	86	68	26[b]	26[b]	60	38	36	28
Weighted	+	–	–	–	–	+	–	–
Graded	0–1	0–1	0–3	0–1	0–3	0–1	0–3	0–1
Tender	+	+	+	+	+	–	+	+
Swollen	–	+	–	–	+	–	+	+
Both tender and swollen	–	–	–	–	–	+	–	–
Joints included								
Cervical spine			+	+				
Temporomandibular	+	+	+	+	+			
Sternoclavicular	+	+	+	+	+			
Acromioclavicular	+	+	+	+	+			
Shoulder	+	+	+	+	+			+
Elbow	+	+	+	+	+	+	+	+
Wrist	+	+	+	+	+	+	+	+
Metacarpophalangeal	+	+	+	+	+	+	+[c]	+
Finger PIP	+	+	+	+	+	+	+	+
Finger DIP	+	+						
Hip	+	+	+	+	+			
Knee	+	+	+	+	+	+	+	+
Ankle	+	+	+	+	+	+	+	
Subtalar	+	+	+	+	+			
Tarsometatarsal	+		+	+				
Metatarsophalangeal	+	+	+	+	+	+	+	
Toe PIP	+	+			+			

ARA, American Rheumatism Association; CSSRD, Cooperative Systematic Studies of Rheumatic Diseases; DIP, distal interphalangeal; PIP, proximal interphalangeal; +, positive; –, negative.

[a]Hips scored for tenderness only.

[b]The following joint areas are considered as a single unit, with the score of the most involved joint recorded: both temporomandibular joints, both sternoclavicular and acromioclavicular joints, all left metacarpophalangeal joints, all right metacarpophalangeal joints, all left finger PIP joints, all right finger PIP joints, all left metatarsophalangeal joints, and all right metatarsophalangeal joints.

[c]Thumb metacarpophalangeal joints are excluded.

ranging from 0.52 to 0.83 (15,16,27). Grading the severity of joint tenderness contributes greatly to differences between examiners. Using ungraded counts and standardizing the methods of examination can improve the reliability of joint counts (16,28–30). The tender joint count has been found to have high or moderate sensitivity to change, although its sensitivity to change is lower than that of measures of pain and global arthritis assessment in many studies (23,25,31–34). Swollen joint counts tend to be less sensitive to change than tender joint counts, as might be expected if synovial thickening or residual pannus remains despite effective treatment (23,31,32).

Recently, patient-reported joint counts have been tested as an efficient and inexpensive way to assess the extent of joint inflammation. The agreement (by intraclass correlation coefficients; possible range, 0–1) between patients' counts and rheumatologists' counts ranged from 0.31 to 0.88 for tender joint counts, and from –0.02 to 0.56 for swollen joint counts, indicating good agreement in some studies but poor agreement in other studies (35–41). Patients tended to report higher tender joint counts than rheumatologists. The summed circumferences of the proximal interphalangeal joints has been abandoned as a measure of RA activity because of poor reliability and validity.

Symptoms

Pain is the major symptom of RA, and relief of pain is the main reason patients seek medical care (42–46). Pain has been recommended as a core measure of RA activity (9–12). Almost universally, measurement of pain in RA refers to quantification of the intensity of pain rather than assessment of the quality of pain, its location or distribution, or its emotional or behavioral impact (47). Pain intensity may be rated by patients; assessed by other observers, including physicians; or judged based on observed pain behaviors. Most often, patient-reported measures of pain intensity have been used because they are simple, reliable, and valid (47,48). Patient-reported pain scores are among the RA activity measures with the highest sensitivity to change in many studies (25,31,33,34) but not all (23,32).

Several self-report scales have been used to measure pain intensity. The most commonly used measure is the horizontal visual analog scale (VAS), a 10-cm or 15-cm line, often labeled at the ends with anchoring descriptors of "No Pain" and "Pain as Bad as It Could Be," on which patients mark the level of pain they have experienced today, in the past week, or in some other specified interval (48). A VAS is used as the measure of pain in the HAQ. Rating scales that use numbers ("Rate your pain on a scale of 0 to 10"), words to describe pain intensity, or faces to depict pain intensity may be simpler, but the ordinal scale of these measures makes it more difficult to interpret changes in such scales. Single-item rating scales are often less sensitive to change than VASs (32,48,49). The pain subscale of the Arthritis Impact Measurement Scales (AIMS) is a composite measure of several verbal rating scales and has been found to be highly sensitive to change (32,34,46,50–54).

Because patients' reports of pain intensity may be affected by their mood, some investigators have advocated use of measures that are less susceptible to such bias (55,56). A method to quantify pain behaviors, such as guarding, grimacing, and rubbing, observed as patients perform a standardized set of maneuvers while being videotaped, has been shown to correlate well with patient-reported pain intensity, independent observers' ratings, and other measures of RA activity (55,57,58). However, the need for trained raters and the complexity and expense of this measurement technique has limited its use.

Although traditionally used as an indicator of inflammatory arthritis, the duration of morning stiffness correlates less well with other measures of RA activity and is only moderately sensitive to change (23–25,31,32). For these reasons, morning stiffness has not been recommended as a core measure of RA activity. Part of the difficulty with this measure is a problem in establishing a precise definition. Patients variably interpret morning stiffness to mean pain, limited movement, tightness, or functional limitation, and its duration may be timed from either awakening or arising to either first improvement or maximal improvement (59–62). Large intrapatient variability likely contributes to its lower sensitivity to change (61). Measurement of the severity of morning stiffness may be more reliable and responsive than measurement of the duration of morning stiffness (60,63).

Fatigue is a common symptom of RA but has not often been studied as a measure of RA activity, likely because it is too nonspecific. Some measures of general health status include subscales that specifically assess fatigue (see below).

Functional Disability

Functional disability refers to the degree of difficulty a person has in performing activities of daily living, such as eating, dressing, personal hygiene, and mobility. Functional disability is less exclusively a measure of RA activity than other measures considered here, because it may develop as a consequence of joint damage, deformity, and muscle weakness, as well as because of reversible inflammatory arthritis. Because functional disability is an integrated measure of damage and inflammation, the relative contribution of these components to functional disability scores may be difficult to discern in an individual patient at a given time. As in the measurement of pain, there can be different reporters of functional disability: self-reported by the patient; judged by other observers, including physicians; or directly tested in performance-based measures. Patient-reported measures have been most commonly used because of their ease of administration and excellent measurement properties and have been recommended as core measures of RA activity (9,10,12).

There are numerous patient-reported measures of functional disability that exist either as stand-alone questionnaires or as components of questionnaires that also ask about other aspects of health status or health-related quality of life (64). In RA, the HAQ Disability Index and the AIMS physical function scales have been used most often. The HAQ Disability Index is a 20-question index that asks respondents to report the degree of difficulty (0 = no difficulty, 1 = some difficulty, 2 = much difficulty, 3 = unable to do) they have experienced performing tasks in eight areas (dressing, arising, eating, walking, hygiene, reaching, gripping, and errands and chores) in the past week (65; available at http://aramis.stanford.edu). The highest scores in each functional area are averaged to compute the Disability Index, which is an ordinal scale with increments of 0.125 and a possible range of 0 to 3. Use of aids or the need for help from another person to perform a task can also be incorporated in the scoring. The reliability and longitudinal construct validity of the HAQ Disability Index have been extensively documented (66,67). In clinical trials and observational studies, the sensitivity to change of the Disability Index has been found to be moderately high, although often lower than that of pain scores and global assessments (22,25,32,34,54,66–68). This lower sensitivity to change is likely due to the fact that measures of functional disability represent irreversible joint damage, as well as joint inflammation. Shorter versions of the HAQ Disability Index have been developed, including the modified HAQ and the RA-HAQ, but these instruments discriminate levels of functional disability less well than the full index and may be less sensitive to change (33,69–71).

The original AIMS has been supplanted by the AIMS2, the physical functioning component of which is a 28-item questionnaire that asks respondents to report how often in the past month they experienced difficulty performing tasks in six functional areas (mobility, walking and bending, hand and finger function, arm function, self-care, and household tasks) (46). Possible responses can range from 0 (no days) to 5 (all days); scores in each functional area are summed, normalized to a 0 to 10 scale, and then scores in the six functional areas are summed, for a possible range of 0 to 60. A shorter version of the AIMS2 has also been developed (72). The reliability, longitudinal construct validity, and sensitivity to change of the AIMS and AIMS2 physical functioning component and its subscales have been established in several clinical trials and observational studies (32,34,51–54,72–75). In some studies, the sensitivity to change of the AIMS physical functioning scale was lower than that of the HAQ Disability Index when these were directly compared (32,34,54,75).

The McMaster Toronto Arthritis Patient Preference Disability Questionnaire (MACTAR) differs from many other functional disability assessment tools by eliciting and measuring changes in five functional tasks nominated by the patient as the ones he or she would most like to improve, rather than rating a set list of tasks as in the HAQ Disability Index or AIMS (76,77). This approach is more relevant for each patient, and, as only problematic tasks are included, the MACTAR may be more sensitive to change than questionnaires that include a standard set of tasks. The MACTAR is administered as a semistructured interview, which reduces its ease of application, and there is some concern about the appropriateness of aggregating results when the tasks that are rated vary greatly among patients.

Patient-reported measures of functional disability may be affected by the mood of the patient but less so than measures of pain (56,78–83). Observer-based measures of functional disability, less susceptible to confounding by mood, have long been used to classify patients. The four-category American Rheumatism Association, or Steinbrocker, classification of functional disability was revised to the ACR 1991 criteria for the classification of global functional status (84,85). This measure retains the four hierarchical categories of the original scale, but the classes are now defined as *no limitations* (class I), *limited in avocational activities only* (class II), *limited in vocational and avocational activities* (class III), and *limited in self-care, vocational and avocational activities* (class IV). Although useful to describe patients' functional status in broad terms, these categories are too crude for this measure to be a useful evaluative measure. The Keitel functional index records limitations in joint motion as well as difficulty performing certain tasks such as walking and rising from a chair (86). Therefore, it assesses a mix of impairments and disabilities, rather than specifically measuring functional disability, and has been rarely used in clinical trials (87).

Performance-based measures of functional disability include measurement of grip strength, walking time, and the button test. As with other measures of functional disability, these measures are influenced by joint damage and deformity, as well as by joint inflammation (88). The ability of these measures to predict long-term outcomes, including mortality, may relate more to their measurement of damage than to the fact that they are markers of RA activity (89). These measures also depend on the effort and enthusiasm of the patient, which can contribute to measurement error. These measures tend to have lower longitudinal construct validity, tend to be less sensitive to change than other measures of functioning, and have not been recommended as core measures of RA activity (23,25,31,32,34,90).

Global Arthritis Assessment

Patient and physician global assessments provide an overall assessment of RA activity, asking the rater to integrate and summarize in a single impression all the ways in which RA is currently impacting the patient. These measures usually have the form of a single VAS on which respondents rate their current overall status. Occasionally, these measures have the form of transition questions, which ask respondents to rate the degree of change in overall RA activity since the last visit or since the start of a new treatment. Patient and physician global assessments have good longitudinal construct validity, reliability, and sensitivity to change and are recommended as core measures of RA activity (9–12,23,25,31–34). Not unexpectedly, global assessments of the transition format are more sensitive to change than those rating current status (32,34).

General Health Status and Health-Related Quality of Life

Pain and functional disability are major consequences of RA, but other aspects of life may also be impacted and be important to patients. These include mental health, fatigue, sleep, social interactions, and ability to perform at work, home, or school (64). Assessment of these additional aspects of health status may provide important information about how RA is affecting an individual, which might not otherwise be discovered by the use of more focused assessments. For example, the impact of extraarticular manifestations of RA may be captured by general health status measures but would not otherwise be considered in the assessment of RA activity.

Many general health status surveys and profiles have been developed, and many have been tested in RA (64,91,92). The most commonly used general health status survey in RA has been the Medical Outcomes Study Short-Form 36 (SF-36), a 36-item questionnaire that asks respondents how often they experience limitations in eight areas (physical functioning, role limitations due to physical problems, pain, general health perceptions, vitality, social functioning, role limitations due to emotional problems, and mental health) (93,94). Summary physical and mental subscales can be computed from the first four categories and the last four categories, respectively. Shorter versions of the SF-36, as well as an arthritis-specific health index derived from the SF-36, have also been developed (95).

Because general health measures include aspects of health that might not be directly affected by RA, the sensitivity to change of these measures may be lower than more targeted measures of RA activity. In a recent clinical trial of methotrexate and leflunomide, the SF-36 physical component demonstrated good sensitivity to change, but mental component scales did not improve (33). However, in a small study of etanercept in RA, the SF-36 mental component scale and several subscales showed improvement (96).

Health-related quality of life is an even broader concept that builds on general health status and health perceptions and includes the impact of health status on a person's life, his or her emotional response to this impact, and his or her satisfaction (64,97). Measures of health-related quality of life include questionnaire- and interview-based assessments, as well as utilities, which measure a person's preference for, or valuation of, a particular state of health (64). How well these measures capture changes in RA activity is uncertain, as few have been tested in longitudinal studies. A recently developed RA-specific quality-of-life measure, the Rheumatoid Arthritis Quality of Life (RAQoL) questionnaire, may be a useful addition if it can be demonstrated to be highly sensitive to change (98–99).

LABORATORY MEASURES

Erythrocyte Sedimentation Rate

The ESR, an indirect measure of the acute phase response, has long been used as a measure of RA activity. Of the several different methods of measuring the ESR, the Westergren method has been most commonly used. In general, the ESR improves along with other RA activity measures with initiation of effective treatment and can predict long-term health outcomes (24,100–104). However, it is less clear how closely the ESR tracks short-term changes in RA activity, with low or only moderately high correlations between changes in the ESR and changes in other RA activity measures. However, the Westergren ESR performed better than other laboratory measures, including the C-reactive protein (CRP) concentration, in these analyses (25,105–107). These low-to-moderate correlations may be due to the influence of factors other than RA activity on the ESR, including anemia, abnormalities in red blood cell morphology, and intercurrent illnesses. Age and gender also affect the ESR, but these would not influence short-term within-patient evaluations using the ESR.

In general, the sensitivity to change of the ESR has been found to be lower than that of many other measures of RA activity (23,25,31,32,34), although some studies found its sensitivity to change to be comparable to that of other measures (33). Recommendations for core measures of RA activity include a laboratory test of the acute phase response, including either the ESR or CRP, but neither test has been specifically recommended (9–12).

Acute Phase Reactants

Many acute phase reactants have been studied as markers of RA activity, but the CRP has been favored based on the abrupt changes in its serum concentration that occur after an inflammatory stimulus, its short serum half-life, and its ability to predict radiologic damage and disability (106–111). Few longitudinal studies have directly compared the construct validity of the CRP and ESR, but the available evidence indicates that short-term changes in both measures correlate equally well with changes in other RA activity measures (105,112). It is difficult to draw firm conclusions about the relative sensitivity to change of the ESR and CRP, because few studies report results for both tests. In most recent controlled trials that reported both tests, effect sizes of the CRP were either similar to or lower than those of the ESR, indicating that the CRP may be less sensitive to change than the ESR (34,113–118).

Rheumatoid Factor

Serum concentrations of immunoglobulin M RF, measured by semiquantitative methods, such as latex fixation or sheep-cell agglutination, have not been useful evaluative tests in RA because changes in titers generally occur slowly and often lag behind other markers of RA activity (119–121). In clinical trials, use of effective antirheumatic treatments has led to decreases in RF concentrations, but the crude gradations of the titer make it poorly sensitive to change (119–125). Use of newer techniques to quantify RF concentrations, such as nephelometry and fluoroimmunoassay, may improve the sensitivity to change of this measure (126,127).

POOLED INDEXES

The diversity of measures of RA activity makes it difficult to categorize the status of patients concisely. Efforts to develop

TABLE 5.2. Pooled Indexes and Their Component Measures

	Lansbury	Mallya-Mace	Van Riel	Index of Disease Activity	Stoke	DAS	Chronic Arthritis Systemic Index	Overall Status in RA	RADAI	ARA Remission
Ritchie index		+			+	+	+			
Tender joint count			+						+	+
Swollen joint count					+	+				+
Tender and swollen joint count				+				+		
Pain		+		+			+	+	+	+
Morning stiffness	+	+	+		+			+	+	+
Grip strength	+	+		+						
HAQ Disability Index				+			+			
Patient global assessment						+		+	+	
Fatigue	+									+
Extraarticular features								+		
Aspirin consumption	+									
ESR	+	+	+	+	+	+	+			+
C-reactive protein					+					
Hemoglobin		+	+	+						

ARA, American Rheumatism Association; DAS, Disease Activity Score; ESR, erythrocyte sedimentation rate; HAQ, Health Assessment Questionnaire; RADAI, Rheumatoid Arthritis Disease Activity Index.

indexes of RA activity that combine the scores of individual activity measures have been motivated by a desire to describe RA activity comprehensively but succinctly. Use of a single pooled measure in clinical trials would help reduce the problems of interpretation that arise when multiple measures are tested and would possibly have greater sensitivity to change than individual measures (128). Pooled indexes have also been reported to have better longitudinal construct validity than individual measures and to be more highly associated with outcomes of RA, including functional disability and radiographic damage (105).

Resistance to the use of pooled measures results from concern about the appropriate choice and weighting of the composite measures, problems with interpretability of a pooled index, and, for some indexes, difficulty computing them. Despite these perceived difficulties, the attractiveness of a single summary measure has led to the development of numerous pooled indexes, which combine clinical measures, or clinical and laboratory measures, into a single scale to describe current RA activity (Table 5.2). These indexes should be distinguished from response criteria, which specifically measure changes in RA activity over time.

The Lansbury systemic index is an ad hoc measure developed to complement the Lansbury articular index (129). It includes grip strength, morning stiffness, and the time to onset of fatigue after awakening, which is difficult to measure. Pain is measured using daily aspirin consumption as a surrogate, making this index of historical interest only (130). The Mallya-Mace index is another ad hoc measure that grades each of six measures into four categories, with the final index being the average grade (131). This index uses the Ritchie articular index, pain scale, and ESR but also includes the poorly responsive measure of morning stiffness and the less-valid measures of grip strength and hemoglobin concentration. The van Riel index and the Index of Disease Activity are modifications of the Mallya-Mace index that delete or substitute some measures of the original index (132,133). These measures have been criticized for using grades, which are arbitrarily defined and convey less information than continuous measures, and for including the hemoglobin concentration (130).

The Stoke index is an ad hoc index that uses a hierarchical combination of five measures in a branching tree algorithm to classify patients into 1 of 17 ranked classes of RA activity (134). The ranking is heavily dependent on the first measure in the algorithm, the degree of proximal interphalangeal synovitis, and on laboratory tests, including both the ESR and CRP, but many other aspects of RA activity are not included. The index was able to detect improvement in patients treated with disease-modifying medications, and time-averaged scores on the Stoke index predicted mortality (135,136). Limited evidence suggests the Stoke index may be more sensitive to change than the Mallya-Mace index (134).

The most carefully developed and widely used pooled index is the Disease Activity Score (DAS) (137). This index was derived from a longitudinal observational study of patients in which 19 clinical and laboratory measures were tested for their ability to discriminate periods of active RA from inactive RA. Periods of active RA were identified using the implicit judgments of treating rheumatologists, based on their decision to begin treatment with a disease-modifying medication or to discontinue a disease-modifying medication because of ineffectiveness. The DAS is a weighted sum of four measures, calculated as

$$(0.53938 \times \sqrt{\text{Richie index}}) + (0.06465 \times \text{swollen joint count}) + (0.33 \times \ln \text{ESR}) + (0.00722 \times \text{patient general health assessment})$$

Alternative forms that exclude the general health scale and that are based on counts of 28 tender and swollen joints have also been developed (138). The DAS reliably detects improvement in patients treated with disease-modifying medications (105,139). The validity of the DAS was comparable to the Mallya-Mace index, but the DAS may be more sensitive to change than other indexes and individual activity measures (140,141). The DAS has been criticized for computational difficulty and low interpretability.

The Chronic Arthritis Systemic Index was developed by factor analysis of 29 individual activity measures (142). This index is a weighted sum of one measure (HAQ Disability Index, pain scale, ESR, and Ritchie index) from each of the four factors that contributed most to interpatient variation in RA activity. In initial studies, the index was reliable and able to detect changes in RA activity over time. More extensive testing of its longitudinal construct validity and sensitivity to change are needed. The Overall Status in Rheumatoid Arthritis activity measure is an ad hoc measure designed as a quick clinical tool for use in practice and includes extraarticular manifestations, as well as patient global assessment, pain, morning stiffness, and tender and swollen joint counts (143). Initial testing demonstrated adequate reliability and the ability of the index to detect improvement in patients after hospitalization and in outpatients, but it may be less sensitive to change than the DAS and Mallya-Mace index (144). The Rheumatoid Arthritis Disease Activity Index is unique in that all items, including joint counts, are patient reported (145–147). In one small study, the Rheumatoid Arthritis Disease Activity Index and the DAS were equally sensitive to change (148); further testing of its responsiveness and longitudinal construct validity is needed.

Remission is the particular state of absence of RA activity. The ACR preliminary criteria for remission were developed as the combination of clinical and laboratory measures that best differentiated patients in remission from those with some RA activity using rheumatologists' assessments as the gold standard (149). The criteria include morning stiffness of 15 minutes or less, no fatigue, no joint pain, no joint tenderness on examination, no swelling in joints or tendon sheaths, and a normal ESR. Among patients who met at least five of these criteria for 2 consecutive months, these criteria had a sensitivity of 0.72 and a specificity of 0.96 for remission. The criteria apply regardless of medication use. The current U.S. Food and Drug Administration definition of *remission* requires both satisfaction of the ACR criteria and absence of radiographic progression for 6 months—while off of all antirheumatic medications (150). Using the ACR criteria as the standard, a DAS score of less than 1.6 indicates clinical remission (151).

RESPONSE CRITERIA AND CRITERIA FOR CLINICALLY IMPORTANT IMPROVEMENT

The purpose of evaluative measurement is to determine if a patient's condition has improved or worsened. Two critical questions are as follows: (a) How much of a change in clinical status is needed before a change is recognized? and (b) How large must the change be before it is recognized as an important or meaningful change? Determining benchmarks for clinically important changes in measures of RA activity is necessary because these provide gauges by which to judge the effectiveness of treatment. Such estimates can be used in the planning of clinical trials to ensure that sufficiently large samples are studied so that improvements of a degree considered to be clinically important can be detected.

Several types of change can be defined (152). First, the minimal potentially detectable change represents the smallest unit change that a measure can register (e.g., one joint in a tender joint count or 1 mm per hour in the ESR). Measures that are more finely graded would be capable of registering smaller changes than crudely graded measures and would permit more subtle changes to be recognized as potentially important. A second type of change, the minimum detectable change, uses statistical estimates of the repeatability of a measure in clinically stable patients to project the degree of change that would need to occur in the measure to be confident that the change did not occur by chance. Using this approach, Greenwood and colleagues estimated an important change in the HAQ Disability Index to be at least 0.48, based on a statistical assessment of variability of the Disability Index over 2 months in 40 patients with stable RA (153). This analysis did not measure changes or include valuations of those changes.

A third type of change is the observed change in a measure that occurs after use of a known effective treatment, which can be used to estimate the typical or modal change in a measure. If the treatment is accepted as effective, the effects of this treatment can be taken to represent an important change. Kosinski and colleagues applied this method to the results of two randomized controlled trials of nonsteroidal antiinflammatory drugs to relate measured changes in the HAQ Disability Index and the SF-36 to changes in other arthritis activity measures (154). For example, they reported that a 1-grade improvement in the patient global assessment was associated with a mean improvement in the HAQ Disability Index (possible range, 0–3) of 0.24, and of 4.4 points in the physical component subscale of the SF-36 (possible range, 0–100). The investigators interpreted these changes as minimal clinically important differences, based on the premise of expected changes with known effective treatments, but their analysis did not include patients' assessments of changes or their judgments of importance.

These three definitions provide a guide to the degree of change detectable or commonly seen in a measure and have been used to establish response criteria. However, these definitions do not include valuation of the change, which is a critical feature of a clinically important change.

A fourth type of change is an observed or measured change that is explicitly valued as an improvement, a worsening, or no appreciable change. This approach typically assesses a patient before and after a treatment is begun or during a period of changing RA activity. The observed change is then related to a retrospective assessment of whether a change in clinical status was recognized. For example, a patient's pain score may have improved by 15 points (on a 0–100 scale) 1 month after treatment with prednisone, and the patient may judge his or her pain to have improved or not improved over the month. This judgment may be further qualified as to whether an important change has occurred and by degree of importance (minimally important, moderately important, very important). The minimal clinically important difference has received attention as a marker. The minimal clinically important difference represents the smallest change in a measure that is recognizable as a change in clinical status and is distinguishable from more minor changes considered only random variation or noise (155).

This last definition captures the essential conceptual feature of a clinically important change as being a normative standard. Normative standards are those based on the beliefs, opinions, and values of those experiencing the change; they represent the norms of this group of patients. As such, they are intrinsic to the group being assessed (156). The judge of whether an important change has occurred may be the patient or clinician. The most appropriate judge may depend on the specific measure being examined. For example, physicians might be the most appropriate judges of the importance of changes in joint swelling, whereas patients may be the most appropriate judges of the importance of changes in pain severity. This distinction is important because patients and physicians often differ in their assessments of changes in RA activity (157,158). Improvement should be assessed separately from worsening and not considered together as "change" versus "no change," because the amount of change needed to be recognized as an improvement is often larger than the change recognized as a worsening (159,160). Changes may be expressed in absolute or relative terms; for example, an important improvement in the tender joint count may be a decrease of eight or more joints or at least a 30% decrease in the number of tender joints. Valid estimates of clinically important changes can also only be made for measures that are sensitive to change. Changes that may be considered important by a patient may not be registered as a change by a poorly responsive measure.

Perhaps the most difficult aspect of determining clinically important changes is determining these judgments for groups of patients. Assessing whether an important change has occurred in an individual patient is done routinely in clinical practice, but for these criteria to be useful in assessing new treatments, summary estimates of the opinions of representative groups of patients must be generated. Mean changes in a measure that are considered important by a group of patients may be used, but determining the degree of change that has the highest sensitivity and specificity of being identified as an important change by a group of patients may be more informative (161–164).

Despite the importance of knowing what constitutes a clinically important improvement in RA, few studies have been performed to define clinically important changes (152,155). In two small studies, Redelmeier and colleagues assessed the minimum clinically important difference in the HAQ Disability Index (possible range, 0–3) to be approximately 0.20 units, in the pain VAS (possible range, 0–10) to be approximately 0.6 units, and in a global assessment (possible range, 0–10) to be approximately 1.0 unit (159,160). These investigators used the unconventional approach of having patients compare themselves to other patients to determine the boundary between feeling "about the same" and "somewhat better." It is not clear how relevant these social comparisons are to intra-individual valuations of changes in one's own health.

Response Criteria

Response criteria define the degree of change in RA activity measures that categorize a patient as improved or not. They have been considered benchmarks of clinically important improvement because they represent the degree of improvement attributable to known effective treatments (third definition in section Response Criteria and Criteria of Clinically Important Improvement). However, response criteria differ in several important conceptual, methodologic, and practical ways from criteria for clinically important improvements (156). These differences include being relative standards rather than normative standards, being estimated from between-patient differences in response to treatment rather than within-patient longitudinal differences, and dependence on the specific data used to estimate responses to active treatment and placebo. Clinically important changes and response criteria are related but distinct concepts. Estimates of clinically important changes set the standards for change. Response criteria use these standards to judge whether patients have improved.

Response criteria typically include more than one evaluative measure and define both the number of measures and the degree of improvement that needs to be met to qualify as improvement. Although based on a combination of measures, response criteria differ from pooled indexes in that they define transitions in RA activity, rather than describing the state of RA activity at a particular time. Although a number of response criteria have been proposed (165–169), three sets have been most widely used: the Paulus criteria, the ACR preliminary criteria, and the EULAR criteria (Table 5.3) (170–172).

TABLE 5.3. Components of the Paulus Response Criteria, the American College of Rheumatology Preliminary Response Criteria, and the European League Against Rheumatism Response Criteria

Paulus Criteria	American College of Rheumatology Preliminary Criteria	European League Against Rheumatism Criteria
≥20% Improvement in four of the following six measures: Tender joint count Swollen joint count Patient global assessment Physician global assessment Morning stiffness ESR	≥20% Improvement in tender joint count ≥20% Improvement in swollen joint count AND ≥20% Improvement in three of the following five measures: Pain score Patient global assessment Physician global assessment Patient-reported functional disability ESR or CRP	Good response: DAS decreases by >1.2, and final DAS is 2.4 or less Moderate response: DAS decreases by >1.2, but final DAS is >2.4 OR DAS improves by 0.6–1.2, and final DAS is 3.7 or less

CRP, C-reactive protein; DAS, Disease Activity Score; ESR, erythrocyte sedimentation rate.

The Paulus criteria were developed using data from four randomized controlled trials of disease-modifying medications to identify the ability of six evaluative measures (tender joint count, swollen joint count, duration of morning stiffness, ESR, patient global assessment, and physician global assessment) to distinguish placebo-treated patients from those who received active treatment. A cut point of 20% improvement in at least four measures resulted in a low proportion of placebo-treated patients being categorized as improved (12% or less), whereas higher proportions of active-treated patients were categorized as responders (24% or more). These criteria have been used as an end-point measure in several clinical trials (173–184). The Paulus criteria have been criticized for not including all measures in the ACR core set; for including the duration of morning stiffness, which is poorly sensitive to change; and for not requiring that the joint count measures improve (171). In an independent assessment in a controlled trial of minocycline, the Paulus criteria did not discriminate placebo-treated and active-treated patients as well as did the ACR preliminary criteria (185).

The preliminary ACR criteria were selected from a field of 40 candidate criteria sets, including modifications of the Paulus and World Health Organization criteria, variations of the ACR core set of measures, and variations of the DAS (171). This field was narrowed based on expert judgment and, in an analysis of data from five placebo-controlled trials, by how well the criteria maximized the difference in the proportions of active-treated and placebo-treated patients categorized as responders. The final selection was based on face validity of the criteria and consistency ratings of rheumatologists who participated in the development exercise. In this exercise, the preliminary ACR criteria classified 7% of placebo-treated patients as improved, as compared to 39% of patients who received the active treatment. The criteria also performed well in discriminating improvement in patients treated with methotrexate compared to those treated with auranofin in a comparison trial (171). The preliminary ACR criteria have been used as the primary end-point measure in several clinical trials (186–198) and have been recommended by the U. S. Food and Drug Administration in the evaluation of antirheumatic medications (150).

The preliminary ACR criteria tested and validated 20% improvements in its component measures, but, in practice, the criteria have been expanded to include responses of 50% and 70%. Maintenance of 70% responses for at least 6 months has been recommended as a definition of major clinical response (150). Although these more stringent criteria identify patients with more marked improvements, these cut points discriminate less well between treatments of different efficacy than the 20% cut point, with consequent decreased statistical power (199). It has also been proposed that these response criteria can be converted into a measure of disease activity, the "numeric ACR" measure, to characterize RA activity at any given time (200). This proposal confuses measures of states and measures of transition. Because the methods of development and qualities of good state and transition measures differ, use of the numeric ACR measure should be discouraged (201).

The EULAR response criteria differ from other response criteria in specifying criteria for both moderate and good responses and in specifying improvement by both the amount of change and the final degree of RA activity present (172). Its developers contended that improvements in RA activity that do not result in low levels of RA activity should be given less credit than improvements that do result in low levels of RA activity. These response criteria are based on the DAS. Meaningful change in the DAS was determined to be changes greater than twice the measurement error in the DAS when repeatedly assessed in stable patients. The EULAR criteria are comparable to the preliminary ACR criteria in differentiating placebo-treated patients from active-treated patients, and responses predict the likelihood of subsequent radiographic damage (202–204). The EULAR response criteria have been used in several clinical trials (205,206). These response criteria bear the criticisms associated with the DAS and require that patients have a DAS of at least 2.2 to be eligible to have a response.

MEASURES IN CLINICAL PRACTICE

The development of sound evaluative measures has provided a cornerstone for clinical research in RA, but the extent to which these measures are used in clinical practice is unclear. Surveys of rheumatologists indicate that tender and swollen joint counts, global assessments of improvement or worsening, and the duration of morning stiffness are the measures they most commonly use to assess RA activity (207,208). The use of validated instruments, such as the HAQ or AIMS, to quantify pain or functional disability was reported by 16% of Canadian rheumatologists and less than 10% of Australian rheumatologists (207,208). Laboratory testing using either the ESR or CRP is much more common: 86% of American rheumatologists use these tests despite their low correlation with other activity measures and lower sensitivity to change (209). One-half of rheumatologists reported measuring the ESR or CRP on 50% or more of patient visits, but most indicated using them to provide corroborative information and did not alter treatment based on changes in the laboratory tests alone (209).

Rheumatologists differ greatly in their use of measures to assess RA activity and to judge the need for a change in treatment (210,211). Testing of explicit and implicit preferences also suggests that the measures rated by rheumatologists as most important in influencing treatment decisions may not be the ones actually used to make these decisions (210,211). The adoption of standardized measures of health status, such as the HAQ, in clinical practice has been advocated to help assess RA activity more accurately and completely, to assess better the need for changes in treatment, and to elicit the patient's assessment and better incorporate his or her perspective in the treatment plan (212–214). However, in a 1-year randomized controlled trial, providing information on patient-reported pain and functional disability from the HAQ or AIMS to rheumatologists did not result in greater clinical improvement (215). The short study duration, inclusion of patients with stable RA, lack of timing of health status assessments with clinic visits, and unfamiliarity with the measures may have impacted the study results. Whether the routine use of formal evaluative measures in clinical practice would improve the health outcomes of patients with RA remains uncertain.

SUMMARY

Much progress has been made in identifying and developing evaluative measures of RA activity that are reliable, valid, and sensitive to change. Individual measures of symptoms, signs, and laboratory tests continue to be preferred to pooled indexes, and health status and health-related quality of life have been increasingly recognized as important aspects of RA to assess. Response criteria, such as the ACR20, have greatly aided interpretation of clinical trials, but response criteria should not be directly equated to clinically important changes. Research to define clinically important changes in measures of RA activity is needed to better evaluate and compare new treatments.

REFERENCES

1. Kirshner B, Guyatt G. A methodological framework for assessing health indices. *J Chron Dis* 1985;38:27–36.
2. Ward MM. Evaluative laboratory testing. *Arthritis Rheum* 1995;38:1555–1563.
3. Guyatt GH, Kirshner B, Jaeschke R. Measuring health status: what are the necessary measurement properties? *J Clin Epidemiol* 1992;45:1341–1345.
4. Streiner DL, Norman GR. *Health measurement scales: a practical guide to their development and use.* New York, Oxford University Press, 1989.
5. Katz JN, Larson MG, Phillips CB, et al. Comparative measurement sensitivity of short and longer health status instruments. *Med Care* 1992;30:917–925.
6. Stucki G, Liang MH, Fossel AH, et al. Relative responsiveness of condition-specific and generic health status measures in degenerative lumbar spinal stenosis. *J Clin Epidemiol* 1995;48:1369–1378.
7. Wright JG, Young NL. A comparison of different indices of responsiveness. *J Clin Epidemiol* 1997;50:239–246.
8. Laupacis A, Wong C. The use of generic and specific quality-of-life measures in hemodialysis patients treated with erythropoietin. The Canadian Erythropoietin Study Group. *Control Clin Trials* 1991;12:168S–179S.
9. Tugwell P, Boers M. Developing consensus on preliminary core efficacy endpoints for rheumatoid arthritis clinical trials. OMERACT Committee. *J Rheumatol* 1993;20:555–556.
10. Felson DT, Anderson JJ, Boers M, et al. The American College of Rheumatology preliminary core set of disease activity measures for rheumatoid arthritis clinical trials. *Arthritis Rheum* 1993;36:729–740.
11. van Riel PLCM. Provisional guidelines for measuring disease activity in clinical trials on rheumatoid arthritis. *Br J Rheumatol* 1992;31:793–796.
12. Boers M, Tugwell P, Felson DT, et al. World Health Organization and International League of Associations for Rheumatology core endpoints for symptom modifying antirheumatic drugs in rheumatoid arthritis clinical trials. *J Rheumatol* 1994;21[Suppl 41]:86–89.
13. Lansbury J, Haut DD. Quantitation of the manifestations of rheumatoid arthritis. 4. Area of joint surfaces as an index to total joint inflammation and deformity. *Am J Med Sci* 1956;232:150–155.
14. The Cooperating Clinics Committee of the American Rheumatism Association. A seven-day variability study of 499 patients with peripheral rheumatoid arthritis. *Arthritis Rheum* 1965;8:302–334.
15. Ritchie DM, Boyle JA, McInnes JM, et al. Clinical studies with an articular index for the assessment of joint tenderness in patients with rheumatoid arthritis. *QJM* 1968;37:393–406.
16. Hart LE, Tugwell P, Buchanan WW, et al. Grading of tenderness as a source of interrater error in the Ritchie Articular Index. *J Rheumatol* 1985;12:716–717.
17. Williams HJ, Ward JR, Reading JC, et al. Low-dose D-penicillamine therapy in rheumatoid arthritis. A controlled, double-blind clinical trial. *Arthritis Rheum* 1983;26:581–592.
18. Thompson PW, Silman AJ, Kirwan JR, et al. Articular indices of joint inflammation in rheumatoid arthritis. Correlation with the acute-phase response. *Arthritis Rheum* 1987;30:618–623.
19. Egger MJ, Huth DA, Ward JR, et al. Reduced joint count indices in the evaluation of rheumatoid arthritis. *Arthritis Rheum* 1985;28:613–619.
20. Fuchs HA, Brooks RH, Callahan LF, et al. A simplified twenty-eight-joint quantitative articular index in rheumatoid arthritis. *Arthritis Rheum* 1989; 32:531–537.

21. Smolen JS, Breedveld FC, Eberl G, et al. Validity and reliability of the twenty-eight-joint count for the assessment of rheumatoid arthritis activity. *Arthritis Rheum* 1995;38:38–43.
22. van der Heide A, Jacobs JWG, Dinant HJ, et al. The impact of endpoint measures in rheumatoid arthritis clinical trials. *Semin Arthritis Rheum* 1992;21:287–294.
23. Anderson JJ, Felson DT, Meenan RF, et al. Which traditional measures should be used in rheumatoid arthritis clinical trials? *Arthritis Rheum* 1989; 32:1093–1099.
24. Hassell AB, Davis MJ, Fowler PD, et al. The relationship between serial measures of disease activity and outcome in rheumatoid arthritis. *QJM* 1993;86:601–607.
25. Ward MM. Clinical measures in rheumatoid arthritis: which are most useful in assessing patients? *J Rheumatol* 1993;21:17–21.
26. Prevoo MLL, van Riel PLCM, van't Hof MA, et al. Validity and reliability of joint indices. A longitudinal study in patients with recent onset rheumatoid arthritis. *Br J Rheumatol* 1993;32:589–594.
27. Lassere MND, van der Heijde D, Johnson KR, et al. Reliability of measures of disease activity and disease damage in rheumatoid arthritis: implications for smallest detectable difference, minimal clinically important difference, and analysis of treatment effects in randomized controlled trials. *J Rheumatol* 2001;28:892–903.
28. Thompson PW, Hart LE, Goldsmith CH, et al. Comparison of four articular indices for use in clinical trials in rheumatoid arthritis: patient, order and observer variation. *J Rheumatol* 1991;18:661–665.
29. Klinkhoff AV, Bellamy N, Bombardier C, et al. An experiment in reducing interobserver variability of the examination for joint tenderness. *J Rheumatol* 1988;15:492–494.
30. Bellamy N, Anastassiades TP, Buchanan WW, et al. Rheumatoid arthritis antirheumatic drug trials. I. Effects of standardized procedures on observer dependent outcome measures. *J Rheumatol* 1991;18:1893–1900.
31. Gotzsche PC. Sensitivity of effect variables in rheumatoid arthritis: a meta-analysis of 130 placebo controlled NSAID trials. *J Clin Epidemiol* 1990;43:1313–1318.
32. Buchbinder R, Bombardier C, Yeung M, et al. Which outcome measures should be used in rheumatoid arthritis clinical trials? Clinical and quality-of-life measures' responsiveness to treatment in a randomized controlled trial. *Arthritis Rheum* 1995;38:1568–1580.
33. Tugwell P, Wells G, Strand V, et al. Clinical improvement as reflected in measures of function and health-related quality of life following treatment with leflunomide compared with methotrexate in patients with rheumatoid arthritis. Sensitivity and relative efficiency to detect a treatment effect in a twelve-month, placebo-controlled trial. *Arthritis Rheum* 2000;43:506–514.
34. Verhoeven AC, Boers M, van der Linden S. Responsiveness of the core set, response criteria, and utilities in early rheumatoid arthritis. *Ann Rheum Dis* 2000;59:966–974.
35. Stewart MW, Palmer DG, Knight RG. A self-report articular index measure of arthritic activity: investigations of reliability, validity and sensitivity. *J Rheumatol* 1990;17:1011–1015.
36. Mason JH, Anderson JJ, Meenan RF, et al. The rapid assessment of disease activity in rheumatology (RADAR) questionnaire. *Arthritis Rheum* 1992;35:156–162.
37. Stucki G, Stucki S, Bruhlmann P, et al. Comparison of the validity and reliability of self-reported articular indices. *Br J Rheumatol* 1995;34:760–766.
38. Hanly JG, Mosher D, Sutton E, et al. Self-assessment of disease activity by patients with rheumatoid arthritis. *J Rheumatol* 1996;23:1531–1538.
39. Escalante A. What do self-administered joint counts tell us about patients with rheumatoid arthritis? *Arthritis Care Res* 1998;11:280–290.
40. Taal E, Abdel-Nasser AM, Rasker JJ, et al. A self-report Thompson articular index: what does it measure? *Clin Rheumatol* 1998;17:125–129.
41. Wong AL, Wong WK, Harker J, et al. Patient self-report tender and swollen joint counts in early rheumatoid arthritis. Western Consortium of Practicing Rheumatologists. *J Rheumatol* 1999;26:2551–2561.
42. Lorig KR, Cox T, Cuevas Y, et al. Converging and diverging beliefs about arthritis: Caucasian patients, Spanish speaking patients, and physicians. *J Rheumatol* 1984;11:76–79.
43. Gibson T, Clark B. Use of simple analgesics in rheumatoid arthritis. *Ann Rheum Dis* 1985;44:27–29.
44. McKenna F, Wright V. Pain and rheumatoid arthritis [Letter]. *Ann Rheum Dis* 1985;44:805.
45. Kazis LE, Meenan RF, Anderson JJ. Pain in the rheumatic diseases. Investigation of a key health status component. *Arthritis Rheum* 1983;26:1017–1022.
46. Meenan RF, Mason JH, Anderson JJ, et al. AIMS2. The content and properties of a revised and expanded Arthritis Impact Measurement Scales health status questionnaire. *Arthritis Rheum* 1992;35:1–10.
47. Bradley LA. Pain measurement in arthritis. *Arthritis Care Res* 1993;6:178–186.
48. Jensen MP, Karoly P. Self-report scales and procedures for assessing pain in adults. In: Turk DC, Melzack R, eds. *Handbook of pain assessment.* New York: The Guilford Press, 1992:135–151.
49. Bellamy N, Campbell J, Syrotuik J. Comparative study of self-rating pain scales in rheumatoid arthritis patients. *Curr Med Res Opin* 1999;15:121–127.
50. Meenan RF, Gertman PM, Mason JH. Measuring health status in arthritis. The Arthritis Impact Measurement Scales. *Arthritis Rheum* 1980;23:146–152.
51. Kazis LE, Anderson JJ, Meenan RF. Effect sizes for interpreting changes in health status. *Med Care* 1989;27[Suppl]:S178–S189.
52. Meenan RF, Anderson JJ, Kazis LE, et al. Outcome assessment in clinical trials. Evidence for the sensitivity of a health status measure. *Arthritis Rheum* 1984;27:1344–1352.
53. Anderson JJ, Rieschein HE, Meenan RF. Sensitivity of a health status measure to short-term clinical changes in arthritis. *Arthritis Rheum* 1989;32:844–850.
54. Fitzpatrick R, Ziebland S, Jenkinson C, et al. A comparison of the sensitivity to change of several health status instruments in rheumatoid arthritis. *J Rheumatol* 1993;20:429–436.
55. Anderson KO, Keefe FJ, Bradley LA, et al. Prediction of pain behavior and functional status of rheumatoid arthritis patients using medical status and psychological variables. *Pain* 1988;33:25–32.
56. Ward MM. Are patient self-report measures of arthritis activity confounded by mood? A longitudinal study of patients with rheumatoid arthritis. *J Rheumatol* 1994;21:1046–1050.
57. McDaniel LK, Anderson KO, Bradley LA, et al. Development of an observational method for assessing pain behavior in rheumatoid arthritis patients. *Pain* 1986;24:165–184.
58. Anderson KO, Bradley LA, McDaniel LK, et al. The assessment of pain in rheumatoid arthritis. Validity of a behavioral observation method. *Arthritis Rheum* 1987;30:36–43.
59. Rhind VM, Unsworth A, Haslock I. Assessment of stiffness in rheumatology: the use of rating scales. *Br J Rheumatol* 1987;26:126–130.
60. Hazes JMW, Hayton R, Silman AJ. A reevaluation of the symptom of morning stiffness. *J Rheumatol* 1993;20:1138–1142.
61. Hazes JMW, Hayton R, Burt J, Silman AJ. Consistency of morning stiffness: an analysis of diary data. *Br J Rheumatol* 1994;33:562–565.
62. Lineker S, Badley E, Charles C, et al. Defining morning stiffness in rheumatoid arthritis. *J Rheumatol* 1999;26:1052–1057.
63. Vliet Vleiland TPM, Zwinderman AH, Breedveld FC, et al. Measurement of morning stiffness in rheumatoid arthritis clinical trials. *J Clin Epidemiol* 1997;50:757–763.
64. Spilker B, ed. *Quality of life and pharmacoeconomics in clinical trials*, 2nd ed. Philadelphia: Lippincott–Raven Publishers, 1996.
65. Fries JF, Spitz P, Kraines RG, et al. Measurement of patient outcomes in arthritis. *Arthritis Rheum* 1980;23:137–145.
66. Ramey DR, Raynauld J-P, Fries JF. The Health Assessment Questionnaire 1992. Status and review. *Arthritis Care Res* 1992;5:119–129.
67. Ramey DR, Fries JF, Singh G. The Health Assessment Questionnaire 1995—status and review. In: Spilker B, ed. *Quality of life and pharmacoeconomics in clinical trials*, 2nd ed. Philadelphia: Lippincott–Raven Publishers, 1996:227–237.
68. Hawley DJ, Wolfe F. Sensitivity to change of the Health Assessment Questionnaire (HAQ) and other clinical and health status measures in rheumatoid arthritis. Results of short-term clinical trials and observational studies versus long-term observational studies. *Arthritis Care Res* 1992;5:130–136.
69. Pincus T, Summey JA, Soraci SA Jr, et al. Assessment of patient satisfaction in activities of daily living using a modified Stanford Health Assessment Questionnaire. *Arthritis Rheum* 1983;26:1346–1353.
70. Callahan LF, McCoy A, Smith W. Comparison and sensitivity to change of self-report scales to assess difficulty, dissatisfaction, and pain in performing activities of daily living over one and five years in rheumatoid arthritis. *Arthritis Care Res* 1992;5:137–145.
71. Wolfe F. Which HAQ is best? A comparison of the HAQ, MHAQ and RA-HAQ, a difficult 8 item HAQ (DHAQ), and a rescored 20 item HAQ (HAQ20): analyses in 2,491 rheumatoid arthritis patients following leflunomide initiation. *J Rheumatol* 2001;28:982–989.
72. Guillemin F, Coste J, Pouchot J, et al. The AIMS2-SF. A short form of the Arthritis Impact Measurement Scales 2. *Arthritis Rheum* 1997;40:1267–1274.
73. Haavardsholm EA, Kvien TK, Uhlig T, et al. A comparison of agreement and sensitivity to change between AIMS2 and a short form of AIMS2 (AIMS2-SF) in more than 1,000 rheumatoid arthritis patients. *J Rheumatol* 2000;27:2810–2816.
74. Hagen KB, Smedstad LM, Uhlig T, et al. The responsiveness of health status measures in patients with rheumatoid arthritis: comparison of disease-specific and generic instruments. *J Rheumatol* 1999;26:1474–1480.
75. HERA study group. A randomized trial of hydroxychloroquine in early rheumatoid arthritis: the HERA study. *Am J Med* 1995;98:156–168.
76. Tugwell P, Bombardier C, Buchanan WW, et al. The MACTAR patient preference disability questionnaire—an individualized functional priority approach for assessing improvement in physical disability in clinical trials in rheumatoid arthritis. *J Rheumatol* 1987;14:446–451.
77. Verhoeven AC, Boers M, van der Linden S. Validity of the MACTAR questionnaire as a functional index in a rheumatoid arthritis clinical trial. *J Rheumatol* 2000;27:2801–2809.
78. Peck JR, Smith TW, Ward JR, et al. Disability and depression in rheumatoid arthritis. A multi-trait, multi-method investigation. *Arthritis Rheum* 1989;32: 1100–1106.
79. Lorish CD, Abraham N, Austin J, et al. Disease and psychological factors related to physical functioning in rheumatoid arthritis. *J Rheumatol* 1991; 18:1150–1157.
80. van den Ende CHM, Hazes JMW, LeCessie S, et al. Discordance between objective and subjective assessment of functional ability of patients with rheumatoid arthritis. *Br J Rheumatol* 1995;34:951–955.
81. Spiegel JS, Leake B, Spiegel TM, et al. What are we measuring? An examination of self-reported functional status measures. *Arthritis Rheum* 1988;31:721–728.
82. Bijlsma JWJ, Huiskes CJAE, Kraaimaat FW, et al. Relation between patients' own health assessment and clinical and laboratory findings in rheumatoid arthritis. *J Rheumatol* 1991;18:650–653.

83. Wolfe F. A reappraisal of HAQ disability in rheumatoid arthritis. *Arthritis Rheum* 2000;43:2751–2761.
84. Steinbrocker O, Traeger CH, Batterman RC. Therapeutic criteria in rheumatoid arthritis. *JAMA* 1949;140:659–662.
85. Hochberg MC, Chang RW, Dwosh I, et al. The American College of Rheumatology 1991 revised criteria for the classification of global functional status in rheumatoid arthritis. *Arthritis Rheum* 1992;35:498–502.
86. Kalla AA, Smith PR, Brown GMM, et al. Responsiveness of Keitel functional index compared with laboratory measures of disease activity in rheumatoid arthritis. *Br J Rheumatol* 1995;34:141–149.
87. Bombardier C, Ware J, Russell IJ, et al. Auranofin therapy and quality of life in patients with rheumatoid arthritis. Results of a multicenter trial. *Am J Med* 1986;81:565–578.
88. Spiegel JS, Paulus HE, Ward NB, et al. What are we measuring? An examination of walk time and grip strength. *J Rheumatol* 1987;14:80–86.
89. Pincus T, Callahan LF. Rheumatology function tests: grip strength, walking time, button tests and questionnaires document and predict longterm morbidity and mortality in rheumatoid arthritis. *J Rheumatol* 1992;19:1051–1057.
90. Grace EM, Gerecz EM, Kassam YB, et al. 50-foot walking time: a critical assessment of an outcome measure in clinical therapeutic trials of antirheumatic drugs. *Br J Rheumatol* 1988;27:372–374.
91. Coons SJ, Rao S, Keininger DL, et al. A comparative review of generic quality-of-life instruments. *Pharmacoeconomics* 2000;17:13–35.
92. Nichols MB, Harada AS. Measuring the effects of medication use on health-related quality of life in patients with rheumatoid arthritis. A review. *Pharmacoeconomics* 1999;15:433–448.
93. Kosinski M, Keller SD, Hatoum HT, et al. The SF-36 health survey as a generic outcome measure in clinical trials of patients with osteoarthritis and rheumatoid arthritis. Tests of data quality, scaling assumptions and score reliability. *Med Care* 1999;37[Suppl]:MS10–MS22.
94. Kosinski M, Keller SD, Ware JE Jr, et al. The SF-36 health survey as a generic outcome measure in clinical trials of patients with osteoarthritis and rheumatoid arthritis. Relative validity of scales in relation to clinical measures of arthritis severity. *Med Care* 1999;37[Suppl]:MS23–MS39.
95. Ware JE Jr, Keller SD, Hatoum HT, et al. The SF-36 Arthritis-Specific Health Index (ASHI). I. Development and cross-validation of scoring algorithms. *Med Care* 1999;37[Suppl]:MS40–MS50.
96. Mathias SD, Colwell HH, Miller DP, et al. Health-related quality of life and functional status of patients with rheumatoid arthritis randomly assigned to received etanercept or placebo. *Clin Ther* 2000;22:128–139.
97. Wilson IB, Cleary PD. Linking clinical variables with health-related quality of life. A conceptual model of patient outcomes. *JAMA* 1995;273:59–65.
98. DeJong Z, van der Heijde D, McKenna SP, et al. The reliability and construct validity of the RAQoL: a rheumatoid arthritis-specific quality of life instrument. *Br J Rheumatol* 1997;36:878–883.
99. Wells G, Boers M, Shea B, et al. Sensitivity to change of generic quality of life instruments in patients with rheumatoid arthritis: preliminary findings in the generic health OMERACT study. OMERACT/ILAR task force on Generic Quality of Life. *J Rheumatol* 1999;26:217–221.
100. McConkey B, Crockson RA, Crockson AP. The assessment of rheumatoid arthritis. A study based on measurements of the serum acute-phase reactants. *QJM* 1972;41:115–125.
101. Clark P, Tugwell P, Bennet K, et al. Injectable gold for rheumatoid arthritis (Cochrane Review). In: The Cochrane Library, 2002. Oxford: Update Software.
102. Suarez-Almazor ME, Belseck E, Shea B, et al. Antimalarials for treating rheumatoid arthritis (Cochrane Review). In: The Cochrane Library, 2002. Oxford: Update Software.
103. Suarez-Almazor ME, Belseck E, Shea B, et al. Sulfasalazine for treating rheumatoid arthritis (Cochrane Review). In: The Cochrane Library, 2002. Oxford: Update Software.
104. Suarez-Almazor ME, Belseck E, Shea B, et al. Methotrexate for treating rheumatoid arthritis (Cochrane Review). In: The Cochrane Library, 2002. Oxford: Update Software.
105. van der Heijde DMFM, van't Hof MA, van Riel PLCM, et al. Validity of single variables and composite indices for measuring disease activity in rheumatoid arthritis. *Ann Rheum Dis* 1992;51:177–181.
106. Bull BS, Levy WC, Westengard JC, et al. Ranking of laboratory tests by consensus analysis. *Lancet* 1986;2:377–380.
107. Bull BS, Westengard JC, Farr M, et al. Efficacy of tests used to monitor rheumatoid arthritis. *Lancet* 1989;2:965–967.
108. Otterness IG. The value of C-reactive protein measurement in rheumatoid arthritis. *Semin Arthritis Rheum* 1994;24:91–104.
109. Emery P, Luqmani R. The validity of surrogate markers in rheumatic disease. *Br J Rheumatol* 1993;32[Suppl 3]:3–8.
110. Plant MJ, Williams AL, O'Sullivan MM, et al. Relationship between time-integrated C-reactive protein levels and radiologic progression in patients with rheumatoid arthritis. *Arthritis Rheum* 2000;43:1473–1477.
111. Devlin J, Gough A, Huissoon A, et al. The acute phase and function in early rheumatoid arthritis. C-reactive protein levels correlate with functional outcome. *J Rheumatol* 1997;24:9–13.
112. Dixon JS, Bird HA, Sitton NG, et al. C-reactive protein in the serial assessment of disease activity in rheumatoid arthritis. *Scand J Rheumatol* 1984;13:39–44.
113. Jeurissen MEC, Boerbooms AMT, van de Putte LBA, et al. Methotrexate verus azathioprine in the treatment of rheumatoid arthritis. A forty-eight-week randomized, double-blind trial. *Arthritis Rheum* 1991;34:961–972.
114. Rau R, Herborn G, Menninger H, et al. Comparison of intramuscular methotrexate and gold sodium thiomalate in the treatment of early erosive rheumatoid arthritis: 12 month data of a double-blind parallel study of 174 patients. *Br J Rheumatol* 1997;36:345–352.
115. Elliott MJ, Maini RN, Feldmann M, et al. Randomised double-blind comparison of chimeric monoclonal antibody to tumour necrosis factor alpha (cA2) versus placebo in rheumatoid arthritis. *Lancet* 1994;344:1105–1110.
116. Smolen JS, Kalden JR, Scott DL, et al. Efficacy and safety of leflunomide compared with placebo and sulphasalazine in active rheumatoid arthritis: a double-blind, randomized, multicentre trial. *Lancet* 1999;353:259–266.
117. Jacobs JWG, Geenen R, Evers AWM, et al. Short term effects of corticosteroid pulse treatment on disease activity and the wellbeing of patients with active rheumatoid arthritis. *Ann Rheum Dis* 2001;60:61–64.
118. Proudman SM, Conaghan PG, Richardson C, et al. Treatment of poor-prognosis early rheumatoid arthritis. A randomized study of treatment with methotrexate, cyclosporin A, and intraarticular corticosteroids compared with sulfasalazine alone. *Arthritis Rheum* 2000;43:1809–1819.
119. Wernick R, Merryman P, Jaffe I, et al. IgG and IgM rheumatoid factors in rheumatoid arthritis. Quantitative response to penicillamine therapy and relationship to disease activity. *Arthritis Rheum* 1983;26:593–598.
120. Withrington RH, Teitsson I, Valdimarsson H, et al. Prospective study of early rheumatoid arthritis. II. Association of rheumatoid factor isotypes with fluctuations in disease activity. *Ann Rheum Dis* 1984;43:679–685.
121. Eberhardt KB, Turedsson L, Pettersson H, et al. Disease activity and joint damage progression in early rheumatoid arthritis: relation to IgG, IgA, and IgM rheumatoid factor. *Ann Rheum Dis* 1990;49:906–909.
122. Ward JR, Williams HJ, Egger MJ, et al. Comparison of auranofin, gold sodium thiomalate, and placebo in the treatment of rheumatoid arthritis. A controlled clinical trial. *Arthritis Rheum* 1983;26:1303–1315.
123. Andersen PA, West SG, O'Dell JR, et al. Weekly pulse methotrexate in rheumatoid arthritis. Clinical and immunological effects in a randomized, double-blind study. *Ann Intern Med* 1985;103:489–496.
124. Australian Multicentre Clinical Trial Group. Sulfasalazine in early rheumatoid arthritis. *J Rheumatol* 1992;19:1672–1677.
125. Alarcon GS, Schrohenloher RE, Bartolucci AA, et al. Suppression of rheumatoid factor production by methotrexate in patients with rheumatoid arthritis. Evidence for differential influences of therapy and clinical status on IgM and IgA rheumatoid factor expression. *Arthritis Rheum* 1990;33:1156–1161.
126. Knijff-Dutmer E, Drossaers-Bakker W, Verhoeven A, et al. Rheumatoid factor measured by fluoroimmunoassay: a responsive measure of rheumatoid arthritis disease activity that is associated with joint damage. *Ann Rheum Dis* 2002;61:603–607.
127. Maini R, St. Clair EW, Breedveld F, et al. Infliximab (chimeric anti-tumour necrosis factor alpha monoclonal antibody) versus placebo in rheumatoid arthritis patients receiving concomitant methotrexate: a randomized phase III trial. *Lancet* 1999;354:1932–1939.
128. Roberts RS. Pooled outcome measures in arthritis: the pros and cons. *J Rheumatol* 1993;20:566–567.
129. Lansbury J. Report of a three-year study on the systemic and articular indices in rheumatoid arthritis. Theoretic and clinical considerations. *Arthritis Rheum* 1958;1:505–522.
130. Boers M, Tugwell P. The validity of pooled outcome measures (indices) in rheumatoid arthritis clinical trials. *J Rheumatol* 1993;20:568–574.
131. Mallya RK, Mace BEW. The assessment of disease activity in rheumatoid arthritis using a multivariate analysis. *Rheumatol Rehab* 1981;20:14–17.
132. van Riel PLCM, Reekers P, van de Putte LBA, et al. Association of HLA antigens, toxic reactions and therapeutic response to auranofin and aurothioglucose in patients with rheumatoid arthritis. *Tissue Antigens* 1983;22:194–199.
133. Corkill MM, Kirkham BW, Chikanza IC, et al. Intramuscular depot methylprednisolone induction of chrysotherapy in rheumatoid arthritis: a 24-week randomized controlled trial. *Br J Rheumatol* 1990;29:274–279.
134. Davis MJ, Dawes PT, Fowler PD, et al. Comparison and evaluation of a disease activity index for use in patients with rheumatoid arthritis. *Br J Rheumatol* 1990;29:111–115.
135. Borg AA, Fowler PD, Shadforth MF, et al. Use of the Stoke index to differentiate between disease-modifying agents and nonsteroidal antiinflammatory drugs in rheumatoid arthritis. *Clin Exp Rheumatol* 1993;11:469–472.
136. Chehata JC, Hassell AB, Clarke SA, et al. Mortality in rheumatoid arthritis: relationship to single and composite measures of disease activity. *Rheumatology* 2001;40:447–452.
137. van der Heijde DMFM, van't Hof MA, van Riel PLCM, et al. Judging disease activity in clinical practice in rheumatoid arthritis: first step in the development of a disease activity score. *Ann Rheum Dis* 1990;49:916–920.
138. Prevoo MLL, van't Hof MA, Kuper HH, et al. Modified disease activity scores that include twenty-eight-joint counts. Development and validation in a prospective longitudinal study of patients with rheumatoid arthritis. *Arthritis Rheum* 1995;38:44–48.
139. Fuchs HA. The use of the Disease Activity Score in the analysis of clinical trials in rheumatoid arthritis. *J Rheumatol* 1993;20:1863–1866.
140. Villaverde V, Balsa A, Cantalejo M, et al. Activity indices in rheumatoid arthritis. *J Rheumatol* 2000;27:2576–2581.
141. Verhoeven AC, Boers M, van der Linden S. Responsiveness of the core set, response criteria, and utilities in early rheumatoid arthritis. *Ann Rheum Dis* 2000;59:966–974.
142. Ferraccioli GF, Salaffi F, Troise-Rioda W, et al. The Chronic Arthritis Systemic Index (CASI). *Clin Exp Rheumatol* 1994;12:241–247.

143. Symmons DPM, Hassell AB, Gunatillaka KAN, et al. Development and preliminary assessment of a simple measure of overall status in rheumatoid arthritis (OSRA) for routine clinical use. *QJM* 1995;88:429–437.
144. Birrell FN, Hassell AB, Jones PW, et al. Why not use OSRA? A comparison of overall status in rheumatoid arthritis (RA) with ACR core set and other indices of disease activity in RA. *J Rheumatol* 1998;25:1709–1715.
145. Stucki G, Liang MH, Stucki S, et al. A self-administered rheumatoid arthritis disease activity index (RADAI) for epidemiologic research. Psychometric properties and correlation with parameters of disease activity. *Arthritis Rheum* 1995;38:795–798.
146. Houssien DA, Stucki G, Scott DL. A patient-derived disease activity score can substitute for a physician-derived disease activity score in clinical research. *Rheumatology* 1999;38:48–52.
147. Fransen J, Langenegger T, Michel BA, et al. Feasibility and validity of the RADAI, a self-administered rheumatoid arthritis disease activity index. *Rheumatology* 2000;39:321–327.
148. Fransen J, Hauselmann H, Michel BA, et al. Responsiveness of the self-assessed Rheumatoid Arthritis Disease Activity Index to a flare of disease activity. *Arthritis Rheum* 2001;44:53–60.
149. Pinals RS, Masi AT, Larsen RA. Preliminary criteria for clinical remission in rheumatoid arthritis. The Subcommittee for Criteria of Remission in Rheumatoid Arthritis of the American Rheumatism Association Diagnostic and Therapeutic Criteria Committee. *Arthritis Rheum* 1981;24:1308–1315.
150. U.S. Department of Health and Human Services, Food and Drug Administration. Clinical development programs for drugs, devices, and biological products for the treatment of rheumatoid arthritis (RA). www.fda.gov/cber/gdlns/rheumcln.htm, accessed on 7/28/02.
151. Prevoo MLL, van Gestel AM, van't Hof MA, et al. Remission in a prospective study of patients with rheumatoid arthritis. American Rheumatism Association preliminary remission criteria in relation to the disease activity score. *Br J Rheumatol* 1996;35:1101–1105.
152. Beaton DE, Bombardier C, Katz JN, et al. Looking for important change/differences in studies of responsiveness. *J Rheumatol* 2001;28:400–405.
153. Greenwood MC, Doyle DV, Ensor M. Does the Stanford Health Assessment Questionnaire have potential as a monitoring tool for subjects with rheumatoid arthritis? *Ann Rheum Dis* 2001;60:344–348.
154. Kosinski M, Zhao SZ, Dedhiya S, et al. Determining minimally important changes in generic and disease-specific health-related quality of life questionnaires in clinical trials of rheumatoid arthritis. *Arthritis Rheum* 2000;43:1478–1487.
155. Wells G, Beaton D, Shea B, et al. Minimal clinically important differences: review of methods. *J Rheumatol* 2001;28:406–412.
156. Ward MM. Response criteria and criteria for clinically important improvement: separate and equal? *Arthritis Rheum* 2001;44:1728–1729.
157. Kwoh CK, O'Connor GT, Regan-Smith MG, et al. Concordance between clinician and patient assessment of physical and mental health status. *J Rheumatol* 1992;19:1031–1037.
158. Kirwan JR, Chaput de Saintonge DM, Joyce CRB, et al. Clinical judgment in rheumatoid arthritis. III. British rheumatologists' judgments of "change in response to therapy." *Ann Rheum Dis* 1984;43:686–694.
159. Redelmeier DA, Lorig K. Assessing the clinical importance of symptomatic improvements. An illustration in rheumatology. *Arch Intern Med* 1993;153:1337–1342.
160. Wells GA, Tugwell P, Kraag GR, et al. Minimum important difference between patients with rheumatoid arthritis: the patient's perspective. *J Rheumatol* 1993;20:557–560.
161. Guyatt GH, Osoba D, Wu AW, et al. Clinical Significance Consensus Meeting Group. Methods to explain the clinical significance of health status measures. *Mayo Clin Proc* 2002;77:371–383.
162. Deyo RA, Inui TS. Toward clinical applications of health status measures: sensitivity of scales to clinically important changes. *Health Serv Res* 1984;19:275–289.
163. Deyo RA, Centor RM. Assessing the responsiveness of functional scales to clinical change: an analogy to diagnostic test performance. *J Chron Dis* 1986;39:897–906.
164. Ward MM, Marx AS, Barry NN. Identification of clinically important changes in health status using receiver operating characteristic curves. *J Clin Epidemiol* 2000;53:279–284.
165. Smythe HA, Helewa A, Goldsmith CH. Selection and combination of outcome measures. *J Rheumatol* 1982;9:770–774.
166. Goldsmith CH, Smythe HA, Helewa A. Interpretation and power of a pooled index. *J Rheumatol* 1993;20:575–578.
167. Scott DL, Dacre JE, Greenwood A, et al. Can we develop simple response criteria for slow acting antirheumatic drugs? *Ann Rheum Dis* 1990;49:196–198.
168. Scott DL. A simple index to assess disease activity in rheumatoid arthritis. *J Rheumatol* 1993;20:582–584.
169. Furst DE. Considerations on measuring decreased inflammatory synovitis. *ILAR Bull* 1994;2:17–21.
170. Paulus HE, Egger MJ, Ward JR, et al. Analysis of improvement in individual rheumatoid arthritis patients treated with disease-modifying antirheumatic drugs, based on the findings in patients treated with placebo. Cooperative Systemic Studies of Rheumatic Diseases Group. *Arthritis Rheum* 1990;33:477–484.
171. Felson DT, Anderson JJ, Boers M, et al. American College of Rheumatology preliminary definition of improvement in rheumatoid arthritis. *Arthritis Rheum* 1995;38:727–735.
172. van Gestel AM, Prevoo MLL, van't Hof MA, et al. Development and validation of the European League Against Rheumatism response criteria for rheumatoid arthritis. Comparison with the Preliminary American College of Rheumatology and the World Health Organization/International League Against Rheumatism criteria. *Arthritis Rheum* 1996;39:34–40.
173. Dougados M, Combe B, Beverideg T, et al. IX 207–887 in rheumatoid arthritis. A double-blind placebo-controlled study. *Arthritis Rheum* 1992;35:999–1006.
174. Wiesenhutter CW, Irish BL, Bertram JH. Treatment of patients with refractory rheumatoid arthritis with extracorporeal protein A immunoadsorption columns: a pilot trial. *J Rheumatol* 1994;21:804–812.
175. Elliott MJ, Maini RN, Feldmann M, et al. Randomised double-blind comparison of chimeric monoclonal antibody to tumour necrosis factor alpha (cA2) versus placebo in rheumatoid arthritis. *Lancet* 1994;344:1105–1110.
176. Matteson EL, Yocum DE, St. Clair EW, et al. Treatment of active refractory rheumatoid arthritis with humanized monoclonal antibody CAMPATH-1H administered by daily subcutaneous injection. *Arthritis Rheum* 1995;38:1187–1193.
177. Gravallese EM, Handel ML, Coblyn J, et al. *N*-[4-hydroxyphenyl] retinamide in rheumatoid arthritis: a pilot study. *Arthritis Rheum* 1996;39:1021–1026.
178. Maksymowych WP, Avina-Zubieta A, Luong M, et al. High dose intravenous immunoglobulin (IVIg) in severe refractory rheumatoid arthritis: no evidence for efficacy. *Clin Exp Rheumatol* 1996;14:657–660.
179. Schnitzer TJ, Yocum DE, Michalska M, et al. Subcutaneous administration of CAMPATH-1H: clinical and biological outcomes. *J Rheumatol* 1997;24:1031–1036.
180. Barnett ML, Kremer JM, St. Clair EW, et al. Treatment of rheumatoid arthritis with oral type II collagen. Results of a multicenter, double-blind, placebo-controlled trial. *Arthritis Rheum* 1998;41:290–297.
181. Maini RN, Breedveld FC, Kalden JR, et al. Therapeutic efficacy of multiple intravenous infusions of anti-tumor necrosis factor alpha monoclonal antibody combined with low-dose weekly methotrexate in rheumatoid arthritis. *Arthritis Rheum* 1998;41:1552–1563.
182. Bresnihan B, Alvaro-Garcia JM, Cobby M, et al. Treatment of rheumatoid arthritis with recombinant human interleukin-1 receptor antagonist. *Arthritis Rheum* 1998;41:2196–2204.
183. Furst DE, Lindsley H, Baethge B, et al. Dose-loading with hydroxychloroquine improves the rate of response in early, active rheumatoid arthritis: a randomized, double-blind six-week trial with eighteen-week extension. *Arthritis Rheum* 1999;42:357–365.
184. Caldwell J, Gendreau RM, Furst D, et al. A pilot study using a Staph protein A column (Prosorba) to treat refractory rheumatoid arthritis. *J Rheumatol* 1999;26:1657–1662.
185. Pillemer SR, Folwer SE, Tilley BC, et al. Meaningful improvement criteria sets in a rheumatoid arthritis clinical trial. *Arthritis Rheum* 1997;40:419–425.
186. Weinblatt ME, Kremer JM, Bankhurst AD, et al. A trial of etanercept, a recombinant tumor necrosis factor receptor: Fc fusion protein, in patients with rheumatoid arthritis receiving methotrexate. *N Engl J Med* 1999;340:253–259.
187. Moreland LW, Schiff MH, Baumgartner SW, et al. Etanercept therapy in rheumatoid arthritis. A randomized, controlled trial. *Ann Intern Med* 1999;130:478–486.
188. Tak PP, Hart BA, Kraan MC, et al. The effects of interferon beta treatment on arthritis. *Rheumatology* 1999;38:362–369.
189. Strand V, Cohen S, Schiff M, et al. Treatment of active rheumatoid arthritis with leflunomide compared with placebo and methotrexate. Leflunomide Rheumatoid Arthritis Investigators Group. *Arch Intern Med* 1999;159:2542–2550.
190. Maini R, St. Clari EW, Breedveld F, et al. Infliximab (chimeric anti-tumour necrosis factor alpha monoclonal antibody) versus placebo in rheumatoid arthritis patients receiving concomitant methotrexate: a randomized phase III trial. ATTRACT Study Group. *Lancet* 1999;354:1932–1939.
191. Bathon JM, Martin RW, Fleischmann RM, et al. A comparison of etanercept and methotrexate in patients with early rheumatoid arthritis. *N Engl J Med* 2000;343:1586–1593.
192. Kavanaugh A, St. Clair EW, McCune WJ, et al. Chimeric anti-tumor necrosis factor-alpha monoclonal antibody treatment of patients with rheumatoid arthritis receiving methotrexate therapy. *J Rheumatol* 2000;27:841–850.
193. Proudman SM, Conaghan PG, Richardson C, et al. Treatment of poor-prognosis early rheumatoid arthritis. A randomized study of treatment with methotrexate, cyclosporin A, and intraarticular corticosteroids compared with sulfasalazine alone. *Arthritis Rheum* 2000;43:1809–1819.
194. Cazzola M, Antivalle M, Sarzi-Puttini P, et al I. Oral type II collagen in the treatment of rheumatoid arthritis. A six-month double blind placebo-controlled study. *Clin Exp Rheumatol* 2000;18:571–577.
195. Furst D, Felson D, Thoren G, et al. Immunoadsorption for the treatment of rheumatoid arthritis: final results of a randomized trial. Prosorba Trial Investigators. *Ther Apher* 2000;4:363–373.
196. Scott DL, Smolen JS, Kalden JR, et al. Treatment of active rheumatoid arthritis with leflunomide: two year follow up of a double blind, placebo controlled trial versus sulfasalazine. *Ann Rheum Dis* 2001;60:913–923.
197. Cohen S, Cannon GW, Schiff M, et al. Two-year, blinded, randomized, controlled trial of treatment of active rheumatoid arthritis with leflunomide compared with methotrexate. Utilization of Leflunomide in the Treatment of Rheumatoid Arthritis Trial Investigators Group. *Arthritis Rheum* 2001;44:1984–1992.

198. Cohen S, Hurd E, Cush J, et al. Treatment of rheumatoid arthritis with anakinra, a recombinant human interleukin-1 receptor antagonist, in combination with methotrexate: results of a twenty-four week, multicenter, randomized, double-blind, placebo-controlled trial. *Arthritis Rheum* 2002; 46:614–624.
199. Felson DT, Anderson JJ, Lange MLM, et al. Should improvement in rheumatoid arthritis clinical trials be defined as fifty percent or seventy percent improvement in core set measures, rather than twenty percent? *Arthritis Rheum* 1998;41:1564–1570.
200. Schiff M, Weaver A, Keystone E, et al. Comparison of ACR response, numeric ACR, and ACR AUC as measures of clinical improvement in RA clinical trials. *Arthritis Rheum* 1999;42[Suppl]:S81.
201. van Riel PLCM, van Gestel AM. Area under the curve for the American College of Rheumatology improvement criteria: a valid addition to existing criteria in rheumatoid arthritis? *Arthritis Rheum* 2001;44:1719–1722.
202. van Gestel, van Gestel AM, Anderson JJ, et al. ACR and EULAR improvement criteria have comparable validity in rheumatoid arthritis trials. *J Rheumatol* 1999;26:705–711.
203. van Gestel AM, Haagsma CJ, van Riel PLCM. Validation of rheumatoid arthritis improvement criteria that include simplified joint counts. *Arthritis Rheum* 1998;41:1845–1850.
204. Svensson B, Schaufelberger C, Teleman A, et al. Remission and response to early treatment of RA assessed by the Disease Activity Score. BARFOT study group. *Rheumatology* 2000;39:1031–1036.
205. Dougados M, Combe B, Cantagrel A, et al. Combination therapy in early rheumatoid arthritis: a randomized, controlled, double blind 52 week clinical trial of sulphasalazine and methotrexate compared with the single components. *Ann Rheum Dis* 1999;58:220–225.
206. Barrera P, van der Maas A, van Ede AE, et al. Drug survival, efficacy and toxicity of monotherapy with a fully human anti-tumour necrosis factor-alpha antibody compared with methotrexate in long-standing rheumatoid arthritis. *Rheumatology* 2002;41:430–439.
207. Bellamy N, Kaloni S, Pope J, et al. Quantitative rheumatology: a survey of outcome measurement procedures in routine rheumatology outpatient practice in Canada. *J Rheumatol* 1998;25:852–858.
208. Bellamy N, Muirden KD, Brooks PM, et al. A survey of outcome measurement procedures in routine rheumatology outpatient practice in Australia. *J Rheumatol* 1999;26:1593–1599.
209. Donald F, Ward MM. Evaluative laboratory testing practice of United States rheumatologists. *Arthritis Rheum* 1998;41:725–729.
210. Kirwin JR, Chaput de Saintonge DM, Joyce CRB, et al. Clinical judgment in rheumatoid arthritis. II. Judging 0 "current disease activity" in clinical practice. *Ann Rheum Dis* 1983;42:648–651.
211. Kirwin JR, Chaput de Saintonge DM, Joyce CRB, et al. Inability of rheumatologists to describe their true policies for assessing rheumatoid arthritis. *Ann Rheum Dis* 1986;45:156–161.
212. Fries JF. Reevaluating the therapeutic approach to rheumatoid arthritis: the "sawtooth" strategy. *J Rheumatol Suppl* 1990;22:12–15.
213. Wolfe F, Pincus T. Standard self-report questionnaires in routine clinical and research practice—an opportunity for patients and rheumatologists. *J Rheumatol* 1991;18:643–646.
214. Wolfe F, Pincus T, O'Dell J. Evaluation and documentation of rheumatoid arthritis disease status in the clinic: which variables best predict change in therapy. *J Rheumatol* 2001;28:1712–1717.
215. Kazis LE, Callahan LF, Meenan RF, Pincus T. Health status reports in the care of patients with rheumatoid arthritis. *J Clin Epidemiol* 1990;43:1243–1253.

CHAPTER 6

Autoantibodies and Other Laboratory Tests

Mark H. Wener

Laboratory tests assist in the care of patients with rheumatoid arthritis (RA) in several important ways. Specifically, laboratory tests help (a) establish a diagnosis, (b) determine prognosis, (c) monitor disease activity, (d) monitor disease progression or damage, (e) monitor drug or therapeutic toxicities, (f) evaluate possible complications of the underlying disease process, and (g) exclude alternative diagnoses. A diagnostic test should be *sensitive* (able to identify a disease when present) and *specific* (able to identify that the disease is not present). Although the perfect diagnostic test should be 100% sensitive and 100% specific, this goal is rarely achieved in clinical practice. An evaluative or monitoring test should be sensitive to change in the disease state over time. Even though not all laboratory tests meet these goals, ideally tests should be inexpensive, standardized, easily performed, and readily available.

ACUTE PHASE RESPONSE: GENERAL INFLAMMATORY DISEASE ACTIVITY MARKERS

In response to most types of inflammation associated with release of proinflammatory cytokines, such as interleukin-6 (IL-6), tumor necrosis factor-α (TNF-α), and IL-1, hepatic protein synthesis undergoes stereotypical changes collectively known as the *acute phase response*. Although circulating cytokines, such as IL-6, can be measured in blood, instability of TNF-α and IL-1 under normal circumstances during clinical phlebotomy, as well as lack of standardization in their measurement, leads to problems in interpretation of blood levels of many cytokines. The changes in hepatic protein synthesis result in elevated plasma concentrations of acute phase reactants such as C-reactive protein (CRP), fibrinogen, alpha-1-antitrypsin, haptoglobin, the complement proteins, etc. Other proteins are synthesized at a lower rate, and therefore their concentrations fall during inflammation. Examples of these negative acute phase reactants include albumin and transferrin; the fall in the iron transport protein transferrin contributes to the low total iron-binding capacity characteristic of the anemia of chronic disease. Gamma globulins [immunoglobulins (Igs)] are elevated in inflammation caused by chronic infections and many autoimmune diseases. These changes in protein concentrations can be detected by serum protein electrophoresis, leading to characteristic patterns associated with acute and chronic inflammation. Changes in plasma protein concentrations also alter the rate at which erythrocytes in plasma fall in the gravitational field [i.e., the erythrocyte sedimentation rate (ESR)]. Elevated concentrations of fibrinogen and many globulins increase the ESR, as does a fall in albumin concentration. In addition, anemia raises the ESR. Thus, in chronic inflammation, the elevated ESR is caused by the protein changes as well as by the associated anemia. Because these protein changes are mostly independent of the type of inflammation, elevations in the ESR are nonspecific.

Erythrocyte Sedimentation Rate

The ESR is not sufficiently sensitive to screen for all kinds of inflammation, but it has long been used as a marker of inflammation in patients with RA. In surveys of rheumatologists, the ESR is the most commonly ordered laboratory test to assess disease activity of patients with RA, used by approximately 85% of rheumatologists in the United States (1) and similar proportions in France (2). Elevation in the ESR is widely used as an entrance criterion for drug intervention studies in patients with RA, as a marker of disease activity, and as an end point for treatment. The ESR (or CRP) is recommended as part of the guidelines for baseline evaluation and for monitoring disease activity in RA patients (3). When formally evaluated by studies, however, changes in the ESR correlate only modestly ($r = 0.10$ to $r = 0.74$) with other measures of disease activity (reviewed in reference 4). Elevations of the ESR at presentation predict persistent synovitis in some studies (5) but not others (6,7). Persistently elevated ESR values in a patient with established RA are associated with progression of radiographic erosions and functional disability (4,8,9). Although an individual ESR value or the ESR at presentation does not correlate well with the long-term development of radiographic erosions, the time-integrated or time-averaged ESR is a strong predictor of long-term radiographic damage over decades. Correlation coefficients between radiographic progression rates and time-integrated levels of acute phase markers are in the range of 0.4 to 0.7 (10–12). In some patients, the ESR is unreliable as an indicator of inflammation because factors unrelated to inflammation can influence the concentrations of factors that determine the ESR. For example, patients with chronic hypoalbuminemia due to nephrotic syndrome, elevated Igs due to multiple myeloma, or anemia due to iron deficiency may have elevated ESR even in the absence of overt inflammation. The presence of anti-erythrocyte antibodies, particularly cold agglutinins, can lead to marked elevations in the ESR that do not reflect a generalized inflammatory response. Because of abnormalities in the red cells, patients with sickle cell anemia, polycythemia, or other erythrocyte abnormalities may have unexpectedly low values of ESR.

In patients with alterations of the ESR related to factors other than inflammation, the CRP is more reliable than the ESR as an indicator of inflammation. The ESR is subject to substantial errors if a specimen is handled incorrectly. If the blood specimen is kept at room temperature for more than a few hours, an elevated ESR may fall into the normal range, yielding incorrect results (13). Therefore, off-site laboratories that analyze older specimens should verify that the blood specimen has been properly handled to provide a reliable ESR result. The ESR cannot be used in multicenter studies requiring that all laboratory assays be performed in the same centralized laboratory. The upper limit of normal of the ESR depends on the age and gender of the patient. For the upper limit of normal, published "in the clinic" formulae (14) that many clinicians find useful if the laboratory does not provide an age-adjusted reference range are

$$\text{Women: ESR (mm/hour)} = \frac{(\text{age in years} + 10)}{2}$$

$$\text{Men: ESR (mm/hour)} = \frac{(\text{age in years})}{2}$$

C-Reactive Protein

The concentration of CRP in the serum can also help evaluate and monitor inflammation. CRP concentrations rise and fall rapidly in response to inflammation, and the concentration of CRP fluctuates with the degree of inflammation in most clinical situations. For most patients and conditions, the ESR and CRP correlate well, but, in some patients, either the ESR or CRP reflects inflammation more reliably than the other test. Both the ESR and CRP are nonspecific measures of inflammation and neither is, by itself, diagnostic of any condition. CRP may be a somewhat better indicator of inflammation in serially followed RA patients than the ESR test (15). CRP has an advantage for multicenter studies in which laboratory tests are performed in a centralized laboratory, because CRP is a stable serum protein whose measurement can be delayed until many hours or days after the blood is drawn.

As with the ESR, the serum level of CRP is a prognostic factor for the development of both disability and radiographic erosions in patients with RA, although its ability to predict the course for an individual patient is only fair (8). If the CRP is persistently low, the likelihood of developing erosive disease is low, whereas the likelihood is much higher if the CRP is persistently elevated or fluctuates (16). In the comparison of the serum levels of CRP and ESR, the prognostic value of the CRP value has been better than that of the ESR in some studies (11,12), whereas the ESR has been superior to serum CRP levels for predicting radiographic changes in other studies (17). Analyses of studies of radiographic progression in randomized controlled clinical trials of potent disease-modifying agents showed disappointingly weak correlations between x-ray changes and CRP levels over the short time frames (18), but longer time-integrated values of CRP that reflect the long-term inflammatory process improve the correlation with measures of radiographic erosion (11).

CRP variation within the normal range has recently been shown to be a useful indicator of cardiovascular risk among patients without identified inflammatory conditions; higher values of CRP are associated with increased risk of myocardial infarction, mortality, stroke, and other cardiovascular end points (19). Higher levels of CRP may predict a response to statin therapy, even in patients without elevations in cholesterol. Because proinflammatory cytokines, such as IL-6, are made by adipose tissue, obesity may cause a mild increase in CRP (20). Within the general population, women have higher values of CRP than men, and older subjects have higher values than younger subjects. Analogous to the formula for calculating the upper limit of the reference range of ESR, the formulae for the upper limit (95th percentile) of the reference range for CRP in the United States are (21)

$$\text{For men: CRP (in mg/L)} = \frac{\text{age}}{5}$$

$$\text{For women: CRP (in mg/L)} = 6 + \frac{\text{age}}{5} \text{ or } \frac{(\text{age} + 30)}{5}$$

In addition, race and ethnicity influence the distribution of CRP values in the U.S. population (21). The American Heart Association and the U.S. Centers for Disease Control and Prevention have recommended that CRP measurement be part of the evaluation for selected patients at intermediate risk for cardiovascular disease, with the CRP value of 3.0 mg per L as the cutoff for the highest tertile of risk (22). As part of that recommendation, patients with overt inflammation (CRP concentrations above 10 mg per L or 1.0 mg per dL) should be excluded from use of CRP as a cardiovascular risk indicator. Whether it is possible to use CRP to assess cardiovascular risk in patients with RA or other active chronic inflammatory diseases is unclear, but it is likely that the inflammation associated with RA contributes to vascular disease (23).

Ferritin

A variety of other nonspecific changes occur as part of the acute phase response. One of the acute phase proteins is the iron transport protein ferritin. Ferritin can be extremely elevated with values greater than 1,000 ng per mL in a variety of types of inflammation (24). The serum ferritin concentration characteristically is highly elevated in patients with the systemic form of juvenile RA (JRA) (25) or adult Still's disease (26). The levels of serum ferritin tend to be significantly more elevated in patients with adult-onset Still's disease than in other inflammatory or febrile diseases with similar presentations (27). Furthermore, the proportion of glycosylated ferritin in the serum of Still's disease patients is abnormally low, and the high proportion of unglycosylated ferritin may be useful as a marker or a classification criterion for adult Still's disease (27,28). Elevation of serum ferritin may be a reflection of elevations in alpha-interferon rather than other inflammatory cytokines (29).

Cytokines, Cytokine Receptors, and Chemokines

Because of the critical role of cytokines in synovial inflammation, investigators have sought to determine if cytokine profiles in peripheral blood could provide diagnostic or prognostic information. Furthermore, because imbalances in cytokines and their inhibitors could play a role in the pathogenesis of RA (30), measuring their levels could allow stratification of patients for prognosis and treatment and might govern choices of therapies. Cytokines and related molecules, such as IL-1β, IL-1 receptor antagonist (IL-1ra), IL-6, soluble IL-2 receptor, IL-8, and soluble TNF receptor (sTNFR) correlate with disease activity and the response to treatment (31–33). Lower ratios of IL-1ra/IL-1β produced by peripheral blood mononuclear cells cultured *in vitro* correlate with a better response to methotrexate; the serum ratio of IL-1ra/IL-1β does not predict the methotrexate response (34). The pattern of cytokine secretion by peripheral blood mononuclear cells also distinguishes early synovitis patients from chronic RA patients, with the early synovitis patients producing larger amounts of IL-2 and interferon γ. In contrast, cells from patients with chronic RA produce larger amounts of IL-6, IL-20, and TNF-α (35).

In children with juvenile chronic arthritis, the cytokine profile may help to differentiate subtypes of the disease. Serum levels of soluble IL-2 receptor, IL-6, and soluble TNF receptors are indicators of inflammation and are higher in children with systemic onset JRA than in other subtypes (36,37). In contrast, the concentrations of IL-1ra are higher in JRA patients with rheumatoid factors (RFs) than in other groups of JRA patients (37). Synovial fluid (SF) IL-6 levels are significantly higher in patients with systemic JRA than in SF from patients with pauciarticular JRA or adults with RA, whereas SF levels of IL-1α are lower in systemic-onset JRA than in other types of JRA (38). SF IL-11 levels are significantly higher in patients with adult RA than patients with JRA. In contrast to the observation that serum levels of sTNFR are different in systemic-onset JRA than other forms of RA, there is no difference in SF sTNFR levels among JRA subtypes. There are no significant differences between groups of JRA patients in SF levels of IL-1β, IL-1ra, TNF-α, or leukemia inhibitory factor (38).

Factors influencing inflammatory cell trafficking through the joint have been measured as a way to characterize and monitor the response to therapy. Soluble forms of adhesion molecules, such as intercellular adhesion molecule-1, E-selectin, and vascular cell adhesion molecule-1, are released from cell surfaces by proteolytic cleavage and can be found in the serum. In RA, concentrations of these adhesion molecules fall in response to effective treatment (39). Serum concentrations of leukocyte-attracting chemokines, such as IL-8, and monocyte chemotactic protein-1 in RA also fall after beneficial treatment interventions (40).

Numerous problems can arise in measuring circulating cytokines. Some cytokines, such as TNF-α, are unstable in blood. Efficient specimen handling with rapid freezing is required to maintain the stability of some cytokines (41). Cytokine concentrations can be measured by immunoassays or bioassays. Antiinflammatory and immunosuppressive medications may interfere with the results of bioassays (31). Assays from different vendors often do not agree with each other, leading to difficulties in interpreting quantitative cytokine data (42).

Immune Complexes

RA has been characterized as an immune complex disease, with SF immune complexes consisting of RFs and other antigen-antibody complexes potentially contributing to the pathogenesis of rheumatoid synovitis (43). Self-associating IgG RFs, in which the IgG RF is both an antigen and antibody, have the potential to be pathogenic (44). Tests for circulating immune complexes have been developed to determine if their detection could be an indicator of disease activity and disease pathogenesis. In a detailed study of several different assays for immune complexes, the C1q fluid-phase binding assay (using radiolabeled C1q as the detector) and the staphylococci-binding assays were demonstrated to be the best indicators of active RA. The tests performed similarly to the ESR and the IgG RF test (the two best markers of many examined) in assessing disease activity (45). Tests for circulating immune complexes contribute little additionally to the assessment of disease activity or prognostication, and those tests are rarely used for monitoring RA patients. Cryoglobulins, which are a special form of immune complex or immune aggregate that precipitates in the cold, are also sometimes present in the sera of patients with RA (see Autoantibodies Associated with Rheumatoid Arthritis).

Autoantibodies to C1q have also been described in sera of patients with rheumatoid vasculitis. Whereas anti-C1q antibodies are common and of the IgG class in patients with systemic lupus erythematosus (SLE), they are rather uncommon in RA. When anti-C1q antibodies are present in RA patients, they are frequently of the IgA class (46,47).

AUTOANTIBODIES ASSOCIATED WITH RHEUMATOID ARTHRITIS

Rheumatoid Factors

BRIEF HISTORICAL REVIEW

RFs were first described in 1940 by Waaler, who noted that sera from some patients with RA caused agglutination of sheep erythrocytes that had been coated with rabbit antibodies to sheep erythrocytes (48). Use of RF measurement as a diagnostic test was promoted in 1949 by Rose et al. (49), and the Waaler-Rose RF test subsequently became part of the routine evaluation of patients with RA (50). Later, other particles, including bentonite particles and latex beads, were substituted for sheep cells to detect agglutination, and latex agglutination (Singer-Plotz assay) (51) and sheep cell agglutination assay (SCAT, Waaler-Rose assay) were for many years the methods of choice in clinical laboratories. In more recent years, nephelometry and enzyme-linked immunosorbent assay (ELISA) have been used for detection of RFs, especially in larger laboratories. RFs may be of the IgM, IgA, IgG, or IgE class. Until ELISAs for RF measurement became available, clinical assays for RF detected only IgM RF.

TARGET DETECTED BY RHEUMATOID FACTORS

The antigen detected by RF is the Fc portion of the IgG molecule. Most RFs bind to amino acid sequences of the Cγ2 and/or Cγ3 domains of IgG, and frequently require both domains for binding, suggesting the binding site on IgG is a conformational epitope (52,53). The Cγ2-Cγ3 binding site for RF has been confirmed by x-ray crystallography studies (54) that indicate that at least some IgM RF Fab fragments bind antigen unusually via the side of the Fab at the edge of the usual antigen-binding site. This type of recognition is unlike the classical antigen-antibody interaction at the central end of the heavy and light chain dimer (55). Other experiments using peptides synthesized with overlapping sequences from the Fc portion of IgG have provided evidence that some RFs may bind to linear epitopes within IgG (56). Most RFs bind preferentially to IgG subclasses IgG1, IgG2, and IgG4, and bind less well or not at all to IgG3. Recognition of the human IgG3 isotype by RFs may be different than the recognition of other IgG subclasses (57). Studies in mice and humans have suggested that IgG becomes immunogenic when in the form of an immune complex, which leads to the formation of RFs (58,59).

The term *advanced glycation end products* (AGEs) refers to stable nonenzymatically glycosylated proteins or possibly other molecules caused by oxidation related to hyperglycemia, hyperlipidemia, or aging. Glycosylated hemoglobin (hemoglobin A_{1c}) is the most commonly measured glycosylation end product. Under oxidative stress, many different proteins, including IgG, can undergo such glycosylation. IgG-AGE are present in the sera of patients with a variety of forms of early synovitis, including RA (60). The continued presence of IgM antibodies directed against IgG-AGE is found almost exclusively in RA patients whose sera also contain RFs (61,62). Other modifications of IgG, such as free radical–induced oxidation, may also make IgG more immmunogenic (63). It is not clear whether the increased immunogenicity of IgG resulting from these modifications promotes the formation of RFs in RA patients.

The genetic origin of RFs has been investigated. Many monoclonal RFs are encoded by a limited number of germ-line genes, which are preferentially expressed in early development (reviewed in reference 64). RFs are preferentially produced by RA synovial B cells and show evidence of an antigen-driven immune response (65). The DNA sequences that encode monoclonal RFs, often seen in patients with malignancies, are not the same as those that encode RFs produced in the synovial tissue of patients with RA. Monoclonal RFs from patients with B-cell malignancies are derived from V-regions that are similar to germ-line, unmutated genes, whereas RFs from the synovium of patients with RA are typically derived from Ig V-genes, which have undergone mutations, suggesting that RF production is an antigen-driven process (66). RFs associated with hepatitis C mixed cryoglobulinemia frequently bear the WA idiotype (67). This public idiotype is frequently found on monoclonal RFs and is encoded in most cases by the 51p1 Ig V_H gene (68). Mixed cryoglobulins, associated with the mixed cryoglobulinemia syndrome, are cold-precipitating immune complexes formed from IgM RFs that recognize serum IgG or IgG-containing immune complexes.

IgG or γ-globulin pools from rabbits, humans, bovine, or, occasionally, other species have been used as the antigen source for RF detection (69). IgG from different species differ in binding by RFs; thus, RF assay results vary when IgG from different species are used as antigens. Assays using rabbit IgG as the antigen source may be less sensitive and more specific for the diagnosis of RA than are assays that use IgG from other species (70). In some patients, RFs may be tightly bound to endogenous human serum IgG, and therefore undetectable by conventional RF assays. These RFs, which are termed *hidden RFs*, occur uncommonly in sera of adult patients with RA, but have been reported in the sera of 60% to 85% of patients with JRA (71). Hidden RFs can be detected by separating the IgM fraction of serum by chromatography under acid conditions or by rapid ion exchange chromatography, followed by RF testing using conventional means.

ANALYTICAL METHODS AND STANDARDIZATION

Traditionally, agglutination methods have been used for the detection of RFs. Commercially available reagents use stabilized preparations of sensitized sheep cells for the sheep cell agglutination test to allow adequate shelf life. The latex agglutination assay typically uses inert polystyrene latex particles coated nonspecifically with human IgG. Manual and visual agglutination techniques are quite dependent on the skill and consistency of the technologists performing the assay and can involve subjective determination of the final titer. The agglutination methods described originally were performed in test tubes, with agglutination promoted by temperature-controlled incubation and centrifugation of the sheep cells or latex particles. A more rapid, but somewhat less consistent, variation is to measure agglutination on glass slides at ambient temperature without a centrifugation step. Substantial differences in results can be found because of different conditions used during performance of agglutination assays. Manual agglutination assays typically are reported as titers, quantified by serial dilutions of serum until agglutination is no longer visualized.

In centralized hospital and commercial laboratories, the most common method for performing the test for RF is by nephelometry. Nephelometry is an analytical method in which light is directed through a cuvette that contains varying amounts of aggregates of suspended immune complexes or aggregated latex particles. The light scattered by the suspended particles is quantified. The amount of light scattered is proportional to the size and amount of aggregates, which is then a measure of the antigen-antibody reaction being studied (72). Many nephelometric assays have been developed for the detection of RF. For the RF tests, the target antigen is typically heat-aggregated human IgG or, occasionally, chemically cross-linked IgG or immune complexes. In the latex-enhanced methods, preparations of human or rabbit IgG, or both, are used to coat latex particles, analogous to the agglutination assays performed manually, with the nephelometer providing a more automated, objective, and precise quantitation of agglutination than is possible by manual methods. The intra-laboratory coefficient of variation of nephelometric methods has been reported to be as low as 2% (73–75).

ELISAs have also been used to assess RF activity by measuring the amount of Ig that binds to the target antigen (IgG or IgG fragments) adsorbed to a solid phase (76). Using ELISAs, the Ig class of the antibody can be determined by using class-specific antibodies as the reagent for detecting human Ig binding (see section Measurement of Rheumatoid Factor Isotypes). Use of IgG from different species may be responsible for different results in the ELISA tests for RF (77). In addition, high background binding (from nonspecifically "sticky" serum Igs that bind to plastic) is relatively common among sera from diseased patients.

Most nephelometric and ELISA assays have used calibrators measured against standard sera established by the World Health Organization (WHO) (78) or, occasionally, the Centers for Disease Control and Prevention (79), with results reported in units rather than titers. Use of the WHO standard tends to promote uniformity in IgM RF quantitation by all methods (80,81); however, consistency in results of RF measurements is still difficult to achieve (82–84). The WHO standard does not contain IgG or IgA RF (85) and, thus, cannot be used as a standard for IgG or IgA RF. The long-term stability of the standard is unknown. When the WHO standard was established in 1970, it was suggested that its activity would decline by 50% in approximately 8 years, although the estimates of the time to 50% reduction ranged from 1 to 250 years (78,86). The correlation between RF agglutination titers and international units is imperfect, but it has been observed that a serum RF level of approximately 50 IU per mL is equivalent to a Singer-Plotz latex agglutination titer of 1:160 (87). The lowest value of clinical significance is approximately 12.5 IU per mL (78), although values as low as 5 IU have been considered significant in some approaches (6).

High titers of serum RF can interfere with other immunoassays (88). For example, experience with measurement of troponin in the evaluation of patients with possible cardiac damage demonstrated that RFs in sera could lead to frequent false-positive results (89,90), although commercial assays have largely corrected that interference. As, in general, RFs are more likely to bind to rabbit IgG than to goat or mouse IgG, this interference may be less frequent in immunoassays using murine monoclonal antibodies in sandwich assays (91). IgM RFs can cause false-positive serologic tests for IgM antibodies in a patient with IgG antibodies to a particular antigen and, thus, can interfere with the interpretation of serologic tests in which the presence of IgM antibodies is used to diagnose a new or recent infection, whereas IgG antibodies alone would signify a remote infection.

MEASUREMENT OF RHEUMATOID FACTOR ISOTYPES

A number of investigators have measured RF activity or concentration associated with different Ig classes or isotypes. These assays use heterologous antibodies directed against human Ig classes or subclasses as the detection reagents. Because human RFs can be both antigens and antibodies, the assays must be designed carefully to prevent the RF from binding to the antihuman Ig reagents. To assure specificity of assay results, various pairs of antigen and detecting antibodies or their fragments can be used. For example, use of intact rabbit IgG or the Fc fragment of human IgG can be used as the target antigen, together with F(ab')2 fragments of the antihuman IgG as the detection antibody. If RFs reacting specifically with human IgG are to be measured, then the antigen can be the Fc fragment of human IgG, and the detection antibody can be F(ab')2 fragments of antibodies to the Fd region [i.e., the heavy-chain portion of the F(ab) fragment] of IgG. Papain digestion of serum and other approaches have been advocated to allow accurate quantitation of IgG RF (92). Also, measurement of IgG RF is complicated by the fact that two or more molecules of IgG RF can self-associate (44), as IgG is both the antigen and antibody in this situation. Furthermore, non-RF serum IgG may be bound with IgM RFs or IgA RFs, thus providing falsely elevated results of IgG RF.

Whereas the utility of measuring IgM RF by agglutination techniques is well documented, the clinical use of IgA RF and IgG RF measurements remains controversial. In general, all isotypes of RF tend to occur together in the same patient, with the titers of the different RF isotypes correlating. Furthermore, some studies suggest that agglutination assays may detect not only IgM RF but also IgA RF (93,94) because IgA RF may exist at least partly in the form of a J-chain–containing polymer capable of cross-linking targets of agglutination assays. Numerous reports suggest that IgA RF may have greater diagnostic and prognostic utility than other RF isotypes (e.g., see references 95–99), whereas others have failed to confirm those findings (e.g., see references 100–102). The presence of multiple classes of RFs, particularly IgM and IgA RF, may have additive prognostic or diagnostic value (103,104). Different conclusions concerning the role of IgA RF may depend in part on the species of IgG used as the target antigen for RF measurement (70). One investigating group observed IgA RF more frequently in patients with primary Sjögren's syndrome than in RA patients (105). When agglutination assays are compared with isotype-specific RF assays, they perform similarly in predicting the long-term course of RA (102).

The reported prevalence of the RF isotypes in RA patient populations varies widely. IgG RF has been reported in 36% to 66% of patients, IgA RF in 19% to 88%, IgM RF in up to 92%, and IgE RF in 16% to 79% (reviewed in reference 101). RFs of all isotypes have been found in subjects who do not develop RA, and smoking has been associated with a higher positive rate of both IgG and IgA RF isotypes in subjects without arthritis (106). If there were a difference in seroprevalence of IgA or IgG RF in patients with chronic hepatitis C or other infections in comparison with RA patients, such a finding would help in differential diagnosis of these common conditions; however, the limited information on this topic does not suggest that the isotype of RF will reliably differentiate these diagnoses (107). Specific RF isotype measurements are not part of formal diagnostic or classification criteria.

CLINICAL INTERPRETATION

Results of RF measurements are used to help diagnose and classify patients with inflammatory polyarthritis. The presence of RF is one of a set of criteria established by the American College of Rheumatology (ACR) for the classification of RA (108). A positive test for RF does not by itself establish a diagnosis, but it increases the probability of the diagnosis of RA. Elderly individuals, especially elderly females, are likely to have low titers of RF even in the absence of RA; thus, clinical interpretation of a given result should consider the age and gender of the patient being evaluated. Nevertheless, testing for RF can be considered to have a sensitivity of approximately 80% with a specificity of 96% to 98% in a rheumatic disease clinic population and a specificity of 95% to 96% relative to other patients with inflammatory rheumatic diseases (109). The presence of RF in the serum often precedes the diagnosis and overt clinical manifestations of RA for many years, as demonstrated by studies in a Pima Native American population (110) and population studies from Finland (111), Iceland (104), and Sweden (112). In these studies, the presence of RF substantially increases the risk of subsequent development of RA.

The concentration of serum RF may change over time. Among patients with RA, RF levels in an individual generally correlate with the degree of inflammation and disease activity in RA. This magnitude of change in RF can be measured using more precise techniques, such as nephelometry and ELISA, rather than less reproducible and precise semi-quantitative agglutination titers quantified by serial twofold dilutions of sera (73,113). In general, other measures of disease activity, including clinical variables and ESR and serum CRP concentrations, are sufficient and probably superior to RF measurement for routinely monitoring disease activity in RA patients (114). Among patients with RA, RF may become positive when originally negative, or vice versa. In a series of 119 patients enrolled in a prospective study of early RA, 46 (39%) were RF-positive on presentation, and an additional 23 (19%) developed RF later, yielding a total positive rate of 58% (97). Other studies have shown substantial variation in RF titer, with reversal of seropositivity and seronegativity. The majority of patients with RF will have a positive test within 6 months of the onset of symptoms, but for some it may be more than a year until the RF test first becomes positive (115). It has been reported that the functional avidity of RF may change over time (116), therefore changes in both the quantity and avidity of RF could contribute to changes in measured RF. Persistently high levels of RF have been shown to be associated with more severe radiologic joint destruction over at least a 3-year follow-up period (117).

Subjects without RA are more likely than RA patients to have serum RFs that do not persist on long-term follow-up (104). Studies from a number of populations indicate that presence of RF tends to occur in a few percent (typically approximately 1.5% to 3.0%) of the apparently healthy population, with a higher frequency in older than younger subjects and in females than males (e.g., see reference 118). Some studies have used a 4% to 5% positive rate in control subjects for establishing the upper limit of normal or threshold for a positive result using ELISA tests for RF (e.g., see reference 98). Some spontaneous fluctuation of RF titer may be seen commonly among apparently healthy individuals, and the intra-subject coefficient of variation of RF measurements in healthy middle-aged volunteers over several months has been measured to be approximately 8.5% (119).

CLINICAL ASSOCIATIONS

RFs are associated most closely with RA but may also be seen in patients with certain other autoimmune diseases. The majority of patients with primary Sjögren's syndrome also have serum RF. Patients with certain forms of vasculitis, particularly those with the syndrome of mixed cryoglobulinemia associated with hepatitis C virus (HCV), also may have high titers of serum RF (120). Patients with B-cell malignancies, particularly lymphomas or Waldenström's macroglobulinemia, may have very high levels of circulating RF produced by the malignant clone. Other associations are summarized in Table 6.1. It has been suggested that smoking is associated with a chronically elevated RF in the absence of rheumatic disease (106), and presence of RF [and antibodies to nuclear antigens (ANAs)] may be associated with a higher risk of cardiovascular disease even in patients without RA (121).

Up to 70% of patients with chronic active hepatitis due to HCV have been reported to have positive RF tests, and the RF titers can be quite elevated in HCV-infected patients (120). The prevalence of RA in the population (approximately 1%) is similar to the prevalence of chronic HCV (0.5% to 2.0% in the general population); thus, if the RF test is performed on an unselected population, a positive RF test is as likely to be caused by chronic HCV infection as by RA. After treatment of

TABLE 6.1. Clinical Associations of Rheumatoid Factor

Autoimmune diseases
- Rheumatoid arthritis
  - Juvenile rheumatoid arthritis subtype
- Sjögren's syndrome
- Systemic lupus erythematosus
- Vasculitis
  - Mixed cryoglobulinemia syndrome
- Idiopathic pulmonary fibrosis

Infectious diseases
- Chronic bacterial diseases
  - Bacterial endocarditis
  - Chronic osteomyelitis
  - Syphilis
- Chronic viral diseases
  - Hepatitis C

Lymphoproliferative disorders
- Waldenström's macroglobulinemia
- B-cell lymphoma
- Chronic lymphocytic leukemia

Environmental exposures
- Smoking

HCV infection, the RF level usually decreases, and a patient whose sera tested positive for RF may become negative (122).

SUMMARY OF CLINICAL UTILITY OF RHEUMATOID FACTOR TESTING

The RF test is most commonly ordered as a diagnostic adjunct in evaluating a patient with possible RA and in establishing the prognosis. In multiple studies, RA patients with RF tend to have a worse prognosis than patients with RA who lack RF, in that deformities, radiographic erosions, and extraarticular manifestations all tend to be more frequent and more severe in patients with serum RF. Excess mortality related to the diagnosis of RA is also associated with the presence of RF (123,124). Furthermore, when RA is treated successfully, the RF titer tends to fall, and loss of RF positive status is associated with a better prognosis (125,126).

Diagnostically, the presence of an RF lends support to a clinical impression of RA when combined with other clinical data, but it should not be considered a test that, by itself, is diagnostic. More important, RF is useful prognostically because the presence of RF in high titer is associated with more severe RA. RF-positive (also known as *seropositive*) RA patients are more likely to have progressive, erosive arthritis with loss of joint function and are also more likely to have extraarticular complications. The tendency toward earlier and more aggressive treatment of severe RA makes identifying patients likely to have severe disease a major goal. Although imperfect, RF is one of the best prognostic indicators currently available. RF remains the single test most used by rheumatologists to support the diagnosis of RA (2,127). Recent studies continue to demonstrate the high prognostic value of RF in prediction of more severe and erosive RA, with the presence of an initial RF at a titer of at least 1:160 associated with more than twice as much progression of radiographic changes over 5 years as observed in patients without RF (128).

Antibodies to Citrullinated Peptides

Antibodies to citrullinated peptides or proteins have been described by several different names, depending on the method of detection and the investigators performing the assays. Using indirect immunofluorescent microscopy, antibodies binding to perinuclear granules of buccal mucosal cells

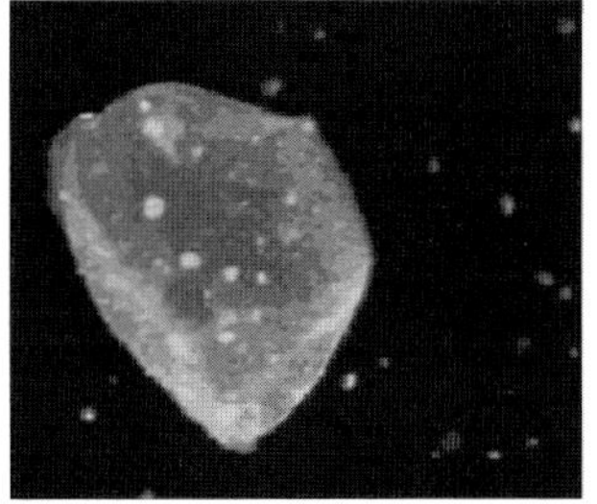

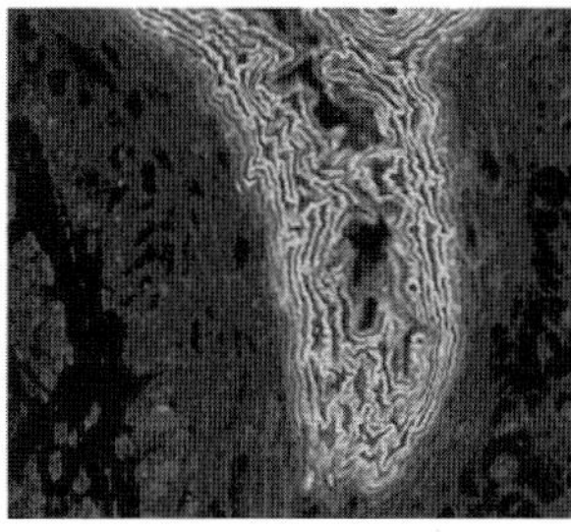

A,B

Figure 6.1. Anti-citrulline antibodies detected by indirect immunofluorescence microscopy. Substrates are allowed to react with rheumatoid arthritis serum containing anticitrulline, then antibodies are detected with fluoresceinated antihuman immunoglobulin G. **A:** Antiperinuclear factor. Buccal mucosal cell substrate. The perinuclear granular staining is characteristic. **B:** Antikeratin antibodies. Substrate is monkey esophagus tissue.

were reported by Dutch investigators in 1964 as a specific finding in sera of patients with RA; those antibodies were descriptively named "anti-perinuclear factor" (129) (Fig. 6.1). Performance of the test required as substrate buccal mucosal cells from selected donors, as not all donors' buccal cells seemed to contain the antigen. The antigen detected by this assay was located in the keratohyalin granules that surround the nucleus of buccal mucosa cells, accounting for the observed staining pattern. Using immunofluorescence microscopy, British investigators in 1979 reported that antibodies from sera of RA patients could bind the mature granular layer of rat esophagus. Those antibodies were called "antikeratin antibodies" (AKAs) (130) (Fig. 6.1). Additional studies reported in 1993 led to the conclusion that AKAs and antiperinuclear factor (APF) were very similar sets of antibodies that both bound to the epidermal matrix intermediate filament–associated protein filaggrin, a protein expressed in keratinizing epithelial cells and involved in cornification of the epidermis (131). Further studies by Schellekens and colleagues found that binding of these antibodies required the presence of the amino acid citrulline for recognition by RA sera (132). The amino acid citrulline is formed by post-translational deimination of the amino acid arginine (Fig. 6.2). In filaggrin contained in mature epithelial cells, approximately 20% of the arginine is normally converted to citrulline by the enzyme peptidylarginine deiminase (133), thus explaining the previous identification of filaggrin as the target antigen.

Another RA-specific autoantigen described in 1994 as "Sa" was originally characterized as a 50-kd antigen detected in an extract from human placenta (134). Subsequently, the antigen was found in extracts from normal human spleen and RA synovial

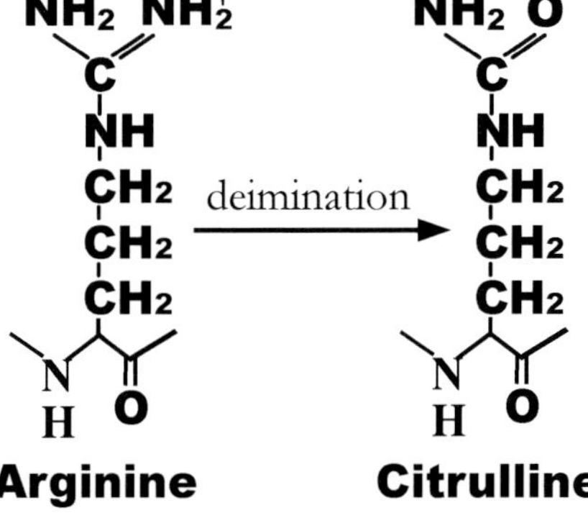

Figure 6.2. Deimination reaction causes post-translational change from residues of arginine to amino acid citrulline.

extracts. The Sa antigen has now been identified as a hapten-carrier complex in which citrulline is the antigenic determinant and vimentin, an intermediate filament protein, is the carrier (135). Antibodies to Sa have been described in approximately 40% of RA patients overall, with detection in close to 50% of patients with long-standing RA and approximately 25% of patients with recent-onset RA (136). Among adults with a variety of inflammatory arthritides besides RA, approximately 8% have anti-Sa. Anti-Sa has also been linked to the presence of RF and HLA DRB1*04 (136). The presence of anti-Sa has been associated with a higher probability of severe, erosive disease. Because anti-Sa and APF assays detect the same family of antibodies, it is not surprising that when both are measured in the same sera, the presence of anti-Sa is strongly associated with the presence of APF.

With the understanding that citrullinated peptides in filaggrin, vimentin, fibrin (137), and other proteins and peptides can be recognized by RA serum antibodies, citrullinated peptides have been synthesized as antigens for the development of diagnostic immunoassays. Investigators in the Netherlands have found that the diagnostic utility of citrullinated peptides can be improved by synthesizing circular peptides using disulfide bonds within the small peptide to form a ring structure (138). This circular peptide may expose or stabilize the citrulline residue, improving the sensitivity of the ELISA assays that have been developed. Using different cyclic citrullinated peptides has led to improvements in the tests sold by commercial diagnostics companies, and testing for antibodies to the cyclic citrullinated peptide (anti-CCP) has been approved for the diagnosis of RA. The test is moderately sensitive (41% to 80%, depending on the cohort studied) and approximately 90% to 98% specific for the diagnosis of RA (138–140). In direct comparison using the same population of patients, a positive test for anti-CCP was found to be somewhat less sensitive but somewhat more specific than tests for IgM RF (138,140). When both RF and anti-CCP are present, the specificity for the diagnosis of RA is more than 99.5%, even when a variety of disease controls are included in the reference population. Furthermore, antibodies to the family of citrullinated antigens are frequently positive early in the course of RA when the diagnosis may be uncertain, as exemplified by finding anti-Sa among the patients who developed RA in an early synovitis cohort (141). In cohorts of patients prospectively followed in Sweden, the anti-CCP test was 25% sensitive for the diagnosis of RA in sera drawn more than 1.5 years before the diagnosis of RA was established. In sera available within 1.5 years before the diagnosis of RA, anti-CCP was present in 52% (112). Anti-CCP was present in sera collected as long as 9 years before the diagnosis of RA, and once anti-CCP antibodies are detected, they almost always remain present in sera collected subsequently from the same individual.

If antibodies to citrullinated peptides are detected in patients diagnosed with RA, the test for those antibodies almost always remains positive, whereas the serum concentration of RF may return to normal over time (142). Anti-CCP can be found in RA patients both with and without IgM RF, although it is more frequent in RA patients with RF. Sera of patients with hepatitis C and cryoglobulinemia, although frequently testing positive for the presence of RF, rarely have anti-CCP, thus demonstrating that there is not a direct connection between the development of RF and development of anti-CCP in patients without RA (143). Anti-CCP has been described in as few as 2% (144) and as many as two out of three (145) children with JRA of a variety of subtypes, suggesting that anti-CCP measurement could be useful in diagnosis of RF-negative JRA.

In addition to use of anti-CCP as a diagnostic test, it may be useful as a prognostic indicator. In long-term follow-up of patients, the presence of anti-CCP is a risk factor for development of erosive arthritis (138,146). In some series, anti-CCP was not as accurate as IgM RF in predicting erosive disease (140,147), whereas in other series anti-CCP was superior to RF testing in predicting erosive disease (6). Use of both anti-CCP and RF tests might improve the ability to predict erosive or disabling disease, or both, but evidence in support of that possibility has been mixed. In general, the additional prognostic accuracy from combining test results for anti-CCP and RF, rather than using either alone, has been modest among patients who already have a diagnosis of RA (147,148). Use of the test combination may be more useful in evaluating patients with early synovitis. In a study of early synovitis patients with a variety of diagnoses, presence of anti-CCP had the highest predictive value of any laboratory test for the development of persistent synovitis and for the development of erosive arthritis at 2 years after presentation (6). The authors of this study proposed a point system for predicting the development of persistent versus self-limited arthritis and for the development of erosive arthritis. In this algorithm, both anti-CCP and IgM RF tests were important early diagnostic and prognostic factors (6).

The biologic significance and mechanism for generation of anti-CCP remains unclear but could provide clues to the pathogenesis of RA (149,150). Of interest, filaggrin, whether in its native state or citrullinated, does not cause T-cell proliferation (151). The cellular regulation and T-cell immunology associated with citrulline-related autoimmunity requires further study. Anti-filaggrin autoantibody (AFA) was reported to be relatively enriched in extracts from synovial pannus compared with the serum of RA patients, but similar concentrations were observed in serum and in SF from RA patients (152). These findings, and the finding that synovial extracts seemed to produce AFA, suggested that AFA is produced in the synovium. The search for citrullinated antigens in rheumatoid synovium that could be recognized by anti-CCP has identified the presence of citrullinated fibrin (137) and an intracellular citrullinated antigen (153). These citrullinated proteins in synovium could be targeted by anti-CCP and promote synovitis. A polymorphism of the PADI4 (peptidyl arginine deiminase 4) gene, which encodes one of the genes responsible for the formation of citrulline within proteins, has been associated with higher risk of developing RA (153a), suggesting that citrullination could have an important role in the development of RA.

With better availability and standardization, CCP antibody testing in evaluation of RA patients is likely to become an increasingly used laboratory measure both for diagnosis of RA and for establishing its prognosis of RA. Overall, testing for anti-CCP can be regarded as similar to but additive to the information provided by RF testing, with similar or somewhat lower sensitivity, higher specificity, and similar prognostic value. Measurement of anti-CCP may be particularly helpful as part of a diagnostic algorithm to classify early synovitis patients (6).

Anti-RA33/Heterogeneous Nuclear Ribonucleoprotein-A2

RA33 was described as a 33-kd autoantigen recognized by IgG in the serum from approximately 35% of patients with RA (154). RA33 was subsequently characterized as the A2 protein of the heterogeneous nuclear ribonucleoproteins (RNPs). Although RA33 was originally described as characteristic of RA, immunoblot testing of sera from patients with a range of rheumatic diseases has demonstrated the presence of the antibody in sera of 35% of RA patients, 38% of mixed connective tissue disease (MCTD) patients, 23% of SLE patients, and, rarely, in patients with other rheumatic disorders (155). The A2 protein is associated with the spliceosome, as are the autoantigens U1-RNP (associated with SLE and MCTD) and Sm (associated with SLE), which are polypeptides that contribute to the small nuclear RNPs. Although patients with SLE and MCTD have antibodies to both RA33/A2 and small nuclear RNPs, patients with RA only have antibodies to RA33/A2 (155). The antigen may be overexpressed in rheumatoid synovium, where it may be a potential target for autoreactive lymphocytes (151).

Chaperone and Heat Shock Proteins

Anti-p68/BiP was first described in 1995 as the predominant antigen recognized by rheumatoid sera in synovial membrane extracts (156). Presence of the antibody is approximately 60% sensitive and 99% specific for the diagnosis of RA. Follow-up studies indicate that the antigen is ubiquitous and that rheumatoid sera preferentially bind the glycosylated form of the p68 protein (157). Subsequent investigations using proteomic approaches to characterize the antigen identified the p68 antigen as the endoplasmic reticulum chaperone BiP (158). The antigen is also recognized by T cells (158). BiP is a glucose-regulated stress protein, also known as *Ig-binding protein*, that plays a critical role in stabilizing proteins, including Ig heavy and light chains, and directing them out of the endoplasmic reticulum for secretion.

Other stress proteins have also been described as targets of antibodies from sera of RA patients. Antibodies from RA patients have been found to recognize unidentified or poorly identified members of the 70-kd family of heat shock proteins (hsp 70) from humans, *Escherichia coli*, and bovine sources (159,160). Measurement of antibodies to heat shock proteins depends on the detection methods; thus, the finding of anti–heat shock proteins should be interpreted cautiously (161).

Glycolytic Enzymes: Anti–Glucose-6-Phosphate Isomerase and Enolase

In 1999, Matsumoto et al. described an animal model of arthritis that initially depended on T cells and at later stages could be passively transferred with serum alone. Both the T-cell and B-cell autoantigen responsible for this disease is the ubiquitous glycolytic pathway enzyme glucose-6-phosphate isomerase (GPI) (162). A subsequent paper described anti-GPI in the sera and SFs of a majority of patients with RA, thus bridging the animal model and human RA (163). Follow-up studies failed to replicate the finding of a high prevalence of anti-GPI in RA sera and also determined that anti-GPI is found with similar low frequency in other conditions (164). The model is of interest, however, because it may result from nonspecific binding of the GPI protein to cartilage and extracellular synovial matrix, with the pathologic reaction caused by an immune response to the planted antigen (165).

Other enzymes in the glycolytic pathway have been implicated as autoantigens in RA. The enzyme alpha-enolase was identified as an autoantigen detected by sera from approximately 25% of RA patients (166). Half of the patients with anti-enolase did not have RF or filaggrin antibodies, yet the presence of anti-enolase was associated with more severe, erosive disease. The recombinant form of the antigen was recognized much less frequently than the native antigen, perhaps reflecting enhanced recognition of translationally modified antigen. The enzyme aldolase A (fructose-bisphosphate aldolase) was also identified as an autoantigen recognized by RA sera (167). In this study, approximately 10% of RA patients (vs. no controls) had antibodies to aldolase A , and the denatured antigen was recognized preferentially.

Calpastatin

Calpastatin is the physiologic inhibitor of calpains, which are calcium-dependent cysteine proteases that are overexpressed in rheumatoid synovial tissue and may contribute to cartilage destruction. In screening for antigens with a nonspecific library, Depres et al. observed that 45% of sera from RA patients contained antibodies to one of their expressed proteins, identified as calpastatin (168). Subsequent studies have found anti-calpastatin in sera of 10% to 50% of RA patients (169). Anti-calpastatin is found in sera from similar proportions of sera from patients with a variety of other rheumatic diseases, including SLE, Sjögren's syndrome, and systemic sclerosis (169), although not in patients with spondylitis (170).

Antibodies to Nuclear Antigens

Although positive tests for ANAs are described in RA, in most series specificity of the antibody has not been identified. Anti-Ro/Sjögren's syndrome antigen A and anti-La/Sjögren's syndrome antigen B are occasionally observed in the sera of patients with RA and coexistent Sjögren's syndrome; unlike the situation with primary Sjögren's syndrome, however, most patients with Sjögren's syndrome secondary to RA have negative tests for those antibodies. After treatment of RA patients with infliximab and other TNF inhibitors, a minority of patients develop antibodies to double-stranded DNA (171).

Positive ANA tests occur in patients with JRA. In particular, JRA patients with serum ANAs are likely to have pauciarticular disease and uveitis and often carry the HLA-DR5 antigen.

Anti-Collagen

Antibodies to type II collagen (CII) and other joint-specific autoantigens could contribute to the pathogenesis of RA. Indeed, animal models have demonstrated that an immune response to collagen can lead to synovitis resembling RA. Antibodies to CII, the major collagen in joint cartilage, were described in SFs and sera from patients with RA many years ago, and recent investigations have attempted to clarify the nature of the antibodies to CII that are present in RA patients. The test for anti-CII is not used clinically as a marker for RA, because, in most studies, a minority of patients with RA have serum antibodies to CII. Also, control groups, including patients with SLE, ankylosing spondylitis, and some normal control sera, contain antibodies to CII (172).

Anti-CII is a marker for relapsing polychondritis, an autoimmune inflammatory disease in which cartilage of the ear, nose, eye, as well as joints become inflamed and destroyed, although the dominant immune response in relapsing polychondritis is to the nonarticular matrix protein matrilin (173,174). Antibodies to the collagen-like regions of C1q are present in the sera of patients with SLE and occasionally also the sera of patients with RA. The antibodies detected in assays for collagen are distinct from the population of antibodies to the collagen-like region of C1q (175).

One of the complexities in evaluating the literature concerning antibodies to CII is that antibody responses have been evaluated using CII from different species (primarily human, bovine, chicken, and rat collagens), as well as different physical forms (i.e., denatured collagen or native collagen). Binding of Igs to native collagen represents a typical antigen-antibody interaction, mediated by binding of antigen via the Fab of an antibody. In contrast, binding of antibodies to denatured collagen may be mediated by less specific binding of high-molecular-weight fibronectin-Ig complexes that adhere to denatured collagen because of the binding of fibronectin to collagen (176). This interaction may contribute to the observation that the levels of anti-collagen antibodies, more than other antibodies, are subject to storage artifacts (177). Studies of antibodies to denatured collagen therefore should be interpreted with caution.

Antibodies to CII in RA may fluctuate over the course of disease. One study described a higher frequency of anti-collagen earlier in the course of RA, which subsequently declined over time (178), whereas another study concluded that these antibodies were present at a lower frequency in early RA than later in the course of disease (179). The frequency of collagen antibodies appears to differ in RA populations from different geographic regions (180).

Anti-collagen antibodies are found in higher concentration in the SF than in the sera of patients with RA, and B cells producing anti-CII are increased in the synovium of RA patients (181). High levels of collagen antibodies are not found in SFs from patients with other diagnoses (182,183). The IgG isotypes of antibodies to CII in RA are typically IgG1 and IgG3 (184,185), whereas IgG4 antibodies constitute the predominant isotype of anti-collagen among patients with SLE (184).

Mapping studies have allowed comparison of the epitopes on collagens recognized by sera from RA patients with those recognized by rodent serum in the collagen-induced arthritis model (186). In some of these studies, peptide fragments produced by cyanogen bromide cleavage of collagen have been used to characterize the binding site on collagen (187). The challenge of determining conformational epitopes on various regions of the native collagen molecule has been approached by inserting specific amino acid sequences containing the epitopes of interest from CII as a cassette into a constant framework of type X collagen (188). Linear epitopes of CII with preserved helical conformation have also been synthesized (188). These approaches preserve the overall triple helical structure of the collagen, while allowing specific linear epitopes from CII to be evaluated and compared with each other with regard to their antibody binding. These studies have led to the conclusion that the dominant epitopes on CII are sterically accessible and represent evolutionally conserved regions. The dominant epitope in RA appears to reside in residues 359 to 369 of CII, whereas other epitopes are also recognized by sera of patients with relapsing polychondritis or osteoarthritis (OA) (188).

TISSUE-SPECIFIC MARKERS

Use of Tissue Biomarkers in Rheumatoid Arthritis

The tissues manifesting the primary pathology in patients with RA are synovium, cartilage, and juxtaarticular bone. In principle, serum, urine, or SF markers that reflect either increased synthesis or breakdown of those tissues could be useful in diagnosis, in establishing the prognosis of disease, in indicating the pathologic or physiologic stage of disease, as indicators of disease activity, or as indicators of the response to therapy. There is considerable interest in effective biomarkers, particularly tissue-specific markers (reviewed in references 189–193). A National Institutes of Health consensus conference on use of biomarkers for evaluation of OA identified several potential biomarkers for evaluation of joint disease (194). In general, markers that are indicative of joint destruction in OA also may be useful in patients with RA. Markers indicative of altered cartilage turnover include CII-C-propeptide (synthesis indicator), CII fragments (degradation indicator), proteoglycan aggrecan 846 epitope (synthesis indicator), and proteoglycan aggrecan keratan sulfate (KS) fragments (degradation indicator). Markers of bone turnover potentially helpful in arthritis include osteocalcin or bone-specific alkaline phosphatase (synthesis indicators) and type I collagen cross-links (resorption indicator). Biologic markers considered as measures of synovial disease included cartilage oligomeric matrix protein (COMP) and hyaluronic acid (synovitis indicators). Table 6.2 summarizes representative results observed in measuring these markers in SF, serum, and urine of patients with RA, in comparison with measurements in normal individuals.

Assessing the utility of biomarkers requires understanding their tissue distribution and molecular expression in a variety of clinical conditions. Some markers may be less specific than originally anticipated. For example, the YKL-40 marker, originally thought to be specific for synovial and articular cartilage, is now known to be associated with a variety of conditions ranging from liver disease to malignancy. Another problem with interpretation of biomarker measurements is that the concentrations of the markers can be substantially affected by physical activity, SF volume, and alterations in clearance of SF, thus leading to substantial inter- and intra-individual variation in measurements (193,195,196). The concentration of these molecules in blood and urine is also influenced by other processes such as liver and kidney clearance or metabolism. Calculation of ratios of markers has been proposed as a mechanism to compensate for some of the variability encountered in biomarker concentrations (192).

Markers of Cartilage and Synovium Turnover

YKL-40

One protein considered a potential indicator of cartilage and synovium turnover is the protein YKL-40, also called *human cartilage glycoprotein 39*. The YKL-40 molecule is a member of the family of 18-glycosyl-hydrolases, or chitinases. YKL-40 was originally described as a mammary protein from cows and later found in large amounts in synoviocytes and chondrocytes (197,198). Concentrations of YKL-40 have been measured in SF and serum of patients with RA and have been found to be elevated compared with concentrations observed in patients without joint disease (199). The levels are higher in SF of affected joints than in serum and are thought to be a reflection of increased synthesis by synoviocytes and or cartilage cells. Serum YKL-40 levels may reflect both inflammation and joint destruction in patients with RA (200,201), as elevated levels of serum YKL-40 in RA patients correlate both with inflammation measures and with the radiologic score. In one study, YKL-40 levels in the serum were highest early in the course of RA and then declined with treatment (202). Serum concentrations correlate with clinical and laboratory features of inflammation and with the baseline Larsen erosion score but do not predict radiographic progression (17,202). Of interest, antibodies to YKL-40 and a homolog, YKL-39, occur in the sera of a minority of RA patients (203).

SF concentrations of YKL-40 are elevated in OA, and serum concentrations may be elevated in patients with advanced OA; thus, elevated levels are not specific for RA (204). In addition, the YKL-40 protein is secreted by activated macrophages, neutrophils, and osteosarcoma cells, as well as by chondrocytes and synoviocytes. Elevated serum levels have been described in patients with cirrhosis of the liver, breast and colorectal cancers, and, acutely, in patients with infection. Serum levels of YKL-40 are not a specific marker of joint or cartilage disease but can be elevated in a variety of inflammatory and neoplastic conditions (205–209).

CARTILAGE OLIGOMERIC MATRIX PROTEIN

COMP is a noncollagenous protein found in the matrix of articular cartilage. COMP is a 525-kd extracellular matrix glycoprotein, a member of the thrombospondin family, consisting of five identical disulfide-linked subunits. Although present in the highest concentration in articular cartilage, COMP is synthesized by synoviocytes, as well as chondrocytes, and is also found in tendons, the meniscus, and in nasal and tracheal cartilage (210). It is not found in skin or lungs. Saxne and Heinegard initially described elevated levels of the protein in blood and SFs from patients with

TABLE 6.2. Tissue-Related Markers and Their Changes in Rheumatoid Arthritis

Site	Molecule	Marker	Mechanism for Release	Synovial Fluid	Serum	Urine
Cartilage	Aggrecan	Chondroitin sulfate Epitopes 846, 3B3, 7D4	S	—	High	—
		Core protein fragments	D	High	—	—
		Keratan sulfate Fragment epitopes 5D4, AN9PI	D ??	Low	Normal or low	—
	CII	PII propeptides PIICP PIIANP	S	High	High	—
		CII telopeptides	D	—	—	High
		CII fragments CII-3/4m CII-1/4N	D	—	—	High
Synovium/ cartilage	Collagens	Pyr Glc-Gal-PYD	D	—	—	High
		Pyr/D-Pyr ratio	D; lower with bone, higher with synovium/cartilage (?)	—	—	High
		Procollagen III N-terminal propeptides	S	High	High	—
	Hyaluronan	Hyaluronan	S	Low	High	—
	Other proteins	YKL-40	S	High > serum	High	—
		Cartilage oligomeric matrix protein	D	High > serum	High	—
Bone	Collagen I	Procollagen I propeptides (PINP, PICP)	S	—	Normal	—
		D-pyridinoline	D	—	—	Normal or high
		Pyridinoline	D	—	—	High
		Telopeptides (NTx, CTx, ICTP)	D	High	High	High
	Other	Bone-specific alkaline phosphatase	S	—	Normal	—
		Osteocalcin	S	Normal or low	D	—
		Bone sialoprotein	D	High	High	—
		Tartrate-resistant acid phosphatase	D	—	High (not from bone)	—

CII, type II collagen; CII-3/4 m, type II collagen peptide 3/4 m; CII-1/4N, type II collagen epitope 1/4; CTx, C-terminal telopeptides; D, mechanism for increase of marker relates to degradation or catabolism; D-Pyr, D-pyridinoline; ICTP, type I collagen C-terminal telopeptide; NTx, N-terminal telopeptides; PICP, procollagen I C-terminal propeptides; PII, procollagen II; PIIANP, procollagen IIA N-terminal propeptides; PIICP, procollagen II C-terminal propeptides; PINP, procollagen I N-terminal propeptides; Pyr, pyridinoline; S, mechanism for increase of marker relates to synthesis.
Note: Entries with dashes indicate missing or incomplete data about the association of the marker in rheumatoid arthritis.

arthritis (211). Levels of COMP are higher in SF than in serum, indicating release from involved joints with subsequent release into the circulation (211). In the SF of patients with RA and inflammatory arthritis, high levels of fragments of COMP are present, whereas fragmented COMP is not prominent in SF of OA patients (210). Serum levels of COMP are higher in those who later develop more aggressive and advanced disease affecting large joints, such as the hip and knee (212,213), but progression of joint destruction in small joints of the hands and feet is not associated with higher levels of COMP (214).

Studies on the use of COMP levels to predict the long-term course of RA have yielded inconsistent results. One report suggested that COMP serum levels had a high predictive value for more severe disease among patients receiving TNF-α antagonists (215), but another 5-year prospective study found no significant prognostic value associated with COMP levels in RA patients (216). The magnitude of COMP elevation may relate to the course of disease, as it has been reported that levels of COMP are lower in patients with more advanced RA (211).

PROTEOGLYCAN MARKERS

Knowledge of the biology of cartilage and synovial proteoglycans has improved the potential for clinical use of measures of proteoglycan turnover. These large macromolecular complexes consist of hyaluronic acid bound via link protein to the proteoglycan, aggrecan. Aggrecan in turn is composed of the aggrecan core protein to which are bound many molecules of the glycosaminoglycans KS and chondroitin sulfate. These proteoglycans are degraded by a number of nonspecific matrix metalloproteinases (MMPs), as well as by more specific aggrecanases. The aggrecanases are members of the family of zinc metalloproteinases named for their structural features as members of the ADAMTS (*a d*isintegrin and *a m*etalloproteinase domain with *t*hrombospondin motif*s*) protein family (217). Because the aggrecanases and nonspecific MMPs cleave aggrecan at specific, different sites, measurements of different aggrecan fragments and glycosaminoglycans can provide clues to the catabolism of these proteoglycans. This approach has been facilitated through use of antibodies directed specifically against novel antigenic determinants created by enzymatic degradation, known as *catabolic neoepitopes* (218). The novel fragments in many instances are named for the designations of the clones used to generate the monoclonal antibodies that detect the fragments.

Concentrations of the core protein are elevated in the SF of patients with acute arthritis, but not usually in SF from RA patients (219). Quantification of aggrecan in SF may help predict which patients with acute arthritis will develop chronic disease (220). Assays have been developed that differentially quantify polypeptides from the central portion of the core protein, and other assays detect metabolites from the N-terminal first globular (G1) domain. The G1 domain of the core protein binds to hyaluronic acid and tends to be retained in cartilage. The ratio of central peptides/G1 decreases in late-stage RA and is a marker for erosive disease (221). Serum levels of aggrecan core protein in RA are similar to those in controls. Antibodies have been generated against C-terminal and N-terminal neoepitopes of the core protein after metalloproteinase cleavage and could prove to be useful markers of cartilage destruction.

Neoepitopes have been revealed on chondroitin sulfate, reflecting degradation or newly synthesized molecules of aggrecan. Chondroitin sulfate epitope 846 is thought to be present only on newly synthesized aggrecan and is therefore a putative marker of cartilage aggrecan synthesis (222). Concentrations of this marker are increased in the serum of RA patients with slow joint destruction, whereas concentrations are not increased in serum of RA patients with rapid joint destruction (212). Elevated serum levels of the 846 epitope were therefore thought to indicate a more favorable prognosis in patients with RA. Concentrations of the marker are higher in SF than in serum (222).

KS epitope AN9PI is thought to be present on intact and degraded molecules of aggrecan. Serum levels are abnormally low in RA patients in most studies (222) and are inversely related to inflammatory markers (222), although other studies have reported elevated values of KS in RA (223,224).

HYALURONAN

Serum levels of hyaluronan (HA) are elevated in patients with RA, and, generally, levels correlate with clinical measures of disease activity (225) and arthritis progression (226). HA, a very-high-molecular-weight molecule, is cleared from the SF through the lymphatics and subsequently removed from the circulation by the liver. Thus, serum concentrations are elevated in patients with significant hepatic disease, as well as with increased synthesis and clearance associated with active synovitis. There is substantial intra-individual circadian variation in circulating HA levels. Serum concentrations may change with eating, possibly reflecting changes in lymphatic drainage related to meals (194).

COLLAGEN FRAGMENTS

CII is found in high concentrations in articular collagen and is nearly specific for that tissue (CII is also found in the eye). As such, there is interest in the potential to measure type CII fragments as an indication of joint turnover. In principle, propeptides derived from procollagen II would be measures of CII synthesis. Elevated levels of the C-propeptide of CII were observed in patients with RA, indicating increased collagen synthesis, but the elevated levels did not correlate with the course or pace of disease (212). High levels of the C-propeptide of CII have been observed in SF of OA patients with a lesser increase in SF of RA patients, suggesting increased cartilage repair in OA compared with RA (227). Cross-linked telopeptides or neoepitopes specific for cleaved CII should serve as indices of cartilage degradation, and such assays are under development. Baseline levels of urinary C-terminal telopeptides have been shown to correlate with radiographic progression of RA (228).

CII propeptide fragments derived from synovium or cartilage, or both, are elevated in blood and SF of patients with RA (229,230). The elevations correlate with disease activity and predict development of radiographic erosions.

METALLOPROTEINASES

Metalloproteinases lead to the breakdown of cartilage, proteoglycans, and other matrix molecules. The MMPs MMP-1 (also known as *collagenase*), MMP-2 (also known as *gelatinase*), and MMP-3 (stromelysin) all have been implicated in the pathogenesis of destructive or erosive arthritis. Imbalance between the levels of these proteinases and their natural inhibitors [tissue inhibitors of metalloproteinases (TIMPs)] may lead to destruction of joint tissues. SF concentrations of MMPs and TIMPs are elevated in RA, and the ratio of the enzymes to the inhibitors is elevated, plausibly suggesting that they may mediate breakdown of synovial cartilage (231). Serum concentrations of MMPs, particularly MMP-3, and TIMPs are also elevated in active RA and have been used as a marker of disease response to therapy (232,233). Some investigators have found that the elevated levels of MMP-3 observed in RA correlate very well with levels of CRP (234), and therefore that measurement of MMP-3 may be more a measure of inflammation. In contrast, measurement of MMP-1 may be linked more closely to development of erosive arthritis (233).

Bone Markers

Because of bone destruction associated with RA, bone synthesis and degradation markers could be useful in monitoring disease. However, as most bone is not periarticular, general markers of bone turnover are not very specific for assessing RA, and both generalized bone disorders and active RA contribute to changes in bone markers (235). Nevertheless, elevated levels of type I collagen telopeptides, a measure of bone degradation and turnover, predict radiographic progression of RA (228). Serum levels of tartrate-resistant alkaline phosphatase, usually considered a bone synthesis marker, are elevated in RA patients, but the isoform of acid phosphatase that is increased is likely to be derived from macrophages rather than from bone (236). Bone sialoprotein (BSP) is a glycoprotein that is enriched at the bone-cartilage interface, and therefore could be more specific as a marker of bone damage or turnover caused by arthritis. BSP levels were increased in the SF of knees of patients with RA and correlated with knee damage (237). BSP levels have also been reported to be increased in sera of patients with RA but did not correlate with progressive disease (212). Further studies may clarify if BSP measurement is likely to have a greater role in monitoring RA patients or in predicting the development of bone erosions.

CLINICAL UTILITY OF LABORATORY TESTS

The utility of a diagnostic laboratory test depends on the performance of the test itself and the pre-test probability or frequency of the disease in the population being evaluated. In general, there is a trade-off between the sensitivity and specificity of diagnostic tests, which can be described by a receiver-operating characteristics curve. By plotting the true-positive rate (= sensitivity) on the ordinate and the false-positive rate (= 1 – specificity) on the abscissa, one can determine the performance of a quantitative test over a range of cut-off values. Furthermore, one can compare two tests or testing algorithms by plotting their curves on the same graph; the superior test is one that is closer to the top left corner of the graph and has a larger area under the curve. These issues are illustrated in Figure 6.3 using data evaluating different models of tests used to discriminate between self-limited and persistent arthritis among patients presenting to an early arthritis clinic (from reference 6). Models 1 and 2 follow curves closer to the top left corner of the graph (the ideal of perfect sensitivity and specificity) and have a larger area under the curve than models 3 and the ACR criteria. The authors of this study demonstrate that their diagnostic criteria for model 1 (scored with symptom duration, duration of morning stiffness, arthritis in at least 3 joints, compression tenderness of the MTPs, IgM RF at least 5 IU, anti-CCP at least 92 IU, and erosions on hand or foot radiographs) are equivalent to model 2

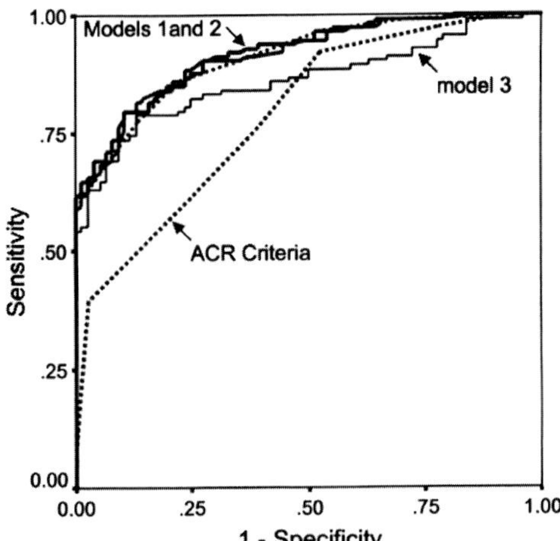

Figure 6.3. Receiver operator characteristics curve demonstrating the trade-off between sensitivity and specificity of diagnostic tests and allowing comparison of diagnostic tests (see text). ACR, American College of Rheumatology.

(with immunogenetic data added to model 1) and superior to an alternative model 3 (use of laboratory tests and x-ray data only) and to the ACR classification criteria for RA. Standards for publishing reports of diagnostic accuracy of laboratory tests have been developed, and could lead to improvement in the quality of such reports (238,239).

COMBINATIONS OF AUTOANTIBODY TESTS AND ROLE IN EVALUATION

Combinations of laboratory tests increase the prognostic value of laboratory tests. In several recent studies, both RF and antibodies to citrullinated peptides (or an equivalent, such as APF) had additive predictive value for the development of erosions (6,17,142). The degree of elevation of ESR and CRP levels also contribute to the ability to prognosticate about the likelihood of development of radiologic progression. Among patients with early synovitis, RF and AKA/APF independently contributed to the diagnosis of RA, and it has been suggested that the presence of both RF and citrulline antibodies should be tested early in the course of disease to maximize the predictive value of laboratory testing (6,142). In a cross-sectional study of RA patients, anti-CCP was found to be more specific for the diagnosis of RA than RF tests, suggesting that the specificity of anti-CCP antibodies makes them useful in establishing the diagnosis of RA, although IgM RF may be a better predictor of disease severity (140). The absence of anti-CCP in a patient with high-titer RF but low likelihood of RA suggests that the RF is related to some other cause (e.g., chronic infection).

Laboratory tests are commonly performed to monitor potential toxicity of treatments of RA. The ACR has released guidelines concerning management of RA that include guidelines for monitoring drug toxicities. Although it is prudent to follow those guidelines in clinical practice, recently, investigators have formally studied the diagnostic yield of laboratory monitoring of disease-modifying antirheumatic drugs used in the treatment of RA (240). The authors of this study observed that important laboratory abnormalities were observed during the first 4 months of therapy only, and they recommended that laboratory tests should be performed in weeks 2 and 4, then monthly for the first 4 months of therapy, then two to four times per year. Using this approach led to detection of more than 98% of laboratory abnormalities in a reasonably timely manner, with a nearly 80% reduction in laboratory costs. The authors recommended that formal guidelines be modified in accord with their data.

What laboratory tests should be done to evaluate the possibility of RA in patients presenting with rheumatic disease complaints? The most important factors are the history and physical, followed by radiographs. If the diagnosis and prognosis of a patient are clear (e.g., if a patient has radiographic changes of erosive RA), there is little value in additional immunologic tests to establish a diagnosis or prognosis, as erosive disease serves as a predictor for further erosive disease. Establishing disease activity may be aided by evaluating simple measures of inflammation, including a complete blood cell count, ESR, and CRP. If a diagnosis of RA is being considered, IgM RF remains the antibody of choice to test clinically, but testing for anti-CCP may be useful, particularly in RF-negative patients for whom the clinician is seeking additional diagnostic support. A positive test for anti-CCP in a synovitis patient with or without RF would provide support for the diagnosis of RA associated with a worse prognosis and would lend support to trying earlier, more aggressive treatment. The role of tissue-specific markers in RA is still being evaluated. They may provide support for tissue-specific effects in clinical trials and in research in patients with RA, but they have not been shown to be of clear benefit in routine clinical practice.

REFERENCES

1. Donald F, Ward MM. Evaluative laboratory testing practices of United States rheumatologists. *Arthritis Rheum* 1998;41:725–729.
2. Saraux A, Maillefert JF, Fautrel B, et al. Laboratory and imaging studies used by French rheumatologists to determine the cause of recent onset polyarthritis without extra-articular manifestations. *Ann Rheum Dis* 2002;61:626–629.
3. American College of Rheumatology Subcommittee on Rheumatoid Arthritis Guidelines. Guidelines for the management of rheumatoid arthritis. 2002 update. *Arthritis Rheum* 2002;46:328–346.
4. Ward MM. Evaluative laboratory testing. Assessing tests that assess disease activity. *Arthritis Rheum* 1995;38:1555–1563.
5. Tunn EJ, Bacon PA. Differentiating persistent from self-limiting symmetrical synovitis in an early arthritis clinic. *Br J Rheumatol* 1993;32:97–103.
6. Visser H, le Cessie S, Vos K, et al. How to diagnose rheumatoid arthritis early: a prediction model for persistent (erosive) arthritis. *Arthritis Rheum* 2002;46:357–365.
7. Wolfe F, Ross K, Hawley DJ, et al. The prognosis of rheumatoid arthritis and undifferentiated polyarthritis syndrome in the clinic: a study of 1141 patients. *J Rheumatol* 1993;20:2005–2009.
8. Scott DL. Prognostic factors in early rheumatoid arthritis. *Rheumatology (Oxford)* 2000;39[Suppl 1]:24–29.
9. Wolfe F, Hawley DJ. The longterm outcomes of rheumatoid arthritis: work disability: a prospective 18 year study of 823 patients. *J Rheumatol* 1998;25:2108–2117.
10. Wolfe F, Sharp JT. Radiographic outcome of recent-onset rheumatoid arthritis: a 19-year study of radiographic progression. *Arthritis Rheum* 1998;41:1571–1582.
11. van Leeuwen MA, van der Heijde DM, van Rijswijk MH, et al. Interrelationship of outcome measures and process variables in early rheumatoid arthritis. A comparison of radiologic damage, physical disability, joint counts, and acute phase reactants. *J Rheumatol* 1994;21:425–429.
12. Amos RS, Constable TJ, Crockson RA, et al. Rheumatoid arthritis: relation of serum C-reactive protein and erythrocyte sedimentation rates to radiographic changes. *BMJ* 1977;1:195–197.
13. Hertzman A, Evans TI, Sanders KM, Mullinax F. Effects of blood storage on the erythrocyte sedimentation rate [Letter]. *J Rheumatol* 1993;20:2178–2179.
14. Miller A, Green M, Robinson D. Simple rule for calculating normal erythrocyte sedimentation rate. *BMJ* 1983;286:266.
15. Wolfe F. Comparative usefulness of C-reactive protein and erythrocyte sedimentation rate in patients with rheumatoid arthritis. *J Rheumatol* 1997;24:1477–1485.
16. Dawes PT, Fowler PD, Clarke S, et al. Rheumatoid arthritis: treatment which controls the C-reactive protein and erythrocyte sedimentation rate reduces radiological progression. *Br J Rheumatol* 1986;25:44–49.
17. Combe B, Dougados M, Goupille P, et al. Prognostic factors for radiographic damage in early rheumatoid arthritis: a multiparameter prospective study. *Arthritis Rheum* 2001;44:1736–1743.
18. Strand V, Sharp JT. Radiographic data from recent randomized controlled trials in rheumatoid arthritis: what have we learned? *Arthritis Rheum* 2003;48:21–34.

19. Ridker P, Rimfain N, Clearfield M, et al. Measurement of C-reactive protein for the targeting of statin therapy in the primary prevention of acute coronary events. *N Engl J Med* 2001;344:2016–2018.
20. Visser M, Bouter L, McQuillan G, et al. Elevated C-reactive protein levels in overweight and obese adults. *JAMA* 1999;282:2131–2135.
21. Wener MH, Daum PR, McQuillan GM. The influence of age, sex, and race on the upper reference limit of serum C-reactive protein concentrations. *J Rheumatol* 2000;27:2351–2359.
22. Pearson TA, Mensah GA, Alexander RW, et al. Markers of inflammation and cardiovascular disease: application to clinical and public health practice: a statement for healthcare professionals from the Centers for Disease Control and Prevention and the American Heart Association. *Circulation* 2003;107:499–511.
23. Wong M, Toh L, Wilson A, et al. Reduced arterial elasticity in rheumatoid arthritis and the relationship to vascular disease risk factors and inflammation. *Arthritis Rheum* 2003;48:81–89.
24. Lee MH, Means RT Jr. Extremely elevated serum ferritin levels in a university hospital: associated diseases and clinical significance. *Am J Med* 1995;98:566–571.
25. Craft AW, Eastham EJ, Bell JI, Brigham K. Serum ferritin in juvenile chronic polyarthritis. *Ann Rheum Dis* 1977;36:271–273.
26. Ohta A, Yamaguchi M, Kaneoka H, et al. Adult Still's disease: review of 228 cases from the literature. *J Rheumatol* 1987;14:1139–1146.
27. Fautrel B, Le Moel G, Saint-Marcoux B, et al. Diagnostic value of ferritin and glycosylated ferritin in adult onset Still's disease. *J Rheumatol* 2001;28:322–329.
28. Fautrel B, Zing E, Golmard J-L, et al. Proposal for a new set of classification criteria for adult-onset Still disease. *Medicine (Baltimore)* 2002;81:194–200.
29. Stam TC, Swaak AJG, Kruit WHJ, Eggermont AMM. Regulation of ferritin: a specific role for interferon-alpha (IFN-alpha)? The acute phase response in patients treated with IFN-alpha-2b. *Eur J Clin Invest* 2002;32[Suppl 1]:79–83.
30. Arend WP. Cytokine imbalance in the pathogenesis of rheumatoid arthritis: the role of interleukin-1 receptor antagonist. *Semin Arthritis Rheum* 2001;30:1–6.
31. Barrera P, Boerbooms AM, Janssen EM, et al. Circulating soluble TNF receptors, interleukin-2 receptors, tumor necrosis factor alpha, and interleukin-6 levels in rheumatoid arthritis. Longitudinal evaluation during methotrexate and azathioprine therapy. *Arthritis Rheum* 1993;36:1070–1079.
32. Crilly A, McInness IB, McDonald AG, et al. Interleukin 6 (IL-6) and soluble IL-2 receptor levels in patients with rheumatoid arthritis treated with low dose oral methotrexate. *J Rheumatol* 1995;22:224–226.
33. Seitz M, Loetscher P, Dewald B, et al. Interleukin 1 (IL-1) receptor antagonist, soluble tumor necrosis factor receptors, IL-1 beta, and IL-8—markers of remission in rheumatoid arthritis during treatment with methotrexate. *J Rheumatol* 1996;23:1512–1516.
34. Seitz M, Zwicker M, Villiger PM. Pretreatment cytokine profiles of peripheral blood mononuclear cells and serum from patients with rheumatoid arthritis in different American College of Rheumatology response groups to methotrexate. *J Rheumatol* 2003;30:28–35.
35. Kanik KS, Hagiwara E, Yarboro CH, et al. Distinct patterns of cytokine secretion characterize new onset synovitis versus chronic rheumatoid arthritis. *J Rheumatol* 1998;25:16–22.
36. Mangge H, Kenzian H, Gallistl S, et al. Serum cytokines in juvenile rheumatoid arthritis. Correlation with conventional inflammation parameters and clinical subtypes. *Arthritis Rheum* 1995;38:211–220.
37. Muzaffer MA, Dayer J-M, Feldman BM, et al. Differences in the profiles of circulating levels of soluble tumor necrosis factor receptors and interleukin 1 receptor antagonist reflect the heterogeneity of the subgroups of juvenile rheumatoid arthritis. *J Rheumatol* 2002;29:1071–1078.
38. De Benedetti F, Pignatti P, Gerloni V, et al. Differences in synovial fluid cytokine levels between juvenile and adult rheumatoid arthritis. *J Rheumatol* 1997;24:1403–1409.
39. Paleolog E, Hunt M, Elliott MJ, et al. Deactivation of vascular endothelium by monoclonal anti-tumor necrosis factor alpha antibody in rheumatoid arthritis. *Arthritis Rheum* 1996;39:1089–1092.
40. Taylor PD, Peters AM, Paleolog E, et al. Reduction of chemokine levels and leukocyte traffic to joints by tumor necrosis factor alpha blockade in patients with rheumatoid arthritis. *Arthritis Rheum* 2000;43:38–47.
41. Riches P, Gooding R, Millar BC, Rowbottom AW. Influence of collection and separation of blood samples on plasma IL-1, IL-6 and TNF-alpha concentrations. *J Immunol Methods* 1992;153:125–131.
42. Kreuzer KA, Rockstroh J, Sauerbruch T, Spengler U. A comparative study of different enzyme immunosorbent assays for human tumor necrosis factor-alpha. *J Immunol Methods* 1996;195:49–54.
43. Mannik M. Rheumatoid factors in the pathogenesis of rheumatoid arthritis. *J Rheumatol* 1992;32[Suppl]:46–49.
44. Mannik M, Nardella FA. IgG rheumatoid factors and self-association of these antibodies. *Clin Rheum Dis* 1985;11:551–572.
45. McDougal JS, Hubbard M, McDuffie FC, et al. Comparison of five assays for immune complexes in the rheumatic diseases. An assessment of their validity for rheumatoid arthritis. *Arthritis Rheum* 1982;25:1156–1166.
46. Siegert CE, Daha MR, van der Voort EA, Breedveld FC. IgG and IgA antibodies to the collagen-like region of C1q in rheumatoid vasculitis. *Arthritis Rheum* 1990;33:1646–1654.
47. Wener MH, Mannik M. C1q Autoantibodies. In: Peter JB, Shoenfeld Y, eds. *Autoantibodies*. Amsterdam: Elsevier, 1996:132–138.
48. Waaler E. On the occurrence of a factor in human serum activating the specific agglutination of sheep blood corpuscles. *Acta Path Microbiol Scand* 1940;17:172–178.
49. Rose HM, Ragan C, Pearce E, Lipman MO. Differential agglutination of normal and sensitized sheep erythrocytes by sera of patients with rheumatoid arthritis. *Proc Soc Exp Biol Med* 1949;68:1–11.
50. Fraser KJ. The Waaler-Rose test: anatomy of an eponym. *Semin Arthritis Rheum* 1988;18:61–71.
51. Singer J, Plotz C. The latex fixation test. I. Application to the serologic diagnosis of rheumatoid arthritis. *Am J Med* 1956;21:888–892.
52. Bonagura VR, Artandi SE, Davidson A, et al. Mapping studies reveal unique epitopes on IgG recognized by rheumatoid arthritis-derived monoclonal rheumatoid factors. *J Immunol* 1993;151:3840–3852.
53. Sasso EH, Barber CV, Nardella FA, et al. Antigenic specificities of human monoclonal and polyclonal IgM rheumatoid factors. The Cg2-Cg3 interface region contains the major determinants. *J Immunol* 1988;140:3098–3107.
54. Corper AL, Sohi MK, Bonagura VR, et al. Structure of human IgM rheumatoid factor Fab bound to its autoantigen IgG Fc reveals a novel topology of antibody-antigen interaction. *Nat Struct Biol* 1997;4:374–381.
55. Sutton B, Corper A, Bonagura V, Taussig M. The structure and origin of rheumatoid factors. *Immunol Today* 2000;21:177–183.
56. Williams RC Jr., Malone CC. Rheumatoid-factor-reactive sites on CH2 established by analysis of overlapping peptides of primary sequence. *Scand J Immunol* 1994;40:443–456.
57. Wong A, Kenny TP, Ermel R, Robbins DL. IgG3 reactive rheumatoid factor in rheumatoid arthritis: etiologic and pathogenic considerations. *Autoimmunity* 1994;19:199–210.
58. Nemazee DA. Immune complexes can trigger specific T cell-dependent autoanti-IgG antibody production in mice. *J Exp Med* 1985;161:242–250.
59. Tarkowski A, Czerkinsky C, Nilsson L-Å. Simultaneous induction of rheumatoid factor- and antigen-specific antibody-secreting cells during the secondary immune response in man. *Clin Exp Immunol* 1985;61:379–387.
60. Newkirk MM, Goldbach-Mansky R, Lee J, et al. Advanced glycation end-product (AGE)-damaged IgG and IgM autoantibodies to IgG-AGE in patients with early synovitis. *Arthritis Res Ther* 2003;5:R82–R90.
61. Lucey MD, Newkirk MM, Neville C, et al. Association between IgM response to IgG damaged by glyoxidation and disease activity in rheumatoid arthritis. *J Rheumatol* 2000;27:319–323.
62. Ligier S, Fortin PR, Newkirk MM. A new antibody in rheumatoid arthritis targeting glycated IgG: IgM anti-IgG-AGE. *Br J Rheumatol* 1998;37:1307–1314.
63. Lunec J, Griffiths HR, Brailsford S. Oxygen free radicals denature human IgG and increase its reactivity with rheumatoid factor antibody. *Scand J Rheumatol Suppl* 1988;75:140–147.
64. Schrohenloher RE, Bridges SLJ, Koopman WJ. Rheumatoid factor. In: Koopman WJ, ed. *Arthritis and allied conditions*, 13th ed. Baltimore: Williams & Wilkins, 1999:1109–1130.
65. Randen I, Pascual V, Victor K, et al. Synovial IgG rheumatoid factors show evidence of an antigen-driven immune response and a shift in the V gene repertoire compared to IgM rheumatoid factors. *Eur J Immunol* 1993;23:1220–1225.
66. Randen I, Thompson KM, Pascual V, et al. Rheumatoid factor V genes from patients with rheumatoid arthritis are diverse and show evidence of an antigen-driven response. *Immunol Rev* 1992;128:49–71.
67. Agnello V, Chung RT, Kaplan LM. A role for hepatitis C virus infection in type II cryoglobulinemia. *N Engl J Med* 1992;327:1490–1495.
68. Sasso EH, Willems van Dijk K, Bull AP, Milner EC. A fetally expressed immunoglobulin VH1 gene belongs to a complex set of alleles. *J Clin Invest* 1993;91:2358–2367.
69. Butler VPJ, Vaughan JH. Hemagglutination by rheumatoid factor of cells coated with animal gamma globulin. *Proc Soc Exp Biol Med* 1964;116:585–593.
70. Houssien DA, Jonsson T, Davies E, Scott DL. Rheumatoid factor isotypes, disease activity and the outcome of rheumatoid arthritis: comparative effects of different antigens. *Scand J Rheumatol* 1998;27:46–53.
71. Moore TL, Dorner RW, Osborn TG, Zuckner J. Hidden 19S IgM rheumatoid factors. *Semin Arthritis Rheum* 1988;18:72–75.
72. Carpeneter AB. Antibody-based methods. In: Rose NR, Hamilton RG, Detrick B, eds. *Manual of clinical laboratory immunology*, 6th ed. Washington, DC: ASM Press, 2002:6–25.
73. Painter PC, Lyon JM, Evans JH, et al. Performance of a new rate-nephelometric assay for rheumatoid factor, and its correlation with tube-titer results for human sera and synovial fluid. *Clin Chem* 1982;28:2214–2218.
74. Roberts Thomson PJ, Wernick RM, Ziff M. Quantitation of rheumatoid factor by laser nephelometry. *Rheumatol Int* 1982;2:17–20.
75. Desjarlais F, Daigneault R. Rheumatoid factors measured in serum with a fully automated laser nephelometer, and correlation with agglutination tube titers [Letter]. *Clin Chem* 1985;31:1077–1078.
76. Aggarwal A, Dabadghao S, Naik S, Misra R. Serum IgM rheumatoid factor by enzyme-linked immunosorbent assay (ELISA) delineates a subset of patients with deforming joint disease in seronegative juvenile rheumatoid arthritis. *Rheumatol Int* 1994;14:135–138.
77. Grunnet N, Espersen GT. Comparative studies on RF-IgA and RF-IgM ELISA—human or rabbit IgG as antigen? *Scand J Rheumatol Suppl* 1988;75:36–39.
78. Anderson SG, Bentzon MW, Houba V, Krag P. International reference preparation of rheumatoid arthritis serum. *Bull World Health Organ* 1970;42:311–318.

79. Taylor RN, Huong AY, Fulford KM, et al. Quality control for immunologic tests. HEW Publication No (CDC) 79-8376 ed. Atlanta: U.S. Dept of Health, Education, and Welfare, 1979.
80. Klein F, Janssens MB, van Romunde LK, Eilers GA. Comparative study of test kits for measurement of rheumatoid factors by the latex fixation test. *Ann Rheum Dis* 1990;49:801–804.
81. Taylor RN, Fulford KM, Jones WL. Reduction of variation in results of rheumatoid factor tests by use of a serum reference preparation. *J Clin Microbiol* 1977;5:42–45.
82. Collins RJ, Neil JC, Wilson RJ. Rate nephelometric determination of rheumatoid factor: comparison between Kallestad QM-300 and Beckman ICS-II (RF) methods. *J Clin Pathol* 1990;43:243–245.
83. Jaspers JP, Van Oers RJ, Leerkes B. Nine rheumatoid factor assays compared. *J Clin Chem Clin Biochem* 1988;26:863–871.
84. Rippey JH, Biesecker JL. Results of tests for rheumatoid factor on CAP survey specimens. *Am J Clin Pathol* 1983;80:599–602.
85. van Leeuwen MA, Westra J, Limburg PC, et al. Quantitation of IgM, IgA and IgG rheumatoid factors by ELISA in rheumatoid arthritis and other rheumatic disorders. *Scand J Rheumatol* 1988;75[Suppl]:25–31.
86. Hay FC, Nineham LJ. Standardization of assays for rheumatoid factors and antiglobulins. In: Dumonde DC, Seward MW, eds. *Laboratory tests in the rheumatic diseases. Standardization in clinical-laboratory investigation.* Baltimore: University Park Press, 1979:101–105.
87. Fulford KM, Taylor RN, Przybyszewski VA. Reference preparation to standardize results of serological tests for rheumatoid factor. *J Clin Microbiol* 1978;7:434–441.
88. Larsson A, Sjöquist J. False-positive results in latex agglutination tests caused by rheumatoid factor. *Clin Chem* 1988;34:767–768.
89. Krahn J, Parry DM, Leroux M, Dalton J. High percentage of false positive cardiac troponin I results in patients with rheumatoid factor. *Clin Biochem* 1999;32:477–480.
90. Dasgupta A, Banerjee SK, Datta P. False-positive troponin I in the MEIA due to the presence of rheumatoid factors in serum. Elimination of this interference by using a polyclonal antisera against rheumatoid factors. *Am J Clin Pathol* 1999;112:753–756.
91. Hamilton RG, Whittington K, Warner NB, Arnett FC. Human IgM rheumatoid factor reactivity with rabbit, sheep, goat, and mouse immunoglobulin. *Clin Chem* 1988;34:1165(abst).
92. Kleveland G, Egeland T, Lea T. Quantitation of rheumatoid factors (RF) of IgM, IgA and IgG isotypes by a simple and sensitive ELISA. Discrimination between false and true IgG-RF. *Scand J Rheumatol Suppl* 1988;75:15–24.
93. Elkon KB, Delacroix DL, Gharavi AE, et al. Immunoglobulin A and polymeric IgA rheumatoid factors in systemic sicca syndrome: partial characterization. *J Immunol* 1982;129:576–581.
94. van Snick JL, Masson PL. Incidence and specificities of IgA and IgM anti-IgG autoantibodies in various mouse strains and colonies. *J Exp Med* 1980; 151:45–55.
95. Teitsson I, Withrington RH, Seifert MH, Valdimarsson H. Prospective study of early rheumatoid arthritis. I. Prognostic value of IgA rheumatoid factor. *Ann Rheum Dis* 1984;43:673–678.
96. Withrington RH, Teitsson I, Valdimarsson H, Seifert MH. Prospective study of early rheumatoid arthritis. II. Association of rheumatoid factor isotypes with fluctuations in disease activity. *Ann Rheum Dis* 1984;43:679–685.
97. Winska Wiloch H, Thompson K, Young A, et al. IgA and IgM rheumatoid factors as markers of later erosive changes in rheumatoid arthritis. *Scand J Rheumatol* 1988;[Suppl 75]:238–243.
98. Jonsson T, Valdimarsson H. Clinical significance of rheumatoid factor isotypes in seropositive arthritis. *Rheumatol Int* 1992;12:111–113.
99. van Leeuwen MA, Westra J, van Riel PL, et al. IgM, IgA, and IgG rheumatoid factors in early rheumatoid arthritis predictive of radiological progression? *Scand J Rheumatol* 1995;24:146–153.
100. Eberhardt KB, Svensson B, Truedsson L, Wollheim FA. The occurrence of rheumatoid factor isotypes in early definite rheumatoid arthritis—no relationship with erosions or disease activity. *J Rheumatol* 1988;15:1070–1074.
101. Gioud-Paquet M, Auvinet M, Raffin T, et al. IgM rheumatoid factor (RF), IgA RF, IgE RF, and IgG RF detected by ELISA in rheumatoid arthritis. *Ann Rheum Dis* 1987;46:65–71.
102. Tuomi T, Aho K, Palosuo T, et al. Significance of rheumatoid factors in an eight-year longitudinal study on arthritis. *Rheumatol Int* 1988;8:21–26.
103. Jonsson T, Steinsson K, Jonsson H, et al. Combined elevation of IgM and IgA rheumatoid factor has high diagnostic specificity for rheumatoid arthritis. *Rheumatol Int* 1998;18:119–122.
104. Halldorsdottir HD, Jonsson T, Thorsteinsson J, Valdimarsson H. A prospective study on the incidence of rheumatoid arthritis among people with persistent increase of rheumatoid factor. *Ann Rheum Dis* 2000;59:149–151.
105. Elkon KB, Caeiro F, Gharavi AE, et al. Radioimmunoassay profile of antiglobulins in connective tissue diseases: elevated level of IgA antiglobulin in systemic sicca syndrome. *Clin Exp Immunol* 1981;46:547–556.
106. Jonsson T, Thorsteinsson J, Valdimarsson H. Does smoking stimulate rheumatoid factor production in non-rheumatic individuals? *Apmis* 1998;106:970–974.
107. Abe Y, Tanaka Y, Takenaka M, et al. Leucocytoclastic vasculitis associated with mixed cryoglobulinaemia and hepatitis C virus infection. *Br J Dermatol* 1997;136:272–274.
108. Arnett FC, Edworthy SM, Bloch DA, et al. The American Rheumatism Association 1987 revised criteria for the classification of rheumatoid arthritis. *Arthritis Rheum* 1988;31:315–324.
109. Wolfe F, Cathey MA, Roberts FK. The latex test revisited. Rheumatoid factor testing in 8,287 rheumatic disease patients. *Arthritis Rheum* 1991;34:951–960.
110. del Puente A, Knowler WC, Pettitt DJ, Bennett PH. The incidence of rheumatoid arthritis is predicted by rheumatoid factor titer in a longitudinal population study. *Arthritis Rheum* 1988;31:1239–1244.
111. Aho K, Heliovaara M, Maatela J, et al. Rheumatoid factors antedating clinical rheumatoid arthritis. *J Rheumatol* 1991;18:1282–1284.
112. Rantapaa-Dahlqvist S, de Jong BAW, Hallmans G, et al. Antibodies against citrullinated peptides (CCP) predict the development of rheumatoid arthritis. *Arthritis Rheum* 2003;48:2741–2749.
113. Hicks MJ, Heick M, Finley P, et al. Rheumatoid factor activity by rate nephelometry correlated with clinical activity in rheumatoid arthritis. *Am J Clin Pathol* 1982;78:342–345.
114. Wolfe F. A comparison of IgM rheumatoid factor by nephelometry and latex methods: clinical and laboratory significance. *Arthritis Care Res* 1998;11:89–93.
115. Jacoby RK, Jayson MI, Cosh JA. Onset, early stages, and prognosis of rheumatoid arthritis: a clinical study of 100 patients with 11-year follow-up. *BMJ* 1973;2:96–100.
116. Saraux A, Bendaoud B, Dueymes M, et al. The functional affinity of IgM rheumatoid factor is related to the disease duration in patients with rheumatoid arthritis. *Ann Rheum Dis* 1997;56:126–129.
117. Paimela L, Palosuo T, Leirisalo-Repo M, et al. Prognostic value of quantitative measurement of rheumatoid factor in early rheumatoid arthritis. *Br J Rheumatol* 1995;34:1146–1150.
118. Allander E, Bjornsson OJ, Kolbeinsson A, et al. Rheumatoid factor in Iceland: a population study. *Int J Epidemiol* 1972;1:211–223.
119. Jimenez CV. Usefulness of reference limits and evaluation of significant differences. An example of the biological variation of serum rheumatoid factors. *Ann Biol Clin Paris* 1994;52:529–533.
120. Pawlotsky JM, Ben Yahia M, Andre C, et al. Immunological disorders in C virus chronic active hepatitis: a prospective case-control study. *Hepatology* 1994;19:841–848.
121. Aho K, Salonen JT, Puska P. Autoantibodies predicting death due to cardiovascular disease. *Cardiology* 1982;69:125–129.
122. Lamprecht P, Moosig F, Gause A, et al. Immunological and clinical follow-up of hepatitis C virus associated cryoglobulinemic vasculitis. *Ann Rheum Dis* 2001;29:296–304.
123. Heliovaara M, Aho K, Knekt P, et al. Rheumatoid factor, chronic arthritis and mortality. *Ann Rheum Dis* 1995;54:811–814.
124. Mikuls TR, Saag KG, Criswell LA, et al. Mortality risk associated with rheumatoid arthritis in a prospective cohort of older women: results from the Iowa Women's Health Study. *Ann Rheum Dis* 2002;61:994–999.
125. Pope RM, Lessard J, Nunnery E. Differential effects of therapeutic regimens on specific classes of rheumatoid factor. *Ann Rheum Dis* 1986;45:183–189.
126. Reilly PA, Cosh JA, Maddison PJ, et al. Mortality and survival in rheumatoid arthritis: a 25 year prospective study of 100 patients. *Ann Rheum Dis* 1990;49:363–369.
127. Aletaha D, Eberl G, Nell VPK, et al. Practical progress in realisation of early diagnosis and treatment of patients with suspected rheumatoid arthritis: results from two matched questionnaires within three years. *Ann Rheum Dis* 2002;61:630–634.
128. Bukhari M, Lunt M, Harrison BJ, et al. Rheumatoid factor is the major predictor of increasing severity of radiographic erosions in rheumatoid arthritis: results from the Norfolk Arthritis Register Study, a large inception cohort. *Arthritis Rheum* 2002;46:906–912.
129. Nienhuis RLF, Mandema EA. A new serum factor in patients with rheumatoid arthritis. The antiperinuclear factor. *Ann Rheum Dis* 1964;23:302–305.
130. Young BJJ, Mallya RK, Leslie RDJ, et al. Antikeratin antibodies in rheumatoid arthritis. *BMJ* 1979;2:97–99.
131. Simon M, Girbal E, Sebbag M, et al. The cytokeratin filament-aggregating protein filaggrin is the target of the so-called "antikeratin antibodies," autoantibodies specific for rheumatoid arthritis. *J Clin Invest* 1993;92:1387–1393.
132. Schellekens GA, de Jong BA, van den Hoogen FH, et al. Citrulline is an essential constituent of antigenic determinants recognized by rheumatoid arthritis-specific autoantibodies. *J Clin Invest* 1998;101:273–281.
133. Girbal-Neuhauser E, Durieux JJ, Arnaud M, et al. The epitopes targeted by the rheumatoid arthritis-associated antifilaggrin autoantibodies are posttranslationally generated on various sites of (pro)filaggrin by deimination of arginine residues. *J Immunol* 1999;162:585–594.
134. Despres N, Boire G, Lopez-Longo FJ, Menard HA. The Sa system: a novel antigen-antibody system specific for rheumatoid arthritis. *J Rheumatol* 1994;21:1027–1033.
135. Menard HA, Boire G, Lopez-Longo FJ, et al. Insights into rheumatoid arthritis derived from the Sa immune system. *Arthritis Res* 2000;2:429–432.
136. Hayem G, Chazerain P, Combe B, et al. Anti-Sa antibody is an accurate diagnostic and prognostic marker in adult rheumatoid arthritis. *J Rheumatol* 1999;26:7–13.
137. Masson-Bessiere C, Sebbag M, Girbal-Neuhauser E, et al. The major synovial targets of the rheumatoid arthritis-specific antifilaggrin autoantibodies are deiminated forms of the alpha- and beta-chains of fibrin. *J Immunol* 2001;166:4177–4184.
138. Schellekens GA, Visser H, de Jong BAW, et al. The diagnostic properties of rheumatoid arthritis antibodies recognizing a cyclic citrullinated peptide. *Arthritis Rheum* 2000;43:155–163.
139. Lee DM, Schur PH. Clinical utility of the anti-CCP assay in patients with rheumatic diseases. *Ann Rheum Dis* 2003;62:870–874.

140. Bas S, Perneger TV, Seitz M, et al. Diagnostic tests for rheumatoid arthritis: comparison of anti-cyclic citrullinated peptide antibodies, anti-keratin antibodies and IgM rheumatoid factors. *Rheumatology (Oxford)* 2002;41:809–814.
141. Goldbach-Mansky R, Lee J, McCoy A, et al. Rheumatoid arthritis associated autoantibodies in patients with synovitis of recent onset. *Arthritis Res* 2000;2:236–243.
142. Cordonnier C, Meyer O, Palazzo E, et al. Diagnostic value of anti-RA33 antibody, antikeratin antibody, antiperinuclear factor and antinuclear antibody in early rheumatoid arthritis: comparison with rheumatoid factor. *Br J Rheumatol* 1996;35:620–624.
143. Wener MH, Hutchinson K, Morishima C. Antibodies to cyclic citrullinated peptide in sera of patients with hepatitis C virus infection and cryoglobulinemia. *Arthritis Rheum* 2002;46:S66(abst).
144. Avcin T, Cimaz R, Falcini F, et al. Prevalence and clinical significance of anti-cyclic citrullinated peptide antibodies in juvenile idiopathic arthritis. *Ann Rheum Dis* 2002;61:608–611.
145. Moore TL, Chung AK, Kietz DA, Pepmueller PH. Anti-cyclic citrullinated peptide antibodies in juvenile rheumatoid arthritis patients. *Arthritis Rheum* 2001(abst).
146. Genevay S, Hayem G, Verpillat P, Meyer O. An eight year prospective study of outcome prediction by antiperinuclear factor and antikeratin antibodies at onset of rheumatoid arthritis. *Ann Rheum Dis* 2002;61:734–736.
147. Kroot EJ, de Jong BA, van Leeuwen MA, et al. The prognostic value of anti-cyclic citrullinated peptide antibody in patients with recent-onset rheumatoid arthritis. *Arthritis Rheum* 2000;43:1831–1835.
148. van Jaarsveld CH, ter Borg EJ, Jacobs JW, et al. The prognostic value of the antiperinuclear factor, anti-citrullinated peptide antibodies and rheumatoid factor in early rheumatoid arthritis. *Clin Exp Rheumatol* 1999;17:689–697.
149. van Boekel MAM, Vossenaar ER, van den Hoogen FHJ, van Venrooij WJ. Autoantibody systems in rheumatoid arthritis: specificity, sensitivity and diagnostic value. *Arthritis Res* 2002;4:87–93.
150. van Venrooij WJ, Pruijn GJ. Citrullination: a small change for a protein with great consequences for rheumatoid arthritis. *Arthritis Res* 2000;2:249–251.
151. Fritsch R, Eselbock D, Skriner K, et al. Characterization of autoreactive T cells to the autoantigens heterogeneous nuclear ribonucleoprotein A2 (RA33) and filaggrin in patients with rheumatoid arthritis. *J Immunol* 2002;169:1068–1076.
152. Masson-Bessiere C, Sebbag M, Durieux JJ, et al. In the rheumatoid pannus, anti-filaggrin autoantibodies are produced by local plasma cells and constitute a higher proportion of IgG than in synovial fluid and serum. *Clin Exp Immunol* 2000;119:544–552.
153. Baeten D, Peene I, Union A, et al. Specific presence of intracellular citrullinated proteins in rheumatoid arthritis synovium: relevance to antifilaggrin autoantibodies. *Arthritis Rheum* 2001;44:2255–2262.
153a. Suzuki A, Yamanda R, Chang X, et al. Functional haplotypes of PADI4, encoding citrullinating enzyme peptidylarginine deiminase 4, are associated with rheumatoid arthritis. *Nat Genet* 2003;34:395–402.
154. Hassfeld W, Steiner G, Hartmuth K, et al. Demonstration of a new antinuclear antibody (anti-RA33) that is highly specific for rheumatoid arthritis. *Arthritis Rheum* 1989;32:1515–1520.
155. Hassfeld W, Steiner G, Studnicka-Benke A, et al. Autoimmune response to the spliceosome. An immunologic link between rheumatoid arthritis, mixed connective tissue disease, and systemic lupus erythematosus. *Arthritis Rheum* 1995;38:777–785.
156. Blass S, Specker C, Lakomek HJ, et al. Novel 68 kDa autoantigen detected by rheumatoid arthritis specific antibodies. *Ann Rheum Dis* 1995;54:355–360.
157. Blass S, Meier C, Vohr HW, et al. The p68 autoantigen characteristic of rheumatoid arthritis is reactive with carbohydrate epitope specific autoantibodies. *Ann Rheum Dis* 1998;57:220–225.
158. Blass S, Union A, Raymackers J, et al. The stress protein BiP is overexpressed and is a major B and T cell target in rheumatoid arthritis. *Arthritis Rheum* 2001;44:761–771.
159. Hayem G, De Bandt M, Palazzo E, et al. Anti-heat shock protein 70 kDa and 90 kDa antibodies in serum of patients with rheumatoid arthritis. *Ann Rheum Dis* 1999;58:291–296.
160. Hirata D, Hirai I, Iwamoto M, et al. Preferential binding with *Escherichia coli* hsp60 of antibodies prevalent in sera from patients with rheumatoid arthritis. *Clin Immunol Immunopathol* 1997;82:141–148.
161. Tishler M, Shoenfeld Y. Anti-heat-shock protein antibodies in rheumatic and autoimmune diseases. *Semin Arthritis Rheum* 1996;26:558–563.
162. Matsumoto I, Staub A, Benoist C, Mathis D. Arthritis provoked by linked T and B cell recognition of a glycolytic enzyme. *Science* 1999;286:1732–1735.
163. Schaller M, Burton DR, Ditzel HJ. Autoantibodies to GPI in rheumatoid arthritis: linkage between an animal model and human disease. *Nat Immunol* 2001;2:746–753.
164. Matsumoto I, Lee DM, Goldbach-Mansky R, et al. Low prevalence of antibodies to glucose-6-phosphate isomerase in patients with rheumatoid arthritis and a spectrum of other chronic autoimmune disorders. *Arthritis Rheum* 2003;48:944–954.
165. Matsumoto I, Maccioni M, Lee DM, et al. How antibodies to a ubiquitous cytoplasmic enzyme may provoke joint-specific autoimmune disease. *Nat Immunol* 2002;3:360–365.
166. Saulot V, Vittecoq O, Charlionet R, et al. Presence of autoantibodies to the glycolytic enzyme alpha-enolase in sera from patients with early rheumatoid arthritis. *Arthritis Rheum* 2002;46:1196–1201.
167. Ukaji F, Kitajima I, Kubo T, et al. Serum samples of patients with rheumatoid arthritis contain a specific autoantibody to "denatured" aldolase A in the osteoblast-like cell line, MG-63. *Ann Rheum Dis* 1999;58:169–174.
168. Despres N, Talbot G, Plouffe B, et al. Detection and expression of a cDNA clone that encodes a polypeptide containing two inhibitory domains of human calpastatin and its recognition by rheumatoid arthritis sera. *J Clin Invest* 1995;95:1891–1896.
169. Mimori T, Suganuma K, Tanami Y, et al. Autoantibodies to calpastatin (an endogenous inhibitor for calcium-dependent neutral protease, calpain) in systemic rheumatic diseases. *Proc Natl Acad Sci U S A* 1995;92:7267–7271.
170. Vittecoq O, Jouen-Beades F, Krzanowska K, et al. Rheumatoid factors, anti-filaggrin antibodies and low in vitro interleukin-2 and interferon-gamma production are useful immunological markers for early diagnosis of community cases of rheumatoid arthritis. A preliminary study. *Joint Bone Spine* 2001;68:144–153.
171. Charles PJ, Smeenk RJ, De Jong J, et al. Assessment of antibodies to double-stranded DNA induced in rheumatoid arthritis patients following treatment with infliximab, a monoclonal antibody to tumor necrosis factor alpha: findings in open-label and randomized placebo-controlled trials. *Arthritis Rheum* 2000;43:2383–2390.
172. Clague RB, Shaw MJ, Holt PJ. Incidence of serum antibodies to native type I and type II collagens in patients with inflammatory arthritis. *Ann Rheum Dis* 1980;39:201–206.
173. Buckner JH, Wu JJ, Reife RA, et al. Autoreactivity against matrilin-1 in a patient with relapsing polychondritis. *Arthritis Rheum* 2000;43:939–943.
174. Hansson AS, Heinegard D, Piette JC, et al. The occurrence of autoantibodies to matrilin 1 reflects a tissue-specific response to cartilage of the respiratory tract in patients with relapsing polychondritis. *Arthritis Rheum* 2001;44:2402–2412.
175. Cook AD, Rowley MJ, Wines BD, Mackay IR. Antibodies to the collagen-like region of C1q and type II collagen are independent non-cross-reactive populations in systemic lupus erythematosus and rheumatoid arthritis. *J Autoimmun* 1994;7:369–378.
176. Mannik M, Kapil S, Merrill CE. In patients with rheumatoid arthritis IgG binding to denatured collagen type II is in part mediated by IgG-fibronectin complexes. *J Immunol* 1997;158:1446–1452.
177. Woodruff T, Cook A, Rowley M, Mackay I. Antibodies to type II collagen in human serum: storage effects and role of IgM antiidiotype in regulation. *J Rheumatol* 1994;21:197–202.
178. Cook AD, Rowley MJ, Mackay IR, et al. Antibodies to type II collagen in early rheumatoid arthritis. Correlation with disease progression. *Arthritis Rheum* 1996;39:1720–1727.
179. Morgan K, Clague RB, Reynolds I, Davis M. Antibodies to type II collagen in early rheumatoid arthritis. *Br J Rheumatol* 1993;32:333–335.
180. Clague RB, Morgan K, Reynolds I, Williams HJ. The prevalence of serum IgG antibodies to type II collagen in American patients with rheumatoid arthritis. *Br J Rheumatol* 1994;33:336–338.
181. Rudolphi U, Rzepka R, Batsford S, et al. The B cell repertoire of patients with rheumatoid arthritis. II. Increased frequencies of IgG+ and IgA+ B cells specific for mycobacterial heat-shock protein 60 or human type II collagen in synovial fluid and tissue. *Arthritis Rheum* 1997;40:1409–1419.
182. Rowley MJ, Williamson DJ, Mackay IR. Evidence for local synthesis of antibodies to denatured collagen in the synovium in rheumatoid arthritis. *Arthritis Rheum* 1987;30:1420–1425.
183. Tarkowski A, Klareskog L, Carlsten H, et al. Secretion of antibodies to types I and II collagen by synovial tissue cells in patients with rheumatoid arthritis. *Arthritis Rheum* 1989;32:1087–1092.
184. Collins I, Morgan K, Clague RB, et al. IgG subclass distribution of antinative type II collagen and antidenatured type II collagen antibodies in patients with rheumatoid arthritis. *J Rheumatol* 1988;15:770–774.
185. Cook AD, Mackay IR, Cicuttini FM, Rowley MJ. IgG subclasses of antibodies to type II collagen in rheumatoid arthritis differ from those in systemic lupus erythematosus and other connective tissue diseases. *J Rheumatol* 1997;24:2090–2096.
186. Iribe H, Kabashima H, Ishii Y, Koga T. Epitope specificity of antibody response against human type II collagen in the mouse susceptible to collagen-induced arthritis and patients with rheumatoid arthritis. *Clin Exp Immunol* 1988;73:443–448.
187. Boissier MC, Chiocchia G, Texier B, Fournier C. Pattern of humoral reactivity to type II collagen in rheumatoid arthritis. *Clin Exp Immunol* 1989;78:177–183.
188. Burkhardt H, Koller T, Engstrom A, et al. Epitope-specific recognition of type II collagen by rheumatoid arthritis antibodies is shared with recognition by antibodies that are arthritogenic in collagen-induced arthritis in the mouse. *Arthritis Rheum* 2002;46:2339–2348.
189. Young-Min SA, Cawston TE, Griffiths ID. Markers of joint destruction: principles, problems, and potential. *Ann Rheum Dis* 2001;60:545–549.
190. Poole AR. Can serum biomarker assays measure the progression of cartilage degeneration in osteoarthritis? *Arthritis Rheum* 2002;46:2549–2552.
191. Garnero P, Rousseau JC, Delmas PD. Molecular basis and clinical use of biochemical markers of bone, cartilage, and synovium in joint diseases. *Arthritis Rheum* 2000;43:953–968.
192. Moller HJ. Connective tissue markers of rheumatoid arthritis. *Scand J Clin Lab Invest* 1998;58:269–278.
193. Simkin PA, Bassett JE. Cartilage matrix molecules in serum and synovial fluid. *Curr Opin Rheumatol* 1995;7:346–351.
194. Poole R. NIH white paper: biomarkers, the osteoarthritis initiative. A basis for discussion. http://www.niams.nih.gov/ne/oi/oabiomarwhipap.htm; 2000.
195. Myers SL, Brandt KD, Eilam O. Even low-grade synovitis significantly accelerates the clearance of protein from the canine knee: implications for mea-

surement of synovial fluid 'markers' of osteoarthritis. *Arthritis Rheum* 1995;38:1085–1091.

196. Manicourt DH, Poilvache P, Nzeusseu A, et al. Serum levels of hyaluronan, antigenic keratan sulfate, matrix metalloproteinase 3, and tissue inhibitor of metalloproteinases 1 change predictably in rheumatoid arthritis patients who have begun activity after a night of bed rest. *Arthritis Rheum* 1999;42:1861–1869.
197. Verheijden GFM, Rijnders AWM, Bos E, et al. Human cartilage glycoprotein-39 as a candidate autoantigen in rheumatoid arthritis. *Arthritis Rheum* 1997;40:1115–1125.
198. Hakala BE, White C, Racklies AD. Human cartilage gp-39, a major secretory product of articular chondrocytes and synovial cells, is a mammalian member of a chitinase protein family. *J Biol Chem* 1993;268:25903–25910.
199. Johansen JS, Jensen HS, Price PA. A new biochemical marker for joint injury: analysis of YKL-40 in serum and synovial fluid. *Br J Rheumatol* 1993;32:949–955.
200. Matsumoto T, Tsurumoto T. Serum YKL-40 levels in rheumatoid arthritis: correlations between clinical and laboratory parameters. *Clin Exp Rheumatol* 2001;19:655–660.
201. Johansen JS, Kirwan JR, Price PA, Sharif M. Serum YKL-40 concentrations in patients with early rheumatoid arthritis: relation to joint destruction. *Scand J Rheumatol* 2001;30:297–304.
202. Peltomaa R, Paimela L, Harvey S, et al. Increased level of YKL-40 in sera from patients with early rheumatoid arthritis: a new marker for disease activity. *Rheumatol Int* 2001;20:192–196.
203. Sekine T, Masuko-Hongo K, Matsui T, et al. Recognition of YKL-39, a human cartilage related protein, as a target antigen in patients with rheumatoid arthritis. *Ann Rheum Dis* 2001;60:49–54.
204. Johansen JS, Hvolris J, Hansen M, et al. Serum YKL-40 levels in healthy children and adults. Comparison with serum and synovial fluid levels of YKL-40 in patients with osteoarthritis or trauma of the knee joint. *Br J Rheumatol* 1996;35:553–559.
205. Cintin C, Johansen JS, Christensen IJ, et al. High serum YKL-40 level after surgery for colorectal carcinoma is related to short survival. *Cancer* 2002;95:267–274.
206. Kronborg G, Ostergaard C, Weis N, et al. Serum level of YKL-40 is elevated in patients with *Streptococcus pneumoniae* bacteremia and is associated with the outcome of the disease. *Scand J Infect Dis* 2002;34:323–326.
207. Johansen JS, Christoffersen P, Moller S, et al. Serum YKL-40 is increased in patients with hepatic fibrosis. *J Hepatol* 2000;32:911–920.
208. Nordenbaek C, Johansen JS, Junker P, et al. YKL-40, a matrix protein of specific granules in neutrophils, is elevated in serum of patients with community-acquired pneumonia requiring hospitalization. *J Infect Dis* 1999;180:1722–1726.
209. Vos K, Steenbakkers P, Miltenburg AM, et al. Raised human cartilage glycoprotein-39 plasma levels in patients with rheumatoid arthritis and other inflammatory conditions. *Ann Rheum Dis* 2000;59:544–548.
210. Neidhart M, Hauser N, Paulsson M, et al. Small fragments of cartilage oligomeric matrix protein in synovial fluid and serum as markers for cartilage degradation. *Br J Rheumatol* 1997;36:1151–1160.
211. Saxne T, Heinegard D. Cartilage oligomeric matrix protein: a novel marker of cartilage turnover detectable in synovial fluid and blood. *Br J Rheumatol* 1992;31:583–591.
212. Mansson B, Carey D, Alini M, et al. Cartilage and bone metabolism in rheumatoid arthritis. Differences between rapid and slow progression of disease identified by serum markers of cartilage metabolism. *J Clin Invest* 1995;95:1071–1077.
213. Mansson B, Geborek P, Saxne T. Cartilage and bone macromolecules in knee joint synovial fluid in rheumatoid arthritis: relation to development of knee or hip joint destruction. *Ann Rheum Dis* 1997;56:91–96.
214. Fex E, Eberhardt K, Saxne T. Tissue-derived macromolecules and markers of inflammation in serum in early rheumatoid arthritis: relationship to development of joint destruction in hands and feet. *Br J Rheumatol* 1997;36:1161–1165.
215. den Broeder AA, Joosten LAB, Saxne T, et al. Long term anti-tumour necrosis factor alpha monotherapy in rheumatoid arthritis: effect on radiological course and prognostic value of markers of cartilage turnover and endothelial activation. *Ann Rheum Dis* 2002;61:311–318.
216. Roux-Lombard P, Eberhardt K, Saxne T, et al. Cytokines, metalloproteinases, their inhibitors and cartilage oligomeric matrix protein: relationship to radiological progression and inflammation in early rheumatoid arthritis. A prospective 5-year study. *Rheumatology (Oxford)* 2001;40:544–551.
217. Nagase H, Kashiwagi M. Aggrecanases and cartilage matrix degradation. *Arthritis Res Therapy* 2003;5:94–103.
218. Caterson B, Flannery CR, Hughes CE, Little CB. Mechanisms involved in cartilage proteoglycan catabolism. *Matrix Biology* 2000;19:333–344.
219. Saxne T, Heinegard D, Wollheim FA, Pettersson H. Difference in cartilage proteoglycan level in synovial fluid in early rheumatoid arthritis and reactive arthritis. *Lancet* 1985;2:127–128.
220. Lindqvist E, Saxne T. Cartilage macromolecules in knee joint synovial fluid. Markers of the disease course in patients with acute oligoarthritis. *Ann Rheum Dis* 1997;56:751–753.
221. Saxne T, Heinegard D. Synovial fluid analysis of two groups of proteoglycan epitopes distinguishes early and late cartilage lesions. *Arthritis Rheum* 1992;35:385–390.
222. Poole AR, Ionescu M, Swan A, Dieppe PA. Changes in cartilage metabolism in arthritis are reflected by altered serum and synovial fluid levels of the cartilage proteoglycan aggrecan. Implications for pathogenesis. *J Clin Invest* 1994;94:25–33.
223. Mehraban F, Finegan CK, Moskowitz RW. Serum keratan sulfate. Quantitative and qualitative comparisons in inflammatory versus noninflammatory arthritides. *Arthritis Rheum* 1991;34:383–392.
224. Haraoui B, Thonar EJ, Martel-Pelletier J, et al. Serum keratan sulfate levels in rheumatoid arthritis: inverse correlation with radiographic staging. *J Rheumatol* 1994;21:813–817.
225. Poole AR, Dieppe P. Biological markers in rheumatoid arthritis. *Semin Arthritis Rheum* 1994;23:17–31.
226. Paimela L, Heiskanen A, Kurki P, et al. Serum hyaluronate level as a predictor of radiologic progression in early rheumatoid arthritis. *Arthritis Rheum* 1991;34:815–821.
227. Nelson F, Dahlberg L, Laverty S, et al. Evidence for altered synthesis of type II collagen in patients with osteoarthritis. *J Clin Invest* 1998;102:2115–2125.
228. Garnero P, Landewe R, Boers M, et al. Association of baseline levels of markers of bone and cartilage degradation with long-term progression of joint damage in patients with early rheumatoid arthritis: the COBRA study. *Arthritis Rheum* 2002;46:2847–2856.
229. Horslev-Petersen K, Saxne T, Haar D, et al. The aminoterminal-type-III procollagen peptide and proteoglycans in serum and synovial fluid of patients with rheumatoid arthritis or reactive arthritis. *Rheumatol Int* 1988;8:1–9.
230. Horslev-Petersen K, Bentsen KD, Engstrom-Laurent A, et al. Serum amino terminal type III procollagen peptide and serum hyaluronan in rheumatoid arthritis: relation to clinical and serological parameters of inflammation during 8 and 24 months' treatment with levamisole, penicillamine, or azathioprine. *Ann Rheum Dis* 1988;47:116–126.
231. Yoshihara Y, Nakamura H, Obata K, et al. Matrix metalloproteinases and tissue inhibitors of metalloproteinases in synovial fluids from patients with rheumatoid arthritis or osteoarthritis. *Ann Rheum Dis* 2000;59:455–461.
232. Brennan FM, Browne KA, Green PA, et al. Reduction of serum matrix metalloproteinase 1 and matrix metalloproteinase 3 in rheumatoid arthritis patients following anti-tumour necrosis factor-alpha (cA2) therapy. *Br J Rheumatol* 1997;36:643–650.
233. Cunnane G, Fitzgerald O, Beeton C, et al. Early joint erosions and serum levels of matrix metalloproteinase 1, matrix metalloproteinase 3, and tissue inhibitor of metalloproteinases 1 in rheumatoid arthritis. *Arthritis Rheum* 2001;44:2263–2274.
234. Keyszer G, Lambiri I, Nagel R, et al. Circulating levels of matrix metalloproteinases MMP-3 and MMP-1, tissue inhibitor of metalloproteinases 1 (TIMP-1), and MMP-1/TIMP-1 complex in rheumatic disease. Correlation with clinical activity of rheumatoid arthritis versus other surrogate markers. *J Rheumatol* 1999;26:251–258.
235. Hall GM, Spector TD, Delmas PD. Markers of bone metabolism in postmenopausal women with rheumatoid arthritis. Effects of corticosteroids and hormone replacement therapy. *Arthritis Rheum* 1995;38:902–906.
236. Janckila AJ, Neustadt DH, Nakasato YR, et al. Serum tartrate-resistant acid phosphatase isoforms in rheumatoid arthritis. *Clin Chim Acta* 2002;320:49–58.
237. Saxne T, Zunino L, Heinegard D. Increased release of bone sialoprotein into synovial fluid reflects tissue destruction in rheumatoid arthritis. *Arthritis Rheum* 1995;38:82–90.
238. Bossuyt PM, Reitsma JB, Bruns DE, et al. The STARD statement for reporting studies of diagnostic accuracy: explanation and elaboration. *Ann Intern Med* 2003;138:W1–W12.
239. Bossuyt PM, Reitsma JB, Bruns DE, et al. Towards complete and accurate reporting of studies of diagnostic accuracy: The STARD Initiative. *Ann Intern Med* 2003;138:40–44.
240. Aletaha D, Smolen JS. Laboratory testing in rheumatoid arthritis patients taking disease-modifying antirheumatic drugs: clinical evaluation and cost analysis. *Arthritis Rheum* 2002;47:181–188.

CHAPTER 7

Radiographic Findings

R. Lee Cothran, Jr., and Salutario Martinez

Radiographic examination of the patient with arthritis is a critical component of the workup to establish diagnosis and prognosis. Radiographs provide an important window into the body to help evaluate the type and degree of arthropathy and to assist in the formulation of a differential diagnosis. Radiographs can also assist in the evaluation of disease progression. Newer modalities, such as magnetic resonance imaging (MRI) and ultrasound (US) imaging, may also provide important diagnostic information, particularly with respect to soft tissue changes. These modalities are discussed elsewhere in this book. This chapter addresses primarily the musculoskeletal radiographic manifestations of rheumatoid arthritis and briefly discusses the characteristics of other inflammatory arthropathies and how they may be differentiated from rheumatoid arthritis.

PATHOPHYSIOLOGY

To understand the radiographic manifestations of rheumatoid arthritis in the musculoskeletal system, an understanding of the pathophysiology and histology of the underlying disease is necessary. This information, of course, is discussed in much more detail in other chapters of this book. However, the following summary provides a basis for predicting the radiographic manifestations of this disease.

Rheumatoid arthritis is a complex inflammatory process that results from the interplay of various immune cell populations in conjunction with activation and proliferation of synovial fibroblasts. This inflammatory response affects the synovium of the articulations, bursae, and tendons, as well as other tissues throughout the body. Patients affected by this disease may have varying clinical presentations and distribution of musculoskeletal involvement (1).

Within the synovial tissues, inflammation occurs prominently, resulting in edema and capillary and mesenchymal cell proliferation. In the synovium and synovial fluid, leukocytes accumulate, releasing lysosomal enzymes and other proinflammatory and toxic mediators (2,3). Along with activated immune cells and synovial fibroblasts, these mediators can destroy the adjacent articular cartilage. If the process continues unchecked, the articular surface is destroyed, with gradual fibrosis of the joint capsule and synovium resulting in fibrous or bony ankylosis.

Histologically, in the early stages of rheumatoid arthritis, there is villous hypertrophy of the synovium with influx of inflammatory cells, creating a structure termed *pannus*. Areas of fibrinoid necrosis and lymphoid follicles are present. In the later stages of the disease, there is cartilage destruction and synovial and capsular fibrosis, with the ultimate end stage being fibrous or bony ankylosis.

RADIOGRAPHIC APPROACH

In view of these steps in pathogenesis, the radiographic examination can be approached according to the effects of the disease on the appearance of the articular structures. An *ABC* approach—*a*rticular space, *b*one density, and *c*apsule—can provide a framework to analyze radiographs. The radiograph can be approached using these letters in reverse to follow the progression of rheumatoid arthritis in the joints.

Rheumatoid arthritis begins as a soft tissue inflammatory process; therefore, the first radiographic clue to the presence of the disease is often soft tissue swelling. The earliest imaging manifestations of rheumatoid arthritis occur in the soft tissues surrounding the joints (4,5), or, in the case of a simplified approach, the *c*apsule. The joints of the hand and wrist can be used as an illustration, but the changes seen here apply to most of the joints affected by rheumatoid arthritis.

The joint capsule comprises the connective tissue that forms the nonarticular margins of the joint and is the nonosseous, noncartilaginous portion of a joint. The capsule is lined by synovium, which is lubricated by a small amount of synovial fluid secreted by the synovial cells. This synovial fluid provides nourishment to the chondrocytes. In the initial stages of the inflammatory process of rheumatoid arthritis, the gross appearance of the radiograph may be completely normal. There may be no visible indication of the underlying disease. Those imaging modalities that can better distinguish differences in the composition of soft tissues (MRI and US imaging, among others) will be able to detect soft tissue changes at an earlier stage.

Radiographically, the earliest manifestation of rheumatoid arthritis is the distention or enlargement of the soft tissue density (representing the capsule and its contents) around the involved joint (5). This swelling is due to a number of factors, including edema of the soft tissues, proliferation of the synovial tissues (synovitis or pannus), and an increase in the amount of fluid within the joint (effusion) (4). As mentioned previously, the degree of disease and distribution of disease may vary significantly between affected individuals.

These soft tissue changes occur not only in the joints but also in other anatomic structures (e.g., tendons and their sheaths) affected by the inflammatory process. Soft tissue swelling may

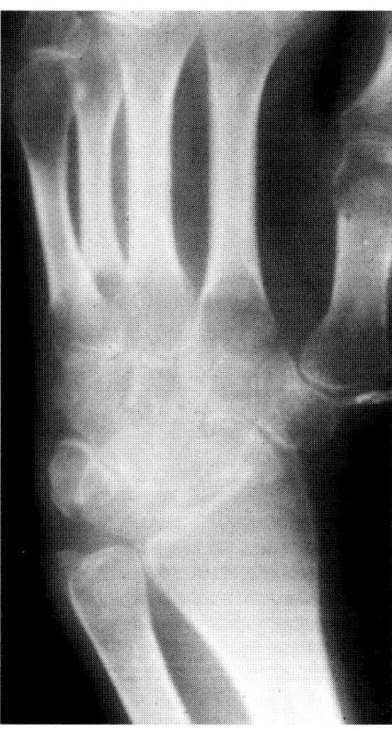

Figure 7.1. Oblique view of the wrist in a patient with rheumatoid arthritis reveals decreased bone density about the carpal joints and the metacarpophalangeal joints (periarticular osteopenia).

manifest along the ulnar styloid as an indicator of involvement of the extensor carpi ulnaris tendon that travels adjacent to this osseous structure (6). As the disease progresses, the capsular support structures and ligaments are weakened, and subluxations or dislocations may occur (7). Also, soft tissue structures not directly related to the joint, such as tendons, may be weakened. Tendon weakening may lead to rupture, as is seen not infrequently in the rotator cuff of the shoulder or in the infrapatellar tendon (8,9).

The inflammation and synovial proliferation that cause enlargement of the soft tissues will also affect the adjacent bony structures, leading to a change in the bone density. The combination of inflammation and disuse (due to pain) results in a greater degree of bone resorption than bone formation, leading to osteopenia. Osteopenia is characteristically periarticular in location (Fig. 7.1). In addition, the proliferation of synovium results in destruction of the bone at the margins of the articular cartilage, producing the erosions that are a prominent feature of this disease. These erosions occur first along the marginal bone of a joint, as this bone is unprotected by articular cartilage (5,10).

Finally, the articular surface becomes involved, with subsequent uniform narrowing of the joint space due to articular cartilage loss. There is eventual complete loss of the articular cartilage if the disease progresses unchecked. In some patients, this inflammation and fibrosis may progress to bony ankylosis, particularly in the small joints of the hands and feet. In other patients, secondary degenerative changes occur with features resembling osteoarthritis.

QUANTIFICATION OF RADIOGRAPHIC FINDINGS

Interpretation of the severity of disease in affected joints can be a relatively subjective process. Radiographic staging systems have been proposed as a method for more precise characterization of radiographic manifestations of rheumatoid arthritis. These systems allow quantification of the changes seen on the radiograph in rheumatoid arthritis for the purposes of assessment of treatment efficacy and progression or stage of disease. Multiple grading systems have been proposed, including the Sharp scoring system (11) and its modifications (12) and the Larsen scoring system (13). These systems involve assessment of erosions and joint space narrowing in multiple joints, typically of the hands and wrists. Studies have compared the Steinbrocker, Larsen, and modified Sharp scoring systems and found highly significant correlation among them. They also found that the scoring systems correlated significantly with the duration of disease, indicating that scores increased with increasing duration of disease (14). The scoring systems are discussed in more detail in Chapter 8.

RADIOGRAPHIC PATTERNS

The patterns of involvement in particular body regions are often helpful in the diagnosis and radiographic assessment of rheumatoid arthritis. Although the disease process occurring in each of these body regions is the same, the manifestations in a particular region may be unique. Given the varying manifestations, a review of the radiographic appearance of rheumatoid arthritis in different body regions is useful.

Hand and Wrist

The radiographic manifestations of rheumatoid arthritis in the musculoskeletal system often present first in the small joints of the hands and feet. The hands and wrists and the feet and ankles are regions that are easily imaged for evaluation of early or subtle imaging characteristics of this disease. Although the disease may begin somewhat asymmetrically (4), the typical distribution is bilaterally symmetric, and the involvement of the hand and wrist joints tends to be more severe proximally in the carpal joints and the metacarpophalangeal (MCP) joints than distally in the interphalangeal joints (15). The disease is initially manifest as periarticular soft tissue swelling or capsular swelling (5), especially around the MCP joints, the proximal interphalangeal (PIP) joints, and the ulnar side of the wrist.

Involvement of the joint capsule is the primary reason for the changes seen at the MCP and PIP joints (4). However, the soft tissue involvement about the ulnar aspect of the wrist is more often due to early involvement of the extensor carpi ulnaris tendon and its synovial sheath (6). These findings are often followed by decreased bone density, or osteopenia, particularly in paraepiphyseal or periarticular distribution (5,15). There are some patients in whom osteopenia is not prominent. These patients may be laborers or people who, for some other reason, continue to have a greater degree of mobility than those with osteopenia. Some investigators have found that the degree of physical activity and the development of large cystic erosions are inversely related to the degree of osteopenia (16).

The next step in the radiographic progression of the disease is the development of erosions, which have been called the most definite radiologic change of rheumatoid arthritis (5). In a radiographic study of patients with rheumatoid arthritis published in 1977, the bones about the wrist were the second most common site of early erosions [behind the metatarsophalangeal (MTP) joints], with a significant proportion of those erosions occurring in the ulnar styloid (15). Indeed, the distal ulna has been considered an important site for the recognition of rheumatoid arthritis early in the disease; joint space loss at the radiocarpal joint and the joints of the scaphoid with the trapezoid and trapezium are also early manifestations of disease, with erosions appearing along the radial aspect of the scaphoid (4). So-called surface or

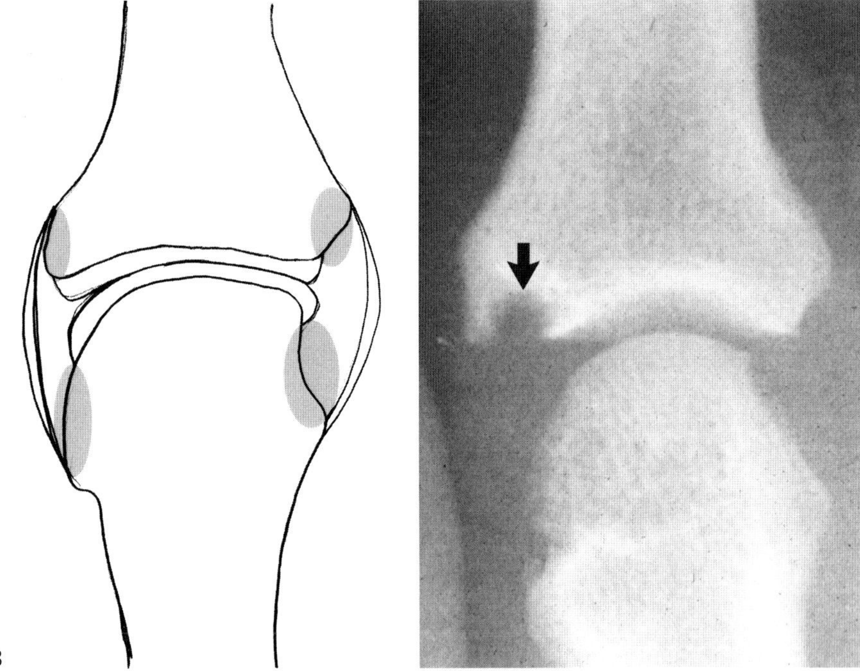

Figure 7.2. **A:** Schematic representation of the marginal areas affected by early rheumatoid erosions. **B:** Magnified view of metacarpophalangeal joint showing marginal erosion (*arrow*).

marginal erosions occur at the margins of the articular space and are the result of synovial proliferation and invasion of the exposed bone unprotected by articular cartilage (Fig. 7.2).

The evaluation of these radiographic findings at baseline in a patient presenting for evaluation of a polyarthropathy, along with serologic studies, may be predictive of future progression of disease. In results from the Norfolk Arthritis Register Study published in 2002 (17), a high-titer rheumatoid factor was found to be a predictor of radiographic severity at first film in a group of patients presenting to a primary care clinic for inflammatory polyarthritis. C-reactive protein levels, the presence of nodules, and the number of swollen joints at baseline were also predictive of radiographic severity at first film. The baseline radiographic score was found to be a predictor of the severity of deterioration over 5 years. A high rheumatoid factor titer was also found to be an independent predictor of radiographic deterioration at 5 years. Other recent studies have supported rheumatoid factor positivity as a predictor of more severe disease activity (18).

Radiographic projection may affect detection of disease in the hands and wrists. The earliest erosions in the MCP joints are often difficult to appreciate on the standard posteroanterior and lateral radiographic views of the hands and wrists. The "halfway supinate" oblique view of the hands is useful for the detection of these small early erosions in the hands (19). These early erosions tend to occur in relatively distinct locations within the wrists and hands, as illustrated in Figure 7.3.

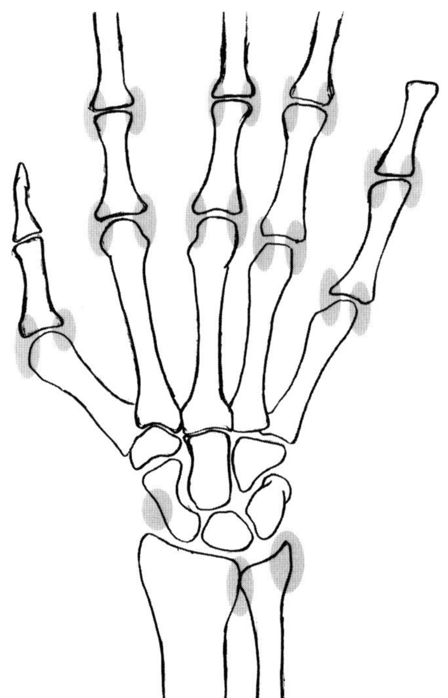

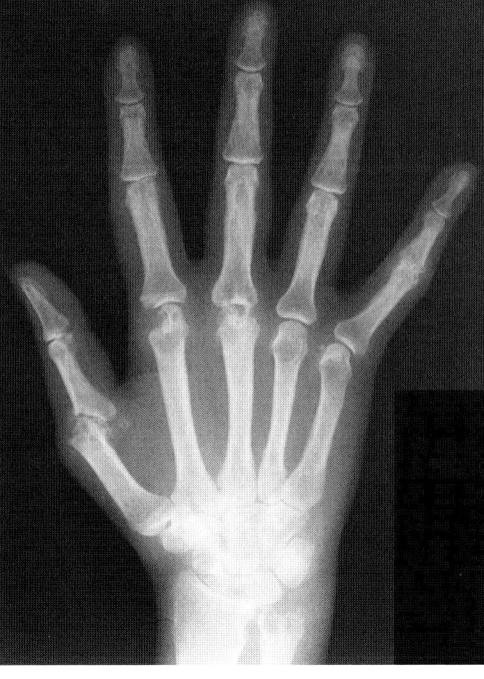

Figure 7.3. **A:** Schematic representation of the sites of early erosions in the hand and wrist in rheumatoid arthritis. **B:** Posteroanterior radiograph of the hand with classic distribution of rheumatoid erosions.

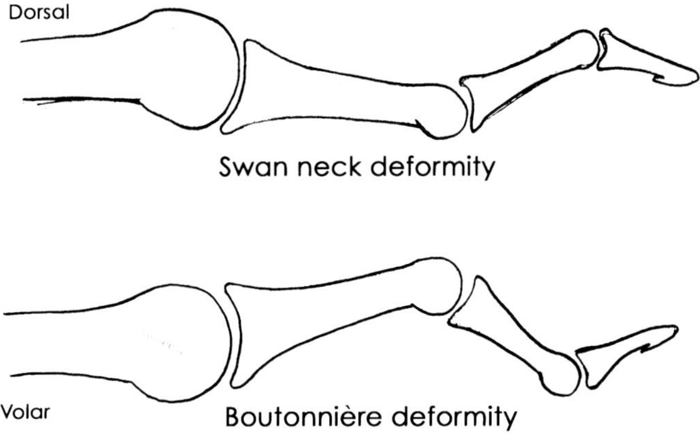

Figure 7.4. Schematic representation of the swan-neck and boutonnière deformities often seen in advanced rheumatoid arthritis.

Pocketed erosions or pseudocysts may occur away from the margins of the articular cartilage and are due to herniation of synovial membrane and synovial fluid along vascular channels. These erosions involve areas of the bone where the overlying cartilage has been destroyed by pannus or by preexisting or coexisting degenerative disease (5). It has been suggested that the pseudocysts present in rheumatoid arthritis progress by becoming filled with hyperplastic synovial tissue, which subsequently undergoes necrosis, liquefication, and hemorrhage causing a *pressure erosion* of the bone (10). Some authors have reported that patients with rheumatoid arthritis who continue to perform heavy labor or who have a high pain tolerance develop larger pseudocysts (5,16). Other authors have suggested that increased activity does not contribute to the development or progression of pseudocysts (20).

Boutonnière and swan-neck deformities (Fig. 7.4), along with ulnar deviation at the MCP joints, are classic clinical and radiographic findings in rheumatoid arthritis. The boutonnière deformity results from the rupture of the central slip of the extrinsic extensor tendon of the finger, causing PIP joint flexion and distal interphalangeal (DIP) joint extension. The base of the proximal phalanx "buttonholes" through the residual lateral slips of the extrinsic extensor tendon (thus the French *boutonnière,* meaning "buttonhole"). Although initially reducible, this deformity may become fixed over time (21). This deformity is readily identifiable on radiographs due to the position of the interphalangeal joints.

The swan-neck deformity consists of PIP joint extension and DIP joint flexion. This deformity is the result of hypertrophied rheumatoid synovium weakening the volar plate and collateral ligaments of the PIP joint or rupturing of the superficial flexor tendon. Hyperextension may occur from unopposed action of the extensor tendons at the PIP joint. The lateral bands then slide dorsally, maintaining a hyperextension force at the PIP joint. The result is "a relative lengthening of the extensor apparatus, relative tightening of the flexor profundus, and superimposed intrinsic contracture" (22), which combine to produce flexion at the DIP joint. The swan-neck deformity is so named because of its resemblance to the neck of a swan when viewed from the lateral position.

Elbow

The earliest radiographic sign of involvement of the elbow by rheumatoid arthritis is the displacement of anterior and posterior fat pads that occurs with the development of a joint effusion or synovitis from any cause. A study in 1970 evaluating the fat pads of the elbow in rheumatoid arthritis found a radiographically evident, positive fat pad sign in 88% of 160 elbows (23). Other fat pads about the elbow are also displaced by the synovial hypertrophy and joint effusion (24). This synovial hypertrophy and effusion occurs along with, or preceding, the periarticular osteopenia and bone destruction that are the sequelae of rheumatoid arthritis in the elbow. It has been reported that the demineralization of the elbow is most likely to occur about the olecranon and coronoid process (23).

Inflammation of the bursae about the elbow may also occur in rheumatoid arthritis. These bursae are typically paraarticular in location. Two of the bursae that may be affected in rheumatoid arthritis are the olecranon bursa on the dorsal aspect of the elbow overlying the olecranon process of the ulna, and the bicipital bursa adjacent to the insertion of the biceps tendon on the radial tuberosity just distal to the elbow joint. Radiographically, these bursae may be difficult to detect but may be visible as soft tissue density masses on the dorsal and volar aspects of the elbow, respectively.

Shoulder

Within the shoulder, synovial proliferation and inflammation with joint effusion develops just as in the other joints. However, there is also damage to the rotator cuff tendons (8), given their intimate association with the joint. In a study of rheumatoid arthritis patients, the clinical symptoms of arthritis, tendonitis, and bursitis of the shoulder were found in 50% of patients, with a large proportion of patients also having pain at the scapulothoracic articulation (25).

Rheumatoid arthritis results in a significantly increased risk of rotator cuff tear (8). Radiographically, a tear is manifest by a decrease in the space between the top of the humeral head and the inferior aspect of the acromion, the so-called acromiohumeral interval. This space is normally occupied by the tendons of the supraspinatus and infraspinatus muscles. Once these tendons rupture and retract, the action of the deltoid muscle elevates the humeral head, resulting in loss of the acromiohumeral interval and, in some cases, formation of a pseudarthrosis between the humeral head and the acromion.

The other joint about the shoulder that is frequently affected by rheumatoid arthritis is the acromioclavicular joint. This articulation may be involved with synovitis, although there is often resorption of bone more focally in the distal or lateral aspect of the clavicle. This finding may be seen on a standard chest radiograph; although not completely specific for rheumatoid arthritis, it provides supporting evidence for the diagnosis. In addition, there may be focal erosion of bone at the attachment sites of the coracoclavicular ligaments.

The subacromial subdeltoid bursa lies just superficial to the rotator cuff tendons and may become inflamed in rheumatoid arthritis, either due to primary inflammation involving the bursa or to adjacent rotator cuff abnormalities. This bursitis is typically not evident on radiographs but may be detected by other imaging modalities, such as MRI.

Foot and Ankle

Within the foot and ankle are multiple joints that may be affected by rheumatoid arthritis. As stated above, a 1952 study reported that radiographs of the feet may provide the most diagnostic information in those patients with clinical symptoms in the feet. The diagnostic yield of foot radiographs in patients in this study was followed closely by the diagnostic yield of radiographs of the hands and wrists (26). More recent studies have also supported the inclusion of foot films in the assessment of treatment effect in rheumatoid arthritis (27).

One of the most commonly affected joints in the foot is the fifth MTP joint (28). Erosions of the fifth metatarsal head are among the

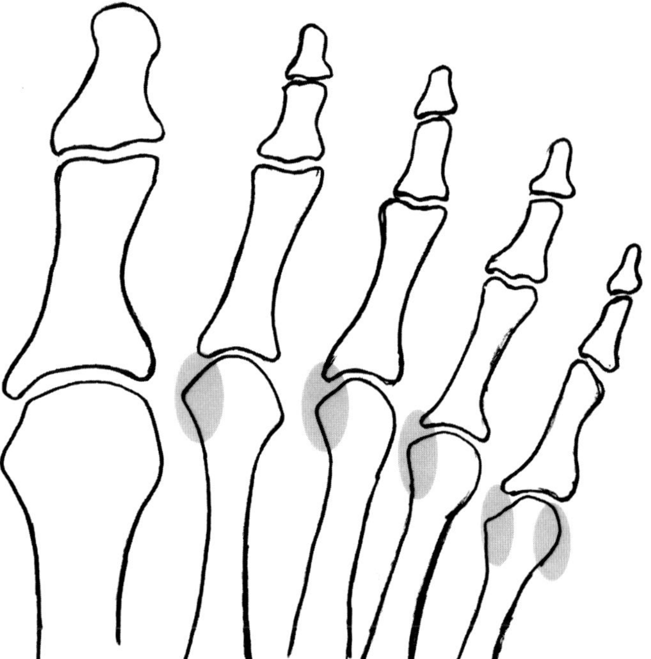

Figure 7.5. Schematic representation of the sites of erosions in the forefoot in rheumatoid arthritis. The first metatarsophalangeal joint is often relatively spared.

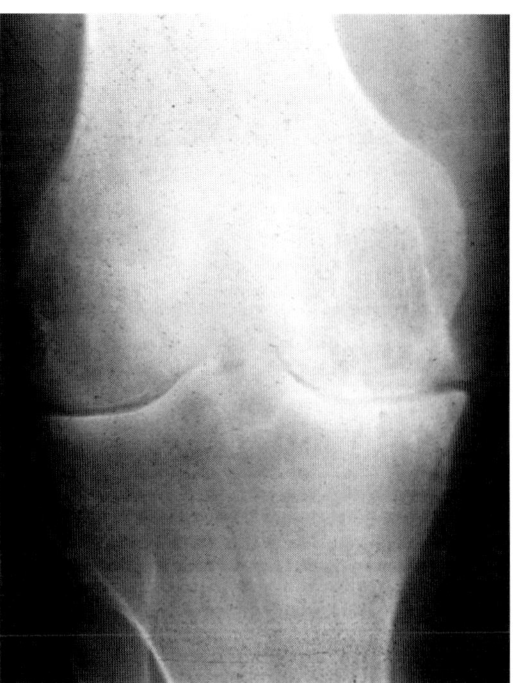

Figure 7.6. Knee radiograph in patient with rheumatoid arthritis. Note the global loss of articular space without significant osteophytosis.

earliest erosions seen in rheumatoid arthritis of the foot and are almost always present when there is any involvement of the foot in rheumatoid arthritis. The second through fourth MTP joints may also be affected, as illustrated in Figure 7.5. Hallux valgus has also been described as an early and frequent manifestation of rheumatoid arthritis in the foot. There also may be fibular deviation of the remainder of the toes, analogous to the ulnar deviation of the fingers, seen in radiographs of the hands. The "cock-up" toe deformity is also a common manifestation of the disease and is attributable to tendon contractures and joint capsule laxity, resulting in flexion deformities and subluxations (29). The midfoot may also be affected by rheumatoid disease, with findings analogous to the carpal bones in the hands—diffuse narrowing of the joint spaces with scattered erosions (4).

The hindfoot is also involved in rheumatoid arthritis, with manifestations including erosions of the calcaneus at the insertion of the Achilles tendon. Achilles tendinitis or tendinopathy is also common in this disease (29) and may be seen on the radiograph as a thickening of the soft tissue silhouette of the tendon near its insertion on the calcaneus. There may also be a bursitis adjacent to this tendon attachment, seen as an increase in the soft tissue density behind the calcaneus (4). This process may eventually erode the calcaneus posteriorly (29).

Tendon rupture and tenosynovitis may become manifest on radiographs of the ankle due to focal areas of swelling, increased soft tissue density, or even adjacent periostitis in the setting of a tenosynovitis. The structure of the ankle and foot may also be altered, as in the acquired pes planus deformity, which results from rupture of the diseased posterior tibial tendon and abnormality of the supporting ligaments of the arch of the foot, including the spring ligament.

Knee

In the larger joints, such as the knee, erosions are a relatively late manifestation, with the primary early features being symmetric global loss of all articular spaces, joint effusion, and periarticular osteopenia (Fig. 7.6). This last characteristic, along with the lack of osteophyte formation, helps to distinguish rheumatoid arthritis radiographically from early osteoarthritis. Erosions, and even geodes, or subchondral cysts, may occur later in the disease. In some cases, pannus formation, or synovial proliferation, may cause large excavations of bone that extend significantly beyond the subchondral bone. Some investigations have suggested that increased fluid and increased intraarticular pressure contribute to the formation of these large subchondral cysts and that patients who maintained a high level of physical exertion, despite their disease, are more prone to the development of these large cysts (16). However, other authors have concluded that these large subchondral cysts are simply the result of invasive synovium and have nothing to do with the degree of physical activity or the amount of intraarticular fluid present (20).

Within the knee, the synovial proliferation and joint effusion may decompress through the posteromedial aspect of the joint into a Baker's cyst. A Baker's cyst may be apparent on the lateral radiograph of the knee as an ovoid area of increased density extending inferiorly from the popliteal fossa. Baker's cysts may also contain loose bodies that can be seen on the radiograph. Leakage of these cysts can result in pain and inflammation that may mimic a cellulitis or deep venous thrombosis clinically. Hemorrhage into these cysts may also cause acute symptoms.

Hip and Pelvis

In the hip, rheumatoid arthritis causes soft tissue swelling and diffuse joint space narrowing with osteopenia and without osteophytosis. This diffuse cartilage loss may result in axial migration of the femoral head within the acetabulum, as opposed to the superior migration of the femoral head seen in osteoarthritis (30). In some patients, the bone of the acetabulum is weakened by the inflammatory process, and there is remodeling of the softened bone, resulting in protrusio acetabuli, in which the medial wall of the acetabulum protrudes into the pelvis. Crabbe (31) proposed a classification of hip involvement with rheumatoid arthritis. Grade Ia disease is early-stage disease with loss of articular cartilage superiorly and medially due to lysis of cartilage; grade Ib is remission of the active synovial disease and, in some cases, the onset of secondary osteoarthritis. Grade II involves bony destruction or loss superiorly in the femoral head. Grade III disease is what Crabbe called the "classical rheumatoid hip" with erosion of the medial acetabular wall and central dislocation of the femoral head. Grade IV disease is joint disintegration resulting in a Charcot-type appearance.

A 1998 study performed in Finland of 96 patients with seropositive rheumatoid arthritis with a 15-year follow-up found that severe radiologic changes occurred in 32% of patients and protrusio acetabuli was seen in 5% during the 15-year follow-up period. Only half of the patients with hip destruction radiographically had symptoms, and nearly half (46%) of patients without radiographic changes had hip symptoms (32). Therefore, the absence of symptoms does not necessarily exclude hip involvement in patients with rheumatoid arthritis.

Another entity that should be considered in the evaluation of hip disease in rheumatoid arthritis is avascular necrosis (AVN). This condition is characterized by infarction of the marrow and bone of the femoral head, resulting from compromise of the blood supply. AVN may be secondary to steroid treatment, which is often a component of the treatment regimen for rheumatoid arthritis and is a known risk factor for the development of AVN. Early in the process of AVN, radiographs remain normal. As the AVN progresses, patchy sclerosis becomes apparent in the femoral heads. If the disease continues to progress, subchondral bone resorption and collapse may occur, with subsequent development of secondary osteoarthritis. AVN may be a bilateral process, even when symptoms are unilateral. If AVN is suspected and initial radiographs are normal, MRI is more sensitive for early diagnosis and is a useful adjunct to radiographs in this disorder. AVN may also occur in the humeral heads, with a similar appearance.

Other portions of the pelvis may also be affected in rheumatoid arthritis. Although very rare, the sacroiliac joints may exhibit erosions and even ankylosis, occurring less commonly than in ankylosing spondylitis. There also may be erosions at the symphysis pubis and the ischial tuberosities in rheumatoid arthritis (33).

Cervical Spine

The cervical spine is an area of particular concern in the patient with rheumatoid arthritis. This disease may affect multiple joints in the cervical spine, which includes as many as 29 synovial articulations between the level of the occiput and T1 (34). As discussed above, the supporting structures of these joints may also be affected by the inflammation of rheumatoid arthritis. Within the cervical spine, this involvement can lead to significant neurologic compromise because of vertebral subluxations (35–38). Rheumatoid arthritis affects the atlanto-occipital articulation, the atlanto-dens articulations, facet and uncovertebral joints, ligaments of the cervical spine, and intervertebral disc spaces.

In a large prospective study of patients with rheumatoid arthritis (39), symptoms referable to the neck occurred in 88% of patients. Radiographic changes were observed in 50% of patients with rheumatoid arthritis, with the most frequent changes being at the apophyseal joints of C2-3. Vertebral end plate erosions were seen in 14% of all patients with rheumatoid arthritis. One of the most concerning factors, however, was the presence of atlantoaxial subluxation in 25% of the 333 patients evaluated.

Anterior atlantoaxial subluxation is the condition in which the space between the posterior aspect of the anterior arch of the C1 vertebral body and the anterior aspect of the odontoid process (dens) of C2 becomes abnormally widened. This diagnosis can be made when, in the lateral radiograph, the space between these two structures exceeds 2.5 mm in the adult. This subluxation is often dynamic and may require a flexion-extension radiographic examination for diagnosis, as the space may be normal in the neutral position but increase in flexion (Fig. 7.7). This subluxation can be due to laxity or disruption of the transverse ligament or to erosion of the dens of C2. Erosion of the dens can become so severe that the dens is completely destroyed, allowing subluxation in the presence of intact transverse ligaments, or the dens fractures, also resulting in subluxation (34). This instability becomes an important clinical problem when the space available

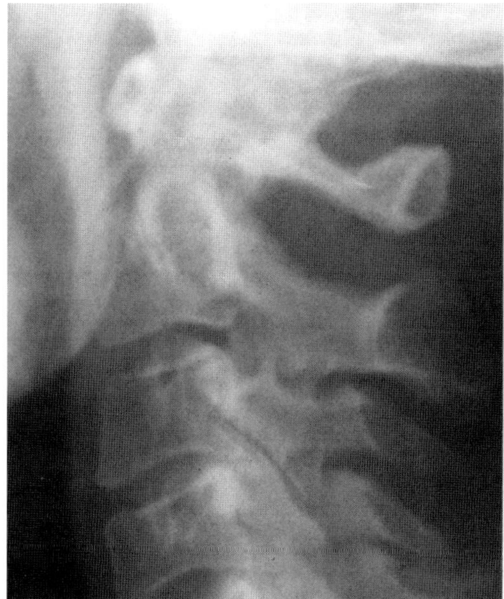

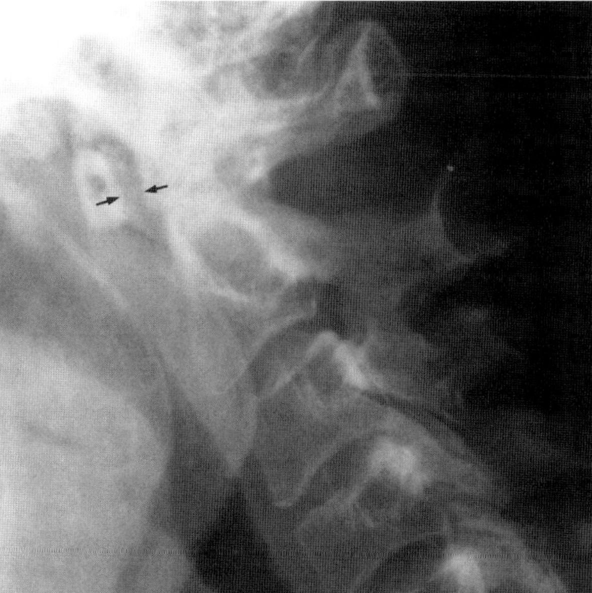

Figure 7.7. Lateral neutral **(A)** and flexion **(B)** views of the cervical spine in patient with rheumatoid arthritis illustrating increase in atlanto-dens interval on flexion (*arrows*), indicating ligament insufficiency.

for the spinal cord decreases, producing a mass effect on the spinal cord. This mass effect can cause weakness and, in extreme cases, paralysis in the setting of superimposed trauma. Many patients with rather striking subluxations, however, are relatively asymptomatic from a neurologic standpoint.

Another potentially devastating complication of rheumatoid arthritis occurs at the level of the craniocervical junction. This process is called *basilar invagination* (also called *atlantoaxial superior subluxation* or *cranial settling*) and results from softening of the bone in the skull base. This bone softening allows the skull to settle onto the cervical spine. Superior migration of the odontoid process into the foramen magnum can be visualized on the lateral cervical spine radiograph. This superior migration of the dens results in a mass effect on the brainstem with the potential for significant neurologic compromise. This complication must be recognized and treated promptly to prevent potentially significant morbidity.

Subluxation within the cervical spine is not limited to the craniocervical junction and the C1-2 level. It is often seen at multiple levels in patients with advanced rheumatoid arthritis. The treatment may involve surgical fusion of the involved levels. Despite the impressive appearance of the radiographs in some patients, the radiographic findings in the cervical spine do not always parallel the neurologic deficits. However, early recognition of these abnormalities will allow correction or stabilization before permanent neurologic damage occurs.

Ankylosis is on the opposite end of the spectrum from subluxation, resulting in loss of motion in the cervical spine. However, ankylosis of the cervical spine does not occur as commonly in the adult with rheumatoid arthritis as it does in juvenile rheumatoid arthritis. In fact, although the apophyseal joints of the cervical spine may become ankylosed in rheumatoid arthritis, the spine changes are predominantly nonankylosing (33). This lack of ankylosis helps distinguish the spine changes of rheumatoid arthritis from the spine changes seen in ankylosing spondylitis and psoriasis.

The thoracic spine and lumbar spine are less affected by rheumatoid arthritis than is the cervical spine, with the predominant abnormality being erosive end plate changes with relatively little sclerosis and osteophyte formation. Patients with rheumatoid arthritis may develop osteoporosis as a result of the disease process, decreased activity, or medications (i.e., steroids). Osteoporosis may result in compression fractures of the thoracic and lumbar spine, with resulting pain and deformity.

EARLY RADIOGRAPHIC FINDINGS

Knowledge of the early progression of radiographic joint damage has evolved with the development of more reliable scoring systems, more effective therapies, as well as a research focus on the identification of patients with early disease. Many of the studies describing the natural history of rheumatoid arthritis were performed before the advent of scoring systems for quantification of radiographic findings. There are also differing definitions of "early" disease. More recent studies involve patients who are undergoing therapies that may alter the radiographic manifestations of the disease; therefore, older studies conducted before the use of these therapies may not provide an accurate picture of the progression of disease likely to be seen with modern therapies.

A study published by Hulsmans et al. in 2000 (27) examined a cohort of patients from the Utrecht region of the Netherlands. All of these patients were randomly assigned to three different pharmacologic therapies, and all had disease duration of less than 1 year at the time of entry into the study. This cohort of patients was followed for a mean of 2.7 years (maximum, 6 years) with radiographs of the hands and feet (posteroanterior views). Radiographs were graded using the van der Heijde modification of the Sharp scoring method. Hulsmans et al. reported that 2% of joints in the hand and 6% of joints in the feet exhibited at least one erosion at the beginning of the study. They reported that 3% of joints in the hand and 6% of joints in the feet at entry showed joint space narrowing. During the follow-up of these patients, the authors found a linear progression of joint damage. They also found that 95% of patients exhibited erosions and joint space narrowing after 6 years and that damage occurred earlier and more often in the joints of the feet than in the joints of the hand and wrist.

This prospective study provides a general idea of the progression of the disease in the hand and foot, but the degree and rate of progression, as well as the distribution of disease, might vary with the type of treatment used, and certainly may vary among individual patients. Other studies (40–42) show a nonlinear progression of disease, with a greater degree of disease progression occurring in the first 1 to 3 years. Therefore, generalization of results from any single study is difficult because of the number of variables potentially involved in the progression of rheumatoid arthritis.

DIFFERENTIATION FROM OTHER ARTHROPATHIES

An important part of the diagnosis of rheumatoid arthritis—a diagnosis often made from radiographs of the hand and wrist—is differentiation from other erosive or inflammatory arthropathies. The distribution of the abnormalities identified in the hand and wrist, the character of the erosions, and the presence or absence of osteopenia are helpful in making this distinction (Table 7.1). Seronegative spondyloarthropathies, including psoriatic arthropathy, are often a differential consideration, as they are also erosive in nature. However, the distribution of the erosions in the seronegative spondyloarthropathies is typically different from that in rheumatoid arthritis. As previously discussed, rheumatoid arthritis tends to affect the hand and wrist more proximally than distally, with changes seen in the wrist, MCP joints, and, occasionally, PIP joints. Seronegative spondyloarthropathies, on the other hand, tend to involve the DIP and PIP joints more than the MCP joints early in the disease (43). The wrist may also be involved in seronegative arthropathies, although this involvement typically occurs later in the course of the disease.

Another difference between seronegative arthropathies and rheumatoid arthritis is the propensity for periosteal new bone formation in the seronegative spondyloarthropathies. This bone formation usually takes the form of periostitis or enthesopathic calcification (calcification at the sites of tendon attachment to bone) along the phalanges, distal radius and ulna, or other sites of hand and wrist involvement. Figure 7.8 shows a comparison of two wrists, one from a patient with rheumatoid arthritis and the other from a patient with psoriatic arthritis, showing the periosteal new bone formation and enthesopathic calcification in affected areas. Seronegative spondyloarthropathies also often have sacroiliac joint erosions and lower thoracic and lumbar spine involvement. These findings are uncommon in rheumatoid arthritis.

Systemic lupus erythematosus (SLE) may cause periarticular osteopenia similar to that in rheumatoid arthritis. The presence of paraarticular calcifications is a helpful sign in the diagnosis of SLE, as these do not occur in rheumatoid arthritis. Hand radiographs of patients with SLE often exhibit dislocations and subluxations without developing erosions; erosions are rela-

TABLE 7.1. Comparison of Radiographic Findings in Erosive or Deforming Arthropathies

	Rheumatoid Arthritis	Psoriasis	Erosive Osteoarthritis	Gout	Systemic Lupus Erythematosus
Soft tissue swelling	Periarticular, symmetric	Fusiform along digits	Intermittent, not as prominent as others	Eccentric, tophi	Periarticular
Subluxation	Yes	Occasional	Occasional	Uncommon	Yes
Mineralization	Decreased periarticularly	Maintained	Maintained	Maintained	Decreased periarticularly
Calcification	No	No	No	Occasionally in tophi	Periarticular, soft tissue
Joint space	Uniform decrease	Decrease, sometimes dramatic	Decreased	Preserved until late	Usually preserved
Erosion	Marginal early, other locations late	Yes, "pencil-in-cup"; "mouse ears"	Yes, intraarticular	"Punched out" with sclerotic margins	Uncommon
Bone production	No	Yes, periosteal new bone and syndesmophytes (spine)	Yes	Overhanging edge of cortex	No
Symmetry	Bilaterally symmetric	Often asymmetric	Bilaterally symmetric	Asymmetric	Bilaterally symmetric
Location	Proximal > distal	Distal > proximal	Distal > proximal	Feet > ankles > hands > elbows	Hand and wrist, hip, knee, shoulder
Distinguishing characteristics	Polyarticular	Monoarticular or oligoarticular, "mouse ear" erosions, spondylitis	"Seagull" appearance to interphalangeal joints	Crystals	Osteonecrosis not uncommon

tively uncommon in SLE. Therefore, such deformities in the absence of erosions would be more suggestive of SLE than rheumatoid arthritis (44).

Erosive osteoarthritis is another erosive arthropathy that might initially be confused with rheumatoid arthritis when evaluating a radiograph of the hand and wrist. However, the erosions present in erosive osteoarthritis will also involve the articular surface in addition to the marginal zones initially affected in rheumatoid arthritis. Also, the distribution of the abnormalities in erosive osteoarthritis tends to be distal, involving the PIP and DIP joints more than the wrist and MCP joints (Fig. 7.9). In contrast to rheumatoid arthritis, erosive arthritis does not typically show a periarticular osteopenia (45).

Finally, gout is an erosive crystal deposition disease that may affect the hand and wrist. Gout may be monoarticular and is often asymmetric, in contrast to the typically more symmetric abnormality seen in rheumatoid arthritis. In addition, the erosions of gout typically have sclerotic margins and often have "overhanging edges" occurring in paraarticular locations. Paraarticular osteopenia is not as prominent as in rheumatoid arthritis (46). Soft tissue nodules or tophi may occur and may be confused with rheumatoid nodules.

MAGNETIC RESONANCE IMAGING AND ULTRASOUND

Continued advances in MRI and US and the increasing availability of these imaging modalities have improved the evaluation of soft tissue processes in a myriad of disease processes, including rheumatoid arthritis. These modalities provide improved visualization of the soft tissue structures within and around the joints and also have the advantage of multiplanar imaging and, in the case of US, easily performed dynamic assessment of joints and tendons. These modalities also do not use ionizing radiation to acquire images.

Although they are advantageous in the assessment of soft tissue changes and have been shown to be more sensitive to early erosions, MRI and US do have disadvantages in comparison to radiographs in the routine assessment of the patient with rheumatoid arthritis. MRI is expensive and is not readily available in all locations. Acquisition of MR images takes longer than acquisition of radiographs, and greater effort and time are required for the interpretation of MRI data than for radiographs. US is more readily available in most locations than MRI, is less costly, and, with newer handheld units, may even be performed at the bed-

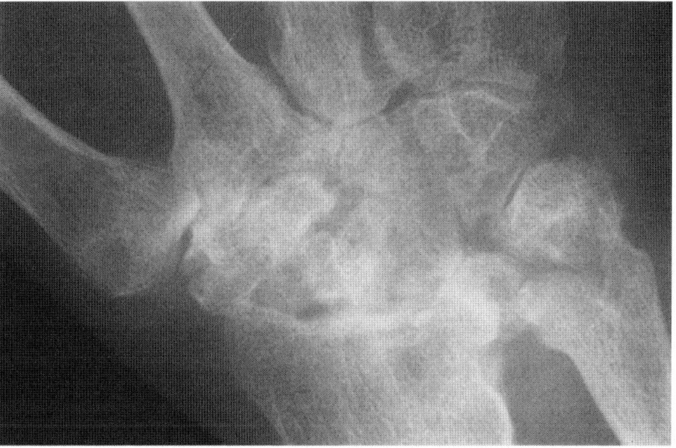

A

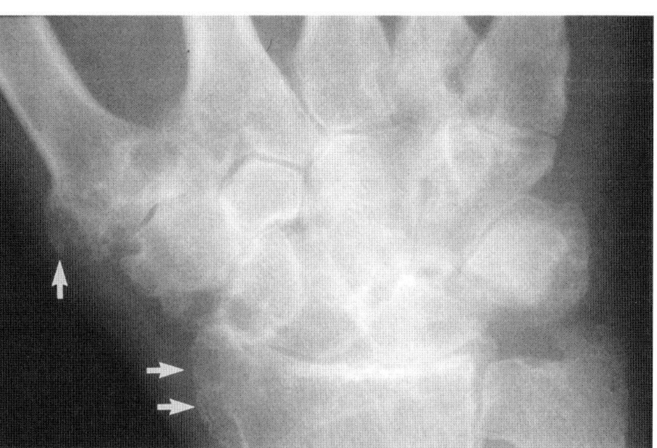

B

Figure 7.8. Posteroanterior views of the wrist in a patient with rheumatoid arthritis **(A)** and a patient with psoriatic arthritis **(B)**. Both wrists exhibit erosion and joint space loss, but note the periosteal new bone formation seen in psoriatic arthritis (*arrows*) but not present in rheumatoid arthritis.

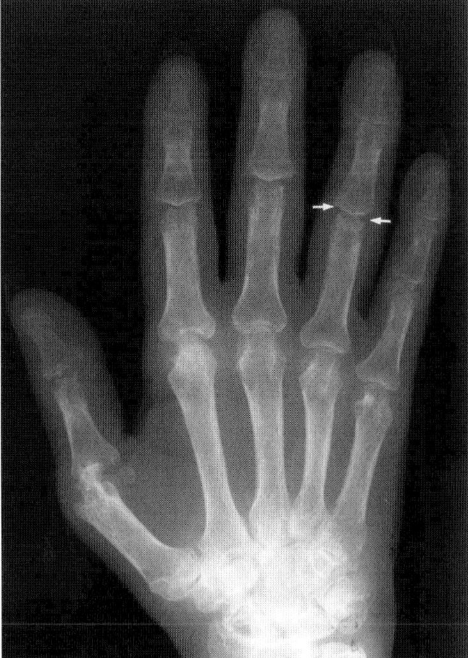
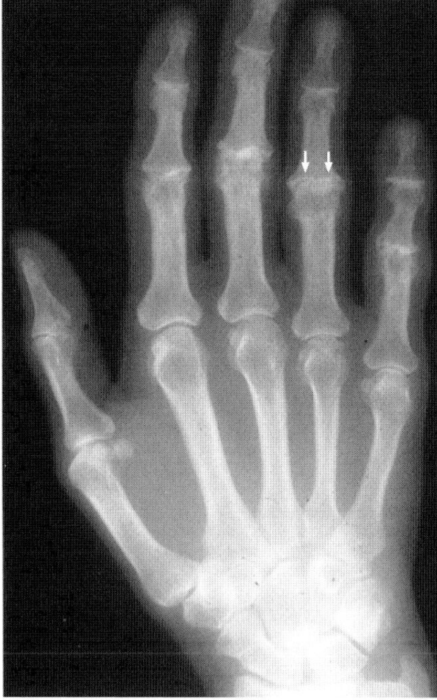

A,B

Figure 7.9. Comparison of posteroanterior radiographs in a patient with rheumatoid arthritis **(A)** and a patient with erosive osteoarthritis **(B)**. Note the predominance of proximal disease in rheumatoid arthritis, involving the carpus and metacarpophalangeal joints to a greater degree than the proximal interphalangeal (PIP) joints. Disease in erosive osteoarthritis predominates more distally in PIP joints. Note also the marginal erosions at PIP in rheumatoid arthritis **(A)** (*arrows*) and intraarticular erosions at PIP in erosive osteoarthritis **(B)** (*arrows*).

side. However, accurate imaging of the musculoskeletal system with US requires a great deal of experience and is much more operator dependent than either radiographs or MRI. US also has limitations in the evaluation of the axial skeleton.

Although it is likely that MRI and US will continue to be used in the assessment of rheumatoid arthritis, the monetary and time costs involved currently would limit them from being as widely and frequently performed as radiographs. These modalities are discussed in detail in Chapter 9.

CONCLUSION

Rheumatoid arthritis is an inflammatory arthropathy whose primary radiographic abnormalities consist of soft tissue swelling, periarticular osteopenia, erosions, and joint space loss. Although not specific for rheumatoid arthritis, these findings, when they occur in a particular distribution—proximal greater than distal in the hands and feet; relatively symmetric; predilection for the ulnar styloid, MCP joints, head of fifth metatarsal, and cervical spine—form a pattern characteristic of this disease. Radiographic assessment can provide valuable information for diagnosis and determination of disease progression, thereby facilitating efforts to prevent consequences of these disorders by early detection of erosions and deformities.

REFERENCES

1. Cush JJ, Lipsky PE. Cellular basis for rheumatoid arthritis. *Clin Orthop* 1991;265:9–22.
2. Lee D, Weinblatt M. Rheumatoid arthritis [Review]. *Lancet* 2001;358:903–911.
3. Katrib A, McNeil H, Youssef P. What can we learn from the synovium in early rheumatoid arthritis? *Inflamm Res* 2002;51:170–175.
4. Berens DL, Lockie LM, Lin R, et al. Roentgen changes in early rheumatoid arthritis. *Radiology* 1964;82:645–653.
5. Bywaters EGL. The early radiological signs of rheumatoid arthritis. *Bull Rheum Dis* 1960;11:231–234.
6. Resnick D. Rheumatoid arthritis of the wrist: why the ulnar styloid? *Radiology* 1974;112:29–35.
7. Collins LC, Lidsky MD, Sharp JT, et al. Malposition of the carpal bones in rheumatoid arthritis. *Radiology* 1972;103:95–98.
8. Resnick D. Rheumatoid arthritis. In: Resnick D, ed. *Diagnosis of bone and joint disorders*, 4th ed. Philadelphia: W.B. Saunders, 2002:891–987.
9. Razzano CD, Wilde AH, Phalen GS. Bilateral rupture of the infrapatellar tendon in rheumatoid arthritis. *Clin Orthop* 1973;91:158–161.
10. Martel W, Hayes JT, Duff IF. The pattern of bone erosion in the hand and wrist in rheumatoid arthritis. *Radiology* 1965;84:204–214.
11. Sharp JT, Lidsky MD, Collins LC, et al. Methods of scoring the progression of radiologic changes in rheumatoid arthritis: correlation of radiologic, clinical and laboratory abnormalities. *Arthritis Rheum* 1971;14:706–720.
12. Sharp JT, Young DY, Bluhm GB, et al. How many joints in the hands and wrists should be included in a score of radiologic abnormalities used to assess rheumatoid arthritis? *Arthritis Rheum* 1985;28:1326–1335.
13. Larsen A, Dale K, Eek M. Radiographic evaluation of rheumatoid arthritis and related conditions by standard reference films. *Acta Radiol Diagn (Stockh)* 1977;18:481–491.
14. Pincus T, Callahan LF, Fuchs HA, et al. Quantitative analysis of hand radiographs in rheumatoid arthritis: time course of radiographic changes, relation to joint examination measures, and comparison of different scoring methods. *J Rheumatol* 1995;22:1983–1989.
15. Brook A, Corbett M. Radiographic changes in early rheumatoid disease. *Ann Rheum Dis* 1977;36:71–73.
16. Castillo BA, El Sallab RA, Scott JT. Physical activity, cystic erosions and osteoporosis in rheumatoid arthritis. *Ann Rheum Dis* 1965;24:522–527.
17. Bukhari M, Lunt M, Harrison B, et al. Rheumatoid factor is the major predictor of increasing severity of radiographic erosions in rheumatoid arthritis. *Arthritis Rheum* 2002;46:906–912.
18. Papadopoulos I, Katsimbri P, Katsaraki A, et al. Clinical course and outcome of early rheumatoid arthritis. *Rheumatol Int* 2001;20:205–210.
19. Norgaard F. Earliest roentgenological changes in polyarthritis of the rheumatoid type: rheumatoid arthritis. *Radiology* 1965;85:325–329.
20. Magyar E, Talerman A, Feher M, et al. The pathogenesis of the subchondral pseudocysts in rheumatoid arthritis. *Clin Orthop* 1974;100:341–344.
21. Coons MS, Green SM. Boutonniere deformity. *Hand Clin* 1995;11:387–402.
22. Rizio L, Belsky MR. Finger deformities in rheumatoid arthritis. *Hand Clin* 1996;12:531–540.
23. Jackman RJ, Pugh DG. The positive elbow fat pad sign in rheumatoid arthritis. *Am J Roentgenol Radium Ther Nucl Med* 1970;108:812–818.
24. Weston WJ. The synovial changes at the elbow in rheumatoid arthritis. *Australas Radiol* 1971;15:170–175.
25. Laine VAI, Vaino KJ, Pekanmaki K. Shoulder affections in rheumatoid arthritis. *Ann Rheum Dis* 1954;13:157–160.
26. Fletcher DE, Rowley KA. The radiological features of rheumatoid arthritis. *Br J Radiol* 1952;25:282–295.
27. Hulsmans H, Jacobs J, van der Heijde D, et al. The course of radiologic damage during the first six years of rheumatoid arthritis. *Arthritis Rheum* 2000;43:1927–1940.
28. Thould AK, Simon G. Assessment of radiological changes in the hands and feet in rheumatoid arthritis: their correlation with prognosis. *Ann Rheum Dis* 1966;25:220–228.
29. Calabro J. A critical evaluation of the diagnostic features of the feet in rheumatoid arthritis. *Arthritis Rheum* 1962;5:19–29.
30. Resnick D. Patterns of migration of the femoral head in osteoarthritis of the

hip. Roentgenographic-pathologic correlation and comparison with rheumatoid arthritis. *Am J Roentgenol Radium Ther Nucl Med* 1975;124:62–74.
31. Crabbe WA. Rheumatoid arthritis affecting the hip. *Guys Hosp Rep* 1968; 117:31–47.
32. Lehtimaki MY, Kautiainen H, Hamalainen MM, et al. Hip involvement in seropositive rheumatoid arthritis. Survivorship analysis with a 15-year follow-up. *Scand J Rheumatol* 1998;27:406–409.
33. Martel W, Duff IF. Pelvospondylitis in rheumatoid arthritis. *Radiology* 1961;77:744–756.
34. Corrigan AB. Radiological changes in rheumatoid cervical spines. *Australas Radiol* 1969;13:370–375.
35. Halla JT, Fallahi S. Cervical discovertebral destruction, subaxial subluxation, and myelopathy in a patient with rheumatoid arthritis. *Arthritis Rheum* 1981;24:944–947.
36. Williams LE, Bland JH, Lipson RL. Cervical spine subluxations and massive osteolysis in the upper extremities in rheumatoid arthritis. *Arthritis Rheum* 1966;9:348–360.
37. Kudo H, Iwano K, Yoshizawa H. Cervical cord compression due to extradural granulation tissue in rheumatoid arthritis. *J Bone Joint Surg Br* 1984; 66:426–430.
38. Hopkins JS. Lower cervical rheumatoid subluxation with tetraplegia. *J Bone Joint Surg Br* 1967;49B:46–51.
39. Conlon PW, Isdale IC, Rose BS. Rheumatoid arthritis of the cervical spine: an analysis of 333 cases. *Ann Rheum Dis* 1966;25:120–126.
40. Fuchs HA, Pincus T. Radiographic damage in rheumatoid arthritis—description by nonlinear models. *J Rheumatol* 1992;19:1655–1658.
41. Salaffi F, Ferraccioli G, Peroni M, et al. Progression of erosion and joint space narrowing scores in rheumatoid arthritis assessed by nonlinear models. *J Rheumatol* 1994;21:1626–1630.
42. Van der Heijde DMFM, van Leeuwen MA, van Riel PLCM, et al. Radiographic progression on radiographs of hands and feet during the first 3 years of rheumatoid arthritis measured according to Sharp's method (van der Heijde modification). *J Rheumatol* 1995;22:1792–1796.
43. Belsky MR, Feldon P, Millender LH, et al. Hand involvement in psoriatic arthritis. *J Hand Surg [Am]* 1982;7:203–207.
44. Weissman BN, Rappaport AS, Sosman JL, et al. Radiographic findings in the hands in patients with systemic lupus erythematosis. *Radiology* 1978; 126:313–317.
45. Kidd KL, Peter JB. Erosive osteoarthritis. *Radiology* 1966;86:640–647.
46. Watt I, Middlemiss H. The radiology of gout. *Clin Radiol* 1975;26:27–36.

CHAPTER 8

Measurement of Radiologic Outcomes

Désirée M. F. M. van der Heijde

Structural damage of joints is an important feature of rheumatoid arthritis (RA). Features visualized on radiographs are considered to be hallmarks of RA. Plain radiography is currently the standard method to assess RA damage. A series of radiographs comprise the simplest and cheapest permanent record of the cumulative joint damage caused by the disease. Plain-film radiography can be used to define single-time-point damage in RA as well as progression of the disease over time. The latter is useful in assessing both disease progression in clinical practice and the effectiveness of interventional therapy. With the availability of new therapies that can substantially retard the progression of structural damage, it is becoming important to assess the progression of damage in individual patients and, if necessary, to adjust therapy accordingly. Although structural damage alone is not an outcome in the sense of "burden of disease," it constitutes an important surrogate. It has high face validity and an established relation with functional capacity (1).

ADVANTAGES AND DISADVANTAGES OF RADIOGRAPHY

Radiography is widely available in all hospitals, and waiting time is negligible. Radiography provides high contrast and resolution for imaging cortical and trabecular bone but has poor contrast for visualizing soft tissue. The technique is not suitable to assess soft tissue structures in detail. Although usually limited, there is radiation exposure. The most obvious disadvantage of radiography is that the three-dimensional anatomy is converted into a two-dimensional image, resulting in superimposition of overlying structures. This problem can only be overcome by using a tomographic technique (e.g., computed tomography scan or magnetic resonance imaging). On the other hand, such tomographic imaging requires a large number of images, as only a small area can be viewed on a single image. Radiography, in contrast, is able to assess a large area, allowing many joints to be projected simultaneously on a single film. Moreover, it is a very fast imaging technique, especially in comparison to magnetic resonance imaging.

RADIOGRAPHIC TECHNIQUE

In imaging joints, it is important to have high-quality films to obtain adequate contrast without blurring of the joint margins. Blurring reduces the contrast and visibility of small anatomic structures, causing a reduction in details. Both overexposed and underexposed images significantly diminish contrast. High-efficiency, single-screen, single-emulsion film-screen combinations produce the highest-quality films. This high-quality imaging is especially important in clinical trials when assessing the effect of drugs on structural damage in therapeutic trials. Conventional radiographs produce analogue images that are stored on radiographic film. The disadvantage of this technique is that it requires considerable space to store films; if copies are needed, the original films must be reproduced, and the reproduction step results in a considerable loss of image quality. Moreover, data cannot be recovered if the original films are lost. Storage of image data in digital format has several advantages. Significant information can be stored in a small space and transferred electronically to multiple sites over long distances, and multiple copies can be made without losing quality. Moreover, the quality of the image can be adjusted by, for example, noise reduction and contrast modification (2).

RADIOGRAPHIC VIEWS

Straight views are the most widely used views for joint radiology. For the hands, a posteroanterior view is used, and, for the feet, knees, pelvis, and shoulders, an anteroposterior view is used. A lateral view of the feet can be used to judge the heel. Both the Nørgaard view and the Brewerton view have been advised for hand radiographs (3,4). Nørgaard recommended a 45-degree supine view of the hands with straight fingers to allow detection of early erosive changes at the dorsoradial aspects of the bases of proximal phalanges in the fingers in patients with RA. Brewerton described a tangential view taken with the metacarpophalangeal (MCP) joints flexed at 65 degrees and with a 15-degree volar beam ("ballcatcher's view"). The rationale for this view is the better demonstration of erosive changes at the MCP joints. Studies give conflicting results regarding whether this indeed leads to increased sensitivity (5–10). Due to problems with positioning, it is difficult to get exactly the same views in a series of radiographs taken over time. This introduces inconsistencies in the comparison of films and causes major problems in scoring such radiographs. Therefore, the best view for both hand and foot radiographs in the follow-up of patients is the straight view.

For the knees, an extra lateral view is warranted. The cervical spine should be imaged in neutral position and during flexion. The latter is to evaluate ligamentous laxity and apophyseal joints. An open-mouth frontal view demonstrates the odontoid.

For the initial assessment of a patient with RA, radiographs of hands and feet should be taken for all patients and further individually tailored to involved joints. For follow-up, radiographs of hands and feet can provide general information on the course of the disease, as damage in radiographs of hands and feet is a good reflection of overall joint damage (11,12). An important finding in a follow-up of an inception cohort of 12 years was that none of the patients without erosions in hands or feet showed erosions in the large joints (12). Joints other than hands and feet should be radiographed only if there is a clinical indication. The cervical spine could be an exception, as this site is frequently involved subclinically with the presence of damage that might have severe clinical consequences—for example, spinal instability during intubation for anesthesia.

RADIOGRAPHIC FEATURES IN RHEUMATOID ARTHRITIS

Several features can be demonstrated in RA, of which some are highly specific. Usually, there is symmetrical joint involvement. Osteoporosis can be present both in a juxtaarticular and generalized distribution. Fusiform swelling of soft tissue around the joint is a characteristic of arthritis. Joint space narrowing is a hallmark of RA and results from loss of cartilage (Figs. 8.1 and 8.2). This cartilage loss is diffuse and has a tendency to be present in all compartments of a complex joint. The presence of joint space narrowing can be helpful in discriminating between RA and gout (destruction with preservation of joint width) and osteoarthritis (mainly a focal joint space narrowing) (13). Bony ankylosis in RA is common only in the wrist and midfoot and rare at other locations (Fig. 8.1). Another hallmark of RA by radiographs is the appearance of bony erosions (Figs. 8.1 and 8.2). Initially, erosions are seen primarily at the bare areas of a joint, which are not covered by cartilage. These are called *marginal erosions*. At other sites, erosions can occur due to the loss of subchondral bone. In areas of osteoporosis, erosions can be compressed, leading to a bone-into-bone formation. This is mostly seen in the hips and MCPs. Erosions as a consequence of surface resorption are frequently reported in bone adjacent to inflamed tendons, for example, in the wrist. A characteristic erosive feature is the focal loss of the continuity of the subchondral bone plate (also called the *dot–dash pattern*), often seen in the radial head of the second and third MCPs. In the feet, the first involved areas are the head of the first (medial site) and fifth metacarpal head (lateral site).

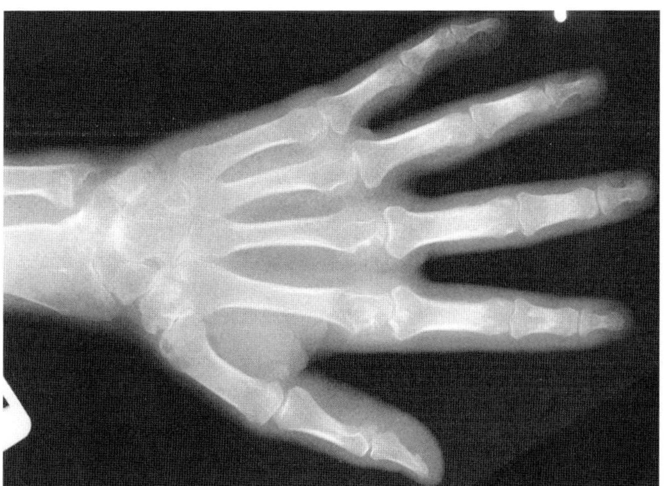

Figure 8.1. Radiograph of the hand showing erosions in the first through third metacarpophalangeal joints, ulna, and various carpal bones. Also seen are joint space narrowing in several carpal joints and ankylosis of the carpus with the radius.

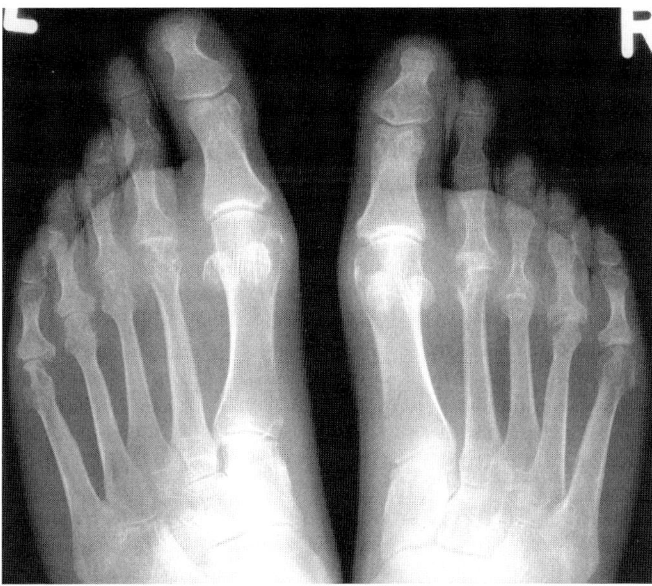

Figure 8.2. Radiograph of the foot showing erosions in the interphalangeal joint and all metatarsophalangeal joints, with joint space narrowing predominantly in the second through fourth metatarsophalangeal joints.

Bony cysts, which are subchondral lesions without a connection to the joint surface, are common in RA. Small cysts can occur in all joints; large cysts can be encountered in large joints such as elbows, hips, and knees. Major destruction can lead to deformities of the joints. However, this deformity is mostly caused by laxity or disruption of tendons and ligaments and, consequently, an alteration of the normal muscle pull. Well-known examples are subluxations in MCPs and metatarsophalangeal (MTP) joints.

SCORING RADIOGRAPHS

Radiographs can be used to establish a diagnosis of RA, give information on the severity of the disease, provide prognostic information, and provide a measure to follow the course of the disease and assess the efficacy of interventional therapy. To use radiographs for longitudinal studies, the amount of damage needs to be expressed quantitatively. Therefore, several scoring methods have been developed to quantify joint damage.

Scoring Methods

Most scoring methods are subjective evaluations of the films using readers. However, a few semiautomated methods are published, although they are not widely used. The methods involving readers can be categorized as follows: (a) global score of the whole patient (e.g., Steinbrocker), (b) global grading per joint (e.g., Larsen), (c) assessment of erosions and joint space narrowing separately (e.g., Sharp), and (d) methods suitable for measuring sequential change (e.g., carpometacarpal index) (14–17). Methods belonging to the first three categories can be used to assess both the damage at a certain point in time as well as the progression in time and thus are suitable for cross-sectional and sequential studies. Methods from the fourth category can be used to measure progression in time only, because they do not give an absolute score but rather a score based on a direct comparison. Progression with the methods from the first three categories is usually assessed in an indirect way, subtracting initial from final scores. These various methods have been reviewed extensively in the literature (18,19). Here, only an overview of the most widely used scoring methods, the Larsen and Sharp methods with their modifications, will be presented (15,16,20–23).

LARSEN AND SHARP SCORING METHODS

The Larsen method is a global grading of joints that is mainly based on erosive damage. Reference films are available for both small and large joints. The wrist is scored as a single joint, and its score is multiplied by five. Scores for the separate joints of the hands and feet are added to obtain the total Larsen score (15). The popular modification by Scott changed the description of early damage, leading to improved reliability (21). Another modification is that by Rau, which grades the extent of the eroded surface of the joints (22).

The Sharp method is a detailed scoring of erosions and joint space narrowing separately (16). Originally, this method was designed for the hands only but was subsequently extended to include the feet by van der Heijde (20). Another modification of the Sharp method, described by Genant, extended the scale for progression from a 6-point scale to an 8-point scale with 0.5 increments from 0 to 3+ for erosions and from a 5-point scale to a 9-point scale with 0.5 increments from 0 to 4 for joint space narrowing (23). Depending on the exact modification used, the range of the Larsen methods is usually from 0 to 200 and for the Sharp method from 0 to 314, up to 448 for the van der Heijde modification. All of these methods have been tested extensively and showed good reliability. There are some indications that the Sharp methods show a greater sensitivity to change (24–28).

Of note, none of the above-mentioned methods explicitly score malalignment, although subluxation is included in the joint space narrowing grading of the van der Heijde modification of the Sharp method, and other features, such as repair (healing), that may be pertinent.

Scoring in Clinical Practice

The above-mentioned scoring methods are appropriate for clinical trials but not for use in clinical practice. Therefore, a simplification of the Sharp–van der Heijde method has been developed for use in clinical practice and large epidemiologic studies. This method consists of adding the number of joints with erosions and the number of joints with joint space narrowing to yield a simple erosion–narrowing score (29). Sensitivity to change is closely related between the original Sharp–van der Heijde method and the simple erosion–narrowing score, at least during the first 5 years of the disease. Further study is required to determine whether sensitivity to change is maintained over longer follow-up periods. Because of the simplicity of the method and the small time involved in scoring, this method is feasible for use in daily clinical practice.

NATURAL PROGRESSION

The progression of structural damage as assessed in longitudinal cohorts does not reflect the natural history of disease but, in fact, progression during treatment. However, data collected before the introduction of aggressive treatment, including biologics, are usually viewed as representing "natural progression." It is important to rely on inception cohorts, as cross-sectional studies are usually hampered by biased samples of patients. Most inception cohorts followed long-term show linear progression on a group level (30–32). This linear progression rate has been shown, for example, by Wolfe and Sharp in a group of 256 patients seen within the first 2 years of disease and followed for 20 years (30). Over the first 6 years of disease, Hulsmans et al. found a similar annual progression rate (31). Scott summarized data of six prospective cohorts that all showed a linear progression (32). Based on these studies, he calculated the annual progression rates for the various scoring methods. This rate was 3.2 to 3.6 units per year for the Larsen method, 3.9 to 5.9 units per year for the Sharp, and 7.2 to 8.5 units per year for the Sharp–van der Heijde method. However, all these data are on a group level, with variable progression among individual patients (33).

Development of Erosions

Approximately 75% of the patients in inception cohorts show erosive changes, and most of them do so within the first year of follow-up (34). Foot joints often become eroded earlier and more extensively than hand joints; it is, therefore, important to take foot films, especially in the early phases of the disease (31,35,36). By individual joints, the fifth MTP joint is the first eroded joint, followed by the other five assessed foot joints and only one of the MCP joints [first MTP, interphalangeal (IP) joint, first MCP, third MTP, fourth MTP, second MTP]. After 5 years of follow-up, the most frequently eroded joints are the fifth MTP, second MCP, first MTP, IP, third MTP, second MTP, and third MCP (31).

Development of Joint Space Narrowing

The pattern is different for the narrowing of joints. The first narrowed joints are the IP, first MTP, multiangular-navicular joint, fourth proximal interphalangeal joint (PIP), radiocarpal joint, fifth PIP, and fifth MTP. After 5 years of follow-up, the most frequently narrowed joints are the IP, radiocarpal joint, fifth MTP, multiangular-navicular joint, first MTP, fifth PIP, and fourth PIP. The joints of the feet are thus the most frequently eroded joints, and the joints of the wrists and PIPs are the most frequently narrowed joints. This pattern of involvement indicates that a variety of joint groups and features comprise the complete spectrum of the disease.

Repair

For a long time, structural damage was assumed to be an irreversible process. However, data from patients during remission with a longer follow-up show that some repair may occur. The reconstitution of an eroded joint into a normal structure is a rare phenomenon and can be seen probably only in early cases with very limited damage. Features assumed to be characteristic of repair are sclerosis, remodeling, filling in of erosions, and recortication. A recent study of an expert panel showed that repair indeed exists, although the specificity of the above-mentioned features was very low (37). During an OMERACT (Outcome Measures in Rheumatology Clinical Trials) workshop devoted to repair of erosions in RA, it became apparent that many questions still need to be addressed, such as the features and scoring of repair, as well as the relation to function (38). One of the essential issues concerns the ability of applied scoring methods to detect repair. In other words, do negative scores in trials represent repair or are they merely due to measurement error (e.g., partly due to differences in positioning)? Studies to address these issues are under way.

USE OF RADIOGRAPHS IN CLINICAL TRIALS

To assess the effect of therapy on structural damage, radiographs are still accepted as the "gold standard" by most investigators and clinicians, as well as drug agencies. Most modern trials include films of hands and feet and apply one of the above-described scoring methods. The minimum follow-up for an agent to be able to demonstrate an effect on structural damage is set at 1 year. However, several studies have shown that effects can already be measured after a follow-up of 6 months. With the availability of drugs that have a beneficial impact on structural damage, it has become tempting to compare data across trials. However, it is difficult, if not impossible, to make these comparisons. Moreover, knowledge of the limitations in studies of radiographic progression of joint damage is essential to correctly interpret the data. Below is an overview based on three published reports (39–41). The limitations that will be discussed are differences in study design, prognostic similarity, duration of follow-up, scoring methodology (method used, readers scoring the films, order in which the radiographs are read), handling of missing data, and presentation of data.

Comparability of Data across Studies

In general, clinical homogeneity is warranted if trials need to be studied in a quantifiable way (as is done in a metaanalysis or by a direct comparison of the results). Clinical homogeneity means that patient characteristics across different studies are comparable, methods are similar, and treatments (kind, dosage, and treatment rules) are the same. A comparison of the homogeneity of the various published drug trials shows that these studies are only homogeneous with respect to the underlying disease (RA) and the kind of drug (disease-modifying agent). However, these studies differ in the populations of patients studied (patients with early RA and with more advanced RA). Importantly, there is also a difference in the radiologic scoring techniques applied in the various studies (modified Larsen score, modified Sharp score, scoring with sequence known or sequence blinded, different readers). Various aspects of the lack of homogeneity among studies on radiographic progression are discussed in more detail.

Study Design

Some trials with the aim to study radiographic progression are performed in patients who receive the drug under investigation (drug A) as the first treatment (trial 1). Other trials require that patients have a suboptimal response to a drug (drug B) and are randomized thereafter to receive the drug under investigation (drug A), with drug B as background therapy (trial 2). In both examples, the comparative arm in the trial can be a placebo or another active drug. The arm of trial 1 with drug A is not directly comparable to the arm with drug A from trial 2. First, the treatment in trial 1 is monotherapy (drug A), whereas, in trial 2, it is combination therapy (drug A + drug B). Even if there were a second arm in trial 1 with drug A + drug B, it would not be comparable to the arm A + B in trial 2, because, in trial 1, patients already had a suboptimal response to drug B, and, in trial 2, drug B would be a new drug. Patients who receive a drug for the first time are more likely to respond to that drug than patients who have not responded to other drugs in general (42,43). This poorer response is even more likely if patients already failed (partially) one of the drugs under study (drug B in this example).

Prognostic Similarity

If arms of different studies are compared, randomization is broken and we are no longer dealing with randomized and, therefore, comparable groups of patients. Several prognostic factors are known to predict an unfavorable outcome with respect to structural joint damage (such as rheumatoid factor, early erosive disease, and rapid joint destruction). But these factors account for only a small part of the variation in structural damage. It is most likely that other unknown factors contribute to the risk of structural joint damage. It is because of these unknown factors that randomization is essential. With randomization, these factors are equally distributed over the two arms. However, if trial arms from various studies are compared, this randomization has not taken place, and many hidden differences between the patient populations may exist. Anderson et al. (42) described the factors that should be specifically considered when interpreting data from clinical trials. These factors were based on the analysis of 14 randomized clinical trials and included disease duration, gender, previous treatment with disease-modifying antirheumatic drugs, functional class, and level of disease activity.

Structural Damage As Prognostic Factor

One of the factors that seems to be of major importance in the evaluation of structural joint damage is the baseline radiographic damage. The extent of damage is, of course, linked to the disease duration. In general, the longer the disease, the more damage exists. However, another measure relating disease duration and damage to each other has been proposed to allow more meaningful comparisons: the predicted (or estimated) yearly progression rate (44). This rate is calculated for each patient as the damage at baseline divided by the disease duration. Within trials, this predicted yearly progression rate shows a relation with the treatment effect. This treatment effect was highest in patients with the highest progression rate before entering the trial. The predicted yearly progression rate is also advocated to serve as an anchor to compare arms across trials. However, more data are needed to know if the predicted yearly progression rate is a valid way to serve as an anchor for comparison of arms across trials. One of the problems is the use in early disease. If patients have a very short disease duration (e.g., a few months) the denominator is uncertain: A small mistake in disease duration has a major impact on the predicted yearly progression rate. Also, measurement error in the score of the radiographs introduces significant uncertainty in the number. The following example illustrates this point. Consider patient A with disease duration of 6 months (0.5 years) and baseline score of 6, and patient B with disease duration of 5 years and baseline score of 60. The measurement error in assessing disease duration is 2 months (patient A, 0.33–0.66 years; patient B, 9.8–10.2 years), and the measurement error in assessing the score is 2 units (patient A, 4–8; patient B, 58–62). The predicted yearly progression rate in patient A is calculated as 12 with a range of 6.1 (4/0.66) to 24.2 (8/0.33) and, for patient B, as 12 with a range of 11.2 (58/5.2) to 12.8 (62/4.8). Even if the measurement error of the radiographic score is expressed as a percentage of 10% (patient A, 0.6 unit; patient B, 6 units)—and, therefore, relatively larger in patients with more damage—the range for patient A (8.2–20.0) is still much larger than for patient B (10.4–13.7). So, in early disease, the predicted yearly progression rate might be an unreliable estimate of the true progression rate.

Duration of Follow-Up

Because radiographs show cumulative damage, differences in trial duration are expected to have a large impact on the results. Results from a trial with 6 months' follow-up cannot be compared directly to a trial with 12 months' follow-up. As explained earlier, the progression rate is linear for cohorts of patients but might vary widely for individual patients. Due to the large patient-to-patient variability in radiologic patterns, scores cannot easily be corrected by dividing progression scores by follow-up duration to calculate, for example, a monthly progression rate. Therefore, it is significant that the duration of follow-up be similar when radiographic progression is compared across trials.

Scoring Methodology

The most widely used scoring methods evaluate different joint features, assess different joints, and have different scoring ranges. Therefore, a score of 5 obtained with the Larsen score, for example, is not equivalent to a score of 5 obtained by the Sharp score. A mathematic way to get around the difference in the maximum possible range is to calculate the percentage of the maximum obtainable score (e.g., $5/200 \times 100\%$ for Larsen, and $5/314 \times 100\%$ for Sharp). But calculating the score as a percentage of a maximum score is dealing only with one aspect of the problem of the differences between the scoring methods. Comparability assumes, for example, that the scales are equally spaced over the entire range and that the entire range is used in both methods, and it neglects the most fundamental differences in evaluated features and joints. Views on the validity of pooling might, however, differ. As Lassere concluded:

> [D]espite differences between the Sharp and Larsen methods, they essentially measure the construct of radiographic damage, and as long as the spectrum of radiographic damage in the pooled series is similar, then the scoring methods are robust to pooling. However, where the spectrum of damage is not similar, for example, studies of radiographic progression of early disease compared with late disease, pooling should be exercised with caution (45).

The last warning is present in many of the trials, which significantly reduces the possibilities of pooling.

Number of Readers

Clinical trials are typically designed to have one or two observers read and score each radiograph. Increasing the number of readers (and using their mean score) reduces random error and increases the sensitivity to change; this increased sensitivity to change reduces the required sample size to demonstrate a difference. However, increasing the number of readers also increases complexity and cost of the assessment. Fries et al. studied the influence of the number of readers on the number of patients needed in a trial and concluded that two readers was the best compromise (46). Interobserver reliability is typically high for progression scores, which is usually the subject of interest in evaluating clinical trial results. However, the absolute scores from reader to reader may be significantly different. In other words, each observer has his or her own reading level (and is consistent with his or her own reading). Although each observer's reading level may be clearly different from that of another observer, the progression seen is fairly consistent between the observers. Therefore, when comparing absolute scores across trials, readers are another source of variability.

Another important issue about scoring films, which has not yet been resolved, is determining the order in which the films should be scored. A series of films can be ordered in several ways for assessment, for example: (a) films can be grouped per patient (e.g., all available radiographs of the hands and feet of one particular patient) and ordered chronologically (*chronological*), (b) films can be grouped per patient but scored in random time order (*paired*), (c) films can be grouped and scored per region (e.g., both hands) from a particular patient at a single point in time (*single-pair*), and, finally, (d) single films can be scored without any grouping or ordering—that is, all films of all patients mixed randomly (*single*). There are advantages and disadvantages for all of these methods. Scoring in chronological order provides the most information to the reader. This may help to reduce measurement error introduced by such factors as the variation in positioning or quality of the films. However, it could also introduce bias, as the observer may expect progression of damage over time. Recent studies have confirmed that chronological reading leads to larger changes than does random reading, even in an observation period of 3 years (47–49). However, it is still unclear whether chronological order really overestimates progression of damage. It is also possible that so much measurement error is introduced by limiting the information the reader gets in random reading that the signal is lost in the noise, resulting in underestimation of change. An indication for this underestimation of change is found in a study comparing scores obtained with paired and chronological reading with those of a panel of rheumatologists. The panel of rheumatologists judged progression to be clinically relevant. Those reading the films in chronological order detected the progression, whereas those reading the films in paired order did not (50). When highest sensitivity to change is the most important factor—for example, in phase II clinical trials to assess the possible impact of a drug on structural joint damage—scoring in chronological order could be the best option. In general, in randomized trials, films are scored without information on treatment and patient identity. If chronological scoring would lead to biased information, this bias would be similar in both treatment arms, while ensuring the highest sensitivity to detect progression. At the moment, trials that are scored for registration purposes of the drug are scored without information on sequence. It should be noted carefully in the method section of a trial in which order the films are scored, and this information should be taken into consideration when comparing results.

Importance of Missing Data

As radiographs show cumulative structural joint damage, missing radiographs are an important issue in the analysis of clinical trial data. This missing information cannot be handled in the same way as is often done for clinical data, which is by imputing the last observation. Using this last-observation-carried-forward technique would underestimate the progression rate in those patients with missing data. Moreover, it is rare that missing data caused by dropouts happen randomly. In general, patients with a worse prognosis (higher disease activity, higher radiologic progression rate) and patients in a placebo arm have a higher prior probability for premature discontinuation in any clinical trial (39). This selective dropout likely plays a role in trials with losses of more than 10% and is, therefore, an important argument to rely on the intention-to-treat analysis. With an intention-to-treat analysis, it is critical to know how the data were handled for those patients who have incomplete data. Radiographic data are always skewed because a high proportion of patients will have no or little progression, whereas only a subset of patients will have substantial progression. Therefore, parametric statistics should be applied. However, skewed data are very sensitive to selective dropout. This is demonstrated with an example by Landewé et al., showing that excluding 10% of the patients with the highest scores leads to an overestimation of the effect, whereas excluding 10% of the patients with the lowest scores leads to an underestimation of the effect (39). It should be stressed that it is crucial to obtain follow-up radiographs in all patients regardless of premature discontinuation and to limit data imputation as much as possible. It is also important to perform sensitivity analyses to check the influence of the missing data on the radiologic outcome.

TABLE 8.1. Guidelines for Presentation of Radiographic Results in Clinical Trials

Radiographs of hands and feet
Smallest detectable difference (SDD) as quality control
Preferably two or more observers
  Kappa and/or intraclass correlations, and SDD for interobserver agreement
Average score of observers
If one observer
  Kappa and/or intraclass correlations for intra- and interobserver agreement
  SDD for intraobserver agreement
Presentation of absolute numbers
Primary end point: total score (erosions and joint space narrowing combined)
Secondary end points for Sharp methods: erosions, joint space narrowing
Primary analysis: group level
  Reporting of mean, standard error, standard deviation
  Box-whisker plot (median, percentiles, outliers)
Secondary analysis: patient level
  Percent of patients with progression >0.5 for two observers, >0.0 for one observer
  Percent of patients with progression >SDD

From van der Heijde D, Simon L, Smolen J, et al. How to report radiographic data in randomized clinical trials in rheumatoid arthritis: guidelines from a roundtable discussion. *Arthritis Rheum* 2002;47:215–218, with permission.

Presentation of Data

Clinical trials present radiographic data in a variety of ways, making the comparison across trials difficult. To minimize this obstacle, a roundtable conference was held to establish a minimum set of radiographic results that should be presented for each trial (51). The results of this roundtable conference are presented in Table 8.1. Some of the recommendations are described earlier in this chapter. These include radiographs of hands and feet; for clinical trials, the use of two (or more) observers (for other studies, such as large epidemiologic studies, one observer is acceptable); average score of the observers; presentation of absolute numbers; and appropriate statistical tests, usually nonparametric tests. For the primary end point, the total joint score of the Sharp methods should be used (or the grading of the Larsen methods). As a secondary end point, the erosions and joint space narrowing scores of the Sharp method should be used (if this method is used to evaluate the trial). The primary analysis should analyze the data on a group level. The data should be presented as mean and standard deviation but also as box-whisker plots presenting the median; the 10th, 25th, 75th, and 90th percentiles; and outliers. The combined information describes the population in detail. The average scores are mainly determined by the subset of patients with high progression scores. The percentiles present the proportion of patients with a certain progression; for example, the 25th percentile shows the progression that is achieved by up to 25% of the patients, whereas the remaining patients show a higher progression. An additional important way to analyze the data is on an individual patient level as a secondary analysis. A cut-off value has to be selected to assess patients that show progression versus those who do not show progression. The most obvious cut-off seems to be 0 (for one observer, or 0.5 if the average of two observers is used). However, this cut-off does not take into account measurement error, which is always present. Therefore, the smallest detectable difference (SDD) beyond measurement error is advised as a more realistic cut-off. This SDD is based on the 95% limits of agreement as described by Bland and Altman (Fig. 8.3) (52). In case of the use of two observers, the SDD is derived from the agreement of the progression scores of the two observers. Figure 8.3 presents the level of agreement in progression scores between two observers who independently scored the same data set.

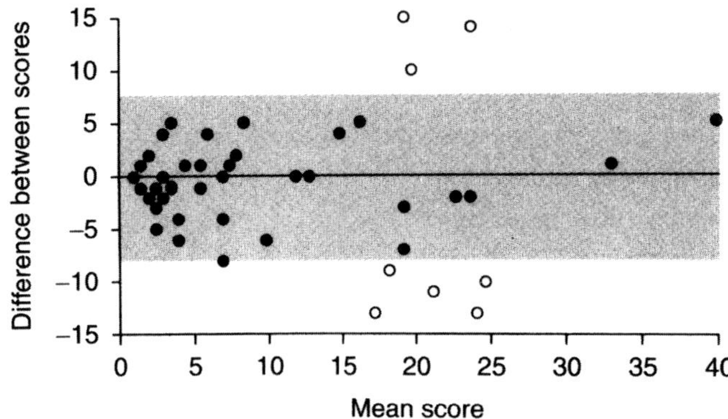

Figure 8.3. Example of a Bland-Altman plot in which the difference of the observers' scores is plotted against the mean of the observers' scores to graphically illustrate whether random measurement error is equal over the total range of the scores.

In a Bland-Altman plot, the mean score of both observers of every patient is plotted against the difference of both scores. Every dot incorporates the results of two separate scorings on the same data, and the greater the distance to the *X*-axis, the greater the interobserver variability or measurement error. This plot visualizes that a cut-off of 0 (or 0.5) is not realistic. The SDD is context specific and depends on the scoring method, readers, baseline damage, and progression observed in the trial and should, therefore, be calculated for each trial separately (53). The 95% limits of agreement should be used, but another percentage of agreement would also be justifiable, such as the 80% limits of agreement. The choice of the cut-off has a major impact on the analysis of a trial, as is demonstrated by applying several cut-offs in a trial (39). Using the cut-off of 0, the difference in percentage of patients showing progression greater than 0 between two trial arms was 11%. However, using the 95% SDD resulted in a difference of 27% between the two trial arms, and the 80% SDD resulted in a difference of 25%. The results based on the 95% and 80% SDDs were in accordance with the analysis of the trial on a group level with continuous data. This example makes clear that it is incorrect to compare results from various trials that use different cut-offs. The SDDs, as well as kappa statistics and intraclass correlations, can be used as a quality control of the readers.

Taking all the different issues together, it is a hazardous exercise to compare data across studies in a quantifiable way. Some of the issues can be overcome by using the same scoring method, observers, and order in which the films are scored; performing the same analyses; and presenting the data in a comparable way. Applying the above recommendations would definitely provide more insight, although several of the fundamental problems would still remain.

Wording of Claims

Reviewing the literature, it is clear that many words are used to describe the results of radiographic progression of trials. Some words give the impression that a drug is having a greater effect than another drug, whereas the truth could be the other way around. Therefore, some guidance on how to describe the results was presented at the same roundtable conference as mentioned earlier (Table 8.2) (51). The words "reduce," "retard," and "slow" can be used if a statistically significant difference is detected on a

TABLE 8.2. Proposed Wording with Minimum Requirements for Using the Wording

Wording	Requirement
Group 1	
Reduce	To be used on a group level
Retard	Every statistically significant result compared to comparator
Slow	
Group 2	
Arrest	To be used on a patient level
Halt	Describes the percentage of patients with progression
Inhibit	<cut-off level *Y*
Prevent	
Stop	

From van der Heijde D, Simon L, Smolen J, et al. How to report radiographic data in randomized clinical trials in rheumatoid arthritis: guidelines from a roundtable discussion. *Arthritis Rheum* 2002;47:215–218, with permission.

group level. The words "arrest," "halt," "inhibit," "prevent," and "stop" can be used to describe the results on a patient level. It could follow the format of *X*% of the patients showed a progression smaller than cut-off *Y*; for example, 56% of the patients showed a progression smaller than the SDD of 8.6 in the active group compared to 22% of the patients in the control group.

CONCLUSION

Radiographs are important to assess structural damage in patients with RA and to study severity and progression of the disease. Standard anteroposterior views are usually sufficient. Compared to other imaging techniques, radiography offers the advantages of accessibility, price, information on a large number of joints, and speed of technique. The main disadvantage is the use of a two-dimensional image for a three-dimensional anatomy. High-efficiency, single-screen, single-emulsion film-screen combinations produce the highest-quality films. Erosions and joint space narrowing are the most specific features in RA. Several reliable and sensitive scoring methods exist to quantify the amount of structural damage in hands and feet. This damage in small joints is, in turn, a good reflection of the overall joint damage. On a group level, progression of structural damage is linear over time. Radiographs are useful in assessing the efficacy of drugs on structural damage. Caveats in comparing data across trials are discussed in detail. These caveats are related to difference in patient population, prognostic similarity, study design, and disease duration and to variation in several aspects of the scoring methodology and statistical analyses. Recommendations on the presentation of the radiographic results of a clinical therapeutic trial are presented.

REFERENCES

1. van der Heijde D. Radiographic progression in rheumatoid arthritis: Does it reflect outcome? Does it reflect treatment? *Ann Rheum Dis* 2001;60[Suppl 3]:iii47–50.
2. Peterfy CG. Imaging techniques. In: Klippel JH, Dieppe PA, eds. *Rheumatology (Oxford)*, 2nd ed. London: Mosby; 1998:2.14.4–2.14.7.
3. Nørgaard F. Earliest roentgenological changes in polyarthritis of the rheumatoid type: rheumatoid arthritis. *Radiology* 1965;85:325–329.
4. Brewerton DA. A tangential radiographic projection for demonstrating involvement of metacarpal heads in rheumatoid arthritis. *Br J Radiol* 1967; 40:233–234.
5. Allander E, Brekkan A, Idbohrn H, et al. Is Nørgaard's radiological sign for early rheumatoid arthritis reliable? An epidemiological approach. *Scand J Rheumatol* 1973;2:161–166.
6. De Smet AA, Martin NL, Fritz SL, et al. Radiographic projections for the diagnosis of arthritis of the hands and wrists. *Radiology* 1981;139:577–581.
7. Edwards JC, Edwards SE, Huskisson EC. The value of radiography in the management of rheumatoid arthritis. *Clin Radiol* 1983;34:413–416.
8. Hartley RM, Liang MH, Weissman BN, et al. The value of conventional views and radiographic magnification in evaluating early rheumatoid arthritis. *Arthritis Rheum* 1984;27:744–751.
9. Mewa AA, Pui M, Cockshott WP, et al. Observer differences in detecting erosions in radiographs of rheumatoid arthritis. A comparison of posteroanterior, Nørgaard and Brewerton views. *J Rheumatol* 1983;10:216–221.
10. Moreland LW, Daniel WW, Alarcon GS. The value of the Nørgaard view in the evaluation of erosive arthritis. *J Rheumatol* 1990;17:614–617.
11. Scott DL, Coulton BL, Popert AJ. Long term progression of joint damage in rheumatoid arthritis. *Ann Rheum Dis* 1986;45:373–378.
12. Drossaers-Bakker K, Kroon H, Zwinderman A, et al. Radiographic damage of large joints in long-term rheumatoid arthritis and its relation to function. *Rheumatology (Oxford)* 2000;39:998–1003.
13. Weissman BN, Resnick D, Kaushik S, et al. Imaging. In: Shaun R, Harris ED, Sledge C, eds. *Kelley's textbook of rheumatology*, 6th ed. Philadelphia: W.B. Saunders Company, 2001:627–634.
14. Steinbrocker O, Traeger C, Batterman R. Therapeutic criteria in rheumatoid arthritis. *JAMA* 1949;140:659–662.
15. Larsen A, Dale K, Eek M. Radiographic evaluation of rheumatoid arthritis and related conditions by standard reference films. *Acta Radiol Diagn Stockh* 1977;18:481–491.
16. Sharp JT, Young DY, Bluhm GB, et al. How many joints in the hands and wrists should be included in a score of radiologic abnormalities used to assess rheumatoid arthritis? *Arthritis Rheum* 1985;28:1326–1335.
17. Trentham DE, Masi AT. Carpo:metacarpal ratio. A new quantitative measure of radiologic progression of wrist involvement in rheumatoid arthritis. *Arthritis Rheum* 1976;19:939–944.
18. van der Heijde DM. Plain X-rays in rheumatoid arthritis: overview of scoring methods, their reliability and applicability. *Baillieres Clin Rheumatol* 1996;10:435–453.
19. Boini S, Guillemin F. Radiographic scoring methods as outcome measures in rheumatoid arthritis: properties and advantages. *Ann Rheum Dis* 2001;60:817–827.
20. van der Heijde D. How to read radiographs according to the Sharp/van der Heijde method. *J Rheumatol* 2000;27:261–263.
21. Scott D, Houssien D, Laasonen L. Proposed modification to Larsen's scoring method for hand and wrist radiographs. *Br J Rheumatol* 1995;34:56.
22. Rau R, Herborn G. A modified version of Larsen's scoring method to assess radiologic changes in rheumatoid arthritis. *J Rheumatol* 1995;22:1976–1982.
23. Genant HK, Jiang YB, Peterfy C, et al. Assessment of rheumatoid arthritis using a modified scoring method on digitized and original radiographs. *Arthritis Rheum* 1998;41:1583–1590.
24. Guth A, Coste J, Chagnon S, et al. Reliability of three methods of radiologic assessment in patients with rheumatoid arthritis. *Invest Radiol* 1995;30:181–185.
25. Plant MJ, Saklatvala J, Borg AA, et al. Measurement and prediction of radiological progression in early rheumatoid arthritis. *J Rheumatol* 1994;21:1808–1813.
26. Cuchacovich M, Couret M, Peray P, et al. Precision of the Larsen and the Sharp methods of assessing radiologic change in patients with rheumatoid arthritis. *Arthritis Rheum* 1992;35:736–739.
27. Wassenberg S, Herborn G, Larsen A, et al. Reliability, precision and time expense of four different radiographic scoring methods. *Arthritis Rheum* 1998;41:S50.
28. Lassere M, Boers M, van der Heijde D, et al. Smallest detectable difference in radiological progression. *J Rheumatol* 1999;26:731–739.
29. van der Heijde D, Dankert T, Nieman F, et al. Reliability and sensitivity to change of a simplification of the Sharp/van der Heijde radiological assessment in rheumatoid arthritis. *Rheumatology (Oxford)* 1999;38:941–947.
30. Wolfe F, Sharp JT. Radiographic outcome of recent-onset rheumatoid arthritis: a 19-year study of radiographic progression. *Arthritis Rheum* 1998;41:1571–1582.
31. Hulsmans HM, Jacobs JW, van der Heijde DM, et al. The course of radiologic damage during the first six years of rheumatoid arthritis. *Arthritis Rheum* 2000;43:1927–1940.
32. Scott D, Pugner K, Kaarela K, et al. The link between joint damage and disability in rheumatoid arthritis. *Rheumatology (Oxford)* 2000;39:122–132.
33. Plant MJ, Jones PW, Saklatvala J, et al. Patterns of radiological progression in early rheumatoid arthritis: results of an 8 year prospective study. *J Rheumatol* 1998;25:417–426.
34. van der Heijde DM. Joint erosions and patients with early rheumatoid arthritis. *Br J Rheumatol* 1995;34[Suppl 2]:74–78.
35. Brook A, Corbett M. Radiographic changes in early rheumatoid disease. *Ann Rheum Dis* 1977;36:71–73.
36. van der Heijde DM, van Leeuwen MA, van Riel PL, et al. Biannual radiographic assessments of hands and feet in a three-year prospective followup of patients with early rheumatoid arthritis. *Arthritis Rheum* 1992;35:26–34.
37. Sharp J, van der Heijde D, Boers M, et al. Repair of erosions in rheumatoid arthritis does occur. Results from two studies by the OMERACT subcommittee on healing of erosions. *J Rheumatol* 2003;30:1102–1107.
38. van der Heijde D, Sharp J, Rau R, et al. OMERACT workshop: repair of structural damage in rheumatoid arthritis. *J Rheumatol* 2003;30:1108–1109.

39. Landewé R, Boers M, van der Heijde D. How to interpret radiologic progression in randomised clinical trials? *Rheumatology (Oxford)* 2003;42:2–5.
40. Boers M, van der Heijde DM. Prevention or retardation of joint damage in rheumatoid arthritis: issues of definition, evaluation and interpretation of plain radiographs. *Drugs* 2002;62:1717–1724.
41. van der Heijde D. Structural damage in rheumatoid arthritis as visualized through radiographs. *Arthritis Res* 2002;4[Suppl 2]:S29–S33.
42. Anderson JJ, Wells G, Verhoeven AC, et al. Factors predicting response to treatment in rheumatoid arthritis: the importance of disease duration. *Arthritis Rheum* 2000;43:22–29.
43. Wijnands MJ, van't Hof MA, van Leeuwen MA, et al. Long-term second-line treatment: a prospective drug survival study. *Br J Rheumatol* 1992;31:253–258.
44. Strand V, Landewé R, van der Heijde D. Using estimated yearly progression rates to compare radiographic data across recent randomised controlled trials in rheumatoid arthritis. *Ann Rheum Dis* 2002;61[Suppl 2]:II64–II66.
45. Lassere M. Pooled metaanalysis of radiographic progression: comparison of Sharp and Larsen methods. *J Rheumatol* 2000;27:269–275.
46. Fries JF, Bloch DA, Sharp JT, et al. Assessment of radiologic progression in rheumatoid arthritis. A randomized, controlled trial. *Arthritis Rheum* 1986; 29:1–9.
47. van der Heijde D, Boers M, Lassere M. Methodological issues in radiographic scoring methods in rheumatoid arthritis. *J Rheumatol* 1999;26:726–730.
48. Ferrara R, Priolo F, Cammisa M, et al. Clinical trials in rheumatoid arthritis: methodological suggestions for assessing radiographs arising from the Grisar study. *Ann Rheum Dis* 1997;56:608–612.
49. Salaffi F, Carotti M. Interobserver variation in quantitative analysis of hand radiographs in rheumatoid arthritis: comparison of 3 different reading procedures. *J Rheumatol* 1997;24:2055–2056.
50. Bruynesteyn K, van der Heijde D, Boers M, et al. Minimal clinically important difference in radiological progression of joint damage over 1 year in rheumatoid arthritis: preliminary results of a validation study with clinical experts. *J Rheumatol* 2001;28:904–910.
51. van der Heijde D, Simon L, Smolen J, et al. How to report radiographic data in randomized clinical trials in rheumatoid arthritis: guidelines from a roundtable discussion. *Arthritis Rheum* 2002;47:215–218.
52. Bland JM, Altman DG. Statistical methods for assessing agreement between two methods of clinical measurement. *Lancet* 1986;1:307–310.
53. Lassere MN, van der Heijde D, Johnson K, et al. Robustness and generalizability of smallest detectable difference in radiological progression. *J Rheumatol* 2001;28:911–913.

CHAPTER 9

Ultrasonography and Magnetic Resonance Imaging for Diagnosis and Management

Richard J. Wakefield, Philip G. Conaghan, and Paul Emery

For more than a century, conventional radiography (CR) has been the most widely used imaging modality for investigating patients with rheumatic diseases. Its use, however, has been limited to the assessment of cumulative joint damage, with no information provided about synovitis and current disease activity. In recent years, however, the position of radiography in the hierarchy of imaging has been challenged.

The rationale for early diagnosis and the recent availability of new, targeted, aggressive therapies, particularly for patients with rheumatoid arthritis (RA), has driven the need for sensitive and accurate imaging techniques that can be used not only to accurately diagnose and provide prognostic information but also to monitor the efficacy of new therapies (1). Technologic advances and increasing availability of new imaging techniques, such as ultrasound (US) (2–7) and magnetic resonance imaging (MRI) (1,8–10), have provided new methods for assessing these diseases.

In this chapter, the role of these new modalities in the management of patients with RA is discussed with regard to a description of the technology, diagnostic abilities, and assessment of treatment responses and future developments.

ULTRASOUND

Technology and Practical Issues

A US machine, in simple terms, consists of a computer system with a monitor and a transducer. The transducer contains a number of specialized elements, which operate according to the principle of piezoelectricity (from the Greek *piezo*, to press, and *electron*, meaning amber, which was the fossilized organic resin used in early studies) (11). An electric voltage generated by the computer is transmitted to the transducer, resulting in deformation of the specialized elements within it, thereby converting electric energy into sound energy. The resultant acoustic waves pass through the skin and penetrate the tissues and are subsequently reflected back to the transducer at an amplitude and frequency dependent on acoustic properties of the examined tissue. The reflected sound waves are then converted back into an electric signal, which is translated by the computer into an image. Each white dot on the screen represents a reflected sound wave. The more reflection from an examined object, the whiter the dot (e.g., bone cortex) and the less reflection, the blacker the image (e.g., synovial fluid).

The two most important properties of a transducer are its surface (footprint) characteristics and frequency. For most musculoskeletal work, the transducer should be linear array and high frequency. A linear array transducer contains parallel elements resulting in a rectangular shape. This arrangement enables a flat scanning surface, ensuring maximum emission and capture of sound waves to and from the transducer, so long as the examined structure and transducer are perpendicular to each other. In some circumstances, however, a curved transducer (curvilinear) is most appropriate, particularly where there is a small acoustic window and full coverage of the joint is not permitted, for example, at the hip. In RA, a small footprint size can be an advantage for examining the small joints of the hands and feet, although examination of larger joints can be assisted by the use of a larger footprint.

The frequency of the transducer is also important. There is a trade-off between frequency and depth of penetration. The higher frequencies produce greater image resolution but have a lower depth of penetration. The frequency range for diagnostic US is between 3.5 and 20 MHz; for instance, 3.5 to 5 MHz may be used for the hips, and greater than 10 MHz is preferred for small joints.

Gray-scale US has been the conventional technique for the detection of joint and soft tissue inflammation for many years. Recently, additional US techniques, including Doppler US, have been introduced, offering the potential to improve the accuracy of clinical examination (12).

Doppler US (12) is a technique for making noninvasive measurements of blood flow and was first described by the Austrian physicist Christian Doppler in 1842. He described the effect of motion on sound when he observed a change in the frequency of a sound wave as a result of movement of either its source or receiver. There are two main types of Doppler US: color flow Doppler and power Doppler (PDS). Both produce a similar color spectral map superimposed onto the gray-scale image [the colors being related to the difference in frequency between the transmitted sound wave and that reflected from the moving interface (the Doppler frequency shift)] but actually encode different information. Color flow Doppler represents an estimate of the mean Doppler frequency shift and relates to velocity and direction of red blood cells, whereas PDS denotes the amplitude of the Doppler signal, which is determined by the volume of blood present. In this way, color flow Doppler is better suited for evaluating high-velocity flow in large vessels (e.g., carotids), whereas PDS is better suited for assessing low-velocity flow in small vessels (e.g., synovium). There are a number of particular advantages for using PDS in musculoskeletal assessment. PDS provides increased sensitivity to low-volume and low-velocity blood flow at the microvascular level. Therefore, it is particularly useful for measuring and detecting changes in joints and soft tissue as a consequence of inflammation. PDS also increases the specificity of a US assessment, as it aids differentiation among tissue debris, blood clot, fibrin, and a complex effusion, which can mimic features of synovial proliferation (13).

Achieving the optimum diagnostic yield from a US examination requires good anatomic and clinical knowledge in addition to technical skills and an understanding of the equipment being used (14). Image artifacts are common, with tissue anisotropy being probably the most important. Anisotropy, which results from the transducer and object not being perpendicular to each other, causes reflection of the beam away from the transducer, resulting in a dramatic reduction in the echogenicity of the tissue. This effect can therefore mimic disease of either bone or soft tissue. It can, however, also aid in the identification of tendons, which change echogenicity, especially when they are inflamed.

Diagnostic Properties

DETECTION OF BONE EROSIONS

Grassi et al. (15) and Lund et al. (16) were the first to describe the use of US for the detection of erosions (Fig. 9.1). These studies were only descriptive studies, and although they did not provide reproducibility or validation data, they nonetheless gave a useful insight into the future potential of US. Subsequent authors have attempted to address these problems.

Alasaarela et al. (17) compared CR, MRI, and computed tomography (CT) with US in a preliminary study assessing erosions of the humeral head in patients with established RA. They found that MRI, CT, and US were all more sensitive than CR, with MRI and US superior to CT in detecting small erosions. In particular, US erosions compared with CT and MRI lesions by site. Backhaus et al. (18) compared CR, MRI, scintigraphy, and US in the finger joints [wrists, metacarpophalangeal (MCP) joint, proximal interphalangeal (PIP) joint] of 60 inflammatory arthritis patients, 36 of whom had RA. This cross-sectional study did not demonstrate a superiority of US over CR, possibly reflecting the analogue technology used (19) or the inclusion of the wrists and PIP joints. These joints may also have degenerative changes, making interpretation of bone damage difficult sometimes. A recently published 2-year follow-up study of these patients did, however, show a benefit of US over x-ray (20).

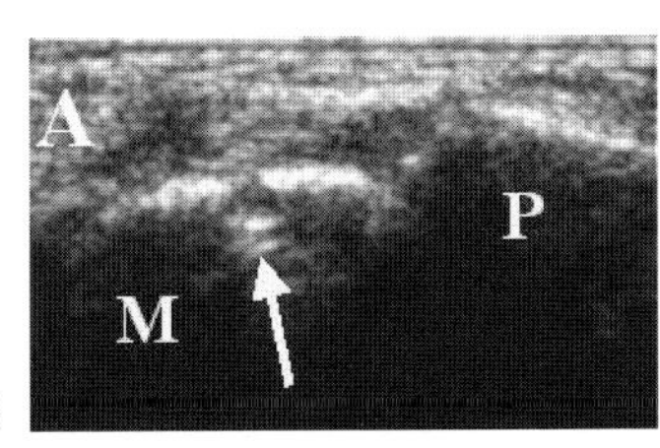

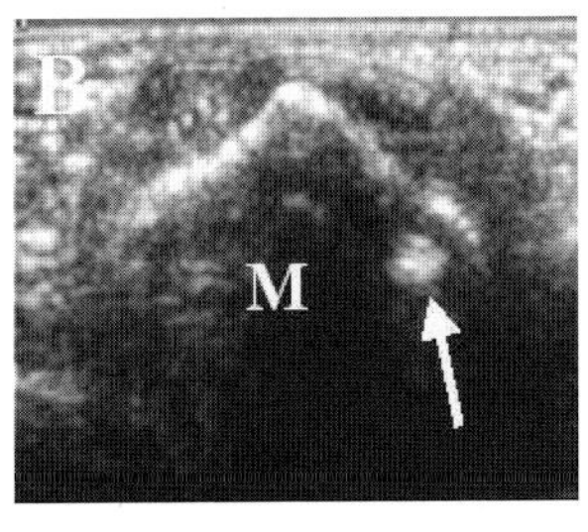

A,B

Figure 9.1. Sections through a metacarpophalangeal joint in a patient with rheumatoid arthritis demonstrating an erosion (*white arrows*) in longitudinal **(A)** and transverse planes **(B)**. M, metacarpal head; P, phalanx.

A study by Wakefield et al. (21) compared US and conventional posteroanterior radiography for the detection of erosions of the MCP joint of 100 patients with RA. The study found that US was a reproducible technique and detected 3.5 times as many erosions as radiography, a difference that was even greater in those 40 patients with early disease (less than 12 months). The superiority of US over plain radiography is explained by the multiplanar capability of US and the fact that US can detect smaller erosions. This latter point may be particularly important in early RA. To help evaluate the pathologic specificity of these additional US erosions, MRI was used to assess the radial aspect of the second MCP heads in 25 patients with early disease. One radiographic erosion, was seen that corresponded exactly with both US and MRI lesions. All ten MRI erosions corresponded exactly with a US erosion, but, interestingly, US detected three additional erosions. These findings can be explained by the superior spatial resolution of US compared to MRI, which, in three patients, depicted two individual US erosions in areas where MRI was only able to depict a diffuse area of edema. This finding has also been confirmed by a more recent study by Alarcón et al. (22). The superiority of US to detect smaller erosions has also been described by Grassi et al. (23) in the hands and Klocke et al. (24) in the feet, both of which also highlight the lateral aspect of the fifth metatarsophalangeal joint as a target in RA. Recently, in a study of 47 patients with RA, Weidekamm et al. (25) found twice as many erosions in the wrists, MCP joint, and PIP joint by US as by conventional posteroanterior radiography. The authors did not comment on how many patients had early disease.

In the authors' own arthritis clinic, US has not replaced radiography for the assessment of bone damage. It is used, instead, as a complementary tool for assessing those patients at high risk of an inflammatory arthritis, in whom radiographs are normal, or for reexamining indeterminate lesions detected on radiography (26).

DETECTION OF SYNOVITIS AND TENOSYNOVITIS

Many studies have highlighted the ability of US to detect synovial disease in both large and small joints (Fig. 9.2) and its superiority over clinical examination (18,27–28). Although most studies have used gray-scale US, more recently, an increasing number have used PDS, with the obvious advantage of being able to assess synovial vascularity.

An early study by Van Holsbeeck et al. (29) compared clinical assessment with thermography and US for the assessment of knee synovitis and joint fluid in patients with RA, pre- and postintraarticular joint injection with corticosteroid. They found that the volume of synovial fluid, as assessed by US, correlated well with clinical assessment, although the synovial fluid took up to 3 months to show any reduction in volume. Rubaltelli et al. compared US synovial thickness with arthroscopic findings in 13 RA (and 14 psoriatic arthritis) knees and found good correlations for the suprapatellar and medial recess compartments (30). Backhaus et al. (18), in a study of 60 patients with inflammatory arthritis, found more synovitis in the joints of the hand and wrist with US than with radiography and clinical examination, and US was comparable to MRI. PDS has been assessed by comparison with histopathology in the knee in RA and osteoarthritis (13,31) and with dynamic MRI in the MCP joint in RA (32) with encouraging results. PDS has also been used successfully to assess inflammatory disease activity in RA (33–36) and monitor response to treatment (37,38).

The sensitivity of PDS may be further enhanced by intravascular bubble contrast agents by raising the intensity of weak signals to a detectable level (39,40). In a study of 40 patients with various arthropathies by Magarelli et al. (41), the use of echo contrast resulted in an increase in the Doppler signal intensity in joints with previously low signal, together with an increased

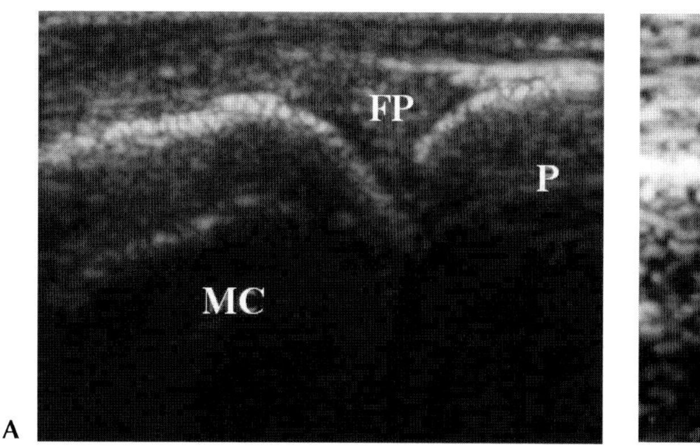

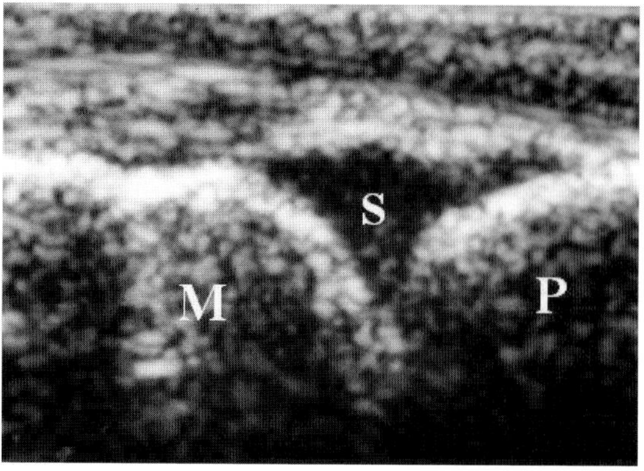

Figure 9.2. Longitudinal sections in a normal **(A)** and synovitic **(B)** metacarpophalangeal joint in patient with rheumatoid arthritis. FP, fat pad; M and MC, metacarpal head; P, phalanx; S, synovitis.

number of joints demonstrating PDS flow that previously had no signal. They also demonstrated concordance with contrast-enhanced MRI in all cases. Other studies have reported a similar increase in detection rate of Doppler signal flow using this technique, but further verification of these findings is required.

A further use of US and MRI in the detection of synovitis has been highlighted by Brown et al. (42). In their study of patients with established RA in clinical remission, as defined by the American College of Rheumatology (ACR) criteria, almost half the patients had signs of subclinical synovitis in joints not thought to have any clinical synovitis. Another group of investigators (43) have used PDS to assess the prognosis of RA patients receiving antitumor necrosis factor therapy. They concluded that the PDS signal predicted the future risk of developing erosive disease.

US has also been used to detect tendon disease in RA, although surprisingly little has been published related to the hand. Grassi et al. (44) described the spectrum of pathologic features seen in 20 patients with RA, including widening of the flexor tendon sheath, loss of the normal fibrillar architecture, tears, and synovial cysts. Swen et al. (45) assessed the use and value of both US and MRI for the detection of partial tears of the extensor tendons of the hand in 21 patients with RA. They concluded that neither had the required sensitivity for routine use when surgical examination was used as the gold standard.

DETECTION OF EXTENT OF DISEASE

In a study of patients with oligoarthritis (46), among those who were rheumatoid factor–positive at baseline, US showed that 83% had evidence of subclinical disease. Of note, only 9% (1 in 12) of patients fulfilled the ACR criteria for RA at baseline, but the addition of US findings (synovitis and erosions) increased this percentage to 50% (6 in 12). These findings demonstrate a potential role for US in the diagnosis of RA and highlights an advantage over MRI because of the ability of US to scan several joints at one time.

Diagnostic and Therapeutic Procedures

US-guided joint aspirations are frequently performed to evaluate the presence of infection or crystal disease (14), assisting in diagnosis. The majority of joints can be aspirated under direct visualization of the needle. The hip is the most common joint requiring US-guided aspiration. On occasion, US examinations can be difficult in the adult, as lower-frequency (3 to 5 MHz) transducers required to achieve the beam penetration result in poorer image quality.

Diagnostic and therapeutic aspirations or injections are of value in the assessment of both joint disease and soft tissue lesions. Diagnostic injections are those performed into or around a structure where local anesthetic is instilled to determine whether the patient's symptoms arise from that area. Two published studies showed extremely poor accuracy of joint injections without imaging guidance and reported an accuracy of 42% to 51% for large joint injection and only 29% for subacromial bursal injections (47,48). For these injections to be of reliable diagnostic and therapeutic value, the exact site of injection must be known. US can and should help clarify this situation by both delineating the abnormality present and recording the site of injection. US allows the operator to dynamically image the needle placement and the distribution of any injection performed (49,50). US-guided synovial biopsy offers another potential use for US. There is as yet little published work in this area (51).

Future Developments

Technologic advances in US are continually improving image quality and contrast between tissues. With respect to RA, identification of patients with a poor prognosis at presentation, differentiation of inactive fibrotic joint tissue from pannus, and quantification of synovitis will all be important areas of investigation. PDS is likely to play an important part in these respects. Additionally, contrast agents may become the equivalent of gadolinium (Gd), allowing the development of transit time curves, bolus arrival times, time to maximum intensity, area under the curve, and wash in–wash out characteristics, which may further improve the characterization of inflammation. Microbubble-specific imaging modes, such as harmonic imaging, as well as three- and four-dimensional US, offer other exciting possibilities for the future.

MAGNETIC RESONANCE IMAGING

As it has for US, interest in the use of MRI in rheumatology has grown dramatically since the 1990s, in part due to the superior imaging of MRI but also to increased access to MRI scanners. This section reviews the application of MRI in relation to rheumatoid arthritis, with special emphasis on its use and on understanding pathogenesis and diagnosis and monitoring response to therapy.

Understanding Magnetic Resonance Imaging Technology

The principles of MRI depend on the alignment of hydrogen protons within tissues when a subject is placed in an external magnetic field provided by the MRI magnet (longitudinal magnetization). An additional alternating or rotating external magnetic pulse is then applied, so that the protons acquire energy, or resonance, with decrease in longitudinal magnetization and increase in transverse magnetization. By rotating these additional fields against the main magnetic field, an electric current is generated. This current is measured as the MRI signal, via a receiving coil, which results in the MRI image. This image comprises volume elements, or voxels, the size of which are determined by MRI parameters of slice thickness, field of view, and the imaging matrix. The physics involved in MRI have been described (52), and, for comprehensive descriptions of MRI terminology and sequences, the reader is referred elsewhere (53).

Given the technology, it is not surprising that technical factors can affect the image quality of scans. The strength of the magnet [measured in tesla (T)], the direction of the sequences acquired (axial, coronal, or sagittal), the nature of the sequences performed, and the coil used to acquire the signal may all be varied and result in different signal-to-resolution ratios. These factors should be kept in mind when reviewing the medical literature and studies using MRI. To further complicate matters, the technology is continuing to change at a rapid rate.

MAGNETS

The most common magnet strengths currently in use are 1.5 T and 1.0 T, and most of the research presented in this chapter used these magnets. Extremity MRI (E-MRI) using smaller, less expensive, and portable magnets with lower field strengths is now available. There may be considerable growth of interest in E-MRI, but, currently, there are few reports using it. One study compared a 0.2 T E-MRI scanner with a 1.5 T scanner in terms of their ability to detect joint effusion, bone edema, and erosions in the small joints of RA patients. This study demonstrated only small differences in agreement (4% or less), and, notably, 64% of the patients preferred the extremity scanner because of more comfortable positioning and less claustrophobia (54).

SEQUENCES

The proton content of tissue and the sequences used for imaging determine the appearance of a tissue on MRI. On a T1-weighted image, fat-containing tissues, such as bone marrow, demonstrate a high signal (i.e., appear white). T1-weighted sequences are useful for demonstrating anatomy, and, in RA, they are especially useful for demonstrating erosions. Because T2-weighted sequences show water as a high signal, they can be used for demonstrating joint effusions and bone marrow edema. Fat-suppression sequences allow the high signal from fat to be reduced, thereby making fluid and, consequently, inflammation more visible. One of the most common tools used for evaluating areas of inflammation, or hypervascularity, is the paramagnetic agent Gd diethylenetriaminepentaacetic acid (Gd-DTPA).

Definitions of Magnetic Resonance Imaging Pathology in Rheumatoid Arthritis

Because of differences in the technology referred to above, it is not surprising that there have been varied definitions for the common MRI RA abnormalities—for example, bone erosions, bone edema, synovitis, and tenosynovitis. As a result, comparison between studies can be difficult. In the last few years, the Outcome Measures in Rheumatology Clinical Trials international consensus group has focused on this issue and provided recommendations for standard definitions (55). These definitions were recently refined and are presented in Table 9.1 (56). It is worth considering these definitions when interpreting MRI studies and in the discussions below.

TABLE 9.1. Definition of Magnetic Resonance Imaging (MRI) Pathological Lesions in Rheumatoid Arthritis

MRI Pathology	Definition
Synovitis	An area in the synovial compartment with above-normal postgadolinium enhancement and thickness greater than the normal synovium
Bone erosion	A sharply marginated lesion with correct juxtaarticular location and typical signal changes, with visibility in two planes and cortical break in at least one plane
Bone edema	A lesion within trabecular bone with ill-defined margins and signal characteristics of increased water content

Adapted from Ostergaard M, Peterfy C, Conaghan P, et al. OMERACT Rheumatoid Arthritis Magnetic Resonance Imaging Studies. Core set of MRI acquisitions, joint pathology definitions, and the OMERACT RA-MRI scoring system. *J Rheumatol* 2003;30:1385–1386.

Magnetic Resonance Imaging Comparisons with Other Imaging Modalities

The earliest studies using MRI in RA examined the sensitivity of MRI in detecting typical RA pathology. Issues of face, content, and construct validity have been addressed by comparison with both clinical examination and other modalities of imaging. These comparison publications have included some longitudinal evaluation of MRI abnormalities.

EROSIONS

A key issue in the use of MRI concerns the relationship between MRI erosions and radiographic erosions (Fig. 9.3). It is important to consider that MRI visualizes protons, not calcified cortex, as in CR. The particular bone abnormality seen on MRI depends on the acquired sequences, and bone edema (Fig. 9.4) can complicate the reader assessment. Most of the early studies compared MRI with CR at the wrist (57–60), knee (61), and shoulder (18) and demonstrated at least a threefold difference in detection of erosions, in favor of MRI. The authors have demonstrated that T1-weighted lesions with loss of trabecular bone correlate 100% with sonographic-determined cortical breaks in the second MCP joint of RA patients, where US has its best access (21). Furthermore, these lesions seem specific for RA. A cross-sectional comparison showed that they are very infrequent in normal controls compared with RA patients (62) and, in a 1-year longitudinal study of RA and

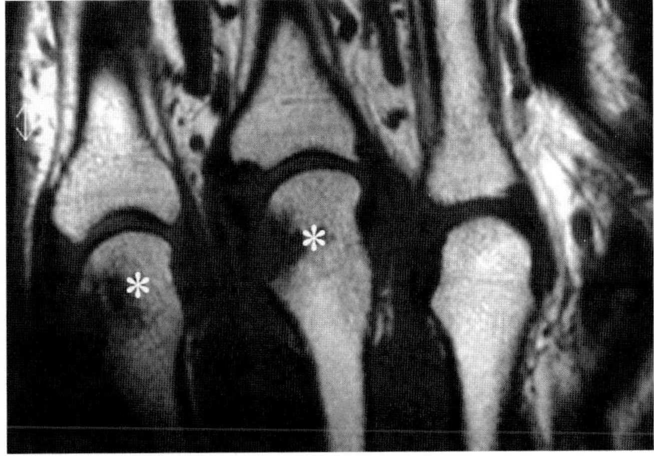

Figure 9.3. Coronal T1-weighted image of the second to fourth metacarpophalangeal joints demonstrating large radial erosions (*white asterisks*) in the second and third metacarpal heads.

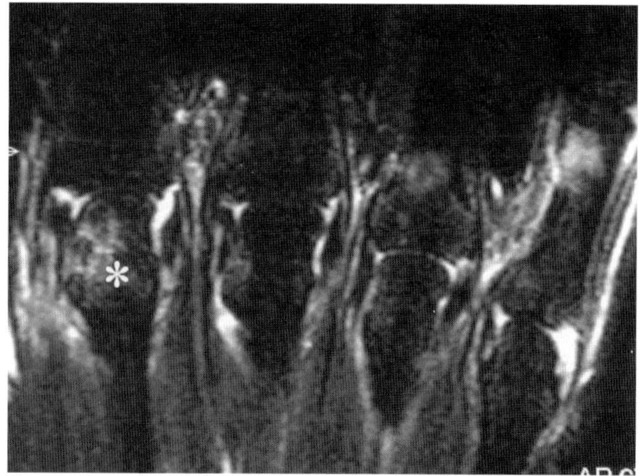

Figure 9.4. Coronal T2-weighted image with fat suppression (low signal intensity from bone marrow) demonstrating bone marrow edema (*white asterisk*) in the radial side of the second metacarpal head.

early unclassified polyarthritis, MRI erosions were only found in patients with baseline RA or those fulfilling ACR RA criteria at 1 year (63). In a study of wrists from 42 early RA patients followed for more than 2 years, McQueen et al. demonstrated that MRI erosions predicted the presence of CR erosions at 1 and 2 years, but only one in four erosions became CR evident over a year (64). It is likely that CR will never detect all MR erosions, due to its lack of tomography. A study compared E-MRI of the second to fifth MCP joints of 25 early RA patients with CR (65). E-MRI detected 9.5 times more erosion than did CR.

SYNOVITIS

RA is primarily a disease of the synovium. It has, therefore, been advantageous to have a tool to image the primary site of disease. Synovitis is probably best imaged using Gd-DTPA, comparing pre- and post-Gd films (Fig. 9.5). Gd-DTPA–enhanced synovial tissue has been positively correlated with macroscopic and microscopic (cellular infiltrates, fibrin deposition, vascular proliferation) changes of inflammation in the knees of RA patients (66–69). Gd-DTPA–enhanced synovitis has also been strongly correlated with mini-arthroscopic synovial scores in RA MCP joints (70). A recent report has demonstrated the advantages of Gd-containing sequences over certain non-Gd sequences in the detection of synovitis in wrists and MCP joint (71). However, moderate inter-reader agreement was still achieved, and the use of Gd must be considered in the context of feasibility.

The quantification of synovitis may be semiquantitative or quantitative. The semiquantitative scoring methods for wrist and MCP joints are suggested in Table 9.1. Quantitative estimation may be:

- Volumetric, using manual outlining on post-Gd scans, or semiautomatic, using subtraction of pre- and post-Gd scans and using thresholding (72). The manual volume methods are probably the nearest to a gold standard but are laborious and time consuming.
- Acquired using dynamic enhanced MRI (DEMRI), which uses postcontrast analysis to determine pharmacodynamic (maximal enhancement, initial rate of enhancement) (73) and even pharmacokinetic (74) parameters.

With respect to detecting synovitis, a growing number of studies has demonstrated the improved sensitivity of MRI over clinical examination in both early (75) and established (76) RA. Goupille et al. reported MRI examination of 12 active RA patients who had both wrists, MCP joints, and PIP joints scanned (77). The clinical swollen joint count was 59, whereas MRI detected synovitis in 162 joints. This sensitivity is similar to data on MCP joints alone in early disease (25) and in patients in clinical remission (42). Goupille et al. also demonstrated significant associations among MRI synovitis and swollen joint count, Ritchie Index, the disease activity score, and early-morning stiffness. E-MRI has also demonstrated more sensitivity than clinical examination in a study of more than 100 MCP joints and demonstrated synovial thickening in 51% of the clinically inactive joints (65).

TENDONS

Flexor and extensor tenosynovitis is an important contributor to hand and foot problems in RA. This area of RA pathology has been less well studied than erosions and synovitis. Both clinical and MRI definitions of tenosynovitis are problematic. However, Hug et al. reported a study of 11 RA patients using fat-suppressed MRI images at the MCP level and defining flexor tenosynovitis as a rim of high signal intensity around the tendon (78). They demonstrated a high frequency of tenosynovitis. A recent study of wrist tendons from 43 established RA patients (with active disease and no clinical tendon tears) and 12 healthy controls studied both intratendon signal and tendon sheath thickness (79). More than one-half of the wrist tendons in the RA group had evidence of increased sheath thickness (presumed tenosynovitis), and only 46% had normal tendons. The greatest degrees of abnormalities were seen in the dorsal and ulnar tendon sheaths. Another study of MCP and PIP joints in early RA demonstrated a high frequency of MRI tenosynovitis (63).

Magnetic Resonance Imaging in Understanding Rheumatoid Arthritis Pathogenesis

One of the major insights derived from MRI of the pathogenesis of inflammatory arthritis has come from studies from McGonagle et al. suggesting two subgroups of patients: a primarily

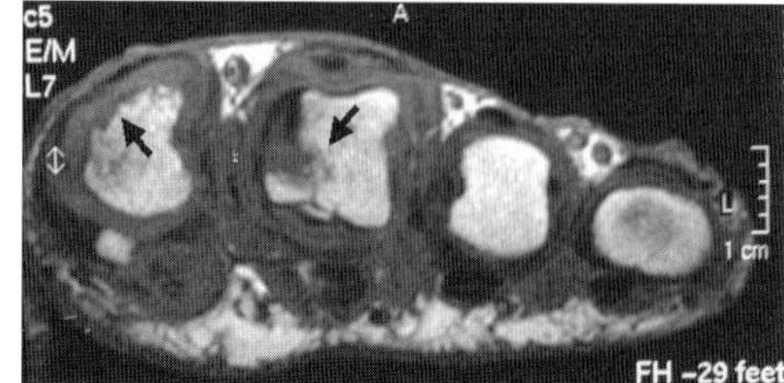

A

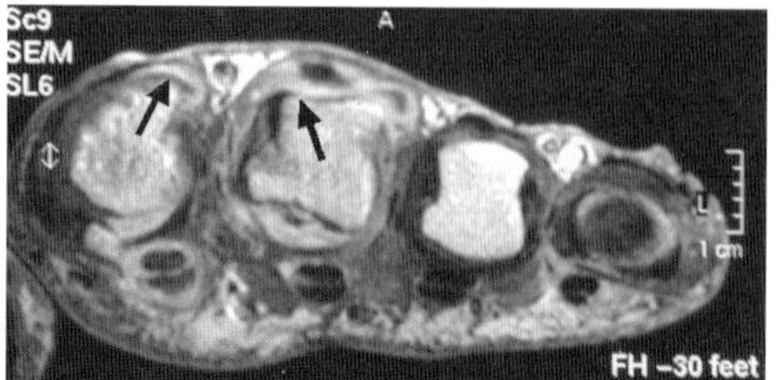

B

Figure 9.5. **A:** Axial section through the second to fifth metacarpal heads, demonstrating small erosion in the second metacarpal head and large erosion in the third metacarpal head (*black arrows*). **B:** Same section as **A** after injection of gadolinium, showing enhancement of synovial tissue in the second and third metacarpal joints (*black arrows*). Flexor tenosynovitis is also demonstrated, most obviously in the second flexor tendon.

intrasynovial group (RA) and an entheseal-based group (for example, the spondyloarthropathies and polymyalgia rheumatica) (80–82). Importantly, further insights into RA pathogenesis have now been gained from the use of MRI.

SYNOVITIS AND BONE DAMAGE

For many years, there was confusion about the relation between synovitis and bone erosions, as CR studies had demonstrated both erosion progression, despite apparent clinical control of inflammation (83–85), and reduced erosion progression, even though there was little change in clinical synovitis (86). Subsequent studies demonstrated that effective disease suppression did reduce bone damage (87,88), and a CR study examining tender and swollen hand joints in early RA patients demonstrated a close relationship between these clinical surrogates and bone erosion progression (89). Studies using MRI have been able to visualize more closely this relationship. Preliminary information on the prognostic value of Gd-enhanced synovitis for predicting erosions in the small finger joints of established RA patients was reported by Jevtic et al. in 1996 (90). In a 12-month duration study of the wrist in 26 RA patients, Ostergaard et al. demonstrated that volumetric measures of synovitis predicted rate of MRI erosion progression (91). Huang et al., using DEMRI in early RA patients, demonstrated the same relationship (92). Using the MCP joints (where the relationship between synovitis and bone damage is easier to visualize at the individual joint level) in 40 early RA patients, Conaghan et al. demonstrated that erosion progression was proportional to the level of synovitis in a given joint and that no erosions occurred in joints without synovitis (93).

The MRI-visualized link between these two pathologic processes, synovitis and MRI erosion, appears to be bone edema. Bone edema is frequently present in new, untreated RA but only infrequently seen in normal controls (94). This finding has been confirmed by the demonstration of bone edema in patients with RA but not polyarthralgia (95). In a cross-sectional study of 31 early RA patients, bone edema was almost exclusively seen in joints with synovitis (94). In a longitudinal evaluation of a different cohort of 40 patients, the synovial thickness was greater in those joints with bone edema than in those without (93). In the same study, bone edema was shown to precede subsequent MRI erosions in approximately 40% of new erosions. A relationship of bone edema to disease duration in the hand joints of RA patients has been reported, probably reflecting the same process—that is, persistence or severity of synovitis causing bone edema and consequent erosion (96). This finding was confirmed in a longitudinal study showing that bone edema in the wrist is predictive for bone erosions at 12 months (97). It is important to note that, at the level of bone edema, bone damage appears reversible (see Magnetic Resonance Imaging As an Outcome Measure in Rheumatoid Arthritis Therapy Evaluation).

JOINT MECHANICS AND ARCHITECTURE

Study of the intrajoint site of erosions with MRI has also increased understanding of the pathogenesis of erosions. A case control study of RA wrists demonstrated that carpal bone damage becomes asymmetric over time, with more damage being evident on the radial, force-bearing side of the wrist (98). A detailed study in 40 early RA patients that scored site of erosions and used DEMRI techniques to ascertain synovitis volumes adjacent to MCP joint collateral ligaments demonstrated a propensity for radial involvement in the second to fourth MCP joints (99). The role of biomechanic factors in relation to synovitis and erosions is thus becoming clear. MRI also opens up the possibility of a highly detailed understanding of joint architecture. Woodburn and colleagues have presented data on three-dimensional reconstructions of rheumatoid subtalar and midtarsal joints compared with normal controls and demonstrated that only subtalar synovitis (with or without erosions) predicted abnormal architectural geometry (100).

Magnetic Resonance Imaging and the Diagnosis of Rheumatoid Arthritis

Early diagnosis with early treatment is now the hallmark of RA management (101). With the reported sensitivity of MRI in detecting erosions and synovitis and the apparent specificity of bone edema changes, it follows that MRI should be an aid in the early diagnosis of RA. There is still only limited work on the impact of MRI in this area. This situation reflects access to MRI, a paucity of knowledge on the critical number or sites of joints to image, and the growing ability of US to easily image multiple joints in real time. Using baseline bilateral total hand contrast-enhanced MRI, Sugimoto and colleagues followed 50 patients with polyarthralgia for more than 2 years and evaluated the ACR diagnostic criteria for RA (102). Comparing MRI-based criteria with the ACR criteria, they reported that MRI had a sensitivity of 96%, a specificity of 86%, and an accuracy of 94%. They then suggested combining imaging criterion with the existing classification tree criteria to improve false-negative diagnosis of RA. Further evaluation of such criteria is required.

Magnetic Resonance Imaging As an Outcome Measure in Rheumatoid Arthritis Therapy Evaluation

The sensitivity of MRI to the key elements in RA pathology suggests that proof-of-concept studies for new therapies could be smaller in size (103). However, as indicated in Definitions of Magnetic Resonance Imaging Pathology in Rheumatoid Arthritis, there has been a great need to address issues of reliability and sensitivity to change before widespread adoption of MRI in clinical trials (104). The Outcome Measures in Rheumatology Clinical Trials RA-MRI group has presented and updated definitions on lesions and has been further involved in exercises to determine inter-reader reliability using these definitions. Although this work is ongoing and iterative, there has generally been excellent agreement when one or two readers are used, with moderate agreement in five-reader studies (105). These reliability studies have evaluated longitudinal scoring and demonstrated intraclass correlation coefficients and smallest detectable difference values similar to those of standard RA outcomes (clinical and CR) (106).

With respect to drug outcome studies, the earliest studies provided proof of MRI's ability to measure change in synovial volume after a known effective therapy, generally corticosteroid injections (107). Other studies involving different disease-modifying drugs (within a study) have demonstrated the efficacy of active treatments (108,109). The Leeds group has reported two studies using DEMRI to assess response in the knee joint in evaluating anti-CD4 and in comparing methotrexate and leflunomide treatments; both studies were performed in patients with established RA (110). In early RA, the Leeds group used semi-quantitative scoring methods to assess the efficacy over 12 months of methotrexate versus methotrexate plus intraarticular corticosteroids (40-patient randomized study) (93), high-dose infliximab with methotrexate (five-patient open study) (97), and methotrexate versus methotrexate and standard-dose infliximab (20-patient randomized trial, preliminary report only) (111). These studies demonstrate that MRI can, with appropriate scientific rigor, be effectively used as an outcome measure.

TABLE 9.2. Advantages and Disadvantages of the Use of Ultrasound

Advantages	Disadvantages
Relatively inexpensive	Operator dependent and slow learning curve
Available in most radiology departments and increasingly available in many rheumatology departments	Limited transducer access—for example, for deep joints such as hip or more superficial joints where adjacent joints lie in close proximity, such as carpal bones
Potential immediate availability in outpatient departments enabling rapid decision making	Limited data on sensitivity to change with treatment
Ability to scan several joints at one time point	Additional time required in clinical setting
Well tolerated	
No ionizing radiation, allowing multiple assessments in time and place	
Relative short scanning time (all joints <40 min; hands and feet, 5 min)	
Allows real-time, dynamic joint assessments	

Magnetic Resonance Imaging in the Detection of Cervical Spine Disease

Cervical spine involvement is common in patients with RA, and atlantoaxial subluxation occurs in up to 40%. Local pannus may result in ligamentous laxity and rupture in addition to erosive damage around the odontoid process. Instability may involve anterior displacement of C1 or posterior displacement of the peg. Until the advent of MRI, CT was the investigation of choice to visualize these changes of the craniocervical region. Pannus, cerebrospinal fluid, and bone erosion and compression of the spinal cord (112) can all be visualized with MRI. Scans can also be obtained in flexion and extension (56,113), but there is probably no advantage to this over a single MRI study, with plain lateral flexion and extension views and tomography to show erosions.

CONCLUSION

Imaging technology continues to change and is improving rapidly. New hardware, software, and falling costs will change the usefulness and availability of both US and MRI. Each modality should be considered complementary to the other, as each has a number of advantages and disadvantages (Tables 9.2 and 9.3). Automated synovitis estimations and the development of dedicated extremity scanners will improve MRI's usefulness to clinicians and researchers. Well-designed validation studies are delineating the role for US in diagnosis and monitoring of early RA, and its real-time advantages make it well suited for use in outpatient settings. The application of new imaging techniques to the early diagnosis and evaluation of treatment response heralds an era in which rheumatologists will be able to better target and reduce synovitis and consequently improve RA patient outcomes.

TABLE 9.3. Advantages and Disadvantages of the Use of Magnetic Resonance Imaging

Advantages	Disadvantages
Multiplanar	Expensive (equipment, running, and personnel costs)
No ionizing radiation	Time consuming (hand and wrist only in 50 min)
Considered gold standard	Limited to one anatomic site per examination
More sensitive than clinical examination, x-ray, and ultrasound for the detection of synovitis and erosions	High level of expertise required
	Not well tolerated by some patients who are anxious and claustrophobic (some may require sedation); have previous metal implants (e.g., heart valves, pacemaker); elderly who find it difficult to lie flat or still
	Motion artifacts
	? Too sensitive (uncertainty about clinical significance)

REFERENCES

1. Emery P. Magnetic resonance imaging: opportunities for rheumatoid arthritis disease assessment and monitoring long-term treatment outcomes. *Arthritis Res* 2002;4[Suppl 2]:S6–S10.
2. Manger B, Kalden J. Joint and connective tissue ultrasonography: a rheumatological bedside tool. *Arthritis Rheum* 1995;38:591–596.
3. Wakefield RJ, Gibbon WW, Emery P. The current status of ultrasonography in rheumatology. *Rheumatology* 1999;38:195–201.
4. Grassi W, Cervini C. Ultrasonography in rheumatology: an evolving technique. *Ann Rheum Dis* 1998;57:268 271.
5. Balint P, Sturrock RD. Musculoskeletal ultrasound imaging: a new diagnostic tool for the rheumatologist? *Br J Rheumatol* 1997;36:1141–1142.
6. Canoso JJ. Ultrasound imaging: a rheumatologists dream. *J Rheumatol* 2000;27:2063–2064.
7. Karim Z, Wakefield RJ, Conaghan PG, et al. The impact of ultrasonography on diagnosis and management of patients with musculoskeletal conditions. *Arthritis Rheum* 2001;44:2932–2933.
8. Peterfy CG. Magnetic resonance imaging in rheumatoid arthritis: current status and future directions. *J Rheumatol* 2001;28:1134–1142.
9. McQueen FM. Magnetic resonance imaging in early inflammatory arthritis: what is its role? *Rheumatology* 2000;39:700–706.
10. Taouli B, Guermazi A, Sack KE, et al. Imaging of the hand and wrist in RA. *Ann Rheum Dis* 2002;61:867–869.
11. Kremkau FW. *Transducers in diagnostic ultrasound,* 5th ed. W.B. Saunders Company, 1998:79–139.
12. Wakefield RJ, Brown AK, O'Connor PJ, et al. Power Doppler sonography: improving disease activity assessment in inflammatory musculoskeletal disease. *Arthritis Rheum* 2003;48:285–288.
13. Schmidt WA, Volker L, Zacher J, et al. Colour Doppler ultrasonography to detect pannus in knee joint synovitis. *Clin Exp Rheumatol* 2000;18:439–444.
14. O'Connor PJ, Wakefield RJ. Musculoskeletal ultrasound in rheumatology. In: Isenberg D, Renton P, eds. *Imaging in rheumatology.* Oxford: Oxford University Press, 2003:25–33.
15. Grassi W, Titarelli E, Pirani O, et al. Ultrasound examination of the metacarpophalangeal joints in rheumatoid arthritis. *Scand J Rheumatol* 1993;22:243–247.
16. Lund PJ, Heikal A, Maricic MJ, et al. Ultrasonographic imaging of the hand and wrist in rheumatoid arthritis. *Skeletal Radiol* 1995;24:591–596.
17. Alasaarela E, Suramo I, Tervonen O, et al. Evaluation of humeral head erosions in rheumatoid arthritis: a comparison of ultrasonography, magnetic resonance imaging, computed tomography and plain radiography. *Br J Rheumatol* 1998;37:1152–1156.
18. Backhaus M, Kamradt T, Sandrock D, et al. Arthritis of the finger joints. A comprehensive approach comparing conventional radiography, scintigraphy, ultrasound, and contrast-enhanced magnetic resonance imaging. *Arthritis Rheum* 1999;42:1232–1245.
19. Schmidt W. Value of sonography in diagnosis of rheumatoid arthritis. *Lancet* 2001;357:1056–1057.
20. Backhaus M, Burmester GR, Sandrock D, et al. Prospective two year follow up study comparing novel and conventional imaging procedures in patients with arthritic finger joints. *Ann Rheum Dis* 2002;61:895–904.
21. Wakefield RJ, Gibbon WW, Conaghan PG, et al. The value of sonography in the detection of bone erosions in patients with rheumatoid arthritis: a comparative study with conventional radiography. *Arthritis Rheum* 2000;43:2762–2770.
22. Alarcón GS, Lopez-Ben R, Moreland LW. High-resolution ultrasound for the study of target joints in rheumatoid arthritis [Letter]. *Arthritis Rheum* 2002;46:1969–1981.
23. Grassi W, Filipucci E, Farina A, et al. Ultrasonography in the evaluation of bone erosions. *Ann Rheum Dis* 2001;60:98–103.
24. Klocke R, Glew D, Cox N, et al. Sonographic erosions of the rheumatoid little toe. *Ann Rheum Dis* 2001;60:896–897.
25. Weidekamm C, Koller M, Weber M, et al. Diagnostic value of high resolution B mode and Doppler sonography for imaging of the hand and finger joints in rheumatoid arthritis. *Arthritis Rheum* 2003;48:325–333.

26. Wakefield RJ, Conaghan PG, O'Connor P, et al. High-resolution ultrasound for the study of target joints in rheumatoid arthritis. *Arthritis Rheum* 2002;46:1969–1981.
27. Conaghan PG, Wakefield RJ, O'Connor P, et al. The metacarpophalangeal joints in early rheumatoid arthritis: a comparison of clinical, radiographic, MRI and ultrasonographic findings. *Ann Rheum Dis* 1999; [Suppl]: 28.
28. Koski JM. Ultrasonographic evidence of hip synovitis in patients with rheumatoid arthritis. *Scand J Rheum* 1989;18:127–131.
29. von Holsbeeck M, Hosbeeck K, Gevers G, et al. Staging and follow-up of rheumatoid arthritis of the knee: comparison of sonography, thermography, and clinical assessment. *J Ultrasound Med* 1988;7:561–566.
30. Rubaltelli L, Fiocco U, Cozzi L, et al. Prospective sonographic and arthroscopic evaluation of proliferative knee joint synovitis. *J Ultrasound Med* 1994;13:855–862.
31. Walther M, Harms H, Krenn V, et al. Correlation of Power Doppler sonography with vascularity of the synovial tissue of the knee joint in patients with osteoarthritis and rheumatoid arthritis. *Arthritis Rheum* 2001;44:331–338.
32. Szkudlarek M, Court-Payen M, Strandberg C, et al. Power Doppler ultrasonography for assessment of synovitis in the metacarpophalangeal joints of patients with rheumatoid arthritis: a comparison with dynamic magnetic resonance imaging. *Arthritis Rheum* 2001;44:2018–2023.
33. Stone M, Whelan B, Bergin D, et al. Power Doppler ultrasonography in metacarpophalangeal joint synovitis. *Ann Rheum Dis* 1999;[Suppl]:29.
34. Qvistgaard E, Røgind H, Torp-Pedersen S, et al. Quantitative ultrasonography in rheumatoid arthritis: evaluation of inflammation by Doppler technique. *Ann Rheum Dis* 2001;60:690–693.
35. Carotti M, Salaffi F, Manganelli P, et al. Power Doppler sonography in the assessment of synovial tissue of the knee joint in rheumatoid arthritis: a preliminary experience. *Ann Rheum Dis* 2002;61:877–882.
36. Klauser A, Frauscher F, Schirmer M, et al. The value of colour-enhanced colour Doppler ultrasound in the detection of vascularisation of finger joints of patients with rheumatoid arthritis. *Arthritis Rheum* 2002;46:647–653.
37. Hau M, Kneitz C, Tony HP, et al. High resolution ultrasound detects a decrease in pannus vascularisation of small finger joints in patients with rheumatoid arthritis receiving treatment with soluble tumour necrosis factor α receptor (etanercept). *Ann Rheum Dis* 2002;61:55–58.
38. Terslev L, Torp-Pedersen S, Qvistgaard E, et al. Effects of treatment with etanercept (Enbrel, TNRF:Fc) on rheumatoid arthritis evaluated by Doppler ultrasonography. *Ann Rheum Dis* 2003;62:178–181.
39. Harvey CJ, Pilcher JM, Eckersley RJ, et al. Advances in ultrasound. *Clin Radiol* 2002;57:157–177.
40. Blomley M, Cosgrove D. Microbubble echo-enhancers: a new direction for ultrasound? *Lancet* 1997;349:1855–1856.
41. Magarelli N, Gugleilmi G, Di Matteo L, et al. Diagnostic utility of an echocontrast agent in patients with synovitis using power Doppler ultrasound: a preliminary study with comparison to contrast-enhanced MRI. *Eur Radiol* 2001;11:1039–1046.
42. Brown AK, Quinn MA, Karim Z, et al. Neither the ACR remission criteria nor the disease activity score accurately define true remission in rheumatoid arthritis. *Arthritis Rheum* 2002;46[Suppl]:S243.
43. Taylor PC. VEGF and imaging of vessels in rheumatoid arthritis. *Arthritis Res* 2002;4[Suppl 3]:S99–107.
44. Grassi W, Tittarelli E, Blasetti P, et al. Finger tendon involvement in rheumatoid arthritis. Evaluation with high-frequency sonography. *Arthritis Rheum* 1995;38:786–794.
45. Swen WA, Jacobs JW, Hubach PC, et al. Comparison of sonography and magnetic resonance imaging for the diagnosis of partial tears of finger extensor tendons in rheumatoid arthritis. *Rheumatology* 2000;39:55–62.
46. Wakefield RJ, Green MJ, Gibbon WW, et al. High resolution ultrasound defined subclinical synovitis—a predictor of response in early oligoarthritis. *Arthritis Rheum* 1998;41:S246.
47. Jones A, Regan M, Ledingham J, et al. Importance of placement of intra-articular steroid injections. *BMJ* 1993;307:1329–1330.
48. Eustace JA, Brophy DP, Gibney RP. Comparison of accuracy of steroid placement with clinical outcomes in patients with shoulder symptoms. *Ann Rheum Dis* 1997;56:59–63.
49. Koski JM. Ultrasound guided injections in rheumatology. *J Rheumatol* 2000;27:2131–2138.
50. Grassi W, Farina A, Filippucci E, et al. Sonographically guided procedures in rheumatology. *Semin Arthritis Rheum* 2001;30:347–353.
51. van Vugt RM, van Dalen A, Bijlsma JW. Ultrasound guided synovial biopsy of the wrist. *Scand J Rheumatol* 1997;26:212–214.
52. Schild HH. *MRI made easy*. Berlin: H Heenemann GmbH & Co, 1990.
53. Kaplan PA, Helms CA, Dussault R, et al. *Musculoskeletal MRI*. Philadelphia: W.B. Saunders, 2001.
54. Savnik A, Malmskov H, Thomsen HS, et al. MRI of the arthritic small joints: comparison of extremity MRI (0.2 T) vs high-field MRI (1.5 T). *Eur Radiol* 2001;11:1030–1038.
55. Conaghan P, Edmonds J, Emery P, et al. Magnetic resonance imaging in rheumatoid arthritis: summary of OMERACT activities, current status, and plans. *J Rheumatol* 2001;28:1158–1162.
56. Ostergaard M, Peterfy C, Conaghan P, et al. OMERACT Rheumatoid Arthritis Magnetic Resonance Imaging Studies. Core set of MRI acquisitions, joint pathology definitions, and the OMERACT RA-MRI scoring system. *J Rheumatol* 2003;30:1385–1386.
57. Gilkeson G, Polisson R, Sinclair H, et al. Early detection of carpal erosions in patients with rheumatoid arthritis: a pilot study of magnetic resonance imaging. *J Rheumatol* 1988;15:1361–1366.
58. Corvetta A, Giovagnoni A, Baldelli S, et al. MR imaging of rheumatoid hand lesions: comparison with conventional radiology in 31 patients. *Clin Exp Rheumatol* 1992;10:217–222.
59. Jorgensen C, Cyteval C, Anaya JM, et al. Sensitivity of magnetic resonance imaging of the wrist in very early rheumatoid arthritis. *Clin Exp Rheumatol* 1993;11:163–168.
60. McQueen F, Stewart N, Crabbe J, et al. Magnetic resonance imaging of the wrist in early rheumatoid arthritis reveals a high prevalence of erosions at four months after symptom onset. *Ann Rheum Dis* 1998;57:350–356.
61. Forslind K, Larsson EM, Johansson A, et al. Detection of joint pathology by magnetic resonance imaging in patients with early rheumatoid arthritis. *Br J Rheumatol* 1997;36:683–688.
62. McGonagle D, Conaghan PG, Gibbon W, et al. The relationship between synovitis and bone changes in early untreated rheumatoid arthritis—a controlled MRI study. *Arthritis Rheum* 1999;42:1706–1711.
63. Klarlund M, Ostergaard M, Jensen KE, et al. Magnetic resonance imaging, radiography, and scintigraphy of the finger joints: one year follow up of patients with early arthritis. *Ann Rheum Dis* 2000;59:521–528.
64. McQueen FM, Benton N, Crabbe J, et al. What is the fate of erosions in early rheumatoid arthritis? Tracking individual erosions using x-rays and magnetic resonance imaging over the first two years of disease. *Ann Rheum Dis* 2001;60:859–868.
65. Lindegaard H, Vallo J, Horslev-Petersen K, et al. Low field dedicated magnetic resonance imaging in untreated rheumatoid arthritis of recent onset. *Ann Rheum Dis* 2001;60:770–776.
66. Ostergaard M, Klarlund M. Importance of timing of post-contrast MRI in rheumatoid arthritis: what happens during the first 60 minutes after IV gadolinium-DTPA? *Ann Rheum Dis* 2001;60:1050–1054.
67. Tamai K, Yamato M, Yamaguchi T, et al. Dynamic magnetic resonance imaging for the evaluation of synovitis in patients with rheumatoid arthritis. *Arthritis Rheum* 1994;37:1151–1157.
68. Gaffney K, Cookson J, Blake D, et al. Quantification of rheumatoid synovitis by magnetic resonance imaging. *Arthritis Rheum* 1995;38:1610–1617.
69. Ostergaard M, Stoltenberg M, Lovgreen-Nielsen P, et al. Magnetic resonance imaging-determined synovial membrane and joint effusion volumes in rheumatoid arthritis and osteoarthritis: comparison with the macroscopic and microscopic appearance of the synovium. *Arthritis Rheum* 1997;40:1856–1867.
70. Ostendorf B, Peters R, Dann P, et al. Magnetic resonance imaging and miniarthroscopy of metacarpophalangeal joints: sensitive detection of morphologic changes in rheumatoid arthritis. *Arthritis Rheum* 2001;44:2492–2502.
71. Ostergaard M. Different approaches to synovial membrane volume determination by magnetic resonance imaging: manual versus automated segmentation. *Br J Rheumatol* 1997;36:1166–1177.
72. Creamer P, Keen M, Zananiri F, et al. Quantitative magnetic resonance imaging of the knee: a method of measuring response to intra-articular treatments. *Ann Rheum Dis* 1997;56:378–381.
73. Ostergaard M, Stoltenberg M, Lovgreeen-Nielsen P, et al. Quantification of synovitis by MRI: correlation between dynamic and static gadolinium-enhanced magnetic resonance imaging and microscopic and macroscopic signs of synovial inflammation. *Magn Reson Imaging* 1998;16:743–754.
74. Reece RJ, Kraan MC, Radjenovic A, et al. Comparative assessment of leflunomide and methotrexate for the treatment of rheumatoid arthritis, by dynamic enhanced magnetic resonance imaging. *Arthritis Rheum* 2002;46:366–372.
75. McQueen FM, Stewart N, Crabbe J, et al. Magnetic resonance imaging of the wrist in early rheumatoid arthritis reveals a high prevalence of erosions at four months after symptom-onset. *Ann Rheum Dis* 1998;57:350–356.
76. Jevtic V, Watt I, Rozman B, et al. Contrast enhanced Dd-DTPA magnetic resonance imaging in the evaluation of rheumatoid arthritis during a clinical trial with DMARDs. A prospective two-year follow-up study on hand joints in 31 patients. *Clin Exp Rheumatol* 1997;15:151–156.
77. Goupille P, Roulot B, Akoka S, et al. Magnetic resonance imaging: a valuable method for the detection of synovial inflammation in rheumatoid arthritis. *J Rheumatol* 2001;28:35–40.
78. Hug C, Huber H, Terrier F, et al. Detection of tenosynovitis by magnetic resonance imaging: its relationship to diurnal variation of symptoms. *J Rheumatol* 1991;18:1055–1059.
79. Valeri G, Ferrara C, Ercolani P, et al. Tendon involvement in rheumatoid arthritis of the wrist: MRI findings. *Skeletal Radiol* 2001;30:138–143.
80. McGonagle D, Gibbon W, Emery P. Classification of inflammatory arthritis by enthesitis. *Lancet* 1998;352:1137–1140.
81. McGonagle D, Gibbon W, O'Connor P, et al. Characteristic magnetic resonance imaging entheseal changes of knee synovitis in spondyloarthropathy. *Arthritis Rheum* 1998;41:694–700.
82. McGonagle D, Pease C, Marzo-Ortega H, et al. Comparison of extracapsular changes by magnetic resonance imaging in patients with rheumatoid arthritis and polymyalgia rheumatica. *J Rheumatol* 2001;28:1837–1841.
83. Mulherin D, Fitzgerald O, Bresnihan B. Clinical improvement and radiological deterioration in rheumatoid arthritis: evidence that the pathogenesis of synovial inflammation and articular erosion may differ. *Br J Rheumatol* 1996;35:1263–1268.

84. Fujii K, Tsuji M, Tajima M. Rheumatoid arthritis: a synovial disease? *Ann Rheum Dis* 1999;58:727–730.
85. Maravic M, Bologna C, Daures JP, et al. Radiologic progression in early rheumatoid arthritis treated with methotrexate. *J Rheumatol* 1999;26:262–267.
86. Kirwan JR and the Arthritis and Rheumatism Council Low-Dose Corticosteroid Study Group. The effect of glucocorticoids on joint destruction in rheumatoid arthritis. *N Engl J Med* 1995;333:142–146.
87. Stenger AAME, van Leeuwen MA, Houtman PM, et al. Early effective suppression of inflammation in rheumatoid arthritis reduces radiographic progression. *Br J Rheumatol* 1998;37:1157–1163.
88. Lipsky PE, van der Heijde DMFM, St Clair EW, et al. Infliximab and methotrexate in the treatment of rheumatoid arthritis. *N Engl J Med* 2000;343:1594–1602.
89. Boers M, Kostense PJ, Verhoeven AC, et al. for the COBRA Trial Group. Inflammation and damage in an individual joint predict further damage in that joint in patients with early rheumatoid arthritis. *Arthritis Rheum* 2001;44:2242–2246.
90. Jevtic V, Watt I, Rozman B, et al. Prognostic value of contrast enhanced Gd-DTPA MRI for development of bone erosive changes in rheumatoid arthritis. *Br J Radiol* 1996;35[Suppl]:26–30.
91. Ostergaard M, Hansen M, Stoltenberg M, et al. Magnetic resonance imaging-determined synovial membrane volume as a marker of disease activity and a predictor of progressive joint destruction in the wrists of patients with rheumatoid arthritis. *Arthritis Rheum* 1999;42:918–929.
92. Huang J, Stewart N, Crabbe J, et al. A 1-year follow-up study of dynamic magnetic resonance imaging in early rheumatoid arthritis reveals synovitis to be increased in shared epitope-positive patients and predictive of erosions at 1 year. *Rheumatology* 2000;39:407–416.
93. Conaghan PG, O'Connor P, McGonagle D, et al. Elucidation of the relationship between synovitis and bone damage: a randomised MRI study of individual joints in patients with early rheumatoid arthritis. *Arthritis Rheum* 2003;48:64–71.
94. McGonagle D, Conaghan PG, Gibbon W, et al. The relationship between synovitis and bone changes in early untreated rheumatoid arthritis. *Arthritis Rheum* 1999;42:1706–1711.
95. Savnik A, Malmskov H, Thomsen HS, et al. Magnetic resonance imaging of the wrist and finger joints in patients with inflammatory joint diseases. *J Rheumatol* 2001;28:2193–2200.
96. Savnik A, Malmskov H, Thomsen HS, et al. MRI of the wrist and finger joints in inflammatory joint diseases at 1-year interval: MRI features to predict bone erosions. *Eur Radiol* 2002;12:1203–1210.
97. Conaghan PG, Quinn M, O'Connor P, et al. Can very high-dose anti-tumor necrosis factor blockade at onset of rheumatoid arthritis produce long-term remission? *Arthritis Rheum* 2002;46:1971–1972.
98. Pierre-Jerome C, Bekkelund SI, Mellgren SI, et al. The rheumatoid wrist: bilateral MR analysis of the distribution of rheumatoid lesions in axial plan in a female population. *Clin Rheumatol* 1997;16:80–86.
99. Tan AL, Tanner SF, Conaghan PG, et al. The influence of metacarpophalangeal joint biomechanical factors on the distribution of synovitis and bone erosion in early rheumatoid arthritis. *Arthritis Rheum* 2003 (*in press*).
100. Woodburn J, Udupa JK, Hirsch BE, et al. The geometric architecture of the subtalar and midtarsal joints in rheumatoid arthritis based on magnetic resonance imaging. *Arthritis Rheum* 2002;46:3168–3177.
101. Quinn MA, Conaghan PG, Emery P. The therapeutic approach of early intervention for rheumatoid arthritis: what is the evidence? *Rheumatology* 2001;40:1211–1220.
102. Sugimoto H, Takeda A, Hyodoh K. Early-stage rheumatoid arthritis: prospective study of the effectiveness of MR imaging for diagnosis. *Radiology* 2000;216:569–575.
103. Peterfy CG. Magnetic resonance imaging of rheumatoid arthritis: the evolution of clinical applications through clinical trials. *Semin Arthritis Rheum* 2001;30:375–396.
104. Lassere MND, Bird P. Measurement of rheumatoid arthritis disease activity and damage using magnetic resonance imaging. Truth and discrimination: does MRI make the grade? *J Rheumatol* 2001;28:1151–1157.
105. Lassere M, McQueen F, Ostergaard M, et al. OMERACT Rheumatoid Arthritis Magnetic Resonance Imaging Studies. Exercise 3: an international multicenter reliability study using the RA-MRI Score. *J Rheumatol* 2003;30:1366–1375.
106. Conaghan P, Lassere M, Ostergaard M, et al. OMERACT Rheumatoid Arthritis Magnetic Resonance Imaging Studies. Exercise 4: an international multicenter longitudinal study using the RA-MRI Score. *J Rheumatol* 2003;30:1376–1379.
107. Ostergaard M, Stoltenberg M, Gideon P, et al. Changes in synovial membrane and joint effusion volumes after intraarticular methylprednisolone. Quantitative assessment of inflammatory and destructive changes in arthritis by MRI. *J Rheumatol* 1996;23:1151–1161.
108. Clunie G, Hall-Craggs MA, Paley MN, et al. Measurement of synovial lining volume by magnetic resonance imaging of the knee in chronic synovitis. *Ann Rheum Dis* 1997;56:526–534.
109. McQueen FM, Stewart N, Crabbe J, et al. Magnetic resonance imaging of the wrist in early rheumatoid arthritis reveals progression of erosions despite clinical improvement. *Ann Rheum Dis* 1999;58:156–163.
110. Veale DJ, Reece RJ, Parsons W, et al. Intra-articular primatised anti-CD4: efficacy in resistant rheumatoid knees. A study of combined arthroscopy, MRI and histology. *Ann Rheum Dis* 1999;58:342–349.
111. Quinn M, Conaghan P, O'Connor P, et al. Rapid and sustained improvement with TNF blockade in early rheumatoid arthritis: results from a double blind placebo-controlled study with MRI outcomes. *Arthritis Rheum* 2002;46 [Suppl]:S519.
112. Einig M, Higer HP, Meairs S, et al. Magnetic resonance imaging of the craniocervical junction in rheumatoid arthritis: value, limitations, indications. *Skeletal Radiol* 1990;19:341–346.
113. Cobby M, Kirwan JRJ. Musculoskeletal ultrasound in rheumatology. In: Isenberg DA, et al., eds. *Imaging in rheumatology*. Oxford: Oxford University Press, 2003:247–277.

CHAPTER 10

Genetic Determinants

Peter K. Gregersen

From a genetic perspective, rheumatoid arthritis (RA) can be grouped with a large number of human diseases that are designated as *complex*. In general, the term *complex disease* implies that the genetic components are not easily understood in terms of classic mendelian segregation. For example, it is not known whether the genes involved in RA act in a dominant or recessive fashion and, with the exception of certain human leukocyte antigen (HLA) alleles, whether they are common or rare. The number of these genes is also uncertain, and it is likely that at least some of the genetic influence on RA involves interactions among several genetic components.

In the simplest formulation, disease susceptibility genes are genes that contain genetic variants, or alleles (A), that confer some degree of risk for disease (D). Risk alleles therefore fulfill the proposition $P(D \mid A) > P(D \mid \text{not } A)$—that is, that the probability of developing the disease is greater when the allele is present than when it is not. The ratio of these probabilities is identical to the relative risk associated with the particular allele. One of the major reasons that the identification of RA susceptibility genes has been so difficult is that this risk ratio is probably quite low for most individual disease susceptibility alleles, although there remains considerable uncertainty on this point. The problem is further complicated by the fact that many of these alleles probably interact with other genes in the background, as well as with environmental factors. Finally, there is undoubtedly a stochastic element to whether a particular combination of genetic and environmental risk factors results in the clinical expression of RA (1).

Within a population of patients with RA, there is likely to be considerable heterogeneity among individuals with respect to the number of genes involved in disease susceptibility and how they interact. To an unknown degree, this genetic heterogeneity probably reflects differences in pathogenesis among patients, since there are numerous levels at which immunity and inflammation are regulated. Therefore, it is highly unlikely that a single gene for RA is waiting to be discovered. Rather, there will be a spectrum of genes, some with relatively modest effects on risk, and perhaps a few rare mutations with strong effects on a subgroup of patients. Whatever the risk profile, identification of these risk alleles should contribute to our understanding of disease pathogenesis.

MEASURING THE STRENGTH OF THE GENETIC COMPONENT IN RHEUMATOID ARTHRITIS

The overall contribution of genes to a disease (or associated phenotypes) can be indirectly assessed by establishing the degree of familial aggregation. This method is indirect because environmental factors (e.g., infectious agents, economic status, or educational status) also aggregate in families and must be controlled for. In addition, the overall extent of genetic variability in the population being studied can have a major effect on the conclusions. For example, if a major risk allele is present in nearly everyone in the population, then there may be only a small increase in familial aggregation due to that allele. Therefore, after correction for environmental factors, familial aggregation is really an indicator of how much of the *variability* of disease expression among individuals is explained by the underlying genetic *variation* in the population under study. For highly outbred (*panmictic*) human populations, such as exists in most modern societies, the overall degree of genetic variation between unrelated individuals is approximately 0.1% of the genome, or approximately 3 million base pair differences on average. Siblings within a family share half of their parental chromosomal material in common; thus, siblings still differ by approximately 1.5 million base pairs over the genome. For the purposes of this discussion, monozygotic (MZ) twins can be assumed to have identical genomes.

A popular method of measuring familial aggregation of complex genetic traits is to calculate the relative risk to siblings of affected subjects, compared with the risk for the trait in the general population (2). This quantity, designated λ_S, is widely used to estimate the extent of genetic risk for complex diseases. The estimates of λ_S for common autoimmune diseases are generally modest, in the range of 10 to 20 (3). For RA, the estimates of λ_S vary considerably, from 2 to 12 (4). A large part of this variation stems from the uncertainty regarding the background population prevalence of the phenotype being analyzed in families. Thus, although the overall prevalence of RA appears to be approximately 0.8% (5), it is not clear if exactly the same phenotype is present in the multiplex families that are used to calculate sibling recurrence rates. This uncertainty is unlikely to be resolved until the heterogeneity of the disease is better understood. However, it seems clear that, for the most broadly defined phenotype of RA, the λ_S is lower than for other autoimmune disorders, such as systemic lupus erythematosus and type 1 diabetes.

One can also calculate the relative risk to individuals who are genetically identical (MZ) twins to affected subjects. This value, the λ_{MZ}, may be as high as 60 for RA (4), again with the same caveats discussed above for the λ_S estimates. Although identical twins have greatly increased risk for disease (high λ_{MZ}), the twin concordance rates for autoimmune diseases are generally in the range of

15% to 30%, depending on the autoimmune disease (6). These relatively low concordance rates are often mistakenly interpreted to mean that the role of genes is minor. Rather, it simply means that nongenetic factors also contribute to the variability of disease expression in the population. Based on twin and family data, heritability estimates of 60% have been suggested for RA (7).

HUMAN LEUKOCYTE ANTIGEN GENES AND MAJOR HISTOCOMPATIBILITY COMPLEX

The association of RA with the HLA-DR4 was originally reported in the 1970s by Stastny (8). This analysis was performed using cellular (9) and antibody reagents (10) that are no longer routinely used for HLA typing, although the nomenclature for HLA alleles still derives from these early typing methods. Our knowledge of the molecular details of HLA structure and genetics has exploded since these original studies. Despite this new information, a definitive causal explanation for the HLA associations with RA remains elusive.

The genes for HLA molecules are located within the major histocompatibility complex (MHC) on chromosome 6. The MHC was originally identified because of the ability of genes in this region to control the strength and pattern of the immune response (11). Thus, both cellular and humoral immunity are regulated by polymorphisms of the HLA molecules encoded within the MHC. As shown in Figure 10.1, a simplified map of the MHC on chromosome 6p21.3 divides this region into three subregions: the HLA class II region (centromeric), the HLA class I region (telomeric), and a region now generally termed the *central MHC*. Figure 10.1 highlights only those genes that have traditionally been associated with immune regulation. However, the MHC extends over 3.6 megabases and contains more than 200 genes (12). Approximately 40% of these genes appear to have a function in the immune system. The full sequence and gene map of the MHC is available at http://www.sanger.ac.uk/HGP/Chr6/MHC.shtml.

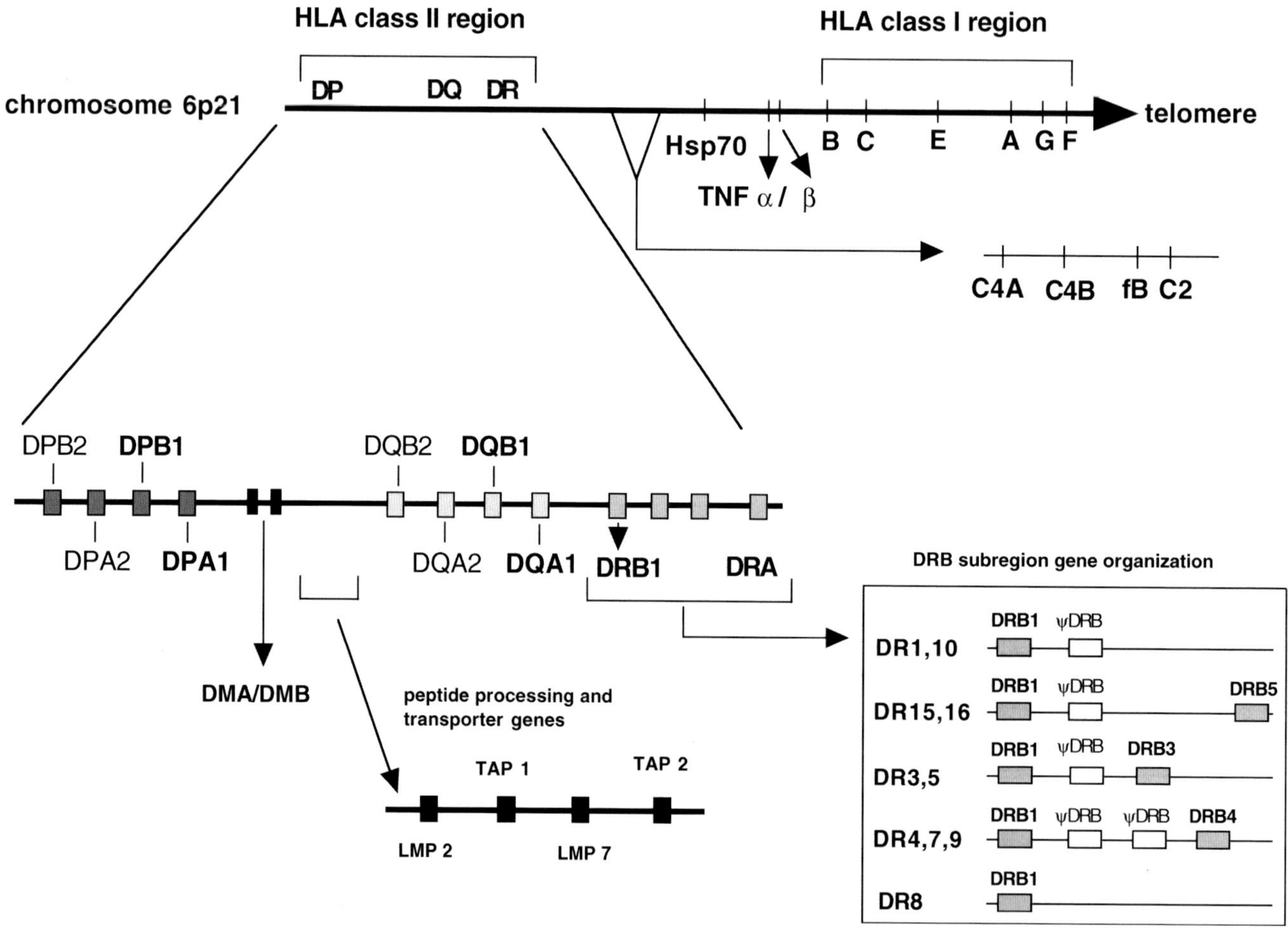

Figure 10.1. Map of the human major histocompatibility complex (MHC). The human leukocyte antigen (HLA) class I and class II molecules are encoded in distinct regions of the MHC. The HLA class II region contains three subregions, DR, DQ, and DP. Each of these contains a variable number of α and β chain genes. HLA class II loci with known functional protein products are labeled in bold. In the case of DR, different numbers of DRB genes are present in different haplotypes. A summary of the most common of these are shown in the box. The DQ and DP subregions each contain one pair of functional α and β chain genes. A number of genes involved in antigen processing and presentation by class I molecules are situated between the DP and DQ subregions.

The HLA class I region contains the three classic class I genes, HLA-A, -B, and -C, as well as other related class I molecules. The gene for familial hemochromatosis resides just telomeric to the HLA class I region. The central MHC also contains a number of genes related to immune function, including the complement components [C4A, C4B, C2, and factor B (fB)], as well as tumor necrosis factor (TNF)-α and -β and several heat shock proteins (Hsp70). The central MHC contains more than 50 genes (12), most of which are not shown on this map. One or more of these may also contribute to rheumatoid arthritis susceptibility (43,51).

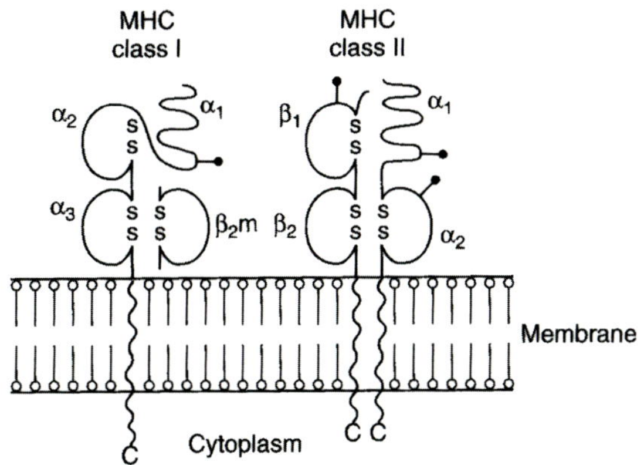

Figure 10.2. A schematic comparison of the structural features of major histocompatibility complex (MHC) class I and class II molecules. MHC class I molecules are anchored in the membrane by a single transmembrane segment contained in the 45-kd α chain. The MHC class I α chain is noncovalently associated with β_2 microglobulin. There are four external domains, three of which contain intramolecular disulfide bonds, as indicated. In contrast, MHC class II molecules consist of noncovalently associated α (32-kd) and β (28-kd) chains, both of which are anchored within the membrane. The overall domain organization of the two molecules is highly similar, however. Glycosylation sites on both molecules are indicated.

A major focus of research on HLA and RA has been to determine precisely which HLA alleles are most strongly associated with disease. This effort has been a massive enterprise carried out by many groups (13–17). The majority, but not unanimous, scientific opinion (see below) is that the HLA-DRB1 locus is highly likely to contain alleles that are somehow directly involved in disease pathogenesis.

The HLA-DRB1 molecule is a cell-surface glycoprotein formed by the noncovalent association of an invariant DR α chain with a highly polymorphic DR β chain. As is typical for all HLA class II isotypes, both the α and β chains are inserted into the cell membrane, in contrast to the situation for HLA class I molecules, where only the α chain possesses a transmembrane segment (see Figure 10.2 for schematic). Following on the pioneering x-ray crystallographic studies of Bjorkman et al. (18), an enormous amount of detailed information on the structure of these molecules has accumulated since the late 1980s. Figure 10.3 shows the x-ray crystallographic structure of a DRB1 molecule with a bound peptide interacting with a T-cell receptor. However, a better way to understand these structures, along with their interactions with T-cell receptor, is to use Web sites that permit rotation of the molecule in three dimensions (for example: http://www.rcsb.org/pdb; see also http://www.imtech.res.in/raghava/mhcbn/tsmhc.html).

HLA molecules are encoded by a highly polymorphic gene family. For example, in the last 2 decades, more than 100 allelic variants of the HLA-DRB1 locus have been described. A compilation of these allelic polymorphisms can be found at http://www.ebi.ac.uk/imgt/hla/. The majority of these polymorphisms lead to amino acid substitutions that are clustered in and around the peptide binding cleft of HLA molecules. These structural polymorphisms are responsible for the functional differences attributed to different HLA alleles with regard to immune recognition. It is assumed, therefore, that these polymorphisms also regulate susceptibility to autoimmune diseases.

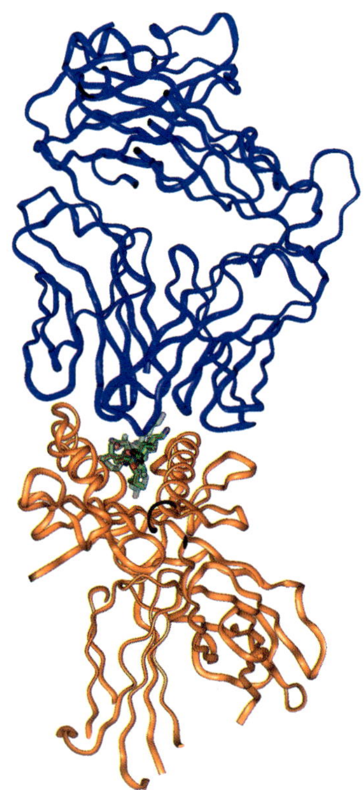

Figure 10.3. Ribbon diagram derived from the three-dimensional crystal structure of the trimolecular complex of a human α/β–T-cell receptor (*top, green*), influenza hemagglutinin antigen peptide, and the major histocompatibility complex class II molecule, HLA-DR1 (115). Note that the peptide is contained with the peptide binding cleft of the HLA-DR molecule. The polymorphisms associated with the shared epitope are located on the α helical rim (DRB1 chain) of the peptide binding cleft.

HLA-DRB1 ASSOCIATIONS WITH RHEUMATOID ARTHRITIS: SHARED EPITOPE HYPOTHESIS

The DRB1*0401 allele [corresponding to the Dw4 type in Stastny's original reports (8,9)] was the first HLA polymorphism to be associated with RA. Numerous studies have generally confirmed that this allele is the most strongly associated with RA, at least in white populations (13,14,17). However, several other HLA-DRB1 alleles have also been associated with RA, although the strength of these associations varies (16,17,19). It is now widely accepted that the following alleles are the major contributors to RA risk at the DRB1 locus: DRB1*0401, -0404, -0405, -0101, and -1001. In addition, minor variants of these alleles, as well as others (DRB1*1402), may also contribute to susceptibility. All of these risk alleles share a common sequence, as shown in Table 10.1. This predicted amino acid sequence ^{70}Q or K-R-R-A-A^{74} has been termed the *shared epitope* (20). (In the case of the DRB1*1001 risk allele, one amino acid varies from this consensus by a conservative change, with an R at position 70.) This structural feature is located on the α helical portion of

TABLE 10.1. Amino Acid Substitutions Comprising the Shared Epitope at Positions 70–74 of DRB1 Alleles Associated with Rheumatoid Arthritis

	Amino Acid Position				
DRB1 Alleles	70	71	72	73	74
0101	Gln	Arg	Arg	Ala	Ala
0401	—	Lys	—	—	—
0404	—	—	—	—	—
0405	—	—	—	—	—
0408	—	—	—	—	—
1402	—	—	—	—	—
1001	Arg	—	—	—	—

the DR β chain in a position where it may influence both peptide binding and T-cell receptor interactions with the DRB1 molecule.

A number of different hypotheses have been advanced to explain the shared epitope association with RA (21,22). Two of these follow directly from knowledge about the role of HLA molecules in antigen presentation and immune regulation. Thus, it has been suggested that a particular peptide antigen, or set of related antigens, may be involved in the initiation or propagation of RA, and that shared epitope–positive DRB1 alleles possess a unique, or enhanced, ability to bind or present these peptides to the immune system (21). It has been difficult to address this hypothesis directly because the identity of these putative disease-causing peptide antigens is unknown. A second hypothesis posits that these risk alleles regulate the formation of the peripheral T-cell repertoire by acting to select for particular T-cell receptors during thymic selection (22). There is elegant experimental evidence in humans to support a role for DR4 alleles in shaping the peripheral T-cell receptor (23). However, it is unclear whether this effect on the T-cell receptor repertoire is responsible for disease risk. In general, attempts to define the T-cell repertoire involved in RA pathogenesis have yielded complex results that are difficult to interpret.

Several alternative hypotheses have also been proposed to explain the shared epitope association with RA. Roudier and colleagues noted the similarity of the shared epitope sequence to viral antigens (24), leading to further proposals of molecular mimicry as a mechanism for the disease association with the shared epitope (25). Murine and human studies have provided evidence that peptides derived from MHC molecules can act as nominal antigen and can play a role in thymic selection and tolerance induction (26,27). There is also evidence that the shared epitope may influence patterns of intracellular trafficking of HLA-DR molecules (28). However, these observations have not yet been supported by definitive experimentation that shows how the shared epitope is actually involved in RA susceptibility.

The shared epitope hypothesis itself been questioned, with some investigators proposing a direct role for HLA-DQ polymorphisms (29,30), in part based on studies in transgenic mice (31). As can be seen in Figure 10.1, the HLA-DQ α and β chains are encoded just centromeric to DRB1, and alleles at this locus are in strong linkage disequilibrium (LD) with DRB1 alleles. (See below for a discussion of LD.) The strong LD between the DR and DQ loci makes it difficult to tease apart the effects of DR versus DQ based solely on population genetic studies; the arguments for a DQ effect generally depend on showing the enrichment of relatively rare genotypes in the RA patient group compared with controls. Overall, a primary role for DQ alleles is not supported by large HLA association studies that have examined this issue (32).

Regardless of whether HLA-DQ alleles are involved in RA susceptibility, it is clear that the shared epitope hypothesis is not a complete explanation for the HLA associations with RA. This has been shown by formal analysis (33) but also is evident from the fact that not all shared epitope–positive alleles carry the same degree of genetic risk, and the strength of the association varies in different populations. In general, DRB1*0101 alleles carry lower levels of relative risk for RA than the DRB1*0401 and 0404 alleles (14), and, yet, DRB1*0101 is the major risk allele in some ethnic groups (34,35). In contrast, the shared epitope itself does not appear to associate with RA in African-American and some Hispanic populations (36,37). Furthermore, certain combinations of DRB1 alleles carry especially high risk, as originally observed by Nepom et al. (38). Thus, the combination of DRB1*0401 with *0404 carries a relative risk of more than 30 in white populations (14). This value compares with relative risk values in the range of 4 or 5 for either allele alone. Some of these relationships are summarized in Table 10.2. It is unclear whether these interactive effects are mediated by the HLA-DR molecules themselves or reflect the action of other genes on these haplotypes. Genetic evidence suggests that the latter explanation is likely for at least some haplotypes (see below).

TABLE 10.2. Genotype Relative Risks of DRB1 Genotypes for Rheumatoid Arthritis

DRB1 Genotype	Relative Risk	*p* Value
0101/DRX	2.3	10^{-3}
0401/DRX	4.7	10^{-12}
0404/DRX	5.0	10^{-9}
0101/0401	6.4	10^{-4}
0401/0404	31.3	10^{-33}

Adapted from Hall FC, Weeks DE, Camilleri JP, et al. Influence of the HLA-DRB1 locus on susceptibility and severity in rheumatoid arthritis. *QJM* 1996;89(11):821–829.

EVIDENCE FOR ADDITIONAL SUSCEPTIBILITY GENES WITHIN MAJOR HISTOCOMPATIBILITY COMPLEX

Given the importance of tumor necrosis factor (TNF) in the pathogenesis of RA and the fact that TNF-α and -β are encoded within the MHC, it was logical for investigators to explore the possibility that TNF polymorphisms might explain some of the MHC associations with RA. Early studies were able to demonstrate evidence of TNF associations with RA (39). However, in the absence of full information on the MHC sequence and gene organization, it was unclear to what extent this association reflected LD with the known HLA-DRB1 susceptibility alleles. The role of TNF polymorphisms in RA susceptibility remains unsettled, particularly with regard to possible influences on disease severity and outcome (40). Nevertheless, it is clear that the central portion of the MHC contains susceptibility genes that are distinct from the DRB1 locus.

Beginning with the report of Mulcahy et al. in 1996 (41), convincing evidence has accumulated that genetic associations with RA in the central portion of the MHC, including TNF, cannot be explained by LD with the known RA-associated DRB1 alleles (42). In fact, it appears that these associations occur most commonly on a DR3 haplotype (41). Of note, the DR3 allele (DRB1*0301) has no similarity to the shared epitope–positive DR alleles and is not itself associated with RA. A comprehensive analysis using 54 markers distributed throughout the HLA complex has led to the conclusion that one or more genes contained within the central portion of the MHC contribute to risk for RA (43). These genes are contained within a DNA segment that is commonly part of a highly conserved DR3 haplotype in many white populations. This haplotype is commonly referred to as the *A1-B8-DR3*, or the *8.1*, haplotype (44).

The A1-B8-DR3 (8.1) haplotype is a striking example of a phenomenon known as LD. Briefly, *LD* refers to the fact that alleles at adjacent loci frequently associate with each other nonrandomly. LD is a characteristic feature of genetic variation in human populations and is particularly prominent within the human MHC (45). For example, in some white populations, the A1 allele is present in approximately 17% of individuals, whereas the B8 allele is present in approximately 12%. If the A1 and B8 alleles were randomly associated in the population, one would expect to find them together in the same individual with a frequency of $0.12 \times 0.17 \sim 0.02$, or approximately 2% of the population. In contrast, they are commonly found together in approximately 10% of northern European whites. The HLA-A and HLA-B genes are more than 1 million base pairs apart (12), yet these particular alleles are found together on the same haplotype much more frequently than expected by chance.

The phenomenon of LD may be due to several different causes. First, the genome is discontinuous with respect to its ability to undergo meiotic recombination; as such, certain segments of the genome tend to remain together as blocks of DNA, even after multiple generations (many rounds of meiotic recombination). This block-like structure of the genome is currently the subject of extensive investigation (46,47). These blocks of conserved haplotypes may be quite variable in length, from a few thousand base pairs to a million base pairs or more in the case of the MHC (48). Overall, the average extent of LD in the human genome frequently extends to 50,000 to 60,000 base pairs (49,50), although this estimate should be viewed as preliminary and may vary among different populations. In some instances, LD may also be due to the recent introduction of founder haplotypes into a population and recent admixture of different ethnic groups, or, alternatively, may reflect selection for certain combinations of alleles at adjacent loci (50). It is likely that all of these factors contribute to the extensive degree of LD observed with the human MHC, at least for some haplotypes (44,48).

Whatever the reason for the high prevalence of the A1-B8-DR3 haplotype in white populations, it is now apparent that one or more genes on this haplotype contribute to risk for RA. These risk genes appear to be contained with a central segment of approximately 500 kilobases (43). This segment contains the TNF-α and -β as well as several complement genes (Fig. 10.1), as well as numerous other genes of potential interest (see http://www.sanger.ac.uk/HGP/Chr6/MHC.shtml). It has been proposed that a gene in the IκB family, IκBL, is the RA risk gene in this region, at least in the Japanese population (51). It remains to be seen whether this observation holds up in other populations.

The fact that one or more genes on the A1-B8-DR3 haplotype contribute to risk for RA is relevant to understanding the pathogenesis of RA. This haplotype is known to be associated with a number of autoimmune disorders, including immunoglobulin deficiency, celiac disease, and dermatitis herpetiformis, among others (44). The A1-B8-DR3 haplotype is also associated with subtle immunologic alterations, many of which are suggestive of immunodeficiency, even in normal individuals. Thus, normal individuals with this haplotype have lower lymphocyte levels (52), lower antibody responses (53,54), lower levels of Th2 cytokine production (55), and defective Fc receptor function (56). In contrast, some reports suggest a higher level of TNF production (57). It will be of interest for future genetic studies to identify which genes on the A1-B8-DR3 haplotype are responsible for these various immunologic traits.

Finally, there may be additional RA susceptibility genes in the class I region of the MHC. The dense mapping studies of Jawaheer et al. provide evidence that a region between HLA-A and HLA-C is associated with RA when present on certain DRB1*0404 haplotypes (43). This is of interest in view of the high relative risks associated with DRB1*0401/0404 compound heterozygosity, as noted above (Table 10.2). Conceivably, complementation between DRB1 alleles and genes in the class I region could account for the especially high risk of this genotype. Weyand and colleagues have also provided evidence for an HLA class I genetic effect in rheumatoid vasculitis (58).

GENETIC DETERMINANTS OUTSIDE OF THE MAJOR HISTOCOMPATIBILITY COMPLEX

It has been estimated that the MHC contributes up to 50% of the total genetic risk for RA (59,60). Genome screens (61,62) have confirmed that the HLA region makes the single largest contribution to the relative risk to siblings (λ_S). This contribution can be estimated by calculating the genotypic risk to siblings due to HLA (λ_{HLA}), which is approximately 1.8 for white populations. Assuming that the total (λ_S) is approximately 5, this leaves a λ of approximately 2.7 (5/1.8) to account for the effects of all other genes combined, assuming that a multiplicative interaction among these genes contributes to the total risk to siblings.

The identification of the non-MHC genes involved in RA is challenging. In the early 1990s, there was optimism that the mapping and sequencing of the human genome would lead to the rapid identification of genes involved in a variety of complex autoimmune, inflammatory, psychiatric, and cardiovascular disorders (63). The experience during that decade has been sobering, and some commentators have expressed outright skepticism concerning the feasibility of positional approaches to mapping complex diseases (64). However, there have been some notable successes (65,66), and there is reason for optimism that positional approaches to gene identification will bear fruit.

The most common method of searching for disease genes in complex disorders has been an approach known as *affected sibling pair* (ASP) analysis (67). This method detects the presence of linkage within families in which multiple siblings are affected with disease. ASP analysis has several advantages over traditional linkage analysis. First, it only uses genetic information from affected individuals and ignores unaffected siblings. This feature is desirable when mapping genes that have low penetrance. Low penetrance means that lack of disease in an individual is a poor indicator of whether an individual is a gene carrier, and this makes these individuals relatively uninformative for linkage analysis. Second, ASP analysis does not require commitment to a particular model (i.e., recessive or dominant); this is an advantage inasmuch as the model is unknown for most complex traits.

In its simplest form, ASP analysis addresses a simple question for a given genetic marker: Do the ASPs share marker alleles more frequently than expected by chance, as predicted by mendelian segregation? This analysis must be done with a large number of families to achieve statistically significant evidence for increased sharing at a marker locus. The basic approach is illustrated in Figure 10.4. In this family, two siblings are affected with RA; the firstborn sibling (sibling 1) has inherited alleles 1 and 3 at a marker locus, X. By the laws of mendelian inheritance, sibling 2 has a 25% chance of inheriting these

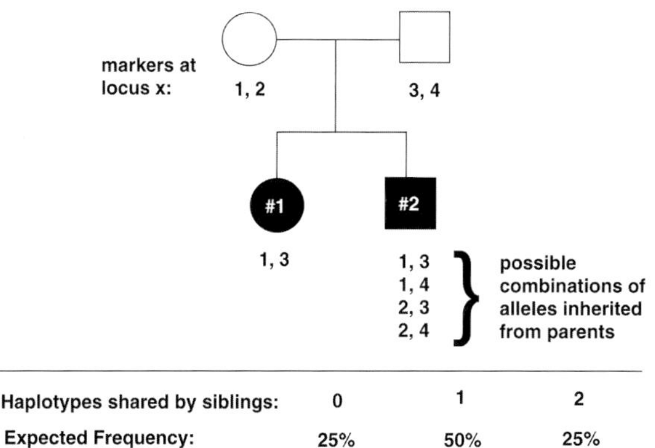

Figure 10.4. A nuclear family with two affected children (affected sibling pair). The possible distribution of alleles at an autosomal locus, X, is shown for sibling 2, along with the predicted frequency of shared haplotypes among the sibs. Such families can be used to detect linkage using affected sibling pair analysis (see text).

TABLE 10.3. Chromosomal Regions Giving *p* Values <.05 in a Combined Screen of 512 North American Rheumatoid Arthritis Consortium Families: Sibling Pair Analysis (SIBPAL)

Locus	Distance (cM)	Screen 1 *p* Values	Screen 2 *p* Values	Combined Screen (*p* Values)	Lambda
Chromosome 1					
D1S1631	136.9	.0141	.0175	.0011	1.22
D1S2141	233.4	.1905	.0701	.0487	1.096
D1S549	239.7	.2477	.0264	.0318	1.133
D1S235[a]	254.6	.0048	.1256	.003	1.151
Chromosome 2					
D2S1353	164.5	.3287	.026	.0453	1.071
Chromosome 4					
D4S2361	93.5	.0639	.0565	.0141	1.05
D4S1647	104.9	.0001	.9198	.0436	1.056
Chromosome 5					
D5S807	19.0	.0789	.1227	.0336	1.078
D5S817	22.9	.0663	.174	.0421	1.073
D5S1462	105.3	.0079	.2887	.0176	1.175
D5S2501	116.9	.0559	.1895	.0382	1.069
Chromosome 6					
D6S1959	34.2	.0135	.0029	1.99×10^{-4}	1.699
D6S265	44.4	2.39×10^{-6}	5.68×10^{-6}	5.33×10^{-11}	1.807
D6S1629	44.9	2.97×10^{-5}	2.76×10^{-7}	5.01×10^{-11}	1.811
D6S273	47.7	3.36×10^{-6}	3.66×10^{-7}	4.19×10^{-12}	1.83
D6S291	49.5	.0013	6.93×10^{-6}	9.90×10^{-8}	1.822
D6S389	53.8	.0126	1.43×10^{-5}	7.99×10^{-7}	1.406
D6S2427	53.8	.031	.0007	1.46×10^{-4}	1.396
D6S1017	63.3	.2764	.0067	.0197	1.503
D6S2410	73.1	.2844	.0004	.0028	1.347
D6S1021[b]	112.2	.0075	.1892	.0083	1.136
Chromosome 8					
D8S264	.7	.0804	.0329	.0115	1.225
D8S277	8.3	.0088	.3713	.026	1.242
D8S1110	67.3	.0187	.0855	.0067	1.088
D8S373	164.5	.0084	.3234	.0224	1.101
Chromosome 9					
D9S1121	44.3	.4972	.001	.01303	1.193
Chromosome 10					
D10S1221	75.6	.1784	.0002	.0006	1.176
D10S1225	80.8	.6662	.0038	.0461	1.149
Chromosome 11					
ATA34E08	33.0	.2418	.0205	.0292	1.087
Chromosome 12					
D12S373	36.1	.0031	.6866	.0499	1.129
D12S1042	48.7	.1247	.0454	.0216	1.183
D12S398	68.2	.0051	.1429	.0048	1.11
D12S1052	83.2	.0227	.2192	.0266	1.041
Chromosome 14					
D14S742[a]	12.5	.1943	.0524	.0433	1.024
Chromosome 16					
D16S403[a]	43.9	.0042	.2083	.0076	1.192
Chromosome 17					
D17S1298	10.7	.0053	.0933	.0031	1
Chromosome 18					
D18S877	54.4	.0635	.0962	.0228	1.128
D18S535	64.5	.1172	.0748	.0309	1.18
D18S858	80.4	.0433	.0098	.002	1.233
D18S1357[c]	88.6	.2631	.0472	.0494	1.12

[a]Indicates nominal (p <.05) evidence of linkage was also observed in a United Kingdom genome screen of 182 affected sibling pair families (70) within 15 cM of this marker.
[b]Indicates "suggestive" (p = .0007) evidence of linkage was also observed in a United Kingdom genome screen of 182 affected sibling pair families (70) within 15 cM of this marker.
[c]Indicates nominal (p <.01) evidence of linkage was also observed in the European Consortium for RA Families genome screen of 261 affected sibling pair families (61) within 15 cM of this marker.
Adapted from Jawaheer D, Seldin MF, Amos CI, et al. Screening the genome for rheumatoid arthritis susceptibility genes: a replication study and combined analysis of 512 multicase families. *Arthritis Rheum* 2003;48(4):906–916.

same two alleles and also has a 25% chance of inheriting neither of these alleles (i.e., sibling 2 inherits 2,4 and shares nothing with sibling 1 at locus X). By a similar reasoning, there is a 50% chance that these two siblings will share one allele in common. This 25:50:25 distribution of sharing 0, 1, or 2 haplotypes is expected if there is no linkage between the disease and the marker locus. However, if a gene that lies very near to the marker locus is involved in disease risk, a significant deviation toward increased sharing among affected siblings will be observed. By examining large numbers of ASPs in this manner, one can develop statistical evidence for linkage using a standard χ^2 analysis, with the null hypothesis being that there is no increased sharing at the marker locus. In general, for an effective genome-wide screen for ASP analysis, at least 300 to 400 markers are required. This means that markers are spaced at intervals of approximately 10 million base pairs across the genome. A more detailed discussion of ASP analysis and related approaches, can be found elsewhere (67,68).

There have been four major genome screens for RA susceptibility genes using ASP families in white populations, each using several hundred ASPs (61,62,69,70). In addition, a smaller study (41 families) has been performed in the Japanese population (71). The first of these genome screens was done in the late 1990s by Cornelis and his colleagues (61) in the European Consortium for RA Families (ECRAF). The results on a total of 261 sibling pair families confirmed that the largest single genetic effect was in the MHC (λ_{HLA} = 1.8) but that numerous other chromosomal regions exhibited some evidence of linkage, with regions on chromosomes 3 and 18 of particular interest. None of these regions achieved accepted levels of significance for definite linkage. Definite evidence for linkage on a genome-wide screen generally requires significance levels of $p = 2.2 \times 10^{-5}$ or better (72).

Subsequently, groups working in the United Kingdom at the University of Manchester and the United States have performed three additional genome screens (62,69,70). Two of these genome screens have been performed in the United States by the North American Rheumatoid Arthritis Consortium (NARAC), and a recent combined analysis of 512 ASP families has been published (69). Again, even with this large combined family collection, definite evidence for linkage outside the MHC has not been achieved. Table 10.3 summarizes the results from this analysis for each chromosomal region that achieved $p < .05$ in support of increased sharing among these ASP (total of 581 independent sibling pairs). Note that multiple regions exhibit evidence of linkage, with six markers achieving significance levels of $p < .005$, on chromosomes 1p (D1S1631), 1q41-43 (D1S235), 10q21.1 (D1S1221), 12q12 (D12S398), 17p13 (D17S1298), and 18q21.2 (D18S858). In contrast to this rather modest evidence of linkage, marker D6S272 within the MHC on chromosome 6p21 displays definite linkage, with $p = 4.19 \times 10^{-12}$.

A comparison of these results with the British and ECRAF genome screens is informative. Evidence for linkage to 1q41-43 has been observed in all studies, and the 18q linkage has been observed in the ECRAF study (61). Interestingly, a candidate region on chromosome 17q is being pursued by Worthington and colleagues at the University of Manchester (73), but linkage to this region was not replicated in the second NARAC screen (69), nor was it reported in the ECRAF study. Other regions exhibit varying degrees of overlap between the various studies, and some of these are indicated in Table 10.3.

This pattern of partial replication of modest evidence for linkage outside the MHC is similar to the experience in type 1 diabetes (74). The ASP analysis in type 1 diabetes has revealed definite linkage to the MHC, with additional modest evidence of linkage regions on other chromosomes. There is a variable degree of replication among different studies (74,75). This variability has led to a major debate in the genetics community about the proper interpretation of these results. The skeptical view emphasizes the occurrence of type 1 error. Undoubtedly, false-positive linkage results account for some of the data. However, it is also likely that none of these studies achieve a sample size that is adequate to detect definite linkage, since each individual genetic region is likely to confer only modest risk. Power calculations in studies of diabetes suggest that several thousand ASPs will be required to achieve definite evidence of linkage (75). This is clearly not feasible for RA at the present time. However, the obvious way to increase the power of the ASP analysis in RA is to combine the data from the various studies; this may lead to more convincing evidence for linkage for at least a few chromosomal regions outside the MHC (76).

Although the results of genome screens in RA are far from definitive, it is of interest that a number of these candidate regions overlap with regions that have been implicated in other autoimmune diseases. This overlap was first pointed out by Becker and colleagues (77) and is consistent with the aggregation of certain autoimmune diseases in families. Thus, RA, autoimmune thyroid disease, type 1 diabetes, and possibly systemic lupus erythematosus may exhibit familial clustering (78). Presumably, this familial clustering reflects in part an overlap in the genetic susceptibility genes involved in these disorders. The presence of linkage at 1q41-43 (as well as other regions) in both systemic lupus erythematosus and RA may be a result of this overlap (79). Likewise, linkage to 18q21 has been reported in both Graves' disease (80) and type 1 diabetes (81), as well as in RA (61,69). It is important to keep in mind that this overlap in linkage results does not necessarily reflect the involvement of the same genes in these diseases.

MOVING FROM LINKAGE TO GENE IDENTIFICATION: NEW APPROACHES TO ASSOCIATION STUDIES

From a practical standpoint, it is not reasonable to require linkage evidence at the $p < 2.2 \times 10^{-5}$ level of significance before moving on to additional studies of particular chromosomal regions. The decision to move forward with association studies in a particular region is complex and to some extent reflects the biases of the research team on the likelihood of success. In the case of the linkage on 18q, for example, the replication of modest evidence for linkage in three of four studies and the presence of a compelling candidate gene in the region (RANK) has led the NARAC investigators (69) to pursue this region in detail. Likewise, the 17q linkage region is of particular interest because of overlap with linkage results in insulin-dependent diabetes mellitus and the existence of a syntenic region in the rat that appears to control susceptibility to experimentally induced arthritis (73).

Whatever chromosomal region is chosen for study, the experimental approach must initially take the form of an association study. A major advantage of association studies is that they have much better statistical power for detecting genetic effects (68). Traditionally, most genetic association studies have been done using a case control design with one, or a few, genetic markers. However, two additional approaches to association are becoming widely used and appear to have significant advantages. First, association can be done using family-based controls, as explained below. Secondly, as alluded to previously in the discussion of the MHC, the analysis of haplotypes, as opposed to single markers, offers more power and efficiency.

To avoid the confounding effects of population stratification in case control studies, family-based controls can be used for association studies. Consider the family shown in Figure 10.5. The affected child carries DR4 and DR3, each of which is inherited from one parent. The laws of mendelian inheritance require

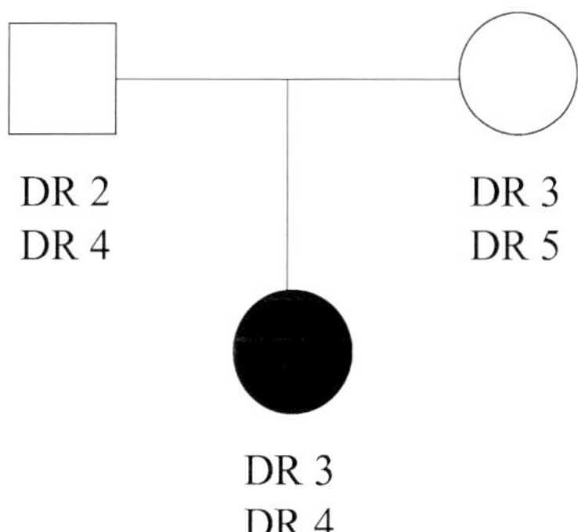

Figure 10.5. A nuclear family with one affected child. The noninherited haplotypes can be thought of as forming a genotype for a control individual (see text).

that one DR haplotype from each parent is not inherited by any given offspring, in this example, DR2 in the father and DR5 in the mother. These two noninherited haplotypes can be thought of as forming a genotype for a control individual. In this manner, issues of population stratification are eliminated because both patients and controls are sampled from the identical (parental) gene pool. This approach to disease association was originally proposed by Falk and Rubinstein and was called the *haplotype relative risk* method (82). Its validity depends on a number of assumptions, including that the genetic marker under study does not influence mating preference or the production of gametes. Because of the potential for recombination between the marker locus and the disease locus, the haplotype relative risk may underestimate the true relative risk. Nevertheless, this disadvantage (implying the need for a somewhat larger study population to achieve statistic significance) is minor, compared to the elimination of artifactual results due to population stratification.

A popular extension of this approach is termed the *transmission disequilibrium test* (83,84). Again, consider the family in Figure 10.5. For a given heterozygous parent (such as the father carrying DR2,4), there is a .5 probability that any given allele—for example, DR4—will be transmitted to the child. Thus, if the DR4 allele has no bearing on disease risk, the probability of transmission (T) to an affected child is equal to the probability of nontransmission (NT). This can be stated simply as $P(T \mid D) = P(NT \mid D)$, where D indicates the presence of disease in the offspring. However, if the allele being examined is associated with disease risk, then $P(T \mid D) > P(NT \mid D)$. If large numbers of heterozygous parents with affected offspring are examined, transmission disequilibrium testing can establish an association between disease and the test allele compared with the (noninherited) control alleles.

Since the late 1990s, there has been renewed interest in the importance of defining haplotypes to carry out association studies, whether case control or family based. The existence of common haplotypes in the population is a direct reflection of linkage disequilibrium, as discussed above. It is now apparent that the overall diversity of the human genome is best described as a patchwork of haplotype blocks, with each block extending from a few thousand base pairs to hundreds of thousands of base pairs, depending on the region (85–87). In some cases, such as the MHC, these haplotype blocks may extend to even larger distances (*vide supra*). Furthermore, for many regions, it appears that most of the haplotypic diversity is contained within a relatively small number of haplotype variants within each block. Thus, for a well-studied region on chromosome 5q31, between 2 and 4 haplotypes account for 90% of the variability in the population for a particular haplotype block (86). It is unclear whether this pattern will hold up for all regions of the genome in all populations.

There are several practical consequences of this pattern of block-like haplotype variation in the genome. First, this pattern implies that the majority of the genetic variation among humans is contained within a limited (although still large) number of relatively conserved blocks of haplotypes. Thus, most of the differences between two individuals can be described by characterizing perhaps several hundred thousand blocks of DNA. In this sense, the average interindividual human genetic diversity of 0.1% can be conceived of as a patchwork of large blocks of DNA, with more limited diversity within each block, rather than consisting of 3 million totally uncorrelated sequence variations. This patchwork simplifies the problem of correlating genetic variation with phenotype by at least an order of magnitude and makes positional gene mapping by genome-wide association a technically approachable problem (88), particularly if one is focusing on a limited number of regions where there is already some evidence of linkage.

One possible negative aspect of this patchwork quality of human genome variation is that once a trait is associated with a particular haplotype block, it may be difficult to determine exactly which gene in the block is responsible for the association. The MHC is a good example of this problem, since the haplotype blocks in the MHC are quite large. For example, as discussed above, it is a major challenge to determine the genes responsible for the immune phenotypes associated with the A1-B8-DR3 haplotype, since all the genetic variants on this haplotype tend to be present together on the same chromosomal segment (44).

COMMON DISEASE—COMMON VARIANT?

In terms of using haplotype blocks for gene mapping by association, there is a critical assumption that underlies this approach. The disease alleles must be reasonably common if they are to be detected as part of these common haplotype blocks. These alleles individually must have relatively low penetrance; otherwise, autoimmunity would be more commonly familial. This common disease–common variant assumption is a topic of great debate in the genetics community (89,90). The linkage signals seen in the genome screens may actually reflect the influence of quite rare alleles with relatively high penetrance in just a few families. If this is the case, it is unlikely that looking for associations with common haplotypes will lead to the identification of these rare alleles. At present, there is really no way to tell whether the genetic risk for autoimmunity is distributed among common low-penetrance genes or uncommon, moderately penetrant genes.

It appears likely that haplotype blocks are a typical feature of genome variation, and, as such, may provide a powerful tool for mapping genes by association, eventually on a genome-wide basis. The technologies for high-throughput single-nucleotide polymorphism typing are evolving rapidly, and it is not unreasonable to expect that, within a few years, an individual can be typed for several hundred thousand single-nucleotide polymorphisms in a few days (91). In addition, strategies for pooling DNA samples are becoming more robust, so that the frequency of large numbers of single-nucleotide polymorphism alleles can be compared quickly among populations of DNA samples (92).

CANDIDATE GENES: END GAME OF GENE IDENTIFICATION

Association studies of candidate genes have been the standard method for investigating susceptibility genes in RA for the last 25 years, beginning with the early HLA associations (10). In general, particular candidate genes are selected because they make sense in terms of the current concepts of disease pathogenesis. Thus, cytokine genes, apoptosis genes, and immunologically relevant cell-surface molecules have been popular targets for study. At present, in addition to considering the biology of candidate genes, investigators also take into account the position of the gene on the genome in making a decision about whether to pursue a full-scale association study. In addition, there is now much more (and rapidly accumulating) information on the number of polymorphisms within any candidate gene, although the functional significance of these polymorphisms is largely unknown for most genes.

Given the large number of plausible candidate genes and even larger number of polymorphisms in the genome, an extremely large number of association studies can be reasonably pursued. This leads to a statistical problem in the interpretation of results, known as *multiple testing*. If one uses the standard cutoff of $p < .05$, then, by chance, 1 out of 20 studies will meet criteria for rejecting the null hypothesis of no association, assuming the a priori probability of association is equivalent for each test. An analysis of candidate gene association studies has shown that the first published reports almost always overestimate the strength of these associations, and subsequent reports often fail to confirm the original findings (93). There is a natural tendency for positive results to be submitted for publication, whereas negative findings may not be written up or published. For this reason, it is prudent for an investigator to include a replication of the original association in the first manuscript. This often means finding collaborators with additional populations to study. Assuming that many genetic effects will be due to common variants, "true" associations are likely to be weak associations with modest relative risks. If expanding the sample size adds to evidence for association, it adds to confidence in the biologic significance of the findings, even if the genetic effects are modest. This has been emphasized by metaanalysis of published association studies in a variety of complex diseases (94).

As noted above, the chromosomal location of a gene can be an important criteria for pursuing a particular candidate gene. If a particular haplotype block shows association with disease, there are likely to be several, or many, genes in the region that are candidates for the disease gene. Indeed, a major advantage of taking a positional approach to gene identification is the elimination of the bias imposed by assumptions about pathogenesis and disease pathways. Thus, an extensive evaluation of all the genes in the associated haplotype is necessary without preconceived notions about the identity of the disease gene. This evaluation will necessarily extend to identifying the function of polymorphisms and developing experiments that address the biology of the various genes and the associated polymorphisms.

USE OF POSITIONAL INFORMATION IN SELECTING CANDIDATE GENES

The absence of linkage evidence in a particular chromosomal region does not mean that genes in that region do not contribute to disease risk. Compared with association methods, ASP analysis and other linkage-based approaches have rather modest statistical power to detect genetic effects in complex disorders, and it is as difficult to exclude a region as it is to prove that it is involved in disease risk (68). Therefore, the absence of linkage evidence should not discourage a well-thought-out candidate gene association study. Most candidate genes studies are unconfirmed, as emphasized by a recent compilation of cytokine gene association studies in autoimmune diseases (95). There are currently no confirmed and definitive genetic associations with RA outside the MHC.

In terms of cytokines and their receptors, association studies of interleukin-3 (IL-3), IL-4, migration inhibitory factor (MIF), and TNF-R2 are of interest. Many of these studies are showing associations only when certain subgroups or disease severity are considered. For example, the association with an IL-3 promoter polymorphism has only been reported in the Japanese population and is strongest in women with an early age of onset (96). In addition, because of linkage disequilibrium, IL-3 itself may not explain the association, since other candidate genes are in the region, such as TGF-β_1 and leukocyte-derived chemotaxin 2 (97). Several reports suggest a role for a VNTR (*v*ariable *n*umber of *t*andem *r*epeats) polymorphism in IL-4 in regulating disease outcome (98,99). The functional effect of this polymorphism has not been demonstrated. In addition, IL-4 lies in the same gene cluster on 5q, as does IL-3. MIF promoter polymorphisms have received attention as a candidate susceptibility genotype in juvenile polyarthritis (100–102), and a study in adult RA suggests a role in disease outcome (103). MIF has numerous biologic activities, one of which is to act as counter-regulator of glucocorticoid action (104). It appears that promoter polymorphisms that lead to high levels of MIF are associated with relative resistance to steroid treatment in the setting of juvenile polyarthritis (105). Finally, two studies have reported an association between TNF-R2 polymorphisms and familial RA (106,107). No associations were observed in sporadic disease, suggesting the existence of subtle differences in disease mechanisms in the familial versus sporadic disease populations.

Very few association studies have examined interactions between candidate genes and other background genes, or the environment. This was formally tested in the IL-3 study in the Japanese population, but with negative results. An interaction between the MHC and killer cell immunoglobulin-like receptor polymorphisms has been reported in rheumatoid vasculitis (58). In addition, Mattey et al. have reported an interaction between smoking (a known environmental risk factor for RA) and the null allele at GSTM-1 (108). GSTM-1 is involved in the detoxification of polycyclic hydrocarbons present in cigarette smoke and is thus a reasonable candidate gene. The difficulty with examining these interactive effects (gene–gene or gene–environment) is that much larger samples sizes are required to detect significant associations. Nevertheless, it is likely that such interactions will be very important for ultimately understanding and confirming these modest genetic effects.

CONCLUSION

Although genes in inflammatory and immunologic pathways are clearly leading candidates for investigation, it is important to consider other areas, such as the neuroendocrine regulation of inflammation (109,110) and the regulation of bone and cartilage metabolism (111). Indeed, it may be possible to define intermediate phenotypes in these systems that can be used to define the genetic influences of candidate genes more clearly. In addition, animal models continue to raise new and unexpected pathways of disease. For example, it has been reported that low production of reactive oxygen species may be a risk factor for inflammatory arthritis in the rat, due to a structural polymorphism in the Ncf1 gene encoding p47phox, a component of the membrane oxidase complex (112). This observation has raised the possibility that signaling, rather than tissue destruction, by reactive oxygen species is involved in disease pathogenesis. Ultimately, it will be the combination of these kinds of novel observations on biology with positional mapping approaches that will allow identification of the genes that control disease susceptibility and outcome. In addition, new techniques such as DNA microarrays and proteomic analysis will likely contribute to this endeavor (113,114). Defining the genetics of RA will be a highly collaborative effort, involving not just geneticists, but statisticians, immunologists, cell biologists, and knowledgeable clinicians, among many others.

ACKNOWLEDGMENTS

This work is supported by the National Institutes of Health (PKG: NO1-AR-7-2232, RO1-AR44222, and NO1-AR-1-2256) and by the Arthritis Foundation. I am grateful to Percio Gulko and Franak Batliwalla for discussions and critical review of the manuscript.

REFERENCES

1. Gregersen PK. Genetics of rheumatoid arthritis: confronting complexity. *Arthritis Res* 1999;1(1):37–44.
2. Risch N. Linkage strategies for genetically complex traits. I. Multilocus models. *Am J Hum Genet* 1990;46(2):222–228.
3. Vyse TJ, Todd JA. Genetic analysis of autoimmune disease. *Cell* 1996;85(3):311–318.
4. Seldin MF, Amos CI, Ward R, et al. The genetics revolution and the assault on rheumatoid arthritis. *Arthritis Rheum* 1999;42(6):1071–1079.

5. Silman AJ. Rheumatoid arthritis. In: Silman AJ, Hochberg MC, eds. *Epidemiology of the rheumatic diseases*. Oxford: Oxford University Press; 1993:7–68.
6. Gregersen PK. Discordance for autoimmunity in monozygotic twins. Are "identical" twins really identical? *Arthritis Rheum* 1993;36(9):1185–1192.
7. MacGregor AJ, Snieder H, Rigby AS, et al. Characterizing the quantitative genetic contribution to rheumatoid arthritis using data from twins. *Arthritis Rheum* 2000;43(1):30–37.
8. Stastny P. Mixed lymphocyte cultures in rheumatoid arthritis. *J Clin Invest* 1976;57(5):1148–1157.
9. Stastny P. HLA-D and Ia antigens in rheumatoid arthritis and systemic lupus erythematosus. *Arthritis Rheum* 1978;21[Suppl 5]:S139–S143.
10. Stastny P. Association of the B-cell alloantigen DRw4 with rheumatoid arthritis. *N Engl J Med* 1978;298(16):869–871.
11. Benacerraf B. Role of MHC gene products in immune regulation. *Science* 1981;212(4500):1229–1238.
12. The MHC Sequencing Consortium. Complete sequence and gene map of a human major histocompatibility complex. *Nature* 1999;401(6756):921–923.
13. Weyand CM, Hicok KC, Conn DL, et al. The influence of HLA-DRB1 genes on disease severity in rheumatoid arthritis. *Ann Intern Med* 1992;117(10):801–806.
14. Hall FC, Weeks DE, Camilleri JP, et al. Influence of the HLA-DRB1 locus on susceptibility and severity in rheumatoid arthritis. *QJM* 1996;89(11):821–829.
15. Moxley G, Cohen HJ. Genetic studies, clinical heterogeneity, and disease outcome studies in rheumatoid arthritis. *Rheum Dis Clin North Am* 2002;28(1):39–58.
16. Ollier W, Winchester R. The germline and somatic genetic basis for rheumatoid arthritis. *Curr Dir Autoimmun* 1999;1:166–193.
17. Nepom GT. Major histocompatibility complex-directed susceptibility to rheumatoid arthritis. *Adv Immunol* 1998;68:315–332.
18. Bjorkman PJ, Saper MA, Samraoui B. Structure of the human class I histocompatibility antigen, HLA-A2. *Nature* 1987;329(6139):506–512.
19. Gregersen PK. T-cell receptor-major histocompatibility complex genetic interactions in rheumatoid arthritis. *Rheum Dis Clin North Am* 1992;18(4):793–807.
20. Gregersen PK, Silver J, Winchester RJ. The shared epitope hypothesis. An approach to understanding the molecular genetics of susceptibility to rheumatoid arthritis. *Arthritis Rheum* 1987;30(11):1205–1213.
21. Buckner JH, Nepom GT. Genetics of rheumatoid arthritis: is there a scientific explanation for the human leukocyte antigen association? *Curr Opin Rheumatol* 2002;14(3):254–259.
22. Roudier J. Association of MHC and rheumatoid arthritis. Association of RA with HLA- DR4: the role of repertoire selection. *Arthritis Res* 2000;2(3):217–220.
23. Walser-Kuntz DR, Weyand CM, Weaver AJ, et al. Mechanisms underlying the formation of the T-cell receptor repertoire in rheumatoid arthritis. *Immunity* 1995;2(6):597–605.
24. Roudier J, Petersen J, Rhodes GH, et al. Susceptibility to rheumatoid arthritis maps to a T-cell epitope shared by the HLA-Dw4 DR beta-1 chain and the Epstein-Barr virus glycoprotein gp110. *Proc Natl Acad Sci U S A* 1989;86(13): 5104–5108.
25. Albani S, Keystone EC, Nelson JL, et al. Positive selection in autoimmunity: abnormal immune responses to a bacterial dnaJ antigenic determinant in patients with early rheumatoid arthritis. *Nat Med* 1995;1(5):448–452.
26. Roudier J, Sette A, Lamont A, et al. Tolerance to a self peptide from the third hypervariable region of the Es beta chain. Implications for molecular mimicry models of autoimmune disease. *Eur J Immunol* 1991;21(9):2063–2067.
27. Salvat S, Auger I, Rochelle L, et al. Tolerance to a self-peptide from the third hypervariable region of HLA DRB1*0401 in rheumatoid arthritis patients and normal subjects. *J Immunol* 1994;153(11):5321–5329.
28. Auger I, Toussirot E, Roudier J. HLA-DRB1 motifs and heat shock proteins in rheumatoid arthritis. *Int Rev Immunol* 1998;17(5–6):263–271.
29. Zanelli E, Huizinga TW, Guerne PA, et al. An extended HLA-DQ-DR haplotype rather than DRB1 alone contributes to RA predisposition. *Immunogenetics* 1998;48(6):394–401.
30. Zanelli E, Gonzalez-Gay MA, David CS. Could HLA-DRB1 be the protective locus in rheumatoid arthritis? *Immunol Today* 1995;16(6):274–278.
31. Taneja V, Griffiths MM, Luthra H, et al. Modulation of HLA-DQ-restricted collagen-induced arthritis by HLA-DRB1 polymorphism. *Int Immunol* 1998;10(10):1449–1457.
32. Milicic A, Lee D, Brown MA, et al. HLA-DR/DQ haplotype in rheumatoid arthritis: novel allelic associations in UK Caucasians. *J Rheumatol* 2002;29(9): 1821–1826.
33. Dizier MH, Eliaou JF, Babron MC, et al. Investigation of the HLA component involved in rheumatoid arthritis (RA) by using the marker association-segregation chi-square (MASC) method: rejection of the unifying-shared-epitope hypothesis. *Am J Hum Genet* 1993;53(3):715–721.
34. Gao X, Gazit E, Livneh A, et al. Rheumatoid arthritis in Israeli Jews: shared sequences in the third hypervariable region of DRB1 alleles are associated with susceptibility. *J Rheumatol* 1991;18(6):801–803.
35. Gao XJ, Brautbar C, Gazit E, et al. A variant of HLA-DR4 determines susceptibility to rheumatoid arthritis in a subset of Israeli Jews. *Arthritis Rheum* 1991;34(5):547–551.
36. Teller K, Budhai L, Zhang M, et al. HLA-DRB1 and DQB typing of Hispanic American patients with rheumatoid arthritis: the "shared epitope" hypothesis may not apply. *J Rheumatol* 1996;23(8):1363–1368.
37. McDaniel DO, Alarcon GS, Pratt PW, et al. Most African-American patients with rheumatoid arthritis do not have the rheumatoid antigenic determinant (epitope). *Ann Intern Med* 1995;123(3):181–187.
38. Nepom BS, Nepom GT, Mickelson E, et al. Specific HLA-DR4-associated histocompatibility molecules characterize patients with seropositive juvenile rheumatoid arthritis. *J Clin Invest* 1984;74(1):287–291.
39. Hajeer AH, Worthington J, Silman AJ, et al. Association of tumor necrosis factor microsatellite polymorphisms with HLA-DRB1*04-bearing haplotypes in rheumatoid arthritis patients. *Arthritis Rheum* 1996;39(7):1109–1114.
40. Mu H, Chen JJ, Jiang Y, et al. Tumor necrosis factor a microsatellite polymorphism is associated with rheumatoid arthritis severity through an interaction with the HLA-DRB1 shared epitope. *Arthritis Rheum* 1999;42(3):438–442.
41. Mulcahy B, Waldron-Lynch F, McDermott MF, et al. Genetic variability in the tumor necrosis factor-lymphotoxin region influences susceptibility to rheumatoid arthritis. *Am J Hum Genet* 1996;59(3):676–683.
42. Ota M, Katsuyama Y, Kimura A, et al. A second susceptibility gene for developing rheumatoid arthritis in the human MHC is localized within a 70-kb interval telomeric of the TNF genes in the HLA class III region. *Genomics* 2001;71(3):263–270.
43. Jawaheer D, Li W, Graham RR, et al. Dissecting the genetic complexity of the association between human leukocyte antigens and rheumatoid arthritis. *Am J Hum Genet* 2002;71(3):585–594.
44. Price P, Witt C, Allcock R, et al. The genetic basis for the association of the 8.1 ancestral haplotype (A1, B8, DR3) with multiple immunopathological diseases. *Immunol Rev* 1999;167:257–274.
45. Huttley GA, Smith MW, Carrington M, et al. A scan for linkage disequilibrium across the human genome. *Genetics* 1999;152(4):1711–1722.
46. Gabriel SB, Schaffner SF, Nguyen H, et al. The structure of haplotype blocks in the human genome. *Science* 2002;296(5576):2225–2229.
47. Phillips MS, Lawrence R, Sachidanandam R, et al. Chromosome-wide distribution of haplotype blocks and the role of recombination hot spots. *Nat Genet* 2003;18:18.
48. Sanchez-Mazas A, Djoulah S, Busson M, et al. A linkage disequilibrium map of the MHC region based on the analysis of 14 loci haplotypes in 50 French families. *Eur J Hum Genet* 2000;8(1):33–41.
49. Abecasis GR, Noguchi E, Heinzmann A, et al. Extent and distribution of linkage disequilibrium in three genomic regions. *Am J Hum Genet* 2001;68(1): 191–197.
50. Reich DE, Cargill M, Bolk S, et al. Linkage disequilibrium in the human genome. *Nature* 2001;411(6834):199–204.
51. Okamoto K, Makino S, Yoshikawa Y, et al. Identification of IkappaBL as the second major histocompatibility complex-linked susceptibility locus for rheumatoid arthritis. *Am J Hum Genet* 2003;72(2):303–312.
52. Caruso C, Bongiardina C, Candore G, et al. HLA-B8,DR3 haplotype affects lymphocyte blood levels. *Immunol Invest* 1997;26(3):333–340.
53. Alper CA, Kruskall MS, Marcus-Bagley D, et al. Genetic prediction of nonresponse to hepatitis B vaccine. *N Engl J Med* 1989;321(11):708–712.
54. Kruskall MS, Alper CA, Awdeh Z, et al. The immune response to hepatitis B vaccine in humans: inheritance patterns in families. *J Exp Med* 1992;175 (2):495–502.
55. Lio D, Candore G, Romano GC, et al. Modification of cytokine patterns in subjects bearing the HLA-B8,DR3 phenotype: implications for autoimmunity. *Cytokines Cell Mol Ther* 1997;3(4):217–224.
56. Lawley TJ, Hall RP, Fauci AS, et al. Defective Fc-receptor functions associated with the HLA-B8/DRw3 haplotype: studies in patients with dermatitis herpetiformis and normal subjects. *N Engl J Med* 1981;304(4):185–192.
57. Lio D, Candore G, Colombo A, et al. A genetically determined high setting of TNF-alpha influences immunologic parameters of HLA-B8,DR3 positive subjects: implications for autoimmunity. *Hum Immunol* 2001;62(7):705–713.
58. Yen JH, Moore BE, Nakajima T, et al. Major histocompatibility complex class I-recognizing receptors are disease risk genes in rheumatoid arthritis. *J Exp Med* 2001;193(10):1159–1167.
59. Deighton CM, Walker DJ, Griffiths ID, et al. The contribution of HLA to rheumatoid arthritis. *Clin Genet* 1989;36(3):178–182.
60. Hasstedt SJ, Clegg DO, Ingles L, et al. HLA-linked rheumatoid arthritis. *Am J Hum Genet* 1994;55(4):738–746.
61. Cornelis F, Faure S, Martinez M, et al. New susceptibility locus for rheumatoid arthritis suggested by a genome-wide linkage study. *Proc Natl Acad Sci U S A* 1998;95(18):10746–10750.
62. Jawaheer D, Seldin MF, Amos CI, et al. A genomewide screen in multiplex rheumatoid arthritis families suggests genetic overlap with other autoimmune diseases. *Am J Hum Genet* 2001;68(4):927–936.
63. Todd JA. La carte des microsatellites est arrivee! [The map of microsatellites has arrived!] *Hum Mol Genet* 1992;1(9):663–666.
64. Weiss KM, Terwilliger JD. How many diseases does it take to map a gene with SNPs? *Nat Genet* 2000;26(2):151–157.
65. Hugot JP, Chamaillard M, Zouali H, et al. Association of NOD2 leucine-rich repeat variants with susceptibility to Crohn's disease. *Nature* 2001;411(6837): 599–603.
66. Ogura Y, Bonen DK, Inohara N, et al. A frameshift mutation in NOD2 associated with susceptibility to Crohn's disease. *Nature* 2001;411(6837):603–606.
67. Risch N. Linkage strategies for genetically complex traits. II. The power of affected relative pairs. *Am J Hum Genet* 1990;46(2):229–241.
68. Risch NJ. Searching for genetic determinants in the new millennium. *Nature* 2000;405(6788):847–856.
69. Jawaheer D, Seldin MF, Amos CI, et al. Screening the genome for rheumatoid arthritis susceptibility genes: a replication study and combined analysis of 512 multicase families. *Arthritis Rheum* 2003;48(4):906–916.
70. MacKay K, Eyre S, Myerscough A, et al. Whole-genome linkage analysis of rheumatoid arthritis susceptibility loci in 252 affected sibling pairs in the United Kingdom. *Arthritis Rheum* 2002;46(3):632–639.

71. Shiozawa S, Hayashi S, Tsukamoto Y, et al. Identification of the gene loci that predispose to rheumatoid arthritis. *Int Immunol* 1998;10(12):1891–1895.
72. Lander E, Kruglyak L. Genetic dissection of complex traits: guidelines for interpreting and reporting linkage results. *Nat Genet* 1995;11(3):241–247.
73. Barton A, Eyre S, Myerscough A, et al. High resolution linkage and association mapping identifies a novel rheumatoid arthritis susceptibility locus homologous to one linked to two rat models of inflammatory arthritis. *Hum Mol Genet* 2001;10(18):1901–1906.
74. Rich SS, Concannon P. Challenges and strategies for investigating the genetic complexity of common human diseases. *Diabetes* 2002;51[Suppl 3]:S288–S294.
75. Cox NJ, Wapelhorst B, Morrison VA, et al. Seven regions of the genome show evidence of linkage to type 1 diabetes in a consensus analysis of 767 multiplex families. *Am J Hum Genet* 2001;69(4):820–830.
76. Jawaheer D, Gregersen PK. The search for rheumatoid arthritis susceptibility genes: a call for global collaboration. *Arthritis Rheum* 2002;46(3):582–584.
77. Becker KG, Simon RM, Bailey-Wilson JE, et al. Clustering of non-major histocompatibility complex susceptibility candidate loci in human autoimmune diseases. *Proc Natl Acad Sci U S A* 1998;95(17):9979–9984.
78. Lin JP, Cash JM, Doyle SZ, et al. Familial clustering of rheumatoid arthritis with other autoimmune diseases. *Hum Genet* 1998;103(4):475–482.
79. Kelly JA, Moser KL, Harley JB. The genetics of systemic lupus erythematosus: putting the pieces together. *Genes Immun* 2002;3[Suppl 1]:S71–S85.
80. Vaidya B, Imrie H, Perros P, et al. Evidence for a new Graves disease susceptibility locus at chromosome 18q21. *Am J Hum Genet* 2000;66(5):1710–1714.
81. Davies JL, Kawaguchi Y, Bennett ST, et al. A genome-wide search for human type 1 diabetes susceptibility genes. *Nature* 1994;371(6493):130–136.
82. Falk CT, Rubinstein P. Haplotype relative risks: an easy reliable way to construct a proper control sample for risk calculations. *Ann Hum Genet* 1987;51:227–233.
83. Spielman RS, Ewens WJ. A sibship test for linkage in the presence of association: the sib transmission/disequilibrium test. *Am J Hum Genet* 1998;62(2):450–458.
84. Schaid DJ, Rowland C. Use of parents, sibs, and unrelated controls for detection of associations between genetic markers and disease. *Am J Hum Genet* 1998;63(5):1492–1506.
85. Daly MJ, Rioux JD, Schaffner SF, et al. High-resolution haplotype structure in the human genome. *Nat Genet* 2001;29(2):229–232.
86. Rioux JD, Daly MJ, Silverberg MS, et al. Genetic variation in the 5q31 cytokine gene cluster confers susceptibility to Crohn disease. *Nat Genet* 2001;29(2):223–228.
87. Jeffreys AJ, Kauppi L, Neumann R. Intensely punctate meiotic recombination in the class II region of the major histocompatibility complex. *Nat Genet* 2001;29(2):217–222.
88. Judson R, Salisbury B, Schneider J, et al. How many SNPs does a genome-wide haplotype map require? *Pharmacogenomics* 2002;3(3):379–391.
89. Pritchard JK, Cox NJ. The allelic architecture of human disease genes: common disease-common variant. . .or not? *Hum Mol Genet* 2002;11(20):2417–2423.
90. Smith DJ, Lusis AJ. The allelic structure of common disease. *Hum Mol Genet* 2002;11(20):2455–2461.
91. Warrington JA, Shah NA, Chen X, et al. New developments in high-throughput resequencing and variation detection using high density microarrays. *Hum Mutat* 2002;19(4):402–409.
92. Wasson J, Skolnick G, Love-Gregory L, et al. Assessing allele frequencies of single nucleotide polymorphisms in DNA pools by pyrosequencing technology. *Biotechniques* 2002;32(5):1144–1146, 1148, 1150 passim.
93. Ioannidis JP, Ntzani EE, Trikalinos TA, et al. Replication validity of genetic association studies. *Nat Genet* 2001;29(3):306–309.
94. Lohmueller KE, Pearce CL, Pike M, et al. Meta-analysis of genetic association studies supports a contribution of common variants to susceptibility to common disease. *Nat Genet* 2003;33(2):177–182.
95. Haukim N, Bidwell JL, Smith AJ, et al. Cytokine gene polymorphism in human disease: on-line databases, Supplement 2. *Genes Immun* 2002;3(6):313–330.
96. Yamada R, Tanaka T, Unoki M, et al. Association between a single-nucleotide polymorphism in the promoter of the human interleukin-3 gene and rheumatoid arthritis in Japanese patients, and maximum-likelihood estimation of combinatorial effect that two genetic loci have on susceptibility to the disease. *Am J Hum Genet* 2001;68(3):674–685.
97. Kameoka Y, Yamagoe S, Hatano Y, et al. Val58Ile polymorphism of the neutrophil chemoattractant LECT2 and rheumatoid arthritis in the Japanese population. *Arthritis Rheum* 2000;43(6):1419–1420.
98. Buchs N, Silvestri T, di Giovine FS, et al. IL-4 VNTR gene polymorphism in chronic polyarthritis. The rare allele is associated with protection against destruction. *Rheumatology (Oxford)* 2000;39(10):1126–1131.
99. Genevay S, Di Giovine FS, Perneger TV, et al. Association of interleukin-4 and interleukin-1B gene variants with Larsen score progression in rheumatoid arthritis. *Arthritis Rheum* 2002;47(3):303–309.
100. Donn R, Alourfi Z, De Benedetti F, et al. Mutation screening of the macrophage migration inhibitory factor gene: positive association of a functional polymorphism of macrophage migration inhibitory factor with juvenile idiopathic arthritis. *Arthritis Rheum* 2002;46(9):2402–2409.
101. Meazza C, Travaglino P, Pignatti P, et al. Macrophage migration inhibitory factor in patients with juvenile idiopathic arthritis. *Arthritis Rheum* 2002;46(1):232–237.
102. Gregersen PK, Bucala R. Macrophage migration inhibitory factor, MIF alleles, and the genetics of inflammatory disorders: incorporating disease outcome into the definition of phenotype. *Arthritis Rheum* 2003;48(5):1171–1176.
103. Baugh JA, Chitnis S, Donnelly SC, et al. A functional promoter polymorphism in the macrophage migration inhibitory factor (MIF) gene associated with disease severity in rheumatoid arthritis. *Genes Immun* 2002;3(3):170–176.
104. Morand EF, Bucala R, Leech M. Macrophage migration inhibitory factor: an emerging therapeutic target in rheumatoid arthritis. *Arthritis Rheum* 2003;48(2):291–299.
105. De Benedetti F, Meazza C, Vivarelli M, et al. Functional and prognostic relevance of the -173 polymorphism of the MIF gene in systemic juvenile idiopathic arthritis. *Arthritis Rheum* 2003;(48(5):1398–1407.
106. Barton A, John S, Ollier WE, et al. Association between rheumatoid arthritis and polymorphism of tumor necrosis factor receptor II, but not tumor necrosis factor receptor I, in Caucasians. *Arthritis Rheum* 2001;44(1):61–65.
107. Dieude P, Petit E, Cailleau-Moindrault S, et al. Association between tumor necrosis factor receptor II and familial, but not sporadic, rheumatoid arthritis: evidence for genetic heterogeneity. *Arthritis Rheum* 2002;46(8):2039–2044.
108. Mattey DL, Hutchinson D, Dawes PT, et al. Smoking and disease severity in rheumatoid arthritis: association with polymorphism at the glutathione S-transferase M1 locus. *Arthritis Rheum* 2002;46(3):640–646.
109. Tracey KJ. The inflammatory reflex. *Nature* 2002;420(6917):853–859.
110. Fife M, Steer S, Fisher S, et al. Association of familial and sporadic rheumatoid arthritis with a single corticotropin-releasing hormone genomic region (8q12.3) haplotype. *Arthritis Rheum* 2002;46(1):75–82.
111. Takayanagi H, Kim S, Taniguchi T. Signaling crosstalk between RANKL and interferons in osteoclast differentiation. *Arthritis Res* 2002;4[Suppl 3]:S227–S232.
112. Olofsson P, Holmberg J, Tordsson J, et al. Positional identification of Ncf1 as a gene that regulates arthritis severity in rats. *Nat Genet* 2003;33(1):25–32.
113. Choubey D, Kotzin BL. Interferon-inducible p202 in the susceptibility to systemic lupus. *Front Biosci* 2002;7:e252–e262.
114. Baechler EC, Batliwalla FM, Karypis G, et al. Interferon-inducible gene expression signature in peripheral blood cells of patients with severe lupus. *Proc Natl Acad Sci U S A* 2003;25:25.
115. Hennecke J, Carfi A, Wiley DC. Structure of a covalently stabilized complex of a human alphabeta T-cell receptor, influenza HA peptide and MHC class II molecule, HLA-DR1. *EMBO J* 2000;19(21):5611–5624.

CHAPTER 11

Pathology

Barton F. Haynes

The pathology of rheumatoid arthritis (RA) reflects the induction and maintenance of immune and inflammatory responses in joints and in extraarticular locations, resulting in multisystem manifestations in many RA patients. Extraarticular disease in RA can affect the skin and subcutaneous tissue, eyes, heart, pericardium, lungs and pleura, central and peripheral nervous systems, spleen and liver, and upper airway, including vocal cords, larynx, and nasal passages. As in other tissues, the normal cells within synovium (synovial cells, fibroblasts, endothelial cells) have functions that become either exaggerated or deficient when perturbed by circulating immune complexes and invading pathogens or activated immune cells. However, the fundamental process that occurs in the joint in RA is the conversion of synovium from its support role in ensuring normal joint function to that of a lymphoid organ.

Evidence is emerging that RA is a genetic disease (see Chapter 10) in which an abnormal antibody and T-cell response is made to an autoantigen (1–6). A number of autoantigens are candidates to trigger RA, including glucose-6-phosphate isomerase (GPI) (2–6), HLA DQ-derived peptide, proteoglycans, immunoglobulins (Igs) [rheumatoid factor (RF)], and collagen (Table 11.1) (1,6) (see Chapter 22). It is likely that immune responses to more than one autoantigen can lead to the clinical syndrome of RA. Regardless of the nature of the triggering antigen or antigens, it has become clear that RA patients have fundamental immune system abnormalities, including premature thymic atrophy (7,8); oligoclonal expansion of autoreactive $CD4^+$, $CD28^-$, $CD7^-$ T cells both in the peripheral blood and in synovium (8–13); and abnormalities in the homeostasis of naïve $CD4^+$ T cells in the periphery (7,8).

Understanding the histopathology of RA can aid in understanding the pathologic mechanisms that cause tissue damage in RA and can help clarify the rationale for the use of treatments for RA, such as inhibitors of the pathogenic cytokines, tumor necrosis factor (TNF)-α, interleukin (IL)-1α, and IL-1β (see Chapters 11, 12, and 20).

PATHOLOGY OF RHEUMATOID ARTHRITIS SYNOVIUM

Normal Synovium and Joint Morphology

Normal synovium forms the lining of the joint capsule and defines the articular space. Within the joint capsule, synovium reflects onto the bone of the joint and tracks up to the articular cartilage within the joint (14) (Fig. 11.1). Normal cartilage is avascular, with a thin layer (approximately 5 mm) of cartilage facing the inner joint. Underneath the noncalcified cartilage layer of articular cartilage is a layer of calcified cartilage followed by subchondral bone.

Normal synovium is comprised of a one- to two-cell layer of lining cells that are superficial to an adipose stroma of connective tissue containing adipocytes, fibroblasts, arterioles, and venules (Fig. 11.2). There is no basement membrane separating synovial lining cells (SLCs) from the stroma and blood vessels beneath. Blood vessels in normal synovium are thin walled and do not generally express the adhesion molecules of blood vessels in inflammatory sites such as intercellular adhesion molecule-1 (ICAM-1) (15). One function of normal synovium is to make synovial fluid and provide cartilage and fibrous tissue within the joint with hyaluronan (a lubricating proteoglycan) and other protein nutrients from the blood. Blood nutrients diffuse from the synovial blood vessels through the intercellular space between SLC into the joint cavity (14).

The SLC are of two types, macrophage-like type A SLC (A-SLC) and fibroblast-like type B SLC (B-SLC) (16–18). A-SLC are bone marrow–derived cells of the myeloid lineage that migrate from bone marrow to the joint space via the blood and are the specialized phagocyte members of the macrophage lineage analogous to Kupffer's cells in the liver and glial cells in the brain. A-SLC display surface markers expressed by macrophages [CD14, CD68, CD33, CD11b, major histocompatibility complex (MHC) class II, and Fc receptors for Ig] and serve to remove debris and pathogens from the joint by phagocytosis and intracellular proteolysis. Like other cells of the myeloid lineage, A-SLC also have the capacity for antigen presentation, which serves the health of the joint when initiating immune responses to eliminate infectious agents within the joint, but serves to promote joint damage and destruction in inflammatory arthritis conditions such as RA. B-SLC are fibroblast-like cells that produce collagen and hyaluronan and, like A-SLC, produce a number of proinflammatory molecules, such as cathepsins, and collagenase, stromelysin, and other metaloproteases (16–18). Unlike A-SLC, B-SLC do not express macrophage markers or MHC class II, and there is no specific marker for B-SLC. B-SLC can be identified morphologically by electron microscopy as a fibroblast-like cellular component of the synovial lining layer. In addition, monoclonal antibodies to procollagen that react with intracellular collagen can identify B-SLC in sections of synovium (Fig. 11.3A) (19).

TABLE 11.1. Autoantigens Defined by Experimental Serum and B-Cell Analysis in Rheumatoid Arthritis Syndromes in Animals and Humans

Type/Nature	Specificity
Self antigen	Citrulline-containing peptides
	Keratin
	Perinuclear factor
	Savoy antigen
	Filaggrin
	Human leukocyte antigen
	Calpastatin
	Immunoglobulin (rheumatoid factor)
	Calreticulin
	Antineutrophil cytoplasmic antibody
	Antinuclear antibody
	Immunoglobulin heavy-chain binding protein/p68
	Heteronuclear ribonucleoprotein A2 (RA33)
	Glucose-6-phosphate isomerase
Cartilage (organ specific)	Collagen type II
	Chondrocyte antigen 65
	Large aggregating chondroitin sulfate proteoglycan (aggrecan)
	Human chondrocyte glycoprotein 39
	Cartilage oligomeric matrix protein
Non-self antigens	Bacterial heat shock protein

Adapted from Magathaes R, Stiehl P, Morawietz L, et al. Morphological and molecular pathology of the B cell response in synovitis of rheumatoid arthritis. *Virchows Arch* 2002;441:415–427.

Histopathology of Synovium in Early Rheumatoid Arthritis

The early changes in synovium in RA are SLC hyperplasia, edema, vessel proliferation, and infiltration of lymphocytes into the sublining area. SLC hyperplasia is due to increased migration of A-SLC to the joint from the bone marrow and by *in situ* proliferation of B-SLC (Fig. 11.3A and Fig. 11.4) (19–24). Upregulation of expression of extracellular matrix and cellular proteoglycans, such as fibronectin (Fig. 11.3B) and cellular CD44, commonly occurs (19).

Within the synovial lining, numerous giant cells appear that are likely induced by the intense production of inflammatory cytokines, including interferon-γ (IFN-γ) (Figs. 11.5A and 11.5B) (see Chapter 12) (20–24). Studies have shown these changes in both new symptomatic joints and in asymptomatic, clinically uninvolved joints of patients with RA (20–24). In asymptomatic joints of RA patients, the pathologic changes include SLC hyperplasia with $CD4^+$ T-cell infiltrations (20–22). Few B cells are seen, and vessel proliferation and fibrin deposition are rare (20).

In symptomatic joints, the histology of the RA synovium shows vascular proliferation, foci of polymorphonuclear cells, and fibrin deposition (Fig. 11.6). Vascular proliferation is driven by production of proangiogenic molecules within synovium, such as vascular endothelial growth factor, basic fibroblast growth factor, IL-8, and monocyte chemotactic protein (MCP)-1 by macrophages, giant cells, and other cell types (25,26). In clinically symptomatic joints, endothelial cells of venules are plump and form high endothelial venules that are identical to those seen in lymph nodes (Fig. 11.7) (27). Inflamed synovial

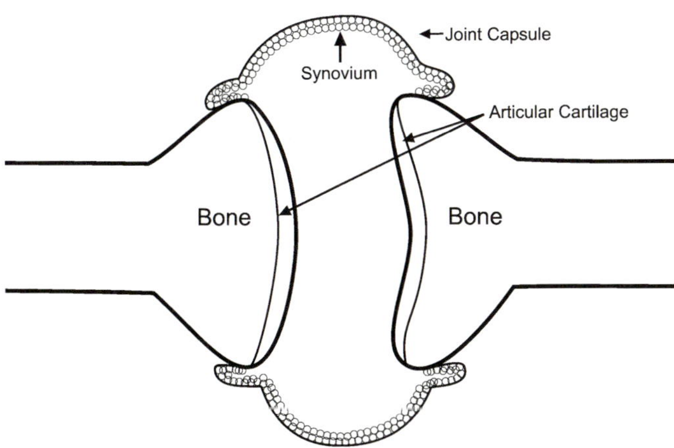

Figure 11.1. Schematic representation of a diarthroidal joint showing the associations of the joint capsule, synovium, bone, and cartilage.

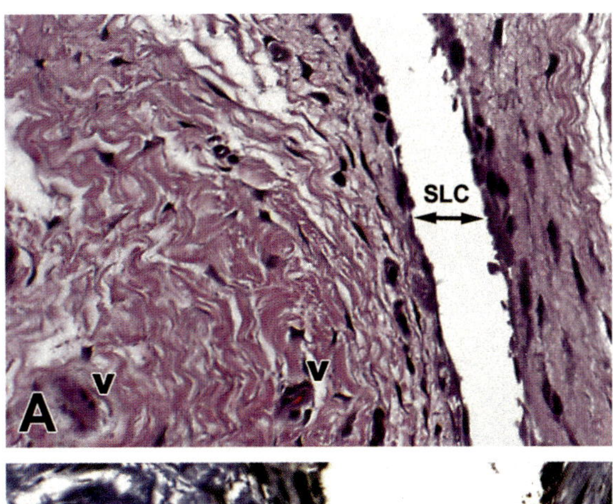

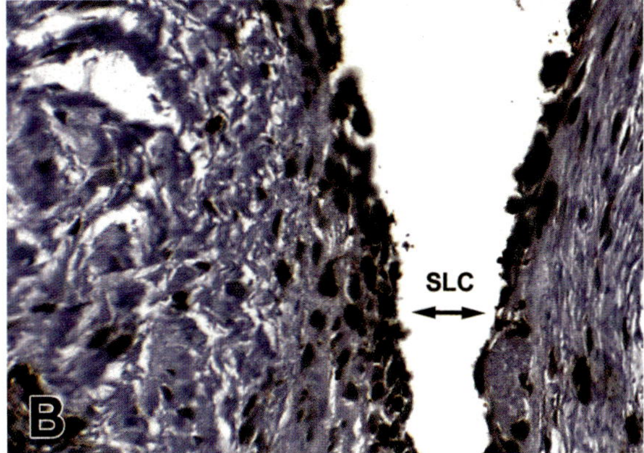

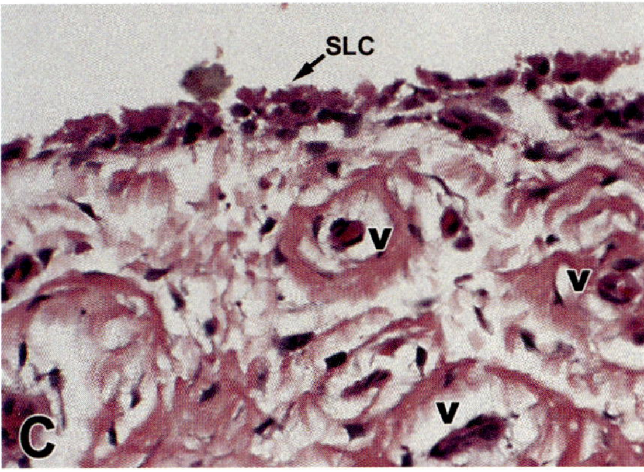

Figure 11.2. Normal synovium. **A,B:** Sequential sections of synovium from a normal joint demonstrating normal one- to two-cell layer of synovial lining cells (SLCs) (panel **A**, hematoxylin and eosin stain; panel **B**, reacted with anti-CD68 monoclonal antibody that identifies tissue macrophages and type A SLC). **B:** CD68 monoclonal antibody binds to the superficial macrophage-derived type A SLCs and also binds to tissue macrophages below the SLC layer. **C:** Another area of normal synovium from the same subject showing multiple thin-walled synovial vessels (v).

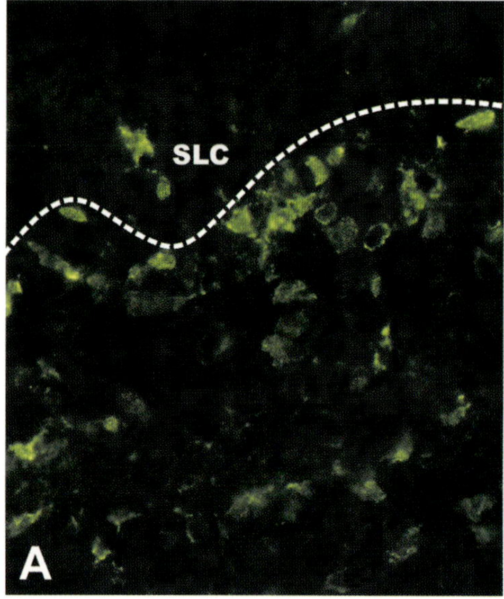

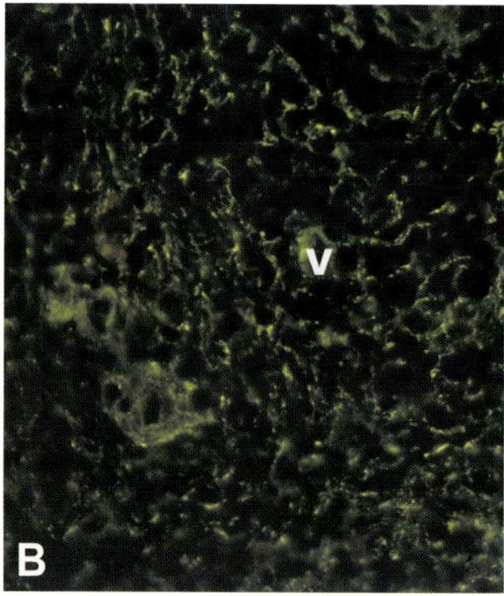

Figure 11.3. Synovium of rheumatoid arthritis reacted with monoclonal antibodies (mabs) to procollagen **(A)** and fibronectin **(B)**. **A:** The synovial lining cells (SLCs) are shown above the dotted line, and B-SLC is shown reacting with a mab against procollagen (decorated with mab and an anti-mab fluorescein isothiocyanate reagent that is green) in the SLC layer. Procollagen-containing synovial fibroblasts can be seen in the sub-SLC layer as well. **B:** The synovium and vessels (v) brightly reacted with an antifibronectin mab demonstrating increased extracellular matrix proteins in active rheumatoid arthritis synovium.

vessels express up-regulated adhesion molecules, such as ICAM-1, that are ligands for molecules on activated circulating leukocytes such as CD11a and CD18 (lymphocyte function–associated antigen-1) (Fig. 11.8). Lymphocyte function–associated antigen-1/ICAM-1 leukocyte–endothelial cell interactions are one of a series of adhesion molecule interactions that mediate leukocyte rolling and extravasation of activated leukocytes in synovium (28,29). Vascular proliferation occurs in other forms of arthritis in addition to RA, including osteoarthritis (OA). However, generally in OA, the proliferating vessels are not "high" and the inflammatory infiltrate in synovium is scant (30) (Fig. 11.9).

Fibrin deposition is a hallmark of severe joint inflammation in RA (31) (Fig. 11.6). Using immunohistologic analysis with specific antibodies, tissue factor (thromboplastin), fibrinogen, factor XIII, tissue transglutaminase, cross-linked fibrin (fibrin D-dimer), and α_2-plasmin inhibitor have all been identified in RA synovium, indicating the presence of activation of the extravascular coagulation cascade during initiation of the inflammatory response in RA (31).

T- and B-Cell Infiltrations in Synovium

T- and B-lymphocyte infiltrations in RA can occur either as diffuse synovial infiltrations with a predominance of $CD4^+$ T cells, scattered $CD8^+$ T cells and few B cells, or classic B-cell germinal centers with either primary follicles present (Fig. 11.10) or, in approximately 20% of RA patients, secondary follicles with germinal centers present (1,30,32–35). Synovial germinal centers have the morphologic and functional characteristics of lymph node germinal centers, except that synovial germinal centers contain higher numbers of T cells (35). T cells in RA synovium have a number of characteristics that likely are relevant to inducing and perpetuating the disease. RA T cells are autoreactive to self MHC class II molecules on RA B cells and are oligoclonal in T-cell receptor (TCR) repertoire with shortened telomeres—all suggesting premature aging of the T-cell arm of the immune system in RA (7–10). In synovium, there is a preponderance of oligoclonal $CD4^+$, $CD28^-$, $CD7^-$, and $CD45RO^+$ (memory) T cells that also express natural killer molecules on their surface and contain intracellular perforin and other molecules used in killing other cell types (11).

The activation of RA synovial T cells depends on the presence of autologous B cells and may explain the response of some patients treated with B-cell–depleting therapies (32–35). B-cell follicles with germinal center formation generally indicate that an antigen-specific immune response is occurring in the synovium. In support of this notion, Takemura et al. have performed microdissections of multiple germinal centers from RA synovium and found identical TCRs from multiple germinal centers, suggesting the same antigen stimulus at each germinal center (34,35).

The role of TCR $\gamma\delta$ T cells in RA remains unclear. TCR $\gamma\delta$ T cells are overexpressed in RA versus other granulomatous tissues, such as tissues from patients with Wegener's granulomatosis, granuloma annulare, and Takayasu's arteritis (36). The number of TCR $\gamma\delta$ T cells in RA synovium is proportional to the degree of inflammation in the synovium by tissue inflammation scores (36). $V\delta2/V\gamma9$ TCR $\gamma\delta$ T cells have been reported to respond to human and bacterial heat shock proteins and have been postulated to be one group of antigens

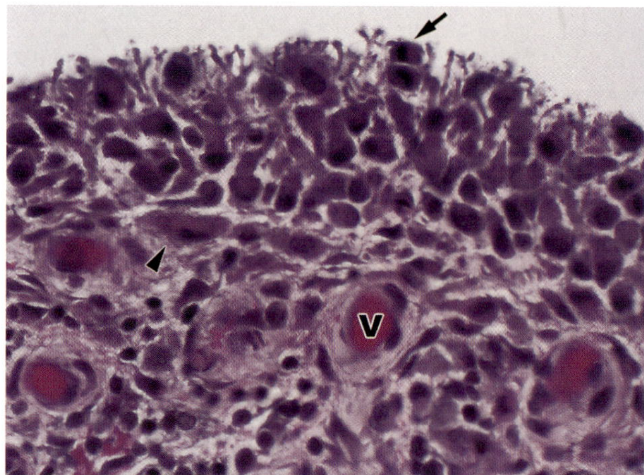

Figure 11.4. Proliferation of synovial lining cells (SLCs) in rheumatoid arthritis (RA). A hematoxylin-and-eosin–stained section of RA synovium with proliferating SLCs (*arrow* points to a SLC with a mitotic figure) and a five- to eight-cell hyperplastic SLC layer. Studies have demonstrated that increase in macrophage-derived type A SLC (A-SLC) in RA synovium is derived from increased migration of A-SLC precursors from bone marrow, whereas increase in fibroblast-like type B SLC (B-SLC) (*arrowhead*) is due to *in situ* proliferation of B-SLC. Also shown are the finger-like projections of B-SLC that are typical of SLC in RA. v, synovial vessel.

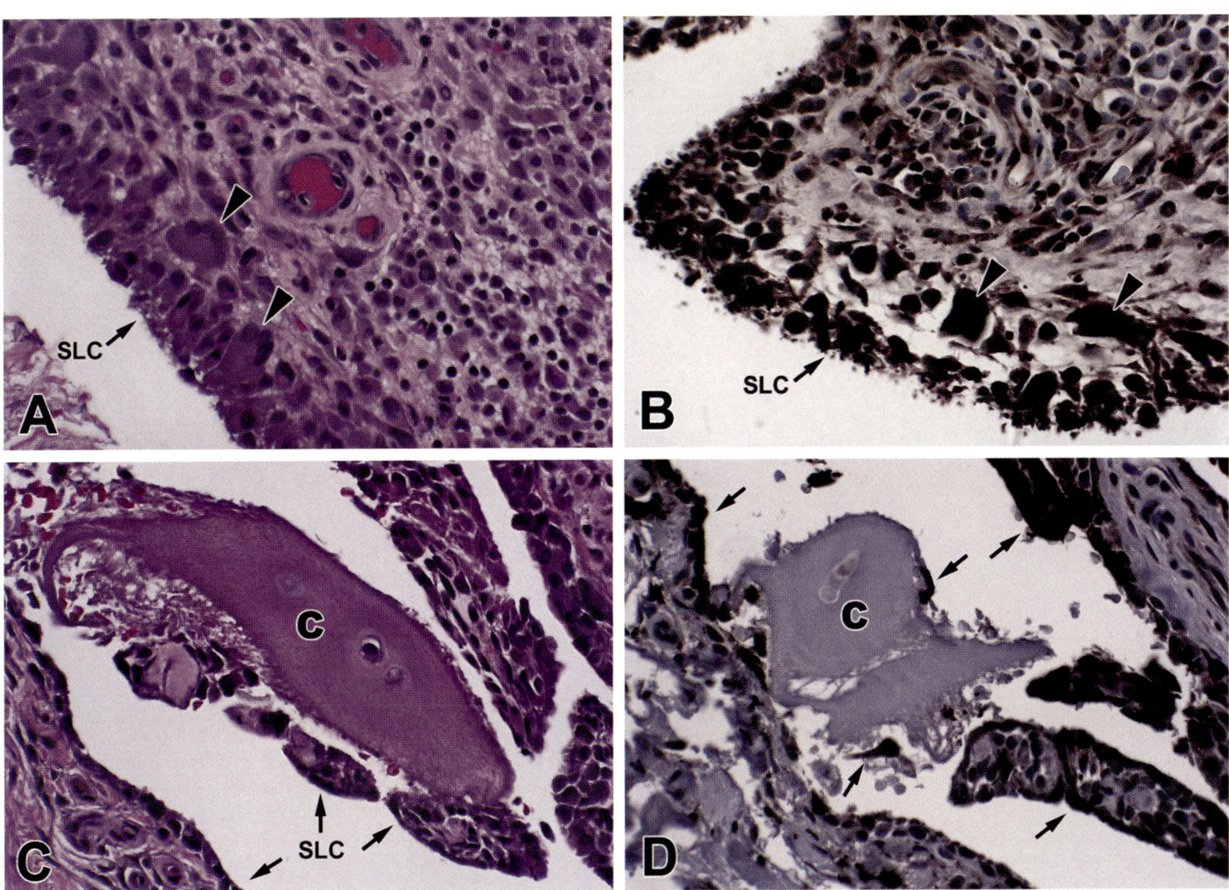

Figure 11.5. Synovial pathology in rheumatoid arthritis (RA). **A:** Hematoxylin-and-eosin–stained section of synovium in RA with multiple multinucleated giant cells in and around the synovial lining cell (SLC) layer (*arrowheads*). **B:** A sequential section of the same synovium in immunohistologic analysis with anti-CD68 monoclonal antibody (mab), showing that the type B SLCs, tissue macrophages, and multinucleated giant cells are all CD68^{+} (i.e., are of macrophage lineage). **C:** Cartilage (c) in an RA joint with adjacent SLC (*arrows*) (hematoxylin and eosin stain). **D:** A sequential section from the same tissue in immunohistologic analysis with anti-CD68 mab, showing invasion of the cartilage (c) by CD68 SLC and tissue macrophages (*arrows*).

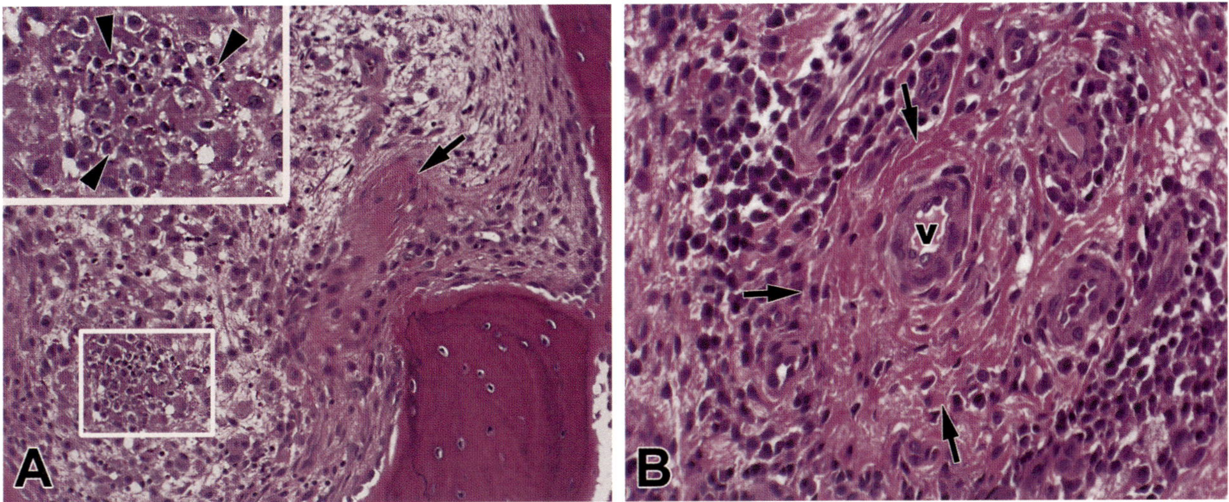

Figure 11.6. Prominent role of fibrin deposition in rheumatoid arthritis synovial pathology. **A:** An area of synovium invading bone with extensive fibrin deposition (*arrow*). White box and insert (*arrowheads*) show an area of focal polymorphonuclear infiltration and cellular debris and necrosis. **B:** A higher-power view of an adjacent area of synovium with a synovial vessel (v) surrounded by fibrin (*arrows*) and lymphocytes (hematoxylin and eosin stain).

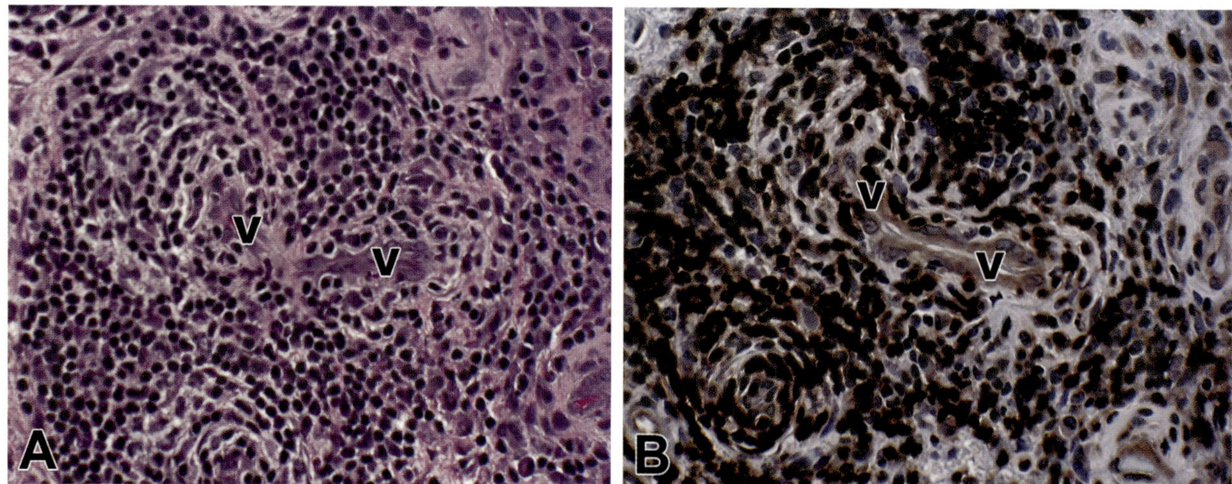

Figure 11.7. High endothelial venules in rheumatoid arthritis (RA) synovium. **A,B:** Sequential sections from the same RA synovial tissue showing, in **A** (hematoxylin and eosin stain), a central high endothelial venule (HEV) surrounded by extravasated lymphocytes forming a synovial lymphoid nodule, and, in **B**, the sequential section reacted in immunohistologic analysis with an anti–T-cell CD3 monoclonal antibody showing a large number of the cells around the HEV are T cells (brown-stained cells). The blue $CD3^-$ lymphocytes are B cells. *v*, synovial vessels.

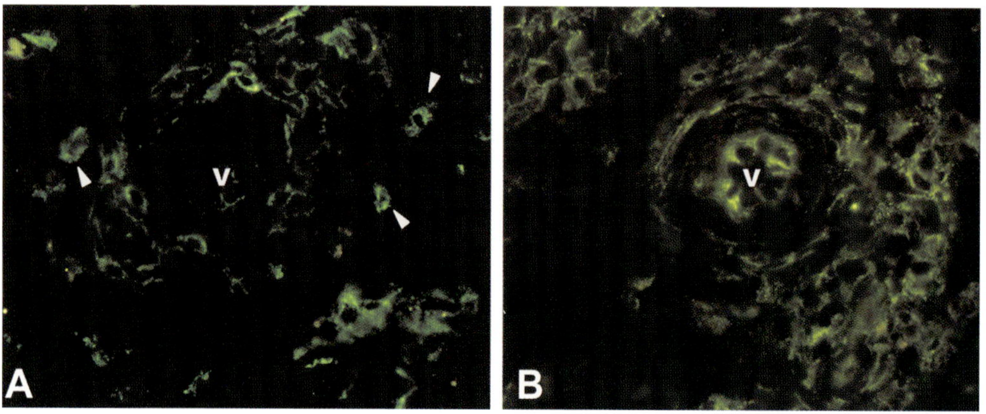

Figure 11.8. Indirect immunofluorescence analysis of expression of lymphocyte function–associated antigen-1 (LFA-1) on extravasated perivascular leukocytes **(A)** and the ligand for LFA-1, intercellular adhesion molecule-1 (ICAM-1) on vessel endothelium **(B)** in rheumatoid arthritis synovium. Although LFA-1 is exclusively expressed on synovial leukocytes (lymphocytes and macrophages) **(A)**, ICAM-1 is expressed (on a sequential section of the same tissue) on vessel high endothelial venule endothelium (*v*) as well as on activated tissue macrophages around the vessel.

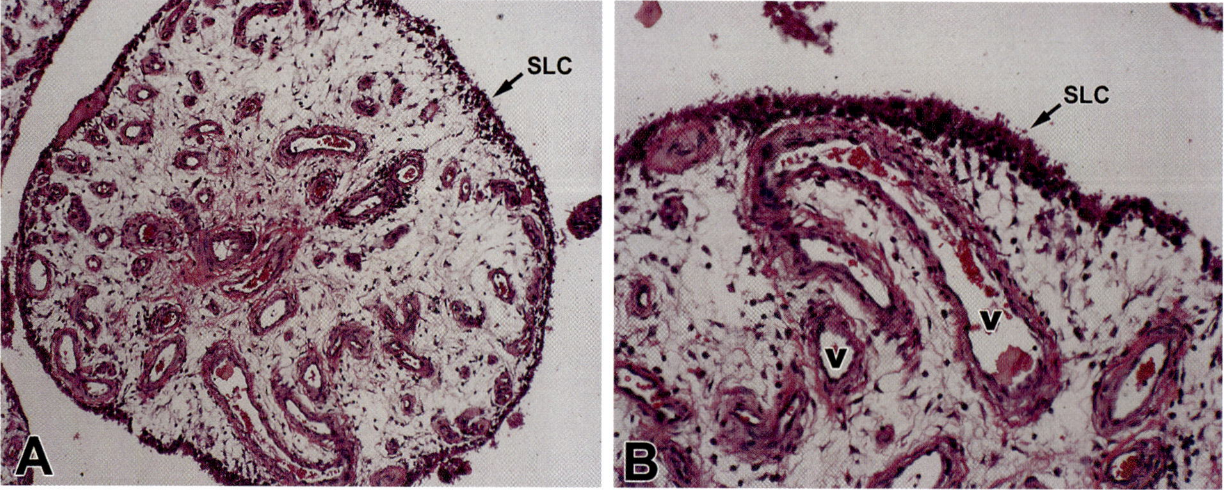

Figure 11.9. Histopathology of osteoarthritis (OA). In OA, the synovial lining cell (SLC) layer is mildly hyperplastic, and the number of synovial vessels (v) is increased, but the cellular infiltrate is scant. The B cells that are present are derived from peripheral B cells that have migrated to the OA synovium from the periphery. **A:** A low-power view of a cross section of a synovial villus. **B:** A higher-power view of the same area (hematoxylin and eosin stain).

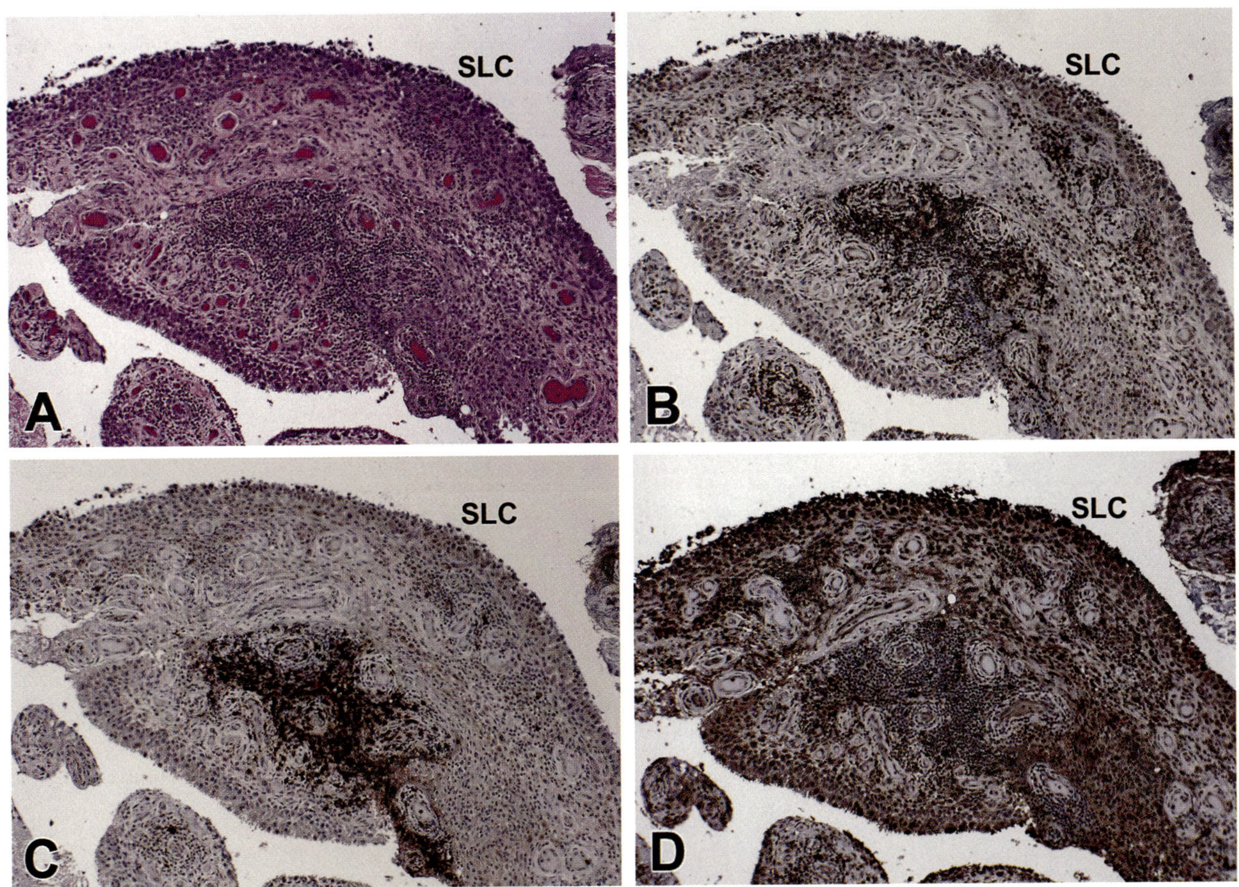

Figure 11.10. Immunohistopathologic analysis of distribution of T cells, B cells, and tissue macrophages in a synovial lymphoid nodule in rheumatoid arthritis (RA). **A–D:** Sequential sections of the same area of RA synovium. **A:** A hematoxylin-and-eosin–stained section showing synovial lining cell (SLC) layer hyperplasia, increased vessels (*red areas*), and a central lymphoid nodule (*central blue area*). **B:** Immunoreactivity of an anti–T-cell CD3 monoclonal antibody (mab) showing scattered T cells below the SLC layer and a cluster of T cells (*brown cells*) in the central lymphoid nodule. **C:** Immunoreactivity of an anti–B-cell CD20 mab demonstrating the distribution of B cells in the central lymphoid nodule (*brown cells*). **D:** Immunoreactivity of an antimacrophage CD68 mab demonstrating the distribution of CD68 type A SLCs and dense infiltrations of synovial macrophages throughout the areas around the lymphoid nodule (*brown cells*).

that can trigger RA (Table 11.1). However, a preponderance of Vδ2/Vγ9 TCR γδ T cells has not been found in RA synovia (36).

The increased numbers of B cells found in RA synovium can be either *accumulative* or *maturational*. B cells can accumulate through infiltration of peripheral B cells that have matured in lymph node, spleen, and other peripheral B-cell development and maturation sites and have migrated to synovium. Alternatively, the expanded B-cell numbers can be *maturational* and originate from B cells that have matured within synovial germinal centers (1). Analysis of VDJ Ig regions from B-cell germinal centers in RA synovium clearly demonstrate the stepwise accumulation of single somatic mutations in Ig VDJ regions characteristic of *in situ* clonal expansion in synovium (1). Thus, RA synovium clearly supports a germinal center reaction normally seen only in peripheral lymphoid tissue. Thus, there are two mechanisms to explain B-cell presence in RA synovium: homing of mature B cells from the periphery and maturation of B cells in synovial germinal centers.

The role of CD8+ T cells in this process has been studied and found to be critical to synovial germinal center formation (32). CD8+ T cells accumulate in the germinal center mantle zone and are characterized by lack of perforin, production of IFN-γ, and expression of CD40 ligand (32). Depletion of CD8+ T cells in the severe combined immunodeficiency disease mouse model of growth of human RA tissue showed that these cells are critical for formation and maintenance of synovial B-cell germinal centers (32).

In contrast to RA, B cells in OA synovial tissues are scattered around in fewer numbers and are derived from migration of B cells from the periphery (Fig. 11.9).

It is of interest that ectopic B-cell germinal center formation is not unique to RA synovium and can occur in the thyroid in autoimmune thyroid disease, in the salivary gland in Sjögren's syndrome, and in thymus in myasthenia gravis, systemic lupus erythematosus, and RA (37).

Synovial Macrophages in Rheumatoid Arthritis

The specialized macrophages of synovium, the A-SLC, are derived from bone marrow precursors, express CD68+ and CD14+, and are replenished by bone marrow cells migrating to synovium (18–20,38) (Figs. 11.5A and 11.5B). The increase in number of A-SLCs comes primarily from migration of more bone marrow precursors to inflamed synovium (23,38,39). Inflammation rating scales, which are based on SLC hyperplasia, vessel proliferation, degree of lymphocyte and macrophage infiltration, and germinal center and pannus formation (19,20,40), have demonstrated that the degree of synovial inflammation correlates both with the degree of bone and cartilage erosions and with clinical symptoms of RA (19,20,40–44).

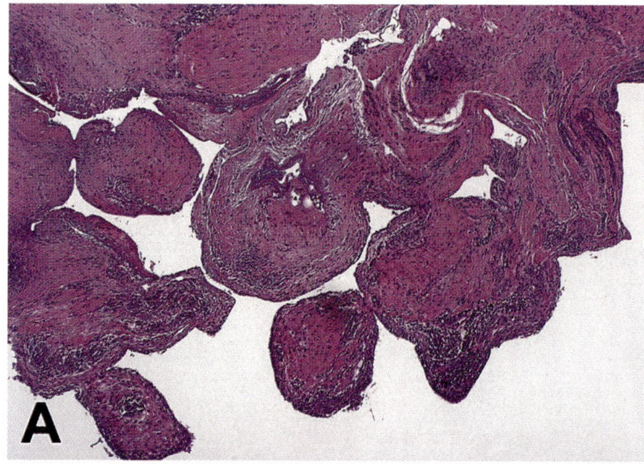

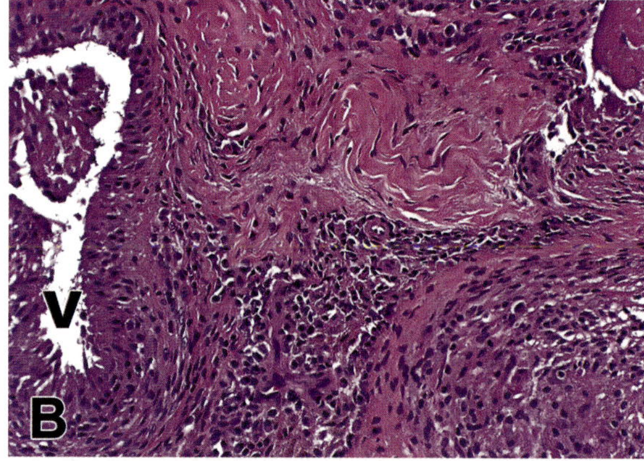

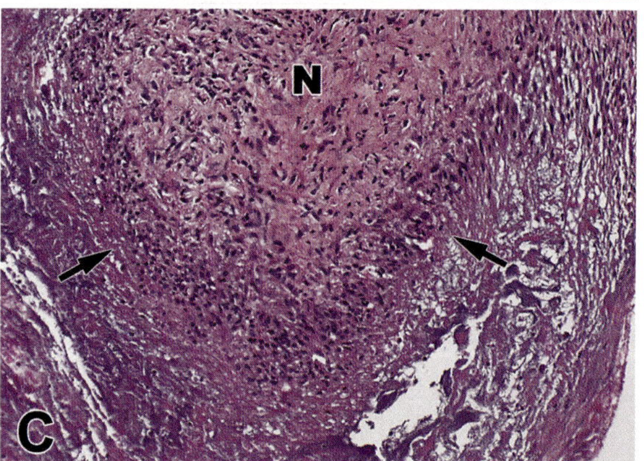

Figure 11.11. Histology of rheumatoid synovial pannus. **A:** A low-power view of hyperplastic rheumatoid arthritis synovium demonstrating pannus formation in synovial villi. **B,C:** Higher-power views of synovium with pannus formation. **B:** A vessel (V) with a luminal clot and vasculitis of the vessel wall adjacent to an intense area of swirls of synovial macrophages, fibroblasts, and lymphocytes. **C:** A typical synovial rheumatoid nodule with palisading macrophages (*arrows*) around a central area of necrosis (N).

Radiologic assessment of bone erosions correlates best with macrophage infiltration of synovium on histologic analysis, not with T-cell infiltration (45). Similarly, clinical disease activity in RA correlates best with SLC hyperplasia and macrophage infiltration into synovium (41,42). Interdigitating dendritic cells and traditional tissue macrophages are present in germinal centers in RA synovium, both of which can present antigen to T cells (33).

Histopathology of Synovium in Late Rheumatoid Arthritis

In late or advanced RA, the inflammatory processes and fibrosis described above progress, and a mass of synovium made up of fibroblasts, macrophages, T cells, and vessels, called *pannus*, develops (Fig. 11.11). The SLC layer is the leading edge of pannus and contains cathepsins, [e.g., collagenase, stromelysin, matrix metalloproteinase (MMP)-3, MMP-13, and cytokines (e.g., TNF-α, IL-1α, IL-1β, IL-6)] (45–50) (Fig. 11.12) (see Chapters 11 and 12). Mutations in oncogenes, such as p53, selectively occur in B-SLC in the SLC areas of synovium compared to the sublining synovial areas and, along with expression of multiple cytokines and chemokines, are thought to confer on pannus the properties for cartilage and bone invasion (Figs. 11.5C, 11.5D, and 11.12) (51).

Bone and Cartilage Erosions in Rheumatoid Arthritis

There are two histologic patterns at the cartilage–pannus junction in RA. One can see pannus adjacent to and invading and eroding cartilage, and one can see a transitional fibroblastic zone overlying the cartilage and separating the cartilage from pannus (23). This transitional fibroblastic zone contains keratin sulfate and type II collagen, suggesting derivation from chondrocytes (23). The transitional fibroblastic zone is more often seen in RA knee and hip joints and less in distal small joints and is associated with fewer bony erosions than when absent (23). Synovial macrophages, B-SLCs, and A-SLCs are mediators of cartilage damage in RA via production of TNF-α, IL-1, IL-6, cathepsins, and metalloproteases at the cartilage–pannus interface (23,46) (Fig. 11.12).

Elegant work in animal models of inflammatory arthritis, as well as histologic and electron microscopic analysis of RA joint tissue, has proven a critical role for osteoclasts in mediation of bone erosions in RA (48,50,52–54). Osteoclasts are multinucleated myeloid lineage cells that are responsible for normal bone resorption and remodeling. Absence or deficiency of osteoclasts leads to the clinical disease osteopetrosis, such as occurs in *c-fos*–deficient homologous recombinant mice (52). Table 11.2 lists the osteoclast-inducing factors that have been detected in RA synovium (50).

In RA, there are two sites of focal bone resorption: the interface of pannus with bone at the joint surface and the interface of invading inflammatory synovium with subchondral bone and bony trabeculae (50) (Fig. 11.12). Inflammatory synovium has abundant numbers of A-SLC and tissue macrophages that are driven by the cytokines and factors in Table 11.2 to become osteoclasts (50) and, in the setting of bone erosion in RA, provides the source of osteoclasts that mediate RA bone destruction. This pathologic process is in contrast to the source of osteoclasts in normal bone resorption, where osteoclasts are derived from bone marrow. Figure 11.12 shows the *in situ* transformation of A-SLCs into osteoclasts, and the location of A-SLC and osteoclasts at the site of "resorption bays" of eroded bone (54).

Recently, investigators have described a pathway where activated synovial T cells produce the cytokine IL-17 and the osteoclast differentiation factor, receptor activator of nuclear factor–κB ligand (RANKL), that synergize to induce osteoclast maturation and activation (50,52,53,55,56). Synovial T cells also induce A-SLC, B-SLC, and synovial tissue macrophages to produce IL-1 and TNF-α. IL-1, TNF-α, IL-17, and RANKL all synergize with the additional osteoclast-activating factors in Table 11.2 to promote intense osteoclast activation and bone destruction in advanced RA.

Correlation of Histopathology with Proposed Pathophysiology of Rheumatoid Arthritis

Chapter 22 discusses many of the interesting and informative animal models of arthritis that have provided considerable

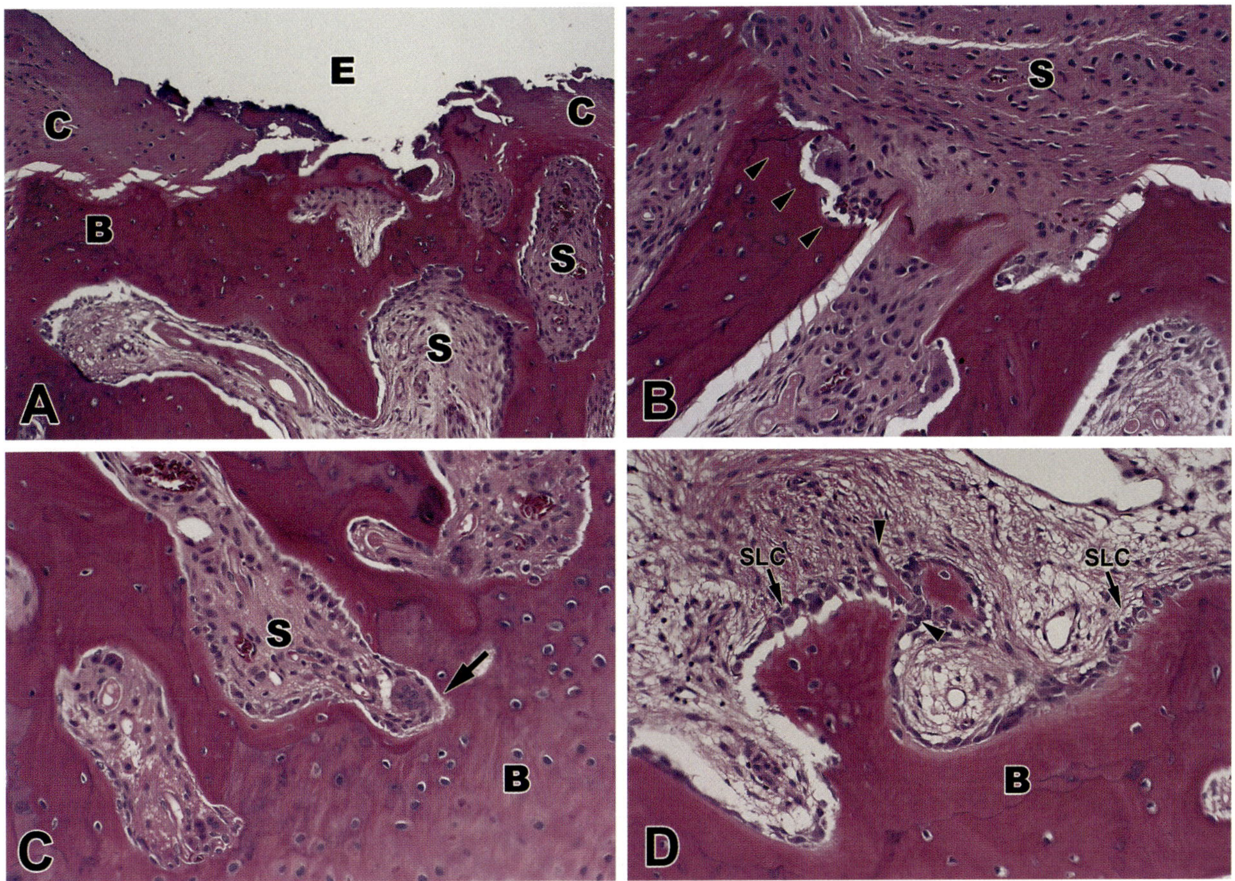

Figure 11.12. Histology of pannus invasion and destruction of cartilage and bone in rheumatoid arthritis (RA). **A:** A low-power view of synovial pannus (S) invading articular bone (B) and cartilage (C). The cartilage has been damaged such that there is a cartilage erosion (E), exposing the bone below. **B:** A higher-power view; arrowheads point out the "resorption bays" in articular bone where the leading edge of synovial pannus is eroding away bone by multinucleated osteoclasts. **C:** A similar lesion with a large multinucleated osteoclast (*arrow*) at the synovial pannus–bone interface. **D:** An area demonstrating the juxtaposition of the synovial lining cell (SLC) layer with bone that is in the process of being resorbed (B). Thus, both multinucleated osteoclasts and activated type A SLCs and type B SLCs participate in bone resorption in RA. (**A–D**, hematoxylin and eosin stain.)

insight into the proposed pathogenesis of human RA. One of these models, called the *K/BxN mouse*, has synovial histopathologic lesions that resemble human RA (2–6). The K/BxN mouse is of particular interest in that the pathogenic T and B cells that cause the disease both recognize GPI, and serum from these mice is sufficient to transfer the disease (2–6). A critical question is how can antibody and CD4$^+$ T-cell responses to a ubiquitous host antigen cause organ-specific autoimmune disease? Recent work has demonstrated in mice that GPI is selectively present in the extracellular space on synovium and cartilage and suggests that autoantibodies to GPI cause disease by binding directly to preexisting extracellular GPI in normal healthy mouse joints (3–5). Some humans with RA have been found to have antibodies against GPI, and GPI has been found in the extracellular space of human joints (4). Table 11.1 lists the pathogenic antigen candidates for animal models of RA and for human RA, and it is likely that several different autoantigens can be pathogenic and cause the RA syndrome in genetically susceptible humans (1).

Figure 11.13 shows, in schematic form, an overall scenario that is one current hypothesis to explain the observed histopathology seen in joint lesions in RA. GPI is shown as the inciting antigen, but one could substitute GPI with any of the potential antigens listed in Table 11.1. Once immune complexes form between the inciting autoantibody and antigen, they bind by Fc receptors to A-SLCs, tissue macrophages, and other cells of the innate immune system with Fc receptors, activate complement, and set up immune complex complement–mediated inflammatory responses. SLCs produce angiogenic factors that induce synovium angiogenesis, and SLCs and tissue macrophages produce IL-1α and IL-1β that activate CD4$^+$ T cells that have homed to inflamed synovium from the periphery. Activated synovial T cells produce osteoclast-inducing factors (Table 11.2) that include IFN-γ, RANKL, and IL-17. Osteoclast-inducing factors act on A-SLC, tissue macrophages, and mye-

TABLE 11.2. Osteoclast-Inducing Factors Detected in Rheumatoid Arthritis Synovium

Interleukin-1α and -β
Interleukin-6
Interleukin-11
Interleukin-15
Interleukin-17
Prostaglandin E_2
Monocyte/macrophage colony-stimulating factor
Tumor necrosis factor-α
Parathyroid hormone–related peptide
Receptor activator of nuclear factor–κB ligand

Adapted from Golding SR. Pathogenesis of bone erosion in rheumatoid arthritis. *Curr Opin Rheumatol* 2002;14:406–410.

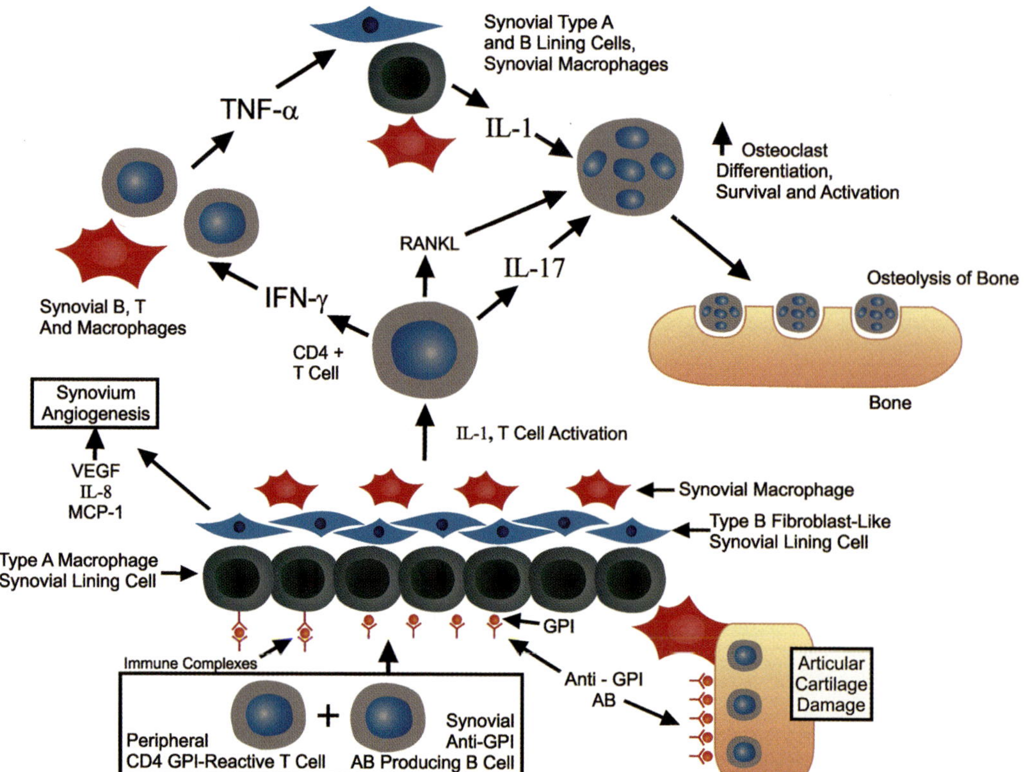

Figure 11.13. Schematic diagram of the overall scenario that is the current hypothesis to explain the observed histopathology seen in joint lesions in rheumatoid arthritis. Glucose-6-phosphate isomerase (GPI) is shown as the inciting antigen, but one could substitute GPI with any of the potential antigens listed in Table 11.1. Once immune complexes form between the inciting autoantibody and antigen, they bind by Fc receptors to type A synovial lining cells (A-SLCs), tissue macrophages, and other cells of the innate immune system with Fc receptors, activate complement, and set up immune complex complement–mediated inflammatory responses. SLCs produce angiogenic factors that induce synovium angiogenesis [vascular endothelial growth factor (VEGF), interleukin (IL)-8, and monocyte chemoattractant protein (MCP)-1], and SLCs and tissue macrophages produce IL-1α and IL-1β that activate CD4+ T cells that have homed to inflamed synovium from the periphery. Activated synovial T cells produce osteoclast-inducing factors (Table 11.2) that include interferon (IFN)-γ receptor activator of nuclear factor–κB ligand (RANKL) and IL-17. Osteoclast-inducing factors act on A-SLCs, tissue macrophages, and myeloid progenitors to induce osteoclast differentiation, survival, and activation. Increased activated osteoclasts at the pannus–bone interface cause osteolysis of bone. AB, antibody; TNF, tumor necrosis factor.

loid progenitors to induce osteoclast differentiation, survival, and activation. Increased activated osteoclasts at the pannus–bone interface cause osteolysis of bone.

PATHOLOGY OF EXTRAARTICULAR MANIFESTATIONS OF RHEUMATOID ARTHRITIS

Cutaneous Lesions in Rheumatoid Arthritis

Cutaneous lesions in RA include rheumatoid nodules, cutaneous vasculitis, and ulcerative lesions, including pyoderma gangrenosum.

Rheumatoid nodules occur in 20% of RA patients and are associated with high RF titers and progressive, severe articular disease and other manifestations of extraarticular disease (57–59). Rheumatoid nodules are found primarily in the subcutaneous tissue, either around pressure points, such as the elbow and Achilles tendon, or at the sites of chronic trauma. Other sites in which rheumatoid nodules have been reported include the sclera, vertebral bodies, vocal cords, lungs, heart, synovium, and skeletal muscles (57–61). The histologic features of the rheumatoid nodule include fibrosis with granulomatous areas of palisading tissue macrophages around a central necrotic area (Fig. 11.14A). Occasional multinucleated giant cells are seen (Fig. 11.14B). These lesions in the presence of typical RA make the diagnosis of rheumatoid nodule. Multiple rheumatoid nodule formation with minimal arthritis in an RF-positive patient is a syndrome called *rheumatoid nodulosis*. The histology of the nodules is the same as described above, and these patients are likely to have mild RA in which the development of rheumatoid nodules is the chief manifestation of the disease. Similar histologically appearing nodules have been reported to occur in normal children (pseudorheumatoid nodules) and in various infectious and noninfectious granulomatous diseases, such as granuloma annulare, necrobiosis lipoidica diabeticorum, and *Mycobacterium tuberculosis* infection (57,59).

Cutaneous vasculitis in RA can be small vessel vasculitis with arterioles and venules involved (hypersensitivity vasculitis) and manifest clinically as palpable purpura and/or livedo reticularis or chronic nonhealing leg ulcers or, rarely, can be medium-sized vessel arteritis and manifest as a systemic necrotizing vasculitis syndrome similar to that seen in polyarteritis nodosa (62). Occasional patients with RA develop cutaneous lesions indistinguishable from pyoderma gangrenosum that, on histology, show necrotizing vasculitis of both small arteries and venules (62). Cryoglobulinemia can occur in RA and can be associated with either hypersensitivity vasculitis and palpable purpura or digital infarcts and digital gangrene (62). Patients with RA vasculitis generally have high

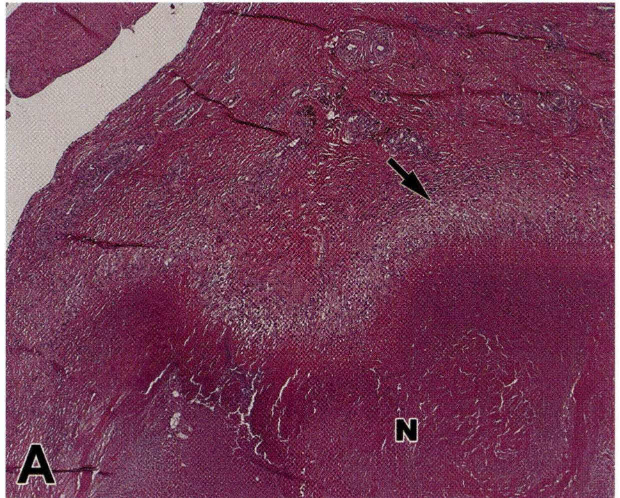

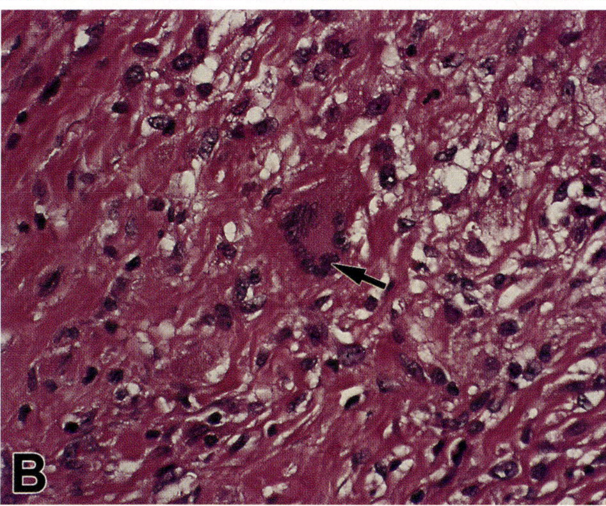

Figure 11.14. Histology of the subcutaneous rheumatoid nodule in rheumatoid arthritis. **A:** A low-power view of a subcutaneous rheumatoid nodule. Arrow points to palisading macrophages that surround a central area of necrosis (N). **B:** A higher-power view of the walls of the rheumatoid nodule with a large central multinucleated giant cell (*arrow*). (**A,B**; hematoxylin and eosin stain.)

titers of RF. The histology of hypersensitivity vasculitis in RA is identical to that in other causes of hypersensitivity vasculitis, with polymorphonuclear infiltrates in and around cutaneous small vessels. Other hallmarks of vasculitis are fibrin deposition, extravasated erythrocytes, and nuclear dust reflective of necrotic cells. In systemic necrotizing vasculitis syndromes in RA, small to medium-sized arteries can be infiltrated with acute and chronic inflammatory cells, often accompanied by fibrinoid necrosis. Vasculitis is frequent in RA and can be seen in synovium (Fig. 11.11B), as well as in any affected extraarticular tissue.

Finally, patients with juvenile RA (JRA) can have all the forms of cutaneous involvement mentioned above that occur in adult RA and, in addition, can manifest the classic "salmon pink" rash of Still's disease. The rash of JRA can be evanescent, and biopsy generally shows only nonspecific and mild perivascular inflammation.

Ocular Disease in Rheumatoid Arthritis

Patients with RA can have multiple forms of eye involvement, including episcleritis, scleritis, anterior uveitis (iridocyclitis),

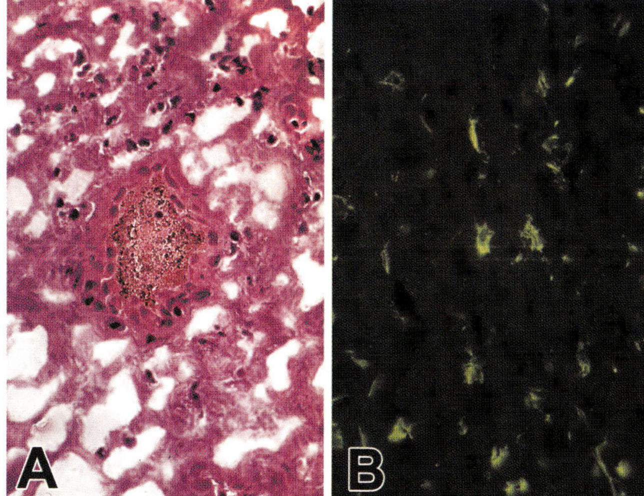

Figure 11.15. Histopathologic findings in inflammatory eye disease in rheumatoid arthritis (RA). **A:** A hematoxylin-and-eosin–stained biopsy of conjunctiva from a patient with severe scleritis and scleromalacia perforans in RA. Central vessel demonstrates vasculitis with inflammatory cells in and around the vessel wall. **B:** Indirect immunofluorescence analysis [with an anti–major histocompatibility complex (MHC) class II monoclonal antibody] of the cornea from an RA patient with corneal stromal loss in the absence of scleral inflammation. In this condition, it is thought that the corneal damage results from infiltration of the avascular cornea with activated MHC class II–positive tissue macrophages (*green cells*) that release collagenases and other metalloproteases and produce corneal stromal loss that leads to corneal ulceration and, in some cases, corneal perforation.

and sterile corneal ulceration in the absence of scleritis (63–66). In severe cases of scleritis associated with RA, inflammation can progress to scleromalacia, or thinning of the sclera, resulting in perforation of the orbit. The histopathology of scleritis in RA is that of a small vessel vasculitis associated with a lymphocytic infiltration in the conjunctiva and sclera (Fig. 11.15A) (63). The pathogenesis of episcleritis and scleritis in RA is presumed to be immune complex–mediated small vessel vasculitis. In corneal ulcerations in RA, the sclera can be uninvolved, and there is scant lymphocytic infiltration in the cornea. Rather, the cornea near the ulcerated area is infiltrated with MHC class II–positive macrophages (Fig. 11.15B), and these cells are thought to be the cells that mediate corneal damage by production of metalloproteases and cytokines (63). Similar ocular complications occur in JRA. In both RA and JRA, cataracts are common complications of both chronic anterior uveitis and steroid use.

Cardiac Disease in Rheumatoid Arthritis

Cardiac disease in RA can manifest as inflammatory pericarditis with effusion, myocarditis, coronary arteritis, accelerated atherosclerosis, aortic and mitral valve inflammation, and cardiac conduction abnormalities (67–70). Cardiac disease is common in RA and accounts for approximately 50% of all deaths in RA patients (69,70). Coronary artery disease has a higher incidence in RA and occurs earlier in life than in non-RA populations (69–71).

The most common cardiac complication of RA is fibrinous pericarditis, and it can be found in up to 30% of patients by echocardiography (72–77). In RA pericarditis and myocarditis, histologic analysis shows chronic inflammation with infiltration of lymphocytes, plasma cells, and macrophages into pericardium or myocardium. Recent study of rheumatoid pericardial tissue with antiimmune cell monoclonal antibodies demonstrated a predominance of $CD8^+$ T cells in RA pericardial tissues, suggesting that these cells play a major role in RA pericarditis (75). Rheumatoid nodules have been reported in all portions of the heart and pericardium, including heart valves and conduction system, and the histology of cardiac rheumatoid nodules is similar to that seen in subcutaneous tissue. Aortic valve inflammation with aortitis is the most common symptomatic valvular disease in RA, with involvement of both the valve and surrounding aorta with granulomatous inflammation. Pathologic studies show that in RA, mitral valve inflammation is greater than aortic valve inflammation, which is greater than other valve involvement (69,70,78,79).

Coronary lesions in RA can either be accelerated atherosclerosis or coronary arteritis, or both (69,70,80–83). As mentioned, RA is an independent risk factor for the development of atherosclerosis, and up to 50% of RA patients have coronary disease at autopsy that is clinically silent. Coronary arteritis is present in 10% to 20% of patients at autopsy (69–71,83). Arterial inflammation is manifested by infiltration of the coronary arteries with lymphocytes, polymorphonuclear leukocytes (PMNs), and tissue macrophages. Fibrinoid necrosis is present in the wall of the vessel, and immunofluorescence studies may reveal Ig and complement deposition in artery walls (69,70).

Lung and Pleural Disease in Rheumatoid Arthritis

Lung and pleural disease in RA is common and, like other extraarticular manifestations of RA, is associated with high titers of RF, hypocomplementemia, circulating immune complexes, and subcutaneous nodules (Table 11.3) (84). It is important to note that respiratory manifestations may precede, coincide with, or follow the onset of articular RA (83). Lung and pleural manifestations of RA are pleuritis with or without effusion, nodular lung disease, rheumatoid pneumoconiosis (Caplan's syndrome), obliterative bronchiolitis, diffuse interstitial lung disease, pulmonary hypertension, and pulmonary arteritis (3,84).

Pleurisy in RA can be asymptomatic or can manifest as pleuritic chest pain, shortness of breath, and audible pleural rub. It may be unilateral or bilateral. Pleural fluid is exudative with large numbers of PMNs and mononuclear cells; glucose is low (<25 mg per dL), and pleural biopsy shows either nonspecific inflammation or granulomatous lesions identical to the histopathology seen in rheumatoid nodules (Figs. 11.11C and 11.14).

Nodular lung disease can manifest either as necrobiotic nodules or as rheumatoid pneumoconiosis. Necrobiotic nodules can either be asymptomatic or manifest as a persistent cough or hemoptysis. If the lesions have cavitated and are infected, fever is common. RA lung nodules are pleural-based masses ranging from 1 mm to several cm; cavitation of these nodules is common. The pathology of necrobiotic nodules is similar to that seen in subcutaneous rheumatoid nodules (84) (Fig. 11.14).

Symptoms in rheumatoid pneumoconiosis (Caplan's syndrome) are related to the underlying pneumoconiosis with shortness of breath and exercise intolerance; with cavitation and infection, fever is common. Distribution of lung nodules is peripheral, and size is similar to that seen in other nodular lung disease with RA. The histopathology is similar to that seen with rheumatoid nodules, with the addition of coal dust particles seen in the necrotic nodules (83).

TABLE 11.3. Pulmonary Manifestations of Rheumatoid Arthritis

Manifestation	Pathologic Features	Radiographic Features	Clinical Correlates of Pathology
Pleurisy with or without effusion	Fluid is exudative with large numbers of polymorphonuclear leukocytes and mononuclear cells; glucose <25 mg/dL; pleural biopsy shows nonspecific inflammation or granulomatous lesions identical to rheumatoid nodules.	Unilateral or bilateral; other intrapulmonary manifestations of rheumatoid arthritis in 33%.	Asymptomatic to pleuritic chest pain to occasional shortness of breath and cough; occasional pleural rub.
Nodular lung disease: necrobiotic nodules	Identical to subcutaneous rheumatoid nodules: central zone of acellular necrosis surrounded by palisading epithelial cells, which are surrounded by lymphocytes, plasma cells, and fibroblasts.	Well-circumscribed, multiple, pleural-based masses ranging in size from 1 mm to 7 cm; other manifestations of rheumatoid lung disease frequently present; cavitation not uncommon.	Asymptomatic; persistent cough and/or hemoptysis, if cavitary; fever if infected.
Rheumatoid pneumoconiosis (Caplan's syndrome)	Similar to above except associated with dust in central necrotic zone.	Single or multiple well-rounded opacities 0.5–5.0 cm in diameter, situated in peripheral lung; lesions may cavitate.	Symptoms generally secondary to underlying pneumoconiosis; occasional fever with cavitation and infection.
Diffuse interstitial lung disease	Early: interstitial lymphocytes, plasma cells, and macrophages. Late: distortion of alveolocapillary units and fibrosis; findings of secondary pulmonary hypertension may be present.	Generalized reticulonodular infiltrates, greatest in lower and middle lung fields; often findings of pulmonary hypertension: pleural abnormalities in 17% and nodules in 20%.	Subacute onset with progressive dyspnea, cough, rales at bases, tachypnea, and occasional clubbing, cyanosis, and pleuritic chest pain; pulmonary hypertension may be present.
Obliterative bronchiolitis	Fibrous narrowing and obliteration of bronchioles and bronchi with infiltration of mononuclear cells; intrabronchiolar polypoid masses of obstructing tissue may be present.	Distended but otherwise normal lungs.	Progressive dyspnea with rales and midinspiratory "squack"; pulmonary function tests reveal irreversible air flow obstruction and air trapping with low lung volumes.
Pulmonary arteritis and hypertension	Features of primary pulmonary hypertension or lymphocytic small muscular arteritis or progressive intimal fibroblastosis.	Pulmonary vascular dilatation and secondary cardiomegaly.	Features of primary hypertension and Raynaud's phenomenon common.

Adapted from McCallum RM, Haynes BF. Management of patients with pulmonary manifestations of collagen-vascular diseases. In: Shelhamer J, Pizzo P, Parrillo J, et al., eds. *Respiratory disease in the immunosuppressed host.* Philadelphia: J.B. Lippincott Co., 1991:664–681.

Diffuse interstitial lung disease in RA presents subacutely with progressive dyspnea, cough, tachypnea, and eventual cyanosis. It may be associated with pleuritic chest pain, and pulmonary hypertension may be present. Chest x-ray shows multiple reticulonodular infiltrates, greatest in lower and middle lung fields, with 15% to 20% of patients having pleural lesions or RA lung nodules, respectively. The histopathology of early diffuse interstitial lung disease in RA shows interstitial lymphocytes, plasma cells, and macrophages in alveolar septae. More advanced disease shows distortion of alveolocapillary units and fibrosis (84).

In obliterative bronchiolitis in RA, progressive dyspnea with rales is present, and pulmonary function tests reveal irreversible air flow obstruction and air trapping with low lung volumes. Histopathology shows fibrous narrowing and obliteration of bronchioles and bronchi with infiltration of mononuclear cells; intrabronchiolar polypoid masses of obstructing granulomatous tissue may be present.

Pulmonary arteritis and hypertension in RA is frequently associated with clinical features of primary pulmonary hypertension; Raynaud's phenomenon is common in this setting as well. On chest x-ray, pulmonary vascular dilatation and secondary cardiomegaly is common. Histopathology shows a lymphocytic muscular arteritis or perivascular fibrosis and intimal fibroelastosis characteristic of pulmonary hypertension.

Rarely spontaneous, pneumothorax can occur in RA due to cavitation of subpleural nodules. Secondary amyloidosis can occur in RA and involve the lungs as well as the kidneys. Finally, stridor secondary to cricoarytenoid joint synovitis can occur and cause a medical emergency due to airway compromise (84) (see Ear, Nose, and Throat Manifestations of Rheumatoid Arthritis).

Neurologic Disease in Rheumatoid Arthritis

Neurologic involvement in RA includes spinal cord compression from cervical spine subluxations, peripheral neuropathies, myopathy and myositis, vasculitis involving the brain or peripheral nerves, dural rheumatoid nodules, and rheumatoid nodule or vasculitis involvement of the brain parenchyma (85,86).

Myelopathy associated with vertebral subluxation in RA can occur from atlantoaxial subluxation when C-1 moves anteriorly on C-2; when C-1 moves posteriorly on C-2, with vertical subluxation of the odontoid; and when there are subluxations at multiple levels, leading to "staircase spine" deformity. RA patients with advanced disease are more likely to develop spine compression, and 30% to 40% of RA patients have radiologic evidence of vertebral subluxation. Instability of C-1 on C-2 results from inflammation and erosions in the transverse ligament of the atlas and the odontoid process itself. In vertical atlantoaxial subluxation, destruction of cartilage and bone allows upward and backward displacement of the odontoid process into the foramen magnum, resulting in compression of the brain stem (85,86). The histopathology of the spinal cord at the level of cord compression in RA shows necrosis throughout the anterior horns with extension of necrosis into the ventral horns, the posterior columns, and the medial portions of the lateral columns (85,86). Upward displacement of the odontoid can compress the vertebral or posterior cerebral artery, leading to thrombosis and ischemic damage to the medulla or cerebellum or both (85,86). Finally, epidural hemorrhage has been described in RA, generally in association with fractures of the cervical spine (85,86), and focal demyelination of nerve roots has been reported with severe atlantoaxial subluxation (85,86).

Peripheral neuropathy in RA can be due to nerve compression leading to entrapment, can be a mild sensory neuropathy with good prognosis, can be a diffuse sensorimotor neuropathy, or can be a fulminant sensorimotor neuropathy due to systemic necrotizing vasculitis (85,86). Nerve conduction studies show evidence of neuropathy in 30% to 40% of patients with RA. In the most common clinical form of RA-associated neuropathy, a mild sensory peripheral neuropathy, patients have paresthesias, dysesthesias, with decrease in vibration sensation. This form of neuropathy can subside when RA disease activity subsides (85,86).

A more severe sensorimotor neuropathy can be present in patients with active RA with symmetric distal weakness in addition to sensory symptoms. Loss of touch sensation is common. Again, this manifestation may improve or slowly progress with control of the RA. In both the more common mild neuropathy and in severe sensorimotor neuropathy in RA, nerve histology is generally not available for evaluation.

In a small number of RA patients, a fulminant sensorimotor syndrome with mononeuritis multiplex can occur and can be associated with a systemic necrotizing vasculitis syndrome (62, 85,86). Serum RF titers are frequently very high, and the neurologic picture is similar to that seen in polyarteritis nodosa. In these patients, an evaluation is warranted to rule out vasculitis, and sural nerve biopsy is performed. Nerve biopsy frequently shows vasculitis of the vasavasorum in the nerve sheath (62,85,86). In the nerves themselves, nerve fiber alterations vary according to the severity of the vasculitis (85,86). Wallerian degeneration of myelinated and unmyelinated fibers can occur, as well as segmental demyelination (85,86).

Three patterns of infiltration by inflammatory cells have been recognized in muscle of RA patients: polymyositis, focal nodular myositis, and vasculitis (62,85,86). In polymyositis type of muscle inflammation in RA, the muscle is infiltrated with lymphocytes, tissue macrophages, and plasma cells associated with muscle fiber degeneration, regeneration, and necrosis (85,86).

Focal nodular myositis occurs most often in RA patients with active, long-standing RA (85,86). The muscle is infiltrated with 1- to 2-mm nodular infiltrations of lymphocytes and plasma cells around or adjacent to muscle vessels (85,86).

Vasculitis of muscle has the same vessel histology as in other affected tissues, with PMN and lymphocyte infiltrations in and around the walls of vessels, perivascular extravasation of erythrocytes, and fibrinoid necrosis of vessel walls (62,85,86). In the setting of denervation due to vasculitis or inflammatory neuropathy, one can see denervation atrophy of muscle with angulated atrophic type II fibers (85,86).

In the setting of nodules, RA, and symptoms of cord compression, the differential diagnosis should include vertebral subluxation as well as the presence of dural rheumatoid nodules. Dural rheumatoid nodules can compress the brain as well. The histopathology of dural rheumatoid nodules is similar to that seen in rheumatoid nodules elsewhere (Fig. 11.14).

Direct involvement of the brain in RA is rare and occurs in the setting of a systemic necrotizing vasculitis syndrome involving central nervous system vessels and via direct formation of rheumatoid nodules in brain parenchyma (62,85,86). Vasculitis can occur in small to medium-sized cerebral and leptomeningeal vessels (62,85,86). Rarely, large arteries, such as the basilar or vertebral arteries, can be involved with aneurysmal formation. Rheumatoid nodules and granulomas most often affect the cranial dura but also have been described in the choroid plexus, vertebral artery, falx cerebri, and cerebral parenchyma.

Renal Disease in Rheumatoid Arthritis

Renal disease in RA can be due to secondary amyloidosis, vasculitis, Sjögren's syndrome, drug toxicity, or nephrosclerosis/mesangial hypercellularity (87). In a study of 132 RA patients at autopsy, 6% had some form of vasculitis, and azotemia was present before death in 23% (88). At autopsy, 90% had nephrosclerosis, 14% had systemic vasculitis, 8% had kidney vasculitis, 11% had kidney amyloidosis, 8% had membranous glomerulopathy, and 8% had focal glomerular disease (88).

The type of amyloidosis in RA is AA amyloidosis and also occurs in other chronic infections and chronic inflammatory conditions. Amyloid is found in 50% of renal biopsies of symptomatic RA patients with renal disease (in particular, proteinuria) (87). The rate of renal failure progression in amyloidosis associated with RA may be related to location of amyloid deposition. Glomerular deposition of amyloid leads to proteinuria, whereas vascular amyloid deposition leads to nephron necrosis and interstitial fibrosis (87,89).

Vasculitis of the kidney in RA is uncommon, with overall incidence of systemic vasculitis during a lifetime with RA of approximately 5% and the incidence of major organ damage due to vasculitis in RA less than 1% (87). As mentioned above, in an autopsy series of RA patients, 14% had systemic vasculitis, whereas 8% had vasculitis of the kidneys (88).

Patients with RA often also have Sjögren's syndrome (keratoconjunctivitis, xerostomia, and a connective tissue disease, usually RA). Although up to 30 percent of primary Sjögren's syndrome patients have renal abnormalities (interstitial nephritis and distal tubular acidosis) (87), it is not known if the association of Sjögren's syndrome with RA (secondary Sjögren's syndrome) is associated with increased incidence of renal disease. Hypergammaglobulinemia in Sjögren's syndrome has been associated with tubular abnormalities (87). In this regard, Boers et al. found glomerular and tubular dysfunction to be present both in RA patients with and without Sjögren's syndrome (87).

Many of the drugs that are used to treat RA patients have renal toxicities (87). Gold and penicillamine are less frequently used today and, when used, cause proteinuria in up to 10% of patients on gold and 30% of patients on penicillamine (87). The pathologic lesion in this setting is membranous glomerulopathy (90).

Nonsteroidal antiinflammatory drugs (NSAIDs) are commonly used and are potent inhibitors of prostaglandin synthesis. The inhibition of vasodilatory prostaglandins can predispose to renal vasoconstriction and exacerbate other situations with decreased renal blood flow, such as salt depletion, hypovolemia, and congestive heart failure. In these settings, acute renal failure can develop with concomitant use of NSAIDs (4). NSAIDs can also cause an acute interstitial nephritis characterized by eosinophilia, eosinophiluria, and proteinuria (86). A more severe NSAID-associated interstitial nephritis is not associated with eosinophilia, and the proteinuria can be at the level to fulfill criteria for nephrotic syndrome (87).

Cyclosporin A in RA alters renal hemodynamics, leading to tubular hypoxia and reduced glomerular filtration rate (87). In high-dose cyclosporin A use (>10 mg per kg), irreversible renal failure can develop with interstitial fibrosis and hyalinization of glomeruli in renal biopsy (87). RA patients are more susceptible to cyclosporin toxicity, likely due to concomitant use of NSAIDs.

A recent prospective study of 235 patients with early RA assessed the type of renal disease that developed over time (91). Renal abnormalities were common, with hematuria the most common (42%) and proteinuria (10%) and elevated creatinine (6%) less common. This study found that proteinuria and elevated creatinine were most likely related to drugs and normalized when the offending drugs were stopped, whereas hematuria was not related to drug use but, rather, was related to RA disease activity. In this study, no renal histology was reported, but other studies have shown mesangioproliferative glomerulonephritis in RA with hematuria (90).

Spleen and Liver Involvement in Rheumatoid Arthritis

The extraarticular manifestations of RA that involve the spleen are primarily those of Felty's syndrome (FS) (RA with neutropenia with or without splenomegaly) and the large granular lymphocyte (LGL) syndrome associated with RA (also called *pseudo-FS*) (92,93).

Splenomegaly is common in RA, occurring in approximately 50% of patients and is usually not associated with neutropenia (92,93). Similarly, neutropenia can occur in RA in the absence of an enlarged spleen. Spleen function in RA as measured by clearance of technetium-99–labeled autologous red blood cells has been reported to be abnormal in approximately 90% of patients (94). The histology of the spleen in RA is either normal or shows foci of granulomatous tissue similar to that seen in rheumatoid nodules (89,92,93). Spontaneous splenic rupture is rare in RA but has been reported, and the splenic histology has shown capsular granulomatous inflammation (92,93).

In the spleen in FS, there is an increase in red pulp, with associated sinus hyperplasia and increased tissue macrophages (92). There is a reduction in sheathed red pulp capillaries associated with an increase in phagocytosis by splenic macrophages in FS. Other changes seen include hyaline arteriosclerosis, endothelial hyperplasia, and increased elastin in the follicular arteries associated with portal hypertension (92). Extramedullary hematopoiesis in splenic cords is common as well (92).

The LGL syndrome that can be associated with RA is characterized by bone marrow infiltration with LGLs, splenomegaly, and neutropenia (92,93). LGLs are lymphocytes with generous cytoplasm containing azurophilic granules (Fig. 11.16) and either express $CD16^+$, $CD56^+$, or $CD8^{+/-}$ (markers of natural killer cells) or are $CD8^+$ TCR $\gamma\delta$ T cells (93–97). Patients with LGL lymphocytosis have associated autoimmune syndromes in 30% of cases of LGL lymphocytosis, one of which is RA. Patients with LGL lymphocytosis can appear to have RA with FS, but the arthritis in LGL-associated disease is reported to be less severe than that with FS and is not associated with extraarticular features (92). Adding confusion to the distinction between LGL lymphocytosis and FS, up to 30% of FS patients have elevated numbers of LGL in peripheral blood (92). Interestingly, Jacobs and Haynes have demonstrated elevated num-

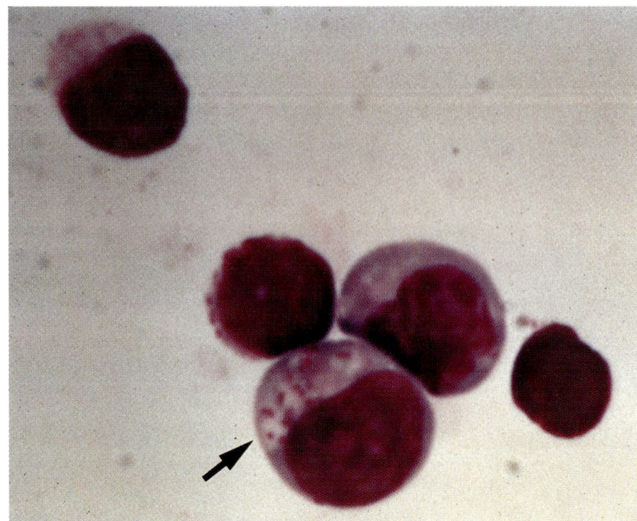

Figure 11.16. Large granular lymphocytes such as those seen in large granular lymphocytosis syndrome associated with rheumatoid arthritis. Arrow points to two large granular lymphocytes.

bers of tissue infiltrating TCR γδ T cells in the synovia of 40% of RA patients (none of whom had FS or LGL with RA) with the highest levels of joint inflammation (36).

Many patients with LGL lymphocytosis have oligoclonal or monoclonal proliferations of LGL, as determined by TCR rearrangement analysis in the T-cell type of LGL (95–99) or determined by polymerase chain reaction–based X-inactivation analysis in LGL with germline TCRs (100). Thus, in RA associated with LGL lymphocytosis, many cases appear to be forms of a T-cell or natural killer cell chronic lymphocytic leukemia with a benign course (99).

Lymph node involvement in RA is manifested most commonly by generalized lymphadenopathy and can occur in 50% to 75% of patients (66). Lymphoid hyperplasia is seen at lymph node biopsy (usually at the time of evaluation of the patient for malignancy), with active germinal centers and follicular hyperplasia and polyclonal B cells (66). B-cell lymphomas can occur in RA patients and, in addition, can be associated with immunosuppressive therapy, such as methotrexate (see Chapter 25).

Nodular regenerative hyperplasia of the liver (NRHL) results from liver regeneration in response to injury or ischemia and can be seen in a variety of autoimmune disease syndromes but is most commonly seen in RA with or without FS (101). NRHL is characterized by nodules of hyperplastic hepatocytes in the absence of fibrosis with some periportal fibrosis (101). Macroscopically, there are diffuse nodules on the liver surface (101). Portal fibrosis in FS can also occur in the absence of NRHL. A rare finding in the liver of FS patients is sinusoidal lymphocytosis, with a diffuse infiltration of the sinusoids with mature-appearing lymphocytes (102).

Ear, Nose, and Throat Manifestations of Rheumatoid Arthritis

The ear, nose, and throat manifestations of RA include involvement of the larynx, the temporomandibular joints, the nose, and, rarely, the ossicular bones of the inner ear (103).

The cricoarytenoid articulations are diarthroidal joints that consist of cartilaginous articular surfaces covered by a synovial lining similar to any other diarthroidal joints that can be affected by inflammation in RA. Occurring in 30% to 50% of patients with RA, cricoarytenoid joint involvement can lead to stridor and loss of airway (103). The pathology of cricoarytenoid inflammation is synovial proliferation, effusions with fibrin deposits, and pannus development. Joint cartilage can be eroded, with obliteration and ankylosis of the joint (103). Vocal cord dysfunction in RA can occur from the development of rheumatoid nodules within the cords themselves and from degenerative changes in laryngeal muscles and nerves (103). Laryngeal nerves can be damaged due to vasculitis of the vasanervorum with obliterative endarteritis or by amyloid infiltration of vessels and nerves (103).

The temporomandibular joint is affected in approximately two-thirds of RA patients and presents with otalgia, pain on chewing and talking (103). In the temporomandibular joint, the pathological processes are likely to be similar to those in other diarthroidal joints, but pathological tissue for analysis is rarely available antemortem.

Involvement of the nose in RA can manifest as nasal ulcers progressing to spontaneous septal perforation from vasculitis (103). Finally, involvement of the ear in RA can rarely involve the diarthroidal joints of the ear, the ossicular chain. RA patients have been described exhibiting hearing loss during the exacerbation of their disease, with subsequent improvement during disease remission (103).

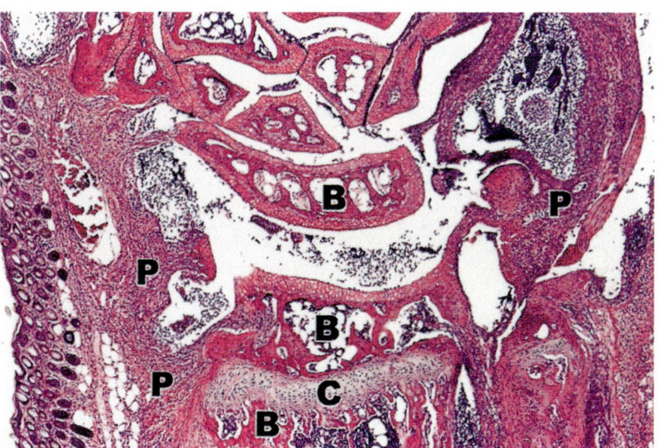

Figure 11.17. Histology of inflamed joint in the human T-cell lymphotropic virus type I (HTLV-I) *tax*-transgenic mouse: the animal model of HTLV-I–associated arthritis (HAA). A hematoxylin-and-eosin–stained section of the hind paw of an HTLV-I *tax*-transgenic mouse. In this model, the animals spontaneously develop a severe rheumatoid arthritis–like syndrome at 2 to 3 months of age. The histology of human HAA is similar to that seen here with pannus (P) invading cartilage (C) and bone (B).

CONDITIONS THAT MAY MIMIC RHEUMATOID ARTHRITIS

It is beyond the scope of this chapter to give a complete differential diagnosis of the arthritis syndromes that can clinically mimic RA (see Chapter 2), but it is of interest to briefly discuss two syndromes that either can mimic or exacerbate RA histopathology [silicone synovitis and human T-cell lymphotropic virus type I (HTLV-I)–associated arthritis (HAA)].

Silicone synovitis occurs in the setting of particulate silicone abraded from carpal implants or other prostheses, most commonly in the hand or wrist, but can occur in any joint with a silicone prosthesis (104–107). Histologic studies of synovium of affected patients demonstrate intracellular and extracellular particular foreign body material 20 to 100 μM in diameter that is refractile under polarized light but is not birefringent. The inflammation seen is histologically similar to that in RA with lymphocytes and plasma cells and foreign body giant cells at the site of silicone particles. Silicone synovitis can exacerbate an underlying inflammatory arthritis such as RA and lead to erosive joint damage.

HAA can take two forms: a leukemia-associated arthritis in patients with frank HTLV-I leukemia (108) and an RA-like syndrome in HTLV-I–positive patients who do not have leukemia (108–110). In the former syndrome, the joint tissue and synovial fluid contain infiltrating HTLV-I–positive malignant T cells (108). In the latter syndrome in humans, and in the animal model of nonleukemia-associated HAA, the *tax*-transgenic mouse (110) (Fig. 11.17), the histology of the arthritis is very similar to that seen in classic (HTLV-I–negative) RA (109–111). Figure 11.17 shows the hind limb diarthrodial joint of an HTLV-I *tax*-transgenic mouse showing pannus (P) infiltrating into bone (B) and cartilage (C), with histologic changes similar to those seen in typical RA. HAA in the absence of leukemia is distinguished by negative RF and positive serologies for HTLV-I (109,110).

CONCLUSION

RA is a systemic disease that can affect multiple tissues throughout the body. The general pathologic process in the joint is outlined in Figure 11.13, leading to SLC proliferation, pannus formation, cartilage and bone erosion, and joint destruction. The formation of granulomatous inflammatory tissue in extraarticular sites frequently has the histologic morphology of rheumatoid nodules, leading to tissue injury and organ dysfunction.

With the advent of microarray technology, sequencing of the human genome, and the automated technology of laser dissection microscopy, it is anticipated that the near future will rapidly produce an understanding of the changes in gene and protein expression that occur in RA tissues during the course of the disease. Further understanding of the changes in gene and protein expression in RA tissues will facilitate better understanding of the pathogenesis of RA and rapidly lead to new and more specific therapeutic strategies for RA. Hopefully, these new studies will also lead to novel strategies to prevent RA from developing in individuals with genes that predispose to the development of RA.

ACKNOWLEDGMENTS

The author acknowledges Kim R. McClammy for her expert secretarial assistance and Robert DeVoe and Steven Conlon for their expert assistance with illustrations.

REFERENCES

1. Magalhaes R, Stiehl P, Morawietz L, et al. Morphological and molecular pathology of the B cell response in synovitis of rheumatoid arthritis. *Virchows Arch* 2002;441:415–427.
2. Matsumoto I, Staub A, Benoist C, et al. Arthritis provoked by linked T and B cell recognition of a glycolytic enzyme. *Science* 1999;286:1732–1735.
3. Matsumoto I, Maccioni M, Lee DM, et al. How antibodies to a ubiquitous cytoplasmic enzyme may provoke joint-specific autoimmune disease. *Nat Immunol* 2002;3:360–365.
4. Schaller M, Burton DR, Ditzel HJ. Autoantibodies to GPI in rheumatoid arthritis: linkage between an animal model and human disease. *Nat Immunol* 2001;2:746–753.
5. Hirano T. Revival of the autoantibody model in rheumatoid arthritis. *Nat Immunol* 2002;3:342–344.
6. Corr M, Firestein GS. Innate immunity as a hired gun: but is it rheumatoid arthritis? *J Exp Med* 2002;195:F33–F35.
7. Koetz K, Bryl E, Spickchen K. T cell homeostasis in patients with rheumatoid arthritis. *Proc Natl Acad Sci U S A* 2000;97:9203–9208.
8. Goronzy JJ, Weyand CM. Thymic function and peripheral T-cell homeostasis in rheumatoid arthritis. *Trends Immunol* 2002;22:251–256.
9. Namekawa T, Wagner UG, Goronzy JJ, et al. Functional subsets of CD4 T cells in rheumatoid synovitis. *Arthritis Rheum* 1998;41:2108–2116.
10. Weyand CM. New insights into the pathogenesis of rheumatoid arthritis. *Rheumatology* 2000;39:3–8.
11. Namekawa T, Snyder MR, Yen J-H, et al. Killer cell activating receptors function as costimulatory molecules on $CD4^+$ $CD28^{null}$ T cells clonally expanded in rheumatoid arthritis. *J Immunol* 2000;165:1138–1145.
12. Vallejo AN, Schirmer M, Weyand CM, et al. Clonality and longevity of $CD4^+$ $CD28^{null}$ T cells are associated with defects in apoptotic pathways. *J Immunol* 2000;165:6301–6307.
13. Warrington KJ, Takemura S, Goronzy JJ. $CD4^+$, $CD28^-$ T cells in rheumatoid arthritis patients combine features of the innate and adaptive immune system. *Arthritis Rheum* 2001;44:13–20.
14. Radin EL. Structure and function of joints in arthritis and allied conditions. In: Koopman WJ, ed. *A textbook of rheumatology*, 14th ed. Philadelphia: Lippincott Williams & Wilkins, 2001.
15. Hale LP, Martin ME, McCollum DE, et al. Immunohistologic analysis of the distribution of cell adhesion molecules within the inflammatory synovial microenvironment. *Arthritis Rheum* 1998;32:22–30.
16. Burmester GR, Dimitriu-Bona A, Waters SJ, et al. Identification of three major synovial lining cell populations by monoclonal antibodies directed to Ia antigens and antigen associated with monocytes/macrophages and fibroblasts. *Scand J Immunol* 1983;17:69–82.
17. Edwards JCW. The origin of type A synovial lining cells. *Immunobiology* 1982;161:227–231.
18. Henderson B, Pettipher ER. A synovial lining cells: biology and pathobiology. *Semin Arthritis Rheum* 1985;15:1–32.
19. Haynes BF, Hale LP, Patton KL, et al. Measurement of an adhesion molecule as an indicator of inflammatory disease activity. *Arthritis Rheum* 1991;34:1434–1443.
20. Soden M, Rooney M, Cullen A, et al. Immunohistological features in the synovium obtained from clinically uninvolved knee joints of patients with rheumatoid arthritis. *Br J Rheumatol* 1989;28:287–292.
21. Kraan M, Versendaal H, Jonker M, et al. Asymptomatic synovitis precedes clinically manifest arthritis. *Arthritis Rheum* 1998;41:1481–1488.
22. Athanasou NA, Quinn J. Immunocytochemical analysis of human synovial lining cells: phenotypic relations to other marrow derived cell. *Ann Rheum Dis* 1991;50:311–315.
23. FitzGerald O, Bresnihan B. Synovial membrane cellularity and vascularity. *Ann Rheum Dis* 1995;54:511–515.
24. Schumacher HR, Kitridou RC. Synovitis of recent onset: a clinicopathologic study during the first month of disease. *Arthritis Rheum* 1972;15:465–485.
25. Yin G, Liu W, An P, et al. Endostatin gene transfer inhibits joint angiogenesis and pannus formation in inflammatory arthritis. *Mol Ther* 2002;5:547–554.
26. Kaiser M, Younge B, Johannes B, et al. Formation of new vasa vasorum in vasculitis: production of angiogenic cytokines by multinucleated giant cells. *Am J Pathol* 1999;155:765–774.
27. FitzGerald O, Soden M, Yanni G, et al. Morphometric analysis of blood vessels in synovial membranes obtained from clinically affected and unaffected knee joints of patients with rheumatoid arthritis. *Ann Rheum Dis* 1991;50:792–796.
28. Liao H-X, Haynes BF. Role of adhesion molecules in the pathogenesis of rheumatoid arthritis. *Rheum Arth* 1995;21:715–741.
29. Patel DD, Haynes BF. Leukocyte homing to synovium. In: Goronzy JJ, Weyand CM, eds. *Current directions in autoimmunity*, vol. 3. New York: Karger, 2001:133–167.
30. Baeten D, Demetter P, Cuvelier C, et al. Comparative study of the synovial histology in rheumatoid arthritis, spondyloarthropathy, and osteoarthritis: influence of disease duration and activity. *Ann Rheum Dis* 2000;59:945–953.
31. Weinberg JB, Pippen AMM, Greenberg CS. Extravascular fibrin formation and dissolution in synovial tissue of patients with osteoarthritis and rheumatoid arthritis. *Arthritis Rheum* 1991;34:996–1005.
32. Kang YM, Zhang X, Wagner WG, et al. CD8 T cells are required for the formation of ectopic germinal centers in rheumatoid synovitis. *J Exp Med* 2002;195:1325 1336.
33. Weyand CM, Kurtin PJ, Goronzy JJ. Ectopic lymphoid organogenesis a fast track for autoimmunity. *Am J Pathol* 2001;159:787–793.
34. Takemura S, Braun A, Crowson C, et al. Lymphoid neogenesis in rheumatoid synovitis. *J Immunol* 2001;167:1072–1080.
35. Takemura S, Klimiuk PA, Braun A, et al. T cell activation in rheumatoid synovial is B cell dependent. *J Immunol* 2001;167:4710–4718.
36. Jacobs MR, Haynes BF. Increase in TCR-γδ T lymphocytes in synovia from rheumatoid arthritis patients with active synovitis. *J Clin Invest* 1992;12:130–138.
37. Kornstein JJ, deBlois GG. Pathology of the thymus and mediastinum. In: *Major problems in pathology*, vol. 33. Philadelphia: W.B. Saunders Co., 1995.
38. Edwards JCW, Willoughby A. Demonstration of bone marrow derived cells in synovial lining by means of giant intracellular granules as genetic markers. *Ann Rheum Dis* 1982;41:177–182.
39. Qu Z, Garcia CH, O'Rourke LM, et al. Local proliferation of fibroblast-like synoviocytes contributes to synovial hyperplasia. *Arthritis Rheum* 1994;37:212–220.
40. Rooney M, Condell D, Quinlau W, et al. Analysis of the histologic variation of synovitis in rheumatoid arthritis. *Arthritis Rheum* 1988;31:956–963.
41. Tak PP, Smeets TJM, Daha MR, et al. Analysis of the synovial cell infiltrate in early rheumatoid synovial tissue in relation to local disease activity. *Arthritis Rheum* 1997;40:217–275.
42. Soden M, Rooney M, Whelan A, et al. Immunohistological analysis of the synovial membrane: search for predictors of the clinical course in rheumatoid arthritis. *Ann Rheum Dis* 1991;50:673–676.
43. Schumacher HR, Bautista BB, Krauser RE, et al. Histological appearance of the synovium in early rheumatoid arthritis. *Semin Arthritis Rheum* 1994;23:3–10.
44. Kraan MC, Haringman JJ, Post WJ, et al. Immunohistological analysis of synovial tissue for differential diagnosis in early arthritis. *Rheumatology* 1999;38:1074–1080.
45. Mulherin D, Fitzgerald O, Bresnihan B. Synovial tissue macrophage populations and articular damage in rheumatoid arthritis. *Arthritis Rheum* 1996;39:115–124.
46. Bromley M, Woolley DE. Histopathology of the rheumatoid lesion. Identification of cell types at sites of cartilage erosion. *Arthritis Rheum* 1984;27:857–863.
47. Yanni G, Whelan A, Feighery C, et al. Synovial tissue macrophage and joint erosion in rheumatoid arthritis. *Ann Rheum Dis* 1994;53:39–44.
48. Zvaifler NJ, Beyle D, Firestein GS. Early synovitis-synoviocytes and mononuclear cells. *Semin Arthritis Rheum* 1994;23:11–16.
49. McCachren SS, Haynes BF, Niedel JE. Localization of collagenase mRNA in rheumatoid arthritis synovium by in situ hybridization histochemistry. *J Clin Immunol* 1990;10:19–27.
50. Goldring SR. Pathogenesis of bone erosion in rheumatoid arthritis. *Curr Opin Rheumatol* 2002;14:406–410.
51. Yamanishi Y, Boyle DL, Rosengren S, et al. Regional analysis of p53 mutations in rheumatoid arthritis synovium. *Proc Natl Acad Sci U S A* 2002;99:10025–10030.
52. Redlich K, Hayer S, Ricci R, et al. Osteoclasts are essential for TNFα-mediated joint destruction. *J Clin Invest* 2002;110:1419–1427.
53. Romas E, Gillespie MT, Martin TJ. Involvement of receptor activator of NFκB ligand and tumor necrosis factor-α in bone destruction in rheumatoid arthritis. *Bone* 2002;30:340–346.
54. Leisen JCC, Duncan H, Riddle JM, et al. The erosive front: a topographic study of the junction between the pannus and the subchondral plate in the macerated rheumatoid metacarpal head. *J Rheumatol* 1988;15:17–22.

55. Pettit AR, Ji H, Stechow D, et al. Trance/Rankl knockout mice are protected from bone erosion in a serum transfer model of arthritis. *Am J Pathol* 2001;159:1689–1699.
56. Lubberts E, Joosten LA, Oppers B, et. al. IL-1 dependent role of IL-17 in synovial inflammation and joint destruction during collagen-induced arthritis. *J Immunol* 2001;167:1004–1013.
57. Sibbitt WL Jr, Williams RC Jr. Cutaneous manifestations of rheumatoid arthritis. *Int J Dermatol* 1982;21:563–572.
58. McGrath MH, Fleischer A. The subcutaneous rheumatoid nodule. *Hand Clin* 1989;5:127–135.
59. Kaye BR, Kaye RL, Bobrove A. Rheumatoid nodules: review of the spectrum of associated conditions and proposal of a new classification, with a report of four seronegative cases. *Am J Med* 1984;76:279–292.
60. Couret M, Combe B, Chuong VT, et al. Rheumatoid nodulosis: report of two new cases and discussion of diagnostic criteria. *J Rheumatol* 1988;15:1427–1430.
61. Pearson ME, Kosco M, Huffer W, et al. Rheumatoid nodules of the spine: case report and review of the literature. *Arthritis Rheum* 1987;30:709–713.
62. Vollertsen RS, Conn DL. Vasculitis associated with rheumatoid arthritis. *Rheum Dis Clin North Am* 1990;16:445–461.
63. Michels ML, Cobo LM, Caldwell DS, et al. Rheumatoid arthritis and sterile corneal ulceration. Analysis of tissue immune effector cells and ocular epithelial antigens using monoclonal antibodies. *Arthritis Rheum* 1984;27:606–614.
64. Legmann A, Foster CS. Noninfectious necrotizing scleritis. *Int Ophthalmol Clin* 1996;36:73–80.
65. Dinowitz K, Aldave AJ, Lisse JR, et al. Ocular manifestations of immunologic and rheumatologic inflammatory disorders. *Curr Opin Ophthalmol* 1994;5:91–98.
66. Hale LP, Haynes BF. Pathology and rheumatoid arthritis and associated disorder. In: Koopman WJ, ed. *Arthritis and allied conditions: a textbook of rheumatology*, 14th ed. Philadelphia: Lippincott Williams & Wilkins, 1995.
67. Sokoloff L. The heart in rheumatoid arthritis. *Am Heart J* 1953;45:635–643.
68. Cathcart ES, Spodick DH. A study of the incidence and nature of cardiac lesions in rheumatoid arthritis. *N Engl J Med* 1962;266:959–964.
69. McCallum RM, Haynes BF. Diagnosis and management of critically ill patients with collagen vascular diseases. In: Parrillo J, Masur H, eds. *The critically ill immunosuppressed patient: diagnosis and management*. Aspen Press, 1987:499–533.
70. Kitas G, Banks MJ, Bacon PB. Cardiac involvement in rheumatoid disease. *Clin Med* 2001;1:18–21.
71. Banks M, Flint J, Gacon PA, et al. Rheumatoid arthritis is an independent risk factor for ischaemic heart disease. American College of Rheumatology National Meeting, Abstract #1909, concurrent session: Cardiovascular Disease and Mortality, 2000.
72. Kelly CA, Bourke JP, Malcolm A, et al. Chronic pericardial disease in patients with rheumatoid arthritis: a longitudinal study. *QJM* 1990;75:461–470.
73. Thould AK. Constructive pericarditis in rheumatoid arthritis. *Ann Rheum Dis* 1986;45:89–94.
74. Burney DP, Martin CE, Thomas CS, et al. Rheumatoid pericarditis: clinical significance and operative management. *J Thorac Cardiovasc Surg* 1979;77:511–515.
75. Travaglio-Encinoza A, Anaya J-M, D'Angeac AD, et al. Rheumatoid pericarditis: new immunopathological aspect. *Clin Exp Rheumatol* 1994;12:313–316.
76. Escalnte A, Kaufman RL, Quismorio FP, et al. Cardiac compression in rheumatoid pericarditis. *Semin Arthritis Rheum* 1990;20:148–163.
77. Hancock EW. Subacute effusive-constructive pericarditis. *Circulation* 1971; XLIII:183–192.
78. Ahern M, Lever JV, Cosh J. Complete heart block in rheumatoid arthritis. *Ann Rheum Dis* 1983;42:389–397.
79. Kleiner RC, Raber IM, Passero FC. Scleritis, pericarditis, and aortic insufficiency in a patient with rheumatoid arthritis. *Ophthalmology* 1984;91:941–946.
80. Chand EM, Freant LJ, Rubin JW. Aortic valve rheumatoid nodules producing clinical aortic regurgitation and a review of the literature. *Cardiovasc Pathol* 1999;8:333–338.
81. Morris PB, Imber MJ, Heinsimer JA, et al. Rheumatoid arthritis and coronary arteritis. *Am J Cardiol* 1986;57:689–690.
82. Slack JD, Waller B. Acute congestive heart failure due to the arteritis of rheumatoid arthritis: early diagnosis by endomyocardial biopsy: a case report. *Angiology* 1986;37:477–482.
83. Voyles WF, Searles RP, Bankhurst AD. Myocardial infarction caused by rheumatoid vasculitis. *Arthritis Rheum* 1980;23:860–863.
84. McCallum RM, Haynes BF. Management of patients with pulmonary manifestations of collagen-vascular diseases. In: Shelhamer J, Pizzo P, Parrillo J, Masur J, eds. *Respiratory disease in the immunosuppressed host*. Philadelphia: J.B. Lippincott Co., 1991:664–681.
85. Kim RC, Collins GH. The neuropathology of rheumatoid disease. *Hum Pathol* 1981;12:5–15.
86. Nakano KK. Neurologic complications of rheumatoid arthritis. *Orthop Clin North Am* 1975;6:861–880.
87. Boers M. Renal disorders in rheumatoid arthritis. *Semin Arthritis Rheum* 1990;20:57–68.
88. Boers M, Croonen AM, Dijkmans BA, et al. Renal findings in rheumatoid arthritis: clinical aspects of 132 necropsies. *Ann Rheum Dis* 1987;46:658–663.
89. Hollingsworth JW, Saykaly RJ. Systemic complications of rheumatoid arthritis. *Med Clin North Am* 1977;61:217–228.
90. Nakano M, Ueda M, Nishi S, et al. Analysis of renal pathology and drug history in 158 Japanese patients with rheumatoid arthritis. *Clin Nephrol* 1998;50:154–160.
91. Koseki Y, Terai C, Moriguchi M. A prospective study of renal diseases in patients with early rheumatoid arthritis. *Ann Rheum Dis* 2001;60:327–331.
92. Fishman D, Isenberg DA. Splenic involvement in rheumatic diseases. *Semin Arthritis Rheum* 1997;27:141–155.
93. Bowman SJ. Hematological manifestations of rheumatoid arthritis. *Scand J Rheumatol* 2002;31:251–259.
94. William BD, Pussell BA, Lockwood CM, et al. Defective reticuloendothelial system function in rheumatoid arthritis. *Lancet* 1979;1:311–314.
95. Vie H, Chevalier S, Garand R, et al. Clonal expansion of lymphocytes bearing the gamma delta T-cell receptor in a patient with large $\gamma\delta$ granular lymphocyte disorder. *Blood* 1989;74:285–290.
96. Nichols GE, Normansell DE, Williams ME. Lymphoproliferative disorder of granular lymphocytes: nine cases including one with features of CD56 (NKH1)-positive aggressive natural killer cell lymphoma. *Mod Pathol* 1994;7:819–824.
97. Sivakumaran M, Richards S. Immunological abnormalities of chronic large granular lymphocytosis. *Clin Lab Haematol* 1997;19:57–60.
98. Friedman HD, Kurec AS, Goldberg J, et al. Large granular lymphocytosis terminating in a polymorphous B-lymphocytic proliferation after low-dose cyclophosphamide therapy: a case report with necropsy findings. *Hematol Pathol* 1992;6:209–218.
99. Samanta A, Grant I, Nichol FE, et al. Large granular lymphocytosis associated with rheumatoid arthritis. *Ann Rheum Dis* 1988;47:873–875.
100. Kelly A, Richards SJ, Sivakumaran M, et al. Clonality of CD3 negative large granular lymphocyte proliferations determined by PCR based X-inactivation studies. *J Clin Pathol* 1994;47:399–404.
101. Ruiz FP, Martinez FJO, Mendoza ACZ, et al. Nodular regenerative hyperplasia of the liver in rheumatic diseases: report of seven cases and review of the literature. *Semin Arthritis Rheum* 1991;21:47–54.
102. Cohen ML, Manier JW, Bredfeldt JE. Sinusoidal lymphocytosis of the liver in Felty's syndrome with a review of the liver involvement in Felty's syndrome. *J Clin Gastroenterol* 1989;1:92–94.
103. Brooker DS. Rheumatoid arthritis: otorhinolaryngological manifestations. *Clin Otolaryngol* 1988;13:239–246.
104. Atkinson RE, Smith RJ. Silicone synovitis following silicone implant arthroplasty. *Hand Clin* 1986;2:291–299.
105. Kleinert JM, Lister GD. Silicone transplant. *Hand Clin* 1986;2:271–290.
106. Christie AJ, Pierret G, Levitan J. Silicone synovitis. *Semin Arthritis Rheum* 1989;19:166–171.
107. Foliart DE. Synovitis and silicone joint implants: a summary of reported cases. *Plast Reconstr Surg* 1996;99:245–252.
108. McCallum RM, Patel DD, Moore JO, et al. Arthritis syndromes associated with human T cell lymphotropic virus type I infection. *Med Clin North Am* 1997;81:261–276.
109. Iwakura Y, Tosu M, Yoshida E, et al. Induction of inflammatory arthropathy resembling rheumatoid arthritis in mice transgenic for HTLV-I. *Science* 1991;253:1026.
110. Nishioka K, Maruyama I, Sato K, et al. Chronic inflammatory arthropathy associated with HTLV-I. *Lancet* 1989;1:441.
111. Sato K, Maruyama I, Maruyama Y, et al. Arthritis in patients infected with human T lymphotropic virus type I. *Arthritis Rheum* 1991;34:714.

CHAPTER 12

Role of Cytokines

Evangelos T. H. Andreakos, Brian M. J. Foxwell, Fionula M. Brennan, and Marc Feldmann

The immune and inflammatory systems use a complex system of cells and proteins to specifically recognize foreign pathogens and generate an immune response to promote their elimination. Central to this process are cytokines, which are small soluble proteins or glycoproteins that act as local messengers of essentially all important biologic processes, including cell growth, development, repair, fibrosis, inflammation, and immunity. Although, in most cases, cytokine production is beneficial for the host, there are increasing numbers of examples in which excess or deregulated cytokine production is involved in mediating pathophysiologic events. This is the case in many autoimmune and inflammatory diseases. In this chapter, the basic biology of cytokines and cytokine receptors, the immune processes controlled by cytokines, and the regulation of cytokine expression are discussed with particular relevance to the pathogenesis and therapy of rheumatoid arthritis (RA).

CYTOKINE FAMILIES

Cytokines can be produced by cells of any type, although they are most frequently and abundantly produced by leukocytes. They signal by binding to cell-surface cytokine receptors on target cells. All cells have receptors for many cytokines (1). Cytokines can be divided into families on the basis of their similarity in amino acid sequence and, most important, in three-dimensional structure (Table 12.1). Thus, the hematopoietin family comprises cytokines that form four α helices, whereas members of the tumor necrosis factor (TNF) family form a jelly-roll motif. Other important families are the interleukin (IL)-1, the interferon α/β (IFN-α/β), the platelet-derived growth factor (PDGF), and the T-cell growth factor β (TGF-β) families. The largest family is probably the chemokine family, which is itself subdivided into two major groups, the cys-x-cys (C-X-C) and the cys-cys (C-X) chemokine families, depending on whether the first two of four conserved cysteine residues are separated by one amino acid.

Most cytokines are single polypeptide chain proteins, but homodimers (IFN-γ, IL-10, TGF-β) or homotrimers (TNF-α and other members of the TNF family) also exist. IL-12 and related proteins (e.g., IL-23) are heterodimers, as is lymphotoxin α/β (LT-α/β). Although cytokines were originally considered and defined as secreted molecules, membrane-bound forms have been documented for many cytokines, including TNF-α, IL-1, IFN-γ, fibroblast growth factor (FGF), TGF-α, TGF-β, macrophage colony-stimulating factor (M-CSF), and stem cell factor (SCF). The cell-surface forms of these proteins are capable of signaling. Some cytokines exist chiefly as a cell-surface form (e.g., LT-β). Cytokines vary widely in function; they can have a proinflammatory, antiinflammatory, or chemotactic role; and all have multiple actions, which differ depending on the target cell. The effects of individual cytokines are summarized in Table 12.2 (1).

CYTOKINE RECEPTOR FAMILIES

Cytokines interact with cells through specific high-affinity cell-surface receptors, the density of which is usually between 10 to 10,000 sites per cell. On the basis of their structural similarity, cytokine receptors can also be subdivided into families. Thus, the largest family is the hematopoietin receptor family, which is characterized by an extracellular region composed of one or more domains containing four conserved cysteines and a tryptophan-serine-X-tryptophan-serine amino acid motif in the membrane proximal domain. Other families include the immunoglobulin (Ig) receptor family that has Ig-like motifs, the TNF receptor family that contains multiple cysteine-rich domains, the IFN receptor family, the TGF-β receptor family, and the chemokine receptor family, which is characterized by the seven-transmembrane segments structure common to the rhodopsin receptor family (Fig. 12.1).

It is apparent that, in most instances, more than one polypeptide is needed to constitute a functional receptor. The IL-2 receptor, for example, consists of three different polypeptide chains, whereas the IL-6 receptor consists of two. This receptor complex probably comprises four chains in total. In many cases, there are chains common to several receptors, such as the IL-2Rγ chain that also associates with the IL-4, IL-7, IL-9, and IL-15 receptors; the glycoprotein-130 (gp130) chain that associates with IL-6, ciliary neurotrophic factor, oncostatin M (OSM), leukemia inhibitory factor (LIF), IL-11, and cardiotropin-1 receptors; and the β chain of the IL-3 receptor that also associates with the granulocyte-macrophage colony-stimulating factor (GM-CSF) and IL-5 receptors. The TNF receptor, on the other hand, consists of trimers of the same chain. In addition to cell-surface receptors, soluble receptors corresponding to the ligand-binding domains of cytokine receptors have been described. Soluble receptors act, in most cases, as inhibitors of cytokines, although the soluble IL-6 receptor family members are co-agonists.

CYTOKINES IN THE CONTROL OF IMMUNE PROCESSES

Cytokines regulate various immunologic processes, the most important of which are summarized here.

TABLE 12.1. Cytokine Families Grouped by Structural Similarity

Family	Cytokines
Hematopoietins	IL-2, IL-3, IL-4, IL-5, IL-6, IL-7, IL-9, IL-11, IL-12, IL-15, IL-16, IL-17, EPO, LIF, GM-CSF, G-CSF, OSM, CNTF, GH, and TPO
TNF family	TNF-α, LT-α, LT-β, CD40L, CD30L, CD27L, 4-1BBL, OX40, OPG, and FasL
IL-1	IL-1α, IL-1β, IL-1ra, IL-18, bFGF, aFGF, and ECGF
PDGF	PDGF A, PDGF B, and M-CSF
TGF-β	TGF-β and BMPs (1, 2, 4, etc.)
C-X-C chemokines	IL-8, Gro-α/β/γ, NAP-2, ENA 78, GCP-2, PF4, CTAP-3, Mig, and IP-10
C-C chemokines	MCP-1, MCP-2, MCP-3, MIP-1α, MIP-1β, RANTES

aFGF, acidic fibroblast growth factor; 4-1 BBL, 4-1 BB ligand; bFGF, basic fibroblast growth factor; BMP, bone morphogenetic proteins; C-C, cysteine-cysteine; CD, cluster of differentiation; CNTF, ciliary neurotrophic factor; CTAP, connective tissue activating peptide; C-X-C, cysteine-x-cysteine; ECGF, endothelial cell growth factor; EPO, erythropoietin; FasL, Fas ligand; GCP-2, granulocyte chemotactic protein-2; G-CSF, granulocyte colony-stimulating factor; GH, growth hormone; GM-CSF, granulocyte colony-stimulating factor; Gro, growth-related gene products; IFN, interferon; IL, interleukin; IP, interferon-γ inducible protein; LIF, leukemia inhibitory factor; LT, lymphotoxin; MCP, monocyte chemoattractant; M-CSF, macrophage colony-stimulating factor; Mig, monokine induced by interferon-γ; MIP, macrophage inflammatory protein; NAP-2, neutrophil activating protein-2; OPG, osteoprotegerin; OSM, oncostatin M; PDGF, platelet-derived growth factor; PF, platelet factor; R, receptor; RANTES, regulated on activation, normal T cell–expressed and –secreted; TGF, transforming growth factor; TNF, tumor necrosis factor; TPO, thyroperoxidase.

Leukocyte Adhesion, Extravasation, and Migration

Leukocyte adhesion, extravasation, and migration are essential for both acute and chronic inflammatory responses. Cytokines regulate this process in a number of different ways. They regulate adhesion molecule expression and production of chemoattractant chemokines. First, the cytokines TNF-α, IL-1α, IL-1β, and IFN-γ, produced mainly by macrophages, neutrophils, or T cells, increase the expression of adhesion molecules endothelial-leukocyte adhesion molecule-1 (ELAM-1), intracellular adhesion molecules-1 and -2 (ICAM-1 and ICAM-2), and vascular adhesion molecule-1 (VCAM-1) in endothelial cells. This increase in adhesion molecule expression facilitates the adhesion of leukocytes to the vascular endothelium and their extravasation into the tissues and is negatively regulated by IL-4 and IL-10, which inhibit many of the effects of TNF-α, IL-1α, IL-1β, and IFN-γ on the endothelium. Second, GM-CSF, produced by macrophages, T cells, fibroblasts, and endothelial cells, and IL-8, produced by macrophages, fibroblasts, endothelial cells, and neutrophils, enhance monocyte and neutrophil migration, respectively, by up-regulating the expression of the adhesion molecules CD11 and CD18. Finally, C-X-C chemokines, produced by activated macrophages, dendritic cells, endothelial cells, fibroblasts, and platelets, act as chemoattractants mostly for neutrophils, whereas the C-C chemokines, produced primarily by activated T cells and macrophages, act as chemoattractants for lymphocytes, monocytes, eosinophils, and basophils but not neutrophils. Endothelial cells are also an important source of chemokines.

Leukocyte Development, Proliferation, Activation, and Differentiation

Cytokines are essential for leukocyte development, proliferation, activation, and differentiation. Thus, T-cell development in the thymus requires IL-7 for pro–T cells to survive and for rearranging the genes encoding the T-cell receptor chains. The proliferation and survival of pro–T cells at early thymocyte stages depends on SCF and Flt-3 ligand. Negative selection of intermediate thymocyte stages is partly mediated by FasL, the Fas ligand, and CD30L, the CD30 ligand. T-cell proliferation and activation requires IL-2, a major TGF secreted by T cells but also dendritic cells. Other cytokines, such as IL-4, IL-7, IL-9, IL-15, and IL-21, whose receptor complex shares the γc chain with the IL-2 receptor, can also induce T-cell proliferation. T-cell proliferation is inhibited by TGF-β and IFNs, whereas it is increased by TNF-α (acutely) and prolactin. FasL induces T-cell death, helping to eliminate unneeded T cells after an immune response has occurred. Finally, the differentiation of activated T cells to particular phenotypes is also under the control of cytokines. Thus, CD4$^+$ T-cell differentiation to the T helper 1 (Th1) phenotype requires the action of IL-12, IL-23, or IFN-γ and can be enhanced by IFN-α, IL-1, or IL-18. Differentiation to the T helper 2 (Th2) phenotype depends on IL-4. Cytotoxic T-cell development seems to require IL-2 and to be favored by IFN-γ, IL-12, and IL-15.

B-cell development in the bone marrow depends on the chemokine stromal cell–derived factor. The proliferation of B cells is promoted by various cytokines, such as IL-2, IL-4, IL-6, IL-10, IL-13, B lymphocyte stimulator (BLyS), and CD40L and inhibited by TGF-β. In mice and humans, B-cell isotype switching to IgE and IgG1 requires IL-4 or IL-13, whereas isotype switching to IgG2a and IgG3 requires IFN-γ. TGF-β promotes IgA isotype switching. All isotype switching in B cells requires CD40L. At the same time, IL-2, IL-10, and IL-15 increase Ig production, whereas TGF-β inhibits it, except for IgA. Memory B-cell development requires CD40L.

The growth and differentiation of monocytes from pluripotent hematopoietic stem cells and myeloid progenitors are also tightly regulated by specific growth factors and cytokines such as IL-3, M-CSF, GM-CSF, IL-4, and IL-13 and growth inhibitors such as IFN-α/β, TGF-β, and LIF. These processes are further modulated by interactions with adjacent stromal and other cells (fibroblasts, endothelial cells, and T cells) through c-kit ligand (SCF), Flt-3 ligand, and other interactions. Once monocytes are generated, their ability to proliferate is very limited. However, their ability to differentiate remains intact and is again controlled by cytokines. Thus, M-CSF and GM-CSF induce monocyte differentiation to a macrophage phenotype. In the presence of IL-4, however, GM-CSF induces monocyte differentiation to an immature dendritic cell phenotype that can become mature potent antigen-presenting cells in the presence of other signals, such as TNF-α, IL-1, or CD40L. TNF-α, IL-1, and CD40L, as well as IFN-γ and IL-3, can also result in monocyte/macrophage activation by stimulating their antigen-presenting, cytotoxic, and inflammatory functions. Monocytes and macrophages, in turn, produce high amounts of various other cytokines and chemokines, including TNF-α, IL-1, IL-6, IL-8, IL-12, IL-18, macrophage inflammatory protein-1 (MIP-1), MIP-1α/β, and RANTES (regulated on activation, normal T cell–expressed and –secreted), amplifying the inflammatory response.

Induction of Acute Phase Proteins

Cytokines regulate the release of acute phase proteins that are involved in the restoration of the body's function towards normality (homeostasis) after infection, inflammation, or other insults. Acute phase proteins C-reactive protein (CRP) and serum amyloid A are produced by hepatocytes and are primarily induced by IL-6 (2). IL-6 stimulates large increases in the production of CRP and serum amyloid A, with smaller increases of ceruloplasmin, complement components C3 and C4, haptoglobin, α-1 antiprotease, ferritin, and fibrinogen also seen. At the same time, IL-6 decreases the production by hepatocytes of other proteins that include albumin, transferrin, transthyretin, and α-fetoprotein. Hepatic acute phase protein production is also influenced by other cytokines, such as TNF-α, IL-1, and TGF-β, that often synergize with IL-6 and other members of the IL-6 family (e.g., IL-11, OSM). Glucocorticoids can also synergize

TABLE 12.2. Properties of Cytokines and Chemokines

Cytokine	MW (kd)	Sources	Inducers	Effects	Inhibited
Proinflammatory cytokines					
IL-1α	33 (membrane bound) 17 (soluble)	Most cells, especially macrophages, keratinocytes, and endothelial cells	Microbial agents, such as LPS; injurious agents, such as TNF, GM-CSF, IL-1, substance P, and IFN-γ	Induces prostaglandin production and metalloproteinases; up-regulates adhesion molecules, cytokines (IL-2, IFN, CSF, TNF, IL-6, IL-8, etc.), acute phase proteins, T- and B-cell activation; and stimulates the hypothalamic-pituitary-adrenal axis.	IL-4, IL-13, IL-10, and TGF-β
IL-1β	33 processed to 17 by IL-1–converting enzyme	Macrophages, neutrophils, astrocytes	As above	As above.	As above
TNF	17 trimeric	Macrophages, neutrophils, astrocytes	Depends on cell type but are mostly similar to IL-1 inducers	As above. In addition, it up-regulates macrophage and neutrophil activation, HLA class I expression, and tumor cytotoxicity.	IL-4 and IL-13, IL-10 and TGF-β
LT	25 trimeric	T and B lymphocytes and NK cells	Antigens and mitogens	As above for TNF.	IL-4 and IL-10
IL-6	20	Macrophages, fibroblasts, and B and T cells	Like IL-1 and TNF	B-cell growth, Ig production, acute phase proteins, stem cell and NK cell activation, platelet production, mesangial cell proliferation, osteolysis, and IFN production.	As above
IFN-γ	20–25 dimer	CD4 and CD8 T cells, CD4 Th1 cells, and NK cells	T-cell activation, IL-12, IL-18, and IL-2	Induces class I and II. Activates monocytes, primes for cytokine production and up-regulates cell-surface protectors. Involved in CTL differentiation, blocks Th2 activity, and promotes the DTH. It inhibits B-cell proliferation and IgE production. Activates neutrophils and NK cells.	IL-10 and TGF-β
Antiinflammatory cytokines					
IL-10	18 dimer	Macrophages, T and B cells, and keratinocytes	LPS for macrophages, others for T-cell activation	Inhibits macrophage cytokine production (IL-1, IL-6, TNF, GM-CSF, IL-12) and antigen presentation; down-regulates cytokine receptor expression and up-regulates cytokine inhibitors (sTNF-R, IL-1ra); and induces strong B-cell activation, Ig production, and MMP expression.	—
TGF-β	25	Most cells	Depends on cell type	Activates connective tissue growth and synthesis of extracellular matrix inhibitor of hemopoiesis, immune cell activity, and inflammation.	—
IL-4	20	T cells and mast cells	T-cell activation and IgE production	T-cell growth factor, inducer of Th2 cells, co-activator of B-cell growth and Ig secretion, and activator of most cells and basophils. Inhibits macrophage proinflammatory cytokine production (IL-1, TNF, IL-6, etc.).	—

(*continued*)

TABLE 12.2. (*continued*)

Cytokine	MW (kd)	Sources	Inducers	Effects	Inhibited
IL-13	—	T cells and mast cells	T-cell activation and IgE production	Co-activator of B-cell growth and Ig secretion, and activator of most cells and basophils. Inhibits macrophage proinflammatory cytokine production (IL-1, TNF, IL-6, etc.).	—
Chemotactic cytokines (chemokines)					
IL-8 (C-X-C)	—	Almost all cells, fibroblasts, macrophages, and neutrophils	Depends on cell type, LPS, and proinflammatory cytokines such as TNF, IL-1	Attracts neutrophils, basophils, eosinophils, and T cells; induces keratinocyte proliferation and neutrophil activation (degranulation, enzyme release, respiratory burst).	—
Gro-α/β/γ (C-X-C)	—	Almost all cells	IL-1, TNF, LPS, etc.	Neutrophil chemotaxis and activation, melanoma cell proliferation, fibroblast proliferation, and basophil chemoattraction.	—
ENA78 (C-X-C)	—	Epithelial cells	IL-1, TNF, etc.	Attracts and activates neutrophils.	—
IP-10 (C-X-C)	—	Most cells	IL-1, TNF, LPS, etc.	Chemoattractant of monocytes and T cells.	—
MCP-1 (C-C)	—	Monocytes and fibroblasts	IL-1, TNF, LPS, etc.	Monocyte and basophil chemotaxis and activation.	—
MCP-2 (C-C)	—	Keratinocytes and endothelium	—	Monocyte and basophil chemotaxis and degranulation.	—
MIP-1α (C-C)	—	Monocytes and lymphocytes	IL-1, TNF, LPS, and T-cell activators	Monocyte chemotaxis, T cells (particularly CD8+), and B cells.	—
MIP-1β (C-C)	—	Monocytes, lymphocytes	IL-1, TNF, LPS, and T-cell activators	Monocyte chemotaxis, T cells (particularly CD8+), and B cells.	—
RANTES (C-C)	—	Lymphocytes	T-cell activators	Monocyte chemotaxis.	—

C-C, cysteine-cysteine; CD, cluster of differentiation; CSF, colony-stimulating factor; CTL, cytotoxic T lymphocyte; C-X-C , cysteine-x-cysteine; ENA, extractable nuclear antigen; GM-CSF, granulocyte colony-stimulating factor; Gro, growth-related gene product; IFN, interferon; Ig, immunoglobulin; IL, interleukin; IL-1ra, interleukin-1 receptor antagonist; IP, interferon-γ inducible protein; LPS, lipopolysaccharide; LT, lymphotoxin; MCP, monocyte chemoattractant; MIP, macrophage inflammatory protein; MMP, matrix metalloproteinase; MW, molecular weight; NK, natural killer; R, receptor; RANTES, regulated on activation, normal T–cell expressed and –secreted; sTNF-R, souluble tumor necrosis factor receptor; TGF, transforming growth factor; Th1, T helper 1; Th2, T helper 2; TNF, tumor necrosis factor; VEGF, vascular endothelial growth factor.

with IL-6. However, the serum levels of these cytokines are poorly correlated with those of the acute phase proteins, highlighting the complexity of regulation.

Induction of Angiogenesis

Cytokines can regulate angiogenesis, an important physiologic process that can contribute to tissue damage in chronic inflammatory diseases such as RA. Thus, vascular endothelial growth factor induces endothelial cell proliferation and increases vascular permeability, facilitating the extravasation of plasma proteins such as fibrinogen. Fibrin, as well as collagen type I and collagen type III in the connective tissue matrix further enhances the growth of new blood vessels by forming a scaffold for proliferating endothelial cells. Cytokines such as TNF-α and IL-8 may also be important in angiogenesis, because neutralizing antibodies to these cytokines inhibit the angiogenic activity of supernatants from cultured rheumatoid fibroblasts (3). Other angiogenic factors in RA fluid include FGF and platelet-derived growth factor and other C-X-C chemokines. Angiogenesis has been extensively reviewed elsewhere (4).

PROPERTIES AND REGULATION OF CYTOKINES

Cytokines induce or suppress the production of other cytokines in a variety of cells, creating a "cytokine network" (5–7). Cells of one type communicate with cells of another type through the production of cytokines. For instance, the cytokines IL-1 and IL-6 made by antigen-presenting cells can signal to a T cell to produce IL-2, up-regulate IL-2 receptors, and augment cytotoxic T-lymphocyte activity. IL-2 produced may then act in both an autocrine and paracrine fashion to induce T-cell proliferation and increase the production of other cytokines, such as IFN-γ and GM-CSF. These latter proteins may then feed back to up-regulate the activities of the antigen-presenting cell, thus illustrating how cytokines can act in networks. Similarly, IL-12 and IL-18 act in conjunction to direct naïve T cells toward the Th1 subtype and to induce cell-mediated immunity (8,9). IFN-γ that is produced by Th1 cells, in turn, activates macrophages to produce more IL-12 and IL-18. This process can be blocked by the Th2 products IL-4, IL-10, and IL-13 that inhibit the generation of IL-12 by human monocytes and macrophages, as well as the differentiation of T cells towards a Th1 phenotype.

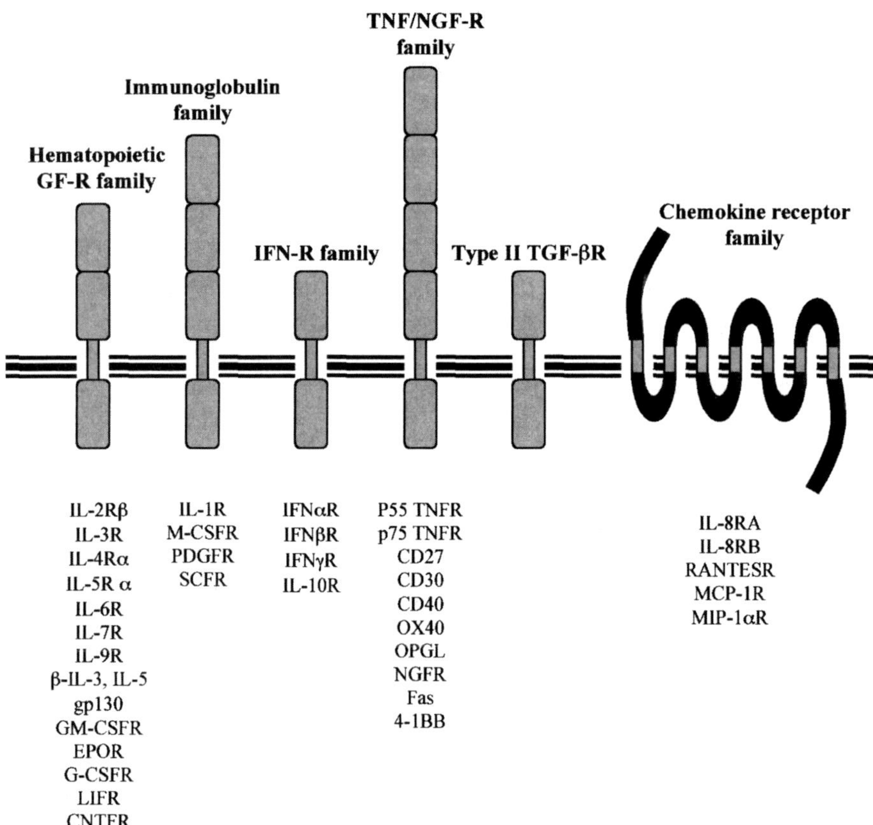

Figure 12.1. Cytokine receptors can be grouped broadly into six families based on their molecular structure. CNTF, ciliary neurotrophic factor; EPO, erythropoietin; G-CSF, granulocyte colony-stimulating factor; GF, growth factor; GM-CSF, granulocyte-macrophage colony-stimulating factor; gp, glycoprotein; IFN, interferon; IL, interleukin; LIF, leukemia inhibitory factor; MCP-1, monocyte chemoattractant protein-1; M-CSF, macrophage colony-stimulating factor; MIP, macrophage inflammatory protein; NGF, nerve growth factor; OPGL, osteoprotegerin ligand; PDGF, platelet-derived growth factor; R, receptor; RANTES, regulated on activation, normal T cell–expressed and –secreted; SCF, stem cell factor; TGF, T-cell growth factor; TNF, tumor necrosis factor. (Adapted from Feldmann M, Dower S, Brennan FM. The role of cytokines in normal and pathological situations. In: Brennan FM, Feldmann M, eds. *Cytokines in autoimmunity*. London: R.G. Landes Company, 1996;1–23.)

Another very important network is characterized by the ability of TNF-α to induce IL-1, both of which can, in turn, induce IL-6 and GM-CSF, which regulate numerous other cytokines and inflammatory mediators (5,7,10). IL-10 acts as a negative regulator of this process. This type of cytokine network is found in the synovium, with its discovery providing the rationale for blockade of TNF-α in RA (7,11). As documented in detail in this book, anti–TNF-α therapy has been shown to reduce the chronic inflammation and ameliorate disease states and protect the joints in RA (12–15).

SIGNALING BY CYTOKINE RECEPTORS

Cytokines signal through their respective receptors. The intracellular signaling pathways induced by cytokines that result in cellular activation and gene expression of various other cytokines and inflammatory mediators have attracted major interest because of their implications for therapy. Some of the most important signaling pathways activated by cytokines are described here.

Tumor Necrosis Factor α Signaling

As with many cytokine receptors, signal transduction through the TNF receptors depends on initial receptor aggregation after ligand binding (16,17). This aggregation results in the recruitment of a number of adapter proteins to the cytoplasmic domain that, in turn, recruit kinases and other downstream signaling molecules. Thus, the p55 TNF receptor (TNF-R) has a death domain (DD) in its intracellular portion that is required for TNF-α–induced apoptosis (Fig. 12.2) (16). The DD mediates homotypic interactions with other DD-containing proteins such as the TNF-R–associated DD (TRADD), the Fas-associated DD (FADD/MORT1), the RIPK1 domain containing adapter with death domain/caspase and RIP adapter with death domain (RAIDD/CRADD) and the serine/threonine kinase receptor interacting protein (RIP). TNF-α signaling through the p55 TNF-R can induce apoptosis, as well as nuclear factor–κB (NF-κB) activation (Fig. 12.2). These signaling pathways have been shown to bifurcate at the level of TRADD, where TRADD interacts with FADD to transduce the apoptotic signal and TNF-R–associated factor 2 (TRAF2) to induce NF-κB activation. In addition to TRAF2, FADD/MORT1 and RIP can also induce NF-κB activation when overexpressed, but the physiologic significance of this pathway is unclear.

The p75 TNF-R, on the other hand, does not possess a DD but forms a heterodimeric complex with TRAF1 and TRAF2 (17). These interactions allow the recruitment of the proteins TRAF-associated NF-κB activator/inhibitor of TRAF (TANK/I-TRAF), cellular inhibitor of apoptosis proteins 1/2 (cIAP1/2) and A20. TANK/I-TRAF has been implicated in the activation of NF-κB by the p75 TNF-R, although this role was questioned in a study showing that TANK/I-TRAF may inhibit NF-κB activation by interacting with TRAF2. The function of cIAP proteins is not known but, because they display homology to the baculovirus inhibitors of IAPs, they may be antiapoptotic. Finally, A20 may function as an inhibitor of NF-κB activation and apoptosis.

Further downstream, TNF-α induces the phosphorylation and activation of a wide variety of proteins that may differ between cell types and that are shared with many other cytokine signal transduction pathways. Thus, TNF-α activates protein kinase C isoforms, protein kinase A, TNF-α, and IL-1 activated kinase, casein kinase I-like enzymes, and mitogen-activated protein kinases (MAPKs). All three types of MAPK—p38, p42/44, and p54 MAPK—become activated in response to TNF-α (17). The p38 MAPK cascade has been implicated in the regulation of many inflammatory genes in response to TNF-α stimulation, including IL-6, IL-8, and TNF-α itself, through its effects on transcription, messenger RNA (mRNA) stability, and translation. The p38 MAPK

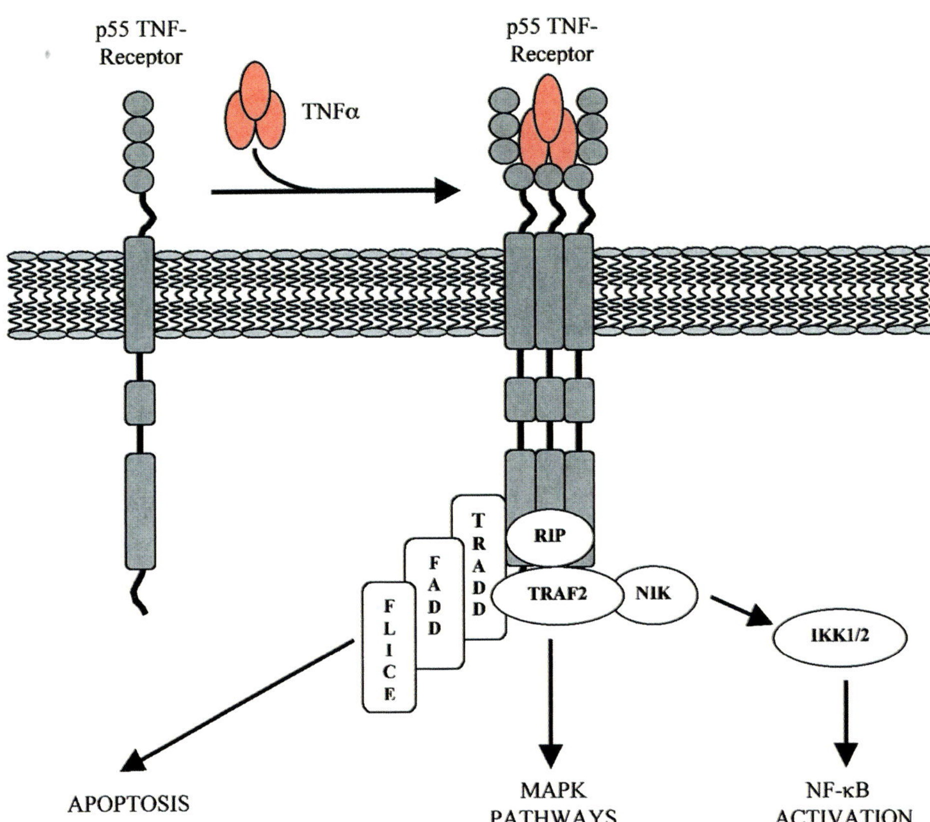

Figure 12.2. On ligand binding and via receptor-associated proteins, the p55 tumor necrosis factor (TNF) receptor induces signaling cascades that lead to mitogen-activated protein kinase (MAPK) and nuclear factor–κB (NF-κB) activation and apoptosis. FADD, Fas-associated death domain; FLICE, FADD-like interleukin-1β–converting enzyme; IKK, IκB kinase; NIK, NF-κB–inducing kinase; RIP, receptor interacting protein; TRADD, TNF receptor–associated death domain; TRAF, TNF receptor–associated factor 6.

pathway modulates activating transcription factor 2 (ATF2), as well as the cytosolic proteins cytoplasmic phospholipase A2 ($cPLA_2$) and heat shock protein 27 (Hsp27). The p42/44 MAPKs [extracellular signal-related kinase (ERK)] are involved in the proliferative and inflammatory effects of TNF-α. They activate transcription factors such as Ets-like protein (Elk)-1 and cytosolic proteins such as $cPLA_2$ and MAPK activated protein kinase (MAPKAP). Finally, p54 MAPK (SAPK/JNK) activates a number of transcription factors such as ATF2, Elk1, cAMP response element binding proteins (CREB), and activator protein-1 (AP-1) (fos/jun). The pathways leading to MAPK activation are summarized in Figure 12.3.

TNF receptor signaling also induces the activation of phosphatidylcholine-phospholipase C and the generation of diacylglycerol. This activates the atypical protein kinase C–ζ and the acid sphingomyelinase that have been implicated in NF-κB activation (18). Activation of acid sphingomyelinase has been shown to map to the DD of the p55 TNF-R. However, individuals defective in acid sphingomyelinase show no defects in TNF-α–induced NF-κB. TNF-α also induces neutral sphingomyelinase activity by using FAN, a p55 TNF-R–associated protein. By inducing ceramide production, TNF-α activates ceramide-activated kinase and phosphatase. Ceramide-activated kinase may be important in the upstream activation of Raf1 and, consequently, p42/44 MAPK, and the insulin-signaling adapter molecule insulin receptor substrate-1 (IRS-1).

IL-1 Signaling

There are two forms of the IL-1 receptor, both of which are members of the Ig superfamily. The type I IL-1 receptor (IL-1RI) is a widely expressed 80-kd transmembrane glycoprotein, comprising a 319–amino acid extracellular region with three Ig-like domains, a 20–amino acid transmembrane region, and a 213–amino acid cytosolic region (19,20). The type II IL-1 receptor (IL-1RII) resembles the type I receptor in that it has an extracellular part of 330 amino acids that comprises three Ig domains and a transmembrane part of 26 amino acids. It differs from the type I IL-1 receptor, however, because of a short intracellular portion of 29 amino acids that is incapable of signaling. Thus, IL-1RII is a decoy receptor that binds to IL-1 and reduces its free concentration.

Both IL-1 receptors associate with the IL-1R accessory protein (IL-1RAcP), but IL-1 signaling occurs only through the type I receptor. This receptor has no kinase, src homology (SH)2- or SH3-domains, but contains a highly conserved cytosolic domain that is homologous to the cytoplasmic domain of the *Drosophila* protein toll and defines it as a member of the Toll-like receptor (TLR family). After ligand binding, IL-1, IL-1RI, and IL-1RAcP form a trimeric complex (21,22), which leads to recruitment of the adapter molecule MyD88 via protein interactions between the Toll domains of the IL-1RI complex and a conserved Toll domain present in the C-terminal region of MyD88. The N-terminal region of MyD88 contains a DD that is involved in the recruitment of the serine/threonine kinases IL-1R–associated kinase 1 and 2. These kinases, in turn, recruit the adapter protein TRAF6, and the signaling cascade progresses further through the IKK complex to the activation of NF-κB. IL-1 signaling also induces the activation of the transcription factors NF-IL-6 and IL-1 nuclear factor and the activation of MAPKs, β-casein kinase, and phosphatidylinositol 3-kinase that appear to associate with the cytoplasmic region of IL-1RAcP and initiate a parallel signaling pathway that leads to the transactivation of NF-κB subunits by phosphorylation.

IL-6 Signaling

The IL-6 receptor (IL-6R) complex is composed of the IL-6R α chain and the protein gp130. After the molecular cloning of the IL-6R α chain, it was realized that signal transduction is mediated by gp130, whereas the IL-6R α chain is only involved in IL-6 binding.

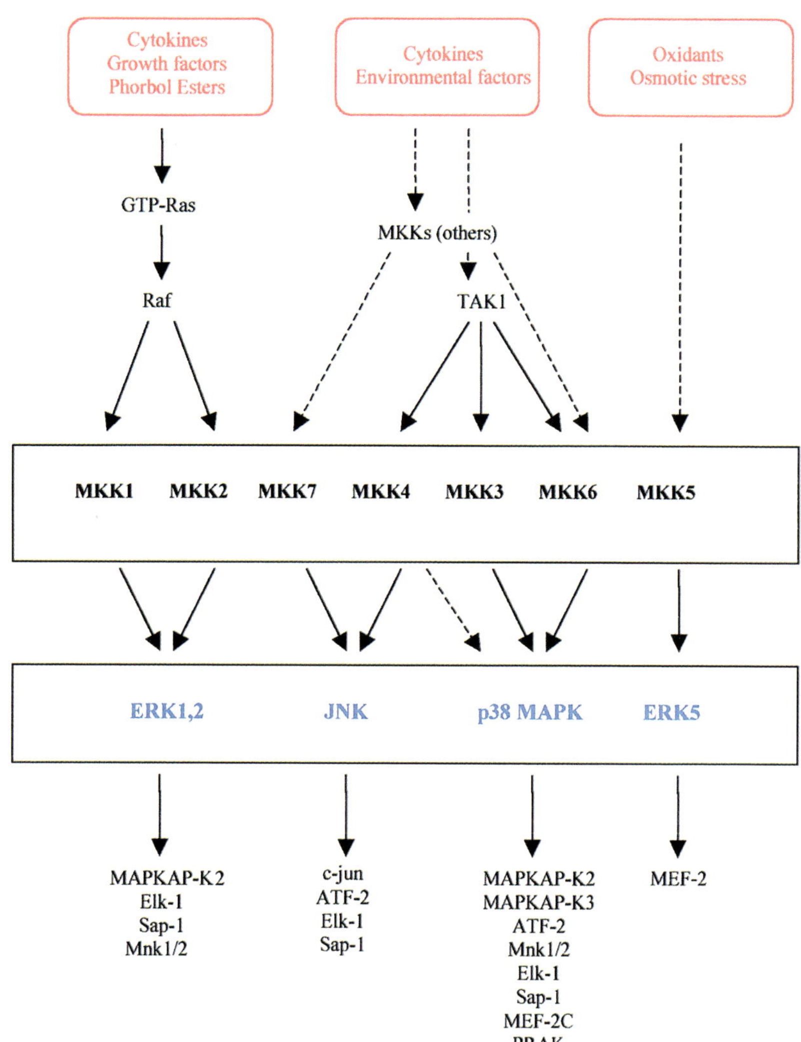

Figure 12.3. Signaling via mitogen-activated protein kinase (MAPK) results in the activation of many molecules and transcription factors that regulate gene expression. ATF, activating transcription factor; Elk, E twenty-six–like protein; ERK, extracellular signal-related kinase; GTP-Ras, guanosine triphosphate-Ras; JNK, c-jun NH(2) terminal kinase; MAPKAP, MAPK activated protein kinase; MEF, myocyte enhancer factor; MKK, MAPK kinase; Mnk, MAP kinase–interacting kinase; PRAK, p38 regulated and activated kinase; Sap, serum response factor accessory protein; TAK1, T-cell growth factor b–activated kinase 1.

It was subsequently found that gp130 is shared with other receptor complexes of structurally related cytokines IL-11, LIF, OSM, ciliary neutrophic factor, and cardiotrophin-1, explaining why these cytokines have very similar biologic activities to IL-6.

Binding of IL-6 to the IL-6R results in its association with gp130, which allows the whole complex to homodimerize (23). The IL-6R does not need to be membrane anchored, as soluble IL-6R can also bind to IL-6 and function through gp130. gp130 has no intrinsic tyrosine kinase domain. However, homo- or heterodimerization of gp130 may trigger the activation of a cytoplasmic tyrosine kinase that is bound to it. Janus kinase 1 (JAK1), JAK2, and tyrosine kinase 2 (TYK2) of the JAK family are associated with gp130 and become activated in response to IL-6 and other structurally related cytokines. IL-6 signaling also results in the activation of the latent cytoplasmic transcription factors STATs (signal transducers and activators of transcription). STAT3 is the most potently activated member of the STAT family, although STAT1 activation is also observed. Interestingly, other cytokines have also been shown to activate JAK and STAT family members. Thus, IFN-γ activates JAK1, JAK2, and STAT1; IL-4 activates STAT6; IL-12 activates STAT3 and STAT4; and IL-10 activates STAT3.

Besides the activation of JAK and STAT members, IL-6R triggering also results in the activation of Ras and MAPKs. Further downstream, the transcription factor NF-IL-6 is activated through a process that requires the phosphorylation of a specific threonine residue through the action of MAPK. The action of NF-IL-6 in conjunction with STAT3 and other as-yet-unidentified factors then accounts for the widespread biologic effects observed after IL-6 stimulation. Other cytokines structurally related to IL-6 have also been shown to signal through similar mechanisms.

Transforming Growth Factor β Signaling

TGF-β is the prototype member of the TGF-β family of cytokines that also includes bone morphogenetic proteins. TGF-β signals through the TGF-β receptor complex that is formed from two distinct single transmembrane proteins known as *type I* and *type II* receptors (24). Both of these receptors contain an intracellular serine/threonine kinase domain. Upon ligand binding, the type I and II receptors associate, leading to the unidirectional phosphorylation of the type I receptor by the type II receptor. This phosphorylation of the type I receptor activates the kinase activity of the type I receptor that induces downstream signaling events. Thus, phosphorylation of the SMAD (vertebrate homologues of *Xenopus* Sma and Mad) family members SMAD2 and SMAD3 is observed, with SMAD3 forming DNA-binding complexes with SMAD4 that recruit transcription factors and modulate gene expression. In addition to these agonistic SMADs, inhibitory SMADs such as SMAD6 and SMAD7 also exist that bind to the activated TGF-β receptor, interfering with the recruitment and activation of SMAD2 and SMAD3. Expression of SMAD7 is induced by TGF-β, suggesting that it acts as a negative-feedback regulator of TGF-β signaling.

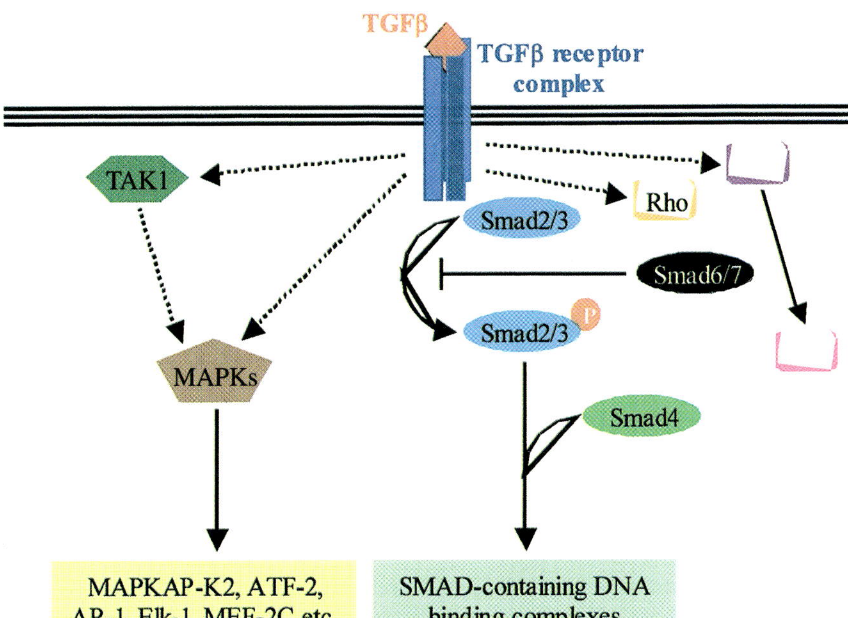

Figure 12.4. Schematic diagram of transforming growth factor β (TGF-β)–mediated downstream signaling. On ligand binding, the type I and type II receptors of TGF-β associate to form the TGF-β receptor complex. This results in the phosphorylation and activation of many intracellular signaling mediators, such as SMAD2 (vertebrate homologues of *Xenopus* Sma and Mad), SMAD3, TGF-β–activated kinase (TAK1), mitogen-activated protein kinases (MAPKs), Rho guanosine triphosphatases, and protein kinase B, modulating transcription factors, DNA binding, and gene expression. AP-1, activator protein-1; ATF, activating transcription factor; Elk-1, E twenty-six–like protein-1; MAPKAP-K2, MAPK activated protein kinase 2; MEF-2C, mycocyte enhancer factor.

The TGF-β pathway also activates other signaling molecules, such as p38, p42/44, and p54 MAPKs. Activated MAPKs may, in turn, directly phosphorylate SMADs, adding to the complexity of the regulation of SMAD activity. In addition, activation of TGF-β–activated kinase 1, protein kinase B, and the Rho family of guanosine triphosphatases has been reported, although no direct link between these pathways to the TGF-β receptor complex has been made. A schematic representation of TGF-β–induced downstream signaling is shown in Figure 12.4. Other TGF-β family members (e.g., bone morphogenetic proteins) signal in a similar manner through the action of distinct type I and II receptors. In vertebrates, seven distinct type I receptors have been described that can bind to five distinct type II receptors to mediate signals of their ligands.

NUCLEAR FACTOR–κB ACTIVATION

A common theme in cytokine signaling shared by many cytokines, including TNF-α and IL-1, is the activation of the transcription factor NF-κB. NF-κB is, perhaps, the most important transcription factor family with proinflammatory effects. Five NF-κB subunits—relA (p65), relB, c-rel, p50, and p52—are known to exist in mammalian cells and form various homo- and heterodimers (25). In the vast majority of cells, NF-κB dimers are sequestered in the cytoplasm in an inactive form complexed with inhibitor of NF-κB proteins (IκB). However, under a large spectrum of chemically diverse agents and cellular stress conditions, including bacterial lipopolysaccharides, microbial and viral pathogens, cytokines such as TNF-α and IL-1, and growth factors, NF-κB gets rapidly activated (26). Activation involves the phosphorylation, polyubiquitination, and subsequent degradation of IκB by the 26S proteasome, a major pathway for the degradation of intracellular proteins in eukaryotic cells. IκB degradation leads to the exposure of a nuclear translocation sequence of the NF-κB dimer, allowing its nuclear translocation and DNA binding. NF-κB interacts with the consensus sequence 5'-GGGPuNNPyPyCC-3', which is present in numerous immunologically relevant genes—for example, cytokines (TNF-α, IL-6, and so forth), chemokines, adhesion molecules, and matrix metalloproteinases (MMPs), but, importantly, not cytokines with inhibitory function or tissue inhibitors of MMPs (TIMPs).

CYTOKINE EXPRESSION IN RHEUMATOID ARTHRITIS

As described in detail elsewhere in this book, the RA synovium shows markedly increased cellularity due to infiltration of leukocytes recruited from the blood. The lining layer of the synovial membrane contains mainly macrophages (also referred to as *type A synoviocytes*) and the underlying layer consists of fibroblast-like cells (*type B synoviocytes*). This layer is normally one or two cells thick, but, in RA, it is enlarged to ten or more cells thick. The deeper layers within the synovium contain follicles of lymphoid cells around vessels and interspersed lymphocytes. Neovascularization is prominent as endothelial cells become activated. The most abundant cells in the RA synovium are macrophages, T cells, and fibroblasts, but plasma cells, dendritic cells, and endothelial cells are also found. In contrast, the RA synovial fluid is enriched predominantly with neutrophils, but macrophages, T cells, and dendritic cells are also present. As many of these cells have an activated phenotype and express high levels of HLA class II and adhesion molecules, the expression of cytokines in the rheumatoid synovium was anticipated and has now been well documented.

The first studies of cytokines in RA were performed using synovial fluid, because of its accessibility. Thus, cytokines such as IL-1α (27) and TNF-α were first documented in this compartment. However, the RA fluid acts as a sink for a large number of molecules, including hyaluronan, other proteoglycans, degradative enzymes, and serum proteins, many of which inhibit or degrade cytokine function. In addition, the mechanisms controlling the influx of cytokines in the synovial fluid are not understood, making the relevance of cytokines found there in the pathogenesis of the disease uncertain. Much more relevant is the synovial membrane, a principal site of immune and inflammatory activity in RA. Thus, subsequent studies of cytokine expression in RA were mainly done in the synovial membrane. Synovial membrane is usually obtained after joint replacement surgery. Although surgical specimens provide large numbers of cells, the tissue reflects a late stage of the disease. Occasionally, small samples of tissue can be obtained from earlier stages of the disease by arthroscopic biopsies.

Initial studies investigated the expression of cytokine mRNA and used that as an index of local synthesis. By using Northern

TABLE 12.3. Cytokines Expressed in Rheumatoid Synovial Tissue

Cytokines	mRNA	Protein
Proinflammatory		
IL-1α,β	+	+
TNF-α	+	+
LT	+	±
IL-6	+	+
GM-CSF	+	+
M-CSF	+	+
LIF	+	+
Oncostatin M	+	+
IL-2	+	±
IL-3	–	–
IL-7	?	?
IL-9	?	?
IL-12	+	+
IL-15	+	+
IFN-α/β	+	+
IFN-γ	+	±
IL-17	+	+
IL-18	+	+
Immunoregulatory		
IL-4	±	–
IL-10	+	+
IL-11	+	+
IL-13	+	±
TGF-β	+	+
Chemokines		
IL-8	+	+
Gro-α	+	+
MIP-1	+	+
MCP-1	+	+
ENA-78	+	+
RANTES	+	+
Growth factors		
FGF	+	+
PDGF	+	+
VEGF	+	+

ENA, epithelial neutrophil-activating peptide; FGF, fibroblast growth factor; GM-CSF, granulocyte colony-stimulating factor; Gro, growth-related gene product; IFN, interferon; IL, interleukin; LIF, leukemia inhibitory factor; LT, lymphotoxin; MCP, monocyte chemoattractant; M-CSF, macrophage colony-stimulating factor; MIP, macrophage inflammatory protein; mRNA, messenger RNA; PDGF, platelet-derived growth factor; RANTES, regulated on activation, normal T cell–expressed and –secreted; TGF, transforming growth factor; TNF, tumor necrosis factor; VEGF, vascular endothelial growth factor.
Adapted from Feldmann M, Brennan FM, Maini RN. Role of cytokines in rheumatoid arthritis. *Annu Rev Immunol* 1996;14:397–440.

blot hybridization and slot blotting techniques, the presence of cytokines such as TNF-α, IL-1, IL-2, and IFN-γ was documented as synthesized in the rheumatoid synovium (28,29). Protein levels of TNF-α and IL-1 were subsequently detected by using immunohistologic localization and demonstrated predominant expression of these molecules in macrophages (30).

The cloning of a number of other cytokines and growth factors allowed more detailed characterization of cytokines that are expressed in the RA synovium, where they may play a role in pathogenicity and serve as potential therapeutic targets. Thus, many proinflammatory cytokines such as IL-6, IL-12, IL-15, IL-18, LIF, IFN-α, GM-CSF, M-CSF, OSM, and others were detected. In addition, many chemokines that include IL-8, growth-related gene product (Gro)-α, MIP-1α, MIP-1β, and RANTES were also present. Similar expression was also observed for antiinflammatory cytokines such as IL-10 and IL-13 and the T-cell cytokines IL-2 and IFN-γ, initially detected only at the mRNA level. Soon, it was realized that the rheumatoid synovium is enriched with almost every cytokine known, as shown in Table 12.3 (14,30,31). This complexity made the identification of potential therapeutic targets difficult. The history of defining TNF-α as the target for RA has been recently reviewed (11).

CYTOKINE RECEPTOR EXPRESSION IN RHEUMATOID ARTHRITIS

With the identification and cloning of cytokine receptor complementary DNAs and the production of relevant antibodies, the study of the presence of cytokine receptors in small samples of RA tissue has become possible. The presence of cytokine receptors was investigated by using mRNA quantification, radioligand binding, and monoclonal antibodies recognizing specific receptors at the cell surface. The expression of many cytokine receptors has now been studied thoroughly. For example, both the p55 and p75 TNF surface receptors are up-regulated in active RA tissues at both the mRNA and protein level (32). Their expression occurs throughout the synovium, including the areas abutting the sites of erosion (33) and the endothelial cells. These are sites of active TNF-α synthesis (Fig. 12.5), suggesting that TNF-α signaling is probably taking place. The presence of NF-κB in the nucleus of cells supports this probability. The expression of many other cytokine receptors such as IL-1, IL-6, and GM-CSF has also been demonstrated in RA (30).

SOLUBLE CYTOKINE RECEPTORS

Soluble cytokine receptors have also been detected in RA both in the serum and synovial fluid. These are usually cleaved from the surface receptors of cells by proteolytic enzymes, although some can be generated by alternative splicing, and some others, such as the IL-18 binding protein, can come from a gene distinct from the receptor (34). Thus, in RA patients' synovial fluid, p55 and p75 soluble TNF receptors (sTNF-R) are elevated above those in the serum, suggesting that synthesis may be chiefly at sites of inflammation. In plasma, the levels of sTNF-R correlate with disease activity. In RA synovial cultures, endogenous sTNF-Rs are capable of neutralizing a significant proportion of the TNF-α generated (35). A soluble IL-1R is also present in RA synovial tissue and fluid and was originally identified as the type II IL-1R that functions as a decoy receptor on the cell surface or as a cytokine inhibitor when in its soluble form. The type II IL-1R binds to proIL-1β, preventing its processing, and mature IL-1β, preventing its signaling, but does not bind to IL-1 receptor antagonist (IL-1ra). Other soluble cytokine receptors identified in RA include soluble IL-6 and IL-11 receptors that can act as agonists rather than antagonists, soluble IFN-γ receptors, as well as abundant IL-18 binding protein.

CYTOKINE NETWORKS IN RHEUMATOID ARTHRITIS

The presence of cytokines in all rheumatoid synovial samples investigated suggested that, in contrast to normal cells in which cytokine expression is transient, in the rheumatoid synovium, cytokine expression is prolonged or even continuous. This finding, in combination with the observation that almost every cytokine assessable is present in the rheumatoid synovium, highlights the difficulty in determining which, if any, of these cytokines are important or rate-limiting for the pathogenesis of the disease. These might be therapeutic targets. This problem has been approached by using short-term cultures from rheumatoid synovial membranes as an *in vitro* model to investigate synovial tissue cytokine production *in vivo*. Short-term (5–6 days) cultures of rheumatoid synovial membranes contain 30% T cells, 30% to 40% macrophages, and fewer fibroblasts, dendritic cells, endothelial cells, plasma cells, and B lymphocytes. In the absence of extrinsic stimulation, these cultured cells pro-

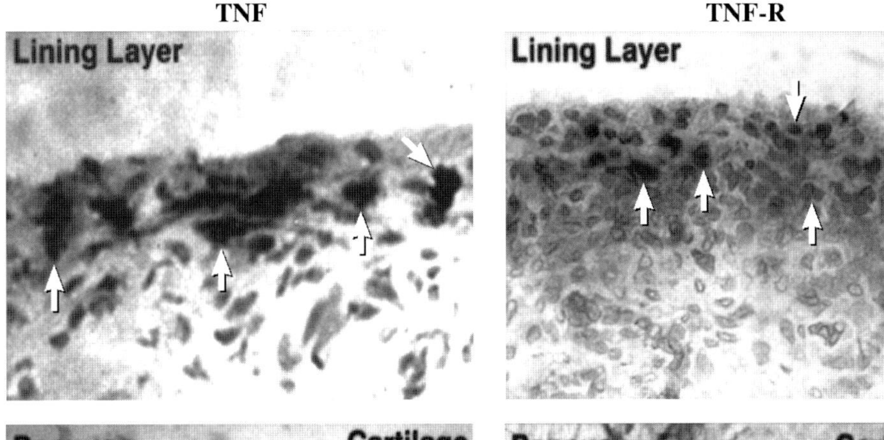

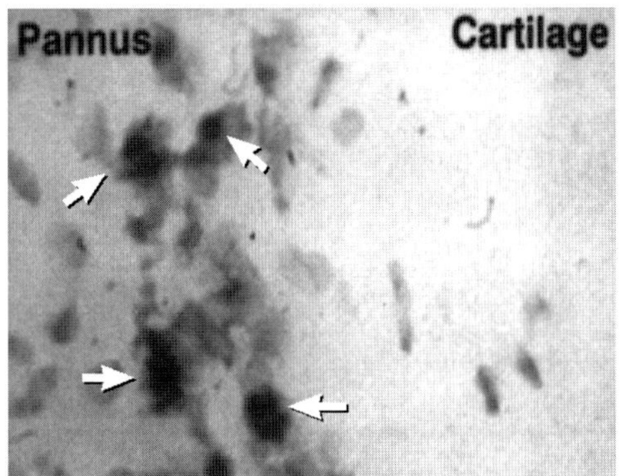

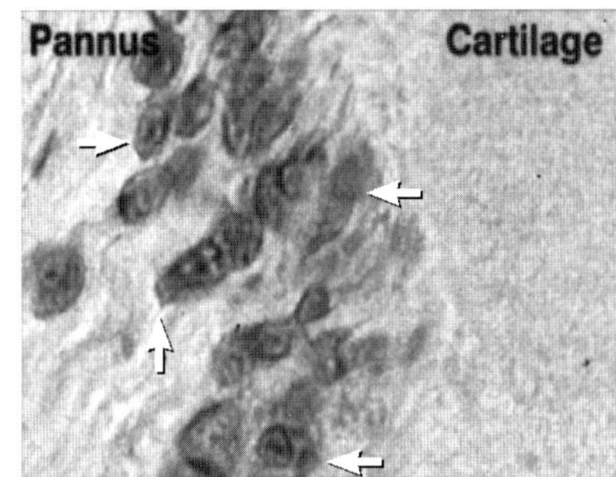

Figure 12.5. Immunolocalization of tumor necrosis factor α (TNF-α) and p55 TNF receptor (TNF-R) in the rheumatoid synovium. Arrows indicate TNF-α–positive cells (*left panels*) and TNF-R–positive cells (*right panels*). [From Deleuran BW, et al. Localization of tumor necrosis factor receptors in the synovial tissue and cartilage-pannus junction in patients with rheumatoid arthritis. Implications for local actions of tumor necrosis factor alpha. Arthritis Rheum 1992;35(10):1170–1178, with permission.]

duce the cytokine mediators that had been detected *in vivo*. This finding indicated that the cytokine and noncytokine signals regulating cytokine production in the rheumatoid synovium also exist in these cultures and encouraged the use of this system as a disease model.

These short-term cultures were used for the investigation of potential cytokine "networks" or "cascades" that could operate in the rheumatoid synovium, up-regulating, down-regulating, or simply prolonging the expression of other cytokines. The first cytokine to be investigated was IL-1 because it had been previously shown that IL-1 is important in cartilage and bone damage. Interestingly, it was found that a neutralizing antibody against TNF-α, a potent inducer of IL-1 in other systems but not against the closely related LTα (that also binds to the p55 and p75 TNF receptors), reproducibly inhibited the production of the great majority of synovial IL-1 (7). This observation is important because it indicates that IL-1 production in the rheumatoid synovium is dependent on TNF-α, despite the presence of many other molecular signals known to potently induce IL-1, such as IL-1 itself, GM-CSF, IFN-γ, immune complexes, and cellular interactions. Blockade of TNF-α also reduces the production of other proinflammatory mediators such as GM-CSF, IL-6, and IL-8 (36,37), as well as the antiinflammatory mediator IL-10 (38). GM-CSF was another important cytokine implicated in the pathogenesis of RA by augmenting hematopoiesis, activating monocytes and macrophages, maintaining or even inducing HLA class II expression in RA synovial cells, and augmenting neutrophil-mediated cartilage degradation and adherence (39).

Because TNF-α production is also known to be up-regulated by IL-1 as well as GM-CSF and IFN-γ, the effect of IL-1 blockade by recombinant IL-1ra was investigated. It was found that IL-1ra does not affect TNF-α or IL-1 production, although it does down-regulate IL-6 and IL-8 production (36). Collectively, these observations indicated that many of the major proinflammatory mediators in the rheumatoid synovium are linked in a "network" or "cascade," with TNF-α at its apex. These data and this concept are supported by the fact that TNF-α is the most rapidly produced cytokine at times of stress; therefore, it is plausible that TNF-α regulates other cytokines and inflammatory mediators. Mice injected with gram-negative bacteria were found to produce serum TNF-α before serum IL-2 and IL-6 (40). Antibody to TNF-α markedly inhibited the IL-2 and IL-6 production in keeping with a TNF-α–dependent cytokine cascade (5,7,10).

The cytokine network is also under the influence of antiinflammatory cytokines. Thus, addition of exogenous IL-10 to the rheumatoid synovial membrane cultures inhibited the production of TNF-α and IL-1 by 50% (38), a finding also reproduced in a similar study using synovial tissue organ cultures (41). Thus, IL-10 acts as an important immunoregulator in this system. It can up-regulate the production of soluble TNF receptors, acting as a TNF-α inhibitor, and, simultaneously, down-regulate the expression of surface TNF-R (42). IL-11 and IL-13 can also function as immunomodulators to down-regulate TNF-α production. The addition of exogenous IL-11 alone or in combination with IL-10 decreases TNF-α production in rheumatoid synovial cultures (43), and the transduction of human RA synovial tissue explants with adenovirus expressing IL-13 decreases the production of TNF-α, IL-1β, IL-8, and MIP-1α (44). Thus, RA may be envisaged as a disease in which there is an imbalance between the production of proinflammatory and antiinflammatory mediators (Fig. 12.6).

CYTOKINES IN ANIMAL MODELS OF ARTHRITIS

A variety of animal models that include collagen-induced arthritis (CIA), streptococcal cell wall arthritis, and adjuvant arthritis in mouse, rats, or even primates have been used to study pathogenic mechanisms as well as therapy (45). The most commonly used of these models is CIA. CIA is induced by

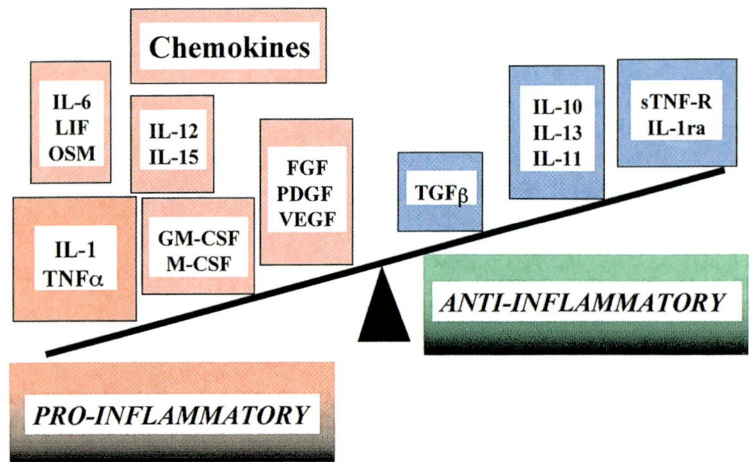

Figure 12.6. Cytokine imbalance in the rheumatoid synovium. FGF, fibroblast growth factor; GM-CSF, granulocyte-macrophage colony-stimulating factor; IL, interleukin; IL-1ra, IL-1 receptor antagonist; LIF, leukemia inhibitory factor; M-CSF, macrophage colony-stimulating factor; OSM, oncostatin M; PDGF, platelet-derived growth factor; TGF, transforming growth factor; TNF, tumor necrosis factor; sTNF-R, soluble TNF receptor; VEGF, vascular endothelial growth factor. (Adapted from Andreakos ET, Foxwell BM, Brennan FM, et al. Cytokines and anti-cytokine biologicals in autoimmunity: present and future. *Cytokine Growth Factor Rev* 2002;13:299–313.)

immunization of genetically susceptible strains of rodents and primates with type II collagen (CII) and leads to the development of a severe polyarticular arthritis that is mediated by an autoimmune response. Like RA, synovitis and erosions of cartilage and bone are hallmarks of CIA, and susceptibility to both RA and CIA is linked to the expression of specific major histocompatibility complex class II molecules. CIA, however, as with other animal models of arthritis, resembles, but does not entirely mimic, human RA. Nevertheless, analysis of animal models of arthritis provides possible insights into the pathogenesis of RA, and animal models can also be used to test therapeutic strategies. Extensive cytokine studies in animal models of arthritis have been performed, and most involve the administration of recombinant cytokines or anticytokine agents. Injection of IL-1 alone or in combination with TNF-α into the joint of a rabbit results in synovitis with proteoglycan degradation (46). Similarly, injection of IL-1 or TNF-α into collagen-immunized mice or rats accelerates the onset and increases the severity of inflammatory arthritis. Subsequently, several studies have shown that blockade of TNF-α through the use of anti–TNF-α neutralizing antibody or other TNF-α inhibitors prevents or even treats established disease (47–49) in the CIA model in mice. Both inflammation assessed by footpad swelling and joint destruction assessed by histologic analysis of the joints is reduced. In addition, blockade of IL-1 signaling by daily administration of IL-1ra delays the onset and reduces the incidence of arthritis (50). The same inhibitory effect is observed after neutralization of IL-1α and IL-1β before or after the onset of arthritis (51,52). In gene therapy studies, administration of a dimeric chimeric human p55 TNF-R–IgG fusion protein through adenoviral gene transfer after disease onset has also resulted in disease improvement.

Similar results have been obtained in a transgenic mouse model of arthritis bearing a deregulated TNF-α transgene with a deletion in the 3' untranslated region of TNF-α essential for the gene's normal regulation (53). This transgene results in increased TNF-α production and an erosive joint disease with histologic features closely resembling human RA that can be prevented by using an anti–TNF-α or an anti–IL-1R neutralizing antibody. The latter result confirms that TNF-α is also important for the generation of IL-1 *in vivo*. This model is of interest because the arthritis does not need T cells or B cells, as shown by persistence in backcrosses with lymphocyte-lacking recombinase-activating gene (RAG)1–deficient mice. This finding verifies that TNF-α, once produced, is sufficient for generating erosive arthritis.

A number of other proinflammatory cytokines have also been examined for their role in arthritis in animal models. Administration of an anti–IL-6R neutralizing antibody in mice or monkeys significantly delayed the onset of CIA and reduced its severity (54,55). A role of IL-6 in this model is also supported by studies of IL-6–deficient mice in which mice were completely protected from the development of CIA (56). Similarly, administration of a soluble form of the IL-15 receptor α chain profoundly suppressed the development of CIA in mice (57). These animal studies have led to clinical trials of IL-6 or IL-15 blockade using an IL-6R or an anti-IL-15 monoclonal antibody, respectively.

The role of antiinflammatory cytokines has also been examined in animal models of arthritis. Thus, subcutaneous administration of IL-4 delayed the onset of arthritis and suppressed the clinical symptoms by down-regulating Th1 responses and TNF-α production (58), whereas intraperitoneal administration of an anti–IL-4 neutralizing antibody before disease onset markedly augmented both the incidence and severity of CIA (59).

Administration of IL-4 after disease onset had only a moderate effect on the inflammatory component of CIA (60,61) but did strongly reduce the histologic damage of cartilage and bone (60). On the other hand, administration of an anti–IL-4 neutralizing antibody after disease onset had no effect on disease activity, although it did increase disease severity when given in combination with an anti–IL-10 neutralizing antibody (61).

Subsequent gene therapy studies have confirmed these findings. Intraarticular or intravenous injection of adenoviral vectors expressing IL-4, intramuscular injection of adeno-associated vectors expressing IL-4, or intravenous administration of IL-4–expressing dendritic cells, all reduced or improved established disease and protected against cartilage and bone destruction in mice. Interestingly, IL-4 production during the CIA disease process seems to require IFN-γ, as IFN-γ–deficient mice or mice treated with an anti–IFN-γ neutralizing antibody develop more severe disease and more readily than their wild-type untreated counterparts (62). Initial phase I studies of IL-4 therapy for RA failed to show evidence of clinical efficacy, so this approach has not been further studied.

Administration of IL-11 has been less well examined with only one study demonstrating significant reduction in the severity of mouse CIA after administration of recombinant IL-11 (63). Delivery of IL-13, a Th2 cytokine, through adenoviral gene transfer, also suppressed the onset and improved established arthritis in rat adjuvant-induced arthritis. In both cases, IL-13 significantly reduced the cellular infiltration, paw swelling, bone damage, and neovascularization (64). Similarly, the constitutive expression of IL-13 via administration of IL-13 complementary DNA–transfected fibroblasts ameliorated established disease both in the murine CIA model and in the transgenic model of arthritis carrying the deregulated TNF-α transgene.

IFN-β administration has also been evaluated in CIA. In mice, the constitutive expression of IFN-β by administration of retrovirally transduced syngeneic fibroblasts prevented disease onset and ameliorated established disease. This treatment reduced paw swelling, improved histologic features, decreased serum levels of anticollagen antibodies, and suppressed cytokine production (65). Similarly, in rhesus monkeys, the systemic administration of recombinant IFN-β-1a produced a remarkable clinical improvement and decreased serum levels of CRP (66). However, the effect of IFN-β-1a therapy in tender joint counts, swollen joint counts, and pain of human RA patients is only moderate.

IL-10 is expressed during the course of arthritis in animal models. Its absence in IL-10–deficient mice or its inhibition by anti–IL-10 neutralizing antibodies accelerates disease onset and severity of CIA in mice (61,67,68), verifying the importance of IL-10 as an immunoregulatory factor. In contrast, exogenous administration of IL-10 protein (61,69–71) or IL-10 complementary DNA through the use of plasmid DNA, transfected antigen-specific T cells, or recombinant adenoviruses significantly reduced both the paw swelling and joint damage, as well as the disease onset or progression in various animal models, such as CIA in mice and rats, streptococcal cell wall arthritis in mice, and adjuvant-induced arthritis in rabbits. Intraarticular administration of recombinant adenovirus expressing IL-10 protects against arthritis not only in the injected joint but also in the contralateral joint. This systemic effect may be due to trafficking of small numbers of adenovirus-transduced cells expressing IL-10 from the injected joint into the circulation, entry of adenovirus particles into the circulation, or IL-10 release from the injected joint into the circulation.

The kinetics of cytokine expression during the early stages of mouse CIA have also been analyzed using immunolocalization techniques. TNF-α, IL-1β, IL-6, and TGF-β expression are mainly found in the synovial lining layer and in the sites of pannus formation and joint erosion (72,73). IFN-γ was found in scattered cells within the deeper layers of the synovium; IL-2, IL-4, or IL-5 could not be detected in any joint (73). TNF-α expression is detectable during the disease onset, whereas IL-1β and IL-6 expression is seen at slightly later stages (1–2 days after disease onset) (72). At later stages of the disease, TNF-α, IL-1β, and IL-6 are still present in the pannus junction, whereas IFN-γ expression disappears (72,73). Lymph node cells isolated from CII-immunized mice have been stimulated *in vitro* with CII and analyzed for cytokine production. TNF-α and IL-1β, as well as IFN-γ, are produced during the induction phase of arthritis, with a rapid decrease in IFN-γ production after disease onset (74). In contrast, IL-10 is not produced by lymph node cells during disease onset; IL-4 production is detectable although markedly suppressed in the presence of CII.

CYTOKINES AND CYTOKINE ANTAGONISTS AS THERAPEUTIC AGENTS IN RHEUMATOID ARTHRITIS

The direct implication from the *in vitro* and *in vivo* studies is that blocking certain cytokines is likely to be beneficial in RA. The first cytokine to be blocked in RA clinical trials was TNF-α, because of evidence placing it at the apex of the proinflammatory cascade operating in the rheumatoid synovium (30). Clinical trials were initiated in 1992 and involved the use of infliximab, initially known as *cA2* (Remicade), a chimeric mouse Fv-human IgG1 monoclonal antibody of high TNF-α–neutralizing capacity produced by Centocor Inc. (75).

In long-standing active RA patients who failed all prior therapy, averaging four disease-modifying drugs, infliximab resulted in the rapid alleviation of pain, morning stiffness and tiredness, and reduction of swollen and tender joints within a week or two. The serum concentration of inflammatory markers such as CRP was also reduced. Re-administration of infliximab after relapse induced repeated benefit (12,76). The efficacy of infliximab was subsequently confirmed in a phase II double-blind, randomized, placebo-controlled clinical trial in which a 60% to 70% reduction in the measures of disease activity (such as swollen or tender joint counts and CRP) was observed. In this study, 79% of patients receiving 10 mg per kg and 44% of patients receiving 1 mg per kg of infliximab reached the required level of improvement (Paulus 20) when compared to 8% of the placebo control patients. This study was the formal proof of efficacy. However, the duration of this trial was very short (4 weeks) in order to reduce the dropouts of the placebo group. Hence, further trials were needed to establish whether longer-term treatment was possible.

Interestingly, in a multidose trial, five doses over 3 months, with a 3-month follow-up, a synergy between low doses of infliximab and low-dose methotrexate (MTX) was also demonstrated with more than 60% to 70% improvement in individual parameters of disease activity achieved (77). In subsequent longer-term phase III studies, joint protection was also observed when hands and feet were examined using a modified Sharp x-ray scoring system (78,79).

Other anti–TNF-α–blocking agents have also been used in subsequent studies. These agents include etanercept (Enbrel) (80), a p75 TNF-R IgG fusion protein; D2E7/adalimumab (81), a human monoclonal antibody; CDP571, a humanized chimeric antibody; a PEGylated p55 TNF-R produced by Amgen; and lenercept, a p55 TNF-R Ig Fc fusion protein (14,31) and are listed in Table 12.4.

All the anti–TNF-α agents seem to be effective at blocking both the inflammatory and destructive processes of RA similarly to infliximab—with the exception of lenercept, for which results have been positive but somewhat variable probably due to immunogenicity of the construct or manufacturing problems related to variations in glycosylation of the protein from one batch to another (82). Etanercept (Enbrel, Immunex/American Home Products) was the first TNF-α inhibitor to be approved for the treatment of RA. In placebo-controlled phase II and phase III trials, etanercept therapy reduced swollen and tender

TABLE 12.4. Tumor Necrosis Factor-α Blocking Agents Used in the Clinic in Rheumatoid Arthritis

Name	Composition	Manufacturer
Monoclonal antibodies		
Infliximab, Remicade	Chimeric (mouse × human)	Centocor, USA
CDP571	Humanized murine CDR3	Celltech, UK
D2E7, Adalimumab	Fully human	Cambridge Antibody Technology/BASF, UK
PEG Fab	Fully human	Celltech, UK
TNF-R: Fc fusion proteins		
Etanercept, Enbrel	p75-TNF-R:Fc	Immunex/American Home Products, USA)
Lenercept	p55-TNF-R:Fc	Roche, Switzerland
	PEGp55-TNF-R	Amgen, USA

PEG, pegylated; TNF, tumor necrosis factor; TNF-R, TNF receptor.
Adapted from Feldmann M, Maini RN. Anti-TNF alpha therapy of rheumatoid arthritis: what have we learned? *Annu Rev Immunol* 2001;19:163–196.

joints and ameliorated disease activity (83–85). Etanercept is also beneficial for patients with active RA despite MTX therapy (84). In a clinical trial of patients with active MTX-resistant RA, etanercept retarded the progression of bone erosions, as assessed by radiography of the hands and feet (80). The consistent beneficial effect of multiple TNF-α–blocking agents in a very large number of patients (more than 300,000 by the end of 2002) confirms the importance of TNF-α in RA.

Anticytokine therapy in RA is most advanced to TNF-α blockade but is not limited to it. Other important proinflammatory cytokines have also been targeted. One such cytokine is IL-1. When IL-1 was blocked by administering IL-1ra (anakinra, Amgen) in clinical trials involving patients with RA, the results were positive but less dramatic than these observed with the anti–TNF-α agents. Treatment with IL-1ra improves clinical disease (86) and reduces joint destruction as determined by radiology (86–88). This finding is indicative of an important role of IL-1 in bone resorption, as suggested by both *in vitro* and *in vivo* studies (89,90). This agent has recently been approved by the U.S. Food and Drug Administration in the United States for the treatment of RA.

IL-6 has also been targeted in RA. In one study, administration of a murine antihuman IL-6 neutralizing antibody resulted in a short-term improvement in clinical disease, although the number of patients tested was small (91). In another open-label study, administration of a humanized monoclonal anti–IL-6 receptor antibody improved the clinical symptoms of RA and normalized acute phase proteins within 2 weeks (54). Although the overall benefit of anti–IL-6 therapy is slower in onset than that of TNF-α blockade, the extent of clinical improvement was significant, and randomized trials are under way to determine its effects on inflammation and joint destruction.

Administration of antiinflammatory cytokines has also been investigated as an alternative approach to inhibit proinflammatory cytokine production. Despite their conceptual appeal, inhibitory cytokines have not shown significant treatment benefit in clinical trials of RA. Thus, in two independent phase I studies, administration of IL-10 or IL-11 to patients with active disease did not result in any significant clinical improvement when compared to placebo in small numbers of patients (85,92,93).

MECHANISM OF ACTION STUDIES

Clinical trials with anticytokine biologic agents, which have a specific mode of action, have provided insight into the pathophysiology of RA. Treatment mechanisms have been evaluated using serum and synovial samples. First, the effect of anti–TNF-α on the expression of cytokines was examined. It was found that anti–TNF-α administration rapidly decreased the levels of cytokines such as IL-1, IL-6, IL-8, MCP-1, and vascular endothelial growth factor in the serum (4,12,94–96). Using synovial tissue biopsies, smaller studies also demonstrated reductions in synovial cytokines by immunohistology. These results verify that TNF-α is, indeed, at the apex of the inflammatory cascade in RA, confirming previous experimental observations. Second, anti–TNF-α reduced the trafficking of leukocytes into the joints, as shown directly in studies using labeled cells (95). This reduced trafficking of leukocytes into the joints was due to down-regulation of the production of multiple chemokines and adhesion molecules (4,95,97). Third, anti–TNF-α inhibited angiogenesis in inflamed joints (98). This may be partly due to the decrease in vascular endothelial growth factor production (4). Finally, anti–TNF-α reduced hematologic abnormalities observed in RA patients, such as anemia and elevated platelet counts, although the mechanisms that account for this finding remain unknown (92).

TNF-α blockade was also effective at blocking structural damage in the joint, indicating that TNF-α plays a major role in the pathogenesis of bone damage. This observation resolves a theoretical discussion based on animal models that predicted that IL-1 blockade would be necessary for the prevention of bone damage. It is not known, however, whether the beneficial effect of TNF-α blockade on joint damage is direct or indirect through the inhibition of other cytokines, such as IL-1. Certainly, IL-1 is also important in mediating joint damage, as clinical studies blocking IL-1 with anakinra have shown. At the moment, it is unclear whether blockade of other cytokines can also affect the radiographic progression of the disease, but it is likely that the widespread clinical effects of anti–TNF-α therapy are due to its ability to interfere with multiple biologic pathways.

FUTURE PROSPECTS OF ANTICYTOKINE THERAPY

The success of anticytokine therapy has stimulated the development of novel therapies with increased efficacy. Two approaches seem to be most promising at the moment: combination therapy and therapy targeting cytokine gene expression.

Combination Therapy

The observation that anti–TNF-α agents work better for the treatment of RA when administered in combination with MTX suggests that combination therapy may produce superior results and forms a basis for building on these treatment advances. Strong evidence to support combination therapy comes from experiments in animal models of arthritis. In these experiments, the benefit from anti–TNF-α therapy can be increased when combined with anti–T-cell therapy. Thus, the co-administration of neutralizing anti–TNF-α antibodies with depleting anti-CD4 or anti-CD3 antibodies, or CTLA-4Ig fusion proteins, ameliorates disease in the CIA model when compared with the administration of anti–TNF-α alone (99) (RO Williams, *unpublished data*). Several antirheumatic agents, including cyclosporin and leflunomide, are inhibitory to T cells (100,101) and may be used as a component of combination therapy. MTX also has anti–T-cell effects (reduction of IFN-γ production, promotion of apoptosis) and is routinely used with infliximab therapy for RA. In addition, in animal models, the administration of TNF-α and IL-1–blocking agents has a synergistic effect in the treatment of arthritis (102). It is possible that a synergistic effect between TNF-α and IL-1–blocking agents is also the case in humans and such clinical trials are in progress (etanercept and anakinra), with the earliest results suggesting that this may increase the risk of bacterial infections. Combination therapy has extensively been reviewed elsewhere (103).

Small Chemical Molecules Targeting Cytokine Gene Expression

Currently the major drawback of anti–TNF-α therapies and other anticytokine biologics is the high cost of treatment. Additional problems include the inconvenience of administering anti–TNF-α biologics by injection and the increased risk of infections with chronic treatment (104). An alternative and perhaps less costly approach involves the use of small chemical molecules that target cytokine gene expression instead of the cytokine product itself. This approach has the potential to specifically inhibit mechanisms involved in the production of cytokines such as TNF-α in pathologic processes without necessarily compromising the mechanisms involved in the expression of the same cytokines under normal physiologic processes. The key problem is to

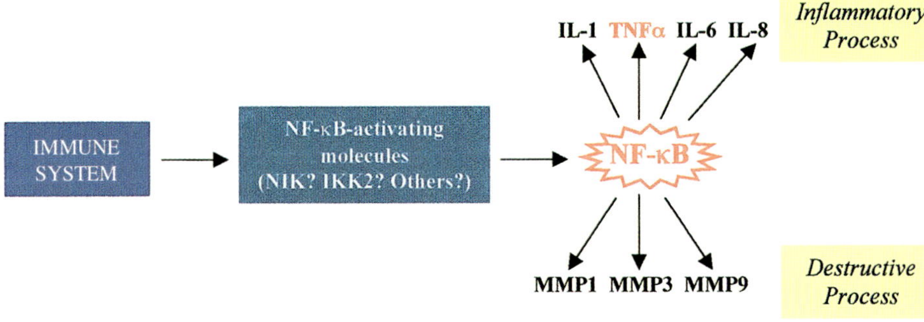

Figure 12.7. Nuclear factor–κB (NF-κB) is central to immune and destructive processes operating in the rheumatoid arthritis synovium. IKK, IκB kinase; IL, interleukin; MMP, matrix metalloproteinase; NIK, NF-κB–inducing kinase; TNF, tumor necrosis factor. [From Andreakos E, et al. Cytokines and anti-cytokine biologicals in autoimmunity: present and future. *Cytokine Growth Factor Rev* 2002;13(4–5):299–313, with permission.]

define the appropriate therapeutic targets that would yield both efficacy and safety.

A significant number of studies have recently investigated the mechanisms involved in gene expression of proinflammatory as well as antiinflammatory cytokines in RA. First, the role of the transcription factor NF-κB has been examined because of its ability to bind to the 5' promoter region of multiple proinflammatory genes, including TNF-α and IL-6. In rheumatoid synovial cells, NF-κB regulates the production of TNF-α, IL-1β, IL-6, and IL-8, as the expression of these cytokines can be blocked by IκBα, the natural inhibitor of NF-κB (105,106). Interestingly, NF-κB is only minimally required for the production of the immunoregulatory cytokines IL-10 and IL-11, or IL-1ra (Fig. 12.7).

Similarly, NF-κB is required for the expression of MMP-1, MMP-3, and MMP-13, enzymes that play a role in the destructive process of RA by breaking down human cartilage (107–109). In contrast, NF-κB does not regulate the expression of TIMP-1, the inducible tissue inhibitor of MMP enzymatic action. These findings demonstrated that NF-κB is essential for both inflammatory and destructive processes of RA. As NF-κB is only minimally involved in the regulation of antiinflammatory cytokines or TIMP-1, blocking NF-κB may be beneficial in RA, as it may restore the cytokine equilibrium in the joint, reducing cartilage and bone damage (Fig. 12.7). Similar data demonstrating the essential role of NF-κB in inflammatory and destructive processes in arthritic joints have also been obtained in animal models of arthritis (110,111), providing compelling evidence about the role of NF-κB in arthritis. Indeed, many conventional antiinflammatory and antiarthritic agents, such as glucocorticoids, sodium salicylate, and sulfasalazine, are inhibitors of NF-κB and TNF-α, suggesting that this property could at least partially explain their therapeutic efficacy (112).

Another major pathway that controls inflammatory gene expression and has attracted major attention in RA involves the MAPKs. In human monocytes/macrophages, p54 MAPK controls TNF-α production at the translational level (113), whereas p42/44 MAPK regulates TNF-α production at the transcriptional levels (105,114). On the other hand, p38 MAPK affects TNF-α expression at multiple levels that involve transcriptional, posttranscriptional, and translational mechanisms (114–116). In rat models of arthritis, PRP200765A, a novel p38 MAPK inhibitor reduces the incidence and progression of arthritis (117), whereas SP600125, a novel p54 MAPK inhibitor, prevents radiologic joint destruction but only modestly decreases paw swelling (118). For optimal therapeutic efficacy, combinations of inhibitors of different MAPKs may be required. Clinical trials of p38 MAPK inhibitors in RA are under way, so their efficacy in humans will be evaluated soon.

CONCLUSION

The identification, cloning, and generation of reagents for cytokines and cytokine receptors over the last 2 decades have provided major insights into the molecular mechanisms of RA. The study of cytokine expression and the elucidation of cytokine networks operating in both the rheumatoid synovium and animal models of arthritis are revealing novel targets of therapeutic potential. This research has already been translated to major therapeutic benefit in the clinic with the advent of TNF-α–blocking biologics (with more than 300,000 patients with RA treated by the end of 2002). The challenge for the near future will be to improve such approaches, possibly by using combinations of anticytokine biologics with already existing therapies, or, in the longer term, by developing small molecule cytokine inhibitors of increased efficiency and specificity. Future developments in the field of anticytokine therapy in RA are eagerly awaited.

REFERENCES

1. Oppenheim JJ, Feldmann M. Cytokine reference. *A compendium of cytokines and other mediators of host defense. Volume I: Ligands*. Academic Press, 2001.
2. Kushner I. The role of IL-6 in regulation of the acute phase response, in IL-6. In: Revel M, ed. *Physiopathology and clinical potentials*. New York: Raven Press, 1992:163–171.
3. Koch AE, et al. Enhanced production of monocyte chemoattractant protein-1 in rheumatoid arthritis. *J Clin Invest* 1992;90:772–779.
4. Paleolog EM, Fava RA. Angiogenesis in rheumatoid arthritis: implications for future therapeutic strategies. *Springer Semin Immunopathol* 1998;20:73–94.
5. Dinarello CA, et al. Tumor necrosis factor (cachectin) is an endogenous pyrogen and induces production of interleukin 1. *J Exp Med* 1986;163:1433–1450.
6. Balkwill FR, Burke F. The cytokine network. *Immunol Today* 1989;10:299–304.
7. Brennan FM, et al. Inhibitory effect of TNF alpha antibodies on synovial cell interleukin-1 production in rheumatoid arthritis. *Lancet* 1989;2:244–247.
8. Scott P. Selective differentiation of CD4+ T helper cell subsets. *Curr Opin Immunol* 1993;5:391–397.
9. Fearon DT, Locksley RM. The instructive role of innate immunity in the acquired immune response. *Science* 1996;272:50–53.
10. Tracey KJ, et al. Anti-cachectin/TNF monoclonal antibodies prevent septic shock during lethal bacteraemia. *Nature* 1987;330:662–664.
11. Feldmann M. Development of anti-TNF therapy for rheumatoid arthritis. *Nature Rev Immunol* 2002;2:364–371.
12. Elliott MJ, et al. Treatment of rheumatoid arthritis with chimeric monoclonal antibodies to tumor necrosis factor alpha. *Arthritis Rheum* 1993;36:1681–1690.
13. Elliott MJ, et al. Randomized double-blind comparison of chimeric monoclonal antibody to tumour necrosis factor alpha (cA2) versus placebo in rheumatoid arthritis. *Lancet* 1994;344:1105–1110.
14. Feldmann M, Maini RN. Anti-TNF alpha therapy of rheumatoid arthritis: what have we learned? *Annu Rev Immunol* 2001;19:163–196.
15. van Dullemen HM, et al. Treatment of Crohn's disease with anti-tumor necrosis factor chimeric monoclonal antibody (cA2). *Gastroenterology* 1995;109:129–135.
16. Chen G, et al. TNF-R1 signaling: a beautiful pathway. *Science* 2002;296:1634–1635.
17. Heyninck K, et al. Crosstalk between NF-kappaB-activating and apoptosis-inducing proteins of the TNF-receptor complex. *Mol Cell Biol Res Commun* 2001;4:259–265.
18. Muller G, et al. PKC zeta is a molecular switch in signal transduction of TNF-alpha, bifunctionally regulated by ceramide and arachidonic acid. *Embo J* 1995;14:1961–1969.
19. Sims JE, et al. Cloning the interleukin 1 receptor from human T cells. *Proc Natl Acad Sci U S A* 1989;86:8946–8950.

20. Saklatvala J, Dean J, Finch A. Protein kinase cascades in intracellular signaling by interleukin-I and tumour necrosis factor. *Biochem Soc Symp* 1999;64:63–77.
21. O'Neill LA, Greene C. Signal transduction pathways activated by the IL-1 receptor family: ancient signaling machinery in mammals, insects, and plants. *J Leukoc Biol* 1998;63:650–657.
22. O'Neill LA, Dinarello CA. The IL-1 receptor/toll-like receptor superfamily: crucial receptors for inflammation and host defense. *Immunol Today* 2000;21:206–209.
23. Taga T, Kishimoto T. Gp130 and the interleukin-6 family of cytokines. *Annu Rev Immunol* 1997;15:797–819.
24. Attisano L, Wrana JL. Signal transduction by the TGF-beta superfamily. *Science* 2002;296:1646–1647.
25. Baeuerle PA, Baltimore D. NF-kappa B: ten years after. *Cell* 1996;87:13–20.
26. Karin M, Ben-Neriah Y. Phosphorylation meets ubiquitination: the control of NF-(kappa)B activity. *Annu Rev Immunol* 2000;18:621–663.
27. Fontana A, et al. Interleukin 1 activity in the synovial fluid of patients with rheumatoid arthritis. *Rheumatol Int* 1982;2:49–53.
28. Buchan G, et al. Detection of activated T cell products in the rheumatoid joint using cDNA probes to interleukin-2 (IL-2) IL-2 receptor and IFN-gamma. *Clin Exp Immunol* 1988;71:295–301.
29. Buchan G, et al. Interleukin-1 and tumour necrosis factor mRNA expression in rheumatoid arthritis: prolonged production of IL-1 alpha. *Clin Exp Immunol* 1988;73:449–455.
30. Feldmann M, Brennan FM, Maini RN. Role of cytokines in rheumatoid arthritis. *Annu Rev Immunol* 1996;14:397–440.
31. Andreakos E, et al. Cytokines and anti-cytokine biologicals in autoimmunity: present and future. *Cytokine Growth Factor Rev* 2002;13:299–313.
32. Brennan FM, et al. Enhanced expression of tumor necrosis factor receptor mRNA and protein in mononuclear cells isolated from rheumatoid arthritis synovial joints. *Eur J Immunol* 1992;22:1907–1912.
33. Deleuran BW, et al. Localization of tumor necrosis factor receptors in the synovial tissue and cartilage-pannus junction in patients with rheumatoid arthritis. Implications for local actions of tumor necrosis factor alpha. *Arthritis Rheum* 1992;35:1170–1178.
34. Novick D, et al. Interleukin-18 binding protein: a novel modulator of the Th1 cytokine response. *Immunity* 1999;10:127–136.
35. Brennan FM, et al. TNF inhibitors are produced spontaneously by rheumatoid and osteoarthritic synovial joint cell cultures: evidence of feedback control of TNF action. *Scand J Immunol* 1995;42:158–165.
36. Butler DM, et al. Modulation of proinflammatory cytokine release in rheumatoid synovial membrane cell cultures. Comparison of monoclonal anti TNF-alpha antibody with the interleukin-1 receptor antagonist. *Eur Cytokine Netw* 1995;6:225–230.
37. Haworth C, et al. Expression of granulocyte-macrophage colony-stimulating factor in rheumatoid arthritis: regulation by tumor necrosis factor-alpha. *Eur J Immunol* 1991;21:2575–2579.
38. Katsikis PD, et al. Immunoregulatory role of interleukin 10 in rheumatoid arthritis. *J Exp Med* 1994;179:1517–1527.
39. Firestein GS, et al. Cytokines in chronic inflammatory arthritis. I. Failure to detect T cell lymphokines (interleukin 2 and interleukin 3) and presence of macrophage colony-stimulating factor (CSF-1) and a novel mast cell growth factor in rheumatoid synovitis. *J Exp Med* 1988;168:1573–1586.
40. Fong Y, et al. Antibodies to cachectin/tumor necrosis factor reduce interleukin 1 beta and interleukin 6 appearance during lethal bacteremia. *J Exp Med* 1989;170:1627–1633.
41. Chomarat P, et al. Balance of IL-1 receptor antagonist/IL-1 beta in rheumatoid synovium and its regulation by IL-4 and IL-10. *J Immunol* 1995;154:1432–1439.
42. Joyce DA, et al. Two inhibitors of pro-inflammatory cytokine release, interleukin-10 and interleukin-4, have contrasting effects on release of soluble p75 tumor necrosis factor receptor by cultured monocytes. *Eur J Immunol* 1994;24:2699–2705.
43. Hermann JA, et al. Important immunoregulatory role of interleukin-11 in the inflammatory process in rheumatoid arthritis. *Arthritis Rheum* 1998;1:1388–1397.
44. Woods JM, et al. Reduction of inflammatory cytokines and prostaglandin E2 by IL-13 gene therapy in rheumatoid arthritis synovium. *J Immunol* 2000;165:2755–2763.
45. Williams RO. Rodent models of arthritis: relevance for human disease. *Clin Exp Immunol* 1998;114:330–332.
46. Henderson B, Pettipher ER. Arthritogenic actions of recombinant IL-1 and tumour necrosis factor alpha in the rabbit: evidence for synergistic interactions between cytokines in vivo. *Clin Exp Immunol* 1989;75:306–310.
47. Williams RO, Feldmann M, Maini RN. Anti-tumor necrosis factor ameliorates joint disease in murine collagen-induced arthritis. *Proc Natl Acad Sci U S A* 1992;89:9784–9788.
48. Thorbecke GJ, et al. Involvement of endogenous tumor necrosis factor alpha and transforming growth factor beta during induction of collagen type II arthritis in mice. *Proc Natl Acad Sci U S A* 1992;89:7375–7379.
49. Piguet PF, et al. Evolution of collagen arthritis in mice is arrested by treatment with anti-tumour necrosis factor (TNF) antibody or a recombinant soluble TNF receptor. *Immunology* 1992;77:510–514.
50. Wooley PH, et al. The effect of an interleukin-1 receptor antagonist protein on type II collagen-induced arthritis and antigen-induced arthritis in mice. *Arthritis Rheum* 1993;36:1305–1314.
51. van den Berg WB, et al. Amelioration of established murine collagen-induced arthritis with anti-IL-1 treatment. *Clin Exp Immunol* 1994;95:237–243.
52. Bessis N, et al. The type II decoy receptor of IL-1 inhibits murine collagen-induced arthritis. *Eur J Immunol* 2000;30:867–875.
53. Keffer J, et al. Transgenic mice expressing human tumour necrosis factor: a predictive genetic model of arthritis. *EMBO J* 1991;10:4025–4031.
54. Takagi N, et al. Blockage of interleukin-6 receptor ameliorates joint disease in murine collagen-induced arthritis. *Arthritis Rheum* 1998;41:2117–2121.
55. Mihara M, et al. Humanized antibody to human interleukin-6 receptor inhibits the development of collagen arthritis in cynomolgus monkeys. *Clin Immunol* 2001;98:319–326.
56. Alonzi T, et al. Interleukin 6 is required for the development of collagen-induced arthritis. *J Exp Med* 1998;187:461–468.
57. Ruchatz H, et al. Soluble IL-15 receptor alpha-chain administration prevents murine collagen-induced arthritis: a role for IL-15 in development of antigen-induced immunopathology. *J Immunol* 1998;160:5654–5660.
58. Horsfall AC, et al. Suppression of collagen-induced arthritis by continuous administration of IL-4. *J Immunol* 1997;159:5687–5696.
59. Yoshino S. Effect of a monoclonal antibody against interleukin-4 on collagen-induced arthritis in mice. *Br J Pharmacol* 1998;123:237–242.
60. Joosten LA, et al. Protection against cartilage and bone destruction by systemic interleukin-4 treatment in established murine type II collagen-induced arthritis. *Arthritis Res* 1999;1:81–91.
61. Joosten LA, et al. Role of interleukin-4 and interleukin-10 in murine collagen-induced arthritis. Protective effect of interleukin-4 and interleukin-10 treatment on cartilage destruction. *Arthritis Rheum* 1997;40:249–260.
62. Vermeire K, et al. Accelerated collagen-induced arthritis in IFN-gamma receptor-deficient mice. *J Immunol* 1997;158:5507–5513.
63. Walmsley M, et al. An anti-inflammatory role for interleukin-11 in established murine collagen-induced arthritis. *Immunology* 1998;95:31–37.
64. Woods JM, et al. Interleukin-13 gene therapy reduces inflammation, vascularization, and bony destruction in rat adjuvant-induced arthritis. *Hum Gene Ther* 2002;13:381–393.
65. Triantaphyllopoulos KA, et al. Amelioration of collagen-induced arthritis and suppression of interferon-gamma, interleukin-12, and tumor necrosis factor alpha production by interferon-beta gene therapy. *Arthritis Rheum* 1999;42:90–99.
66. Tak PP, et al. The effects of interferon beta treatment on arthritis. *Rheumatology (Oxford)* 1999;38:362–369.
67. Cuzzocrea S, et al. Absence of endogenous interleukin-10 enhances the evolution of murine type-II collagen-induced arthritis. *Eur Cytokine Netw* 2001;12:568–580.
68. Kasama T, et al. Interleukin-10 expression and chemokine regulation during the evolution of murine type II collagen-induced arthritis. *J Clin Invest* 1995;95:2868–2876.
69. Walmsley M, et al. Interleukin-10 inhibition of the progression of established collagen-induced arthritis. *Arthritis Rheum* 1996;39:495–503.
70. Tanaka Y, et al. Effect of IL-10 on collagen-induced arthritis in mice. *Inflamm Res* 1996;45:283–288.
71. Persson S, et al. Interleukin-10 suppresses the development of collagen type II-induced arthritis and ameliorates sustained arthritis in rats. *Scand J Immunol* 1996;44:607–614.
72. Marinova-Mutafchieva L, et al. Dynamics of proinflammatory cytokine expression in the joints of mice with collagen-induced arthritis (CIA). *Clin Exp Immunol* 1997;107:507–512.
73. Mussener A, et al. Cytokine production in synovial tissue of mice with collagen-induced arthritis (CIA). *Clin Exp Immunol* 1997;107:485–493.
74. Mauri C, et al. Relationship between Th1/Th2 cytokine patterns and the arthritogenic response in collagen-induced arthritis. *Eur J Immunol* 1996;26:1511–1518.
75. Knight DM, et al. Construction and initial characterization of a mouse-human chimeric anti-TNF antibody. *Mol Immunol* 1993;30:1443–1453.
76. Cope AP, et al. Chronic exposure to tumor necrosis factor (TNF) in vitro impairs the activation of T cells through the T cell receptor/CD3 complex; reversal in vivo by anti-TNF antibodies in patients with rheumatoid arthritis. *J Clin Invest* 1994;94:749–760.
77. Maini RN, et al. Therapeutic efficacy of multiple intravenous infusions of anti-tumor necrosis factor alpha monoclonal antibody combined with low-dose weekly methotrexate in rheumatoid arthritis. *Arthritis Rheum* 1998;41:1552–1563.
78. Maini R, et al. Infliximab (chimeric anti-tumour necrosis factor alpha monoclonal antibody) versus placebo in rheumatoid arthritis patients receiving concomitant methotrexate: a randomized phase III trial. ATTRACT Study Group. *Lancet* 1999;354:1932–1939.
79. Lipsky PE, et al. Infliximab and methotrexate in the treatment of rheumatoid arthritis. Anti-Tumor Necrosis Factor Trial in Rheumatoid Arthritis with Concomitant Therapy Study Group. *N Engl J Med* 2000;343:1594–1602.
80. Bathon JM, et al. A comparison of etanercept and methotrexate in patients with early rheumatoid arthritis. *N Engl J Med* 2000;343:1586–1593.
81. Kempeni J. Update on D2E7: a fully human anti-tumour necrosis factor alpha monoclonal antibody. *Ann Rheum Dis* 2000;59[Suppl 1]:i44–i45.
82. Sander O, et al. Neutralization of TNF by Lenercept (TNFR55-IgG1, Ro 45–2081) in patients with rheumatoid arthritis treated for three months: results of a European phase II trial [abstract]. *Arthritis Rheum* 1996;39[Suppl]:S242.
83. Maini RN, et al. rhuIL-10 in subjects with active rheumatoid arthritis (RA): a phase I and cytokine response study [abstract]. *Arthritis Rheum* 1997;40:S224.

84. Weinblatt ME, et al. A trial of etanercept, a recombinant tumor necrosis factor receptor: Fc fusion protein, in patients with rheumatoid arthritis receiving methotrexate. *N Engl J Med* 1999;340:253–259.
85. Moreland LW, et al. Phase I/II study evaluating the safety and potential efficacy of recombinant interleukin-11 in patients with refractory rheumatoid arthritis. *Arthritis Rheum* 1999;42[Suppl]:224.
86. Bresnihan B, et al. Treatment of rheumatoid arthritis with recombinant human interleukin-1 receptor antagonist. *Arthritis Rheum* 1998;41:2196–2204.
87. Jiang Y, et al. A multicenter, double-blind, dose-ranging, randomized, placebo-controlled study of recombinant human interleukin-1 receptor antagonist in patients with rheumatoid arthritis: radiologic progression and correlation of Genant and Larsen scores. *Arthritis Rheum* 2000;43:1001–1009.
88. Watt I, Cobby M. Treatment of rheumatoid arthritis patients with interleukin-1 receptor antagonist: radiologic assessment. *Semin Arthritis Rheum* 2001;30[5Suppl 2]:21–25.
89. Boyce BF, et al. Effects of interleukin-1 on bone turnover in normal mice. *Endocrinology* 1989;125:1142–1150.
90. Gowen M, et al. An interleukin 1 like factor stimulates bone resorption in vitro. *Nature* 1983;306:378–380.
91. Wendling D, Racadot E, Wijdenes J. Treatment of severe rheumatoid arthritis by anti-interleukin 6 monoclonal antibody. *J Rheumatol* 1993;20:259–262.
92. Davis D, et al. Anaemia of chronic disease in rheumatoid arthritis: in vivo effects of tumour necrosis factor alpha blockade. *Br J Rheumatol* 1997;36:950–956.
93. Moreland L, et al. Results of a phase-I/II randomized, masked, placebo-controlled trial of recombinant human interleukin-11 (rhIL-11) in the treatment of subjects with active rheumatoid arthritis. *Arthritis Res* 2001;3:247–252.
94. Lorenz HM, et al. In vivo blockade of TNF-alpha by intravenous infusion of a chimeric monoclonal TNF-alpha antibody in patients with rheumatoid arthritis. Short term cellular and molecular effects. *J Immunol* 1996;156:1646–1653.
95. Feldmann M, et al. Future prospects for anti-cytokine treatment. *Ann Rheum Dis* 2000;59[Suppl 1]:i119–i122.
96. Charles P, et al. Regulation of cytokines, cytokine inhibitors, and acute-phase proteins following anti-TNF-alpha therapy in rheumatoid arthritis. *J Immunol* 1999;163:1521–1528.
97. Tak PP, et al. Decrease in cellularity and expression of adhesion molecules by anti-tumor necrosis factor alpha monoclonal antibody treatment in patients with rheumatoid arthritis. *Arthritis Rheum* 1996;39:1077–1081.
98. Ballara S, et al. Raised serum vascular endothelial growth factor levels are associated with destructive change in inflammatory arthritis. *Arthritis Rheum* 2001;44:2055–2064.
99. Kumar A, et al. Double-stranded RNA-dependent protein kinase activates transcription factor NF-kappa B by phosphorylating I kappa B. *Proc Natl Acad Sci U S A* 1994;91:6288–6292.
100. Zeidler HK, et al. Progression of joint damage in early active severe rheumatoid arthritis during 18 months of treatment: comparison of low-dose cyclosporin and parenteral gold. *Br J Rheumatol* 1998;37:874–882.
101. Sharp JT, et al. Treatment with leflunomide slows radiographic progression of rheumatoid arthritis: results from three randomized controlled trials of leflunomide in patients with active rheumatoid arthritis. Leflunomide Rheumatoid Arthritis Investigators Group. *Arthritis Rheum* 2000;43:495–505.
102. Feige U, et al. Anti-interleukin-1 and anti-tumor necrosis factor-alpha synergistically inhibit adjuvant arthritis in Lewis rats. *Cell Mol Life Sci* 2000; 57:1457–1470.
103. Bondeson J, et al. Effective adenoviral transfer of IkappaBalpha into human fibroblasts and chondrosarcoma cells reveals that the induction of matrix metalloproteinases and proinflammatory cytokines is nuclear factor-kappaB dependent. *J Rheumatol* 2000;27:2078–2089.
104. Keane J, et al. Tuberculosis associated with infliximab, a tumor necrosis factor alpha-neutralizing agent. *N Engl J Med* 2001;345:1098–1104.
105. Foey AD, et al. Regulation of monocyte IL-10 synthesis by endogenous IL-1 and TNF-alpha: role of the p38 and p42/44 mitogen-activated protein kinases. *J Immunol* 1998;160:920–928.
106. Bondeson J, et al. Selective regulation of cytokine induction by adenoviral gene transfer of IkappaBalpha into human macrophages: lipopolysaccharide-induced, but not zymosan-induced, proinflammatory cytokines are inhibited, but IL-10 is nuclear factor-kappaB independent. *J Immunol* 1999;162:2939–2945.
107. Knauper V, et al. The role of the C-terminal domain of human collagenase-3 (MMP-13) in the activation of procollagenase-3, substrate specificity, and tissue inhibitor of metalloproteinase interaction. *J Biol Chem* 1997;272:7608–7616.
108. Matrisian LM. Metalloproteinases and their inhibitors in matrix remodeling. *Trends Genet* 1990;6:121–125.
109. Cowell S, et al. Induction of matrix metalloproteinase activation cascades based on membrane-type 1 matrix metalloproteinase: associated activation of gelatinase A, gelatinase B and collagenase 3. *Biochem J* 1998;331[Pt 2]:453–458.
110. Miagkov AV, et al. NF-kappaB activation provides the potential link between inflammation and hyperplasia in the arthritic joint. *Proc Natl Acad Sci U S A* 1998;95:13859–13864.
111. Palombella VJ, et al. Role of the proteasome and NF-kappaB in streptococcal cell wall-induced polyarthritis. *Proc Natl Acad Sci U S A* 1998;95:15671–15676.
112. Epinat JC, Gilmore TD. Diverse agents act at multiple levels to inhibit the Rel/NF-kappaB signal transduction pathway. *Oncogene* 1999;18:6896–6909.
113. Swantek JL, Cobb MH, Geppert TD. Jun N-terminal kinase/stress-activated protein kinase (JNK/SAPK) is required for lipopolysaccharide stimulation of tumor necrosis factor alpha (TNF-alpha) translation: glucocorticoids inhibit TNF-alpha translation by blocking JNK/SAPK. *Mol Cell Biol* 1997; 17:6274–6282.
114. Rutault K, Hazzalin CA, Mahadevan LC. Combinations of ERK and p38 MAPK inhibitors ablate tumor necrosis factor-alpha (TNF-alpha) mRNA induction. Evidence for selective destabilization of TNF-alpha transcripts. *J Biol Chem* 2001;276:6666–6674.
115. Dean JL, et al. p38 mitogen-activated protein kinase regulates cyclooxygenase-2 mRNA stability and transcription in lipopolysaccharide-treated human monocytes. *J Biol Chem* 1999;274:264–269.
116. Ridley SH, et al. A p38 MAP kinase inhibitor regulates stability of interleukin-1-induced cyclooxygenase-2 mRNA. *FEBS Lett* 1998;439:75–80.
117. McLay LM, et al. The discovery of RPR 200765A, a p38 MAP kinase inhibitor displaying a good oral anti-arthritic efficacy. *Bioorg Med Chem* 2001;9:537–554.
118. Farzaneh-Far A, et al. A polymorphism of the human matrix gamma-carboxyglutamic acid protein promoter alters binding of an activating protein-1 complex and is associated with altered transcription and serum levels. *J Biol Chem* 2001;276:32466–32473.

CHAPTER 13

Angiogenesis and Leukocyte Recruitment

Zoltán Szekanecz and Alisa E. Koch

A number of factors, including inflammatory cells, soluble mediators, cellular adhesion molecules (CAMs), proteolytic enzymes, and others, are involved in the pathogenesis of synovitis associated with rheumatoid arthritis (RA). In RA, inflammatory leukocytes invade the synovium by transmigrating through the vascular endothelium (Fig. 13.1). Several CAMs interacting with soluble inflammatory mediators, such as cytokines and chemokines, are involved in this process (1–8). Angiogenesis, the formation of new blood vessels (also associated with RA), further perpetuates leukocyte extravasation and thus the formation of inflammatory infiltrates within the synovium (7,8).

The vascular endothelium is involved in inflammatory cell adhesion and migration, as well as angiogenesis. Endothelial cells (ECs) line the lumina of arteries, veins and capillaries, thus separating and also connecting the blood and the extravascular tissues. It has become clear that in inflammatory reactions, such as RA synovitis, ECs are not only passive bystanders but interact with cells and soluble mediators found in the surrounding tissues. ECs are active responders to external stimuli, being targets for leukocytes and their soluble products. On the other hand, these cells themselves produce a number of inflammatory mediators, express CAMs, and thus directly influence the action of leukocytes and the outcome of the inflammatory response (9,10).

Angiogenesis is a crucial process in a number of physiologic processes, such as reproduction, development, and tissue repair, as well as in disease states, including, among others, RA and other inflammatory diseases. The angiogenic process, its mediators and inhibitors, cellular and molecular interactions underlying neovascularization, as well as the role of angiogenesis and the possibilities of angiostatic targeting in RA are extensively discussed in numerous reviews (7,8,11–17). The RA synovium is rich in newly formed vessels. Increased angiogenesis found in RA further perpetuates the extravasation of leukocytes and thus synovitis, which leads to the progression of RA. Therefore, RA is considered an important candidate for "angiogenic diseases" (7,14–16). Several growth factors, proinflammatory cytokines, chemokines, CAMs, extracellular matrix (ECM) components, proteolytic enzymes, and other factors, which may induce angiogenesis, have been detected in the RA synovium. These mediators interact with each other, leading to the perpetuation of neovascularization within and increased leukocyte extravasation into the RA synovial tissue (7,14–16) (Fig. 13.1). Numerous angiostatic compounds may also be able to control synovial inflammation and thus may be used in antirheumatic therapies (7,8,11–17).

In this chapter, we review the role of blood vessels in the pathogenesis of RA. Two major processes, such as leukocyte extravasation and angiogenesis, are discussed. The involvement of soluble inflammatory mediators, including cytokines and chemokines, in the regulation of these processes is being reviewed. Studies of leukocyte-endothelial adhesion and angiogenesis in RA are important, because molecules involved in these processes may be targeted in biologic therapy and may provide future alternatives to antirheumatic therapy. Therefore, data on the clinical relevance of cell adhesion and angiogenesis in RA are also presented here.

CHANGES IN ENDOTHELIAL MORPHOLOGY AND FUNCTION IN SYNOVITIS

The endothelium as well as the affected vessel itself may undergo various morphologic changes during inflammation (Fig. 13.2). These changes include vasodilatation, a key feature of inflammation, as well as increased vascular permeability (vascular leakage). The latter can result from several mechanisms, including endothelial contraction and retraction, as well as leukocyte or antiendothelial antibody–mediated vascular (endothelial) injury and endothelial regeneration (10). Leukocytes interacting with the vascular wall may themselves cause endothelial injury, leading to increased vascular permeability. The key mediators in this process are leukocyte-derived reactive oxygen intermediates and some proteolytic enzymes such as matrix metalloproteinases (MMPs) (18) (Table 13.1).

Antiendothelial cell antibodies occur in various pathologic conditions. These antibodies have been described in several autoimmune and inflammatory diseases including RA (19–21). The presence of these antibodies in the sera may be a marker of vascular damage. Antiendothelial cell antibodies are found more frequently in the sera of patients with rheumatoid vasculitis than RA without this manifestation (20,21).

The process of endothelial proliferation during the regeneration of capillaries after vascular injury and angiogenesis is also associated with leakage. The increased permeability of newly formed vessels is due to open intercellular junctions and the incomplete basement membranes of differentiating ECs (17,22,23). Furthermore, in some cases endothelial regeneration may occur without the formation of new blood vessels. In the latter situation, regeneration is accompanied by increases in capillary permeability. Such events may transpire in the vicinity of necrotic or infarcted tissues (24).

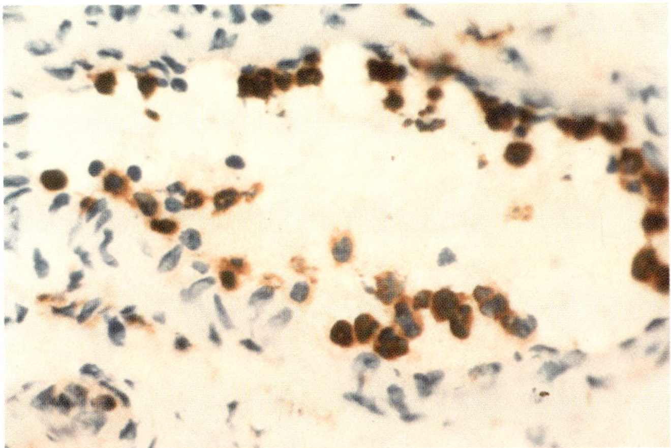

Figure 13.1. Leukocyte extravasation in the synovium of rats with adjuvant-induced arthritis. The inflamed synovium is rich in vessels. Indirect immunoperoxidase staining indicates CD18 (β_2 integrin) expression on leukocytes as indicated by the brown color. (Magnification, ×696.)

TABLE 13.1. Endothelial-Derived Inflammatory Mediators

Cytokines
Interleukin-1 (IL-1)
IL-6
IL-8
Chemokines
Monocyte chemoattractant protein-1
Growth-regulated oncogene-α
Growth factors
Endothelial cell-derived growth factor
Transforming growth factor-β
Colony-stimulating factors
Granulocyte colony-stimulating factor
Granulocyte-macrophage colony-stimulating factor
Others
Platelet-activating factor
Nitric oxide
Prostacyclin

CELLULAR ADHESION MOLECULES IN INFLAMMATION

Adhesion of peripheral blood inflammatory leukocytes to endothelium is a key event in inflammation, leading to the process of leukocyte transendothelial emigration into inflammatory sites (25–28) (Figs. 13.1, 13.2, and 13.3). The adhesion of ECs to the surrounding ECM is also important for endothelial activation, proliferation, migration, and angiogenesis. Leukocyte-endothelial as well as endothelial-ECM adhesion is mediated by CAMs. CAMs have been classified into a number of superfamilies. However, most CAMs involved in endothelial adhesion belong to three families, the integrins, selectins, and immunoglobulin superfamily (reviewed in references 25–28). Although there are several exceptions, integrins are mainly involved in endothelial cell (EC) adhesion to ECM macromolecules, whereas members of the immunoglobulin superfamily and selectins play a role in endothelial adhesion to other cells (25–28) (Table 13.2).

Selectins contain an extracellular N-terminal domain related to lectins, an epidermal growth factor–like domain, and moieties related to complement regulatory proteins (reviewed in references 25–28). This superfamily of CAMs include E-, P-, and L-selectin. Among these CAMs, only E- and P-selectin are present on endothelia (25–28).

E-selectin is not expressed on resting cultured ECs. However, on stimulation with interleukin-1 (IL-1) or tumor necrosis factor α (TNF-α) for even less than 1 hour, ECs begin to express this CAM on their surface. Maximal endothelial E-selectin expression is seen after 4 to 6 hours of cytokine treatment followed by down-regulated expression (29). Thus, E-selectin is a marker of cytokine-dependent endothelial activation. Furthermore, cytokine treatment of ECs results in the shedding of this CAM and the release of soluble E-selectin from the endothelial surface (3,30). E-selectin mediates the adhesion of neutrophils and, to a lesser extent, eosinophils, monocytes, and some memory T cells to endothelia (31). Ligands for E-selectin, such as E-selectin ligand-1, P-selectin ligand-1 (PSGL-1), and cutaneous leukocyte antigen, contain sialylated glycan motifs, such as sialyl Lewis-X (32–34). E-selectin is a marker of endothelial activation in lymphocyte-rich areas in inflammatory sites (35). Abundant expression of E-selectin in RA synovial tissues and increased production of soluble E-selectin in RA synovial fluids were described (30,36). In addition, soluble E-selectin mediates monocyte chemotaxis (37). Antibodies to E-selectin reduce neutrophil influx in animal models of airway and skin inflammation (28,34,38,39).

P-selectin is constitutively present on the membrane of endothelial Weibel-Palade bodies. Its expression on the plasma

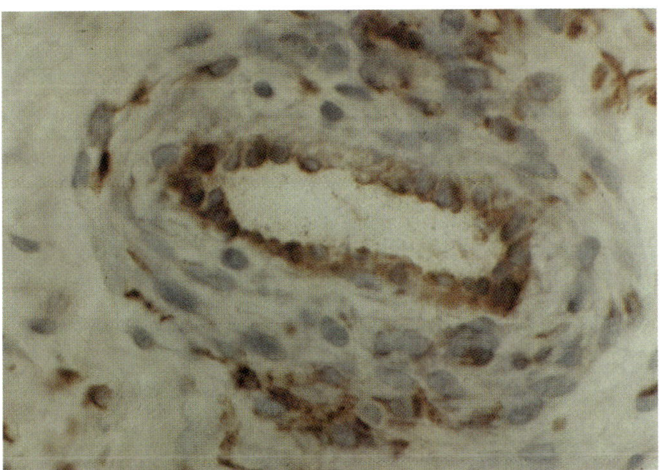

Figure 13.2. Indirect immunoperoxidase staining of frozen rheumatoid synovial tissue showing endothelial intercellular adhesion molecule-1 expression as indicated by the brown color. (Magnification, ×696.)

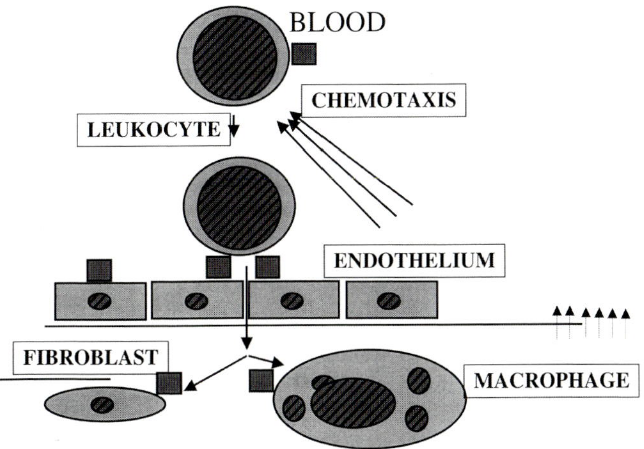

Figure 13.3. Leukocyte extravasation into the synovium. Squares indicate adhesion molecules. Inflammatory mediators, such as cytokines and chemokines, are involved in leukocyte adhesion as well as adhesion molecule expression.

TABLE 13.2. Most Relevant Endothelial Adhesion Molecules in Arthritis

Adhesion Molecule Superfamily	Receptor on Endothelium	Ligand(s)
Integrins	β_1 integrins (most)	ECM components (laminin, fibronectin, collagen, vitronectin, etc.)
	$\alpha_4\beta_1$ integrin	VCAM-1, fibronectin
	$\alpha_V\beta_3$ integrin	ECM components (fibronectin, fibrinogen, thrombospondin)
Immunoglobulins	Intercellular adhesion molecule-1	β_2 integrins: LFA-1, Mac-1
	VCAM-1	$\alpha_4\beta_1$ and $\alpha_4\beta_7$
	LFA-3	CD2
	Platelet-endothelial cell adhesion molecule-1 (CD31)	Homophilic, $\alpha_V\beta_3$
Selectins	E-selectin	E-selectin ligand-1, PSGL-1, cutaneous leukocyte antigen
	P-selectin	PSGL-1
Cadherins	Vascular endothelial-cadherin	Homophilic
Others	CD44	Hyaluronic acid
	Endoglin	Transforming growth factor-β
	Vascular adhesion protein-1	?

ECM, extracellular matrix; LFA, lymphocyte function–associated antigen; PSGL-1, P-selectin ligand-1; VCAM-1, vascular cell adhesion molecule-1.

membrane of ECs is rapidly up-regulated by histamine or thrombin (40). P-selectin is involved in neutrophil and monocyte adhesion to endothelium *in vitro* (41). PSGL-1 is a known ligand for P-selectin (33,34). In contrast to E-selectin, the induction of P-selectin on ECs is an example of endothelial stimulation rather than activation. The up-regulation of P-selectin expression occurs within seconds. Thus, this CAM is thought to be involved in the very early phases of adhesion (42). P-selectin is expressed on RA synovial ECs (43). In addition, soluble P-selectin concentrations are increased in RA versus osteoarthritic synovial fluids (44). Anti-PSGL-1 antibody blocked the migration of T cells into inflammatory sites (34).

L-selectin is absent from ECs, but present on lymphocytes and neutrophils. L-selectin serves as a lymphocyte homing receptor, where it mediates the recirculation of naive cells. L-selectin ligands, including CD34, MadCAM-1, and GlyCAM-1, are present on the specialized endothelia of high endothelial venules (25,26). These ligands, termed *addressins*, are mostly involved in lymphocyte homing. However, there is an increasing body of evidence that L-selectin is also involved in leukocyte-endothelial interactions (28,45). Studies using E- and P-selectin–deficient, L-selectin–transfected cell lines revealed that L-selectin itself is able to mediate leukocyte rolling (46). Nevertheless, as L-selectin expression on leukocytes is down-regulated on cytokine activation (47), the exact role of this CAM in inflammation remains to be elucidated.

Integrins are $\alpha\beta$ heterodimers and are classified into families with respect to their common β subunits. At least eight common β chains (β_1 to β_8) have been identified. Each of these β subunits is associated with one or more α chains (25–28). Among these CAMs, β_1 and β_3 integrins are expressed on ECs. These integrins ($\alpha_{1-9}\beta_1$, $\alpha_V\beta_3$) mediate cell adhesion to ECM components, including various types of collagen, laminin, fibronectin, fibrinogen, tenascin, vitronectin, and thrombospondin. The $\alpha_1\beta_1$ and $\alpha_2\beta_1$ heterodimers mediate EC adhesion to types I and IV collagen, as well as to laminin (25–27,48). The main EC laminin receptor, however, is $\alpha_6\beta_1$. There are two important receptors for fibronectin: $\alpha_5\beta_1$ recognizes the RGD (arginyl-glycyl-aspartyl-) motif in fibronectin, whereas $\alpha_4\beta_1$ is RGD-independent (25–27,48). Both integrins, as well as another fibronectin, laminin, and collagen receptor, $\alpha_3\beta_1$, are also present on ECs (48,49). Integrins containing the β_3 subunit are involved in EC adhesion to fibronectin, vitronectin, thrombospondin, von Willebrand's factor, and fibrinogen. The α_V integrin subunit can be associated with several β chains (β_1, β_3, β_5, β_6, β_8) and mediates EC adhesion to a variety of ECM components, depending on the β subunit (25,27,48,49).

ECM-binding integrins can be classified into subgroups of "basement membrane" (collagen-laminin)–binding integrins ($\alpha_1\beta_1$, $\alpha_2\beta_1$, $\alpha_3\beta_1$, and $\alpha_6\beta_1$) and "inflammatory matrix" integrins (fibronectin-fibrinogen receptors: $\alpha_4\beta_1$, $\alpha_5\beta_1$, α_V, and β_3). Although microvessels express the former but not the latter type of integrins *in situ*, CAMs belonging to both subgroups are present on capillary ECs *in vitro*. These data suggest that ECs have a potential to alter their CAM profile during vascular morphogenesis (49). Most β_1 integrins, as well as $\alpha_V\beta_3$, are highly involved in EC migration on various substrata, angiogenesis (see Angiogenesis: Its Mediators and Inhibitors in Rheumatoid Arthritis), and they are required for the survival and maturation of new blood vessels (48,50).

Integrins are not only involved in EC adhesion to ECM, but sometimes they are able to mediate cell-to-cell contacts. In the latter situation, integrins bind to CAMs belonging to the immunoglobulin superfamily. The two most relevant receptor-counterreceptor pairs are $\alpha_4\beta_1$ integrin recognizing vascular cell adhesion molecule-1 (VCAM-1) and β_2 integrins [lymphocyte function–associated antigen (LFA)-1 and Mac-1] binding to intercellular adhesion molecule-1 (ICAM-1) (25,27) (Table 13.2). Here, VCAM-1 and ICAM-1 are expressed by ECs, whereas integrins are found on the adhering leukocytes. There is abundant expression of endothelial integrins in synovial inflammation (3,43,51–54). Antibodies to β_1 and β_2 integrins abrogated animal models of arthritis (55,56). Antibodies to the common β_2 integrin subunit attenuated meningitis, glomerulonephritis, and arthritis in various animal models (39).

VCAM-1, a ligand for the integrins $\alpha_4\beta_1$ and $\alpha_4\beta_7$, is constitutively expressed on resting ECs. However, its expression is markedly up-regulated by IL-1 and TNF-α, as well as IL-4 (3,57). In EC cultures, a relatively slow increase in VCAM-1 expression reaches its maximum in approximately 24 hours of cytokine treatment (10,57). Antibodies to VCAM-1 inhibit leukocyte-endothelial adhesion (10). *In situ* VCAM-1 expression is associated with sites of lymphocytic infiltration in various types of inflammation (58). There is abundant expression of VCAM-1 on synovial ECs in RA (3,36,59). VCAM-1 may also shed from the cellular surface under inflammatory conditions. There is an increased soluble VCAM-1 concentration in RA sera and synovial fluids of RA patients compared to controls (60). Antibodies to VCAM-1 attenuate inflammation in various animal models (61,62).

ICAM-1 serves as a ligand for the β_2 integrins LFA-1 ($\alpha_L\beta_2$), Mac-1 ($\alpha_M\beta_2$), and p150,95 ($\alpha_X\beta_2$) (25–27). ICAM-1 shows basal expression on ECs; however, its expression can be further stimulated by IL-1, TNF-α, and interferon-γ (IFN-γ) (63). The maximal expression of ICAM-1 on endothelia is observed later (more than 24 hours) than that of E-selectin or VCAM-1 (9). The ICAM-1/β_2 integrin–dependent adhesion pathway is highly important in inflammation, as patients with leukocyte-adhesion deficiency having mutations in the β_2 integrin subunit show marked suppression of the inflammatory response (64). ICAM-1 is highly expressed on ECs in various inflammatory sites, including RA synovium (3,36,65) (Figs. 13.2 and 13.4). There are

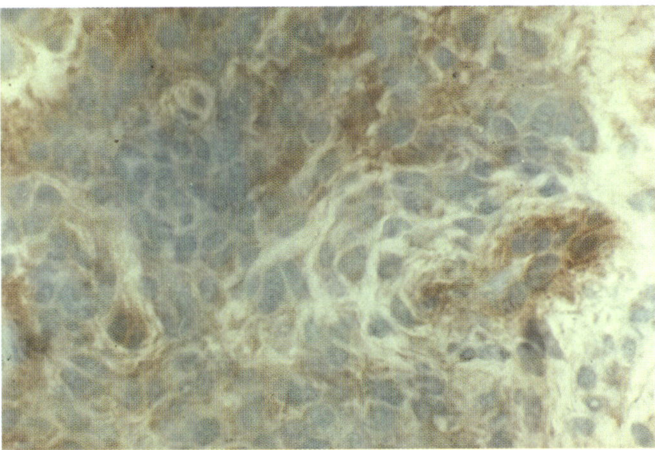

Figure 13.4. Indirect immunoperoxidase staining of frozen rheumatoid synovial tissue showing heavy leukocytic infiltration around vessels. Intercellular adhesion molecule-1 expression on mononuclear leukocytes and vascular endothelium is indicated by brown color. (Magnification, ×696.)

elevated levels of soluble ICAM-1 in the synovia of RA patients (66,67). Anti-ICAM-1 antibodies administered *in vivo* were able to prevent experimental arthritis (28,39,68). A monoclonal antibody to ICAM-1 (enlimomab) was also tried to treat patients with refractory RA. This antibody exerted only temporary effect on the clinical symptoms (69).

Other CAMs mediating EC adhesion to other cells in inflammation include LFA-3, platelet-EC adhesion molecule-1 (PECAM-1; CD31), CD44, vascular adhesion proteins (VAP-1 and VAP-2), endoglin, vascular endothelial (VE)-cadherin, and, possibly, ICAM-3 (25–27,70–73). LFA-3 and its counterreceptor, CD2, are members of the immunoglobulin superfamily. Although CD2 is a T-cell marker, LFA-3 is present on ECs. The CD2/LFA-3 adhesion pathway is involved in various inflammatory responses, including synovitis (3,70,74). PECAM-1, another member of the immunoglobulin superfamily, mediates homotypic adhesion by binding to PECAM-1 as well as heterotypic adhesion by recognizing the $\alpha_V\beta_3$ integrin (25–27,75). PECAM-1 is a marker of activated endothelium and is present in large quantities in the RA synovium (43,76). CD44 is a receptor for hyaluronate (25,27). CD44 is present on activated ECs in inflammation, including RA (43,77,78). VAP-1 has originally been isolated from synovial ECs. The expression of VAP-1 is increased in inflammation (71). Endoglin is a receptor for transforming growth factor-β_1 (TGF-β_1) and TGF-β_3, and is involved in endothelial adhesion. Endoglin is expressed on most ECs in the RA synovium (73). VE-cadherin, a major constituent of this junction, mediates homophilic binding between ECs. It shows co-localization with many other CAMs, including PECAM-1 and endoglin. VE-cadherin is involved in endothelial migration and polarization (79). ICAM-3 is a leukocyte CAM, which is a known ligand for LFA-1. It is absent from most resting ECs. However, ICAM-3 is present on a portion of RA synovial ECs (72,80), which suggests the possible role of endothelial ICAM-3 in inflammation. Thus, a number of CAMs may play a role in the adhesive interactions of ECs (Figs. 13.2 and 13.4; Table 13.2).

LEUKOCYTE-ENDOTHELIAL INTERACTIONS AND THEIR REGULATION BY INFLAMMATORY MEDIATORS

Leukocyte extravasation into inflamed tissues, including synovia, occurs in at least four distinct steps. First, relatively weak adhesion termed *rolling* occurs within 1 to 2 hours after the stimulus, which is mediated by endothelial E- and P-selectins, leukocyte L-selectin, and their counterreceptors. Leukocyte activation and triggering occurs next due to the interactions between chemokine receptors on leukocytes and proteoglycans on ECs. This is followed by activation-dependent, firm $\alpha_4\beta_1$ integrin/VCAM-1 and $\alpha_L\beta_2$ integrin (LFA-1)/ICAM-1 interactions. Intercellular adhesion is accompanied by the secretion of several chemokines. Transendothelial migration or diapedesis occurs when secreted chemokines bind to endothelial heparan sulphate glycosaminoglycans. Chemokines preferentially attract endothelium-bound leukocytes. $\alpha_4\beta_1$ and $\alpha_5\beta_1$ integrins recognize endothelial fibronectin, whereas $\alpha_6\beta_1$ binds to laminin. These adhesive interactions enable leukocyte ingress into the synovium (81) (Fig. 13.3; Table 13.3).

TABLE 13.3. Distinct Steps during Leukocyte Emigration: Role of Adhesion Molecules

Step	Factors on Endothelium	Factors on Leukocytes
Rolling	P-selectin E-selectin L-selectin ligand ?	PSGL-1 ESL-1 Sialyl Lewis-X Cutaneous leukocyte antigen L-selectin
Activation	Chemokines (interleukin-8, monocyte chemoattractant protein-1, etc.) Platelet-activating factor PECAM-1 E-selectin	Cytokine and chemokine receptors PECAM-1 PSGL-1, ESL-1
Firm adhesion	ICAM-1 VCAM-1	β_1, β_2, and β_7 integrins
Diapedesis	ICAM-1 VCAM-1 PECAM-1	β_1, β_2, and β_7 integrins PECAM-1

ESL-1, E-selectin ligand-1; ICAM-1, intercellular adhesion molecule-1; PECAM-1, platelet-endothelial cell adhesion molecule-1; PSGL-1, P-selectin ligand-1; VCAM-1, vascular cell adhesion molecule-1.

Leukocyte-endothelial interactions are regulated by a number of factors (Fig. 13.3). Physical factors, such as altered shear stress, stimulate the rolling and adhesion of neutrophils to endothelium (42). The state of activation of neutrophils is also important for rolling, adhesion, and migration. Resting neutrophils readily adhere to E-selectin and VCAM-1 but not to ICAM-1. In contrast, activated neutrophils prefer to adhere to ICAM-1 (82). This observation is in concordance with the fact that the rolling of resting leukocytes involves selectins, whereas β_2 integrin/ICAM-1–dependent transmigration occurs after neutrophil activation (28,81). As described above, exogenous cytokines, including IL-1, TNF-α, and, in some cases, IL-4 and IFN-γ may up-regulate endothelial CAM expression and stimulate leukocyte-endothelial adhesion (3,57,63). ECs themselves also produce a number of inflammatory mediators, including IL-1, IL-6, IL-8, granulocyte colony-stimulating factor, and granulocyte-macrophage colony-stimulating factor, as well as the chemokines monocyte chemoattractant protein-1 (MCP-1) and growth-related gene product α (Gro-α) (Table 13.1). Some of these endogenous mediators may also be involved in these adhesive processes [e.g., the role of platelet-activating factor in P-selectin–dependent rolling (83) and that of chemokines in integrin-dependent firm adhesion (81)]. ECs produce IL-1, and endogenous IL-1, similarly to exogenous IL-1, induces CAM expression (84). However, the role of endogenous cytokines in neutrophil-endothelial interactions is somewhat controversial. For example, IL-8 enhances neutrophil adhesiveness to ECs (85), although another study indicates exactly the opposite (86). Thus, the exact role of endogenous endothelial-derived cytokines needs to be clarified. Certain CAMs can also crosstalk with each other, resulting in strengthened intercellular adhesion. For example, E- and P-selectin stimulate the adhesive activity of β_2 integrins on neutrophils (83,87). It has been reported that endothelial E- and P-selectin are not only CAMs but also signaling receptors (88). The crosstalk between selectins and integrins is crucial for the transition from rolling to firm adhesion. Finally, intercellular contact itself may result in increased cytokine release and CAM expression (89). These regulatory mechanisms may synchronize the sequence of events described above, and they may be important in the escalation of leukocyte extravasation and the inflammatory process (Figs. 13.2 and 13.4).

ANGIOGENESIS: ITS MEDIATORS AND INHIBITORS IN RHEUMATOID ARTHRITIS

Angiogenesis is pathologically enhanced in a number of inflammatory diseases, such as RA, psoriasis, and malignancies. Inflammation is associated with an increased turnover of capillaries. The neovascularization process and the outcome of "angiogenic diseases" are dependent on the balance or imbalance between angiogenic mediators and inhibitors. A number of cytokines, growth factors, chemokines, and other mediators can stimulate or inhibit neovascularization. The suppression of neovascularization by blocking the action of angiogenic mediators, or by the administration of angiostatic compounds, may be useful in controlling the progression of inflammation (reviewed in references 7,8,14–17,23,90–94) (Table 13.4).

New vessels are generated following a program of several distinct steps. First, ECs are activated by different angiogenic stimuli. In response, the endothelium secretes proteases, which degrade the underlying basement membrane and ECM. The linear emigration of ECs results in the formation of primary capillary sprouts. ECs then further proliferate, migrate, and synthesize new basement membrane. This process is followed by sprout lumen formation. Two sprouts then link to form capillary loops. Finally, the emigration of ECs out of these sprouts results in the development of second and further generation of capillary sprouts (16,17,90,91) (Fig. 13.5).

Recent studies revealed that preferential endothelial precursor cells may exist within the population of blood stem cells. These reports suggest that a distinct subpopulation of $CD34^+$ cells carrying vascular endothelial growth factor (VEGF) receptors may, under certain circumstances, develop into ECs (95–97). Deletion of endothelial-specific VEGF receptor 2 by gene targeting in mice results in the absence of these EC precursors (97). These cells may be important in the induction and perpetuation of angiogenesis, and they may also be used for the induction of neovascularization in future therapeutic trials carried out in patients with certain vascular disorders (98–100). VEGF and basic fibroblast growth factor have been introduced into animal models as well as into human trials to induce angiogenesis by stimulating endothelial morphogenesis from stem cells in ischemic heart disease (98) as well as obliterative arteriosclerosis (99,100).

A number of *in vitro* and *in vivo* models are available to study angiogenesis. *In vitro* systems include endothelial cultures grown on ECM, such as the laminin-containing Matrigel, tissue culture systems, or endothelial chemotaxis assays (7,14–17,101–104). *In vivo* neovascularization has been investigated using the rat, murine, rabbit, or guinea pig corneal micropocket; the chick

TABLE 13.4. Some Angiogenic Mediators and Angiogenesis Inhibitors in Rheumatoid Arthritis

	Mediators	Inhibitors
Growth factors	Basic FGF, acidic FGF Vascular endothelial growth factor Hepatocyte growth factor Platelet-derived growth factor, platelet-derived endothelial cell growth factor Epidermal growth factor Insulin-like growth factor-1 TGF-β[a]	TGF-β[a]
Cytokines	Tumor necrosis factor-α IL-1[a] IL-6[a] IL-13 IL-15 IL-18	IL-1[a] IL-4 IL-6[a] Interferon-α, -γ
Chemokines	IL-8 Epithelial-neutrophil activating protein-78 Growth-regulated oncogene α Connective tissue–activating protein-III Monocyte chemoattractant protein-1 Fractalkine Stromal cell–derived factor-1	Platelet factor-4 Interferon-γ-inducible protein-10 Monokine induced by interferon-γ
Matrix molecules	Type I collagen Fibronectin, laminin Heparin, heparan sulphate	RGD sequence Thrombospondin
Proteolytic enzymes/ inhibitors	Matrix metalloproteinases Plasminogen activators	Metalloproteinase inhibitors Plasminogen activator inhibitors
Adhesion molecules	β_1, β_3 integrins Soluble E-selectin Soluble vascular cell adhesion molecule-1 Endoglin CD31 (platelet-endothelial cell adhesion molecule-1) Lewis-y/H MUC18	RGD sequence
Others	Angiogenin PAF Substance P Prolactin Prostaglandin E_2	Some antirheumatic drugs Some antibiotics SPARC (secreted protein acidic and rich in cysteine) Angiostatin Endostatin

FGF, fibroblast growth factor; IL, interleukin; TGF, transforming growth factor.
[a]Mediators with both pro- and antiangiogenic effects.

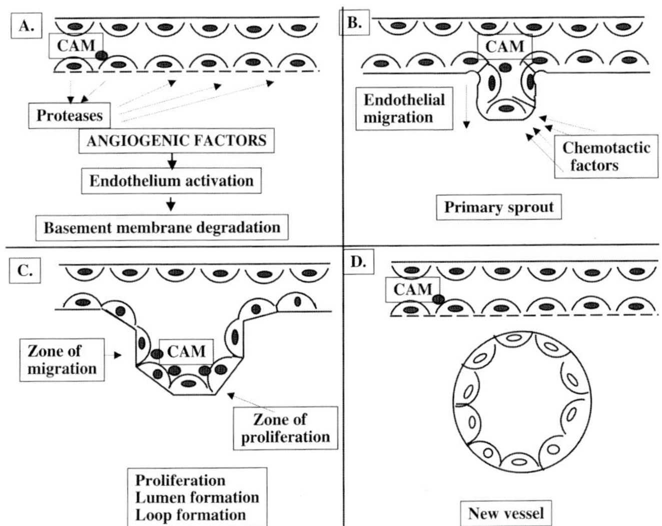

Figure 13.5. The angiogenesis process. Several distinct steps can be distinguished **(A–D)**. CAM, cellular adhesion molecule.

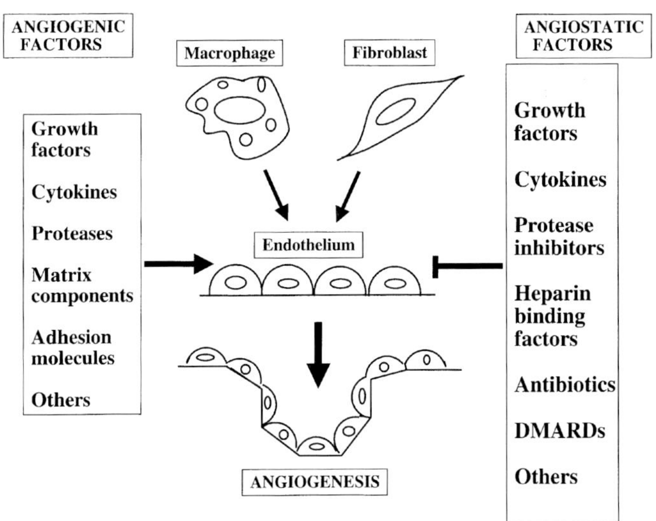

Figure 13.7. Angiogenic mediators and angiostatic factors in rheumatoid arthritis. There is an imbalance toward angiogenic factors. DMARDs, disease-modifying antirheumatic drugs.

embryo chorioallantoic membrane; the hamster cheek pouch; the mesenteric, implanted matrix assays; sponge models; and other systems (7,14–17). These models are suitable to test soluble or cell-bound mediators for their capacity to induce or suppress angiogenesis. Using these assays may be important to investigate the role of angiogenesis in the pathogenesis of certain diseases but also to design strategies for antiangiogenesis therapies (7,8).

Angiogenic factors may act directly on EC proliferation and migration (Fig. 13.6). ECs express receptors for these mediators (5,7,17,23). In contrast, indirect angiogenic mediators act by stimulating macrophages or other cells to release angiogenic growth factors (7,15,90,91). Soluble forms of certain endothelial CAMs can also induce angiogenesis (23,50,103). Only those angiogenic and angiostatic factors that may be involved in inflammatory reactions such as RA are discussed (Figs. 13.6 and 13.7).

Angiogenic mediators involved in the progression of RA include a wide variety of growth factors, cytokines, chemokines, CAMs, ECM components, proteolytic enzymes, and several other factors. Most of these mediators are released by ECs and macrophages; cells present in high quantities in the RA synovium (7,8,12–17) (Fig. 13.7; Table 13.4).

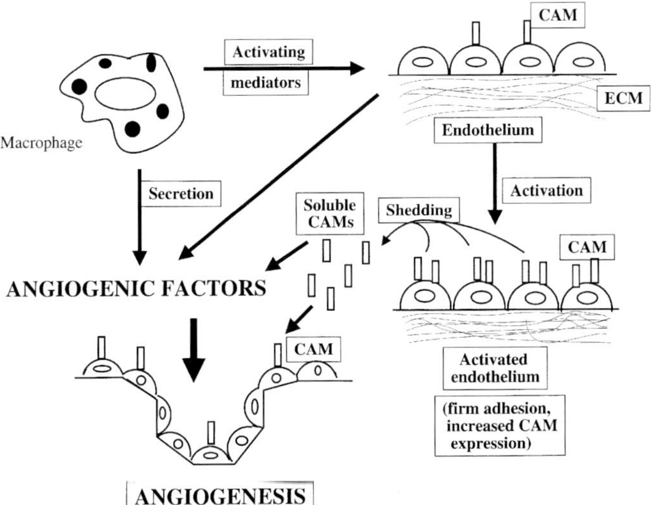

Figure 13.6. The involvement of soluble mediators, as well as soluble and surface-bound adhesion molecules in angiogenesis. CAM, cellular adhesion molecule; ECM, extracellular matrix.

Among growth factors, basic and acidic fibroblast growth factor, VEGF, and hepatocyte growth factor/scatter factor are bound to heparin or heparan sulfate in the interstitial matrix. During the process of angiogenesis, these mediators are released from the matrix by endothelial-derived heparinase and plasmin (7,14–17,105). Recent studies revealed that VEGF, at least in part, stimulated angiogenesis via cyclooxygenase-2 induction (106). The role of VEGF receptor 2–expressing CD34$^+$ stem cells in vascular morphogenesis was discussed above (95–100). Hypoxia-inducible factor 1α is an important regulator of hypoxia-induced VEGF production. This molecule may be involved in synovitis-associated angiogenesis (107).

Other growth factors that mediate neovascularization, such as platelet-derived growth factor, platelet-derived EC growth factor, epidermal growth factor, insulin-like growth factor-1, and TGF-β, do not bind to heparin. However, these growth factors may also promote capillary formation (7,14–16,108,109).

Among proinflammatory cytokines, which also play a role in RA, TNF-α, IL-1, IL-8, IL-13, IL-15, IL-18, and, possibly, IL-6 are involved in angiogenesis (7,8,14–17,110,111).

Chemotactic cytokines termed *chemokines* may be involved in RA-associated angiogenesis (5,7,8,112). Among C-X-C chemokines, IL-8 (CXCL8), epithelial-neutrophil activating protein-78 (ENA-78; CXCL5), Gro-α (CXCL1), and connective tissue–activating protein-III (CTAP-III; CXCL6) promote angiogenesis (8,113,114). It has been shown that IL-8, ENA-78, Gro-α, and CTAP-III contain the ELR (glutamyl-leucyl-arginyl) amino acid sequence. The ELR motif is responsible for their angiogenic activity (113–115). The only ELR-lacking, still angiogenic C-X-C chemokine is stromal cell–derived factor-1 (8,115). In the RA synovium, chemokine-expressing cells were localized in the proximity of factor VIII–related antigen expressing ECs. RA synovial tissue homogenates produced significantly more ENA-78 and IL-8, exhibited increased chemotactic activity toward ECs, and were more angiogenic in the rat cornea assay than homogenates prepared from normal synovial tissues (116). There is relatively little information available on the possible role of C-C chemokines in RA-associated angiogenesis. MCP-1 induces endothelial chemotaxis *in vitro* as well as angiogenesis in the chick chorioallantoic membrane assay *in vivo*. MCP-1–induced neovascularization has been associated with abundant endothelial expression of CCR2 (117). Fractalkine is the only characterized C-X3-C chemokine. This chemokine is expressed on cytokine-activated endothelia (118–120). Fractalkine enhances neovascularization both *in vitro* and *in vivo* (119,120).

Regarding the possible role of chemokine receptors in angiogenesis, a number of these receptors may be detected on ECs, thus playing a role in chemokine-derived angiogenesis. There is a growing body of evidence that CXCR2 may be the most important endothelial receptor for angiogenic C-X-C chemokines containing the ELR amino acid sequence, including IL-8, ENA-78, and groα (114,115,121–124).

In addition to growth factors, cytokines, and chemokines, ECM components, including type I collagen, fibronectin, heparin, laminin, and tenascin; proteolytic enzymes, such as MMPs and plasminogen activators; as well as some CAMs, including soluble E-selectin and soluble VCAM-1, some endothelial β_1, β_3, and β_5 integrins, PECAM (CD31), and endoglin (CD105), have been implicated in angiogenesis. These molecules play an important role in cell adhesion and migration underlying synovial inflammation (reviewed in references 7,8,12–17). Certain glycoconjugates may also serve as angiogenic mediators. Lewis-y/H, which is structurally related to the E-selectin ligand sialyl-Lewis-x, promoted neovascularization using both *in vitro* and *in vivo* models. This glycoconjugate is present in the RA synovium (125). MUC18 (CD146) is a marker for melanoma metastatic potential. This molecule has adhesive properties. Levels of MUC18 in RA synovial fluids correlate with synovial angiogenesis (126). The role of most MMPs has been widely studied in RA. A novel family of metalloproteinases termed *ADAMTS proteinases* includes aggrecanase-1 and -2. These aggrecanases are expressed in the RA synovium, mostly at sites of neovascularization (127).

The COX/prostaglandin system is also involved in angiogenesis. Prostaglandin E_2 is angiogenic (7,17). Cyclooxygenase-2 has been implicated in VEGF-dependent neovascularization (106,128).

Other angiogenic molecules, also produced by synovial cells, including angiogenin, platelet-activating factor, and substance P have been suggested to play a role in RA-associated angiogenesis (7,8,14–17). Recently, prolactin and prolactin-like polypeptides were detected in RA synovial tissues. Prolactin was found to play an important role in T-cell activation, cell communication, and synovial angiogenesis (129).

Angiogenesis inhibitors in RA include some cytokines and growth factors, some of which may also stimulate neovascularization under different circumstances, such as TGF-β, IL-1α, IL-1β, IL-4, IL-6, IL-12, IFN-α , IFN-γ, and leukemia inhibitory factor (reviewed in references 7,8,14–17,92). C-X-C chemokines lacking the ELR motif, such as platelet factor-4 (PF4; CXCL4), monokine induced by IFN-γ (MIG; CXCL9), and IFN-γ–inducible protein (IP-10; CXCL10) also inhibit neovascularization (113–115). Regarding chemokine receptors, as angiostatic chemokines, such as IP-10, MIG, and the recently described SLC, all bind to CXCR3, CXCR3 may play a role in chemokine-mediated angiogenesis inhibition (5,112,130).

In addition to these angiostatic factors, a number of antirheumatic drugs currently used in the treatment of RA inhibit angiogenesis. These drugs include corticosteroids, as well as most disease-modifying antirheumatic drugs, including chloroquine, sulfasalazine, cyclosporin, gold salts, methotrexate, and anti-TNF agents. Neovascularization may also be blocked by protease inhibitors, including tissue inhibitors of metalloproteinases and plasminogen activator inhibitors; thrombospondin-1; derivatives of antibiotics, including fumagillin and minocycline; some cartilage-derived inhibitors; tumor-derived angiostatic agents, including angiostatin and endostatin; cytoskeleton-dissembling agents, including paclitaxel (Taxol); SPARC (*s*ecreted *p*rotein *a*cidic and *r*ich in *c*ysteine)/osteonectin; as well as several other compounds (reviewed in references 7,8,14–17,92). Low endostatin levels occur in RA peripheral blood and synovial fluid samples (131). Endostatin, as well as angiostatin gene transfer inhibits murine arthritis and arthritis-associated angiogenesis (132,133). According to some studies, thalidomide, a TNF-α antagonist compound, which has currently been reintroduced as an immunosuppressive therapy, inhibits neovascularization (134–136). Troponin I is present in the joint and inhibits neovascularization (137). Many of these factors influence the progression of RA, and, thus, they may be useful for the management of this disease.

The angiogenic process and the outcome of angiogenesis, and thus the extent of leukocyte ingress into the synovium, depends on the balance between angiogenic and angiostatic mediators mostly produced by synovial macrophages, ECs, and fibroblasts (7,8,14–17) (Figs. 13.6 and 13.7; Table 13.4). Several intermolecular interactions and feedback loops exist in the RA synovial tissue, as well as in other inflamed tissues, which regulate capillary formation.

Angiogenesis research has important practical clinical, prognostic, and therapeutic relevance. The number of synovial blood vessels in biopsy specimens may reflect the progression of the disease, similarly to the correlation between angiogenesis and the metastatic potential of tumors (reviewed in references 7,8,14–17) (Figs. 13.2 and 13.4). Increased vascularity has been demonstrated in arthritic compared to normal synovial tissues (43,72). The elevated concentration of the angiogenic soluble E-selectin in the synovial fluid of RA patients may also be a useful marker of increased endothelial activation and neovascularization (30,60).

INFLAMMATORY MEDIATORS IN THE REGULATION OF CELLULAR ADHESION AND ANGIOGENESIS

The inflamed synovium contains a regulatory network of proinflammatory cytokines, such as TNF-α and IL-1, chemokines, CAMs, and several other angiogenic factors, such as matrix components, proteolytic enzymes, and other mediators (5,7,8,14). These molecular interactions may be important in leukocyte adhesion, migration, and angiogenesis, and thus the onset and perpetuation of inflammatory synovitis. As several angiogenic mediators are present in the inflamed synovium, and RA is a representative "angiogenic disease," there are complex interactions between endothelium and soluble mediators during angiogenesis. As described above, a number of cytokines, chemokines, and growth factors have been associated with angiogenesis. The proliferating synovium is rich in ECM components. These macromolecules and adhesion molecules regulated by cytokines and chemokines play an important role in the adhesive interactions of ECs during emigration. A number of endothelial CAMs show upregulated expression in the RA synovial tissue (Figs. 13.2 and 13.4). Angiogenic cytokines are proinflammatory and may also include the expression of some CAMs. The interactions between cytokines, chemokines, and CAMs may have additive stimulatory effects on neovascularization. There is evidence for direct interactions between several other angiogenic mediators, which could further perpetuate angiogenesis (7,16,92) (Figs. 13.6 and 13.7).

ANTIADHESION MOLECULE AND ANTIANGIOGENESIS TARGETING

Clinical trials using antiadhesion therapy have provided an important perspective on the role of cell adhesion and CAM in the pathogenesis of RA. In one trial, an antihuman ICAM-1 antibody (enlimomab) was used to treat refractory RA. Many patients reported improvement in their status. A transient increase in the number of circulating T cells after the administration of the antibody suggested that leukocyte extravasation into the RA synovium was inhibited (3,69). Anti–ICAM-1 antibodies may activate blood neutrophils, evidenced by increased β_2 integrin and decreased L-selectin expression on these cells, which may, at least in part, account for the side effects observed during antibody treatment (138). In addition, anti–ICAM-1 and anti-β_2 integrin antibodies prevent the development of arthritis in rats and rabbits, respectively. RGD (arginyl-glycyl-aspartate) peptide, a motif recognized by several integrins, suppresses arthritis in rats (3,7). There have been several attempts in studies of arthritis treatment using animal models, as well as studies of treatment for human RA, to target CAMs involved in the pathogenesis of synovitis, usually with limited success (3).

Angiogenesis research may also have important therapeutic relevance in rheumatology. For example, two central mechanisms may be targeted when developing antiangiogenic therapy. First, switch from the resting to the angiogenic endothelial phenotype could be inhibited by blocking the secretion, transport, and ECM binding of angiogenic factors. Alternatively, vascular EC response to these mediators could be suppressed that regulate migration, proliferation, basement membrane production, and degradation, and expression of endothelial adhesion molecules could be suppressed (101).

As discussed above, a number of antirheumatic drugs currently used in RA, including corticosteroids, nonsteroidal antiinflammatory drugs, or disease-modifying agents, inhibit angiogenesis or the production of macrophage-derived angiogenic mediators (7,8,16,92). For example, sulfasalazine and sulfapyridine inhibited endothelial chemotaxis and tube formation on the laminin-containing matrix Matrigel (139).

The inhibition of several soluble cytokines, growth factors, and chemokines can suppress the pathologic angiogenesis underlying RA. At this moment, TNF-α seems to be a primary target for therapeutic trials, although IL-1, IL-6, IL-8, and other angiogenic mediators have recently been targeted in biologic therapy trials (140). For example, trials with infliximab showed that blocking of TNF-α reduced synovial VEGF expression (141). A humanized anti-VEGF antibody successfully suppressed neovascularization (141).

CAMs could also be targeted in the context of angiogenesis inhibition. For example, fibronectin peptides containing the RGD sequence, which is recognized by several β_1 and β_3 integrins, suppress angiogenesis (142). An $\alpha_v\beta_3$ integrin antagonist inhibited synovial angiogenesis in rats (143).

Other angiostatic compounds could also be used to target arthritis-associated neovascularization. Collagen-induced arthritis in rats was suppressed by a fumagillin-derivative antibiotic angiogenesis inhibitor as well as by the microtubule stabilizer Taxol. Cartilage-derived tissue inhibitors of angiogenesis may also be useful in the treatment of arthritis (7,8,92). MMP inhibitors have been tried in several models of angiogenesis (144). Theoretically, most angiogenesis inhibitors described above may undergo trials in arthritis models.

CONCLUSION

In this chapter, we discussed the putative role of vascular endothelium, including leukocyte-endothelial adhesion and angiogenesis in the pathogenesis of RA. ECs play a central role in leukocyte extravasation, a key feature of inflammatory synovitis. A number of adhesion molecules regulate the sequence of distinct steps. These CAMs interact with soluble inflammatory mediators, such as cytokines and chemokines. The presence of various CAM pairs and the existence of distinct steps of rolling, activation, adhesion, and migration account for the diversity and specificity of leukocyte-endothelial interactions. ECs are active participants in new vessel formation termed *angiogenesis*. A number of soluble and cell-bound factors, including growth factors, cytokines, some chemokines, proteolytic enzymes, ECM components, CAMs, and others may stimulate, whereas others may inhibit, angiogenesis. The outcome of inflammatory and other "angiogenic diseases" depends on the imbalance between angiogenic and angiostatic mediators. There have been several attempts to therapeutically interfere with the cellular and molecular mechanisms described above. Specific targeting of pathologic vascular function, such as increased adhesion and angiogenesis, may be useful for the future management of RA and possibly other inflammatory rheumatic conditions.

REFERENCES

1. Klareskog L, Ronnelid J, Holm G. Immunopathogenesis and immunotherapy in rheumatoid arthritis: an area in transition. *J Int Med* 1995; 238:191–206.
2. Szekanecz Z, Koch AE. Cytokines. In: Ruddy S, Harris ED Jr, Sledge CB, et al., eds. *Textbook of rheumatology*, 6th ed. Philadelphia: WB Saunders, 2001: 275–290.
3. Szekanecz Z, Szegedi G, Koch AE. Cellular adhesion molecules in rheumatoid arthritis. Regulation by cytokines and possible clinical importance. *J Invest Med* 1996;44:124–135.
4. Szekanecz Z, Strieter RM, Koch AE. Cytokines in rheumatoid arthritis: potential targets for pharmacological intervention. *Drugs Aging* 1998;12:377–390.
5. Szekanecz Z, Kunkel SL, Strieter RM, et al. Chemokines in rheumatoid arthritis. *Springer Semin Immunopathol* 1998;20:115–132.
6. Dayer JM, Arend WP. Cytokines and growth factors. In: Kelley WN, Harris ED Jr, Ruddy S, Sledge CB, eds. *Textbook of rheumatology*, 5th ed. Philadelphia: WB Saunders, 1997:267–286.
7. Szekanecz Z, Szegedi G, Koch AE. Angiogenesis in rheumatoid arthritis: pathogenic and clinical significance. *J Invest Med* 1998;46:27–41.
8. Szekanecz Z, Koch AE. Chemokines and angiogenesis. *Curr Opin Rheumatol* 2001;13:202–208.
9. Pober JS, Cotran RS. Cytokines and endothelial cell biology. *Physiol Rev* 1990;70:427–434.
10. Cotran RS. Endothelial cells. In: Kelley WN, Harris ED Jr, Ruddy S, Sledge CB, eds., *Textbook of rheumatology*, 4th ed. Philadelphia: WB Saunders, 1993:327–336.
11. Brenchley PE. Angiogenesis in inflammatory joint disease: a target for therapeutic intervention [editorial]. *Clin Exp Immunol* 2000;121:426–429.
12. Walsh DA. Angiogenesis and arthritis. *Rheumatology* 1999;38:103–112.
13. Paleolog EM, Fava RA. Angiogenesis in rheumatoid arthritis: implications for future therapeutic strategies. *Springer Semin Immunopathol* 1998;20:73–94.
14. Szekanecz Z, Koch AE. Angiogenesis in rheumatoid arthritis. In: Rubanyi GM, ed. *Angiogenesis in health and disease*. New York, Basel: Marcel Dekker, 2000:429–450.
15. Koch AE. Angiogenesis: implications for rheumatoid arthritis. *Arthritis Rheum* 1998;41:951–962.
16. Colville-Nash PR, Scott DL. Angiogenesis in rheumatoid arthritis: pathogenic and therapeutic implications. *Ann Rheum Dis* 1992;51:919–925.
17. Szekanecz Z, Halloran MM, Haskell CJ, et al. Mediators of angiogenesis: the role of cellular adhesion molecules. *Trends Glycosci Glycotechnol* 1999;11:73–93.
18. Varani J, Ginsburg I, Schuger L, et al. Endothelial cell killing by neutrophils. Synergistic interaction of oxygen products and proteases. *Am J Pathol* 1989; 135:435–438.
19. Editorial. Antibodies to endothelial cells. *Lancet* 1991;337:649–650.
20. Van der Zee JM, Heurkens AHM, van der Voort EAM, et al. Characterization of anti-endothelial antibodies in patients with rheumatoid arthritis complicated with vasculitis. *Clin Exp Immunol* 1991;9:589–594.
21. Westphal JR, Boerbooms AMT, Schalkwijk CJM, et al. Anti-endothelial cell antibodies in sera of patients with autoimmune diseases: comparison between ELISA and FACS analysis. *Clin Exp Immunol* 1994;96:444–449.
22. Schoefl G. Studies on inflammation. III. Growing capillaries. *Virchows Arch* 1963;A337:97–100.
23. Szekanecz Z, Koch AE. Adhesion molecules: potent inducers of endothelial cell chemotaxis. In: Zilla PP, Greisler HP, eds. *Tissue engineering of prosthetic vascular grafts*. Austin: RG Landes, 1999:271–277.
24. Joris I, Cuenoud HF, Doern GV, et al. Capillary leakage in inflammation. A study by vascular labeling. *Am J Pathol* 1990;137:1353–1363.
25. Albelda SM, Buck CA. Integrins and other cell adhesion molecules. *FASEB J* 1990;4:2868–2880.

26. Springer TA. Adhesion receptors of the immune system. *Nature* 1990; 346:425–433.
27. Szekanecz Z, Szegedi G. Cell surface adhesion molecules: structure, function, clinical importance. *Orv Hetil* 1992;133:135–142.
28. Carlos TM, Harlan JM. Leukocyte-endothelial adhesion molecules. *Blood* 1994;84:2068–2101.
29. Bevilacqua MP, Pober JS, Mendrick DL, et al. Identification of an inducible endothelial-leukocyte adhesion molecule. *Proc Natl Acad Sci U S A* 1987;84:9238–9242.
30. Koch AE, Turkiewicz W, Harlow LA, et al. Soluble E-selectin in arthritis. *Clin Immunol Immunopathol* 1993;69:29–35.
31. Bochner BS, Luscinskas FW, Gimbrone MA Jr, et al. Adhesion of human basophils, eosinophils, and neutrophils to interleukin 1-activated human vascular endothelial cells: contributions of endothelial cell adhesion molecules. *J Exp Med* 1991;173:1553–1557.
32. Walz G, Aruffo A, Kolanus W, et al. Recognition by ELAM-1 of the sialyl-Lex determinant on myeloid and tumor cells. *Science* 1990;250:1132–1135.
33. Asa D, Raycroft L, Ma L, et al. The P-selectin glycoprotein ligand functions as a common human leukocyte ligand for P- and E-selectins. *J Biol Chem* 1995;270:11662–11670.
34. Borges E, Tietz W, Steegmaier M, et al. P-selectin glycoprotein ligand-1 (PSGL-1) on T helper 1 but not on T helper 2 cells binds to P-selectin and supports migration into inflamed skin. *J Exp Med* 1997;185:573–578.
35. Ishikawa H, Nishibayashi Y, Kita K, et al. Adhesion molecules in the lymphoid cell distribution in rheumatoid synovial membrane. *Bull Hosp Jt Dis* 1993;53:23–28.
36. Koch AE, Burrows JC, Haines GK, et al. Immunolocalization of leukocyte and endothelial adhesion molecules in human rheumatoid and osteoarthritic synovial tissue. *Lab Invest* 1991;64:313–320.
37. Kumar P, Hosaka S, Koch AE. Soluble E-selectin induces monocyte chemotaxis through Src family of tyrosine kinases. *J Biol Chem* 2001;276:21039–21045.
38. Mulligan MS, Varani J, Dame MK, et al. Role of endothelial-leukocyte adhesion molecule 1 (ELAM-1) in neutrophil-mediated lung injury in rats. *J Clin Invest* 1991;88:1396–1406.
39. Kavanaugh A. Adhesion molecules as therapeutic targets in the treatment of allergic and immunologically mediated diseases. *Clin Immunol Immunopathol* 1996;80:S15–S22.
40. McEver RP, Beckstead JH, Moore KL, et al. GMP-140, a platelet alpha-granule membrane protein, is also synthesized by vascular endothelial cells and is localized in Weibel-Palade bodies. *J Clin Invest* 1989;84:92–99.
41. Geng JG, Bevilacqua MP, Moore KL, et al. Rapid neutrophil adhesion to activated endothelium mediated by GMP-140. *Nature* 1990;343:757–760.
42. Lawrence MB, Springer TA. Leukocytes roll on a selectin at physiologic flow rates: distinction from and prerequisite for adhesion through integrins. *Cell* 1991;65:859–873.
43. Johnson B, Haines GK, Harlow LA, et al. Adhesion molecule expression in human synovial tissues. *Arthritis Rheum* 1993;36:137–146.
44. Hosaka S, Shah MR, Pope RM, et al. Soluble forms of P-selectin and intercellular adhesion molecule-3 in synovial fluids. *Clin Immunol Immunopathol* 1996;78:276–282.
45. Von Andrian UH, Chambers JD, McEvoy LM, et al. Two-step model of leukocyte-endothelial cell interaction in inflammation: distinct roles for LECAM-1 and the leukocyte beta 2 integrins in vivo. *Proc Natl Acad Sci U S A* 1991;88:7538–7542.
46. Ley K, Tedder TF, Kansas GS. L-selectin can mediate leukocyte rolling in untreated mesenteric venules in vivo independent of E- or P-selectin. *Blood* 1993;82:1632–1638.
47. Ichikawa Y, Shimizu H, Yoshida M, et al. Accessory molecules expressed on the peripheral blood or synovial fluid T lymphocytes from patients with Sjögren's syndrome or rheumatoid arthritis. *Clin Exp Rheumatol* 1992;10:447–454.
48. Bischoff J. Approaches to studying cell adhesion molecules in angiogenesis. *Trends Cell Biol* 1995;5:69–74.
49. Albelda SM. Differential expression of integrin cell-substratum adhesion receptors on endothelium. *EXS* 1991;59:188–192.
50. Brooks PC, Clark RA, Cheresh DA. Requirement of vascular integrin alpha v beta 3 for angiogenesis. *Science* 1994;264:569–571.
51. Allen CA, Highton J, Palmer DG. Increased expression of p150,95 and CR3 leukocyte adhesion molecules by mononuclear phagocytes in rheumatoid synovial membranes. *Arthritis Rheum* 1989;32:947–954.
52. Laffon A, Garcia-Vicuna R, Humbria A, et al. Upregulated expression and function of VLA-4 fibronectin receptors on human activated T cells in rheumatoid arthritis. *J Clin Invest* 1991;88:546–552.
53. El Gabalawy H, Wilkins J. Beta 1 (CD29) integrin expression in rheumatoid synovial membranes. *J Rheumatol* 1993;20:231–237.
54. Haskard DO. Cell adhesion molecules in rheumatoid arthritis. *Curr Opin Rheumatol* 1995;7:229–234.
55. Jasin HE, Lightfoot E, Davis LS, et al. Amelioration of antigen-induced arthritis in rabbits treated with monoclonal antibodies to leukocyte adhesion molecules. *Arthritis Rheum* 1992;35:541–549.
56. Barbadillo C, Arroyo A, Salas C. Anti-integrin immunotherapy in rheumatoid arthritis: protective effect of anti-alpha 4 antibody in adjuvant arthritis. *Springer Semin Immunopathol* 1995;16:427–436.
57. Thornhill MH, Haskard DO. IL-4 regulates endothelial cell activation by IL-1, tumor necrosis factor, or IFN-gamma. *J Immunol* 1990;145:865–872.
58. Rice GE, Munro M, Corless C, et al. Vascular and non-vascular expression of INCAM-110. *Am J Pathol* 1991;138:385–390.
59. Wilkinson LS, Edwards JC, Poston RN, et al. Expression of vascular cell adhesion molecule-1 in normal and inflamed synovium. *Lab Invest* 1993; 68:82–88.
60. Wellicome SM, Kapahi P, Mason JC, et al. Detection of a circulating form of vascular cell adhesion molecule-1: raised levels in rheumatoid arthritis and systemic lupus erythematosus. *Clin Exp Immunol* 1993;92:412–418.
61. Sans M, Panes J, Ardite E, et al. VCAM-1 and ICAM-1 mediate leukocyte-endothelial cell adhesion in rat experimental colitis. *Gastroenterology* 1999;116:874–883.
62. Orosz CG, Ohye RG, Pelletier RP, et al. Treatment with anti-vascular cell adhesion molecule 1 monoclonal antibody induces long-term murine cardiac allograft acceptance. *Transplantation* 1993;56:453–460.
63. Pober JS, Gimbrone MA Jr, Lapierre LA, et al. Overlapping patterns of activation of human endothelial cells by interleukin 1, tumor necrosis factor, and immune interferon. *J Immunol* 1986;137:1893–1896.
64. Anderson R, Springer TA. Leukocyte adhesion deficiency. *Annu Rev Med* 1978;38:175–190.
65. Munro JM, Pober JS, Cotran RS. Tumor necrosis factor and interferon-gamma induce distinct patterns of endothelial activation and associated leukocyte accumulation in skin of *Papio anubis*. *Am J Pathol* 1989;135: 121–133.
66. Cush JJ, Rothlein R, Lindsley HB, et al. Increased levels of circulating intercellular adhesion molecule 1 in the sera of patients with rheumatoid arthritis. *Arthritis Rheum* 1993;36:1098–1102.
67. Koch AE, Shah MR, Harlow LA, et al. Soluble intercellular adhesion molecule-1 in arthritis. *Clin Immunol Immunopathol* 1994;71:208–215.
68. Iigo Y, Takashi T, Tamatani T, et al. ICAM-1-dependent pathway is critically involved in the pathogenesis of adjuvant arthritis in rats. *J Immunol* 1991;147:4167–4171.
69. Kavanaugh AF, Davis LS, Nichols LA, et al. Treatment of refractory rheumatoid arthritis with a monoclonal antibody to intercellular adhesion molecule-1. *Arthritis Rheum* 1994;37:992–999.
70. Hale LP, Martin ME, McCollum DE, et al. Immunohistologic analysis of the distribution of cell adhesion molecules within the inflammatory synovial microenvironment. *Arthritis Rheum* 1989;32:22–30 .
71. Salmi M, Kalimo K, Jalkanen S. Induction and function of vascular adhesion protein-1 at sites of inflammation. *J Exp Med* 1993;178:2255–2260.
72. Szekanecz Z, Haines GK, Lin TR, et al. Differential distribution of ICAM-1, ICAM-2 and ICAM-3, and the MS-1 antigen in normal and diseased human synovia. *Arthritis Rheum* 1994;37:221–231.
73. Szekanecz Z, Haines GK, Harlow LA, et al. Increased synovial expression of transforming growth factor (TGF)-β receptor endoglin and TGF-β1 in rheumatoid arthritis: possible interactions in the pathogenesis of the disease. *Clin Immunol Immunopathol* 1995;76:187–194.
74. Haynes BF, Hale LP, Denning SM, et al. The role of leukocyte adhesion molecules in cellular interactions: implications for the pathogenesis of inflammatory synovitis. *Springer Semin Immunopathol* 1989;11:163–185.
75. Piali L, Hammel P, Uherek C, et al. CD31/PECAM-1 is a ligand for alpha v beta 3 integrin involved in adhesion of leukocytes to endothelium. *J Cell Biol* 1995;130:451–460.
76. Szekanecz Z, Haines GK, Harlow LA, et al. Increased synovial expression of the adhesion molecules CD66a, CD66b and CD31 in rheumatoid and osteoarthritis. *Clin Immunol Immunopathol* 1995;76:180–186.
77. Haynes BF, Hale LP, Patton KL, et al. Measurement of an adhesion molecule as an indicator of inflammatory disease activity. Up-regulation of the receptor for hyaluronate (CD44) in rheumatoid arthritis. *Arthritis Rheum* 1991; 34:1434–1443.
78. Salmi M, Andrew DP, Butcher EC, et al. Dual binding capacity of mucosal immunoblasts to mucosal and synovial endothelium in humans: dissection of the molecular mechanisms. *J Exp Med* 1995;181:137–149.
79. Dejana E. Endothelial adherens junctions: implications in the control of vascular permeability and angiogenesis. *J Clin Invest* 1996;98:1949–1953.
80. Szekanecz Z, Koch AE. Intercellular adhesion molecule (ICAM)-3 expression on endothelial cells. *Am J Pathol* 1997;151:313–314.
81. Butcher EC. Leukocyte-endothelial cell recognition: three (or more) steps to specificity and diversity. *Cell* 1991;67:1033–1036.
82. Jutila MA, Berg EL, Kishimoto TK, et al. Inflammation-induced endothelial cell adhesion to lymphocytes, neutrophils, and monocytes. Role of homing receptors and other adhesion molecules. *Transplantation* 1989;48:727–731.
83. Lorant DE, Patel KD, McIntyre TM, et al. Coexpression of GMP-140 and PAF by endothelium stimulated by histamine or thrombin: a juxtacrine system for adhesion and activation of neutrophils. *J Cell Biol* 1991;115:223–234.
84. Swerlick RA, Lawley TJ. Role of microvascular endothelial cells in inflammation. *J Invest Dermatol* 1993;100:111S–115S.
85. Carveth HJ, Bohnsack JF, McIntyre TM, et al. Neutrophil activating factor (NAF) induces polymorphonuclear leukocyte adherence to endothelial cells and to subendothelial matrix proteins. *Biochem Biophys Res Commun* 1989; 162:387–393.
86. Gimbrone MA Jr, Obin MS, Brock AF, et al. Endothelial interleukin-8: a novel inhibitor of leukocyte-endothelial interactions. *Science* 1989;246: 1601–1603.
87. Lo SK, Lee S, Ramos RA, et al. Endothelial-leukocyte adhesion molecule 1 stimulates the adhesive activity of leukocyte integrin CR3 (CD11b/CD18, Mac-1) on human neutrophils. *J Exp Med* 1991;173:1493–1500.
88. Lorenzon P, Vecile E, Nardon E, et al. Endothelial cell E- and P-selectin and vascular cell adhesion molecule-1 function as signaling receptors. *J Cell Biol* 1998;142:1381–1391.

89. Bombara MP, Webb DL, Conrad P, et al. Cell contact between T cells and synovial fibroblasts causes induction of adhesion molecules and cytokines. *J Leuk Biol* 1993;54:399–406.
90. Folkman J, Klagsbrun M. Angiogenic factors. *Science* 1987;235:442–447.
91. Klagsbrun M, D'Amore PA. Regulators of angiogenesis. *Annu Rev Physiol* 1991;53:217–239.
92. Auerbach W, Auerbach R. Angiogenesis inhibition: a review. *Pharmacol Ther* 1994;63:265–311.
93. Diaz-Flores L, Gutierrez R, Varela H. Angiogenesis: an update. *Histol Histopathol* 1994;9:807–843.
94. Schweigerer L. Antiangiogenesis as a novel therapeutic concept in pediatric oncology. *J Mol Med* 1995;73:497–508.
95. Peichev M, Naiyer AJ, Pereira D, et al. Expression of VEGFR-2 and AC133 by circulating human CD34(+) cells identifies a population of functional endothelial precursors. *Blood* 2000;95:952–958.
96. Gehling UM, Ergun S, Schumacher U, et al. In vitro differentiation of endothelial cells from AC133-positive progenitor cells. *Blood* 2000;95:3106–3112.
97. Eichmann A, Corbel C, Nataf V, et al. Ligand-dependent development of the endothelial and hemopoetic lineages from embryonic mesodermal cells expressing vascular endothelial growth factor receptor 2. *Proc Natl Acad Sci U S A* 1997;94:5141–5146.
98. Freedman SB, Isner JM. Therapeutic angiogenesis for ischemic cardiovascular disease. *J Mol Cell Cardiol* 2001;33:379–393.
99. Shyu KG, Manor O, Magner M, et al. Direct intramuscular injection of plasmid DNA encoding angiopoietin-1 but not angiopoietin-2 augments revascularization in the rabbit ischemic hindlimb. *Circulation* 1998;98:2081–2087.
100. Isner JM, Baumgartner I, Rauh G, et al. Treatment of thromboangiitis obliterans (Buerger's disease) by intramuscular gene transfer of vascular endothelial growth factor: preliminary clinical results. *J Vasc Surg* 1998;28:964–973.
101. Folkman J. Angiogenesis—retrospect and outlook. *EXS* 1991;59:4–13.
102. Jackson CJ, Jenkins K, Schrieber L. Possible mechanisms of type I collagen-induced vascular tube formation. *EXS* 1991;59:198–204.
103. Koch AE, Halloran MM, Haskell CJ, et al. Angiogenesis mediated by soluble forms of E-selectin and vascular cell adhesion molecule-1. *Nature* 1995;376:517–519.
104. Koch AE, Polverini PJ, Kunkel SL, et al. Interleukin-8 as a macrophage-derived mediator of angiogenesis. *Science* 1992;258:1798–1801.
105. Grant DS, Kleinman HK, Goldberg ID, et al. Scatter factor induces blood vessel formation in vivo. *Proc Natl Acad Sci U S A* 1993;90:1937–1941.
106. Hernandez GL, Volpert OV, Iniguez MA, et al. Selective inhibition of vascular endothelial growth factor-mediated angiogenesis by cyclosporin A: roles of the nuclear factor of activated T cells and cyclooxygenase 2. *J Exp Med* 2001;193:607–620.
107. Hollander AP, Corke KP, Freemont AJ, et al. Expression of hypoxia-inducible factor 1 alpha by macrophages in the rheumatoid synovium: implications for targeting of therapeutic genes to the inflamed joint. *Arthritis Rheum* 2001;44:1540–1544.
108. Koch AE, Harlow LA, Haines GK, et al. Vascular endothelial growth factor. A cytokine modulating endothelial function in rheumatoid arthritis. *J Immunol* 1994;152:4149–4156.
109. Sato N, Beitz JG, Kato J, et al. Platelet-derived growth factor indirectly stimulates angiogenesis in vitro. *Am J Pathol* 1993;142:1119–1130.
110. Angiolillo AL, Kanegane H, Sgadari C, et al. Interleukin-15 promotes angiogenesis in vivo. *Biochem Biophys Res Commun* 1997;233:231–237.
111. Park CC, Morel JC, Amin MA, et al. Evidence of IL-18 as a novel angiogenic mediator. *J Immunol* 2001;167:1644–1653.
112. Koch AE, Kunkel SL, Strieter RM. Chemokines in arthritis. In: Koch AE, Strieter RM, eds. *Chemokines in disease*. Austin: RG Landes, 1996:103–116.
113. Strieter RM, Polverini PJ, Kunkel SL, et al. The functional role of the ELR motif in CXC chemokine-mediated angiogenesis. *J Biol Chem* 1995;270:27348–27357.
114. Strieter RM, Kunkel SL, Shanafelt AM, et al. The role of C-X-C chemokines in regulation of angiogenesis. In: Koch AE, Strieter RM, eds. *Chemokines in disease*. Austin: RG Landes, 1996:195–209.
115. Moore BB, Keane MP, Addison CL, et al. CXC chemokine modulation of angiogenesis: the importance of balance between angiogenic and angiostatic members of the family. *J Invest Med* 1998;46:113–120.
116. Koch AE, Volin MV, Woods JM, et al. Regulation of angiogenesis by the C-X-C chemokines interleukin-8 and epithelial neutrophil activating peptide-78 in the rheumatoid joint. *Arthritis Rheum* 2001;44:31–40.
117. Salcedo R, Ponce ML, Young HA, et al. Human endothelial cells express CCR2 and respond to MCP-1: direct role of MCP-1 in angiogenesis and tumor progression. *Blood* 2000;96:34–40.
118. Bazan JF, Bacon KB, Hardiman G, et al. A new class of membrane bound chemokine with a CX3C motif. *Nature* 1997;385:640–644.
119. Ruth JH, Volin MV, Haines III GK, et al. Fractalkine, a novel chemokine in rheumatoid arthritis and rat adjuvant-induced arthritis. *Arthritis Rheum* 2001;44:1568–1581.
120. Volin MV, Woods JM, Amin MA, et al. Fractalkine: a novel angiogenic chemokine in rheumatoid arthritis. *Am J Pathol* 2001;159:1521–1526.
121. Walz A, Kunkel SL, Strieter RM. C-X-C chemokines—an overview. In: Koch AE, Strieter RM, eds. *Chemokines in disease*. Austin: RG Landes, 1996:1–25.
122. Schonbeck U, Brandt E, Petersen F, et al. IL-8 specifically binds to endothelial but not to smooth muscle cells. *J Immunol* 1995;154:2375–2383.
123. Keane MP, Strieter RM. The role of CXC chemokines in the regulation of angiogenesis. *Chem Immunol* 1999;72:86–101.
124. Rinaldi N, Schwarz-Eywill M, Weis D, et al. Increased expression of integrins on fibroblast-like synoviocytes from rheumatoid arthritis in vitro correlates with enhanced binding to extracellular matrix proteins. *Ann Rheum Dis* 1991;56:45–51.
125. Halloran MM, Carley WW, Polverini PJ, et al. Ley/H: an endothelial-selective, cytokine-inducible, angiogenic mediator. *J Immunol* 2000;164:4868–4877.
126. Neidhart M, Wehrli R, Bruhlmann P, et al. Synovial fluid CD146 (MUC18), a marker for synovial membrane angiogenesis in rheumatoid arthritis. *Arthritis Rheum* 1999,42:622–630.
127. Vankemmelbeke MN, Holen I, Wilson AG, et al. Expression and activity of ADAMTS-5 in synovium. *Eur J Biochem* 2001;268:1259–1268.
128. Leahy KM, Koki AT, Masferrer JL. Role of cyclooxygenases in angiogenesis. *Curr Med Chem* 2000;7:1163–1170.
129. Neidhart M, Gay RE, Gay S. Prolactin and prolactin-like polypeptides in rheumatoid arthritis. *Biomed Pharmacother* 1999;53:218–222.
130. Vicari AP, Ait-Yahia S, Chemin K, et al. Antitumor effects of the mouse chemokine 6Ckine/SLC through angiostatic and immunological mechanisms. *J Immunol* 2000;165:1992–2000.
131. Nagashima M, Asano G, Yoshino S. Imbalance in production between vascular endothelial growth factor and endostatin in patients with rheumatoid arthritis. *J Rheumatol* 2000;27:2339–2342.
132. Yin G, Liu W, An P, et al. Endostatin gene transfer inhibits joint angiogenesis and pannus formation in inflammatory arthritis. *Mol Ther* 2002;5:547–554.
133. Kim JM, Ho SH, Park EJ, et al. Angiostatin gene transfer as an effective treatment strategy in murine collagen-induced arthritis. *Arthritis Rheum* 2002;46:793–801.
134. Calabrese L, Fleischer AB. Thalidomide: current and potential clinical applications. *Am J Med* 2000;108:487–495.
135. Fishman SJ, Feins NR, D'Amoto RJ, et al. Thalidomide for Crohn's disease. *Gastroenterology* 2000;119:596.
136. Oliver SJ, Cheng TP, Banquerigo ML, et al. The effect of thalidomide and two analogs on collagen induced arthritis. *J Rheumatol* 1998;25:964–969.
137. Moses MA, Wiederschain D, Wu I, et al. Troponin I is present in human cartilage and inhibits angiogenesis. *Proc Natl Acad Sci U S A* 1999;96:2645–2650.
138. Vuorte J, Lindsberg PJ, Kaste M, et al. Anti-ICAM-1 monoclonal antibody R6.5 (enlimomab) promotes activation of neutrophils in whole blood. *J Immunol* 1999;162:2353–2357.
139. Volin MV, Harlow LA, Woods JM, et al. Treatment with sulfasalazine or sulfapyridine, but not 5-aminosalicyclic acid, inhibits basic fibroblast growth factor–induced endothelial cell chemotaxis. *Arthritis Rheum* 1999;42:1927–1935.
140. Strand CV, Keystone E. Biologic agents for the treatment of rheumatoid arthritis. In: Ruddy S, Harris ED Jr, Sledge CB, et al., eds., *Kelley's textbook of rheumatology*, 6th ed. Philadelphia: WB Saunders, 2001:899–912.
141. Lin YS, Nguyen C, Mendoza JL, et al. Preclinical pharmacokinetics, interspecies scaling, and tissue distribution of a humanized monoclonal antibody against vascular endothelial growth factor. *J Pharmacol Exp Ther* 1999;288:371–378.
142. Nicosia RF, Bonanno E. Inhibition of angiogenesis in vitro by Arg-Gly-Asp-containing synthetic peptide. *Am J Pathol* 1991;138:829–833.
143. Storgard CM, Stupack DG, Jonczyk A, et al. Decreased angiogenesis and arthritic disease in rabbits treated with an alphavbeta3 antagonist. *J Clin Invest* 1999;103:47–54.
144. Skotnicki JS, Zask A, Nelson FC, et al. Design and synthetic considerations of matrix metalloproteinase inhibitors. *Ann N Y Acad Sci* 1999;878:61–72.

CHAPTER 14

Neutrophils and Small Molecule Mediators

Michael H. Pillinger, Nathalie D. Burg, and Steven B. Abramson

The neutrophil is a key element of the innate immune system. In the absence of functioning neutrophils, humans would be subject to chronic infections and early death. However, the mechanisms neutrophils use to defend the host against infection also contribute to host tissue destruction in various disease states, including rheumatoid arthritis (RA) and other forms of inflammatory arthritis. In this chapter, we review the structure and basic biology of neutrophils and describe the roles of neutrophils in cartilage destruction and the propagation of rheumatoid synovitis.

BASIC NEUTROPHIL BIOLOGY

Neutrophil Development and Morphology

Neutrophils are terminally differentiated effector cells that have lost the capacity for cell division and must therefore be replenished via production of additional neutrophils in the bone marrow. Neutrophil development proceeds from myeloid stem cells and progresses through the promyelocyte, myelocyte, metamyelocyte, band cell, and mature neutrophil stages. Neutrophil development is regulated by a complex interaction of the bone marrow microenvironment and cytokines, the best appreciated of which include granulocyte-macrophage colony-stimulating factor (GM-CSF) and granulocyte colony-stimulating factor (G-CSF). The ability of GM-CSF and G-CSF to stimulate the production and release of neutrophils from the marrow has been exploited clinically in the treatment of sepsis and neutropenia, including in patients with hereditary neutropenia or neutropenia induced by chemotherapy (1,2).

Neutrophils can be recognized on peripheral blood smears by their unique anatomic features. Neutrophils are noteworthy for their unusual multilobar (3 to 5 lobes) nuclei, leading to their designation as *polymorphonuclear leukocytes* (PMNs). In vitamin B_{12} and folate deficiencies, the number of neutrophil lobes may increase to as many as seven, a clinically useful marker whose significance is not entirely clear. Neutrophils may also be recognized by the presence of a large number of granules of multiple functional classes. Thus, neutrophils are considered to be *granulocytes*, a grouping that also includes eosinophils and basophils, as well as macrophages and mast cells. Neutrophilic granules may be distinguished from those of other cells by their distinct tinctorial properties that are midway (neutral, hence, *neutrophil*) between eosinophilic (pink) and basophilic (blue) granules on hematoxylin and eosin staining. Finally, neutrophils may also be thought of as *phagocytes*, a role they share most prominently with macrophages. As discussed below, the ability to phagocytose and destroy foreign particles is the critical and defining function of neutrophils in host innate immunity (3).

Neutrophil Activation and Signal Transduction

CHEMOATTRACTANT RECEPTOR SIGNALING

Chemoattractants, including interleukin-8 (IL-8), formyl-methionyl-leucyl-phenylalanine (FMLP), C5a, and leukotriene B_4 (LTB_4), are generated at infectious or inflammatory sites (Table 14.1) and trigger activation of neutrophil signal transduction pathways (Fig. 14.1). Each chemoattractant binds its own specific seven transmembrane domain, heterotrimeric G protein–coupled receptor. Engagement of these receptors results in G protein activation, with subsequent activation of phospholipase C, adenyl cyclase, and others. Phospholipase C catalyzes the hydrolysis of membrane phospholipids, resulting in the formation of inositol trisphosphate and diacylglycerol. Inositol trisphosphate induces Ca^{2+} release from intracellular stores; diacylglycerol, in conjunction with Ca^{2+}, then activates protein kinase C (4).

MITOGEN-ACTIVATED PROTEIN KINASES

Mitogen-activated protein kinases are serine/threonine kinases, including p38, Erk1 and 2, and Jnk, that participate in cell signaling for growth, differentiation, and responses to stress. p38 activation is required for tumor necrosis factor α (TNF-α)– and FMLP-mediated signaling, and inhibition of p38 abrogates both FMLP-stimulated chemotaxis and TNF-α stimulation of neutrophil oxygen consumption (5). Accumulating evidence points to Erk as a key signaling molecule in neutrophils (6,7) (Fig. 14.1). Erk activation is necessary but not sufficient for neutrophil homotypic aggregation in response to FMLP, LTB_4, C5a, and IL-8 (8). FMLP induces Erk activation through a cascade including the signaling molecules Ras, Raf-1, and MEK (mitogen-activated protein kinase or Erk kinase) (9,10). Exogenously added arachidonic acid also activates Erk through Raf-1 and MEK and stimulates homotypic aggregation. Careful delineation of this pathway reveals that arachidonic acid serves as a substrate for the generation of 5-hydroperoxyeicosatetraenoic acid (5-HPETE) and 5-hydroxyeicosatetraenoic acid (5-HETE) by 5-lipoxygenase; these bioactive lipids then appear to engage G protein–coupled receptors in an autacoid manner (11).

TABLE 14.1. Diversity of Mediators Chemotactic for Neutrophils

Mediator	Source	Activities
C5a	Complement activation product	Chemotaxin, stimulates PMN mediator release, anaphylotoxin, increased vasopermeability
Fibrinopeptides	Plasmin activation of the fibrinolytic system	Chemotaxin, increased vasopermeability
FMLP	Bacterial soluble factor	Chemotaxin, stimulates PMN mediator release
IL-8	C-X-C chemokine product of macrophages, fibroblasts, chondrocytes	Chemotaxin, stimulates PMN mediator release
LTB_4	5-lipoxygenase product of neutrophils, macrophages	Chemotaxin, stimulation of PMN mediator release, inhibits neutrophil apoptosis

FMLP, formyl-methionyl-leucyl-phenylalanine; IL, interleukin; LTB_4, leukotriene B_4; PMN, polymorphonuclear leukocyte.

PHOSPHATIDYLINOSITOL 3-KINASE

Phosphatidylinositol 3-kinase (PI 3-K) has several isoforms and is activated by small GTP binding proteins, Rho and Ras, among others; it in turn phosphorylates both lipids and proteins (Fig. 14.1). The use of the specific PI 3-K inhibitors has elucidated some of the signaling pathways in which PI 3-K is required: PI 3-K is necessary for the chemoattractant-induced respiratory burst, adhesion, and chemotaxis. Independent laboratories have shown that PI 3-K–deficient mice show pronounced neutrophilia (suggesting impaired transmigration), impaired respiratory burst in response to FMLP and C5a, and impaired chemotaxis (12–17). Hii et al. have demonstrated that PI 3-K, but not Erk or PKC, regulates human neutrophil-mediated degradation of cartilage proteoglycan, suggesting an important role for this signaling cascade in the progression of joint destruction (18).

Migration to Inflammatory Sites

NEUTROPHIL ADHESION

Neutrophils are the most populous leukocytes in peripheral blood, making up 60% to 90% of the total white cell count. During an acute infection, large numbers of neutrophils are released from the bone marrow into the circulation, raising the white count dramatically, and, in some cases, leading also to the release of immature forms (bandemia). Neutrophils thus released target capillaries and postcapillary venules, where they respond to bacterial and inflammatory signals by extravasating through the vessels and migrating across tissues to encounter and eradicate microbes. This migration is a multistage process characterized by rolling, firm adhesion, diapedesis, and transmigration (Figs. 14.2 and 14.3).

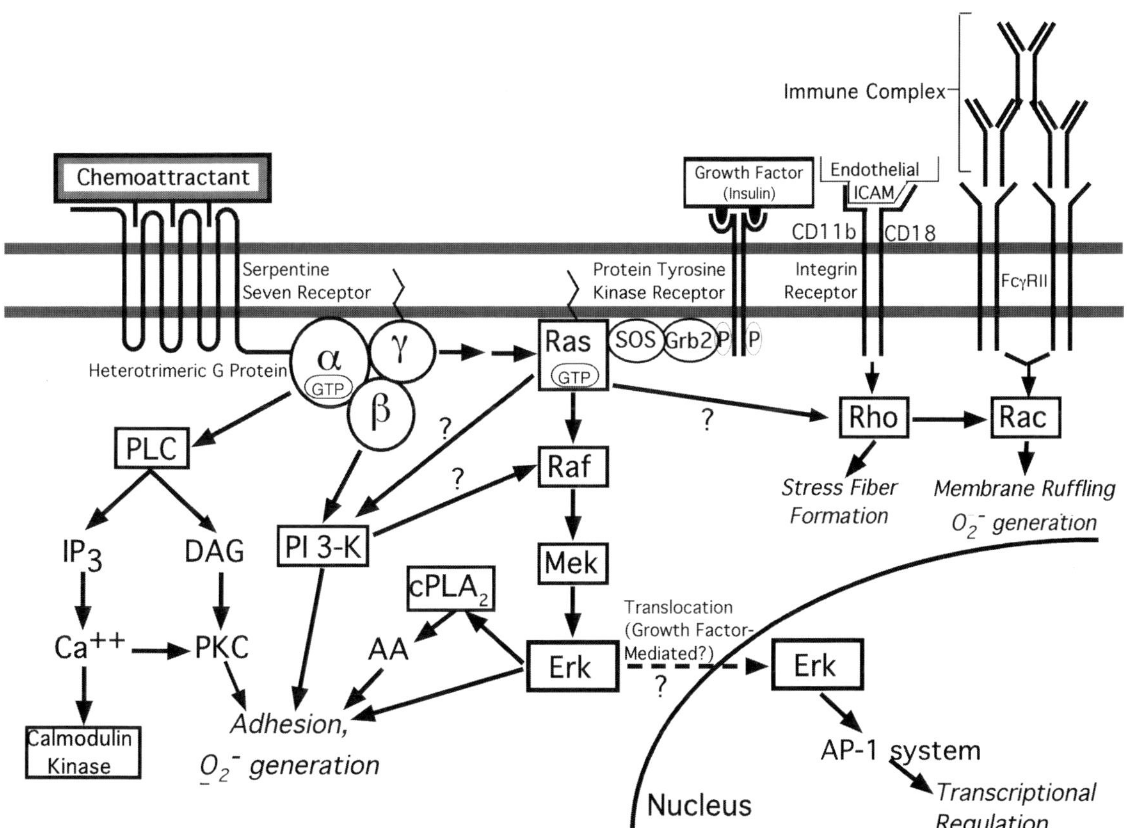

Figure 14.1. Signal transduction pathways in neutrophils. Shown are a number of the signaling pathways in neutrophils activated in response to stimulation by chemoattractants, growth factors, adhesion molecules, and Fcγ receptors. Pathways extrapolated from studies in other cell types are indicated by a question mark. AA, arachidonic acid; cPLA, cytosolic phospholipase A; DAG, diacylglycerol; GTP, guanosine triphosphate; ICAM, intercellular adhesion molecule; IP, inositol triphosphate; PI 3-K, phosphatidylinositol 3-kinase; PKC, protein kinase C; PLC, phospholipase C.

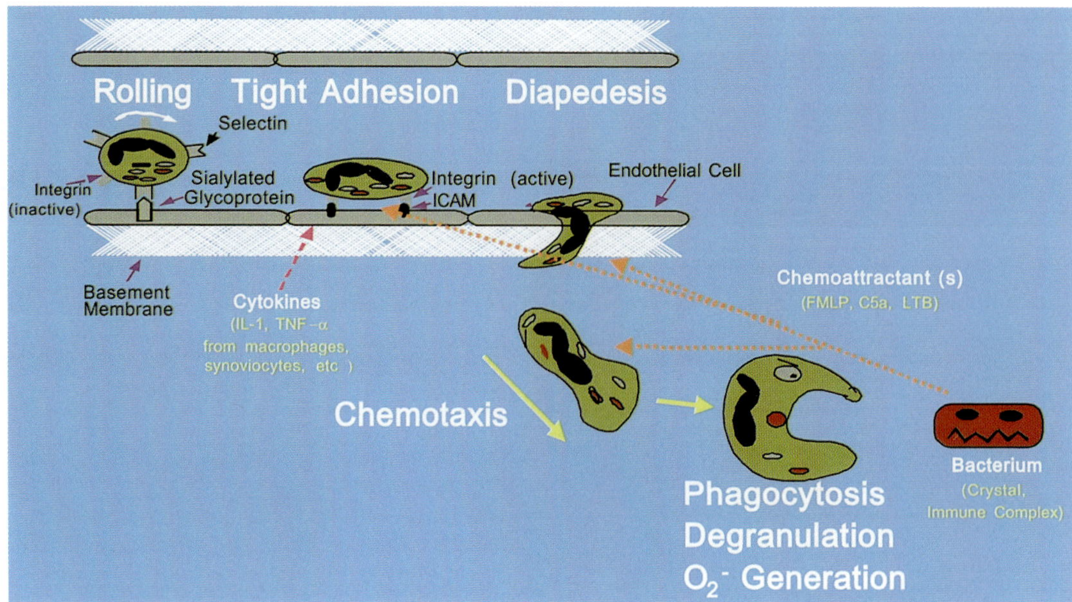

Figure 14.2. Neutrophil rolling, adhesion, and transmigration through the vascular endothelium. By virtue of transient interactions between selectins and sialylated glycoproteins, unstimulated neutrophils in the bloodstream loosely and transiently roll along the vascular endothelium. Chemoattractants, originating at sites of infection or inflammation, stimulate the activation of neutrophil integrins, even as cytokines stimulate the expression of endothelial intercellular adhesion molecules (ICAMs); these processes result in tight adhesions of neutrophils to the vascular wall. Neutrophils subsequently diapedese across the endothelium and migrate up the chemoattractant gradient to the site of inflammation. Interaction between neutrophils and complement and/or immunoglobulins either in immune complexes or on the surface of bacteria leads to phagocytosis of the target and the activation of neutrophil processes, including degranulation and superoxide anion generation. FMLP, formyl-methionyl-leucyl-phenylalanine; ICAM, intercellular adhesion molecule; IL, interleukin; LTB, leukotriene B; TNF, tumor necrosis factor. (Adapted from Pillinger MH, Abramson S. Neutrophils and eosinophils. In: Ruddy S, Harris ED, Jr., Sledge CB, eds. *Kelley's textbook of rheumatology*, 6th ed. Philadelphia: WB Saunders, 2001:195–209.)

Even in the absence of inflammatory signals, neutrophils undergo a process of intermittent rolling and release along the vascular endothelium (Fig. 14.2). This process is mediated by the selectins (P-, E-, and L- for platelet, endothelial, and leukocyte), type 1 membrane glycoproteins that have highly conserved lectin, and endothelial growth factor–like domains. Selectins bind fucosylated and sialylated oligosaccharides such as sialyl Lewis X (sLe^x) (19). Selectin bonds are characterized by their relative resistance to shear stress and their rapid "on" and "off" rates, allowing transient and reversible adhesive contacts. Under conditions of inflammatory stimulation, selectin-mediated adhesion is enhanced. For example, P-selectin, stored in endothelial cell and platelet secretory granules, is rapidly expressed on the cell surface in response to inflammatory stimuli; E-selectin expression is inducible and peaks at 4 to 6 hours after endothelial cell stimulation with TNF-α and IL-1β (20).

A second class of adhesion molecules important for neutrophil function is the β_2 integrins. β_2 integrins are heterodimers composed of one of three distinct subunits (CD11a, b, or c) in combination with a common β (CD18) subunit. The two most important β_2 integrins on the neutrophil are CD11a/CD18 (LFA-1) and CD11b/CD18 (MAC-1, CR3). Chemoattractant stimulation of neutrophils induces modification of the cytoplasmic domains of the β_2 integrins and subsequent conformational changes in the extracellular domains of these molecules (inside-out signaling), enabling them to bind ligands with high affinity (21,22). Unlike selectins, the integrins cannot bind under shear conditions. Once bound, however, they can resist up to 200 times more shear stress than selectins (23). Thus, chemoattractants generated at an extravascular inflammatory site lead to a progression from weak to strong neutrophil adhesion to endothelium. Ligands for integrins include the immunoglobulin (Ig) superfamily members intercellular adhesion molecules-1 and -2. These classic ligands are expressed on vascular endothelium in response to stimuli such as IL-1 and TNF-α, thus permitting the coordinate regulation of neutrophil and vascular adhesion molecules during inflammatory events (Fig. 14.2).

NEUTROPHIL DIAPEDESIS AND TRANSMIGRATION

Neutrophils exit the circulation either between or directly through endothelial cells to arrive at sites of inflammation (24,25) (Fig. 14.3). Receptors involved in this process include platelet–endothelial cell adhesion molecule-1 (PECAM-1), an Ig superfamily member found at endothelial cell junctions. Antibody blockade of endothelial PECAM-1 inhibits transendothelial migration *in vitro* (26–28). PECAM-1 is also expressed on neutrophils themselves, and homotypic PECAM-1/PECAM-1 interactions between neutrophils and endothelial cells may play a role in transmigration. Another potential endothelial cell ligand for neutrophil PECAM-1 is the integrin $\alpha_V\beta_3$, although a role for PECAM-1–$\alpha_V\beta_3$ interactions during transmigration remains to be confirmed (24,27,28). Integrin-associated protein (IAP, CD47), expressed on both neutrophils and endothelial cells, also participates in neutrophil transmigration (29,30). Although IAP has been shown to control the rate of neutrophil transmigration, its presence may not be absolutely required for transmigration to occur (30).

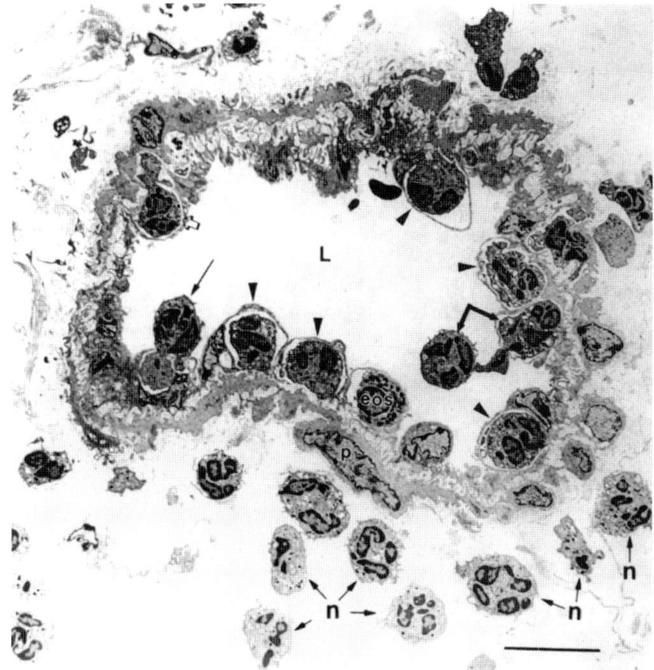

Figure 14.3. Neutrophil adhesion and transmigration through the vascular endothelium. Electron micrograph of a large guinea pig venule 1 hour after intradermal injection of formyl-methionyl-leucyl-phenylalanine. Neutrophils at various stages of transmigration can be seen, including a neutrophil projecting into an endothelial cell (*long arrow*); a pair of neutrophils, including one penetrating the endothelium and a second in the vessel lumen (L) adhering directly to the first (*double arrow*); several neutrophils that have penetrated the endothelium but not the underlying pericytes (p) (*arrowheads*); a neutrophil under the endothelium that is in the process of penetrating a pericyte (*open arrow*); and several neutrophils that have completely exited the vessel and are in the surrounding tissue (n). eos, eosinophil. [From Feng D, Nagy JA, Pyne K, et al. Neutrophils emigrate from venules by a transendothelial cell pathway in response to FMLP. *J Exp Med* 1998;187(6):903–915, with permission.]

ADHESION MOLECULES AND DISEASE

In leukocyte adhesion deficiency-I (LAD-I), patients lack CD18 and, therefore, all β_2 integrins; their neutrophils can neither tightly adhere to endothelium nor exit the circulation in response to infection. LAD-I patients have recurrent skin and mucosal infections, with most patients dying before the age of 10 (31). Another class of patients lacks expression of sLe^x ligands important for selectin binding (32). These LAD-II patients have decreased neutrophil motility *in vitro*, neutrophilia, and recurrent bacterial infections (Table 14.2).

Phagocytosis

FC AND COMPLEMENT RECEPTORS

Microbes opsonized by IgG or complement are engulfed by neutrophils via Fc and CD11b/CD18 receptors, respectively. A study by Caron and Hall suggests that Fc and CD11b/CD18 receptors may modulate distinct aspects of phagocytosis via discrete signaling pathways (33) (Fig. 14.1). Nonetheless, cross-linking of either CD11b/CD18 or Fc receptors results in cocapping both molecules on the neutrophil surface, suggesting that each class of receptors has the capacity to involve the other in signaling responses (34). Neutrophils constitutively express the low-affinity immune globulin receptors FcγRII and RIII and can be induced to express high-affinity FcγRI by incubation with interferon-γ (IFN-γ) (35) (Table 14.3). Extracellular cross-linking of FcγRII triggers protein tyrosine kinase activity of the cytoplasmic tail, leading to autophosphorylation of the FcγRII ITAM (*i*mmunoreceptor *t*yrosine-based *a*ctivation *m*otif) and subsequent signaling for phagocytosis (36).

FcγRIII is attached to the membrane via a lipid anchor and has neither a transmembrane segment nor a cytoplasmic tail. Nevertheless, cross-linking FcγRIII enhances FcγRII-mediated phagocytosis by increasing actin filament assembly and stimulating production of oxidants, which augment the avidity and efficiency of FcγRII (37–39). In an *in vitro* study, FcγRIII was

TABLE 14.2. Heritable Disorders of Neutrophils

Disorder	Defect	Inheritance	Clinical Presentation	Therapy	Typical Prognosis
Neutropenia					
Severe congenital neutropenia (Kostmann's syndrome)	Maturation arrest ($<0.5 \times 10^9$ PMN/L)	AR	Bacterial infections (omphalitis, abscesses, gingivitis, UTIs)	rhG-CSF	Improved with treatment
Adhesion deficiency					
LAD-I	Absent or abnormal CD18; defects of PMN/eosinophil adhesion	AR	Leukocytosis; recurrent infections (skin, mucous membranes, gastrointestinal tract)	Marrow transplant	Fair to poor, on degree of defect
LAD-II	Absent sialyl Lewis X	AR	Neutrophilia; infection; retardation, short stature	—	Poor
Granule disorders					
Chediak-Higashi syndrome	Abnormal and giant granules	AR	Albinism, infection	Marrow transplant	Poor
Specific granule deficientcy	Abnormal/reduced specific and azurophilic granules	AR?	Infection of skin, mucous membranes, lungs	Antibiotics	Fair to good
Oxidase defects					
Chronic granulomatous disease	Oxidase component deficiencies	X-linked and AR	Early childhood infections of skin, mucous membranes	Interferon-γ	Improved with treatment

AR, autosomal recessive; LAD, leukocyte adhesion deficiency; PMN, polymorphonuclear leukocyte; rhG-CSF, recombinant human granulocyte colony-stimulating factor; UTI, urinary tract infection.

TABLE 14.3. Neutrophil Immunoglobulin G (IgG) Receptors

Receptor	Neutrophil Expression	Affinity for IgG	Association with Cell Membrane
FcγRI (CD64)	Not usually present; expression induced by interferon-γ	Binds monomeric IgG with high affinity.	Transmembrane receptor; associates with γ subunit, which contains an ITAM
FcγRIIa (CD32)	Constitutively present	Low-affinity receptor; binds IgG immune complexes. Polymorphism at amino acid position 131 (H vs. R) determines binding to IgG2 opsonized particles (131-His efficiently interacts with IgG2; 131-Arg does not).	Transmembrane, monomeric receptor; cytoplasmic portion contains an ITAM
FcγRIIIb (CD16)	Constitutively present; can be shed during neutrophil activation	Low-affinity receptor; binds IgG immune complexes. Polymorphisms at neutrophil antigens (NA1/NA2) determines binding to IgG subclasses; NA1 cross-linking potentiates FcγRIIa-mediated phagocytosis.	Glycosylphosphatidylinositol linked; not associated with an ITAM

ITAM, immunoreceptor tyrosine kinase-based activation motif.

found to specifically mediate tethering of neutrophils to surfaces coated with immune complexes. CD11b/CD18 was not required for initial neutrophil contact with immune complexes but enhanced firm adhesion to immune complexes under shear rates up to 30 times the physiologic level (40). In another study, FcγRIII was shown to be necessary for neutrophil responses to immune complexes but not absolutely required for bacterial phagocytosis and killing (41). Thus, suppression of FcγRIII signaling represents a potential strategy to reduce undesirable neutrophil function in RA (where immune complexes are primarily responsible for complement generation), while leaving innate immunity intact.

Neutrophil Granules: Content, Function, and Transport

GRANULE DEVELOPMENT AND VARIETY

The earliest (primary) neutrophil granules appear at the promyelocyte stage; they contain myeloperoxidase (MPO) and are called *azurophilic* due to their affinity for azure dye. Later in neutrophil maturation, specific (secondary) granules appear, containing, among other proteins, collagenase, lactoferrin, and gelatinase. Gelatinase (tertiary) granules resemble specific granules but have higher concentrations of gelatinase. At maturity, neutrophils develop highly mobilizable secretory vesicles with cytochrome b_{558} (cyt b_{558}) (see below) and adhesion molecules (including CD11b/18) on their vacuolar membrane surface. Neutrophil stimulation causes extracellular granule secretion in the following order: secretory, gelatinase, specific, and azurophilic (42) (Table 14.4).

GRANULE CONTENT AND HOST DEFENSE

Neutrophil granule enzymes are the cornerstone of innate immunity in host defense. In addition to granule fusion with the plasma membrane, neutrophil stimulation allows fusion of specific and azurophilic granules with the phagocytic vacuole. These fusion events allow for the production of oxygen metabolites within the phagocytic vacuole (see below), as well as the intravacuolar release of a range of cationic proteinases that break down negatively charged bacterial surfaces (Table 14.4).

TABLE 14.4. Neutrophil Granules

Granule	Azurophilic Granules	Specific Granules	Gelatinase Granules	Secretory Vesicles
Relative size	●	●	●	●
Membrane-associated components	CD63, CD68	CD66, CD67 FMLP receptor CD11b/CD18 Cytochrome b_{558} Fibronectin receptor TNF-α receptor	FMLP receptor CD11b/CD18 Deacylating enzyme	FMLP receptor CD11b/CD18 Cytochrome b_{558} Alkaline phosphatase Uroplasminogen activator CD10, CD13, CD16, CD45 CR1 Decay accelerating factor
Cytosolic components	Myeloperoxidase Glucuronidase Elastase Lysozyme Proteinase 3 α_1-Antitrypsin Defensins Cathepsin BPI	Gelatinase Collagenase Lactoferrin β_2 microglobulin	Gelatinase Acetyltransferase	Plasma proteins

BPI, bactericidal/permeability-increasing protein; FMLP, formyl-methionyl-leucyl-phenylalanine; TNF, tumor necrosis factor.

Bactericidal/permeability-increasing protein (BPI) is cytotoxic to many gram-negative bacteria at nanomolar concentrations. One end of the protein binds to lipopolysaccharide, and the other mediates bacterial attachment and phagocytosis (43). Binding of BPI to the outer membrane of gram-negative bacteria increases membrane permeability and enhances bacterial killing. The *defensins* are major components of the azurophilic granules and render target cell membranes more permeable (44). The defensins act synergistically with BPI against gram-negative bacteria, probably by altering the quality of BPI binding or by increasing signaling (45).

Proteinase 3 (PR3) is found both in azurophilic and secretory granules. Membrane-associated PR3 is bioactive and insensitive to α-1 proteinase inhibitor. Although the precise role of PR3 in neutrophil function remains to be elucidated, the presence of anti-PR3 antibodies (cANCA) is a marker for Wegener's granulomatosis.

Elastase is another potent serine protease, mostly known for its destructive potential in patients with α-1 proteinase inhibitor deficiency. However, its physiologic role in host defense has been demonstrated. Elastase degrades an outer membrane protein that is highly conserved among gram-negative bacteria (46). The possible role of this serine protease in inflammation is discussed below.

Secretory phospholipase A_2 (sPLA_2) is a neutrophil granule protein that has very potent bactericidal activity against *Streptococcus aureus*. sPLA_2 synergizes with BPI for intracellular bacterial killing (47). The *cathelicidins*, found in the highly mobilizable specific granules, play an important role in extracellular killing upon their release into inflammatory fluids. Like PLA_2, they synergize with BPI in bacterial phospholipid hydrolysis (45).

Metalloproteinases are zinc-requiring enzymes that are released in inactive forms and include collagenases, gelatinases, and others. They may be required for the migration of neutrophils through basement membranes (42). Enzyme function depends on hypochlorous acid (HOCl)-mediated oxidation; neutrophils from patients with chronic granulomatous disease (CGD) cannot activate collagenase (48). Gelatinase degrades denatured collagen, as well as type IV and V collagen (49). Activation of pro-gelatinase occurs by both oxidative and nonoxidative mechanisms (48). Gelatinase has been shown to truncate several chemokines, notably IL-8, rendering them more biologically active (50).

NEUTROPHILS AND SMALL MOLECULE MEDIATORS

Reactive Oxygen Intermediates

SUPEROXIDE ANIONS

NADPH Oxidase System. Neutrophils produce toxic metabolites from O_2^- in the defense against microorganisms. The enzyme that generates O_2^-, the reduced nicotinamide adenine dinucleotide phosphate (NADPH) oxidase, has multiple cytosolic and membrane-bound components that assemble only on cell activation, permitting regulation of a potentially autotoxic mechanism (Fig. 14.4). There are at least six components of the oxidase: $p47^{phox}$ (for *ph*agocyte *ox*idase), $p67^{phox}$, and $p40^{phox}$, found in the resting state as a cytosolic complex; Rac-2, a cytosolic ras-related protein; and $p22^{phox}$ and $gp91^{phox}$, membrane components that together comprise cyt b_{558}. Translocation of the cytoplasmic components to the membrane and their association with cyt b_{558} renders the complex functional, resulting in the transfer of electrons from NADPH to O_2 to create O_2^-:

$$2O_2 + NADPH \rightarrow 2O_2^- + NADP^+ + H^+$$

Cyt b_{558} is a flavohemoprotein localized predominantly in the membranes of specific granules and secretory vesicles. The flavin group is critical for electron transport to O_2 (51).

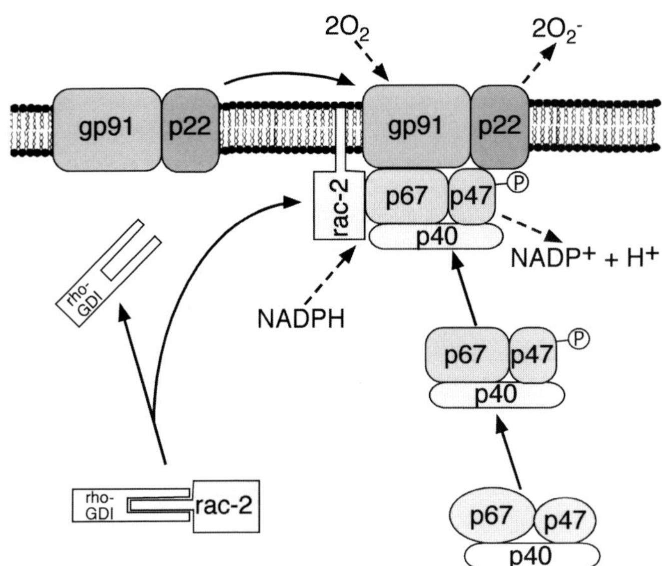

Figure 14.4. Reduced nicotinamide adenine dinucleotide phosphate (NADPH) oxidase system. Neutrophil oxidase components include $gp91^{phox}$ and $p22^{phox}$, membrane components making up the cyt b_{558}; the cytoplasmic components $p47^{phox}$, $p67^{phox}$, and $p40^{phox}$, typically existing complexed within the cytoplasm, and Rac-2, which exists in the cytoplasm complexed to its chaperone, rho-GDI. With appropriate stimulation, the cytosolic components translocate to the plasma membrane, the oxidase complex is assembled, and O_2^- is generated from O_2 and electrons contributed by NADPH. [Adapted from Burg N, Pillinger MH. The neutrophil: function and regulation in innate and humoral immunity. *Clin Immunol* 2001;99(1):7–17.]

$p47^{phox}$ is vital for oxidase function, as demonstrated both *in vitro* and in patients who lack the molecule (see below). Its main role appears to lie in the chaperoning of $p67^{phox}$ to the membrane. $p47^{phox}$ phosphorylation is required for its translocation to the plasma membrane and subsequent O_2^- production (52). $p67^{phox}$ is phosphorylated by PKC and remains complexed with $p47^{phox}$ after phosphorylation (53). $p67^{phox}$ has an activation domain that is critical for NADPH oxidase function and may regulate electron transfer from NADPH to O_2 within cyt b_{558} (54).

Rac-2 also plays a critical role in the activation of the NADPH oxidase. Activation-dependent GTP binding on Rac-2 frees it from its complex with rho-GDI and permits its interaction with $p67^{phox}$, as well as its translocation from cytosol to plasma membrane (55,56). Rac-2's interaction with the N-terminal region of $p67^{phox}$ is required for oxidase function (54–56). In contrast, Rac-2 translocation per se has not been correlated with oxidase activity (57).

Although much is known about activation of the NADPH oxidase, relatively little is known about the way it is deactivated. Clearly, deactivation of this enzyme is an important step in the resolution of inflammation. An ubiquitous serine-threonine kinase CK2 has been shown to phosphorylate $p47^{phox}$, inhibiting its translocation to the membrane. In one study, this phosphorylation was enhanced by arachidonate, probably by inducing conformational changes in $p47^{phox}$, rather than enhancing CK2 activity (58).

Chronic Granulomatous Disease. Genetic defects in $p47^{phox}$, $p67^{phox}$, $p22^{phox}$, and $gp91^{phox}$ are the cause of CGD, a rare disease with an incidence of approximately 1 in 200,000 (59) (Table 14.2). The majority of cases are secondary to genetic deficiencies in $gp91^{phox}$. CGD neutrophils can migrate to and phagocytose bacteria but are deficient in bacterial killing. As a result, patients develop recurrent infections characterized by the pres-

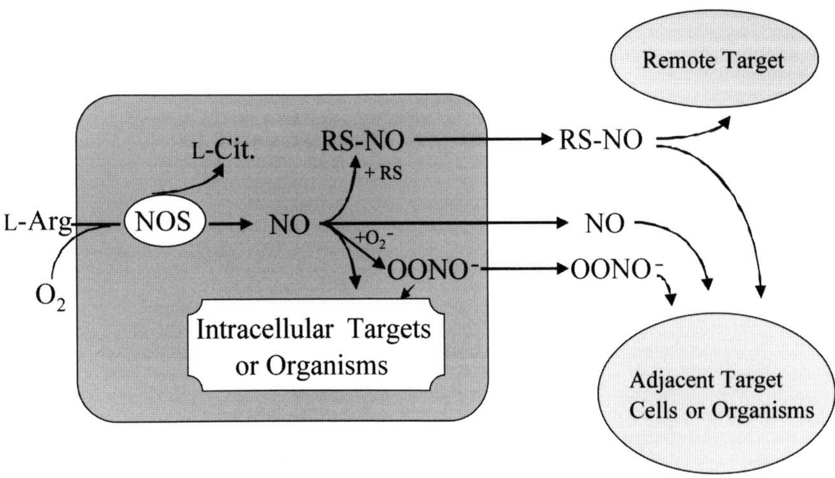

Figure 14.5. Nitric oxide, produced from L-arginine (L-Arg) by nitric oxide synthase (NOS), is a diffusible, highly reactive free radical that can act on both intracellular and extracellular targets. The biologic properties of NO vary with the predominant reaction product in the microenvironment. The reaction with free thiols leads to the formation of *S*-nitrosothiol compounds (RS-NO), which are significantly more stable and retain NO-like vasodilating properties but are less cytotoxic. At sites of inflammation, the reaction of NO with superoxide anion yields peroxynitrite ($OONO^-$), a highly toxic-free radical.

ence of suppurative lymph nodes and granulomas. Untreated, CGD is often fatal, but the use of prophylactic antibiotics and IFN-γ has reduced the frequency of serious infections in CGD patients (60).

NITRIC OXIDE PRODUCTION AND ACTION

Nitric oxide (NO) is synthesized via L-arginine oxidation by a family of three NO synthases (NOS) (61–66). NOS isoforms are typically either calcium dependent and constitutively expressed (neuronal ncNOS, or NOS-1; endothelial ecNOS, or NOS-3) or calcium independent and inducible (iNOS, or NOS-2). NO, a gaseous free radical, is labile (half-life less than 15 seconds) and in the presence of oxygen is rapidly metabolized to nitrate and nitrite (67,68). The chemistry of NO, however, involves interrelated redox forms. The most important reactions are believed to be those with oxygen, with transitional metal ions, and with free thiols (68) (Fig. 14.5). Examples of NO-target interactions include (a) binding of NO to the heme group of soluble guanylate cyclase, leading to cyclase activation and cyclic guanosine monophosphate (cGMP) generation (69–71), (b) reaction of NO with superoxide anion to yield the toxic hydroxyl radical peroxynitrite (72), and (c) reaction of nitric oxide with free thiols to form *S*-nitrosothiol compounds (73–76). *S*-nitrosothiol derivatives, formed both extra- and intracellularly, are significantly more stable than NO and retain NO-like properties (73,74,76,77).

NO production by leukocytes serves as a first-line defense against invading microbial organisms, including parasites, bacteria, and viruses (78–80). However, the cytotoxic effects of NO can also promote tissue injury in a variety of rheumatic diseases, including RA (71,81–84). There is contention over whether human neutrophils produce physiologically significant levels of NO during inflammatory reactions (85–87). NO synthesis by human neutrophils has been detected by functional NO activity by stimulus-induced elevations of cGMP and by adenosine diphosphate (ADP) ribosylation of proteins (88–90). Moreover, human blood neutrophils stimulated *in vitro* with monocyte-derived cytokines and neutrophils from inflamed exudates are reported to express iNOS (91–93). In experiments from our own laboratory, we could not detect significant increases in total nitrate/nitrite production in response to the bacterial peptide FMLP stimulation of human neutrophils, whereas a significant NO-dependent (i.e., prevented by specific NO inhibitors) increase in cGMP levels and ADP ribosylation of actin was observed (94,95).

Although there is general agreement that synthesis of NO by human neutrophils *in vitro* is limited, compared to other cell types exposed to comparable stimuli, it is nonetheless clear that NO exerts important regulatory effects on neutrophil functions. There is considerable evidence that NO acts as an endogenous mediator of the chemotactic response of neutrophils. NOS inhibitors, such as *N*-monomethyl-arginine, inhibit neutrophil chemotaxis induced by FMLP (96). It is likely that NO induces chemotaxis through the synthesis of cGMP, because inhibition of guanylate cyclase activity also inhibits neutrophil chemotaxis. Although experiments indicate that NO produced by activated neutrophils can promote cell migration, there is evidence that NO acts to inhibit other neutrophil functions, such as adherence and superoxide anion production. Moreover, the addition of exogenous NO donors results in the inhibition of neutrophil adhesion to endothelial cells induced by lipopolysaccharide or TNF-α (97,98).

Although excessive NO production is generally associated with tissue injury, it is important to note that NO constitutively produced by endothelium is believed to play a protective role in the microvasculature (71,76,99). This protection is afforded by NO's capacity to inhibit platelet and neutrophil adhesion to endothelial lining cells, as well as to inhibit leukocyte superoxide anion production (71,99–102). It has been postulated that the ability of NO to inhibit neutrophil adhesion to the endothelium results from its ability to inactivate superoxide anions (103). NO added exogenously can also directly inhibit neutrophil superoxide generation. This effect is reported to be due to direct inhibition of the NADPH oxidase occurring before the assembly of the activated complex (100,104). We have demonstrated that NO promotes the ADP ribosylation of G-actin in human neutrophils and inhibits actin polymerization in neutrophils, chondrocytes, and endothelial cell chondrocytes (95,105–107). ADP ribosylation may be an important mechanism by which NO regulates the state of actin polymerization, and thereby cell adhesion, signaling from the extracellular matrix, migration, and phagocytosis (95,106,107).

MYELOPEROXIDASE REGULATES BOTH THE OXIDASE AND NITRIC OXIDE SYNTHASE SYSTEMS

O_2^-, the immediate product of NADPH oxidase activity, is rapidly converted to hydrogen peroxide (H_2O_2) by the enzyme superoxide dismutase. The presence of bacterial catalase can inactivate H_2O_2 via reduction to O_2 and water. However, in the presence of neutrophil MPO, H_2O_2 undergoes conversion to HOCl, the most bactericidal of all neutrophil oxidants (108). HOCl can oxidize amino acids, nucleotides, and hemoproteins and inactivates α-1 antiproteinase, the major circulating inhibitor of serine proteinases (109).

Although NO donors reduce the production of superoxide anion by neutrophils, as noted above, new evidence indicates that HOCl can also oxidize nitrite to produce the active oxidant nitryl chloride, which has toxic bactericidal actions (110). Because iNOS is colocalized with MPO in neutrophil primary granules, NO formation may regulate the bactericidal system of neutrophils (111).

Lipid Mediators of Inflammation

PHOSPHOLIPASES AND ARACHIDONIC ACID GENERATION

Stimulated neutrophils metabolize arachidonic acid to a variety of eicosanoid end products, including thromboxanes, prostaglandins, leukotrienes, and lipoxins. The activation process begins with the liberation of arachidonate from the sn-2 position of membrane phospholipids through activation of PLA_2. Two main classes of PLA_2 have been cloned: $sPLA_2$ (14–18 kd) and cytosolic PLA_2 ($cPLA_2$) (31–110 kd) (112). In addition to catalytic functions, sPLAs act through cell-surface receptors on neutrophils and other cells as autocrine or paracrine amplifiers of inflammation. There is considerable interest in a particular subgroup, group II $sPLA_2$, because its levels are increased in serum and inflammatory exudates in conditions such as septic shock and RA (112).

LEUKOTRIENES

Neutrophils can produce significant amounts of LTB_4 as well as secrete its precursor, LTA_4. These enzyme reactions are catalyzed by 5-lipoxygenase (5-LO), which converts arachidonic acid into 5-HETE, an intermediate rapidly converted to LTA_4. The 5-LO of PMN appears unique among lipoxygenases because, on cell activation, it translocates and interacts with a membrane-associated protein (18 kd) termed *5-LO–activating protein* (FLAP). 5-LO translocation and association with FLAP results in the full activity of the "5-LO complex" (113). Although several enzymatic pathways can process LTA_4, neutrophils possess a single LTA_4 convertase that exclusively converts LTA_4 to LTB_4. LTB_4 is a neutrophil autocoid; namely, it is both released from and acts on the neutrophil. At nanomolar concentrations, LTB_4 is a potent chemoattractant for other neutrophils, as well as for eosinophils, monocytes, and fibroblasts (114,115). At higher concentrations, LTB_4 provokes degranulation and superoxide anion generation. LTB_4 also promotes the synthesis of IL-5, IL-6, and IL-8 and enhances IgE synthesis in B cells (116,117). The normal fate of the neutrophil is to undergo apoptosis and then phagocytosis by macrophages. Studies suggest a critical role for LTB_4 in mediating neutrophil survival *in vitro* (118). Both corticosteroids and cytokines, such as TNF-α and IL-8, have been reported to promote neutrophil survival by up-regulating endogenous synthesis of LTB_4. An LTB_4 antagonist, SB201146, promotes neutrophil apoptosis *in vitro* and blocks the survival-enhancing effects of steroids (119).

LIPOXINS

Neutrophils also contribute to the production of a novel class of lipoxygenase products, the lipoxins (LX) (120). LX are generated by two main routes, each requiring lipoxygenase–lipoxygenase (LO-LO) interactions of neutrophils with other cells (Fig. 14.6). The first involves initial lipoxygenation of arachidonic acid by epithelial cell 15-LO, followed by the action of neutrophil 5-LO. This route is particularly relevant when PMNs interact with mucosal surfaces, as may occur in asthma. A second route, which occurs predominantly within the vasculature, involves the 5-LO–mediated release of LTA_4 from neutrophils and the subsequent conversion of this compound to LX by platelets. Human platelets alone do not generate LX but become an important source as a result of their interactions with neutrophils (121). In contrast to the effects of LTB_4, LXs such as LXA_4 inhibit neutrophil chemotaxis and adhesion. *In vivo* temporal analyses of these eicosanoids in experimental exudates show early coordinate appearance of leukotrienes and prostaglandins with PMN recruitment (122). These results indicate that first-phase eicosanoids promote a shift to antiinflammatory lipids: functionally distinct lipid-mediator profiles switch during acute exudate formation to reprogram the exudate PMNs to resolve inflammation (122).

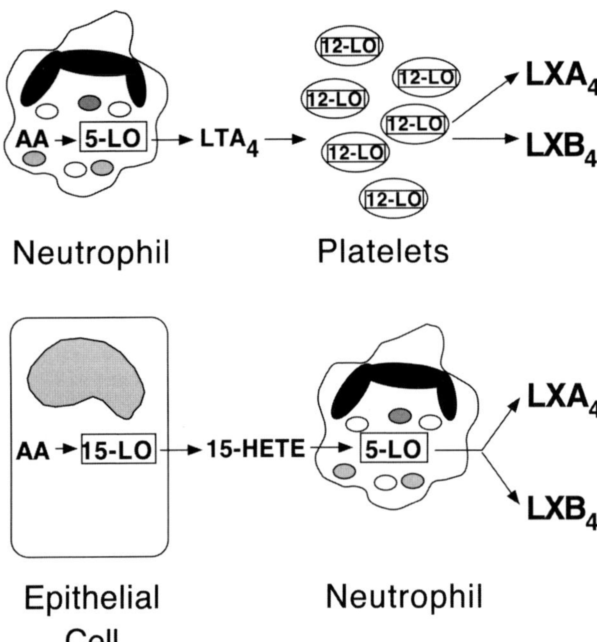

Figure 14.6. Lipoxin formation requires interaction of neutrophils with either platelets or epithelial cells. **Top:** Neutrophil 5-lipoxygenase (5-LO) converts arachidonic acid (AA) to leukotriene A_4 (LTA_4); 12-LO in platelets then converts LTA_4 into the antiinflammatory lipoxins LXA_4 and LXB_4. **Bottom:** Epithelial cell 15-LO converts AA into 15-hydroxyeicosatetraenoic acid (15-HETE); neutrophil 5-LO then converts 15-HETE into LXA_4 and LXB_4.

CYCLOOXYGENASE PRODUCTS

In addition to lipoxygenase products, neutrophils also produce eicosanoids derived from the cyclooxygenase (COX) pathway, such as thromboxane A_2 and E series prostaglandins. Although resting neutrophils exhibit little COX activity, stimulation with proinflammatory cytokines causes the up-regulation of COX-2. Although COX-2–derived prostanoids are traditionally considered proinflammatory, the effects of prostaglandin Es (PGEs) on neutrophil function are inhibitory, as shown in classic studies by Weissmann and Zurier (123,124).

PGE_2, as well as specific EP2- and IP-receptor agonists, inhibit a variety of FMLP-induced neutrophil activities, including calcium translocation, LTB_4 release, superoxide anion generation, and homotypic aggregation (124–126). In contrast, $PGF_{2\alpha}$, EP1-, and EP3-receptor agonists have no inhibitory activity. The mechanisms by which PGEs inhibit neutrophil activation are unclear. As noted earlier, neutrophil Erk is activated in response to chemoattractants, and this activation is critical for homotypic adhesion (8). Erk activation in neutrophils can be inhibited by PGE, indicating a mechanism by which PGE may act to modulate neutrophil activation (127).

NEUTROPHILS IN RHEUMATOID ARTHRITIS

The past decade has seen an emphasis on the cellular and, to a lesser extent, the humoral immune system in RA. Nonetheless, research in humans and animals suggests an important role for the neutrophil in both tissue damage and the stimulation of acquired immunity in RA. Wipke and Allen, for example, have demonstrated an essential role for neutrophils in the initiation and progression of a murine model of RA (128).

Neutrophils and Cartilage Destruction

RA can be considered a two-compartment disease. Rheumatoid synovium (pannus) constitutes the first of the two compartments. Pannus is characterized histologically by hyperplasia of synovial fibroblasts and the infiltration of large numbers of B and T cells and macrophages, as well as dendritic cells (129). Neutrophils are conspicuously underrepresented in synovium, suggesting that they play a small role in synovial responses. However, a number of studies have examined the localization of neutrophils in synovium, and most of these have concluded that the few neutrophils present are concentrated at the cartilage-pannus border and, therefore, are positioned to have effects on cartilage greater than their numbers (130–133). Because neutrophils have been shown to degrade cartilage proteoglycan at a rate up to 28 times that of either synovial fibroblasts or macrophages, their limited numbers may nonetheless produce significant destruction (134).

Neutrophils present in synovium are likely to have direct effects on the ability of other pannus cells to cause joint destruction or stimulate autoimmunity. For example, McCurdy et al. have shown that the presence of stimulated but not unstimulated neutrophils enhanced by up to fivefold the ability of synovial fibroblasts to adhere to cartilage, a necessary step in the degradation of cartilage by these cells (135). Supporting a role for neutrophil–fibroblast interactions, Hashida et al. have demonstrated in a rat model that a negatively charged, 80-kd protein elicited from neutrophils enhances IL-l–induced collagenase and prostaglandin production by synovial fibroblasts, again suggesting that the presence of even small numbers of neutrophils in rheumatoid synovium may enhance the chondrodestructive capacities of their neighboring cells (136). Although the topographic localization of pannus around the joint may lead to the so-called marginal erosion typical of RA, it may not entirely account for the fact that, in RA, the contacting cartilage surfaces of the apposed bones also undergo symmetric destruction and joint space narrowing.

The second compartment of RA is the synovial fluid itself. In contrast to the synovium, neutrophils are by far the most populous leukocyte in rheumatoid synovial fluid, typically comprising more than 90% of the present cells. The rate of neutrophil turnover in the joint is truly astonishing—as many as one billion cells per day in a 30 cc effusion—and the life of rheumatoid synovial neutrophils is prolonged, in part due to the presence of antiapoptotic factors in rheumatoid synovial fluid (137–139). As a result, as many as 100,000 neutrophils per cc may be found in the rheumatoid joint. These neutrophils are susceptible to activation, owing to the presence of both cytokines and immune complexes (including rheumatoid factor) in the synovial fluid (140). Activation may lead to degranulation, which occurs not into lysosomes, as in the case of bacterial phagocytosis, but into the extracellular space. Thus, proteases, toxic oxygen radicals, and other granule antibacterial systems are released directly into the synovial fluid. Although high-molecular-weight hyaluronic acid in synovial fluid has the capacity to inhibit neutrophil inflammatory reactions, superoxide anions and other oxygen metabolites produced by neutrophils can degrade hyaluronic acid, presumably negating the antiinflammatory effect (141–143).

Neutrophils can potentially degrade or damage cartilage through the release of multiple enzymes, including neutrophil collagenase (MMP-8), gelatinase B (MMP-9), stromelysin (MMP-3), and elastase (144–148). Of these, elastase may be primarily responsible for cartilage damage, whereas cleavage of type II collagen by gelatinase B may generate antigenic peptides capable of perpetuating an autoimmune process (149,150). Interestingly, stimulated neutrophils, as well as neutrophil elastase, have the capacity to activate latent stomelysin-1 intrinsic to the cartilage, and so may indirectly as well as directly effect cartilage degradation (151) (Fig. 14.7).

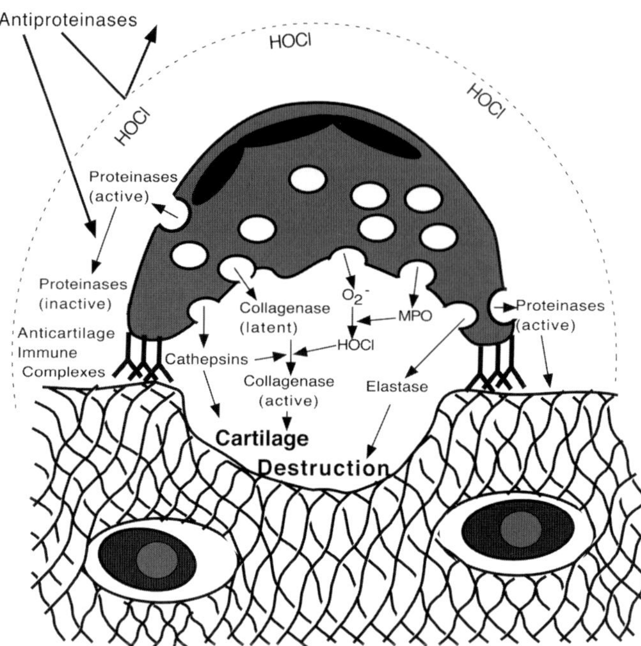

Figure 14.7. Neutrophil adherence and destruction of cartilage—a model. According to this model, adherence of neutrophils to cartilage, mediated in part by immune complexes embedded in or directed against cartilage, establishes a protective space resistant to the actions of antiproteinases, in which multiple neutrophil granule products, as well as superoxide anions, can interact, resulting in activation of multiple chondrodestructive enzymes. (Adapted from Pillinger MH, Abramson SB. The neutrophil in rheumatoid arthritis. *Rheum Dis Clin North Am* 1995;21:691–714.)

Theoretical and practical concerns raise questions, however, about the ability of neutrophil contents, expressed directly into the synovial fluid, to induce joint destruction. Optimal activation of neutrophil proteases requires coordinated interaction between the proteinases and oxygen metabolites. For example, neutrophil collagenase is released in a latent form and requires interaction with either cathepsin G, stromelysin, or MPO-generated HOCl for activation. Whether such activation is favored in a situation in which each constituent is freely diffusible is unclear (48,152–156). Similarly, stromelysin is secreted as an inactive zymogen and must undergo activation by neutrophil elastase (157,158). Moreover, synovial fluid contains antiproteinases—including α-1 antiproteinases—capable of inactivating neutrophil enzymes. Although HOCl has the capacity to inhibit these antiproteinases, its rapid diffusion, as well as the fact that synovial fluid possesses MPO-inhibiting factors, suggest that free-floating synovial neutrophils may have less chondrodestructive potential than their biology would indicate (159). On the other hand, several studies indicate that at least some form of neutrophil proteinases may survive the antiproteinases of the joint space. For example, Moore et al. have demonstrated that neutrophil elastase in the synovial joint may form complexes with α_2 macroglobulin, and that these complexes may maintain their proteolytic activity even in the presence of antiproteinases (160). Similarly, elastase complexed to the cartilage surface appears to be resistant to antiproteinases (161).

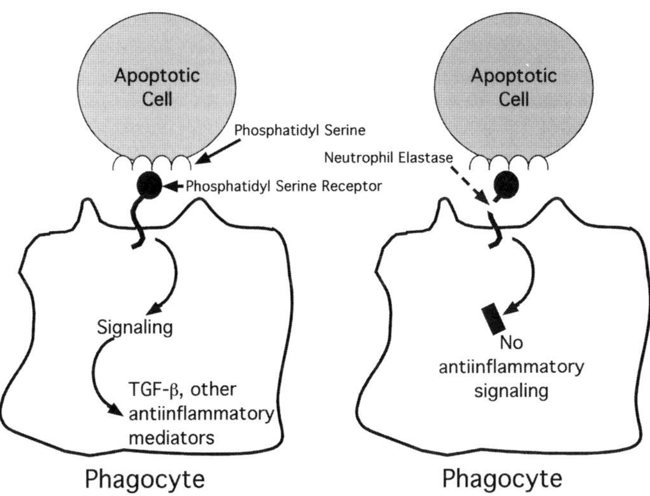

Figure 14.8. Neutrophil elastase and effects on phosphatidyl serine receptor activation. **Left:** Phosphatidyl serine on an apoptotic cell interacts with a phosphatidyl serine receptor on a phagocyte, initiating an antiinflammatory program, including production of transforming growth factor (TGF-β). **Right:** The presence of neutrophil elastase results in cleavage of the phosphatidyl serine receptor and disruption of the antiinflammatory program. (Adapted from Henson PM, Bratton DL, Fadok VA. The phosphatidyl serine receptor: a crucial molecular switch? *Nat Rev Mol Cell Biol* 2001;2:627–633.)

In addition, Weiss has proposed a mechanism by which neutrophils may circumvent synovial fluid defenses (162) (Fig. 14.8). Neutrophils adherent to cartilage may attempt to engulf the cartilage surface and, in so doing, may discharge their contents into the subjacent space (frustrated phagocytosis). Because this space is sealed by the neutrophil membrane itself, it is protected from synovial fluid antiproteinases and other synovial factors. Moreover, the limited space circumscribed by the neutrophil–cartilage interaction provides a reaction crucible in which neutrophil enzymes and oxygen products can interact to maximum activation and in which the activated enzymes are directly apposed to their cartilage targets (163). Additionally, HOCl released into the synovial fluid may be effective as an antiproteinase shield under these circumstances, since the area for its diffusion is limited by the presence of the cartilage surface.

However, this model requires a mechanism by which neutrophils can migrate toward, and adhere to, cartilage. A gradient of IL-8 originating from chondrocytes (and in turn stimulated by neutrophil-derived oxidant stress) may serve to activate and draw neutrophils toward the cartilage surface, but Mitani et al. have demonstrated that the surface macromolecules of intact articular cartilage actually inhibit neutrophil adhesion (164–167). This resistance may be overcome by the neutrophils themselves, to the extent that neutrophil proteases can disrupt the outer cartilage layer and expose the type II collagen beneath. In the setting of a disrupted cartilage surface, the attraction and adherence of neutrophils may be further facilitated by the presence of immune complexes that are found embedded in the cartilage superficial layers. These complexes, which contain rheumatoid factor as well as anti–type II collagen antibodies, may activate complement and serve as de facto cartilage opsonins. Indeed, multiple studies both *in vitro* and in animal models have documented the ability of immune complexes to amplify neutrophil binding, cartilage destruction, or both. However, the interaction between neutrophils and Igs may not be entirely proinflammatory. Data indicate that exposure of human IgG to neutrophil HOCl results in a decreased ability of the IgG to fix complement or stimulate inflammation in rabbit knees, suggesting that neutrophils may demonstrate some antiinflammatory, or at least counterregulatory, activities.

Neutrophils and the Propagation of the Rheumatoid Inflammatory Response

In addition to their capacity to destroy cartilage, neutrophils may play an important role in RA pathogenesis by stimulating or propagating inflammation, immunity, and the development of rheumatoid pannus.

NEUTROPHILS AND CYTOKINE PRODUCTION

Although neutrophils have limited capacity for protein synthesis, their abundance in synovial fluid suggests that any synthesized proteins reaching the extracellular space can achieve potentially significant concentrations. Among the proteins produced by neutrophils are a wide variety of proinflammatory cytokines, including IL-1, IL-12, TNF-α, TNF-β, and Gro-α (87). Hatano et al. have demonstrated that synovial fluid neutrophils in RA secrete the C-C chemokine MIP-1α in a manner concordant with disease activity. Cytokines secreted by neutrophils variously have the capacity to attract additional neutrophils and to stimulate endothelial adhesiveness and synoviocyte activation in the synovial lesion. Rheumatoid, but not nonrheumatoid, neutrophils have also been shown to express oncostatin M, a cytokine that affects a range of cells, including synovial fibroblasts, chondrocytes, and osteoblasts. Oncostatin M shows a variety of pro- and antiinflammatory effects, including stimulation of neutrophil chemotaxis, transcription of collagen, increased expression of COX-2, and inhibition of RANTES (regulated on activation, normal T cell–expressed and –secreted) release.

Yamashiro et al. have emphasized neutrophil heterogeneity and a possible role for specific classes of neutrophils in the modulation of adaptive immunity. In particular, they observed that neutrophils that have been primed by exposure to a 60-kd product of peripheral blood mononuclear cells before stimulation with TNF-α behave differently than cells stimulated with TNF-α alone. Both classes of neutrophils produced IL-1, MIP-1, TNF-α, and TNF-β, as well as the antiapoptotic protein A1, the cyclin-dependent kinase inhibitor $p21^{Waf1/Cip1}$, and the receptor tyrosine discoidin domain receptor. However, only the neutrophils that were first primed with the 60-kd peripheral blood mononuclear cell product before TNF-α stimulation produced significant amounts of monocyte chemoattractant protein-1 (MCP-1, also known as *CCL2*). MCP-1 is a CC-chemokine that has potent monocyte-chemotactic capacity both *in vitro* and *in vivo* and has been implicated as a critical factor in the recruitment of monocytes and lymphocytes in animal models of delayed-type hypersensitivity. Thus, the ability of neutrophils, under proper conditions of priming and stimulation, to elicit MCP-1 suggests one mechanism through which these cells may regulate the transition from innate to adaptive immunity. Perhaps relating to the need for additional signals for its production, MCP-1 production *in vivo* was associated with neutrophils from chronic, but not acute, inflammation.

Another possible role for neutrophils in RA relates to regulation of the vascular bed of the synovium. Studies by Koch et al. have emphasized the role of the vasculature as a necessary support for the influx of inflammatory cells and the hyperproliferation of synovium, and Lattun et al. have demonstrated the ability of an antibody to the vascular endothelial growth factor receptor FLT1 to block arthritic joint destruction. Kasama et al. have demonstrated that synovial fluid neutrophils produce vascular endothelial growth factor in amounts proportional to the level of RA disease activity and that the interaction of fibroblast-like synovial cells with activated neutrophils isolated from RA synovial fluid results in synergistic up-regulation of the production of vascular endothelial growth factor, as well as endothelial cell proliferation.

NEUTROPHIL GRANULE CONTENTS AND THE PROPAGATION OF PANNUS

The ability of neutrophil granule contents to stimulate the propagation of inflammation and synovitis was first appreciated by Weissmann et al. Injection of isolated neutrophil granules (lysosomes) into the joint space of rabbits resulted in the production of synovitis histologically indistinguishable from pannus. These experiments suggest that the contents of neutrophil granules may have a direct effect on pannus formation. Subsequent studies have confirmed that a wide range of neutrophil granule proteins have inflammatory or immune-modulating effects beyond their ability to destroy bacteria or connective tissue. MPO, for example, has been shown to perpetuate experimentally induced arthritis in rats via the up-regulation of cytokine production. This effect requires functional macrophages but can be reproduced by inactivated MPO, indicating that inactivated MPO serves a previously unrecognized, nonenzymatic function as an immunoregulatory molecule.

Another class of granule proteins with a wide range of effects are the defensins. Neutrophil defensins, which were first recognized for their ability to directly kill bacteria, have subsequently been shown to be chemotactic for resting and memory T cells, as well as immature, but not mature, dendritic cells. Defensins are also capable of enhancing phagocytosis by macrophages and of stimulating the production of IL-1 and TNF-α, while suppressing production of the antiinflammatory cytokine IL-10. Furthermore, defensins can stimulate the activation and degranulation of mast cells, a particularly interesting observation in light of a report by Lee et al. that strains of mice deficient in mast cells are resistant to the development of erosive inflammatory arthritis. Defensins may also interact with Toll-like receptors on T cells to coordinate and enhance acquired immune responses (168).

Proteinase 3 (PR3) is a neutral serine proteinase expressed by neutrophils and probably best known as the antigen target of the cytoplasmic antineutrophil cytoplasm response seen commonly in Wegener's granulomatosis. In contrast, the actual physiologic role of PR3 remains speculative. Coeshott et al. have demonstrated that co-incubation of a human monocytic cell line with activated neutrophils resulted in a two- to fivefold increase in the release of TNF-α and IL-1β from the former cells. This effect is unusual, because it does not depend on standard processing of cell membrane–associated TNF-α and IL-1β precursors by TNF-α–converting enzyme and IL-1–converting enzyme. Rather, the neutrophil effect was found to be dependent specifically on the capacity of neutrophils to discharge PR3 (169). Thus, PR3 may play an important role in RA via the cleavage and release of active cytokines from the surface of monocytic cells. Consistent with this hypothesis, Witko-Sarsat et al. have used population studies to demonstrate that the presence of a large proportion of neutrophils expressing PR3 on the cell surface, probably as a genetically determined phenotype, represents a risk factor for RA .

As noted above, neutrophil elastase is a matrix metalloproteinase that appears to play a critical role in cartilage degradation. However, it is likely that elastase may have other effects that relate directly to the propagation of inflammation and autoimmunity. For example, data suggest that elastase may regulate mannose-binding lectin (MBL). MBL is a transmembrane protein with an extracellular lectin, or carbohydrate binding, domain (170). MBL is an important part of the innate immune system by virtue of its ability to bind the surface of microbes via mannose and *N*-acetylglucosamine residues and subsequently destroy the microbes by recruiting the complement cascade via the action of MBL-associated serine proteinases (171). However, low levels of MBL result in immune disruption, and MBL mutations have been associated with both systemic lupus and disease severity in RA. The mechanism by which these mutations affects immunity is not clear. However, Butler et al. have demonstrated that, in contrast to normal MBL, the presence of several MBL mutations renders the lectins susceptible to degradation by neutrophil elastase. Neutrophil collagenase (MMP-8) can also degrade MBL. Thus, the combination of MBL mutations and neutrophil proteases may result in MBL deficiencies and abnormalities of innate immunity.

Another role of neutrophil elastase may be to cleave and inactivate phosphatidyl serine receptors on phagocytic cells (172). Cellular apoptosis results in redistribution of plasma membrane lipids and expression of phosphatidyl serine on the extracellular membrane leaflet. Fadok et al. have identified a phosphatidyl serine receptor on phagocytic cells, including macrophages, B cells, dendritic cells, and others (173). On interaction of apoptotic cells with phagocytes, engagement of the phosphatidyl serine receptor results in potent antiinflammatory and immunosuppressive effects, including the production of TGF-β, down-regulation of the production of TNF-α and other cytokines, reduction of leukocyte infiltration into inflamed areas, as well as decreased leukocyte trafficking into lymph nodes and down-regulation of antibody production (174). Exposure to PMN elastase results in cleavage of phosphatidyl serine receptors and blockade of the antiinflammatory–autoimmune response (172) (Fig. 14.8). If these effects occurred in the rheumatoid joint, neutrophil-elastase–mediated cleavage of the phosphatidyl serine receptors could stimulate inflammation and promote the aggregation of lymphocytes and antigen-presenting cells into structures resembling germinal centers (175).

The importance of neutrophil elastase in RA can be studied on the basis of whether enzyme inhibition ameliorates inflammation or joint destruction. A number of inhibitors of neutrophil elastase have been developed and several have been tested in animal models of arthritis (176). For example, Kakimoto et al. observed that the novel neutrophil elastase inhibitor ONO-5046 inhibited the incidence, severity and cartilage destruction of collagen-induced arthritis in both rat and mouse models. Similarly, Janusz and Durham demonstrated the ability of neutrophil elastase inhibitor MDL-101,146 to inhibit cartilage degradation in rat collagen–induced arthritis (177). Whether the benefits of elastase inhibition in animal models will translate into similar benefits in human RA remains to be determined.

NEUTROPHIL AND ANTIGEN PRESENTATION

A small but growing body of literature suggests that, under certain circumstances, neutrophils may serve as antigen-presenting cells. Exposure of neutrophils to GM-CSF, IFN-γ, or IL-3 results in surface expression of major histocompatibility complex (MHC) class II molecules (178,179). Subsequent studies demonstrated that neutrophils stimulated to express MHC class II can stimulate the proliferation of T cells in the presence of superantigen and present staphylococcus enterotoxin to peripheral T cells, leading to IL-2 induction and T-cell proliferation (180,181). Controversy exists as to whether MHC class II–expressing neutrophils are also able to present tetanus toxoid (180,181). Cross-linking of neutrophil MHC class II receptors by superantigen also results in neutrophil stimulation and induction of IL-8 production (182). Moreover, treatment of immediate precursors of end-stage neutrophils with a cocktail of cytokines drives these cells to acquire certain characteristics of dendritic cells and to present soluble antigen to T cells at least 10,000 times more efficiently than isolated monocytes (183). Taken together, these data suggest the possibility that neutrophils may serve in the propagation, not only of inflammation, but also of acquired autoimmunity.

The studies on antigen presentation by neutrophils must be interpreted with caution, since the experiments were conducted entirely *in vitro*. However, Iking-Konert et al. have demonstrated that neutrophils from patients with Wegener's granulomatosis acquire characteristics of antigen-presenting cells, including the expression of not only MHC class II, but also the dendritic cell costimulatory markers CD80 and CD86 (184). More pertinently, Cross et al. have examined the capacity of neutrophils from patients with RA to express MHC class II. Their data suggest that the expression of MHC class II by neutrophils may be regulated in a stepwise fashion. In particular, they observed that peripheral blood neutrophils from patients with RA expressed messenger RNA, but not protein, for MHC class II, whereas peripheral blood neutrophils from normal controls expressed neither messenger RNA nor protein for this surface molecule. Proceeding further, neutrophils from rheumatoid synovial fluid expressed both MHC class II message and protein (185).

In contrast to their apparent capacity to present antigen directly, neutrophils may also have the capacity to reduce T-cell stimulation by classic antigen-presenting cells. Taurine chloramine (TauCl) is a major product of the neutrophil MPO-halide system and is formed from the reaction of HOCl and taurine, the most abundant free amino acid in cytosol (186). Marcinkiewicz et al. have demonstrated that exposure of dendritic cells to TauCl resulted in down-regulation of MHC class II and the costimulatory molecule B7-2 and inhibition of inflammatory mediator (TNF-α, IL-6, IL-10, IL-12, PGE_2, NO) release and reactive oxygen species from dendritic cells. Exposure of $CD4^+$ T cells to dendritic cells pretreated with TauCl resulted in inhibition of T-cell production of IL-10 as a marker of T-cell activation (187). The balance of effects between the neutrophils' ability to stimulate or present antigen to T cells, and their ability to down-regulate T-cell responses, will clearly require further study and clarification.

NEUTROPHIL AND ANTIRHEUMATIC DRUGS

Many antirheumatic drugs have been used empirically, without a solid understanding of their mechanisms of action. Nonetheless, many of these agents have been shown, experimentally, to have direct or indirect effects on neutrophils. For example, a number of antiinflammatory medications have been shown to inhibit MPO *in vitro*. Dapsone both scavenges HOCl and causes accumulation of an inactive redox intermediate of MPO (188,189). Indomethacin, as well as other nonsteroidal antiinflammatory drugs, inhibit HOCl production *in vitro* by inhibiting the chlorinating activity of MPO (190).

Other medications in the rheumatologist's armamentarium may be antiinflammatory, at least in part, because of their negative effects on neutrophil adhesion molecules. Low concentrations of colchicine alter the distribution of E-selectin and higher concentrations inhibit L-selectin expression on neutrophils (191). Methotrexate augments adenosine release from fibroblasts, inhibiting neutrophil adhesion (192). Corticosteroids lower adhesion molecule expression on both endothelium and neutrophils (193,194). Salicylates also inhibit neutrophil adhesion, probably by blocking activation of CD11b/CD18 via inhibition of Erk (195).

Other antirheumatic agents that target specific aspects of the disease may also have both direct and indirect effects on neutrophils. Both IL-1 and TNF-α enhance neutrophil vascular adhesion and neutrophil trafficking via effects on cytokine production and endothelial stimulation (196,197). Direct effects of TNF-α on neutrophils include priming for stimulus-induced responses such as superoxide generation, cartilage destruction, and the production of cytokines such as IL-8 and LTB_4 (198). At higher concentration, TNF-α may directly stimulate neutrophils, particularly adherent neutrophils. Thus, it is possible that anti–TNF-α biologics, such as etanercept, infliximab, and adalimumab, act in part through effects on neutrophils. Nonetheless, a single study showed little or no difference in a variety of stimulated neutrophil functions tested *ex vivo* (phagocytosis, microbicidal activity, and toxic oxygen radical generation) in patients treated with etanercept for 6 months (199). Thus, systemic blockade of TNF-α may serve to reduce the stimulation of neutrophils *in vivo*, rather than intrinsically altering the neutrophils themselves. Consistent with this suggestion, Cornillie et al. have demonstrated that patients receiving infliximab experience decreases in peripheral blood neutrophil, but not lymphocyte or monocyte, populations (200).

CONCLUSION

The 1990s have seen notable advances in the understanding of basic neutrophil biology and in the role of neutrophils in RA. Not only are neutrophils capable of enzymatic and oxidative damage to cartilage, but they have the capacity to stimulate inflammation and suppress antiinflammatory signals. Moreover, neutrophils appear to play important and proactive roles in the propagation of pannus, and may even, under select circumstances, have the capacity to act as antigen-presenting cells. The next few years will surely see additional advances in the study of neutrophils, and possibly the development of neutrophil-selective antirheumatic therapies.

ACKNOWLEDGMENTS

The authors thank Ms. Madeline Rios for her editorial and technical support. We also thank the Arthritis Foundation, New York Chapter, and the American College of Rheumatology for their ongoing support of our research and educational efforts.

REFERENCES

1. Uzel G, Holland SM. White blood cell defects: molecular discoveries and clinical management. *Curr Allergy Asthma Rep* 2002;2(5):385.
2. Pillinger MH, Rosenthal PB, Cronstein BN. Polymorphonuclear cells. In: Tsokos GC, ed. *Current molecular medicine: principles of molecular rheumatology*. Totowa, NJ: Human Press Inc., 2000:243–257.
3. Pillinger MH, Abramson S. Neutrophils and eosinophils. In: Ruddy S, Harris ED, Jr., Sledge CB, eds. *Kelley's textbook of rheumatology*. Philadelphia: W.B. Saunders Co., 2001:195–209.
4. Bokoch GM. Chemoattractant signaling and leukocyte activation. *Blood* 1995;86:1649.
5. Zu Y, Qi LJ, Gilchrist A, et al. p38 mitogen-activated protein kinase activation is required for human neutrophil function triggered by TNF-alpha or FMLP stimulation. *J Immunol* 1998;160:1982.
6. Grinstein S, Furuya W. Chemoattractant-induced tyrosine phosphorylation and activation of microtubule-associated protein kinase in human neutrophils. *J Biol Chem* 1992;267:18122.
7. Torres M, Hall FL, O'Neill K. Stimulation of human neutrophils with formyl-methionyl-leucyl-phenylalanine induces tyrosine phosphorylation and activation of two distinct mitogen-activated protein-kinases. *J Immunol* 1993;150:1563.
8. Pillinger MH, Feoktistov AS, Capodici C, et al. Mitogen-activated protein kinase in neutrophils and enucleate neutrophil cytoplasts: evidence for regulation of cell–cell adhesion. *J Biol Chem* 1996;271(20):12049.
9. Reference deleted.
10. Worthen GS, Avdi N, Buhl AM, et al. FMLP activates Ras and Raf in human neutrophils. Potential role in activation of MAP kinase. *J Clin Invest* 1994;94(2):815.
11. Capodici C, Pillinger MH, Han G, et al. Integrin-dependent homotypic adhesion of neutrophils. Arachidonic acid activates Raf-1/Mek/Erk via a 5-lipoxygenase-dependent pathway. *J Clin Invest* 1998;102:165.
12. Hirsch E, Katanaev VL, Garlanda C, et al. Central role for G protein-coupled phosphoinositide 3-kinase gamma in inflammation. *Science* 2000;287:1049.

13. Li Z, Jiang H, Xie W, et al. Roles of PLC-beta2 and beta3 and PI3Kgamma in chemoattractant-mediated signal transduction. *Science* 2000;287:1046.
14. Sasaki T, Irie-Sasaki J, Jones RG, et al. Function of P13Kgamma in thymocyte development, T cell activation, and neutrophil migration. *Science* 2000;287: 1040.
15. Ahmed MU, Hazeki K, Hazeki O, et al. Cyclic AMP-increasing agents interfere with chemoattractant-induced respiratory burst in neutrophils as a result of the inhibition of phosphatidylinositol 3-kinase rather than receptor-operated Ca2+ influx. *J Biol Chem* 1995;270:23816.
16. Capodici C, Hanft S, Feoktistov M, et al. Phosphatidylinositol 3-kinase mediates chemoattractant-stimulated, CD11b/CD18-dependent cell-cell adhesion of human neutrophils: evidence for an ERK-independent pathway. *J Immunol* 1998;160:1901.
17. Knall C, Worthen GS, Johnson GL. Interleukin 8-stimulated phosphatidylinositol-3-kinase activity regulates the migration of human neutrophils independent of extracellular signal-regulated kinase and p38 mitogen-activated protein kinases. *Proc Natl Acad Sci U S A* 1997;94:3052.
18. Hii CST, Marin LA, Halliday D, et al. Regulation of human neutrophil-mediated cartilage proteoglycan degradation by phosphatidylinositol. *Immunology* 2001;102:59.
19. McEver RP, Moore KL, Cummings RD. Leukocyte trafficking mediated by selectin-carbohydrate interactions. *J Biol Chem* 1995;270:11025.
20. Bevilacqua MP, Stengelin S, Gimbrone MA Jr., et al. Endothelial leukocyte adhesion molecule 1: an inducible receptor for neutrophils related to complement regulatory proteins and lectins. *Science* 1989;243:1160.
21. Philips MR, Buyon JP, Winchester R, et al. Up-regulation of the iC3b receptor (CR3) is neither necessary nor sufficient to promote neutrophil aggregation. *J Clin Invest* 1988;82:495.
22. Buyon JP, Abramson SB, Philips MR, et al. Dissociation between increased surface expression of gp165/95 and homotypic neutrophil aggregation. *J Immunol* 1988;140:3156.
23. Lawrence MB, Springer TA. Leukocytes roll on a selectin at physiologic flow rates: distinction from and prerequisite for adhesion through integrins. *Cell* 1991;65:859.
24. Del Maschio A, Zanetti A, Corada M, et al. Polymorphonuclear leukocyte adhesion triggers the disorganization of endothelial cell-to-cell adherens junctions. *J Cell Biol* 1996;135:497.
25. Feng D, Nagy JA, Pyne K, et al. Neutrophils emigrate from venules by a transendothelial cell pathway in response to FMLP. *J Exp Med* 1998;187:903.
26. Muller WA, Weigl SA, Deng X, et al. PECAM-1 is required for transendothelial migration of leukocytes. *J Exp Med* 1993;178:449.
27. Thompson RD, Wakelin MW, Larbi KY, et al. Divergent effects of platelet-endothelial cell adhesion molecule-1 and beta 3 integrin blockade on leukocyte transmigration in vivo. *J Immunol* 2000;165(1):426.
28. Piali L, Hammel P, Uherek C, et al. CD31/PECAM-1 is a ligand for alpha v beta 3 integrin involved in adhesion of leukocytes to endothelium. *J Cell Biol* 1995;130:451.
29. Cooper D, Lindberg FP, Gamble JR, et al. Transendothelial migration of neutrophils involves integrin-associated protein (CD47). *Proc Natl Acad Sci U S A* 1995;92:3978.
30. Liu Y, Merlin D, Burst SL, et al. The role of CD47 in neutrophil transmigration. Increased rate of migration correlates with increased cell surface expression of CD47. *J Biol Chem* 2001;276(43):40156.
31. Lekstrom-Himes JA, Gallin JI. Review articles: advances in immunology immunodeficiency diseases caused by defects in phagocytes. *N Engl J Med* 2000;343:1703.
32. Phillips ML, Schwartz BR, Etzioni A, et al. Neutrophil adhesion in leukocyte adhesion deficiency syndrome type 2. *J Clin Invest* 1995;96:2898.
33. Caron E, Hall A. Identification of two distinct mechanisms of phagocytosis controlled by different Rho GTPases. *Science* 1998;282:1717.
34. Zhou M, Todd RFD, van de Winkel JG, et al. Cocapping of the leukoadhesin molecules complement receptor type 3 and lymphocyte function-associated antigen-1 with Fc gamma receptor III on human neutrophils. Possible role of lectin-like interactions. *J Immunol* 1993;150:3030.
35. Perussia B, Dayton ET, Lazarus R, et al. Immune interferon induces the receptor for monomeric IgG1 on human monocytic and myeloid cells. *J Exp Med* 1983;158:1092.
36. Samelson LE, Klausner RD. Tyrosine kinases and tyrosine-based activation motifs. Current research on activation via the T cell antigen receptor. *J Biol Chem* 1992;267:24913.
37. Salmon JE, Brogle NL, Edberg JC, et al. Fc gamma receptor III induces actin polymerization in human neutrophils and primes phagocytosis mediated by Fc gamma receptor II. *J Immunol* 1991;146:997.
38. Salmon JE, Millard SS, Brogle NL, et al. Fc gamma receptor IIIb enhances Fc gamma receptor IIa function in an oxidant-dependent and allele-sensitive manner. *J Clin Invest* 1995;95:2877.
39. Zhou MJ, Brown EJ. CR3 (Mac-1, alpha M beta 2, CD11b/CD18) and Fc gamma RIII cooperate in generation of a neutrophil respiratory burst: requirement for Fc gamma RIII and tyrosine phosphorylation. *J Cell Biol* 1994;125:1407.
40. Coxon A, Cullere X, Knight S, et al. Fc gamma RIII mediates neutrophil recruitment to immune complexes. A mechanism for neutrophil accumulation in immune-mediated inflammation. *Immunity* 2001;14:693.
41. Fossai G, Moots RJ, Bucknal RC, et al. Differential role of neutrophil FcγRIII (CD16) in phagocytosis, bacterial killing, and responses to immune complexes. *Arthritis Rheum* 2002;46:1351.
42. Borregaard N, Cowland JB. Granules of the human neutrophilic polymorphonuclear leukocyte. *Blood* 1997;89:3503.
43. Iovine NM, Elsbach P, Weiss J. An opsonic function of the neutrophil bactericidal/permeability increasing protein depends on both its N and C terminal domains. *Proc Natl Acad Sci U S A* 1997;94:10973.
44. Ganz T, Selsted ME, Lehrer RI. Defensins. *Eur J Haematol* 1990;44:1.
45. Levy O, Ooi CE, Weiss J, et al. Individual and synergistic effects of rabbit granulocyte proteins on *Escherichia coli*. *J Clin Invest* 1994;94:672.
46. Belaaouaj A, Kim KS, Shapiro SD. Degradation of outer membrane protein A in *Escherichia coli* killing by neutrophil elastase. *Science* 2000;289:1185.
47. Weiss J, Inada M, Elsbach P, et al. Structural determinants of the action against *Escherichia coli* of a human inflammatory fluid phospholipase A2 in concert with polymorphonuclear leukocytes. *J Biol Chem* 1994;269:26331.
48. Weiss SJ, Peppin G, Ortiz X, et al. Oxidative autoactivation of latent collagenase by human neutrophils. *Science* 1985;227(4688):747.
49. Weiss SJ, Peppin GJ. Collagenolytic metalloenzymes of the human neutrophil. Characteristics, regulation and potential function in vivo. *Biochem Pharmacol* 1986;35:3189.
50. Van Den Steen PE, Proost P, Wuyts A, et al. Neutrophil gelatinase B potentiates interleukin-8 tenfold by aminoterminal processing, whereas it degrades CTAP-III, PF-4, and GRO-alpha and leaves RANTES and MCP-2 intact. *Blood* 2000;96:2673.
51. Babior GL, Rosin RE, McMurrich BJ. Arrangement of the respiratory burst oxidase in the plasma membrane of the neutrophil. *J Clin Invest* 1981;67:1724.
52. Park JW, Hoyal CR, Benna JE, et al. Kinase-dependent activation of the leukocyte NADPH oxidase in a cell-free system. Phosphorylation of membranes and p47(PHOX) during oxidase activation. *J Biol Chem* 1997;272:11035.
53. Benna JE, Dang PM, Gaudry M, et al. Phosphorylation of the respiratory burst oxidase subunit p67(phox) during human neutrophil activation. Regulation by protein kinase C-dependent and independent pathways. *J Biol Chem* 1997;272:17204.
54. Han CH, Freeman JL, Lee T, et al. Regulation of the neutrophil respiratory burst oxidase. Identification of an activation domain in p67(phox). *J Biol Chem* 1998;273:16663.
55. Diekmann D, Abo A, Johnson C, et al. Interaction of Rac with p67(phox) and regulation of phagocytic NADPH oxidase activity. *Science* 1994;265:531.
56. Kago H, Terasawa H, Nunoi H, et al. Tetratricopeptide repeat (TPR) motifs of p67(phox) participate in interaction with the small GTPase Rac and activation of the phagocyte NADPH oxidase. *J Biol Chem* 1999;274:25051.
57. Philips MR, Feoktistov A, Pillinger MH, et al. Translocation of p21rac2 from cytosol to plasma membrane is neither necessary nor sufficient for neutrophil NADPH oxidase activity. *J Biol Chem* 1995;270:11514.
58. Park HS, Lee SM, Lee JH, et al. Phosphorylation of the leucocyte NADPH oxidase subunit p47(phox) by casein kinase 2: conformation-dependent phosphorylation and modulation of oxidase activity. *Biochem J* 2001;358:783.
59. Segal BH, Leto TL, Gallin JI, et al. Genetic, biochemical, and clinical features of chronic granulomatous disease. *Medicine* 2000;79:170.
60. International Chronic Granulomatous Disease Cooperative Study Group. A controlled trial of interferon gamma to prevent infection in chronic granulomatous disease. *N Engl J Med* 1991;324:509.
61. Bredt DS, Hwang PM, Glatt CE, et al. Cloned and expressed nitric oxide synthase structurally resembles cytochrome P-450 reductase. *Nature* 1991;351:714.
62. Xie QW, Cho HJ, Calaycay J, et al. Cloning and characterization of inducible nitric oxide synthase from mouse macrophages. *Science* 1992;256:225.
63. Lamas S, Mardsden PA, Li GK, et al. Endothelial nitric oxide synthase: molecular cloning and characterization of a distinct constitutive enzyme isoform. *Proc Natl Acad Sci U S A* 1992;89:6348.
64. Janssens SP, Shimouchi A, Quertermous T, et al. Cloning and expression of a cDNA encoding human endothelium derived relaxing factor/nitric oxide synthase. *J Biol Chem* 1992;267:14519.
65. Lyons CR, Orloff GJ, Cunningham JM. Molecular cloning and functional expression of an inducible nitric oxide synthase from a murine macrophage cell line. *J Biol Chem* 1992;267:6370.
66. Nathan C. Perspectives series: nitric oxide and nitric oxide synthases. Inducible nitric oxide synthase: what difference does it make? *J Clin Invest* 1997;100:2417.
67. Marletta MA. Nitric oxide synthase: aspects concerning structure and catalysis. *Cell* 1994;78:927.
68. Stamler JS, Singel DJ, Loscalzo J. Biochemistry of nitric oxide and its redox-activated forms. *Science* 1992;258:1898.
69. Ignarro LJ, Degnan JN, Baricos WH, et al. Activation of purified guanylate cyclase by nitric oxide requires heme: comparison of heme-deficient, heme reconstituted, and heme-containing forms of soluble enzyme from bovine lung. *Biochim Biophys Acta* 1982;718:49.
70. Waldman SA, Murad F. Biochemical mechanisms underlying vascular smooth muscle relaxation: the guanylate cyclase-cyclic GMP system. *J Cardiovasc Pharmacol* 1988;12:S115.
71. Clancy RM, Abramson SB. Nitric oxide: a novel mediator of inflammation. *Proc Soc Exp Biol Med* 1995;210:93.
72. Pryor WA, Squadrito GL. The chemistry of peroxynitrite: a product from the reaction of nitric oxide with superoxide. *Am J Physiol* 1995;268:L-699.
73. Clancy RM, Abramson SB. Novel synthesis of S-nitrosoglutathione and degradation by human neutrophils. *Anal Biochem* 1992;204:365.
74. Myers PR, Minor RL Jr., Guerra R Jr., et al. Vasorelaxant properties of the endothelium-derived relaxing factor more closely resemble S-nitrosocysteine than nitric oxide. *Nature* 1990;345:161.

75. Gow A, Buerk DG, Ischiropoulos H. A novel reaction mechanism for the formation of S-nitrosothiol in vivo. *J Biol Chem* 1997;272:2841.
76. Stamler JS, Jaraki O, Osborne J, et al. Nitric oxide circulates in mammalian plasma primarily as an S-nitroso adduct of serum albumin. *Proc Natl Acad Sci U S A* 1992;89:7674.
77. Clancy RM, Levartovsky D, Leszczynska-Piziak J, et al. Nitric oxide reacts with intracellular glutathione and activates the hexose monophosphate shunt in human neutrophils: evidence for S-nitrosoglutathione as a bioactive intermediary. *Proc Natl Acad Sci U S A* 1994;91:3680.
78. Fang FC. Perspective series: first host/pathogen interactions. Mechanisms of nitric oxide related antimicrobial activity. *J Clin Invest* 1997;99:2818.
79. Farrell AJ, Blake DR. Nitric oxide. *Ann Rheum Dis* 1996;55:7.
80. Nathan C, Hibbs JB. Role of nitric oxide synthesis in macrophage antimicrobial activity. *Curr Opin Immunol* 1991;3:65.
81. Amin AR, Di Cesare PE, Vyas P, et al. The expression and regulation of nitric oxide synthase in human osteoarthritis-affected chondrocytes: evidence for up-regulated neuronal nitric oxide synthase. *J Exp Med* 1995;182:2097.
82. St. Clair EW, Wilkinson WE, Lang T, et al. Increased expression of blood mononuclear cell nitric oxide synthase type 2 in rheumatoid arthritis patients. *J Exp Med* 1996;184:1173.
83. Weyand CM, Wagner AD, Bjornsson J, et al. Correlation of the topographical arrangement and the functional pattern of tissue-infiltration macrophages in giant cell arteritis. *J Clin Invest* 1996;98:1642.
84. Kontinnen YT, Platts LA, Tuominen S, et al. Role of nitric oxide in Sjogren's syndrome. *Arthritis Rheum* 1997;40:875.
85. Amin AR, Attur M, Vyas P, et al. Expression of nitric oxide synthase in human peripheral blood mononuclear cells and neutrophils. *J Inflamm* 1995; 47:190.
86. Yan L,Vandivier RW, Suffredini AF, et al. Human polymorphonuclear leukocytes lack detectable nitric oxide synthase activity. *J Immunol* 1994;153:1825.
87. Sharma P, Raghavan SA, Dikshit M. Role of ascorbate in the regulation of nitric oxide generation by polymorphonuclear leukocytes. *Biochem Biophys Res Commun* 2003;309:12.
88. Clancy R, Leszczynska J, Amin A, et al. Nitric oxide stimulates ADP ribosylation of actin in association with the inhibition of actin polymerization in human neutrophils. *J Leukoc Biol* 1995;58:196.
89. Clements MK, Siemsen DW, Swain SD, et al. Inhibition of actin polymerization by peroxynitrite modulates neutrophil functional responses. *J Leukoc Biol* 2003;73:344.
90. Clancy RM, Amin AR, Abramson SB. The role of nitric oxide in inflammation and immunity. *Arthritis Rheum* 1998;41:1141.
91. Baskic D, Acimovic L, Djukic A, et al. Phagocytic activity and nitric oxide production of circulating polymorphonuclear leukocytes from patients with peritoneal carcinomatosis. *Acta Oncol* 2003;42:846.
92. Sanchez de Miguel L, Arriero MM, Farre J, et al. A nitric oxide production by neutrophils obtained from patients during acute coronary syndromes: expression of the nitric oxide synthase isoforms. *J Am Coll Cardiol* 2002;6:818.
93. Bogdan C. Nitric oxide and the immune response. *Nat Immunol* 2001;2:907.
94. Abramson SB, Amin AR, Clancy RM. The role of nitric oxide in tissue destruction. *Best Pract Res Clin Rheumatol* 2001;15:831.
95. Clancy R, Leszczynska J, Amin A, et al. Nitric oxide stimulates ADP ribosylation of actin in association with the inhibition of actin polymerization in human neutrophils. *J Leukoc Biol* 1995;58:196.
96. Belenky SN, Robbins RA, Rennard SI, et al. Inhibitors of nitric oxide synthase attenuate human neutrophil chemotaxis in vitro. *J Lab Clin Med* 1993;122:388.
97. Secco DD, Paron JA, de Oliveira SH, et al. Neutrophil migration in inflammation: nitric oxide inhibits rolling, adhesion and induces apoptosis. *Nitric Oxide* 2003;9:153.
98. Kosonen O, Kankaanranta H, Malo-Ranta U, et al. Nitric oxide-releasing compounds inhibit neutrophil adhesion to endothelial cells. *Eur J Pharmacol* 1999;382:111.
99. Kubes PM, Suzuki M, Granger DN. Nitric oxide: an endogenous modulator of leukocyte adhesion. *Proc Natl Acad Sci U S A* 1991;88:4651.
100. Clancy RM, Leszczynska-Piziak J, Abramson SB. Nitric oxide, an endothelial cell relaxation factor, inhibits neutrophil superoxide anion production via direct action on the NADPH oxidase. *J Clin Invest* 1992;90:1116.
101. Masini E, Pistelli A, Gambassi F, et al. The role of nitric oxide in anaphylactic reaction of isolated guinea pig hearts and mast cells. In: Moncada S, Nishko G, eds. *Nitric oxide: brain and immune system*. London: Portland Press, 1996: 277.
102. Gutierrez HH, Nieves B, Chumley P, et al. Nitric oxide regulation of superoxide-dependent lung injury: oxidant-protective actions of endogenously produced and exogenously administered nitric oxide. *Free Radic Biol Med* 1996;21:43.
103. Zhuang D, Ceacareanu AC, Lin Y, et al. Nitric oxide attenuates insulin- or IGF1-stimulated aortic smooth muscle cell motility by decreasing hydrogen peroxide levels: essential role of cyclic GMP. *Am J Physiol Heart Circ Physiol* 2004 (*in press*).
104. Coles B, Bloodsworth A, Clark SR, et al. Nitrolinoleate inhibits superoxide generation, degranulation, and integrin expression by human neutrophils: novel antiinflammatory properties of nitric oxide-derived reactive species in vascular cells. *Circ Res* 2002;91:375.
105. Clancy RM, Leszczynska-Piziak J, Abramson SB. Nitric oxide stimulates the ADP-ribosylation of actin in human neutrophils. *Biochem Biophys Res Commun* 1993;191(3):847.
106. Frenkel SR, Clancy RM, Ricci JL, et al. Effects of nitric oxide on chondrocyte migration, adhesion and cytoskeletal assembly. *Arthritis Rheum* 1996;39:1905.
107. Clancy R, Rediske J, Tang X, et al. Outside-in signaling in the chondrocyte: nitric oxide disrupts fibronectin-induced assembly of a subplasmalemmal actin/Rho A/focal adhesion kinase signaling complex. *J Clin Invest* 1997;100(7):1789.
108. Babior BM. Phagocytes and oxidative stress. *Am J Med* 2000;109:33.
109. Weiss SJ. Tissue destruction by neutrophils. *N Engl J Med* 1989;320:365.
110. Whiteman M, Hooper DC, Scott GS, et al. Inhibition of hypochlorous acid-induced cellular toxicity by nitrite. *Proc Natl Acad Sci U S A* 2002;99:12061.
111. Marcinkiewicz J, Chain B, Nowak B, et al. Antimicrobial and cytotoxic activity of hypochlorous acid: interactions with taurine and nitrite. *Inflamm Res* 2000;49:280.
112. Bingham CO 3rd, Austen KF. Phospholipase A2 enzymes in eicosanoid generation. *Proc Assoc Am Physicians* 1999;111:516.
113. Woods JW, Evans JF, Ethier D, et al. 5-lipoxygenase and 5-lipoxygenase-activating protein are localized in the nuclear envelope of activated human leukocytes. *J Exp Med* 1993;178(6):1935.
114. Ford-Hutchinson AW, Bray MA, Doig MV, et al. Leukotriene B_4, a potent chemokinetic and aggregating substance released from polymorphonuclear leukocytes. *Nature* 1980;286:264.
115. Tager AW, Dufour JH, Goodarzi K, et al. BLTR mediates leukotriene B_4-induced chemotaxis and adhesion and plays a dominant role in eosinophil accumulation in a murine model of peritonitis. *J Exp Med* 2000;192(3):439.
116. Feinmark SJ, Lindgren JA, Claesson HE, et al. Stimulation of human leukocyte degranulation by leukotriene B_4 and its omega-oxidized metabolites. *FEBS Lett* 1981;136(1):141.
117. Omann GM, Traynor AE, Harris AL, et al. LTB_4 induced activation signals and responses in neutrophils are short-lived compared to formylpeptide. *J Immunol* 1987;138(8):2626.
118. Hebert MJ, Takano T, Holthofer H, et al. Sequential morphologic events during apoptosis of human neutrophils. Modulation by lipoxygenase-derived eicosanoids. *J Immunol* 1996;157(7):3105.
119. Lee E, Lindo T, Jackson N, Meng-Choong L, et al. Reversal of human neutrophil survival by leukotriene B(4) receptor blockade and 5-lipoxygenase and 5-lipoxygenase activating protein inhibitors. *Am J Respir Crit Care Med* 1999; 160(6):2079.
120. Serhan CN, Fiore S, Levy BD. Cell-cell interactions in lipoxin generation and characterization of lipoxin A4 receptors. *Ann N Y Acad Sci* 1994;744:166.
121. Serhan CN, Sheppard KA. Lipoxin formation during human neutrophil-platelet interactions. Evidence for the transformation of leukotriene A_4 by platelet 12-lipoxygenase in vitro. *J Clin Invest* 1990;85(3):772.
122. Levy BD, Clish CB, Schmidt B, et al. Lipid mediator class switching during acute inflammation: signals in resolution. *Nat Immunol* 2001;2(7):612.
123. Rossetti RG, Braithwaite K, Zurier RB. Suppression of acute inflammation with liposome associated prostaglandin E_1. *Prostaglandins* 1994;48(3):187.
124. Kitsis EA, Weissmann G, Abramson SB. The prostaglandin paradox: additive inhibition of neutrophil function by aspirin-like drugs and the prostaglandin E1 analog misoprostol. *J Rheumatol* 1991;18(10):1461.
125. Sedgwick JB, Berube ML, Zurier RB. Stimulus-dependent inhibition of superoxide generation by prostaglandins. *Clin Immunol Immunopathol* 1985;34(2):205.
126. Tamura DY, Moore EE, Partrick DA, et al. Prostaglandin E1 attenuates cytotoxic mechanisms of primed neutrophils. *Shock* 1998;9(3):171.
127. Pillinger MH, Philips MR, Feoktistov A, et al. Crosstalk in signal transduction via EP receptors: prostaglandin E_1 inhibits chemoattractant-induced mitogen-activated protein kinase activity in human neutrophils. *Adv Prostaglandin Thromboxane Leukot Res* 1995:23:311.
128. Wipke BT, Allen PM. Essential role of neutrophils in the initiation and progression of a murine model of rheumatoid arthritis. *J Immunol* 2001;167:1601.
129. Firestein GS. Rheumatoid synovitis and pannus. In: Maini RN, Zvaifler NJ, Klippel JH, et al., eds. *Rheumatology*. Mosby: London, 1998:5.13.1–5.13.24.
130. Bromley M, Woolley DE. Histopathology of the rheumatoid lesion: identification of cell types at sites of cartilage erosion. *Arthritis Rheum* 1984;27:857.
131. Mohr W, Wessinghage D. The relationship between polymorphonuclear granulocytes and cartilage destruction in rheumatoid arthritis. *Z Rheumatol* 1978;37:81.
132. Mohr W, Westerhellweg H, Wessinghage D. Polymorphonuclear granulocytes in rheumatic tissue destruction III. An electron microscopic study of PMNs at the pannus-cartilage junction in rheumatoid arthritis. *Ann Rheum Dis* 1981;40:396.
133. Mohr W, Wild A, Wolf HP. Role of polymorphs in inflammatory cartilage destruction in adjuvant arthritis of rats. *Ann Rheum Dis* 1981;40:171.
134. Halliday DA, Clemente G, Rathjen DA, et al. Rapid degradation of articular cartilage proteoglycan by neutrophils: comparison with macrophages and synovial fibroblasts. *Inflamm Res* 2000;49:441.
135. McCurdy L, Chatham WW, Blackburn WD Jr. Rheumatoid synovial fibroblast adhesion to human articular cartilage. Enhancement by neutrophil proteases. *Arthritis Rheum* 1995;38:1694.
136. Hashida R, Kuwada M, Chiba KI, et al. A factor derived from polymorphonuclear leukocytes enhances interleukin-1-included synovial cell collagenase and prostaglandin E2 production in rats. *Eur J Biochem* 1996;236:517.
137. Hollingsworth JW, Siegel ER, Creasy WA. Granulocyte survival in synovial exudate of patients with rheumatoid arthritis and other inflammatory joint diseases. *Yale J Biol Med* 1967;39:289.
138. Ottonello L, Frumento G, Arduino N, et al. Delayed neutrophil apoptosis induced by synovial fluid in rheumatoid arthritis: role of cytokines, estrogens, and adenosine. *Ann N Y Acad Sci* 2002;966:226.

139. Hotta K, Niwa M, Hara A, et al. The loss of susceptibility to apoptosis in exudated tissue neutrophils is associated with their nuclear factor-kappa B activation. *Eur J Pharmacol* 2001;433:17.
140. Haruta K, Kobayashi S, Tajima M, et al. Effect of immune complexes in serum from patients with rheumatoid vasculitis on the expression of cell adhesion molecules on polymorphonuclear cells. *Clin Exp Rheum* 2001;19:59.
141. Greenwald RA, Moi WW. Effect of oxygen-derived free radicals on hyaluronic acid. *Arthritis Rheum* 1980;23:455.
142. Schenk P, Schneider S, Miehlke R, et al. Synthesis and degradation of hyaluronate by synovia from patients with rheumatoid arthritis. *J Rheumatol* 1995;22:400.
143. Ghosh, P. Osteoarthritis and hyaluronan—palliative or disease-modifying treatment? *Semin Arthritis Rheum* 1993;22:1.
144. Arner EC, Decicco CP, Cherney R, et al. Cleavage of native cartilage aggrecan by neutrophil collagenase (MMP-8) is distinct from endogenous cleavage by aggrecanase. *J Biol Chem* 1997;272:9294.
145. Grillet B, Dequeker J, Paemen L, et al. Gelatinase B in chronic synovitis: immunolocalization with a monoclonal antibody. *Br J Rheumatol* 1997;36:744.
146. Matsuno H, Yudoh K, Watanabe Y, et al. Stromelysin-1 (MMP-3) in synovial fluid of patients with rheumatoid arthritis has potential to cleave membrane bound Fas ligand. *J Rheumatol* 2001;28:22.
147. Gaudin P, Razakaboay M, Surla A, et al. A study of metalloproteinases in fifty joint fluid specimens. *Rev Rheum Engl Ed* 1997;64:375.
148. Ekerot L, Ohlsson K. Immunoreactive granulocytes elastase in rheumatoid synovial fluid and membrane. *Scand J Plast Reconstr Surg* 1982;16:117.
149. Van Den Steen PE, Proost P, Grillet B, et al. Cleavage of denatured natural collagen type II by neutrophil gelatinase B reveals enzyme specificity, post-translational modifications in the substrate, and the formation of remnant epitopes in rheumatoid arthritis. *FASEB J* 2002;16(3):379.
150. Hilbert N, Schiller J, Arnhold J, et al. Cartilage degradation by stimulated human neutrophils: elastase is mainly responsible for cartilage damage. *Bioorg Chem* 2002;30:119.
151. van Meurs J, van Lent P, Holthuysen A, et al. Active matrix metalloproteinases are present in cartilage during immune complex-mediated arthritis: a pivotal role for stromelysin-1 in cartilage destruction. *J Immunol* 1999; 163:5633.
152. Hasty KA, Hibbs MS, Kang AH, et al. Secreted forms of human neutrophil collagenase. *J Biol Chem* 1986;261:5645.
153. Macartney HW, Tschesche H. Latent and active human polymorphonuclear leukocyte collagenases: isolation, purification and characterization. *Eur J Biochem* 1983;130:71.
154. Chatham WW, Blackburn WD Jr., Heck LW. Additive enhancement of neutrophil collagenase activity by HOCL and cathepsin G. *Biochem Biophys Res Commun* 1993;191:847.
155. Sorsa T, Konttinen YT, Lindy O, et al. Collagenase in synovitis of rheumatoid arthritis. *Semin Arthritis Rheum* 1992;22(1):44.
156. Weiss SJ, Klein R, Slivka A, et al. Chlorination of taurine by human neutrophils. Evidence for hypochlorous acid generation. *J Clin Invest* 1982;70(3):598.
157. Okada Y, Harris ED Jr, Nagase H. The precursor of a metalloendopeptidase from human rheumatoid synovial fibroblasts. Purification and mechanisms of activation by endopeptidases and 4-aminophenylmercuric acetate. *Biochem J* 1988;254:731.
158. Nagase H, Enghild JJ, Suzuki K, et al. Stepwise activation mechanisms of the precursor of matrix metalloproteinase 3 (stromelysin) by proteinases and (4-aminophenyl) mercuric acetate. *Biochemistry* 1990;29:5783.
159. Dularay B, Yea CM, Elson CJ. Inhibition of myeloperoxidase by synovial fluid and serum. *Ann Rheum Dis* 1991;50:383.
160. Moore AR, Appelboam A, Kawabata K, et al. Destruction of articular cartilage by alpha$_2$ macroglobulin elastase complexes: role in rheumatoid arthritis. *Ann Rheum Dis* 1999;58:109.
161. Kawabata K, Moore AR, Willoughby DA. Impaired activity of protease inhibitors towards neutrophil elastase bound to human articular cartilage. *Ann Rheum Dis* 1996;55:248.
162. Weiss SJ. Tissue destruction by neutrophils. *N Engl J Med* 1989;320:365.
163. Janusz MJ, Doherty NS. Degradation of cartilage matrix proteoglycan by human neutrophils involves both elastase and cathepsin G. *J Immunol* 1991;146:3922.
164. Mitani Y, Honda A, Jasin HE. Polymorphonuclear leukocyte adhesion to articular cartilage is inhibited by cartilage surface macromolecules. *Rheumatol Int* 2001;20:180.
165. Pillinger MH, Abramson SB. The neutrophil in rheumatoid arthritis. In: Kremer JM, ed. *Rheumatic disease clinics of North America*. Philadelphia: W.B. Saunders Company, 1995:691–714.
166. DeForge LE, Preston AM, Takeuchi E, et al. Regulation of interleukin 8 gene expression by oxidant stress. *J Biol Chem* 1993;268:25568.
167. Lotz M, Terkeltaub R, Villiger PM. Cartilage and joint inflammation: regulation of IL-8 expression by human articular chondrocytes. *J Immunol* 1992;148:466.
168. Biragyn A, Ruffini PA, Leifer CA, et al. Toll-like receptor 4-dependent activation of dendritic cells by beta-defensin 2. *Science* 2002;298(5595):1025.
169. Coeshott C, Ohnemus C, Pilyavskaya A, et al. Converting enzyme-independent release of tumor necrosis factor-α and IL-1β from a stimulated human monocytic cell line in the presence of activated neutrophils or purified proteinase 3. *Proc Natl Acad Sci U S A* 1999;96:6261.
170. Thiel S, Reid KB. Structures and functions associated with the group of mammalian lectins containing collagen-like sequences. *FEBS Lett* 1989; 250:78.
171. Walport MJ. Complement: first of two parts. *N Engl J Med* 2001;344(14):1058.
172. Vandiver RW, Fadok VA, Hoffmann PR, et al. Elastase-mediated phosphatidylserine receptor cleavage impairs apoptotic cell clearance in cystic fibrosis and bronchiectasis. *J Clin Invest* 2002;109(5):661.
173. Fadok VA, Bratton DL, Rose DM, et al. A receptor for phosphatidylserine-specific clearance of apoptotic cells. *Nature* 2000;405:85.
174. Huynh MLN, Fadock VA, Henson PM. Phosphatidylserine-dependent ingestion of apoptotic cells promotes TGF-α 1 secretion and the resolution of inflammation. *J Clin Invest* 2002;109(1):41.
175. Henson PM, Bratton DL, Fadok VA. The phosphatidylserine receptor: a crucial molecular switch? *Nat Rev Mol Cell Biol* 2001;2:627.
176. Siedle B, Cisielski S, Murillo R, et al. Sesquiterpene lactones as inhibitors of human neutrophil elastase. *Bioorg Med Chem* 2002;10(9):2855.
177. Janusz MJ, Durham SL. Inhibition of cartilage degradation in rat collagen-induced arthritis but not adjuvant arthritis by the neutrophil elastase inhibitor MDL 101,146. *Inflamm Res* 1997;46:503.
178. Gosselin EJ, Wardwell K, Rigby WF, et al. Induction of MHC class II on human polymorphonuclear neutrophils by granulocytes/macrophage colony-stimulating factor, IFN-gamma, and IL-3. *J Immunol* 1993;151(3):1482.
179. Mudezinski SP, Christian TP, Guo TL, et al. Expression of HLA-DR (major histocompatibility complex class II) on neutrophils from patients treated with granulocytes-macrophage colony-stimulating factor for mobilization of stem cells. *Blood* 1995;86(6):2452.
180. Fanger NA, Liu C, Guyre PM, et al. Activation of human T cells by major histocompatibility complex class II expressing neutrophils; proliferation in the presence of superantigen, but not tetanus toxoid. *Blood* 1997;89(11):4128.
181. Radsak M, Iking-Konert C, Stegmaier S, et al. Polymorphonuclear neutrophils as accessory cells for T-cell activation: major histocompatibility complex class II restricted antigen-dependent induction of T-cell proliferation. *Immunology* 2000;101:521.
182. Lei L, Altstaedt J, von der Ohe M, et al. Induction of interleukin-8 in human neutrophils after MHC class II cross-linking with superantigens. *J Leukoc Biol* 2001;70:80.
183. Oehler L, Majdic O, Pickl WF, et al. Neutrophil granulocyte-committed cells can be driven to acquire dendritic cell characteristics. *J Exp Med* 1998;187(7):1019.
184. Iking-Konert C, Vogt S, Wagner C, et al. Polymorphonuclear neutrophils in Wegener's granulomatosis acquire characteristics of antigen presenting cells. *Kidney Int* 2001;60(6):2247.
185. Cross A, Bucknall RC, Edwards SW, et al. Expression of MHC class II molecules by synovial fluid neutrophils. *Arthritis Rheum* 2001;44(9):S303.
186. Wright CE, Tallan HH, Lin YY, et al. Taurine: biological update. *Annu Rev Biochem* 1986;55:427.
187. Marcinkiewicz J, Nowak B, Grabowska A, et al. Regulation of murine dendritic cell functions in vitro by taurine chloramine, a major product of the neutrophil myeloperoxidase-halide system. *Immunology* 1999;9:371.
188. Kettle AJ, Winterbourn CC. Mechanism of inhibition of myeloperoxidase by anti-inflammatory drugs. *Biochem Pharmacol* 1991;41:1485.
189. van Zyl JM, Basson K, Kriegler A, et al. Mechanisms by which clofazimine and dapsone inhibit the myeloperoxidase system. A possible correlation with their anti-inflammatory properties. *Biochem Pharmacol* 1991;42:599.
190. Shacter E, Lopez RL, Pati S. Inhibition of the myeloperoxidase-H202-C1 system of neutrophils by indomethacin and other non-steroidal anti-inflammatory drugs. *Biochem Pharmacol* 1991;41:975.
191. Cronstein BN, Molad Y, Reibman J, et al. Colchicine alters the quantitative and qualitative display of selectins on endothelial cells and neutrophils. *J Clin Invest* 1995;96:994.
192. Cronstein BN, Eberie MA, Gruber HE, et al. Methotrexate inhibits neutrophil function by stimulating adenosine release from connective tissue cells. *Proc Natl Acad Sci U S A* 1991;88:2441.
193. Cronstein BN, Kimmel SC, Levin RI, Martiniuk F, et al. A mechanism for the antiinflammatory effects of corticosteroids: the glucocorticoid receptor regulates leukocyte adhesion to endothelial cells and expression of endothelial-leukocyte adhesion molecule 1 and intercellular adhesion molecule 1. *Proc Natl Acad Sci U S A* 1992;89:9991.
194. Filep JG, Delalandre A, Payette Y, et al. Glucocorticoid receptor regulates expression of L-selectin and CD11/CD18 on human neutrophils. *Circulation* 1997;96:295.
195. Pillinger MH, Capodici C, Rosenthal P, et al. Modes of action of aspirin-like drugs: salicylates inhibit erk activation and integrin-dependent neutrophil adhesion. *Proc Natl Acad Sci U S A* 1998;95:14540.
196. Taylor PC, Peters AM, Paleolog E, et al. Reduction of chemokine levels and leukocyte traffic to joints by tumor necrosis factor alpha blockade in patients with rheumatoid arthritis. *Arthritis Rheum* 2001;44(1):38.
197. Calkins CM, Bensard DD, Shames BD, et al. Il-1 regulates in vivo C-X-C chemokine induction and neutrophil sequestration following endotoxemia. *J Endotoxin Res* 2002;8(1):59.
198. Kowanko IC, Ferrante A, Clemente G, et al. Tumor necrosis factor priming of peripheral blood neutrophils from rheumatoid arthritis patients. *J Clin Immunol* 1996;16(4):216.
199. Moreland LW, Bucy RP, Weinblatt ME, et al. Immune function in patients with rheumatoid arthritis treated with etanercept. *Clin Immunol* 2002;103(1): 13.
200. Cornillie F, Shealy D, D'Haens G, et al. Infliximab induces potent anti-inflammatory and local immunomodulatory activity but no systemic immune suppression in patients with Crohn's disease. *J Endotoxin Res* 2001;15(4):463.

CHAPTER 15

Complement and Other Aspects of Innate Immunity

John Patterson Atkinson

In the study of both normal and pathologic immune response, there is an increasing emphasis on innate immunity to understand phenomena not explained by focusing exclusively on adaptive immunity. Skin and the respiratory, genitourinary, and gastrointestinal tracts are at the interface with the environment. Thus, at these locations, the innate immune system is on the firing line from birth to death (Table 15.1). How many infections are prevented by the innate immune system? Epithelial barriers with their Toll receptors, secretions, natural antibodies, lectins, cytokines, and complement all engage foreign substances at these interfaces. Not only must these systems separate self from nonself but also dangerous from nondangerous pathogens. Innate immunity provides these initial critical separations and, moreover, subsequently instructs how the adaptive immune system responds. The separation of these two systems of immunity is artificial and conceptual. Many of the cells, receptors, and mediators (especially cytokines) overlap, contributing vitally to both systems (Table 15.2).

This chapter focuses on the role played by innate immunity in rheumatoid arthritis (RA) and employs the complement system as an example. It begins with a brief update on the function of complement cascades, followed by a summary of data accumulated since the 1950s on complement's role in RA. The chapter then highlights data about complement's role in two animal models of RA. RA is not likely caused by a deficiency of the complement activating system, because individuals with complement deficiency (e.g., C1q) present with bacterial infections (1) or autoimmunity [usually in the form of systemic lupus erythematosus (SLE)] (2–6). However, in RA, complement activation likely contributes to tissue damage, and a deficiency of complement regulators may play a more direct or causative role in allowing such tissue damage to occur (6,7). This latter scenario has been illustrated by a new mouse model of RA, K/BxN (8), discussed below.

COMPLEMENT SYSTEM

In the 1890s, experimental pathologists were astonished to observe bacteria imploding on exposure to a thermostable blood substance (still worked after being left on the bench top overnight) and a thermolabile blood substance (did not work the next day). The former was antibody (Ab), which is specific and acquired, and the latter was complement, which is nonspecific and innate, because almost everybody has it in abundance. Neither part of this two-component system could independently accomplish the job. Indeed, the labile serum factor was felt to complement the specific substance, hence its name. A few years later, the first autoimmune disease that was understood as such was described. In this form of autoimmune hemolytic anemia (Donath-Landsteiner Ab), the same combination of players was responsible for lysis of the human red blood cells. This scenario was in part responsible for Ehrlich's famous dictum "horror autotoxicus." In Ehrlich's words, "It would be exceedingly dysteleology, if in this situation self poisons, autotoxins, were formed" (9a). In view of these remarkable observations, it is not surprising that the study of Ab and complement dominated immunology for the next 70 years. "Today the complement system still rivals the coagulation system in complexity, although it has also been described as a 'simple little proteolytic cascade'" (9).

The next section provides a few details what is now known about the system, to facilitate interpretation of complement's role in human RA and in mouse models of RA. There are multiple differences between mouse and human complement in their activation schemes and also in their receptors and regulators. This "nasty little secret" (first used by Charles Janeway in his discussions of complete Freund's adjuvant as an immunologist's "dirty little secret") may also apply to the complement system. It seems self-evident but bears repeating that a mouse's immune system has evolved to handle a set of pathogens distinct from those facing humans.

Function

The complement system modifies membranes and soluble antigens to which its larger activation fragments become bound. As part of this process, smaller fragments are liberated in the local milieu to promote the inflammatory response (Figs. 15.1–15.3).

MEMBRANE MODIFICATION

Activated complement proteins deposit in large amounts on microbes and immune complexes (ICs). For example, several

TABLE 15.1. Characteristics of the Innate Immune System

Phylogenetically older than the adaptive immune system and found in both invertebrates and vertebrates.
Cells include macrophages, dendritic cells, natural killer cells, and $\gamma\delta$ T cells.
Carries out a non–antigen-specific response to infectious agents.
Pattern recognition receptors recognize repeating molecular structures on pathogenic agents.
Effector mechanisms include antimicrobial peptides, complement activation fragments, natural killer cell cytotoxicity, and cytokine release.
Initiates an inflammatory response and activates the adaptive immune response.

Adapted from Arend WP. The innate immune system in rheumatoid arthritis. *Arthritis Rheum* 2001;44:2224–2234.

million C3b molecules can attach in clusters to a bacterial surface in less than 2 to 3 minutes. The critical function of these deposited complement proteins is to opsonize the target. C3b and C4b are ligands for complement receptors (CRs) on peripheral blood cells and tissue macrophages. Complement ligands and receptors are particularly adept at this joining process, known as *immune adherence*. On phagocytotic cells, this leads to ingestion of the particle or IC. Additionally, the membranes of some (gram negative, for example) microorganisms and host cells can be disrupted by the terminal complement components (C5b-C9), resulting in lysis. In many cases, though, microbes are resistant to lysis, but the insertion of membrane attack complex (MAC) alters their cellular milieu by triggering signaling pathways.

PROMOTION OF INFLAMMATION BY CELL ACTIVATION

During complement activation, mediators are released that elicit an inflammatory response. These fragments (C4a, C3a, C5a) are termed *anaphylatoxins* because, if released in excessive amounts, they induce a reaction resembling anaphylaxis. C3a and C5a bind to their respective receptors at sites of complement activation, producing histamine release from mast cells and phagocytic cell influx. With improved reagents and newer technology, receptors for C3a and C5a have now been shown to be much more widely expressed than initially thought; for example, by epithelial cells, hepatocytes, endothelial cells, neurons, and many other cell types.

Complement Activation Pathways

There are three pathways of complement activation (Figs. 15.2 and 15.3). Although triggered differently, the early parts of each represent a proteolytic cascade, resulting in an amplification process whereby large amounts of C3b are generated. Also common to all three pathways is the liberation of anaphylatoxins and formation of the MAC.

TABLE 15.2. Cytokines of the Innate Immune System

Signals that mediate the inflammatory response
IL-1, TNF-α, IL-6, IFN-α, IFN-β
Signals that regulate effector functions
IFN-γ, TGF-β, IL-4, IL-5, IL-10, IL-12, IL-15, IL-18

IFN-α, interferon α; IL, interleukin; TGF-β, transforming growth factor β; TNF-α, tumor necrosis factor α.
Adapted from Arend WP. The innate immune system in rheumatoid arthritis. *Arthritis Rheum* 2001;44:2224–2234.

CLASSIC PATHWAY

In the classic pathway (CP), antibodies select the target. This occurs by an interaction between the C1q subcomponent of C1 and the Fc portion of immunoglobulin (Ig) G or IgM, which has become bound to an antigen. IgG subclasses 1, 2, and 3 activate the CP, whereas IgA, IgD, IgE, and IgG4 do not. C-reactive protein (CRP) also activates the CP on binding to its polysaccharide ligand (10,11).

The C1s subunit of C1 is a serine protease that cleaves the next two components, C4 and C2. The C4b generated binds to the target to serve as an opsonin, and a fraction engages C2a to form a C3 convertase. In an example of complement activation by a polyclonal Ab to a membrane antigen of nucleated cells (12), the cells became coated with 2.4×10^6 C4b fragments and 0.67×10^6 C2a molecules (attached to the C4b), followed by 2.1×10^7 molecules of C3b (approximately ten times more C3b than C4b was deposited). These steps all occurred in less than 5 minutes. 1×10^6 MACs (C5b-C9) were attached to cells in the same time period. C4a, C3a, and C5a fragments, equal to the number of C4, C3, and C5 proteins cleaved, were simultaneously liberated. The robustness and speed of this process on cells or microbes are remarkable. However, the process, especially C4b and C3b attachment and, therefore, convertase formation, is not as efficient on a soluble protein.

LECTIN PATHWAY

In the lectin pathway (LP), lectins select the target. Lectins are carbohydrate-binding proteins synthesized by the liver (7,13,14). Initially described as proteins capable of agglutinating red blood cells, lectins are now known to be important players in innate immunity and in rheumatic diseases. In particular, mannan binding lectin (MBL) binds to repeating sugars, such as repeating mannoses on certain pathogens. This protein is also called *mannose binding lectin* and *mannan binding protein*. Structurally and functionally, MBL resembles the C1q subcomponent of C1. It is an oligomer with a collagenous domain on one end and a globular domain on the other. The main structural difference between MBL and C1q is that the carboxyl terminus of MBL possesses a carbohy-

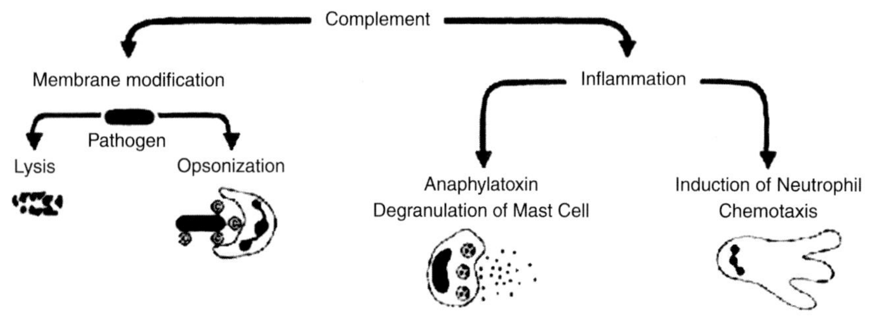

Figure 15.1. Function of the complement system. The most important function of complement is to alter the membrane of a pathogen by coating its surface with clusters of complement components (the phenomenon of opsonization). These, in turn, facilitate interactions with complement receptors and, in some cases, such as with certain gram-negative bacteria and viruses, induce lysis. The second function of complement is to promote the inflammatory response. The complement fragments C3a and C5a (termed *anaphylatoxins*) activate many cell types, such as mast cells, to release their contents, and phagocytic cells, to migrate to an inflammatory site (chemotaxis). (Adapted from Liszewski et al. *Fundamental immunology*, 3rd ed., 1993:917–939.)

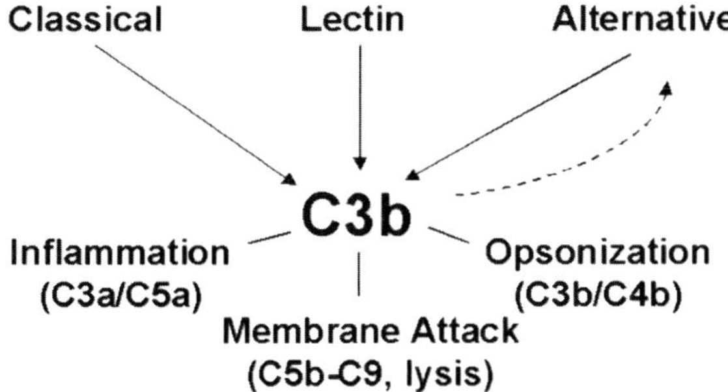

Figure 15.2. The three pathways of complement activation. Deposition of clusters of C3b on a target is the primary goal. As shown by the broken line, the alternative pathway also serves as a feedback loop to amplify C3b deposition.

TABLE 15.3. Complement Receptors for C3 and C4[a]

Name	Primary Ligand	Location	Function
CR1	C3b/C4b	Peripheral blood cells, FDCs	Immune adherence, phagocytosis, antigen localization
CR2	C3dg/C3d iC3b	B lymphocytes, FDCS	Co-receptor for B-cell signaling; antigen localization
CR3/CR4	iC3b	Myeloid lineage	Phagocytosis, adherence

FDCs, follicular dendritic cells.
[a]The CD numbers are CR1, CD35; CR2, CD21; CR3, CD11b/CD18; CR4, CD11c/CD18. Adapted from Klippel JH, ed. *Primer on the rheumatic diseases,* 12th ed. Atlanta: Arthritis Foundation, 2001:66–72.

drate-recognition domain, whereas C1q has an Ig-binding domain. Like C1q, MBL engagement with its sugar ligand leads to the activation of the serine proteases, similar to the C1r and C1s subcomponents of C1, termed *MASP-1* and *MASP-2*. MASP-2, like C1s in the CP, cleaves C4 and C2. Although congenital MBL deficiency states are associated with recurrent infections early in life, accumulating evidence points to this deficiency state as also being related to the development and severity of RA (7).

ALTERNATIVE PATHWAY

The alternative pathway (AP) does not require Ab for its activation. Instead, C3 is continuously turning over (like a car idling) at low level (so-called C3 tickover). If this activated C3 binds to the microbe, it then serves as the nidus for engagement of the AP. Although this process seems like a wasteful or shot-gun approach to host defense, it provides an important surveillance or sentry-like role in the nonimmune host. Amplification of complement activation only occurs if C3b is bound to a target that is deficient in complement regulators. The process is as efficient as the CP, except that there is a delay of several minutes while the feedback loop is set in motion. The end result, however, is the same—that is, the deposition of large amounts of C3b on a target. Of note, the K/BxN model of RA suggests that C3b deposition is an AP-dependent process (15). In addition to this self-triggering capability, a second major role of the AP is to amplify, via the feedback loop, C3b deposition on a target. Initial C3b deposition may be via the CP or LP, but the feedback loop is responsible for depositing the majority of the C3b. This scheme for amplifying C3b deposition is likely to be particularly important in the nonimmune host (LP or natural Ab activation of CP) as is the case early in an immune response to a pathogen.

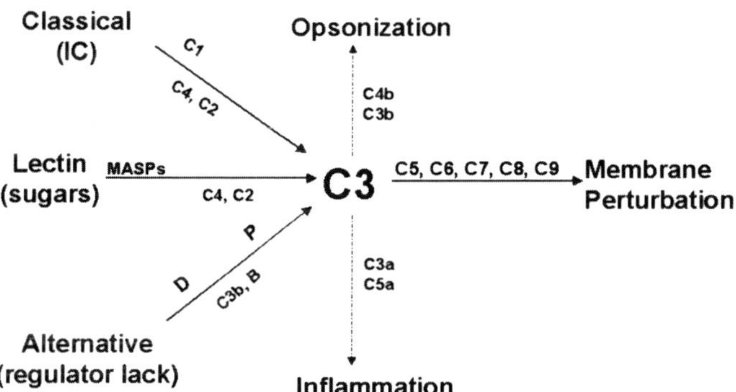

Figure 15.3. Three pathways of complement activation. A deficiency of C1, C4, or C2 predisposes to autoimmunity, especially systemic lupus erythematosus. (Adapted from Barilla-LaBarca ML, Atkinson JP. Rheumatic syndromes associated with complement deficiency. *Curr Opin Rheumatol* 2003;15:55–60.)

Complement Receptors

The complement system exerts much of its effector activity through receptors (Table 15.3). CRs are of two general categories—those for the target-bound opsonic fragments (C3b, C4b, and their degradation fragments) and those for the liberated C3a and C5a fragments. CR1 (CD35) mediates clearance of IC. CR1 on erythrocytes serves as a taxi, or performs a shuttle-like function, by binding C3b/C4b-coated ICs and then transporting them to the liver and spleen. In these organs, the ICs are transferred from the erythrocyte to tissue macrophages, allowing the erythrocyte to return to the circulation for another round of clearance. CR1 on granulocytes and monocytes promotes IC adherence and phagocytosis. On B lymphocytes, tissue macrophages, and follicular dendritic cells (FDCs), CR1 facilitates trapping and processing of IC in lymphoid organs.

CR2 (CD21) binds iC3b and C3d. This receptor is expressed on B lymphocytes and FDCs, where it facilitates antigen localization and is a co-receptor for activation through B-cell antigen receptor. Coating of an antigen with several C3d fragments may enhance its immunogenicity up to 10,000-fold because of the above interactions (16). CR3 (CD11b/CD18) and CR4 (CD11c/CD18) bind to the cleavage fragment iC3b, formed by limited proteolytic degradation of C3b. Finally, the vasomodulatory and chemotactic effects of C3a and C5a (CD88) are due to their interaction with their respective typical G protein–coupled seven-transmembrane receptors.

Control of the Complement System

When unregulated, the complement system fires to exhaustion, a point well illustrated by inborn errors of several regulatory proteins such as the C1-inhibitor (hereditary angioedema with exhaustion of C4 and C2) and factor I (exhaustion of C3) deficiencies. Checks and balances occur at each of the major steps in the pathway (17–19). This regulation is designed to prevent excessive activation on one target, fluid-phase activation (i.e., no target) and activation on self (i.e., wrong target) but does not interfere with appropriate activation such as by Abs or lectins. The C1 inhibitor prevents chronic fluid-phase C1 activation. The C3 and C5 convertases are a focal point of regulation mediated by a family of proteins. These proteins include membrane proteins, decay-accelerating factor (CD55) and MCP (CD46) (Fig. 15.4), and plasma inhibitors, C4 binding protein (C4bp)

A. DAF: Decay Accelerating Activity

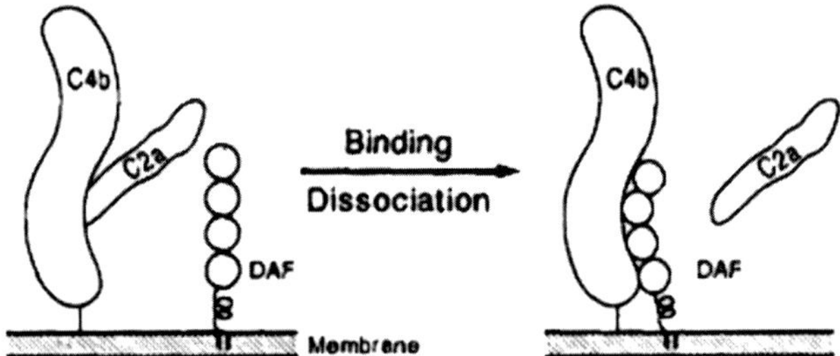

B. MCP: Cofactor Activity

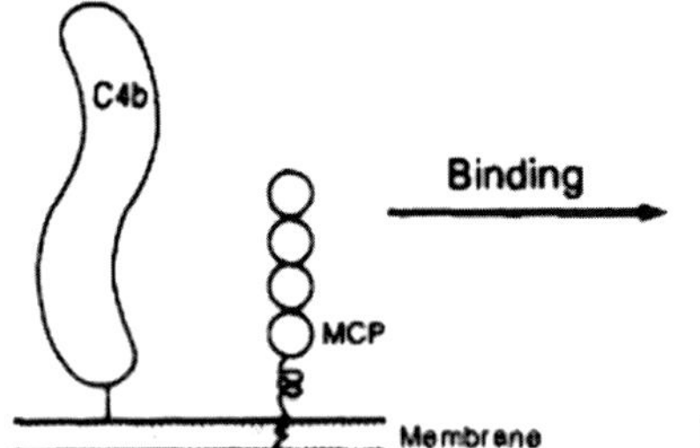

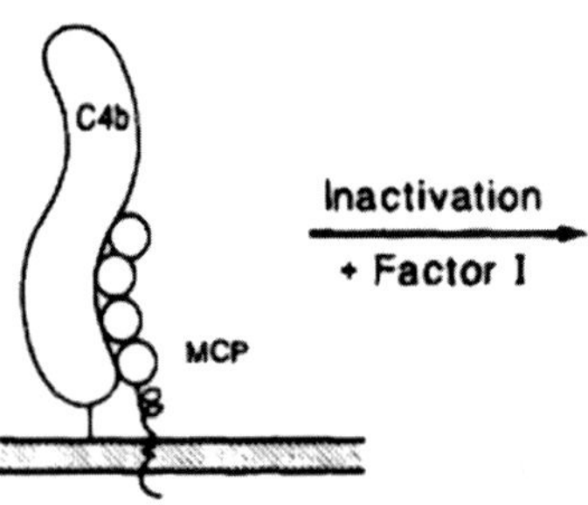

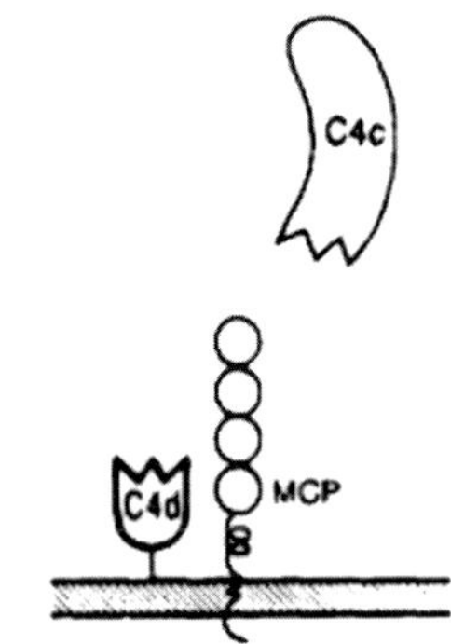

Figure 15.4. A,B: The classic pathway (CP) C3 convertase is shown. Decay-accelerating factor (DAF) displaces the protease, C2a, from C4b, and this C2a cannot rebind. To prevent C4b from interacting with a newly formed C2a, C4b is cleaved by membrane cofactor protein (MCP). The residual C4d has no known biologic activity. CPC5 convertase can be similarly inactivated. Moreover, alternative pathway C3 and C5 convertases are also disassembled in an identical fashion by DAF and MCP, except C3b is cleaved to iC3b rather than to C3dg. (Adapted from Liszewski MK, Farries TC, Lublin DM, et al. Control of the complement system. *Adv Immunol* 1996;61:201–283.)

and factor H. They function by dissociating the convertases (decay-accelerating activity) or by serving as a cofactor for limited proteolytic inactivation of C4b or C3b (cofactor activity) (Fig. 15.4). Microorganisms have captured complement regulators (e.g., pox viruses) or have evolved proteins (e.g., herpes viruses) that mimic these regulatory activities for the convertases. The MAC is also regulated by both a plasma and a cell-anchored protein. CD59, attached by a lipid anchor, or *greasy foot*, binds C8 and C9 to prevent MAC insertion. The plasma protein vitronectin (S-protein) binds and inactivates fluid-phase MAC. A consequence of these activities is that complement attack is focused on foreign surfaces (which usually lack complement regulators) but yet held in check on normal host cells and in body fluids.

It should be recalled, though, that the activation of the CP by Ab is so efficient that the inhibitors have modest effects on limiting damage by high-titer complement-fixing autoantibodies (20). In contrast, the regulators are very efficient at preventing the AP or its feedback loop from being engaged in plasma or on self-tissue.

After the complement system is activated, the regulators become the critical players relative to the magnitude of the local inflammatory reaction. Complement activation occurs in sepsis, ischemia-reperfusion injury, and IC syndromes. A complete or partial deficiency of a complement inhibitor has the potential to produce excessive and undesirable tissue injury secondary to inadequate complement regulation. In paroxysmal nocturnal hemoglobinuria, two complement regulators are deficient on human red blood cells. This leads to complement-mediated intravascular hemolysis (21). In sporadic and familial hemolytic uremic syndrome, there is a deficiency of either a fluid-phase (factor H) or a cell-tethered (MCP, CD46) inhibitor that predisposes to vascular injury (22,23). Surprisingly, and of great interest, heterozygotes are affected, implying that 50% of the normal expression level is not sufficient to regulate complement activation at sites of vascular injury in hemolytic uremic syndrome (24). In multiple animal models of ischemia-reperfusion injury, sepsis, and humoral autoimmunity, complement inhibition can reduce the magnitude of the tissue damage (25–27).

Participation of Complement in Adaptive Immunity

Complement activation is instrumental in the generation of a humoral immune response (28) (Table 15.4). Also, the CP likely is involved in maintenance of tolerance, as evidenced by analysis of C1q-, C4-, or C2-deficient individuals (who commonly present with SLE) and animals (who also have a predisposition to autoimmunity) (2–4,29,30). However, it is not understood how deficiency of these early components of the CP predispose to systemic lupus erythematosus.

Pepys in the 1970s showed that mice depleted of C3 by cobra venom factor had markedly impaired primary Ab responses (31). Similar results were then obtained in other animals and humans with deficiencies of C4, C2, or C3, as well as in animals with defective CR1 and CR2 (28). The major consequences of complement deficiency in these models were a variable but often low primary IgM response, a failure to class switch, and, on a second antigenic challenge, a lack of recall (memory). The defective response could, however, be overcome with larger doses of antigen.

To elaborate, Abs to mouse CR1/CR2 or a competing soluble CR2 (CD21) protein caused a similar defective immune response (32–35). Even more convincing, CR1/CR2 knockout mice had the same immune defect of a decreased primary Ab response, failure

TABLE 15.4. Physiologic Processes in Which Complement Plays an Instrumental Role

Initiation of an inflammatory response
Recruitment of phagocytes to the site of infection
Direct destruction of gram-negative bacteria
Assistance in phagocytosis
Promotion of phagocyte oxidative burst activity and granule release
Generation of a humoral immune response
Collaboration with antibodies in a range of the above-mentioned activities
Clearance of soluble immune complexes from the circulation
Regulation of self-tolerance/autoimmunity

Adapted from Nielsen CH, Leslie RG. Complement's participation in acquired immunity. *J Leukocyte Biol* 2002;72:249–261.

to class switch, and absent memory (28,36,37). In other studies, the immunization of mice in which C3 fragments (C3d) were coupled to a protein antigen (hen egg lysozyme) enhanced the immune response dramatically (10,000-fold greater than to antigen and 100-fold greater than to antigen in complete Freund's adjuvant) (16). These studies have been refined, confirmed, and extended by the use of knockout animals and reconstitution experiments (28).

Based on these results, two theories have arisen to explain these defects in the immune response in complement-deficient animals. The first is an abnormality in clearance of antigens—that is, inefficient transmittal of the antigen to a local lymph node or spleen for processing and retention by FDCs in germinal centers. The second explanation centers on the role of CR2 (C3dg receptor) in signaling through the B-lymphocyte antigen receptor. These hypothesized abnormalities overlap in part and may both contribute to the immune deficiency. The contributions of CR2 on B cells versus FDCs have also begun to be dissected by reconstitution studies. In such studies, B-cell deficiency of CD21 (CR2) most closely resembled the knockout, although a contribution of FDC to long-term memory was apparent (28,38–40).

In summary, C3b binding to an antigen enhances the immune response through at least three mechanisms: (a) the promotion of antigen uptake, processing, and presentation by antigen-presenting cells, (b) direct activation of B cells, and (c) facilitation of B-cell interactions with FDCs. The role of complement in promoting adaptive immunity is the subject of a detailed review by Nielsen and Leslie (28). These authors and others (4,6,29) also provide an analysis of the complement system in autoimmunity.

COMPLEMENT ACTIVATION IN HUMAN RHEUMATOID ARTHRITIS

B cells, antibodies, and complement activation were postulated to play a critical role in mediating synovial inflammation in the early days (1950–1975) of investigations into the immune basis of RA (41,42). However, from approximately 1975 until the turn of the century, T-cell–mediated immunity (the so-called type IV delayed hypersensitivity response) was thought to be the predominant system responsible for the synovial-based reaction in RA (43). A more prominent role for B cells, Ab, and complement has arisen again with the recognition that two animal models of RA are Ab and complement dependent (44,45). Further, C5 deficiency and a monoclonal Ab that inhibits C5 block collagen-induced arthritis (46,47). A humanized monoclonal Ab to C5 was modestly effective in a human RA trial (*personal communication*, 2000). The data on this trial are yet to be published, except in abstract form. However, with the success of methotrexate and tumor necrosis factor α and interleukin-1 inhibitors, the bar has been raised as to how efficacious a novel therapeutic agent needs to be in RA.

What is the evidence that complement mediates inflammation in human RA? A major observation has been that complement is activated locally, in synovial fluid and joint tissue (41,42,48–50). Thus, when the functional activity of joint fluid C4, C2, or C3 was determined, it was low compared to that obtained for a simultaneous antigenic measurement. These data and others established that complement components in RA joint fluid are often antigenically intact but functionally inactive. In other words, the components have been engaged in an immune reaction and are now nonfunctional. Further, complement activation fragments such as C3a, C5a, C4b, C3b, C3bi, C3d, C5b, C5b-C9, and others are elevated in RA joint fluid (41,48,51–54). Also, when synovial tissue is stained for complement, C1q and fragments derived from C4, factor B, and C3, as well as terminal components, are detected. The activation profile is primarily that of the CP (low C4 and C2), but there is substantial evidence for an AP contribution (41,49).

The clinical correlations with complement activation in RA (also in juvenile RA) were seropositivity and a more severe disease process. Rheumatoid factors (RFs) were present in the joint fluid as in the serum of these RF-positive individuals, possibly enriched by local synthesis (as are complement components) (50). ICs containing IgG, RF, and complement fragments have been repeatedly identified in joint fluid of such patients (41,42). In the 1960s and 1970s, immune reactants in RA were assessed with the techniques of protein chemistry. ICs of multiple sizes and shapes, many with potent complement-fixing capabilities, were characterized. These complexes contained RFs of both the IgM and IgG variety. Because RFs only bind to IgG when IgG is fixed to an antigen, it was postulated that the immunopathology of RA was as follows: an autoantibody (IgG) binds to an unknown joint antigen to form an IC, which in turn activates complement and binds RF. This hypothesis remains viable, as there is no definitive evidence to refute this type of an autoimmune process in RA. This proposal is even more attractive today because of increasing data pointing to IC binding to Fcγ receptors, contributing to the inflammatory process (more critical than complement in the mouse models of IC-mediated inflammation) (42,55–57). What is missing in this story is the identification of the alleged specific autoantibody and its joint centered target. Despite much effort, no candidate has withstood rigorous assessment.

Because of a failure to identify the target antigen, the pathogenesis of RA may be more akin to a serum sickness reaction. In other words, it is not an autoimmune attack on the synovial tissue per se, but synovial tissue is an innocent bystander or, perhaps, more appropriately, a sump for ICs. The ICs deposit (for largely unexplained reasons) in joints and then produce the inflammatory response. In addition to traditional serum sickness, SLE, essential mixed cryoglobulinemia, vasculitic syndromes, and subacute bacterial endocarditis are clinical examples in which circulating ICs deposit in joints. However, in contrast to RA, the synovitis in these conditions is usually transient and nondestructive.

Another hypothesis that would explain the joint findings in RA is that of an infectious agent (dead or alive) residing in joint tissue. The immunopathogenesis of RA would be relatively straightforward if either a foreign or self-antigen were identified to which the humoral immune system was responding. To date, neither has been found, but the experience with Lyme disease should keep us vigilant for this possibility.

ANIMAL MODELS

Immune Complex Deposition and Role of Rheumatoid Factors

In the usual serum sickness model in the rabbit using the bovine serum albumin/anti–bovine serum albumin, synovitis develops that is mediated by the deposition of IC and complement activation in joints. In the pre-antibiotic era, a serum sickness reaction was observed in children receiving horse serum containing antibodies to infectious agents, such as diphtheria. The human or rabbit clinical illness lasted 1 to 2 weeks, resolving as the host went into Ab excess and thereby cleared the foreign protein. If additional antigen was injected, an accelerated serum sickness reaction developed. In the case of SLE or mixed cryoglobulinemia secondary to chronic hepatitis B or C infection, chronic antigenemia is present.

In the Arthus model, Abs to a foreign antigen are raised, and then the antigen is reinjected into the immune host. If the antigen is injected in a joint, ICs form in the joint space, complement is activated, Fc receptors engaged, and an inflammatory reaction ensues. It is a transient process, unless more antigen is injected.

In the mouse, Fcγ receptors, not complement receptors, are responsible for most of the downstream effects of ICs, such as in the Arthus reaction (55–58). The argument, though, that one or the other is all important is an oversimplification and is not consistent with a large amount of data. Often, the development of inflammatory reaction requires both of these effector pathways to be engaged (for example, see K/BxN mouse model of RA described below). The contributions of Fcγ receptors versus those of complement depend, as has been demonstrated, on the species, the tissue site, the nature of the IC, and other to-be-defined factors (55–59).

In both clinical and experimental studies, RF is often called an *autoantibody*. This designation belies the biologic role it plays in a normal, healthy immune system. The purpose of RF is to amplify the interaction between IgG and an antigen—both by agglutination of the IgG-coated microbe and by further complement activation. This is particularly critical for the neonate, in whom RF amplifies effects of the maternal IgG that has crossed the placenta. This line of reasoning also explains why 10% to 15% of cord lymphocytes are making RFs. This scheme is also likely to be important in early aspects of an immune response where RF augments low levels of specific IgG. RF augments the effects of an IgG response to control a parasitic infection.

One line of investigation that led to the discovery of RF was, in retrospect, based on this amplification effect of RF on a low-level IgG response. Thus, serum from patients with RA containing RFs agglutinated streptococcal organisms, whereas control sera did not. Thus, the proposal arose that RA is caused by a streptococcal infection. As the phenomenon was further studied, it became apparent that the aggregation of the bacteria was caused by the presence of IgM RF. RF in the serum or joint fluid enhanced the low-level IgG response normally made in response to prior contact with these organisms. Thus, the agglutination observed was secondary to RF cross-linking IgGs bound to the organisms and not due to high levels of IgG Abs to streptococci. This ability of RF to amplify via agglutination particles bearing IgG became the basis of laboratory tests to detect this Ab. Two clinical points worthy of emphasis arise from this historic vignette. One is that RF can augment IgG-mediated reactions and it therefore could be contributing to tissue damage by this same mechanism in human RA, including causing additional complement activation. The second is that serologic tests to detect IgG antibodies to an antigen must be performed with caution in RF-positive sera. Most first-generation tests of this type do not take this issue into account so that false-positive serologic tests are common with sera of patients containing RF.

Collagen-Induced Arthritis

In the collagen-induced mouse and rat model of RA, the experimental animal is immunized with bovine type II collagen in complete Freund's adjuvant (47,49,60). After several weeks, an Ab response develops that cross-reacts with the animal's type II collagen in the joint. The inflammatory arthritis is predominantly in the small joints of the hind and frontpaws. Histopathologically, the synovitis resembles that of RA in humans, and, in the past, collagen was a leading candidate for the autoantigen of human RA. Most investigators presently do not believe this to be the case but, rather, that low levels of such Abs develop in RA patients secondary to cartilage damage.

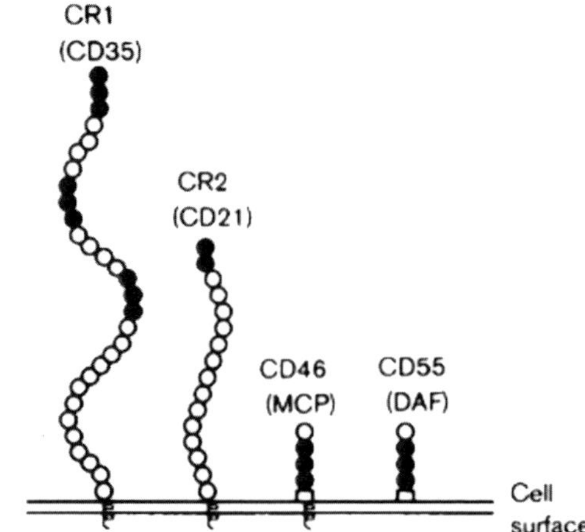

Figure 15.5. The structure of human complement membrane regulators and receptors in the regulator of complement activation family. The circles represent the approximately 60 amino acid repeating modules that are a prominent feature of the extramembranous portion of these proteins and contains the ligand-binding domains (*filled circles*). Filled circles indicate domains required for complement regulation or for binding of complement components. The open boxes at the juxtamembranous segment of CD46 and CD55 represent serine/threonine-rich regions that are extensively *O*-glycosylated. Decay-accelerating factor (DAF) is linked by a glycophospholipid, whereas CR1, CR2, and membrane cofactor protein (MCP) are type 1 transmembrane proteins. (Modified from Lindahl G, Sjobring U, Johnsson E. Human complement regulators: a major target for pathogenic organisms. *Curr Opin Immunol* 2000;12:44–51.)

Two overlapping and internally consistent types of data have established that complement is involved in the synovitis of collagen-induced arthritis. In the first, much as in human RA, complement activation products are prominent in the joint fluid and synovial tissue (49). In the second, disease is milder or absent in (a) C5-deficient mice (47), (b) mice treated with a monoclonal Ab to C5 (46), and (c) mice treated with the potent complement inhibitor known as *soluble CR1* (61). The C5 monoclonal Ab treatment also ameliorated established disease (46). Several issues require elaboration relative to these results. These results imply that C5a or C5b-C9 (MAC) or some combination of the two is responsible for the synovitis. A major contribution to disease pathogenesis from C3 activation products could also be anticipated as well, but this was not observed. In the case of the use of soluble CR1, it was delivered by gene therapy. CR1 blocks at the sequential steps of the C3 and C5 convertase formation, analogous to a combination of MCP and decay-accelerating factor (Figs. 15.4 and 15.5).

Mouse Model (K/BxN)

Since its original description (8), this spontaneous mouse model of RA has provided an important perspective of the pathogenesis of RA (15,44,45,62–74). It was generated by crossing the T-cell receptor (TCR) transgenic mouse line (officially known as *KRNxC56B1/6*) with the nonobese diabetic mouse strain. The original TCR recognized a bovine ribonuclease peptide presented by major histocompatibility complex class II molecule I-A^{g7}. In the context of nonobese diabetic derived I-A^{g7} major histocompatibility complex class II molecule, however, the K/BxN TCR recognizes the ubiquitously expressed glucose-6-phosphate isomerase (GPI) (a glycolytic pathway enzyme expressed by all cells). The important points are as follows: (a) the arthritis arises spontaneously, (b) the pathogenic autoantibodies are directed to GPI, (c) a destructive small joint arthritis not unlike human RA develops in these mice, (d) the synovitis can be transferred to other strains by Ab alone (the transfer model), and (e) the development of arthritis requires complement (15). Surprisingly, the CP is not the perpetrator, as mice deficient in C1q or C4 are as susceptible as wild type. In contrast, mice deficient in C3 or AP component factor B do not develop arthritis. Moreover, C5-deficient mice or mice treated with a monoclonal Ab to C5 do not develop arthritis in the transfer model. To locate the causative complement factors (C5b-C9 vs. C5a), C5a receptor knockout mice were studied (15), and they were protected from disease development. Interestingly, the CR1/CR2 or CR3 knockout mice were as susceptible as wild type. In summary, in this model, AP activation produces C5a, which interacts with its receptor to mediate the complement effect that is required for the disease to develop.

These data raise several interesting questions. Why does the autoantibody to GPI develop? Why does this Ab localize to the joint? Relative to the first question, a definitive answer is not yet available. For the latter, it can be shown that GPI is on the surface of synovial cells or cartilage (71,75). A few minutes after injection, the Abs bind directly to preexisting sources of exposed GPI in the joints of normal, healthy mice (75). C3 fragments colocalize to the site of the Ab binding in the front and rear limb joints. The disease process is then triggered at this location by subsequent AP activation and liberation of C5a.

Another important lesson from this model is the potential role of the complement regulatory proteins in allowing the disease to occur (15,44,45,71). For example, the pathogenic Ab also binds to the kidney glomerulus, but there was no concomitant C3b deposition or subsequent glomerulonephritis. The likely explanation for this finding is that local tissue inflammation requires not only the antigen accessibility to Ab but also a permissive local environment for complement activation. It is postulated that cartilage is relatively devoid of complement regulatory proteins so that the AP can be engaged. The CP is not activated in this model, presumably because most of the Ab is of the IgG1 subclass, which in the mouse is poorly complement fixing (in humans, IgG subclasses 1, 2, and 3 fix complement). Nevertheless, Abs bound to an antigen can protect the cascade from regulation by inhibitors (76). Therefore, although the basis for the autoantibody response is not known, this model has provided important insights into the role of the complement system and about how an autoantibody-mediated inflammatory arthritis could occur.

Another question raised by this model featuring GPI autoantibodies concerns the possibility that these same Abs are pathogenic in human RA. After the initial reports on this model, it was soon reported that 64% of RA patients had GPI antibodies in their serum, versus less than a few percent in non-RA patients or patients with Lyme disease or Sjögren's syndrome (72). These results, suggesting that the autoantigen of RA had finally been found, were not confirmed by two independent groups (63,68,71). One group detected only a very low level of reactivity (2 per 61 and less than 10 cases out of 461 in a survey of many types of rheumatic diseases, including approximately 200 with RA) (63). Both of these groups also pointed out several technical concerns in the original report, especially the use of a commercial preparation of GPI that may have been contaminated (63,68). The first-reporting group defended their data in a rebuttal and reported new data in which approximately 50% of RA sera reacted with a recombinant preparation of human GPI (63,72). The GPI Ab story in humans thus requires more investigation before concluding that it is the elusive autoantigen of human RA.

The differences between this mouse model and human RA should also be kept in mind: (a) the disease arises from an inbred mouse strain bearing a highly skewed population of TCRs that has been crossed to an autoimmune-prone mouse that gets spontaneous diabetes mellitus; (b) RFs are not present; (c) a more important role for innate immunity has been suggested than is the case for human RA; (d) although the presence of GPI Abs in RA is controversial, it seems doubtful at this juncture that GPI is the dominant autoantigen of human RA.

TABLE 15.5. Role of the Innate Immune System in the Initiation of Rheumatoid Arthritis

Nonspecific inflammatory conditions in the synovium may stimulate cytokine release from macrophages, leading to differentiation of dendritic cells into potent antigen-presenting cells.
Mature dendritic cells may present antigens to memory T cells in the synovium with induction of the T helper 1 or T helper 2 response.
Macrophages may carry fragments of bacteria, including immunostimulatory DNA, from mucosal surfaces of the body to the joints.
Local cytokine production by macrophages stimulated by bacteria secondarily activates dendritic cells, B cells, T cells, and natural killer cells.
Activation of the complement system in the joint enhances local inflammation and B-cell responses.

Adapted from Arend WP. The innate immune system in rheumatoid arthritis. *Arthritis Rheum* 2001;44:2224–2234.

Other Aspects of Innate Immunity and Rheumatoid Arthritis

This discussion has focused on the complement system as an example of innate immunity's involvement in RA. Other players in innate immunity—epithelial barriers and their Toll receptors, natural Abs, lectins such as CRP and MBL, $\gamma\delta$ T cells, natural killer cells, monocytes/macrophages, mast cells, granulocytes, cytokines, and dendritic cells—also contribute (Table 15.5). The important role of cytokines (Table 15.2), whether triggered by innate or acquired (or both) immune systems, is perhaps best exemplified by the success of anti–tumor necrosis factor therapies in the treatment of human RA. Granulocytes, mast cells, and monocytes/macrophages are prominent in joint tissues of RA patients. Granulocytes (73) and mast cells (77) are necessary in the GPI mouse model. As pointed out earlier, natural Abs and lectins trigger the complement system. CRP and MBL bind to damaged tissue and in so doing activate complement (10,11,78). The AP would then serve as feedback loop to amplify the initial deposition of C3b produced by these cascades. CRP and many other (as-yet-undiscovered) lectins could bind to infected or otherwise abnormal synovial/cartilage tissue and initiate the complement cascade (7). The potential role of most of these factors has been reviewed by Arend (79).

CONCLUSION

The study of the complement system has undergone a renaissance since the 1980s in part due to the identification of novel complement regulators and receptors (17) and the rediscovery of its important role in innate immunity and in instructing adaptive immunity (28). It has also undergone a reawakening as a mediator of tissue damage in RA (15). In this case, it is largely thanks to the discovery of a new spontaneous model of RA (15), as well as a reevaluation of older models in which knockout animals bearing targeted gene deletion provide more definitive data relative to the complement system causing joint pathology. Whether RA is a reaction to a not particularly dangerous foreign pathogen, an autoimmune process, or some other as-yet-undefined immunologic phenomenon, complement activation appears to be a key mediator in RA. One plausible scenario is that the antigen under attack in RA is located in a microenvironment relatively devoid of complement regulators.

In summary, from the complement system's point of view, one can envision two general scenarios as to how an RA-like illness could develop. In the first, the individual inherits a defective system to regulate complement system. The patient then develops autoantibodies to a joint antigen or another type of joint-damaging process. Excessive tissue damage (i.e., disease) may then occur in this individual who lacks a full set of these regulators. In the other, the immune attack overwhelms the complement inhibitors, especially if the site of inflammation is one with a relative deficiency of such regulatory proteins.

REFERENCES

1. Figueroa JE, Densen P. Infectious diseases associated with complement deficiencies. *Clin Microbiol Rev* 1991;4:359–395.
2. Barilla-LaBarca ML, Atkinson JP. Rheumatic syndromes associated with complement deficiency. *Curr Opin Rheumatol* 2003;15:55–60.
3. Sullivan KE. Complement deficiency and autoimmunity. *Curr Opin Pediatr* 1998;10:600–606.
4. Pickering MC, Botto M, Taylor PR, et al. Systemic lupus erythematosus, complement deficiency, and apoptosis. *Adv Immunol* 2000;76:227–324.
5. Carroll MC. A protective role for innate immunity in autoimmune disease. *Clin Immunol* 2000;95:S30–S38.
6. Ochsenbein AF, Zinkernagel RM. Natural antibodies and complement link innate and acquired immunity. *Immunol Today* 2000;21:624–630.
7. Garred P, Madsen HO, Marquart H, et al. Two edged role of mannose binding lectin in rheumatoid arthritis: a cross sectional study. *Rheumatol* 2000;27:26–34.
8. Kouskoff V, Korganow AS, Duchatelle V, et al. Organ-specific disease provoked by systemic autoimmunity. *Cell* 1996;87:811–822.
9. Atkinson JP. The complement system rises again. *Cell* 1999;98:722–724.
9a. Silverstein AM. *A history of immunology*. San Diego: Academic Press, 1989.
10. DuClos TW. Function of C-reactive protein. *Ann Med* 2000;32:274–278.
11. Atkinson JP. C-reactive protein: a rheumatologist's friend revisited. *Arthritis Rheum* 2001;44:995–996.
12. Ollert MW, Kadlec JV, David K, et al. Antibody-mediated complement activation on nucleated cells. A quantitative analysis of the individual reaction steps. *J Immunol* 1994;153:2213–2221.
13. Fujita T. Evolution of the lectin-complement pathway and its role in innate immunity. *Nat Rev Immunol* 2002;2:346–353.
14. Turner MW. Mannose-binding lectin: the pluripotent molecule of the innate immune system. *Immunol Today* 1996;17:532–540.
15. Ji H, Ohmura K, Mahmood U, et al. Arthritis critically dependent on innate immune system players. *Immunity* 2002;16:157–168.
16. Dempsey PW, Allison ME, Akkaraju S, et al. C3d of complement as a molecular adjuvant: bridging innate and acquired immunity. *Science* 1996;271:348–350.
17. Liszewski MK, Farries TC, Lublin DM, et al. Control of the complement system. *Adv Immunol* 1996;61:201–283.
18. Morgan BP, Harris CL. *Complement regulatory proteins*. San Diego: Harcourt Brace & Company, 1999.
19. Parker CM. *Membrane defenses against attack by complement and perforins*. Berlin: Springer-Verlag, 1992.
20. Barilla-LaBarca ML, Liszewski MK, Lambris JD, et al. Role of membrane cofactor protein (CD46) in regulation of C4b and C3b deposited on cells. *J Immunol* 2002;168:6298–6304.
21. Atkinson JP, Bessler M. Paroxysmal nocturnal hemoglobinuria. In: Stamatoyannopoulos G, ed. *The molecular basis of blood disease*, 3rd ed. Philadelphia: W.B. Saunders Company, 2000:564–577.
22. Zipfel PF, Skerka C, Caprioli J, et al. Complement factor H and hemolytic uremic syndrome. *Int Immunopharmacol* 2001;1:461–468.
23. Caprioli J, Bettinaglio P, Zipfel PF, et al. The molecular basis of familial hemolytic uremic syndrome: mutation analysis of factor H gene reveals a hot spot in short consensus repeat 20. *J Am Soc Nephrol* 2001;12:297–307.
24. Richards A, Kemp EJ, Liszewski MK, et al. Mutations in human complement regulator, membrane cofactor protein (CD46), predispose to development of familial hemolytic uremic syndrome. *Proc Natl Acad Sci U S A* 2003;28:12966–12971.
25. Bhole D, Stahl GL. Therapeutic potential of targeting the complement cascade in critical care medicine. *Crit Care Med* 2003;31:S97–S104.
26. Liszewski MK, Atkinson JP. Novel complement inhibitors. *Exp Opin Investig Drugs* 1998;7:323–332.
27. Klickstein LB, Moore FD Jr., Atkinson JP. Therapeutic inhibition of complement activation with emphasis on drugs in clinical trials. In: Austen KF, Burakoff SJ, Strom TB, et al., eds. *Therapeutic immunology*. Malden, MA Blackwell Science, Inc., 2000:287–301.
28. Nielsen CH, Leslie RG. Complement's participation in acquired immunity. *J Leukoc Biol* 2002;72:249–261.
29. Carroll MC. A protective role for innate immunity in autoimmune disease. *Clin Immunol* 2000;95:S30–S38.
30. O'Neil KM. Complement deficiency. *Clin Rev Allergy Immunol* 2000;19:83–108.
31. Pepys MB. Role of complement in induction of antibody production *in vivo*: effect of cobra venom factor and other C3-reactive agents on thymus dependent and thymus independent antibody responses. *J Exp Med* 1974;140:126–145.
32. Hebell T, Ahearn JM, Fearon DT. Suppression of the immune response by a soluble complement receptor of B lymphocytes. *Science* 1991;254:102–105.
33. Gustavsson S, Kinoshita T, Heyman B. Antibodies to murine complement receptor 1 and 2 can inhibit the antibody response in vivo without inhibiting T helper cell induction. *J Immunol* 1995;154:6524–6528.
34. Thyphronitis G, Kinoshita T, Inoue K, et al. Modulation of mouse complement receptors 1 and 2 suppresses antibody responses in vivo. *J Immunol* 1991;147:224–230.
35. Heyman B, Wiersma EJ, Kinoshita T. In vivo inhibition of the antibody response by a complement receptor-specific monoclonal antibody. *J Exp Med* 1990;172:665–668.
36. Ahearn JM, Fischer MB, Croix D, et al. Disruption of the CD21 locus results in a reduction in B-1a cells and in an impaired B cell response to T-dependent antigen. *Immunity* 1996;4:251–262.
37. Molina H, Holers VM, Li B, et al. Markedly impaired humoral immune response in mice deficient in complement receptors 1 and 2. *Proc Natl Acad Sci U S A* 1996;93:3357–3361.
38. Croix D, Ahearn J, Rosengard A, et al. Antibody response to a T-dependent antigen requires B cell expression of complement receptors. *J Exp Med* 1996;183:1857–1864.
39. Fang Y, Xu C, Fu YX, et al. Expression of complement receptors 1 and 2 on follicular dendritic cells is necessary for the generation of a strong antigen-specific IgG response. *J Immunol* 1998;160:5273–5279.
40. Applequist SE, Dahlstrom J, Jiang N, et al. Antibody production in mice deficient for complement receptors 1 and 2 can be induced by IgG/Ag and IgE/Ag, but not IgM/Ag complexes. *J Immunol* 2000;165:2398–2403.
41. Zvaifler NJ. The immunopathology of joint inflammation in rheumatoid arthritis. *Adv Immunol* 1973;16:265–336.
42. Moxley G, Ruddy S. Immune complexes and complement. In: Kelley WN, Harris ED, Ruddy S, et al., eds. *Textbook of rheumatology*, 5th ed. Philadelphia: W.B. Saunders Company, 1997:228–240.
43. Firestein GS, Zvaifler NJ. How important are T cells in chronic rheumatoid synovitis? *Arthritis Rheum* 1990;33:768–773.
44. Corr M, Firestein GS. Innate immunity as a hired gun: but is it rheumatoid arthritis? *J Exp Med* 2002;195:F33–F35.
45. Hirano T. Revival of the autoantibody model in rheumatoid arthritis. *Nat Immunol* 2002;3:342–344.
46. Wang Y, Rollins SA, Madri JA, et al. Anti-C5 monoclonal antibody therapy prevents collagen-induced arthritis and ameliorates established disease. *Proc Natl Acad Sci U S A* 1995;92:8955–8959.
47. Wang Y, Kristan J, Hao L, et al. A role for complement in antibody-mediated inflammation: C5-deficient DBA/1 mice are resistant to collagen-induced arthritis. *J Immunol* 2000;164:4340–4347.
48. Brodeur JP, Ruddy S, Schwartz LB, et al. Synovial fluid levels of complement SC5b-9 and fragment Bb are elevated in patients with rheumatoid arthritis. *Arthritis Rheum* 1991;34:1531–1537.
49. Linton SM, Morgan BP. Complement activation and inhibition in experimental models of arthritis. *Mol Immunol* 1999;36:905–914.
50. Neumann E, Barnum SR, Tarner IH, et al. Local production of complement proteins in rheumatoid arthritis synovium. *Arthritis Rheum* 2002;46:934–945.
51. Davies ET, Nasaruddin BA, Alhaq A, et al. Clinical application of new technique that measures C4d for assessment of activation of classical complement pathway. *J Clin Pathol* 1988;41:143–147.
52. Hogasen K, Mollnes TE, Harboe M, et al. Terminal complement pathway activation and low lysis inhibitors in rheumatoid arthritis synovial fluid. *J Rheumatol* 1995;22:24–28.
53. Konttinen YT, Ceponis A, Meri S, et al. Complement in acute and chronic arthritides: assessment of C3c, C9, and protectin (CD59) in synovial membrane. *Ann Rheum Dis* 1996;55:888–894.
54. Petersen NE, Elmgreen J, Teisner B, et al. Activation of classical pathway complement in chronic inflammation. Elevated levels of circulating C3d and C4d split products in rheumatoid arthritis and Crohn's disease. *Acta Med Scand* 1988;223:557–560.
55. Ravetch JV. A full complement of receptors in immune complex diseases. *J Clin Investig* 2002;110:1759–1761.
56. Shushakova N, Skokowa J, Schulman J, et al. C5a anaphylatoxin is a major regulator of activating versus inhibitory FcgammaRs in immune complex-induced lung disease. *J Clin Investig* 2002;110:1823–1830.
57. Baumann U, Chouchakova N, Gewecke B, et al. Distinct tissue site-specific requirements of mast cells and complement components C3/C5a receptor in IgG immune complex-induced injury of skin and lung. *J Immunol* 2001;167:1022–1027.
58. Takai T. Roles of Fc receptors in autoimmunity. *Nat Rev Immunol* 2002;2:580–592.
59. Ravetch JV, Bolland S. IgG Fc receptors. *Ann Rev Immunol* 2001;19:275–290.
60. Terato K, Hasty KA, Reife RA, et al. Induction of arthritis with monoclonal antibodies to collagen. *J Immunol* 1992;148:2103–2108.

61. Dreja H, Annenkov A, Chernajovsky Y. Soluble complement receptor 1 (CD35) delivered by retrovirally infected syngeneic cells or by naked DNA injection prevents the progression of collagen-induced arthritis. *Arthritis Rheum* 2000;43:1698–1709.
62. Basu D, Horvath S, Matsumoto I, et al. Molecular basis for recognition of an arthritic peptide and a foreign epitope on distinct MHC molecules by a single TCR. *J Immunol* 2000;164:5788–5796.
63. Schubert D, Schmidt M, Zaiss D, et al. Autoantibodies to GPI and creatine kinase in RA. *Nat Immunol* 2002;3:411–413.
64. Mangialaio S, Ji H, Korganow AS, et al. The arthritogenic T cell receptor and its ligand in a model of spontaneous arthritis. *Arthritis Rheum* 1999;42:2517–2523.
65. Matsumoto I, Staub A, Benoist C, et al. Arthritis provoked by linked T and B cell recognition of a glycolytic enzyme. *Science* 1999;286:1732–1735.
66. Ji H, Gauguier D, Ohmura K, et al. Genetic influences on the end-stage effector phase of arthritis. *J Exp Med* 2001;194:321–330.
67. Corr M, Crain B. The role of FcgammaR signaling in the K/BxN serum transfer model of arthritis. *J Immunol* 2002;169:6604–6609.
68. Kassahn D, Kolb C, Solomon S, et al. Few human autoimmune sera detect GPI. *Nat Immunol* 2002;3:411–413.
69. Kyburz D, Carson DA, Corr M. The role of CD40 ligand and tumor necrosis factor alpha signaling in the transgenic K/BxN mouse model of rheumatoid arthritis. *Arthritis Rheum* 2000;43:2571–2577.
70. Maccioni M, Zeder-Lutz G, Huang H, et al. Arthritogenic monoclonal antibodies from K/BxN mice. *J Exp Med* 2002;195:1071–1077.
71. Matsumoto I, Maccioni M, Lee DM, et al. How antibodies to a ubiquitous cytoplasmic enzyme may provoke joint-specific autoimmune disease. *Nat Immunol* 2002;3:360–365.
72. Schaller M, Burton DR, Ditzel HJ. Autoantibodies to GPI in rheumatoid arthritis: linkage between an animal model and human disease. *Nat Immunol* 2001;2:746–753.
73. Wipke BT, Allen PM. Essential role of neutrophils in the initiation and progression of a murine model of rheumatoid arthritis. *J Immunol* 2001;167:1601–1608.
74. Pettit AR, Ji H, von Stechow D, et al. TRANCE/RANKL knockout mice are protected from bone erosion in a serum transfer model of arthritis. *Am J Pathol* 2001;159:1689–1699.
75. Wipke BT, Wang Z, Kim J, et al. Dynamic visualization of a joint-specific autoimmune response through positron emission tomography. *Nat Immunol* 2002;3:366–372.
76. Ratnoff WD, Fearon DT, Austen KF. The role of antibody in the activation of the alternative complement pathway. *Springer Semin Immunopathol* 1983;6:361–371.
77. Lee DM, Friend DS, Gurish MF, et al. Mast cells: a cellular link between autoantibodies and inflammatory arthritis. *Science* 2002;297:1689–1692.
78. Garred P, Madsen HO, Halberg P, et al. The association of variant mannose-binding lectin genotypes with radiographic outcome in rheumatoid arthritis. *Arthritis Rheum* 2000;43:515–521.
79. Arend WP. The innate immune system in rheumatoid arthritis. *Arthritis Rheum* 2001;44:2224–2234.

CHAPTER 16

T Cells in the Pathogenesis of Rheumatoid Arthritis

Hendrik Schulze-Koops and Peter E. Lipsky

Sustained specific immunity against self-antigens is the pathogenetic basis of many rheumatic diseases. As a consequence of persistent autoimmune responses, local inflammation and cellular infiltration occur, and, subsequently, tissue damage results. Whereas the specific autoantigen(s) eliciting the detrimental immune reactions have rarely been defined, it has become clear that the mechanisms resulting in the destruction of tissue and the loss of organ function during the course of an autoimmune disease are essentially the same as in protective immunity against invasive microorganisms. Of fundamental importance in initiating, controlling, and driving these specific immune responses are CD4 T cells. Currently available data provide compelling evidence for a major role of CD4 T cells in the initiation and perpetuation of chronic inflammation in rheumatoid arthritis (RA). Moreover, appropriate T-cell–directed therapies have been used with clinical success in the treatment of RA.

T CELLS, T-CELL DEVELOPMENT, AND T-CELL SUBSETS

T cells are lymphocytes that originate from the common lymphoid progenitor in the bone marrow and migrate as immature precursor T cells via the bloodstream into the thymus. Here, T cells pass through a series of maturation steps that include the rearrangement of their antigen receptor [*T-cell receptor* (TCR)] genes and distinct changes in the expression of cell-surface receptors, such as the CD3 signaling complex and the co-receptors CD4 and CD8 (1). During maturation, more than 98% of the thymocytes die by apoptosis, as the developing T cells undergo positive selection for their TCR's compatibility with self–major histocompatibility (MHC) molecules, and negative selection against those T cells that express TCRs reactive to autoantigenic peptides (2). T cells that survive selection lose expression of either CD4 or CD8, increase the level of expression of the TCR, and leave the thymus to form the peripheral T-cell repertoire. Thus, mature postthymic T cells are characterized by the expression of a disulfide-linked heterodimeric TCR, the CD3 complex consisting of four invariant transmembrane polypeptides (designated γδεε), and one of the co-receptors, CD4 or CD8 (1–3). Whereas the TCR confers antigen specificity to the T cell, the CD3 complex mediates signaling and is also necessary for the surface expression of the TCR. The TCR/CD3 complex is associated with a largely intracytoplasmic homodimer of ζ chains that are critical for maximum signaling (4). The co-receptors, CD4 and CD8, bind to invariant sites of the MHC class II or I molecules on antigen-presenting cells (APC), respectively, stabilize the MHC-peptide-TCR complex during T-cell activation and, thus, increase the sensitivity of a T cell for activation by MHC-presented antigen by approximately 100-fold (5). The cytoplasmic domains of CD4 and CD8 are constitutively associated with the src-family tyrosine kinase $p56^{lck}$, which phosphorylates particular recognition motifs within the CD3 complex (denoted *immunoreceptor tyrosine-based activation motifs*), thereby promoting T-cell activation.

In humans, the vast majority of peripheral blood T cells expresses TCRs consisting of α and β chains (αβ *T cells*). The TCR α and β polypeptide chains each consists of a variable (V) region, a joining region, and a carboxyl terminal constant region. Extensive somatic DNA recombination of V and joining region gene segments is responsible for the enormous structural TCR diversity that is required for reactivity to the huge arsenal of potential antigens. The TCR loci are organized in a way that TCR diversity is concentrated on the third hypervariable regions [*complementarity determining region*-3 (CDR3)] of the TCR α and β chains. The CDR3 regions of the TCR α and β chains form the center of the antigen-binding site of the TCR. An αβ TCR, however, does not bind antigen directly (in contrast to a B-cell receptor) but recognizes small peptide fragments that have been generated from protein antigens. Those small peptides are presented by MHC molecules on the surface of an APC. MHC molecules are membrane glycoproteins that are encoded by several closely linked, highly polymorphic genes. The MHC molecules display great genetic variation within the population. The expression of polymorphic MHC molecules defines immunologic identity of an individual and increases the range of pathogen-derived peptides that can be bound by MHC and presented to T cells. The phenomenon that T cells simultaneously recognize peptide antigen and parts of the particular presenting MHC molecule is referred to as *MHC restriction*. Whereas MHC class I molecules are virtually expressed on all nucleated cells, MHC class II expression is restricted to APC and activated T cells in humans. MHC class I molecules bind antigens that are generated by the particular cells themselves, as well as antigens from intracellular pathogens that reside in the cytoplasm; they present their antigens to CD8 T cells. MHC class II molecules, in contrast, present antigens derived from ingested extracellular bacteria or proteins to CD4 T cells.

A small group of peripheral T cells bears an alternative TCR composed of γ and δ chains (γδ *T cells*). αβ and γδ T cells diverge early in T-cell development in the thymus. Whereas αβ T cells are responsible for the classic helper or cytotoxic T-cell responses, the function of the γδ T cells within the immune system is largely unknown. In contrast to αβ TCRs, γδ TCRs appear to recognize antigen directly, similar to immunoglobulins (Igs), but do not require presentation by an MHC protein or other molecules and do not depend on antigen processing. In fact, some γδ T cells may recognize nonpeptide molecules, such as lipoglycans derived from bacteria or phosphorylated lipid derivatives of mycobacteria. The diversity of the γδ TCR is limited, suggesting that the ligands for the γδ TCR are conserved and invariant. Some γδ T cells do not express CD8 or CD4, whereas others express the CD8 α chain but not CD8 β. Because of their distinct antigen recognition pattern, their preferential localization in the epithelium, and their ability to secrete a variety of cytokines and to mount cytolytic responses, γδ T cells may contribute to the first line of host defense, arguably at the intersection between innate and adaptive immunity. On the other hand, γδ T cells have also been shown to recognize self-peptides, such as stress-associated antigens expressed on epithelial cells, tumor lines, and primary carcinomas. Recognition of self-peptides and the production of cytokines early during an immune response indicate that γδ T cells might play a role in the development of an immune response against self-tissue. In fact, recent studies have indicated that γδ T cells promote B-cell–mediated systemic autoimmune diseases in MRL/lpr mice, a model system for systemic lupus erythematosus (6). On the other hand, γδ T cells may also play a role in controlling immunity, as mice deficient in γδ T cells have exaggerated responses to pathogens and, notably, to self-tissues (7). Moreover, γδ T cells can tolerize pathogenic autoimmune αβ T cells in the nonobese diabetic mouse (8) and in a rat autoimmune uveitis model (9). Together, the data suggest that γδ T cells might play a role in regulating an autoimmune response, although the precise outcome appears to depend on the particular γδ T-cell clone.

γδ T Cells in Rheumatoid Inflammation

γδ T cells have been implicated in the pathogenesis of RA by several observations. In RA patients, circulating γδ T cells show an activated phenotype, as indicated by reduced expression of the CD3 complex and the Fcγ receptor III (CD16) and elevated levels of MHC class II (10,11). This phenotype, however, is not unique to RA, as the majority of peripheral γδ T cells also has an activated phenotype in healthy individuals (6). However, whereas the data regarding the frequencies of peripheral γδ T cells in RA and their association with disease activity are highly controversial (12–15), an increase in γδ T cells in the synovial infiltrates appears to be a characteristic of rheumatoid synovial inflammation (16,17). In one study, up to 14% of the infiltrating synovial T cells were identified as γδ T cells, and synovia with increased γδ TCR cells had an increased tissue inflammation score, compared to RA synovia with few γδ T cells (16). Importantly, the inflamed synovium of RA patients contained γδ T cells, which expressed particular V chains, for example, Vγ3 or Vδ1. As the frequencies of Vγ3 or Vδ1 expressing γδ T cells in the peripheral circulation of the same patients were lower than in the synovium, these data suggest that γδ T cells are clonally expanded in the joints, presumably in response to their locally expressed specific antigen. Alternatively, Vγ3 or Vδ1 expressing γδ T cells might have preferentially migrated into the synovium, where they could have contributed to inflammation (17–19). Taken together, some phenotypic abnormalities might suggest a role of γδ T cells in the pathogenesis of RA. However, the function of γδ T cells, in particular of synovial γδ T cells, and their contribution to rheumatoid inflammation is still as elusive as the nature of their specific antigen(s).

αβ T-Cell Subsets

For the remainder of this chapter, we refer to αβ T cells when using the term *T cell*, unless explicitly mentioned otherwise. αβ TCR expressing T cells that survive dual selection in the thymus can be divided into two major subgroups, characterized by the expression of either CD4 or CD8. Mature CD4 T cells recognize peptides presented by MHC class II on professional APC, such as B cells, dendritic cells, and macrophages. CD4 T cells primarily function as regulators of other immune cells either by direct cell–cell contact or through secreted cytokines. For their function, CD4 T cells are termed *T helper (Th) cells*. CD8 T cells, on the other hand, respond to antigens bound on MHC class I molecules and are programmed to become cytotoxic effector cells that kill infected target cells. CD8 T cells are, therefore, named *cytotoxic T cells*. Both CD4 and CD8 T cells continuously recirculate through the body from the peripheral blood to secondary lymphoid organs as they search for the presentation of their specific antigen. T cells that emerge from the thymus belong to the naïve T-cell pool that consists of T cells that have never encountered their specific antigen. Naïve T cells are long lived, have a restricted function [for example, CD4-naïve T cells only produce interleukin (IL)-2], but have stringent requirements for activation. In humans, naïve T cells are characterized phenotypically by the expression of the long isoform of CD45, CD45RA. Naïve T cells are normally restricted to recirculate between the blood and secondary lymphoid tissues, although, in some autoimmune diseases, they may also accumulate in chronically inflamed tissues.

In a simplified view of T-cell activation, the recognition of the peptide-MHC complex by a TCR induces clustering of the TCR in concert with other cell-surface receptors. Engagement of the TCR induces the activation of signaling cascades that are transmitted into the nucleus to cause changes in the transcriptional program of the T cell. Naïve T cells, however, require a second signal for activation, which is generally contributed by professional APC in secondary lymphoid organs. The second signal provides an independent stimulus that is triggered by ligation of nonpolymorphic cell-surface receptors. Extensive work has demonstrated that the 44-kd glycoprotein, CD28, is the major co-stimulatory molecule involved in T-cell activation (20). CD28 co-stimulation lowers the threshold required for T-cell activation, increases the expression of lymphokine messenger RNAs (mRNAs), in particular those for IL-2 and IL-4 (21–23), and regulates the expression of Bcl-x_L (24), CD152 [*cytolytic T lymphocyte–associated antigen* (CTLA)-4] (25), the high-affinity receptor for IL-2 (26), and CD154 (CD40 ligand) (27), all of which contribute to successful progression of T-cell responses. On proper activation, naïve T cells proliferate and differentiate into specialized effector cells. Differentiation of T cells is characterized by a number of phenotypic and functional alterations, such as a reduction in activation requirements, alteration in migratory capacities, changes in life span, and secretion of effector cytokines [for example, IL-4 and interferon (IFN) γ] or expression of other effector functions. Most activated naïve T cells become short-lived effector cells, but some enter the long-lived memory T-cell pool. Memory T cells, in humans, can be characterized by the expression of the short isoform of CD45, CD45RO. Memory cells respond more rapidly to antigen challenge, express a diverse array of effector functions, and do not require co-stimulation for activation. Thus, memory T cells do not depend on the interaction with professional APC for activation, provided their specific antigen can be presented in the context of the appropriate MHC molecules by nonprofessional APC.

CYTOTOXIC (CD8 αβ) T CELLS IN RHEUMATOID INFLAMMATION

CD8 T cells play a major role in immune responses. Their natural function is related to protection against viral infections and tumors. CD8 T cells perform this function by cytotoxic damage of target cells expressing MHC class I molecules and the relevant antigenic peptide. As almost all cells express MHC class I molecules, it is clear that there is great potential for tissue damage. In addition, activated CD8 T cells can produce very high levels of tumor necrosis factor (TNF) and IFN-γ, which may contribute directly or indirectly to target cell destruction in autoimmune diseases.

Although the importance of CD8 T cells in the pathogenesis of RA has not extensively been evaluated, some recent evidence suggests that autoreactive CD8 T cells might contribute to rheumatoid inflammation. Whereas the number of CD8 T cells in the peripheral blood of RA patients is not substantially different compared to healthy controls, the population of circulating CD8 T cells shows a remarkable alteration in their TCR repertoire. This alteration is particularly evident in a subgroup of CD8 cells expressing CD57 (28–30). CD57$^+$CD8 T cells accumulate with the duration of the disease in the peripheral blood and the synovial fluid and show especially high levels in knee joint fluid and joint adjacent bone marrow (29). Although oligoclonal expansion is a common feature of the CD57$^+$CD8 T-cell population (31), the extent of oligoclonality involving Vβ3 TCR gene segments in RA is striking: 50% of the RA patients have evidence for oligoclonality in the Vβ3 TCR family, compared with 4% of healthy controls (30). In addition, unrelated RA patients were identified as carrying clonally dominant CD8 T-cell β receptors that were identical in their amino acid sequence, suggesting selection by a common antigen (30). Predominant CD8 T-cell clones from the synovial membrane could be followed in serial samples over almost 1 year (32). As the identity of the antigen(s) has not been defined, it remains to be shown whether these CD8 cells were selected, for example, by self-antigen relevant to the pathogenesis of RA or by an environmental antigen independent of the disease. In fact, enrichment of CD8 T cells specific for epitopes from the Epstein-Barr virus lytic cycle proteins was seen within the synovial fluid from patients with RA and also from patients with psoriatic arthritis and osteoarthritis (33). CD8 T cells specific for cytomegalovirus, Epstein-Barr virus, and influenza virus were enriched in the synovial fluid, compared with peripheral blood in RA patients (34). Clonal or oligoclonal populations of CD8 T cells were found to dominate the responses to these viral epitopes in the synovial fluid from RA patients. These observations may support the hypothesis that restricted TCR usage by large populations of virus-specific T cells provides one explanation for the presence of clonally expanded CD8 T cells within the joints of patients with inflammatory arthritis. Therefore, T-cell clonality at a site of inflammation may reflect enrichment for memory T cells specific for foreign antigens, rather than proliferation of autoreactive T cells specific for self-antigen. Thus, the precise function of oligoclonally expanded CD8 T cells in RA remains to be determined. Of interest, oligoclonally expanded CD8 T cells expressing TCRs encoded by the Vα12 gene were shown to be autoreactive, since they recognized autologous, but not allogeneic, APCs (35). However, as these autoreactive CD8 T cells secreted IL-4 and IL-10, they might be involved in regulation of immunity, rather than aggravation.

Regardless of the antigen specificity of clonally expanded CD8 T cells in RA, synovial CD8 T cells have been implicated in disease progression by two different observations. CD8 T cells from the synovial fluid of RA patients include significant amounts of IFN-γ–producing effectors cell that might contribute to sustained inflammation by secreting proinflammatory cytokines (36). It has also been shown that CD8 T cells may regulate the structural integrity and functional activity of germinal center–like structures in ectopic lymphoid follicles within the synovial membrane (37,38). Activated CD8 T cells might, therefore, be involved in aggravating pathologic responses in rheumatoid synovitis.

Although the accumulated data may indicate a role of CD8 T cells in rheumatoid inflammation, studies in animals deficient in CD4 or CD8 have clearly demonstrated limited importance for CD8 T cells in initiating and maintaining autoimmune inflammatory arthritis. Whereas B10.Q mice lacking CD4 are less susceptible to collagen-induced arthritis (CIA), but not completely resistant, the CD8 deficiency has no significant impact on the disease. No difference in the development of late-occurring relapses was noted (39). Moreover, in mice transgenic for the RA susceptibility gene HLA-DQ8, CD4-deficient mice were resistant to developing CIA, whereas CD8-deficient mice developed disease with increased incidence and greater severity (40). These data indicate that CD8 T cells are not only incapable of initiating CIA but may have a regulatory or protective effect on autoimmune inflammation.

HELPER (CD4 αβ) T CELLS IN RHEUMATOID INFLAMMATION

RA is a chronic systemic autoimmune disease that is characterized by persistent intense immunologic activity, local destruction of bone and cartilage, the accumulation of activated leukocytes within the inflamed synovium, and a variety of systemic manifestations (41–43). It has become clear that the mechanisms resulting in the destruction of tissue and the loss of organ function during the course of an autoimmune disease are essentially the same as in protective immunity against invasive microorganisms. Of fundamental importance in initiating, controlling, and driving these specific immune responses are CD4 T cells. CD4 T cells are activated by an antigen (i.e., peptide), recognized specifically by their TCR if presented in the context of a specific MHC class II molecule on the surface of an APC. Once activated, CD4 T cells differentiate into specialized effector cells and become the central regulators of specific immune responses. CD4 T cells, therefore, have been implicated in playing a central role in RA for a number of reasons (Table 16.1). For example, activated CD4 T cells can be found in the inflammatory infiltrates of the rheumatoid synovium (Figs. 16.1 and 16.2) (44). Moreover, T-cell–directed therapies have provided some clinical benefit in RA (45–47). The most compelling data, however, implying a central role for CD4 T cells in propagating rheumatoid inflammation, remain the association of aggressive forms of the disease with particular MHC class II alleles, such as subtypes of HLA-DR4, that contain similar amino acid motifs in the CDR3 region of the DRβ chain (48,49). Although the exact meaning of this association has not been resolved, all interpretations imply that CD4 T cells orchestrate the local inflammation and cellular infiltration, after which a large number of subsequent inflammatory events occur. The induction of tissue-damaging autoimmunity in animal models of autoimmune diseases by transfer of CD4 T cells from sick animals into healthy syngeneic recipients can be regarded as further evidence of the importance of CD4 T cells in autoimmunity (50,51).

Great efforts have been undertaken to delineate the nature of the CD4 T cells involved in rheumatoid inflammation. Whereas the specific antigen(s) eliciting the detrimental autoimmune response is still unknown, much progress has been made in defining the phenotype and function of CD4 T cells in RA. In 1986, Mosmann and colleagues discovered that repeated antigen-specific

TABLE 16.1. Evidence for the Contribution of CD4 T Cells to Rheumatoid Inflammation

Association with HLA-DR4 and DR1 subtypes (*shared epitope*)
Enrichment of CD4 memory T cells in peripheral blood, synovial membrane, and synovial fluid
Important role in disease initiation in several animal models of inflammatory arthritis
Clinical efficacy of T-cell–directed therapies
Amelioration of disease activity in human immunodeficiency virus–infected patients

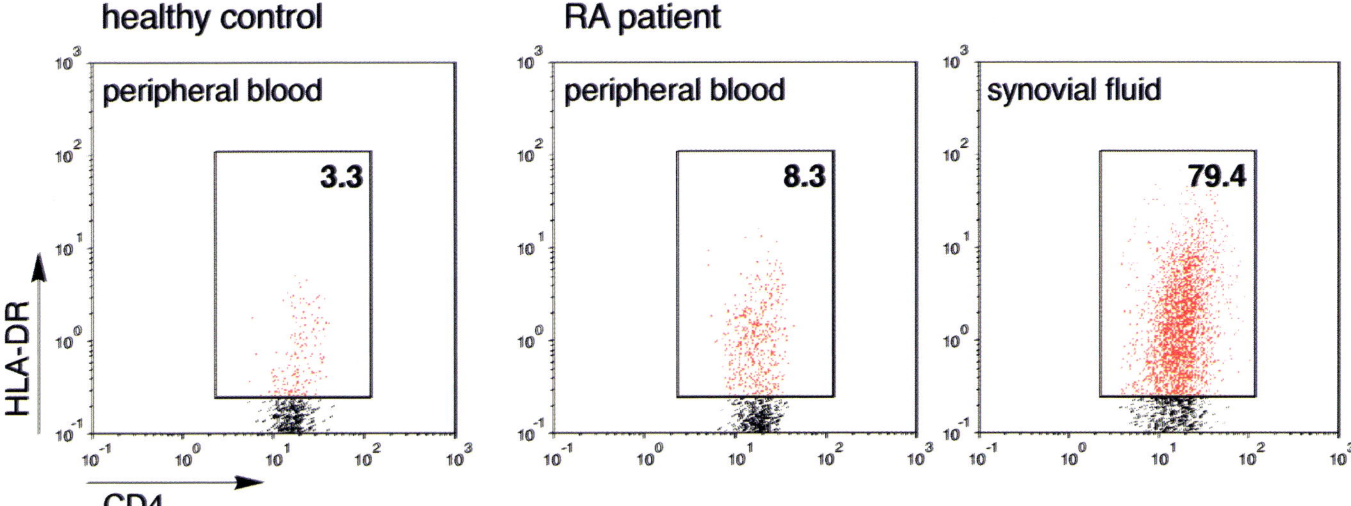

Figure 16.1. Rheumatoid inflammation is characterized by an accumulation of activated CD4 T cells. Mononuclear cells from the peripheral blood of a healthy individual and from the peripheral blood and the synovial fluid from a patient with active rheumatoid inflammation were stained with fluorochrome-labeled monoclonal antibodies to CD4 and HLA-DR as an indicator of T-cell activation. Activated (HLA-DR–positive) cells within the gated population of $CD4^+$ T cells are indicated in red. The numbers indicate the frequencies of activated $CD4^+$ T cells. RA, rheumatoid arthritis.

stimulation of murine CD4 T cells *in vitro* results in the development of restricted and stereotyped patterns of cytokine secretion profiles in the resultant T-cell populations (52). Subsequently, it was observed that many experimental models of autoimmune diseases in animals are characterized by a dominant activation of a particular Th subtype expressing proinflammatory cytokines (Th1 cells) (53). These findings have fostered investigations to categorize the pathogenesis of inflammatory arthritis with respect to the polarized Th effector subsets. Although dichotomizing complex diseases, such as RA, in terms of Th1 or Th2 patterns may be an oversimplification, the concept allows a better understanding of the mechanisms involved in the pathogenesis of the disease and can provide the basis for the development of novel strategies for the treatment of rheumatoid inflammation.

Th1-Th2 Dichotomy. Based on their distinctive cytokine secretion pattern and effector functions, CD4 T cells can be divided into at least three different subsets. Th1 cells develop preferentially during infections with intracellular bacteria. On activation, Th1 cells secrete the proinflammatory cytokines IL-2, IFN-γ, and lymphotoxin (TNF-β). They activate macrophages to produce reactive oxygen intermediates and nitric oxide (NO), stimulate their phagocytic functions, and enhance their ability for antigen presentation by up-regulation of MHC class II molecules. Moreover, Th1 cells promote the induction of complement fixing, opsonizing antibodies, and the induction of antibodies involved in antibody-dependent cell cytotoxicity (e.g., IgG1 in humans and IgG2a in mice). Consequently, Th1 cells are involved in cell-mediated immunity. Immune responses driven by Th1 cells are exemplified by the delayed-type hypersensitivity reaction (52,53). Th2 cells predominate after infestations with gastrointestinal nematodes and helminths. They produce the antiinflammatory cytokines IL-4 and IL-5 and provide potent help for B-cell activation and Ig class switching to IgE and subtypes of IgG that do not fix complement (e.g., IgG2 in humans and IgG1 in the mouse). Th2 cells mediate allergic immune responses and have been associated with down-modulation of macrophage activation, which is conferred to largely by the antiinflammatory effects of IL-4 (52,53). Th2 cells can also secrete IL-6, IL-10, and IL-13. However, in contrast to mice, those cytokines in humans are not confined to the Th2 subset but can also be produced by Th1 cells (53).

It has been shown that the different functional Th subsets do not derive from different precommitted lineages but, rather, may develop from the same uncommitted precursor cell under the influence of environmental and genetic factors (Fig. 16.3) (54). Cytokines are the most important regulators of Th subset differentiation. Whereas IL-2 is required for the differentiation of naïve cells into either Th subset without imposing a functional bias, priming of naïve CD4 T cells in the presence of IL-4 induces differentiation of Th2 effector cells. In contrast, Th1 cell development occurs in the absence of IL-4 and is greatly enhanced by IL-12 (53). Other factors that control Th subset polarization include the nature and intensity of co-stimulatory signals, in particular via CD28 and OX40, the intensity of TCR ligation during priming, the type of APC, the MHC class II genotype, minor histocompatibility complex genes, and corticosteroids or endogenous hormones (53).

Importantly, Th1 and Th2 cells antagonize each other by blocking the generation of the antipodal cell type and by blocking each other's effector functions (Fig. 16.3). For instance, the

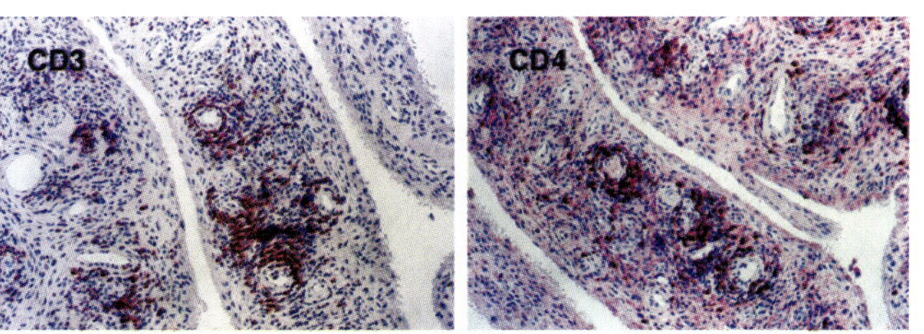

Figure 16.2. $CD4^+$ T cells infiltrate the rheumatoid synovium. Sections from the inflamed synovium from a patient with active disease are illustrated after staining with a monoclonal antibody to CD3 **(A)** or CD4 **(B)**. The cellular infiltrate consists of $CD3^+$ and $CD4^+$ T helper cells. Original magnification: ×200.

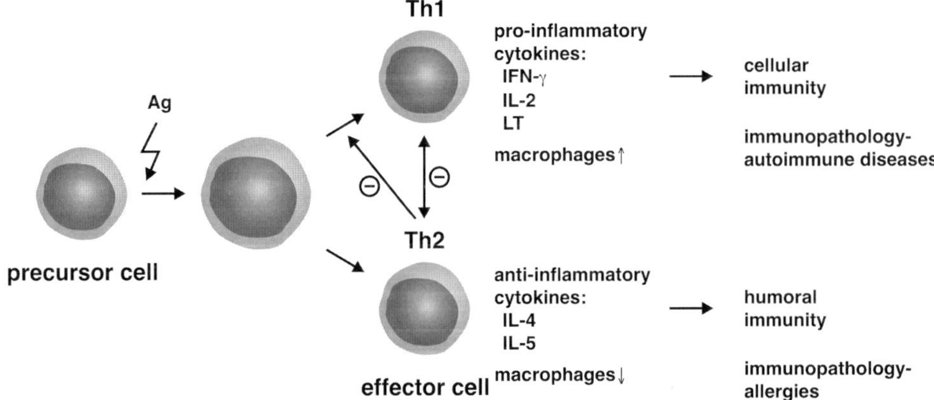

Figure 16.3. Differentiation of CD4 T cells into specialized T helper 1 (Th1) or Th2 effector cells. On activation with specific antigen (Ag), CD4 T cells proliferate and differentiate into either the Th1 or the Th2 subset. The cytokine milieu and the signals received during priming determines differentiation to proinflammatory Th1 or immunomodulatory Th2 effectors. Th1 cells promote cellular immunity and are involved in the development of autoimmune diseases; Th2 cells mediate humoral immunity and are involved in allergic immune responses. Th1 and Th2 cells antagonize each other at the levels of development and effector functions through the effects of their signature cytokines, interferon γ (IFN-γ) and interleukin-4 (IL-4), respectively. LT, lymphotoxin.

generation of Th1 cells can be effectively blocked by high concentrations of IL-4, even in the presence of IL-12 (55). At the level of effector functions, IL-4 antagonizes much of the proinflammatory effects of IFN-γ and inhibits the proliferation of Th1 cells. Conversely, IFN-γ secreted by Th1 cells blocks the proliferation of Th2 cells.

Differentiation of the appropriate Th subset is of crucial importance to the host in mounting protective immunity against exogenous microorganisms. However, it is apparent that immune responses driven preferentially by activated Th subsets are also involved in the development of pathologic immune disorders. Whereas atopic diseases result from Th2-dominated responses to environmental allergens, Th1-mediated immunity is involved in the generation of several organ-specific experimental autoimmune diseases in animals, such as experimental allergic encephalomyelitis, insulin-dependent diabetes mellitus, or CIA (53). Moreover, evidence is accumulating to suggest that human autoimmune diseases, such as RA, might also be driven by preferentially activated Th1 cells without sufficient Th2 cell development to down-regulate inflammation.

A third subset of T cells, designated *T regulatory cells*, has recently been described, first in mice and subsequently in humans. These T cells produce large amounts of IL-10 but not IL-4. It is speculated that T regulatory cells might play a significant role in maintaining peripheral tolerance (56). The precise function of those cells in immune homeostasis and, moreover, in autoimmunity, however, has only begun to be addressed.

IFN-γ. Production of IFN-γ is the hallmark of Th1 cells. In its biologically active form, IFN-γ is a 34-kd homodimer that possesses two *N*-glycosylation sites. IFN-γ is produced mainly by activated T cells and natural killer (NK) cells and has receptors on virtually all cells of the human body. Thus, IFN-γ exerts a multitude of biologic functions. The ability of IFN-γ to activate endothelial cells and macrophages is the basis for defining IFN-γ as a proinflammatory cytokine. IFN-γ stimulates the production of NO and potentiates the respiratory burst responsiveness of macrophages. It increases the expression of MHC class II molecules and thereby enhances the cells' ability to present foreign antigens. IFN-γ up-regulates the expression of the high-affinity Fcγ receptor I on monocytes and neutrophils, which, on binding to Ig, stimulates their phagocytic effector functions. On endothelial cells, IFN-γ augments the expression of the adhesion molecule, intercellular adhesion molecule-1 (ICAM-1, CD54), which increases their adhesiveness for leukocytes. IFN-γ production by T cells can be elicited by various stimuli, such as trauma or antigen-specific activation during infections or autoimmune diseases. It has been documented that monocyte-derived IL-12 is one of the most potent inducers of IFN-γ secretion. Recently, IL-18 has been found to induce IFN-γ production from T cells, and numerous studies have demonstrated the critical role of IL-12 and IL-18 for optimal *in vivo* induction of IFN-γ by exogenous agents (4). Several experimental autoimmune diseases are aggravated by exogenous IFN-γ, although this effect is not uniform in the different models. Nevertheless, the potent proinflammatory effects of IFN-γ, combined with its inhibitory potential for the development of Th2 cells, make IFN-γ a central mediator of the signs and symptoms of chronic autoimmune inflammation.

IL-4. IL-4 was discovered as a T-cell product distinct from IL-2 that could stimulate anti-IgM–treated B cells to proliferate and to differentiate into IgG-secreting plasma cells. IL-4 is a 20-kd secreted glycoprotein that elicits a number of diverse biologic responses in many different cell types. IL-4 is produced by activated T cells, mast cells, NK1.1 T cells, basophils, and eosinophils. Its main functions are to direct T-cell differentiation into the Th2 subset and to mediate Ig class switching to the IgG1 and IgE isotypes in mice and to the IgG4 and IgE isotypes in humans. IL-4 is the signature cytokine of Th2 cells and suppresses Th1 development while promoting Th2 generation. IL-4 is an important growth factor for T and B cells and increases the survival of cultured human lymphocytes. Overproduction of IL-4 has been associated with elevated IgE production and allergic diseases *in vivo*. Of importance in regulating immune responses is its ability to down-modulate the activation and the inflammatory functions of monocytes and macrophages. IL-4 increases the expression of MHC class II molecules and of several cytokine inhibitors, such as IL-1 receptor antagonist (IL-1RA), soluble IL-1 receptor type II, and TNF receptors, while down-regulating the production of the proinflammatory cytokines IL-1, TNF, IL-6, IL-8, and IL-12. The ability of Th2 effectors to control Th1-mediated inflammatory responses has been attributed largely to these antiinflammatory effects of IL-4. Consequently, IL-4 has been used *in vivo* as a treatment for experimental autoimmune diseases in animals and in patients with psoriasis (57). In animal models, IL-4 is the most successful means to ameliorate autoimmune disorders that are caused by activated Th1 cells. For example, IL-4 improves experimental allergic encephalomyelitis, delays the onset and diminishes clinical symptoms of CIA, and prevents joint damage and bone erosion in this experimental autoimmune disease (58). *In vitro*, IL-4 suppresses metalloproteinase production and stimulates tissue inhibitor of metalloproteinase-1 production in human mononuclear phagocytes and cartilage explants, indicating a protective effect of IL-4 toward extracellular matrix degradation. Furthermore, IL-4 inhibits bone resorption through an effect on both osteoclast activity and survival (59) and reduces the spontaneous secretion of proinflammatory cytokines and Ig in *ex vivo* cultured pieces from the rheumatoid synovial membrane (60). Finally, IL-4 down-regulates the surface expression of CD5 on B cells and inhibits spontaneous Ig and IgM rheumatoid factor production in patients with RA (61). Together, IL-4 is a pleiotropic cytokine with potent immunomodulatory functions that affects different cellular targets and is capable of ameliorating signs and symptoms of chronic arthritis.

IL-10. IL-10 is a homodimeric cytokine of 17 kd that was discovered as a potent inhibitor of macrophage effector functions. It is produced by activated monocytes, NK cells, B cells, and T cells. In mice, IL-10 is clearly a Th2 cytokine; however, in humans, IL-10 can be produced by both the Th1 and the Th2 subset. IL-10 is able to ameliorate potential pathologic autoimmune inflammation through the inhibition of various facets of the immune response. IL-10 inhibits the production by macrophages of proinflammatory cytokines, such as IL-1β, IL-6, IL-8, IL-12, and TNF, and up-regulates the production of IL-1RA, soluble p55, and p75 TNF-receptors. IL-10 down-regulates the expression of activating and co-stimulatory molecules on monocytes and dendritic cells, such as MHC class II molecules, ICAM-1, CD80, and CD86. It also reduces the generation of NO, superoxide, and prostaglandin E_2 in macrophages. In T cells, IL-10 inhibits production of IL-2 and IFN-γ and also blocks T-cell proliferation. Thus, IL-10 has potent antiinflammatory functions and has, consequently, been successfully used in the treatment of experimental autoimmune diseases. For example, IL-10 reduces joint swelling, cellular infiltration, proinflammatory cytokine production, and cartilage degradation in CIA (62). Most interestingly, IL-4 and IL-10 synergistically reduce joint inflammation in acute and chronic arthritis models (63). Thus, IL-10 might be an effective means to down-regulate human chronic autoimmune inflammation by counteracting IFN-γ–mediated proinflammatory activities. It should be emphasized, however, that, in humans, IL-10 cannot be assigned to a particular Th subset. Moreover, and of potential interest for human autoimmune diseases, it has been shown in animals that IL-10 is produced by, and induces the development of, regulatory T cells that appear to be most important in maintaining peripheral tolerance.

Evidence for a Dominant Pathogenic Th1 Drive in RA. Different experimental strategies have been pursued to test the hypothesis of a Th1-dominated inflammation in RA. Although categorizing RA as a Th1- or Th2-mediated disease is probably too simplistic, considerable evidence suggests that rheumatoid inflammation can be characterized by the presence of activated Th1 effector cells. For example, T cells cloned from the human rheumatoid synovial membrane functionally represent the Th1 subset. From a panel of 19 synovial membrane–derived T-cell clones, 18 produced large amounts of IFN-γ, whereas IL-4 was absent or present in minimal amounts only (64). In a different study, 15 out of 26 CD4 αβ T-cell clones from the rheumatoid synovial fluid, the synovial membrane, and the peripheral blood from five RA patients produced IFN-γ but not IL-4 on challenge with their specific antigens. Some of those clones produced various amounts of IL-10. Among 11 clones with unknown antigen specificity, seven showed a Th1-like pattern (65).

Analysis of synovial biopsies by *in situ* hybridization, immunohistochemistry, or reverse transcriptase polymerase chain reaction revealed that IFN-γ can be detected in the majority of specimens, whereas IL-4 was rarely found (66,67). Interestingly, a significant frequency of those IFN-γ–producing synovial CD4 T cells apparently has a distinct cytokine secretion profile, as shown by their ability to produce IL-10 (68). Importantly, however, synovial fluid– and synovial tissue–derived T cells express activation markers on their surface, indicating their contribution to tissue inflammation. The frequency of IFN-γ–producing CD4 T cells is significantly increased in the synovial fluid, compared to the peripheral blood (69), resulting in a markedly elevated Th1 to Th2 ratio in the synovial fluid that correlates with disease activity (70). Likewise, drastically reduced synthesis of IL-4 and IL-10 mRNA by synovial fluid mononuclear cells of RA patients correlates with disease activity (71). Finally, when synovial fluid T cells were cultured in the presence of IL-4, they were remarkably stable and resistant to Th2-inducing priming conditions (69). Together, these data strongly suggest that CD4 T cells from the inflamed rheumatoid synovium represent activated Th1 cells, secreting IFN-γ, which, in turn, might orchestrate synovial inflammation.

Analysis of the *in vivo* cytokine profile from CD4 T cells in the peripheral blood of RA patients revealed that 7 out of 14 patients had increased mRNA levels for IL-2, compared with healthy controls, and 5 of 14 for IFN-γ (72). The data imply the presence of activated Th1 cells in the peripheral circulation of patients with RA. Of note, 3 of the 14 patients had elevated levels of IL-4 (72). Most interestingly, when reentry of circulating T cells into sites of inflammation was blocked by a monoclonal antibody (mAb) to ICAM-1, a significant increase in IFN-γ mRNA levels in the peripheral blood was detected that might reflect a redistribution of activated Th1 cells from sites of inflammation into the peripheral circulation (72). In the peripheral blood of patients with new-onset synovitis (less than 1-year duration), increased numbers of cells secreting IFN-γ and IL-2 were found (73). Most interestingly, the frequencies of IFN-γ–secreting peripheral blood T cells in early arthritis correlated with disease activity, emphasizing the role of Th1 cells in the initiation of the disease.

Various epidemiologic and clinical observations also suggest a pathogenic Th1 drive in rheumatoid inflammation. For several decades, clinical observations have highlighted an ameliorating effect of pregnancy on the course of RA (74). In fact, the effect of pregnancy on RA activity is greater than the effect of some of the newer therapeutic agents. Pregnancy improves the symptoms of RA in approximately 75% of the patients, leading to a significant resolution of inflammation and a relief of symptoms, which enables the patients to taper or even stop the use of medications. The mechanisms for this phenomenon are still unclear. However, a marked decrease in Th1-mediated immunity during pregnancy has been firmly established. For example, pregnant women have a higher incidence of infections, compared to nonpregnant females—in particular, infections with intracellular pathogens. The characteristic Th1 immune reaction, delayed-type hypersensitivity, is diminished during pregnancy. In mice, antigen-specific activation of spleen and popliteal lymph node cells yielded reduced IFN-γ and increased IL-4 and IL-5 responses in pregnant animals, compared to controls. Moreover, after *in vivo* challenge with *Leishmania* antigens, serum levels of the Th2-associated IgG1 were elevated in the pregnant mice, as opposed to an increase of the Th1-mediated IgG2a in infected, but nonpregnant, controls (75). Together, the data support the hypothesis that pregnancy induces a shift from Th1 to Th2 immune responses, increasing antiinflammatory cytokines, which may contribute to the gestational amelioration of RA. Interestingly, relapses of RA occur within 6 months postpartum in 90% of the cases. At that time, pregnancy-associated alterations in Th subset activation can no longer be found (74), suggesting that the beneficial Th2 shift has resolved and has allowed the Th1-dominated autoimmune inflammation to reoccur.

Patients with RA have a decreased prevalence of allergic diseases. For example, the prevalence of hay fever in patients with RA is significantly lower than in appropriate controls (4% vs. 8%) (76). Moreover, those patients with RA who have hay fever have less severe disease compared with control patients with RA (without hay fever), as determined by the erythrocyte sedimentation rate, C-reactive protein level, joint score, and radiographic joint damage score (76). As expected, the atopic RA patients had higher levels of serum IgE and peripheral blood eosinophils, but their T cells produced less IFN-γ after maximum *in vitro* stimulation (76). In a different study, the incidence and point prevalence of atopy was lower among patients with RA than in control subjects (3.5% vs. 16.2%), and the cumulative incidence of atopy was significantly lower for patients with RA (7.5%) than for controls (18.8%) (77). As allergy is the prototype Th2 disease and activated Th2 cells are able to inhibit the generation and the function of Th1 effectors, these studies support the contention that the occurrence of a Th2-mediated immune response might be beneficial in RA by inhibiting Th1-driven immunity.

Exogenous cytokines have been used increasingly in recent years for treatment of several different malignancies and viral infections. These therapies, some of which are still experimental, provide the opportunity to explore the effect of cytokines on T-cell function and differentiation after *in vivo* application and the effect on autoimmunity. IL-12 is a strong inducer of Th1 cell development, subsequent IFN-γ production, and, thus, cellular immunity. Therefore, in an attempt to enhance antitumor cellular cytotoxicity, IL-12 has recently been used as an experimental treatment for different forms of cancer. When IL-12 was given to a woman with metastatic cervical cancer, a severe exacerbation of her RA was noted (78). IFN-α has been widely used because of its antiviral and antitumor properties. Like IL-12, IFN-α is a potent inducer of Th1 differentiation in humans. The incidence of autoimmune diseases associated with IFN-α treatment ranges between 4% and 19%, and several authors have noticed the first onset of a newly established or an exacerbation of preexisting RA (79). Together, these observations on the effects of administration of Th1-inducing cytokines into patients with malignancies or viral infections strongly emphasize the role of differentiated Th1 effectors in the pathogenesis of RA.

A final argument for the dominant role of Th1 effectors in RA derives from a study to correlate the Th1 to Th2 ratio in the peripheral blood from patients with RA with the clinical course. Although no apparent correlation was detected with disease activity score or C-reactive protein at baseline, the initial Th1 to Th2 ratio correlated well with the disease activity score 9 months after the beginning of treatment with disease-modifying antirheumatic drugs (DMARDs) (80).

The arguments depicted here in detail demonstrate that Th1 cells and their cytokines are not only present in RA but contribute to the perpetuation of chronic inflammation. However, the data do not yet allow a conclusion about whether Th1 cells are the initiators of rheumatoid inflammation or, rather, appear as a consequence of it. To delineate the mechanisms underlying the dominant Th1 drive in RA, studies were carried out to assess the functional capability of T cells in RA patients. Isolated memory CD4 T cells from the majority of patients with early RA manifested a profound inability to mount Th2 responses (81). Thus, those patients cannot generate immunoregulatory Th2 cells that might down-modulate ongoing Th1-mediated inflammation. Failure to down-regulate activated Th1 cells might allow Th1 inflammation to persist and evolve into chronic inflammation, characterized by the continuous activation of T cells, macrophages, fibroblasts, and osteoclasts and, subsequently, the destruction of tissue. As this functional abnormality of CD4 T cells in RA is evident at the time of initial clinical symptoms of arthritis (81), the data strongly suggest that the Th1-dominated immunity is the basis of rheumatoid inflammation and is not merely its consequence.

An interesting finding has been made that might shed light on the mechanisms contributing to the Th1 drive in RA. T cells from mice transgenic for the human RA-associated MHC class II allele, DRB1*0401, produced significantly more IFN-γ and TNF in response to stimulation with the same specific antigen, gp39, than did T cells from mice transgenic for another MHC class II allele, DRB1*0402, that is not associated with RA (82). These data indicate that disease-associated MHC class II molecules may in fact favor increased Th1-driven immune responses. As T cells recall expression of cytokines that they had been instructed to express as a result of previous activation by somatic imprinting of cytokine genes (83), it is possible that antecedent recognition of antigen presented in the context of disease-associated HLA alleles primed the responding T cells to modify their functional repertoire, predisposing to Th1 cell differentiation after subsequent stimulations.

Together, these data indicate that Th1 cells and their cytokines promote many aspects of synovial inflammation. Moreover, evidence is accumulating that dysregulated T-cell differentiation with impaired Th2 cell generation is instrumental in allowing the initial Th1-driven autoimmune response in RA to evolve into chronic inflammation. Interference with the activation and generation of Th1 cells and with the activity of their secreted cytokines might, therefore, be beneficial in the treatment of RA.

T-CELL FUNCTION IN RHEUMATOID SYNOVITIS

Interaction with Synoviocytes

RA synovitis is characterized by new blood vessel formation, thickening of the lining layer, and an inflammatory infiltrate consisting mainly of mononuclear cells. Approximately 30% to 50% of the synovial cells are T cells, the majority of which are CD4, CD45RO memory T cells that express activation markers on their surface and functionally belong to the Th1 type (44,64–67,84,85). In close proximity with the T cells are MHC class II positive APCs, such as macrophages and dendritic cells (86–88). T cell–macrophage interactions in the synovium are crucial for the stimulation of macrophages (87,89,90). In fact, direct cell–cell contact with stimulated T cells is the main pathway triggering activation of monocytes to produce IL-1 and TNF in the absence of infection (87). Contact-mediated activation of macrophages by stimulated T cells is as potent as optimal stimulation by lipopolysaccharides in inducing IL-1 and TNF production. In RA, TNF production by macrophages in the synovium is T-cell dependent, as removal of $CD3^+$ T cells from the RA synovial mononuclear cells resulted in a significant reduction of macrophage TNF production (91). T-cell–mediated macrophage activation is potentiated by many other factors, including IFN-γ, IL-15, and IL-18. In contrast, Th2 cytokines, such as IL-4, IL-10, IL-13, and TGF-β, are inhibitory (87).

Importantly, activated Th1 clones induced the monocytic cell line, THP-1, to secrete IL-1β and low amounts of the antiinflammatory IL-1RA, whereas Th2 clones induced high amounts of IL-1RA, but little IL-1β (92). Thus, as infiltrating T cells are predominantly Th1, they might exert inflammatory effector functions by direct contact with synovial macrophages. The molecules, however, involved in T-cell–mediated macrophage activation are not yet well-defined. Cytokines bound to the T-cell membrane, such as TNF, IL-1, IL-2, or IFN-γ, appeared to be irrelevant in activating macrophages (87). Moreover, interactions involving CD40/CD40L, leukocyte function–associated antigen (LFA)-1/ICAM-1, and CD69 are of some importance in different experimental systems for inducing proinflammatory cytokine secretion from macrophages after contact with T cells, but not in others (93–95). Regardless of the mode of action, however, direct T cell–macrophage contact in the synovium appears to be important in rheumatoid inflammation. Inhibiting T cell–macrophage interaction might, therefore, provide a novel, promising therapeutic approach. In this regard, it is of interest that a specific inhibitor of contact-mediated macrophage activation (apolipoprotein A-I) has been identified (96). Future work will have to examine whether interference with T-cell–mediated macrophage activation is a suitable therapeutic intervention in RA.

Intimate interaction of T cells and synovial APC promotes macrophage activation to produce proinflammatory cytokines and also provides a mechanism for continuous activation of synovial T cells. For example, the CD68$^+$ synovial macrophages express MHC class II and CD86 and CD80, the ligands for the co-stimulatory T-cell molecule CD28 (97,98), thereby providing the optimal requirement for T-cell activation. Surprisingly, however, freshly isolated dendritic cells from the synovial membrane do not express either CD80 or CD86 (99). *In vitro* culturing of synovial dendritic cells, in contrast, results in spontaneous up-regulation of both T-cell co-stimulatory ligands. The significance of this phenomenon for T-cell activation *in vivo* remains to be determined. CD80 and CD86 also bind to CTLA-4, an activation-induced T-cell surface molecule with T-cell inhibitory activity, and they do so with higher affinity than they bind CD28. As the infiltrating T cells show up-regulation of CTLA-4, enhanced interaction of CD80/CD86 with CTLA-4 might down-regulate T-cell activation, rather than enhance it. On the other hand, as all synovial T cells are memory T cells, they do not require co-stimulation for activation but can be stimulated by engagement of their TCR alone. Thus, the CD80/CD86–CD28 interaction might be of minor importance in T-cell activation in the rheumatoid synovium. In contrast, ligation of CD40 with its receptor, CD154 (CD40 ligand), appears to be crucial for several aspects of rheumatoid inflammation. Expression of CD154 is induced on T cells on stimulation through the TCR. Interaction of CD154 on T cells with its receptor, CD40, on B cells, macrophages, and fibroblasts has important consequences for the regulation of T-cell activation, its cytokine production, the up-regulation of adhesion molecules, the production of NO by synovial macrophages, and Ig class switching by B cells (100). Moreover, ligation of CD40 has been shown to be obligatory in inducing autoimmune inflammation in CIA (101). Together, there is considerable evidence that the interaction between synovial T cells and synovial APC promotes activation of both partner cells and contributes to sustained inflammation. Table 16.2 summarizes those interactions between T cells and synoviocytes involving engagement of co-stimulatory molecules.

TABLE 16.2. Membrane Molecules Implicated in Synovial Interactions of T cells

Co-Stimulatory Molecule on T Cells	Ligand	Ligand Tissue Distribution
CD28	B7.1 (CD80), B7.2 (CD86)	Macrophages, activated T cells, DC
CTLA-4 (CD152)	B7.1 (CD80), B7.2 (CD86)	Macrophages, activated T cells, DC
CD40L (CD154)	CD40	B cells, macrophages, DC, fibroblasts
LFA-2 (CD2)	LFA-3 (CD58)	Fibroblasts, macrophages, activated T cells, B cells, DC, NK cells
LFA-3 (CD58)	LFA-2 (CD2)	NK cells, activated T cells
LFA-1 (CD11a/CD18)	ICAM-1(CD54)	B cells, macrophages, activated T cells, fibroblasts
ICAM-1(CD54)	LFA-1 (CD11a/CD18)	B cells, NK cells, macrophages, activated T cells

CD40L, CD40 ligand; CTLA-4, cytolytic T lymphocyte–associated antigen-4; DC, dendritic cell; ICAM, intercellular adhesion molecule; LFA, leukocyte function–associated antigen; NK, natural killer.
Note: The molecules are denoted by the most common use in immunology. The CD systematic nomenclature is given in parentheses, where indicated.

Regulation by Migration

A prerequisite for any cell from the peripheral circulation to enter inflamed tissue is migration from the bloodstream through endothelial cell layers. Migration of T cells, as of other cells, from the blood into tissue is facilitated by a coordinate expression and sequential interaction of adhesion molecules on the surface of the migrating cells and on endothelial cells. Activated memory T cells in RA express a distinct array of adhesion receptors [for example, members of the *very late activation* (VLA) family, such as VLA-1, VLA-3, VLA-4, VLA-5, and VLA-6, LFA-1, CD2, and ICAM-1], that confer to them an increased migratory capacity (102–104). The ligands for these molecules are the extracellular matrix proteins, collagen, fibronectin, laminin, and molecules expressed on fibroblasts and endothelial cells (105). Synovial fluid memory T cells, when compared with peripheral blood memory T cells from the same patient, express a higher binding to endothelial adhesion receptors, such as the endothelial adhesion molecules endothelial-leukocyte adhesion molecule-1 and vascular cell adhesion molecule-1, suggesting a regulation of synovial T-cell migration at the level of adhesion receptor expression (104). Whereas T cells up-regulate their adhesion receptors on activation, cytokines, such as TNF and IL-1, strongly up-regulate adhesion receptor expression on endothelial cells (106). Together, in RA, adhesion receptor expression on peripheral blood memory T cells and on endothelial cells within the inflamed synovium provides a path for continuous T-cell migration into the synovium and sustained synovial inflammation.

Migration of leukocytes into inflamed tissue is also regulated by chemotactic cytokines, termed *chemokines*. Chemokines are secreted polypeptides that bind to specific surface receptors, which transmit signals through G proteins. Chemokines are divided into four subfamilies on the basis of the position of a pair of cysteine residues. Some chemokines trigger intravascular adhesion, whereas others direct the migration of leukocytes into and within the extravascular space (106). The chemokine receptors exhibit a nonspecific affinity for their ligands (107). In RA, selective chemokine receptor expression on leukocyte subsets has been demonstrated, suggesting a role in the selective inflammatory cell recruitment into the joint (108). With regard to T cells, chemokine receptors have been suggested to play a role in directing particular T-cell subsets into sites of inflammation. Thus,

TABLE 16.3. Chemokines and Their Receptors Expressed on T Cells with Importance in Rheumatoid Arthritis

Chemokine Receptors	Ligand /Chemokine	References
CXCR3	MIG (CXCL9) IP-10 (CXCL10) I-TAC (CXCL11)	Qin et al., 1998 (109); Patel et al., 2001 (112); Mohan et al., 2002 (113)
CXCR4	SDF-1 (CXCL12)	Nanki et al., 2000 (114); Buckley et al., 2000 (115)
CCR4	TARC (CCL17) MDC (CCL22)	Ruth et al., 2001a (108); Thompson et al., 2001 (117)
CCR5	RANTES (CCL5) MIP-1α (CCL3) MIP-1β (CCL4)	Qin et al., 1998 (109); Robinson et al., 1995 (118); Koch et al., 1994 (119)
CX3CR1	Fractalkine (CX3CL1)	Ruth et al., 2001a (108); Ruth et al., 2001b (116)

IP-10, interferon-inducible protein-10; I-TAC, interferon-inducible T cell α-chemoattractant; MDC, macrophage-derived chemokine; MIG, monokine induced by γ interferon; MIP, macrophage inflammatory protein; RANTES, regulated on activation, normal T cell–expressed and –secreted; SDF-1, stromal cell–derived factor-1; TARC, thymus- and activation-regulated chemokine.
Note: The chemokines are denoted by the most common name in current use. The systematic chemokine nomenclature is given in parentheses.

CCR3 appears to be expressed on Th2 effectors, but not on Th1 cells, whereas CCR5 is thought to be present on most Th1, but not on Th2 effectors (107). Accordingly, CCR5 has been detected in the rheumatoid synovial fluid and synovial membrane (108,109). In contrast to the results from *in vitro* culture and from animal experiments, analysis of CD4 memory T cells from the rheumatoid synovium at the single cell level failed to show a clear association of chemokine receptor expression and cytokine production, suggesting that specific surface markers for a cell population might not exist *in vivo* in humans (110). Nevertheless, chemokines and their receptors are involved in a number of inflammatory mechanisms in RA, including cell activation, intercellular adhesion, angiogenesis, and formation of germinal center, like follicles in the synovial membrane (107,111). Table 16.3 summarizes the chemokines and chemokine receptors with importance to T-cell migration and function in RA.

T-CELL–DIRECTED THERAPIES

Based on the concept that activated T cells are the key mediators of chronic autoimmune inflammation, T-cell–directed therapeutic interventions have been introduced for the treatment of RA. Extensive reviews have discussed the concepts and the clinical efficacy of T-cell–directed therapy in RA (120–123). In this chapter, different treatment approaches designed to target T cells in RA will be discussed (Table 16.4).

In an attempt to control disease progression by reducing the number or the activation of T cells, total lymphoid irradiation (47) and thoracic duct drainage (46) have been used in rheumatic diseases. These approaches, however, have provided only modest and inconsistent clinical benefit and have been associated with a number of side effects. Significant advances in the understanding of T-cell biology in recent years has led to the development of novel compounds designed to interfere with T-cell activation specifically. Cyclosporine and FK506 (tacrolimus), for example, inhibit T-cell activation by interfering with calcineurin-mediated transcriptional activation of a number of cytokine genes, such as IL-2, IL-3, IL-4, IL-8, and IFN-γ. Leflunomide is a potent noncytotoxic inhibitor of the enzyme dihydroorotate dehydrogenase, a key enzyme in the *de novo* synthesis of uridine monophosphate (124). In contrast to resting cells, activated T lymphocytes depend on the pyrimidine *de novo* synthesis to fulfill their metabolic needs for clonal expansion and terminal differentiation into effector cells. Thus, by limiting *de novo* pyrimidine biosynthesis, leflunomide inhibits the activation and proliferation of T cells that are important in the inflammation and degradation of synovial tissues.

TABLE 16.4. T-Cell–Targeted Therapies in Rheumatoid Arthritis

- Reduction of T-cell number or function
  - Total lymphoid irradiation
  - Thoracic duct drainage
- Immunosuppressive drugs
  - Glucocorticoids
  - Methotrexate
  - Leflunomide
  - Cyclosporine
  - FK506 (tacrolimus)
  - Rapamycin (sirolimus)
- Biologics
  - T-cell receptor vaccination
  - Monoclonal antibodies to T-cell surface receptors
  - Monoclonal antibodies to surface receptors on cells interacting with T cells
  - Cytokines

Whereas cyclosporine, FK506, and leflunomide exert their antiinflammatory activity by inhibiting T-cell activation, the precise mechanisms of action of other DMARDs are not completely understood. Interestingly, several studies indicate DMARDs might affect rheumatic diseases, at least in part because of their immunomodulatory effects on T-cell subsets. As RA appears to be driven by proinflammatory Th1 cells with impaired differentiation of immunoregulatory Th2 cells (64,72,81,125), a shift in the balance of Th1-Th2 effector cells toward antiinflammatory Th2 cells would be expected to induce clinical benefit. The concept of modulating the Th1-Th2 balance as a treatment for chronic autoimmunity has been successfully applied in a number of animal models of autoimmune diseases (126,127). It is, therefore, of interest to note that DMARDs appear to be able to modulate the Th1-Th2 balance. For example, leflunomide selectively decreases the activation of proinflammatory Th1 cells, while promoting Th2 cell differentiation from naïve precursors (128). Sulfasalazine potently inhibits the production of IL-12 in a dose-dependent manner in mouse macrophages stimulated with lipopolysaccharides. Importantly, pretreatment of macrophages with sulfasalazine either *in vitro* or *in vivo* reduces their ability to induce the Th1 cytokine IFN-γ and increases the ability to induce the Th2 cytokine IL-4 in antigen-primed CD4 T cells (129). Methotrexate significantly decreases the production of IFN-γ and IL-2 in *in vitro* stimulated peripheral blood mononuclear cells, while increasing the concentration of IL-4 and IL-10 (130). Likewise, clinical efficacy of cyclosporine is associated with decreased serum levels of IFN-γ, IL-2, and IL-12 and with significant increases in IL-10 (131). Bucillamine decreases the frequency of IFN-γ–producing CD4 T cells among CD4 T cells generated after a priming culture of mononuclear cells from the peripheral blood (132). Finally, reports have suggested that glucocorticoids inhibit cytokine expression indirectly through promotion of a Th2 cytokine secretion profile, presumably through their action on monocyte activation (133). Together, the data suggest that a number of current treatment modalities in RA exerts their antiinflammatory effects by inhibiting Th1 cell activation or differentiation and by favoring Th2 differentiation, thereby shifting the Th1-Th2 balance toward the Th2 direction.

Despite the immense progress in the treatment of rheumatic diseases, however, current therapy with immunosuppressive drugs is still associated with a number of side effects related to general immunosuppression. Therefore, it cannot be considered optimal therapy. An ideal form of therapy would be one that specifically targets only those cells perpetuating the chronic inflammation with minimal effects on other aspects of the immune or inflammatory systems. The substantial progress in our understanding of molecular and cellular biology has permitted the design of therapeutic tools (*biologics*) with defined targets and effector functions. Based on the increased knowledge of pathogenetic mechanisms of rheumatic diseases, biologics have been developed that are aimed to target only those cells mediating the disease process, with few or no side effects, while maintaining the integrity of the remainder of the immune system. As CD4 T cells are central in initiating and perpetuating the chronic autoimmune response in rheumatic diseases, a large number of biologics has aimed to interfere with T-cell activation or migration.

A major advance in the understanding of T-cell activation has been the identification of the critical co-stimulatory molecules on T cells, such as CD28, LFA-1, CD2, CD4, CD30, CD44, and CD40L, and their interacting ligands on APC or B cells. Although these molecules act through different mechanisms, some delivering co-stimulatory biochemical signals to the T cell, some enhancing adhesion to target tissues, they all have the ability to augment the T-cell proliferative responses to antigenic stimuli. Biologics designed to interfere with co-stimulation via inhibiting engagement of co-stimulatory ligands have been used in several animal models of inflammatory arthritis and in treatment trials in RA. In experimental autoimmune diseases in animals, mAbs to CD4 have been used to prevent the induction of the disease (134,135). Of relevance to human disease, mAbs to CD4 were also able to inhibit further progression when given after the initial inflammation has already become manifest (135,136), although, with one notable exception (137), controlled human trials have largely failed to demonstrate favorable results to date (120). Interaction of CD2 with its ligand, CD58, has been blocked by application of a soluble, fully human, recombinant fusion protein comprising the first extracellular domain of CD58 and the hinge, CH2 and CH3 sequences of human IgG1 (LFA-3-IgG1, *alefacept*). Alefacept has been given to patients with moderate to severe plaque psoriasis with substantial clinical response (138). Interestingly, alefacept selectively binds to and reduces circulating levels of the memory T-cell population, while sparing the naïve T-cell subset (138). Inhibition of CD28-mediated co-stimulatory signals is a potent means of immunosuppression that can be achieved by blocking either CD28 or CD80 and CD86. Currently, humanized anti-B7 mAbs are in phase II clinical trials for solid organ transplantation, graft-versus-host disease, and mild to severe plaque psoriasis. An alternative approach to block CD28 co-stimulation is by coating CD80 and CD86 with a soluble Ig fusion protein of the extracellular domain of CTLA-4 (CD152). As mentioned above, CTLA-4 is a homologue to CD28 and is expressed by activated T cells. It can bind both CD80 and CD86 with higher affinity than CD28. Because CD152 has a high affinity for CD80 and CD86, soluble forms of CTLA-4 inhibit the interaction of CD28 with its ligands. In clinical trials, CTLA4-Ig demonstrated favorable effects in patients with psoriasis vulgaris (139) and in patients with RA (140). The adhesion receptor-counterreceptor pair, LFA-1 (CD11α/CD18) and ICAM-1, is critical for transendothelial migration of T cells and their subsequent activation (141). Therefore, mAbs to LFA-1 and ICAM-1 have been used in autoimmune diseases in an attempt to block migration of T cells into sites of inflammation and their subsequent stimulation by locally expressed antigenic peptides *in vivo* (72,142). Significant clinical benefit was achieved with the mAb to ICAM-1 in patients with active RA (142). It is of interest that clinical benefit was restricted to those patients who showed a marked increase in the levels of Th1 cytokine-producing T cells in their circulation immediately after the administration of the mAb (72). Thus, it can be reasoned that in the responding patients, the circulatory pattern of activated Th1 cells was altered by inhibiting their migration into the inflamed synovium. These data argue for a pathogenic Th1 drive in those patients responding to therapy.

Together, T-cell–directed therapy in RA is based on the idea that CD4 T cells initiate and continuously drive systemic rheumatoid inflammation. T-cell–directed DMARDs and some of the recently used mAbs have been successful in ameliorating signs and symptoms of the diseases, and some also seem to be able to slow disease progression. Thus, although sustained clinical improvement has not been achieved with the biologics, the idea that targeting the CD4 T cells as the controllers of rheumatoid inflammation will interrupt chronic autoimmune inflammation and subsequent tissue destruction has been strongly supported.

CONCLUSION

Strong evidence has been provided for a central role of T cells in the pathogenesis of rheumatoid inflammation. Whereas clinical and epidemiologic observations have indicated that T-cell–mediated cellular immunity is involved in several aspects of RA, experimental data have revealed phenotypic and functional alterations of T cells in the peripheral circulation and the synovial infiltrates that are sufficient to mediate continuous up-regulation of proinflammatory effector functions. The data suggest that T cells play an important role in initiating the autoimmune disease and maintaining inflammation by activating synovial macrophages to produce inflammatory mediators. Alterations in the activity and frequency of proinflammatory T cells are associated with the clinical course of the disease, further emphasizing the role of T cells in RA. Finally, T-cell–directed therapies that modulate T-cell function or activity have been successfully used in modern therapy of RA. The clinical efficacy of T-cell–directed therapies have firmly established the central role of T cells in autoimmune rheumatoid inflammation.

ACKNOWLEDGMENTS

The authors thank Alla Skapenko for stimulating and critical discussions and for her help with the figures and the tables. The work of HSK is supported in part by the Deutsche Forschungsgemeinschaft (Schu 786/2-3), the German Federal Ministry of Education and Research (Network for Competence Rheumatology, Project C2-5), and the Interdisciplinary Center for Clinical Research in Erlangen (Project B27).

REFERENCES

1. Spits H. Development of alphabeta T cells in the human thymus. *Nat Rev Immunol* 2002;2:760–772.
2. Germain RN. T-cell development and the CD4-CD8 lineage decision. *Nat Rev Immunol* 2002;2:309–322.
3. Chan AC, Iwashima M, Turck CW, et al. ZAP-70: a 70 kd protein-tyrosine kinase that associates with the TCR zeta chain. *Cell* 1992;71:649–662.
4. Billiau A, Vandenbroeck K. Interferon-gamma. In: Oppenheim J, Feldmann M, Durum SK, eds. *Cytokine reference: compendium of cytokines and other mediators of host defense*. San Diego: Academic Press, 2001:641–688.
5. Weiss A. T cell antigen receptor signal transduction: a tale of tails and cytoplasmic protein-tyrosine kinases. *Cell* 1993;73:209–212.

6. Peng SL, Madaio MP, Hughes DP, et al. Murine lupus in the absence of alpha beta T cells. *J Immunol* 1996;156:4041–4049.
7. Peng SL, Madaio MP, Hayday AC, et al. Propagation and regulation of systemic autoimmunity by gammadelta T cells. *J Immunol* 1996;157:5689–5698.
8. Harrison LC, Dempsey-Collier M, Kramer DR, et al. Aerosol insulin induces regulatory CD8 gamma delta T cells that prevent murine insulin-dependent diabetes. *J Exp Med* 1996;184:2167–2174.
9. Wildner G, Hunig T, Thurau SR. Orally induced, peptide-specific gamma/delta TCR+ cells suppress experimental autoimmune uveitis. *Eur J Immunol* 1996;26:2140–2148.
10. Bodman-Smith MD, Anand A, Durand V, et al. Decreased expression of FcgammaRIII (CD16) by gammadelta T cells in patients with rheumatoid arthritis. *Immunol* 2000;99:498–503.
11. Lamour A, Jouen-Beades F, Lees O, et al. Analysis of T cell receptors in rheumatoid arthritis: the increased expression of HLA-DR antigen on circulating gamma delta+ T cells is correlated with disease activity. *Clin Exp Immunol* 1992;89:217–222.
12. Hassan J, Yanni G, Hegarty V, et al. Increased numbers of CD5+ B cells and T cell receptor (TCR) gamma delta+ T cells are associated with younger age of onset in rheumatoid arthritis (RA). *Clin Exp Immunol* 1996;103:353–356.
13. Lunardi C, Marguerie C, Walport MJ, et al. T gamma delta cells and their subsets in blood and synovial fluid from patients with rheumatoid arthritis. *Br J Rheumatol* 1992;31:527–530.
14. Smith MD, Broker B, Moretta L, et al. T gamma delta cells and their subsets in blood and synovial tissue from rheumatoid arthritis patients. *Scand J Immunol* 1990;32:585–593.
15. Meliconi R, Pitzalis C, Kingsley GH, et al. Gamma/delta T cells and their subpopulations in blood and synovial fluid from rheumatoid arthritis and spondyloarthritis. *Clin Immunol Immunopathol* 1991;59:165–172.
16. Jacobs MR, Haynes BF. Increase in TCR gamma delta T lymphocytes in synovia from rheumatoid arthritis patients with active synovitis. *J Clin Immunol* 1992;12:130–138.
17. Olive C, Gatenby PA, Serjeantson SW. Evidence for oligoclonality of T cell receptor delta chain transcripts expressed in rheumatoid arthritis patients. *Eur J Immunol* 1992;22:2587–2593.
18. Doherty PJ, Inman RD, Laxer RM, et al. Analysis of T cell receptor gamma transcripts in right and left knee synovial fluids of patients with rheumatoid arthritis. *J Rheumatol* 1996;23:1143–1150.
19. Kageyama Y, Koide Y, Miyamoto S, et al. The biased V gamma gene usage in the synovial fluid of patients with rheumatoid arthritis. *Eur J Immunol* 1994;24:1122–1129.
20. June CH, Bluestone JA, Nadler LM, et al. The B7 and CD28 receptor families. *Immunol Today* 1994;15:321–331.
21. Lindsten T, June CH, Ledbetter JA, et al. Regulation of lymphokine messenger RNA stability by a surface-mediated T cell activation pathway. *Science* 1989;244:339–343.
22. Fraser JD, Irving BA, Crabtree GR, et al. Regulation of interleukin-2 gene enhancer activity by the T cell accessory molecule CD28. *Science* 1991;251:313–316.
23. Li-Weber M, Giasi M, Krammer PH. Involvement of Jun and Rel proteins in up-regulation of interleukin-4 gene activity by the T cell accessory molecule CD28. *J Biol Chem* 1998;273:32460–32466.
24. Boise LH, Minn AJ, Noel PJ, et al. CD28 costimulation can promote T cell survival by enhancing the expression of Bcl-XL. *Immunity* 1995;3:87–98.
25. Alegre ML, Noel PJ, Eisfelder BJ, et al. Regulation of surface and intracellular expression of CTLA4 on mouse T cells. *J Immunol* 1996;157:4762–4770.
26. Cerdan C, Martin Y, Courcoul M, et al. Prolonged IL-2 receptor alpha/CD25 expression after T cell activation via the adhesion molecules CD2 and CD28. Demonstration of combined transcriptional and post-transcriptional regulation. *J Immunol* 1992;149:2255–2261.
27. Yin D, Zhang L, Wang R, et al. Ligation of CD28 in vivo induces CD40 ligand expression and promotes B cell survival. *J Immunol* 1999;163:4328–4334.
28. Wang EC, Lawson TM, Vedhara K, et al. CD8high+ (CD57+) T cells in patients with rheumatoid arthritis. *Arthritis Rheum* 1997;40:237–248.
29. Arai K, Yamamura S, Seki S, et al. Increase of CD57+ T cells in knee joints and adjacent bone marrow of rheumatoid arthritis (RA) patients: implication for an anti-inflammatory role. *Clin Exp Immunol* 1998;111:345–352.
30. Hingorani R, Monteiro J, Furie R, et al. Oligoclonality of V beta 3 TCR chains in the CD8+ T cell population of rheumatoid arthritis patients. *J Immunol* 1996;156:852–858.
31. Morley JK, Batliwalla FM, Hingorani R, et al. Oligoclonal CD8+ T cells are preferentially expanded in the CD57+ subset. *J Immunol* 1995;154:6182–6190.
32. Masuko-Hongo K, Sekine T, Ueda S, et al. Long-term persistent accumulation of CD8+ T cells in synovial fluid of rheumatoid arthritis. *Ann Rheum Dis* 1997;56:613–621.
33. Tan LC, Mowat AG, Fazou C, et al. Specificity of T cells in synovial fluid: high frequencies of CD8(+) T cells that are specific for certain viral epitopes. *Arthritis Res* 2000;2:154–164.
34. Fazou C, Yang H, McMichael AJ, et al. Epitope specificity of clonally expanded populations of CD8+ T cells found within the joints of patients with inflammatory arthritis. *Arthritis Rheum* 2001;44:2038–2045.
35. Behar SM, Roy C, Lederer J, et al. Clonally expanded Valpha12+ (AV12S1),CD8+ T cells from a patient with rheumatoid arthritis are autoreactive. *Arthritis Rheum* 1998;41:498–506.
36. Berner B, Akca D, Jung T, et al. Analysis of Th1 and Th2 cytokines expressing CD4+ and CD8+ T cells in rheumatoid arthritis by flow cytometry. *J Rheumatol* 2000;27:1128–1135.
37. Kang YM, Zhang X, Wagner UG, et al. CD8 T cells are required for the formation of ectopic germinal centers in rheumatoid synovitis. *J Exp Med* 2002;195:1325–1336.
38. Wagner UG, Kurtin PJ, Wahner A, et al. The role of CD8+ CD40L+ T cells in the formation of germinal centers in rheumatoid synovitis. *J Immunol* 1998;161:6390–6397.
39. Ehinger M, Vestberg M, Johansson AC, et al. Influence of CD4 or CD8 deficiency on collagen-induced arthritis. *Immunol* 2001;103:291–300.
40. Taneja V, Taneja N, Paisansinsup T, et al. CD4 and CD8 T cells in susceptibility/protection to collagen-induced arthritis in HLA-DQ8-transgenic mice: implications for rheumatoid arthritis. *J Immunol* 2002;168:5867–5875.
41. Cush JJ, Lipsky PE. Cellular basis for rheumatoid inflammation. *Clin Orthop* 1991;265:9–22.
42. Cush JJ, Lipsky PE. The immunopathogenesis of rheumatoid arthritis: the role of cytokines in chronic inflammation. *Clin Aspects Autoimmun* 1987;1:2–12.
43. Harris ED. Rheumatoid arthritis: pathophysiology and implications for treatment. *N Engl J Med* 1990;322:1277–1289.
44. Van Boxel JA, Paget SA. Predominantly T-cell infiltrate in rheumatoid synovial membranes. *N Engl J Med* 1975;293:517–520.
45. Panayi GS, Tugwell P. The use of cyclosporin A in rheumatoid arthritis: conclusions of an international review. *Br J Rheumatol* 1994;33:967–969.
46. Paulus HE, Machleder HI, Levine S, et al. Lymphocyte involvement in rheumatoid arthritis. Studies during thoracic duct drainage. *Arthritis Rheum* 1977;20:1249–1262.
47. Strober S, Tanay A, Field E, et al. Efficacy of total lymphoid irradiation in intractable rheumatoid arthritis. A double-blind, randomized trial. *Ann Intern Med* 1985;102:441–449.
48. Calin A, Elswood J, Klouda PT. Destructive arthritis, rheumatoid factor, and HLA-DR4. Susceptibility versus severity, a case-control study. *Arthritis Rheum* 1989;32:1221–1225.
49. Winchester R. The molecular basis of susceptibility to rheumatoid arthritis. *Adv Immunol* 1994;56:389–466.
50. Banerjee S, Webber C, Poole AR. The induction of arthritis in mice by the cartilage proteoglycan aggrecan: roles of CD4+ and CD8+ T cells. *Cell Immunol* 1992;144:347–357.
51. Breedveld FC, Dynesius-Trentham R, de Sousa M, et al. Collagen arthritis in the rat is initiated by CD4+ T cells and can be amplified by iron. *Cell Immunol* 1989;121:1–12.
52. Mosmann TR, Cherwinski H, Bond MW, et al. Two types of murine helper T cell clone. I. Definition according to profiles of lymphokine activities and secreted proteins. *J Immunol* 1986;136:2348–2357.
53. Abbas AK, Murphy KM, Sher A. Functional diversity of helper T lymphocytes. *Nature* 1996;383:787–793.
54. Rocken M, Saurat JH, Hauser C. A common precursor for CD4+ T cells producing IL-2 or IL-4. *J Immunol* 1992;148:1031–1036.
55. Hsieh CS, Macatonia SE, Tripp CS, et al. Development of TH1 CD4+ T cells through IL-12 produced by *Listeria*-induced macrophages. *Science* 1993;260:547–549.
56. Groux H, O'Garra A, Bigler M, et al. A CD4+ T-cell subset inhibits antigen-specific T-cell responses and prevents colitis. *Nature* 1997;389:737–742.
57. Ghoreschi K, Thomas P, Breit S, et al. Interleukin-4 therapy of psoriasis induces Th2 responses and improves human autoimmune disease. *Nat Med* 2003;9:40–46.
58. Horsfall AC, Butler DM, Marinova L, et al. Suppression of collagen-induced arthritis by continuous administration of IL-4. *J Immunol* 1997;159:5687–5696.
59. Miossec P, Chomarat P, Dechanet J, et al. Interleukin-4 inhibits bone resorption through an effect on osteoclasts and proinflammatory cytokines in an ex vivo model of bone resorption in rheumatoid arthritis. *Arthritis Rheum* 1994;37:1715–1722.
60. Miossec P, Briolay J, Dechanet J, et al. Inhibition of the production of proinflammatory cytokines and immunoglobulins by interleukin-4 in an ex vivo model of rheumatoid synovitis. *Arthritis Rheum* 1992;35:874–883.
61. Hidaka T, Kitani A, Hara M, et al. IL-4 down-regulates the surface expression of CD5 on B cells and inhibits spontaneous immunoglobulin and IgM-rheumatoid factor production in patients with rheumatoid arthritis. *Clin Exp Immunol* 1992;89:223–229.
62. Persson S, Mikulowska A, Narula S, et al. Interleukin-10 suppresses the development of collagen type II-induced arthritis and ameliorates sustained arthritis in rats. *Scand J Immunol* 1996;44:607–614.
63. Joosten LA, Lubberts E, Durez P, et al. Role of interleukin-4 and interleukin-10 in murine collagen-induced arthritis. Protective effect of interleukin-4 and interleukin-10 treatment on cartilage destruction. *Arthritis Rheum* 1997;40:249–260.
64. Miltenburg AM, van Laar JM, de Kuiper R, et al. T cells cloned from human rheumatoid synovial membrane functionally represent the Th1 subset. *Scand J Immunol* 1992;35:603–610.
65. Quayle AJ, Chomarat P, Miossec P, et al. Rheumatoid inflammatory T-cell clones express mostly Th1 but also Th2 and mixed (Th0) cytokine patterns. *Scand J Immunol* 1993;38:75–82.
66. Kusaba M, Honda J, Fukuda T, et al. Analysis of type 1 and type 2 T cells in synovial fluid and peripheral blood of patients with rheumatoid arthritis. *J Rheumatol* 1998;25:1466–1471.
67. Canete JD, Martinez SE, Farres J, et al. Differential Th1/Th2 cytokine patterns in chronic arthritis: interferon gamma is highly expressed in synovium

of rheumatoid arthritis compared with seronegative spondyloarthropathies. *Ann Rheum Dis* 2000;59:263–268.

68. Morita Y, Yamamura M, Kawashima M, et al. Flow cytometric single-cell analysis of cytokine production by CD4+ T cells in synovial tissue and peripheral blood from patients with rheumatoid arthritis. *Arthritis Rheum* 1998;41:1669–1676.
69. Davis LS, Cush JJ, Schulze-Koops H, et al. Rheumatoid synovial CD4+ T cells exhibit a reduced capacity to differentiate into IL-4-producing T-helper-2 effector cells. *Arthritis Res* 2001;3:54–64.
70. van der Graaff WL, Prins AP, Niers TM, et al. Quantitation of interferon gamma- and interleukin-4-producing T cells in synovial fluid and peripheral blood of arthritis patients. *Rheumatology* 1999;38:214–220.
71. Miyata M, Ohira H, Sasajima T, et al. Significance of low mRNA levels of interleukin-4 and -10 in mononuclear cells of the synovial fluid of patients with rheumatoid arthritis. *Clin Rheumatol* 2000;19:365–370.
72. Schulze-Koops H, Lipsky PE, Kavanaugh AF, et al. Elevated Th1- or Th0-like cytokine mRNA in peripheral circulation of patients with rheumatoid arthritis: modulation by treatment with anti-ICAM-1 correlates with clinical benefit. *J Immunol* 1995;155:5029–5037.
73. Kanik KS, Hagiwara E, Yarboro CH, et al. Distinct patterns of cytokine secretion characterize new onset synovitis versus chronic rheumatoid arthritis. *J Rheumatol* 1998;25:16–22.
74. Da Silva JA, Spector TD. The role of pregnancy in the course and aetiology of rheumatoid arthritis. *Clin Rheumatol* 1992;11:189–194.
75. Krishnan L, Guilbert LJ, Russell AS, et al. Pregnancy impairs resistance of C57BL/6 mice to *Leishmania* major infection and causes decreased antigen-specific IFN-gamma response and increased production of T helper 2 cytokines. *J Immunol* 1996;156:644–652.
76. Verhoef CM, van Roon JA, Vianen ME, et al. Mutual antagonism of rheumatoid arthritis and hay fever; a role for type 1/type 2 T cell balance. *Ann Rheum Dis* 1998;57:275–280.
77. Allanore Y, Hilliquin P, Coste J, et al. Decreased prevalence of atopy in rheumatoid arthritis. *Lancet* 1998;351:497.
78. Peeva E, Fishman AD, Goddard G, et al. Rheumatoid arthritis exacerbation caused by exogenous interleukin-12. *Arthritis Rheum* 2000;43:461–463.
79. Ioannou Y, Isenberg DA. Current evidence for the induction of autoimmune rheumatic manifestations by cytokine therapy. *Arthritis Rheum* 2000;43:1431–1442.
80. van der Graaff WL, Prins AP, Dijkmans BA, et al. Prognostic value of Th1/Th2 ratio in rheumatoid arthritis. *Lancet* 1998;351:1931.
81. Skapenko A, Wendler J, Lipsky PE, et al. Altered memory T cell differentiation in patients with early rheumatoid arthritis. *J Immunol* 1999;163:491–499.
82. Cope AP, Patel SD, Hall F, et al. T cell responses to a human cartilage autoantigen in the context of rheumatoid arthritis-associated and nonassociated HLA-DR4 alleles. *Arthritis Rheum* 1999;42:1497–1507.
83. Agarwal S, Rao A. Modulation of chromatin structure regulates cytokine gene expression during T cell differentiation. *Immunity* 1998;9:765–775.
84. Kingsley G, Pitzalis C, Panayi GS. Immunogenetic and cellular immune mechanisms in rheumatoid arthritis: relevance to new therapeutic strategies. *Br J Rheumatol* 1990;29:58–64.
85. Lipsky PE. Immunopathogenesis and treatment of rheumatoid arthritis. *J Rheumatol* 1992;32:S92–S94.
86. Agostini C, Basso U, Semenzato G. Cells and molecules involved in the development of sarcoid granuloma. *J Clin Immunol* 1998;18:184–192.
87. Burger D, Dayer JM. The role of human T-lymphocyte-monocyte contact in inflammation and tissue destruction. *Arthritis Res* 2002;4 S3:S169–S176.
88. Liu MF, Kohsaka H, Sakurai H, et al. The presence of costimulatory molecules CD86 and CD28 in rheumatoid arthritis synovium. *Arthritis Rheum* 1996;39:110–114.
89. McInnes IB, Leung BP, Liew FY. Cell-cell interactions in synovitis. Interactions between T lymphocytes and synovial cells. *Arthritis Res* 2000;2:374–378.
90. Burmester GR, Stuhlmuller B, Keyszer G, et al. Mononuclear phagocytes and rheumatoid synovitis. Mastermind or workhorse in arthritis? *Arthritis Rheum* 1997;40:5–18.
91. Brennan FM, Hayes AL, Ciesielski CJ, et al. Evidence that rheumatoid arthritis synovial T cells are similar to cytokine-activated T cells: involvement of phosphatidylinositol 3-kinase and nuclear factor kappaB pathways in tumor necrosis factor alpha production in rheumatoid arthritis. *Arthritis Rheum* 2002;46:31–41.
92. Chizzolini C, Chicheportiche R, Burger D, et al. Human Th1 cells preferentially induce interleukin (IL)-1beta while Th2 cells induce IL-1 receptor antagonist production on cell/cell contact with monocytes. *Eur J Immunol* 1997;27:171–177.
93. Wagner DHJ, Stout RD, Suttles J. Role of the CD40-CD40 ligand interaction in CD4+ T cell contact-dependent activation of monocyte interleukin-1 synthesis. *Eur J Immunol* 1994;24:3148–3154.
94. Vey E, Zhang JH, Dayer JM. IFN-gamma and 1,25(OH)2D3 induce on THP-1 cells distinct patterns of cell surface antigen expression, cytokine production, and responsiveness to contact with activated T cells. *J Immunol* 1992;149:2040–2046.
95. McInnes IB, Leung BP, Sturrock RD, et al. Interleukin-15 mediates T cell-dependent regulation of tumor necrosis factor-alpha production in rheumatoid arthritis. *Nat Med* 1997;3:189–195.
96. Hyka N, Dayer JM, Modoux C, et al. Apolipoprotein A-I inhibits the production of interleukin-1beta and tumor necrosis factor-alpha by blocking contact-mediated activation of monocytes by T lymphocytes. *Blood* 2001; 97:2381–2389.
97. Balsa A, Dixey J, Sansom DM, et al. Differential expression of the costimulatory molecules B7.1 (CD80) and B7.2 (CD86) in rheumatoid synovial tissue. *Br J Rheumatol* 1996;35:33–37.
98. Ranheim EA, Kipps TJ. Elevated expression of CD80 (B7/BB1) and other accessory molecules on synovial fluid mononuclear cell subsets in rheumatoid arthritis. *Arthritis Rheum* 1994;37:1637–1646.
99. Summers KL, O'Donnell JL, Williams LA, et al. Expression and function of CD80 and CD86 costimulator molecules on synovial dendritic cells in chronic arthritis. *Arthritis Rheum* 1996;39:1287–1291.
100. Stout RD, Suttles J. The many roles of CD40 in cell-mediated inflammatory responses. *Immunol Today* 1996;17:487–492.
101. Tellander AC, Michaelsson E, Brunmark C, et al. Potent adjuvant effect by anti-CD40 in collagen-induced arthritis. Enhanced disease is accompanied by increased production of collagen type-II reactive IgG2a and IFN-gamma. *J Autoimmun* 2000;14:295–302.
102. Cush JJ, Pietschmann P, Oppenheimer-Marks N, et al. The intrinsic migratory capacity of memory T cells contributes to their accumulation in rheumatoid synovium. *Arthritis Rheum* 1992;35:1434–1444.
103. Takahashi H, Soderstrom K, Nilsson E, et al. Integrins and other adhesion molecules on lymphocytes from synovial fluid and peripheral blood of rheumatoid arthritis patients. *Eur J Immunol* 1992;22:2879–2885.
104. Postigo AA, Garcia-Vicuna R, Diaz-Gonzalez F, et al. Increased binding of synovial T lymphocytes from rheumatoid arthritis to endothelial-leukocyte adhesion molecule-1 (ELAM-1) and vascular cell adhesion molecule-1 (VCAM-1). *J Clin Investig* 1992;89:1445–1452.
105. Dustin ML, de Fougerolles AR. Reprogramming T cells: the role of extracellular matrix in coordination of T cell activation and migration. *Curr Opin Immunol* 2001;13:286–290.
106. von Andrian UH, Mackay CR. T-cell function and migration. Two sides of the same coin. *N Engl J Med* 2000;343:1020–1034.
107. Rocken M, Racke M, Shevach EM. IL-4-induced immune deviation as antigen-specific therapy for inflammatory autoimmune disease. *Immunol Today* 1996;17:225–231.
108. Ruth JH, Rottman JB, Katschke KJ Jr, et al. Selective lymphocyte chemokine receptor expression in the rheumatoid joint. *Arthritis Rheum* 2001;44:2750–2760.
109. Qin S, Rottman JB, Myers P, et al. The chemokine receptors CXCR3 and CCR5 mark subsets of T cells associated with certain inflammatory reactions. *J Clin Investig* 1998;101:746–754.
110. Nanki T, Lipsky PE. Cytokine, activation marker, and chemokine receptor expression by individual CD4(+) memory T cells in rheumatoid arthritis synovium. *Arthritis Res* 2000;2:415–423.
111. Loetscher P, Moser B. Homing chemokines in rheumatoid arthritis. *Arthritis Res* 2002;4:233–236.
112. Patel DD, Zachariah JP, Whichard LP. CXCR3 and CCR5 ligands in rheumatoid arthritis synovium. *Clin Immunol* 2001;98:39–45.
113. Mohan K, Ding Z, Hanly J, et al. IFN-gamma-inducible T cell alpha chemoattractant is a potent stimulator of normal human blood T lymphocyte transendothelial migration: differential regulation by IFN-gamma and TNF-alpha. *J Immunol* 2002;168:6420–6428.
114. Nanki T, Hayashida K, El-Gabalawy HS, et al. Stromal cell-derived factor-1-CXC chemokine receptor 4 interactions play a central role in CD4+ T cell accumulation in rheumatoid arthritis synovium. *J Immunol* 2000;165:6590–6598.
115. Buckley CD, Amft N, Bradfield PF, et al. Persistent induction of the chemokine receptor CXCR4 by TGF-beta 1 on synovial T cells contributes to their accumulation within the rheumatoid synovium. *J Immunol* 2000;165:3423–3429.
116. Ruth JH, Volin MV, Haines GK 3rd, et al. Fractalkine, a novel chemokine in rheumatoid arthritis and in rat adjuvant-induced arthritis. *Arthritis Rheum* 2001;44:1568–1581.
117. Thompson SD, Luyrink LK, Graham TB, et al. Chemokine receptor CCR4 on CD4+ T cells in juvenile rheumatoid arthritis synovial fluid defines a subset of cells with increased IL-4:IFN-gamma mRNA ratios. *J Immunol* 2001;166:6899–6906.
118. Robinson E, Keystone EC, Schall TJ, et al. Chemokine expression in rheumatoid arthritis (RA): evidence of RANTES and macrophage inflammatory protein (MIP)-1 beta production by synovial T cells. *Clin Exp Immunol* 1995;101:398–407.
119. Koch AE, Kunkel SL, Harlow LA, et al. Macrophage inflammatory protein-1 alpha. A novel chemotactic cytokine for macrophages in rheumatoid arthritis. *J Clin Investig* 1994;93:921–928.
120. Schulze-Koops H, Lipsky PE. Anti-CD4 monoclonal antibody therapy in human autoimmune diseases. *Curr Dir Autoimmun* 2000;2:24–49.
121. Schulze-Koops H, Kalden JR. Targeting T cells in rheumatic diseases. In: Smolen JS, Lipsky PE, eds. *Biological therapy in rheumatology*. Martin Dunitz Publishers, 2003:3–24.
122. Panayi GS. Targeting of cells involved in the pathogenesis of rheumatoid arthritis. *Rheumatology* 1999;38S2:8–10.
123. Yocum DE. T cells: pathogenic cells and therapeutic targets in rheumatoid arthritis. *Semin Arthritis Rheum* 1999;29:27–35.
124. Bruneau JM, Yea CM, Spinella-Jaegle S, et al. Purification of human dihydroorotate dehydrogenase and its inhibition by A77 1726, the active metabolite of leflunomide. *Biochem J* 1998;336:299–303.

125. Simon AK, Seipelt E, Sieper J. Divergent T-cell cytokine patterns in inflammatory arthritis. *Proc Natl Acad Sci U S A* 1994;91:8562–8566.
126. Joosten LA, Lubberts E, Helsen MM, et al. Protection against cartilage and bone destruction by systemic interleukin-4 treatment in established murine type II collagen-induced arthritis. *Arthritis Res* 1999;1:81–91.
127. Bessis N, Boissier MC, Ferrara P, et al. Attenuation of collagen-induced arthritis in mice by treatment with vector cells engineered to secrete interleukin-13. *Eur J Immunol* 1996;26:2399–2403.
128. Dimitrova P, Skapenko A, Herrmann ML, et al. Restriction of de novo pyrimidine biosynthesis inhibits Th1 cell activation and promotes Th2 cell differentiation. *J Immunol* 2002;169:3392–3399.
129. Kang BY, Chung SW, Im SY, et al. Sulfasalazine prevents T-helper 1 immune response by suppressing interleukin-12 production in macrophages. *Immunology* 1999;98:98–103.
130. Constantin A, Loubet-Lescoulie P, Lambert N, et al. Antiinflammatory and immunoregulatory action of methotrexate in the treatment of rheumatoid arthritis: evidence of increased interleukin-4 and interleukin-10 gene expression demonstrated in vitro by competitive reverse transcriptase-polymerase chain reaction. *Arthritis Rheum* 1998;41:48–57.
131. de Groot K, Gross WL. Wegener's granulomatosis: disease course, assessment of activity and extent and treatment. *Lupus* 1998;7:285–291.
132. Morinobu A, Wang Z, Kumagai S. Bucillamine suppresses human Th1 cell development by a hydrogen peroxide-independent mechanism. *J Rheumatol* 2000;27:851–858.
133. Almawi WY, Melemedjian OK, Rieder MJ. An alternate mechanism of glucocorticoid anti-proliferative effect: promotion of a Th2 cytokine-secreting profile. *Clin Transplan* 1999;13:365–374.
134. Ranges GE, Sriram S, Cooper SM. Prevention of type II collagen-induced arthritis by in vivo treatment with anti-L3T4. *J Exp Med* 1985;162:1105–1110.
135. Waldor MK, Sriram S, Hardy R, et al. Reversal of experimental allergic encephalomyelitis with monoclonal antibody to a T-cell subset marker. *Science* 1985;227:415–417.
136. Wofsy D, Seaman WE. Reversal of advanced murine lupus in NZB/NZW F1 mice by treatment with monoclonal antibody to L3T4. *J Immunol* 1987; 138:3247–3253.
137. Schulze-Koops H, Davis LS, Haverty TP, et al. Reduction of Th1 cell activity in the peripheral circulation of patients with rheumatoid arthritis after treatment with a non-depleting humanized monoclonal antibody to CD4. *J Rheumatol* 1998;25:2065–2076.
138. Ellis CN, Krueger GG. Treatment of chronic plaque psoriasis by selective targeting of memory effector T lymphocytes. *N Engl J Med* 2001;345:248–255.
139. Abrams JR, Lebwohl MG, Guzzo CA, et al. CTLA4Ig-mediated blockade of T-cell costimulation in patients with psoriasis vulgaris. *J Clin Invest* 1999; 103:1243–1252.
140. Moreland LW, Alten R, Van Den Bosch F, et al. Costimulatory blockade in patients with rheumatoid arthritis: a pilot, dose-finding, double-blind, placebo-controlled clinical trial evaluating CTLA-4Ig and LEA29Y eighty-five days after the first infusion. *Arthritis Rheum* 2002;46:1470–1479.
141. Kavanaugh AF, Lightfoot E, Lipsky PE, et al. The role of CD11/CD18 in adhesion and transendothelial migration of T cells: analysis utilizing CD18 deficient T cell clones. *J Immunol* 1991;146:4149–4156.
142. Kavanaugh AF, Davis LS, Nichols LA, et al. Treatment of refractory rheumatoid arthritis with a monoclonal antibody to intercellular adhesion molecule 1. *Arthritis Rheum* 1994;37:992–999.

CHAPTER 17

Autoimmunity

Anne Davidson and S. Louis Bridges, Jr.

Multiple mechanisms have been postulated to underlie the pathogenesis of rheumatoid arthritis (RA). Among these are aberrant immune responses directed at self-antigens. The most highly studied autoimmune phenomenon in RA is the presence of antibodies reactive with epitopes in the Fc portion of immunoglobulin G (IgG), referred to as *rheumatoid factor* (RF) (Fig. 17.1). Although the focus of this chapter is on insights into RA gleaned from studies of RF, other autoantibodies that have been implicated in the disease process are also discussed.

CLINICAL ASPECTS OF RHEUMATOID FACTOR

Waaler first reported the presence of a serum autoantibody in patients with RA in the late 1930s (1), and these studies were extended by Rose et al. (2). Later, it was shown that serum RF activity was contained in a soluble 22S complex that could be split into an active IgM fraction and an inactive IgG fraction. Advantage was taken of the multiple specificities of RF to identify Ig allotypes, genetic markers on the IgG Fc region. Further studies of RA patients subsequently revealed that RFs were present in synovial fluid and that large numbers of RF-producing plasma cells could be detected in inflamed rheumatoid synovium (3).

Because of the strong association between RA and the presence of high titers of serum RF, researchers interested in the pathogenesis of RA focused on the properties and generation of serum RF. Because there is a relatively small amount of serum RF in most RA patients' sera, isolation of RF in amounts necessary for analysis was initially problematic. However, it had been previously noted that paraproteins expressed in patients with cryoglobulinemia or Waldenström's macroglobulinemia often exhibited RF activity, were present in large amounts in serum of affected individuals, and were typically monoclonal. Thus, analysis of paraproteins from diseases other than RA yielded the first important insights into the binding specificity, biologic properties, and genetic origins of RFs. The development of molecular techniques allowed subsequent isolation and analysis of RFs from patients with RA. RFs also arise routinely in healthy individuals after infection or immunization (4). Comparison of the features of RFs derived from RA patients and the "physiologic" RFs of healthy individuals or the monoclonal RFs that are associated with B-cell disorders has yielded further insight into the dysregulation of RF production that occurs in RA patients.

Significance of Rheumatoid Factor in Rheumatoid Arthritis

RFs are found in the sera of approximately 80% of RA patients (5). Initially, their presence was thought to be specific for the diagnosis of RA. Later studies, however, showed that they may be present in a variety of chronic inflammatory and infectious diseases (Table 17.1) and may occur in the sera of healthy individuals. Although the presence of serum RF is not required for the diagnosis of RA, substantial data support its contribution to the pathogenesis of the disease. Immune complexes composed of RF and IgG are found in the target of inflammation in RA, the synovial tissue (6). In addition, seropositive (RF-positive) and seronegative (RF-negative) RA exhibit clinical differences. Seropositive RA is consistently reported to be more severe, both radiographically and functionally (7–11). Furthermore, patients with seropositive RA have a significantly higher frequency of extraarticular involvement (including subcutaneous nodules, vasculitis, leg ulcers, and neuropathy) than patients with seronegative RA (5,12). RF positivity is also one of several risk factors for increased mortality from RA (13–15).

Time of Expression with Respect to Disease Onset

Several longitudinal studies have reported that the presence of significantly elevated levels of serum RF identifies healthy individuals at increased risk for subsequently developing RA. A British study found that 7 of 19 asymptomatic individuals with elevated serum RF followed for 5 years developed evidence of RA (16). Aho et al. (17) examined sera from 30 individuals who developed RA during a Finnish cardiovascular disease survey and found that 12 exhibited positive tests for RF from 4 months to 5 years before disease diagnosis. In a longitudinal study of 2,712 Pima Indians conducted over a 19-year period, a convincing correlation between RF titer (as measured by the sheep cell agglutination test) and the development of RA was observed (18). Finally, in a cohort of nearly 14,000 participants in a population study performed in Iceland, 135 previously RF-positive persons were identified and evaluated (19). After observation for a mean of 16.5 years, seven participants developed RA, and all had persistently raised RF. Six of the 54 participants with more than one RF isotype developed RA, corresponding to an annual incidence of 0.67%, 7.5 times higher than observed in other participants. Taken together, these results indicate that significantly elevated serum-RF levels provide a marker for increased susceptibility to developing RA and may play a role in its pathogenesis.

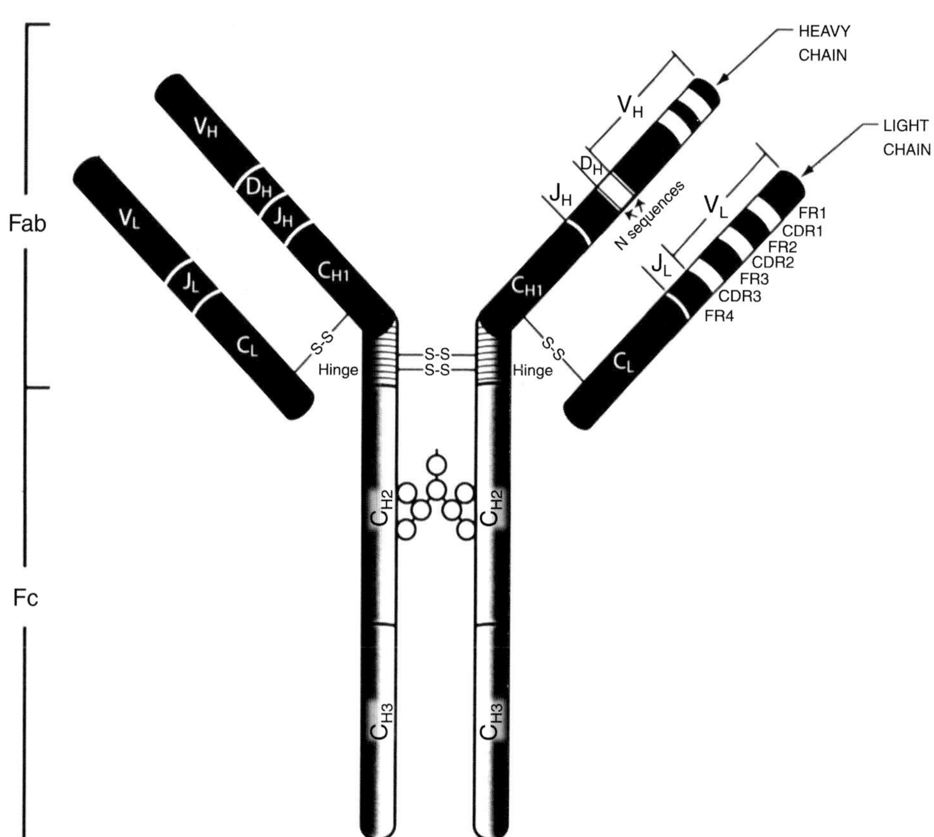

Figure 17.1. Schematic representation of human immunoglobulin G. Each molecule consists of two identical heavy chains and two identical light chains. The antigen-binding domain resides within the antigen-binding fragment (Fab) region and is formed by folding and apposition of six complementarity determining regions (CDRs). The epitopes that bind rheumatoid factor are within the Fc region. The sugar residue at Asn 297 in CH2 is shown.

Other Diseases with Rheumatoid Factor

IgM RFs are found in many diseases other than RA (Table 17.1), including systemic lupus erythematosus (SLE) (20–23). RF appears to be associated with cryoglobulinemia in SLE patients (24), but the role of RF in SLE, if any, remains unclear. RF activity is common among antibodies associated with essential mixed cryoglobulinemia (EMC). EMC is a systemic vasculitis characterized by the production of cold-precipitable Igs and manifested clinically by purpura, arthralgias, and weakness (25). More than 80% of patients with EMC have chronic infection with the hepatitis C virus (HCV). Hepatic lymphoid follicles (LFs), seen in up to 90% of HCV patients, are potential sites of generation of antibodies with RF and cryoglobulin activity. These LFs are rich in T and B cells and resemble germinal centers (GCs), the sites of affinity maturation of the B-cell response. In HCV infection, hepatic LFs contain B cells that are predominantly monoclonal, consistent with an antigen-driven response (26). Such LFs, which are also seen in nonlymphoid tissue in other chronic inflammatory conditions, are known sites of antigen-driven B-cell affinity maturation. The precise pathogenetic role of RF in patients with chronic HCV infection and cryoglobulinemia remains to be elucidated.

Patients with primary Sjögren's syndrome often have serum RF. This syndrome is associated with an increased incidence of monoclonal B-cell non-Hodgkin's lymphoma, which often develops in the salivary glands. In a study of 103 patients with primary Sjögren's syndrome, six of seven patients (86%) who developed lymphoma during a 5-year period had mixed cryoglobulinemia before the appearance of lymphoma, compared with 12 of 96 (12.4%) of the patients who did not develop lymphoma (27). Furthermore, the presence of RF-associated cross-reactive idiotypes on the kappa light chain (17.109) and heavy chain (G6) also correlated with lymphoma development (27).

Martin et al. (28) cloned Igs from monoclonal B-cell lymphomas that arose in the salivary glands of two patients with primary Sjögren's syndrome. They tested recombinant antibodies against a panel of antigens potentially implicated in Sjögren's syndrome and found that the antibodies produced by the neoplastic B cells had RF activity. Thus, RF-expressing B cells may

TABLE 17.1. Diseases Associated with Elevated Serum Rheumatoid Factor

Rheumatic diseases
Rheumatoid arthritis
Systemic lupus erythematosus
Sjögren's syndrome
Scleroderma
Polymyositis/dermatomyositis
Chronic bacterial infections
Subacute bacterial endocarditis
Leprosy
Tuberculosis
Syphilis
Lyme disease
Viral diseases
Rubella
Cytomegalovirus
Infectious mononucleosis
Influenza
Acquired immunodeficiency syndrome
Parasitic diseases
Chronic inflammatory diseases—causes uncertain
Sarcoidosis
Periodontal disease
Pulmonary interstitial disease
Liver disease
Mixed cryoglobulinemia
Hyper γ-globulinemic purpura

undergo malignant transformation, leading to salivary gland lymphomas in patients with Sjögren's syndrome.

STRUCTURAL FEATURES OF RHEUMATOID FACTOR

Antigenic Specificity

The specificity of RFs from healthy individuals and from RA patients has been extensively studied. In general, the range of specificities of the RFs from healthy individuals that arise as part of the physiologic immune response to antigen exposure is much narrower than that of RA patients. There is less cross-reactivity of physiologic RFs with animal IgG; for this reason, the Rose-Waaler test that uses rabbit IgG to coat red cells in an agglutination assay is highly sensitive for the diagnosis of RA. RA-derived RFs are also more likely to cross-react with collagen type II. Physiologic RFs rarely bind IgG3, whereas some subsets of RF from RA patients preferentially bind this isotype (3). Finally, the range of Ig genes that encodes the RFs of RA patients is broader than those of healthy individuals, and somatic mutations leading to amino acid replacements are more likely to have accumulated in the RFs of RA patients than in those of healthy individuals (29,30).

Using a set of chimeric IgG antibodies, Artandi et al. (31) and Bonagura et al. (32,33) mapped the binding sites of monoclonal RFs derived from healthy immunized individuals, from patients with Waldenström's macroglobulinemia, and from patients with RA. The first difference seen was that most RFs from healthy individuals or from macroglobulinemia patients bind to the IgG1, IgG2, and IgG4 isotypes, the so-called Ga specificity. The Ga-binding specificity is, in part, dependent on the amino acid residue at position 435 in the CH3 region, which is His in IgG1, IgG2, and IgG4 but Arg in IgG3 (Fig. 17.2). In contrast, RFs from patients with RA have a broader range of specificities, with more frequent binding to IgG3 and the presence of several novel specificities, such as binding to only one isotype. Many RFs from healthy individuals bind to the same site on IgG as does staphylococcal protein A (SPA) (34,35). The SPA binding site is at the CH2-CH3 border of the Fc region and is formed mostly by the apposition of two loops from the CH2 region at amino acids 252 to 254 and 309 to 311 (32,36). SPA was able to inhibit binding of RFs of the Ga specificity to Fc. In contrast, the Fc binding region of many RA-derived RFs lies outside of this area and is not inhibited by SPA. These structural data suggest a greater diversity of RFs from RA patients than from healthy individuals. The monoclonal RFs derived from patients with Waldenström's macroglobulinemia are restricted in specificity and resemble those from healthy individuals.

Genetic Origins and Idiotypes

An initial understanding of the molecular origins of RFs evolved from idiotypic analysis of paraprotein RFs (37,38). The idiotype of an Ig molecule is formed by a series of structural determinants on its variable region. Antibody molecules that share idiotypes, particularly those that identify isolated heavy or light chain determinants, are often encoded by homologous genes. Thus, identification of idiotypic determinants that are widely expressed by specific autoantibodies can yield important information about their molecular genetic origins.

Kunkel et al. (37,39), using polyclonal antiidiotypic antibodies, identified two major cross-reactive idiotypes on Waldenström's macroglobulinemia–derived monoclonal RFs called *Wa* and *Po*. Subsequently, it was shown that Wa is also the major determinant expressed by the RFs derived from patients with HCV infection (40). Other researchers generated monoclonal antiidiotypes 17.109 and 6B6.6 that recognize almost 80% of paraprotein RFs (38,41–43).

A 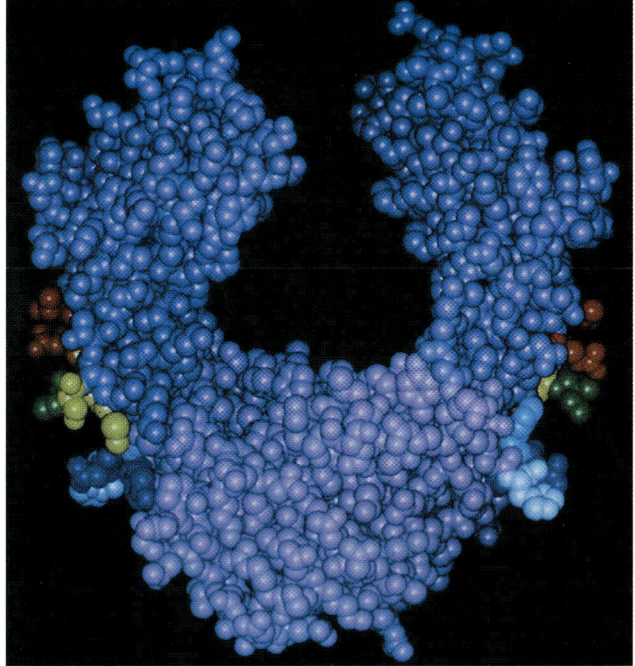

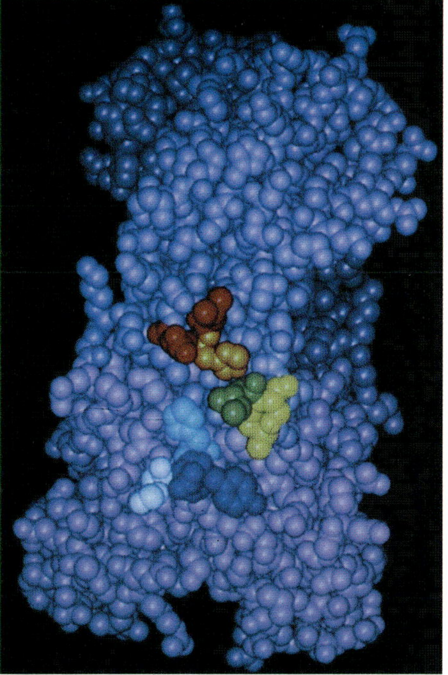 B

Figure 17.2. A: Space-filling model of the entire Fc fragment of immunoglobulin G1. Residues in the three loops contributing to binding of monoclonal rheumatoid factor are highlighted as follows: CH2 loop proximal: Met-252 (*yellow*), Ile 253 (*green*), Ser 254 (*yellow*). CH2 loop distal: Leu 309 (*red*), His 310 (*orange*), Gln 311 (*red*). CH3 loop: His 433 (*gray*), Asn 434 (*blue*), His 435 (*aqua*), Tyr 436 (*blue*). **B:** Model is rotated 90 degrees. (From Artandi SE, Calame KL, Morrison SL, Bonagura VR. Monoclonal IgM rheumatoid factors bind IgG at a discontinuous epitope comprised of amino acid loops from heavy-chain constant-region domains 2 and 3. *Proc Natl Acad Sci U S A* 1992;89:94–98, with permission.)

By sequencing of idiotype-positive RFs, it was shown that at least 60% of monoclonal RFs from patients with B-cell malignancies use a highly restricted germline-encoded light chain repertoire derived from the VκIII gene family (38,44). All 17.109 and Wa-positive proteins use light chains encoded by a Humkv325-related gene (41). Wa-positive RFs use a combination of a VH1-derived heavy chain and a Humkv325-derived light chain (40). The 6B6.6 antiidiotype recognizes RFs whose light chain is encoded by the Humkv328 gene (43). The molecular basis for Po expression is still not clear.

Using the monoclonal 6B6.6 and 17.109 idiotypes, it was shown that polyclonal RFs from RA patients appear to have greater idiotypic diversity than either monoclonal paraprotein RFs or polyclonal RFs derived from healthy individuals or even from patients with Sjögren's syndrome. These idiotypes are expressed on only 1% to 2% of IgM RFs from adult classic RA patients, and their levels do not correlate with RF titers (41,42). Thus, the polyclonal RFs found in patients with RA are clearly structurally different from monoclonal RFs of B-cell malignancies. The low levels of expression of these germline-encoded idiotypes on polyclonal RFs from patients with RA suggests that RFs in RA patients may be encoded by different genes or gene combinations from those used to encode monoclonal RFs, and/or that the genes in RA patients have undergone extensive somatic mutation that has altered the idiotypic determinant (45).

A number of investigators were subsequently able to generate antiidiotypes to conformational, heavy, or light chain determinants that cross-react with polyclonal and monoclonal human RFs (46–50). Davidson et al. identified a cross-reactive idiotype named *4C9* that preferentially recognizes RFs from RA patients but not from healthy individuals (51). Up to 25% of IgM RF from individual RA patients expresses the 4C9 determinant (51). Molecular studies have shown a complex basis for expression of RF-related idiotypes. Several of the heavy chain antiidiotypes have been characterized at the molecular level; two antiidiotypes recognize an overlapping population of heavy chains encoded by the VH1 gene family, and one recognizes VH3-encoded heavy chains (52). Both of these heavy chains can associate with Humkv325-encoded light chains to form RF (53). Comparative molecular analysis of the 6B6.6 and 4C9 light chain idiotypes showed that both recognize the Humkv328 gene as well as the somatically generated light chain third complementarity determining region (CDR3). The 4C9, but not the 6B6.6 antiidiotype, recognizes a determinant that is expressed by the highly related VκIII gene V3g; in this case, 4C9 expression depends on the associated heavy chain in that some heavy chains can mask idiotype expression. The ability of 4C9 to recognize the V3g light chain explains the broader specificity of the 4C9 idiotype compared with the 6B6.6 idiotype (54).

The idea that RFs from RA patients use a wider repertoire of genes than the more restricted RFs that are found in healthy individuals or among paraproteins was confirmed by the analysis of a large number of RF-secreting lines derived from healthy individuals and RA patients. In healthy individuals, as in patients with B-cell malignancies, the gene repertoire that encodes RF is quite restricted, with VκIII genes accounting for approximately 60% of the RFs (55). Preferential pairings of heavy and light chain gene products are also seen, especially that of VH1 with Humkv325 (40) and VH4 with Humkv328 (56). In contrast, sequence analysis of the Ig genes from RFs associated with RA revealed a more diverse repertoire of both heavy and light chains with increased use of VH3 genes and lambda genes (55,57–60).

Molecular analysis of RFs derived from human B-cell lines was then used to determine whether RFs are encoded by unmutated germline genes or by somatically mutated genes. A germline origin of an autoantibody gene would suggest that the autoantibody has been secreted by a naïve B cell that has not been driven by antigen or T-cell factors or, alternatively, from a B-cell subset such as the CD5^{+} subset that does not undergo extensive hypermutation. Demonstration of preferential replacement mutations in the CDRs of an autoantibody gene, which are the antigen contact regions, would suggest the influence of antigen and T-cell factors in eliciting the autoantibody response. Sequence analysis of RF-positive lines from healthy individuals has revealed that somatic mutations leading to replacement of amino acids in the CDRs are infrequent. In contrast, RA-derived RFs show an overall increase in frequency of replacement mutations in the CDRs (57,60). Somatic mutation may increase affinity for the Fc region of IgG. In one case, it was shown for a clonally related pair of IgM RFs derived from rheumatoid synovium that somatic mutation resulted in higher affinity Fc binding (61). However, somatic mutation does not always result in an increase in autoantibody affinity. In another study, back mutation of genes encoding RA synovium–derived RF revealed that the germline-encoded RF had a higher affinity for Fc (62).

Molecular analysis of both heavy and light chain genes encoding RF coupled with site-directed mutagenesis and heavy and light chain mixing studies have shown that the heavy chain makes a major contribution to Fc binding. Furthermore, the major determinant involved is the heavy chain CDR3 region (63,64). The light chain is able to modify the affinity for Fc, with the VJ junction contributing to the refinement of RF specificity and affinity (54). These studies suggest that high-affinity RF specificity is not necessarily germline encoded or generated by somatic mutation but may also be generated during Ig gene recombination in the bone marrow.

The relationship between IgM and IgG RFs remains to be determined. Idiotypic similarity between IgM and IgG RFs has been described in a single RA patient (50). In a study of the 4C9 idiotype, however, no 4C9 activity could be demonstrated on IgG RF (51). Although this finding could be ascribed to loss of idiotypic reactivity by the mechanism of somatic mutation or to interference by the gamma constant region, it is possible that IgG RFs might derive from a B-cell population that is not normally stimulated during a primary response. Williams et al. (65) cloned more than 250 genes from synovial Fc-binding B cells and showed that IgM and IgA RFs derived from the synovium appeared to be clonally related to each other but that IgG RFs used a different gene repertoire.

In sum, these studies show that RFs from RA patients use a more diverse gene repertoire and different heavy and light chain combinations than the more restricted RFs of healthy individuals. High-affinity RF activity may be generated by Ig gene recombination or by somatic mutation. Whether IgM and IgG RFs are genetically related remains to be determined.

Crystal Structure of a Rheumatoid Arthritis–Derived Rheumatoid Factor

Sutton et al. (36) and Corper et al. (66) have solved the crystal structure of an RA-dervied RF (RF-AN) co-crystallized with the Fc region of IgG4 (Fig. 17.3A). This RF has the Ga specificity and is of low relative avidity. The heavy chain is derived from the VH3 gene family, and the light chain is of the lambda isotype. The structure confirms that residues 252 to 254 and residue 435 are important contact residues for RF-AN but residues 309 to 311 are not important for this RF. There is partial overlap with the SPA binding site, as expected. The unusual feature of the crystal structure of this RF is the involvement of only four of the six CDR loops in the binding of the RF variable region to the Fc region in such a way as to leave most of the conventional antigen-binding site free and potentially able to bind a second antigen (Fig. 17.3B). The authors postulate that inclusion of another

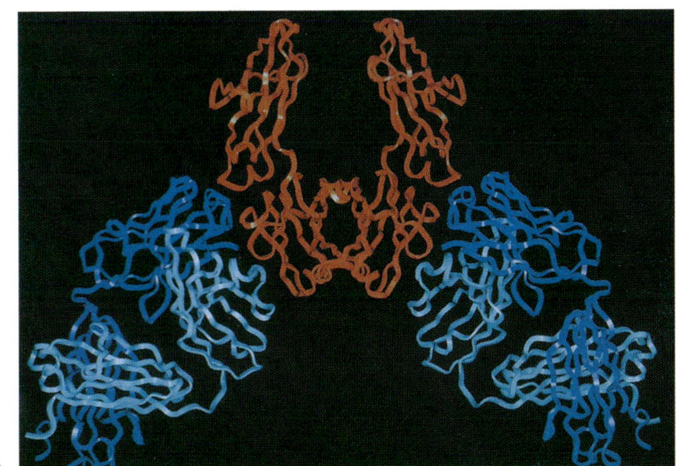

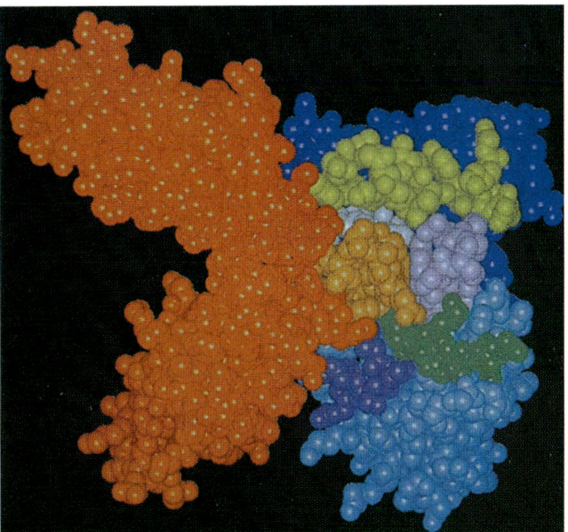

Figure 17.3. **A:** Crystal structure of monoclonal immunoglobulin (Ig) M rheumatoid factor (RF) AN complexed to IgG4 Fc. Two Fabs of AN [heavy chain (*dark blue*), light chain (*light blue*)] bind symmetrically, one to each heavy chain of IgG4 Fc (*red*). The ribbons represent the polypeptide backbone. The epitope on Fc involves both the CH2 and CH3 domains. **B:** The recognition of IgG Fc involves an unconventional use of the RF-combining site. Space-filling model has complementarity determining regions (CDRs) coded as follows: L1 (*green*), L2 (*purple*), L3 (*pink*), H1 (*white*), H2 (*yellow*), H3 (*orange*). All the CDRs are accessible even in the complex. (From Sutton B, Corper A, Bonagura V, et al. The structure and origin of rheumatoid factors. *Immunol Today* 2000;21:177–183, with permission.)

antigen in the RF-IgG complex could potentially stabilize an immune complex, particularly if the affinity for antigen is low. Presence of autoantibody and autoantigens in an immune complexed form could result in increased immunogenicity of self-antigens to which the host is normally tolerant, better fixation of complement, and increased stimulation of the RF-producing B cell. It is of interest, in light of the molecular analyses described above, that the light-chain CDR3 region of RF-AN is not a contact site for Fc, but four of the nine contact residues are from the heavy-chain CDR3. Furthermore, four of the eight contact residues of RF-AN are derived by somatic events, either recombination or mutation. Although this structure may be representative of low-affinity RF of the Ga specificity, it may not be representative of higher-affinity RFs found in RA patients. Further structural information is needed to determine whether the unusual binding characteristics of RF-AN are typical of most low-affinity RFs.

SITES OF PRODUCTION OF RHEUMATOID FACTOR

Location of Rheumatoid Factor–Secreting B Cells in Lymphoid Tissue

The majority of RF-secreting B cells from patients with RA appear to originate in the bone marrow. In one study of RA, mononuclear cells from bone marrow were able to produce IgG, IgA, and IgM RFs (67). Furthermore, the amounts of RF produced by bone marrow cells were similar to those produced by dissociated RA synovial cells. These data suggest that, as with the majority of Igs circulating in the periphery, RFs are mainly derived from the bone marrow.

Extralymphoid Generation of Autoantibodies

Although the majority of RFs appear to be generated in the bone marrow, especially in early RA, other organs or ectopic B-cell infiltrates may contribute as well. Large numbers of RF-producing plasma cells are found in the RA synovium, constituting up to 50% of synovial plasma cells (68). The synovium in patients with long-standing RA contains lymphoid aggregates; these infiltrates can secrete Ig levels approaching that of the spleen (69). In approximately 10% to 30% of patients, these subsynovial infiltrates contain structures histologically similar to GC of normal lymphoid organs (70,71). Although the follicular mantle and other well-defined regions of GCs are often absent from GC-like structures in RA synovia, the cell types and structures necessary for affinity maturation of the B-cell response are present. These include high endothelial venules (72), specialized blood vessels that facilitate entry of lymphocytes into the cortex of lymph nodes, and follicular dendritic cells (FDCs). FDCs function as antigen-presenting cells (APCs) (71,73–75) and can be arranged in networks similar to those seen in healthy lymphoid organs (71). The dependence of these GC-like structures on an unusual population of $CD8^+$ helper T cells has been recently described (76).

The presence of GC-like structures is not unique to RA. Lymphoid neogenesis has been reported in nonlymphoid tissues from individuals with other chronic infectious or inflammatory diseases not necessarily associated with RF production, such as chronic hepatitis B and C (77,78), Lyme disease (79), reactive arthritis (80,81), and autoimmune thyroid disease (82). Thus, the formation of ectopic lymphoid structures in inflammatory tissue may be a common response to tissue injury in autoimmune diseases (83,84).

There has been considerable interest in analyzing the B-cell response in synovial follicular structures to determine whether mature B cells that secrete autoantibodies are generated *in situ*. Plasma cells that secrete RF are abundant within the rheumatoid synovium, and the concentration of RF in synovial fluid is higher than in the serum, suggesting that the synovium can be a source of secreted RF (68). The origin of these plasma cells is still unknown. Although GCs can form within synovial tissue, molecular analysis of synovial GC cells and plasma cells has shown that they express different Ig gene repertoires (85,86). Furthermore, clonal expansion of IgM and IgA RFs has been demonstrated within the synovium, but these RFs do not appear to be clonally related to IgG RFs from the same patient (65). Limited selection of developing B cells within the joint might lead to the repertoire differences observed between synovial GC B cells and plasma cells and between IgM and IgG RFs (86). Alternatively, because rheumatoid synovial tissue expresses high levels of the chemokine CXCL12 that can act as a chemoattractant for plasma cells, it is possible that some preformed plasma cells migrate to the joint (87–89).

A second issue that has been investigated is whether there is loss of tolerance in the synovial lymphoid tissue that results in autoantibody formation. This issue has been explored in a number of ways. First, it was demonstrated by sequencing of complementary DNA libraries generated from rheumatoid synovium that light chain genes derived from this tissue had unusual CDR3 regions that were longer than those normally observed (90), suggesting an alteration in regulation or selection of B cells within the synovium. Second, it has been demonstrated that alterations in antibody specificity that could predispose to autoimmunity may occur in peripheral lymphoid organs such as the spleen or lymph node. RAG-1 and RAG-2 are responsible for Ig gene rearrangements and were initially thought to be expressed only during the period of Ig gene rearrangement in B-cell precursors that occurs in the bone marrow. Recently, however, these enzymes were also found to be expressed in some GC B cells of healthy peripheral lymphoid organs of mice (91–94). Studies of transgenic mice have shown that the expression of RAG in B cells of peripheral lymphoid organs can potentially result in deletion of autoreactive Ig gene sequences, so-called receptor revision (95,96). On the other hand, this process may function to salvage B cells that bear low-affinity antigen receptors, and, as a consequence, autoreactive antibodies may be generated (97). RAG expression occurs in the rheumatoid synovium (98–100), but whether this peripheral RAG expression is beneficial or detrimental in the setting of autoimmunity is still not known. Finally, an unusual B-cell subset has been identified in the synovia of some patients with RA. This subset of B cells expresses two light chains. One of these chains is conventional and the other is the prelight chain that is usually expressed on developing B cells or B cells undergoing receptor revision (101). The heavy and light chains of these B cells are unusual in that they express long CDR3 regions and have structural features that have been described in autoantibodies (102). Whether these cells are indicative of a B-cell regulatory defect within the synovium is not yet known.

REGULATION OF RHEUMATOID FACTOR PRODUCTION

Genetic Predisposition to Rheumatoid Arthritis and Rheumatoid Factor

Predisposition to seropositive RA is associated with inheritance of particular major histocompatibility complex (MHC) class II HLA-DR4 or DR1 alleles, whereas the association of DR4 with seronegative RA is generally less striking (or absent) (103–106). Although the pathogenetic mechanism(s) underlying the association between certain MHC alleles and seropositive RA remains to be unraveled, molecular analysis has revealed a common amino acid motif shared by disease-susceptible DR alleles in the third hypervariable region of their β chains, the so-called shared epitope (107). The possibility that these MHC class II alleles favor enhanced responsiveness to determinants in the Fc portion of IgG cannot be excluded; however, DR4 does not associate with increased levels of RF in the sera of healthy individuals (108). On the other hand, DR4 correlates with RF expression in unaffected first-degree relatives of patients with seropositive RA, suggesting that DR4 may directly predispose to RF production (109). HLA-DR4 alleles have been reported to be strongly associated with RF positivity in RA (110), although this association has not been noted in all studies (111). In a study of women with recent-onset RA, RF positivity was found more frequently among $DR4^+$ individuals with the shared epitope than among $DR1^+$ individuals with the epitope (112). This finding suggests that DR4 or genes linked to DR4, rather than the susceptibility epitope itself, is associated with RF positivity. Further evidence supporting an association between DR4 and RF responses is derived from the finding that polyclonally activated peripheral blood lymphocytes obtained from DR4-positive healthy individuals elaborate higher levels of IgM RF *in vitro* than peripheral blood lymphocytes from their DR4-negative counterparts (113).

There are likely to be other genetic influences on RF production. For example, a 32-base-pair deletion allele in the CC chemokine receptor 5 gene seems to be associated with the absence of IgM RF (114), suggesting that cell migration plays a role in RF production in RA.

The possibility that DR4 may also confer increased risk for more severe disease, unrelated to the presence of RF, has also been suggested by several studies (106,111,115,116). In a recent study of RF-positive patients with RA and erosive disease, individuals with two DRB1 genes containing the susceptibility epitope were more likely to have nodules, extraarticular manifestations, and joint surgery than those with a single susceptibility allele (117).

Differences between Rheumatoid Factors from Healthy Individuals and Rheumatoid Arthritis Patients

B-cell precursors bearing surface RF are commonly found in healthy human lymphoid tissues and in fetal cord blood (118,119). Furthermore, up to 20% of healthy elderly individuals have measurable titers of serum RF. The "physiologic" RFs produced by healthy individuals after infections or immunizations or during chronic inflammatory states have a number of important differences from those of RA patients (Table 17.2). Physio-

TABLE 17.2. Differences between "Physiologic" Rheumatoid Factor and the Rheumatoid Factor Found in Rheumatoid Arthritis Patients

	Physiologic	Rheumatoid Arthritis–Related
Immunoglobulin (Ig) isotype	Predominantly IgM.	All five isotypes.
Affinity	Relatively low. Avidity is increased by pentameric structure.	Variable. Some high affinity.
Somatic mutations	Few.	May occur.
Idiotype specificity	Narrow.	Broad. Many private idiotypes.
Ig gene usage	Restricted. Overuse of VκIII and VH1 genes.	Broad.
Affinity maturation	Does not occur.	Has been reported.
Site of origin	Extraarticular.	Large numbers of rheumatoid factor–producing plasma cells are found in synovial tissue.
Binding specificity	Narrow. Many have Ga specificity.	Broad. Many unique specificities.

logic RFs tend to be only of the IgM isotype and are on average of tenfold lower relative affinity than RFs derived from RA patients. Furthermore, physiologic RFs are more restricted, both in their V region usage and in the range of Fc epitopes that they recognize, than the RFs from RA patients. Finally, unlike most antibodies that arise during the course of a T-cell–dependent response to foreign antigen, physiologic RFs do not undergo isotype switching or affinity maturation. These features of physiologic RFs suggest that they arise in the absence of T-cell help. Alternatively, physiologic RFs may be derived from a subset of B cells (such as B1 cells or marginal zone B cells) that mature outside GCs and tend not to enter the memory B-cell compartment.

In patients with active RA, RFs undergo class switching and, in some instances, affinity maturation, and on switch to IgG can self-associate and generate large aggregates of stable immune complexes that fix complement and are potentially pathogenic (3). Unlike responses to foreign antigen, however, and for reasons that are not well understood, a large component of the RF response remains of the IgM isotype even in patients with longstanding disease.

Elicitation of Rheumatoid Factor by Polyclonal Activators

In healthy lymphoid tissues, cells that stain positively for RF-associated idiotypes are found outside the GC in the mantle zone of the follicle (Fig. 17.4) (119). Mantle zone cells are typically CD5 positive (120). Cord blood RF-producing cells also belong to the CD5-positive B1 subset. In patients with RA, both CD5-positive and -negative B cells contribute to RF secretion. RFs may be produced by peripheral blood B cells *in vitro* as a response to a number of different stimuli. For example, Epstein-Barr virus (EBV) induces B cells from both RA patients and healthy individuals to secrete RF *in vitro* in a T-cell independent fashion (121). This RF derives predominantly from the CD5 B-cell subset (38,122,123). On the other hand, pokeweed mitogen has been shown to induce RF production by peripheral B cells of RA patients only in the presence of T cells (124). Other T-dependent stimuli of RF production include tetanus toxoid (125), SPA (126), activated T cells and T-cell factors (118), and immune complexes (127).

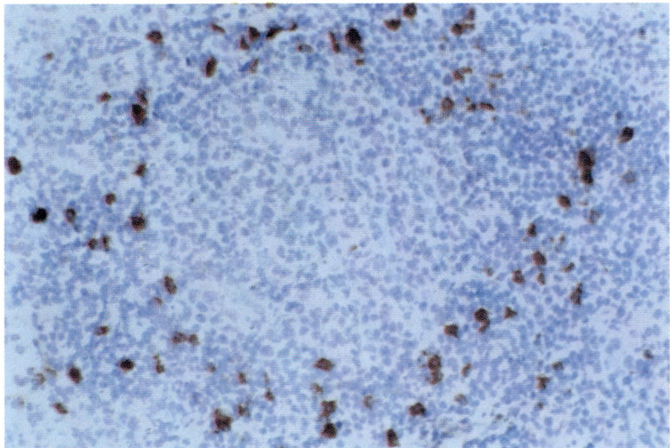

Figure 17.4. Staining of human tonsil with monoclonal antiidiotype 17.109 that recognizes a light chain determinant on human rheumatoid factor. Idiotype-positive cells (*stained red*) are frequent and are confined to the mantle zone surrounding the germinal center. (From Kipps TJ, Fong S, Tomhave E, et al. High-frequency expression of a conserved kappa light-chain variable-region gene in chronic lymphocytic leukemia. *Proc Natl Acad Sci U S A* 1987;84:2916–2920, with permission.)

The RFs induced by EBV share cross-reactive idiotypes with physiologic and paraprotein RFs (53), suggesting that these RFs may derive from the CD5$^+$ B-cell subset. In contrast, in two individual RA patients, RFs produced *in vitro* by T-dependent activation using pokeweed mitogen were idiotypically similar to serum RFs of each patient, but the RFs induced *in vitro* by EBV in a T-independent manner were dissimilar (121). Together, these experiments show that RF production can follow stimulation with a variety of different B-cell activators, and that B-cell origin and Ig gene repertoire may vary depending on the stimulus for production.

Transgenic Models of Rheumatoid Factor Production

An enhanced understanding of the regulation of RF-producing B cells has developed from the analysis of mice transgenic for high- and low-affinity RF. A transgenic mouse expressing a high-affinity human IgM RF that does not cross-react with mouse IgG was generated by Tighe et al. (128). In these mice, as in healthy humans, RF-producing B cells localize to primary follicles and to the mantle zones of secondary follicles in the spleen but do not spontaneously enter the GC. Levels of IgM RF in the serum of these mice are low despite the fact that a large percentage of the B-cell population expresses the transgene. The transgenic cells cannot be induced to secrete antibody by immunization with aggregated IgG, although they proliferate effectively to mitogens *in vitro*. Infusion of soluble deaggregated IgG, on the other hand, results in partial activation followed by deletion of the naïve RF-producing cells located in the primary follicles and mantle zones of the spleen but not of plasma cells established in the red pulp. If nonspecific T-cell help is given in the form of allogeneic T cells, some of the B cells are rescued from deletion, enter the GC, and differentiate into plasma cells (129–131). Although it is unclear whether the transgenic B cells are being regulated by endogenous self-antigen in this system, the studies clearly show that RF production is T-cell dependent *in vivo* and that in the absence of T-cell help, high-affinity RFs can be deleted by soluble Ig. The deletion of these B cells by soluble Ig was shown to be independent of Fas (132) and of T-cell contact and may be due to apoptosis induced by B-cell receptor (BCR) cross-linking in the absence of sufficient T-cell help and co-stimulation.

Mice transgenic for murine RF were generated by Shlomchik et al., who introduced two murine RFs, one of high affinity and one of lower affinity into nonautoimmune mice (132a). This system was designed so that the RFs only recognize a particular Fc allotype (IgG2a^a), and the transgene can be bred onto genetic backgrounds that either do or do not bear the IgG2a^a allotype. In mice transgenic for the high-affinity RF, breeding onto the IgG2a^a background but not onto the IgG2a^b background results in deletion or receptor editing of RF-producing B cells, showing normal central regulation of high-affinity RFs (133). The deletion of RF-producing B cells in this model is a dynamic process, depending on the amount of antigen present in the serum. The deleting antigen is initially derived from maternal Ig and after weaning; once IgG2a^a levels drop in the weanlings, RF-positive B cells begin to emerge. Later in life, as endogenous IgG2^a levels increase, deletion of RF-positive B cells occurs again in some mice, although, in others, tolerance cannot be reestablished (134). In the mice bearing a transgenic RF of lower-affinity, RF-producing B cells are clonally ignorant and can only be induced to secrete large amounts of autoantibody if the mouse is bred onto the autoimmune MRL/lpr background where T-cell help can be provided (135,136). In this setting, RF B cells proliferate at the border of the splenic T zone and the red pulp, not in GCs (137). Most light chain gene segments are highly mutated and, in many cases, genealogic trees can be constructed, suggesting antigen-driven selection of B cells. The authors speculate that there may be an unusually long duration of RF B-cell proliferation in the T-zone red pulp border in these mice. In addition, CD11c$^+$ dendritic cells interact with RF B cells and may support their survival and differentiation. Somatic mutation may be induced whenever B cells are stimulated to undergo a substantial number of cell cycles under conditions in which antigen and T-cell–derived signals required for mutation are present. Thus, extrafollicular B-cell mutation in healthy lymphoid organs or nonlymphoid organs, such as RA synovium, may allow B cells to escape healthy regulatory mechanisms that censor autoreactive B cells in the GC environment.

The studies described above show unequivocally that both antigen and T-cell help are required for activation of RF-secreting B cells. Two further important contributors to the regulation of RF production are evident. The first is the requirement for co-stimulation. It was first shown that deficiency of CD40 in the MRL/lpr mouse (that spontaneously develops RF and arthritis) results in the inability of these mice to generate RFs. In contrast, autoantibodies to SnRNP appear independent of either T-cell help or co-stimulation in the CD40-deficient MRL/lpr mouse (138). In the human RF transgenic model, co-stimulation through CD40 can substitute for T-cell help in the induction of RF production by soluble antigen (131). Similarly, proliferation of murine RF–producing transgenic B cells can be achieved by cross-linking of the BCR together with CD40 ligation (139). Subsequently, the myeloid cell–derived B-cell co-stimulatory molecule BAFF has been shown to induce RF production. BAFF transgenic mice have high levels of circulating immune complexes (CICs) and high levels of RFs. The finding that patients with RA have higher levels of BAFF than healthy controls suggests a mechanism by which RF production could be perpetuated (140).

Another important contributor to the RF response is the presence of antigen in the form of immune complexes (127). In healthy mice, activation of RF-producing cells by immune complexes is T-cell dependent (127). Soulas confirmed this finding using a transgenic model in which the RF is specific for human IgG. In nonautoimmune transgenic mice, aggregated human IgG can effectively delete RF-producing B cells as long as T-cell help is not provided (141).

Immune complexes have the opposite effect in the setting of autoimmunity in which T-cell help is available, such as in the autoimmune MRL/lpr mouse made transgenic for low-affinity RF. Immune complexes bearing Ig of the IgG2a^a allotype were found to be potent stimulators of proliferation of RF-positive B cells derived from these mice, whereas monomeric IgG2a^a was ineffective (139). Furthermore, the nature of the antigen in the immune complex appeared to influence the degree of stimulation of B-cell proliferation. The ability of immune complexes containing nuclear antigens to act as potent stimulators of RF B-cell proliferation has recently been attributed to cross-linking of the BCR by the Fc region with Toll-like receptor 9 by the nuclear antigen (142). Signaling through the Toll-like receptors may lead to altered localization or differentiation of B cells and may be a unifying feature of dominant autoantigens (137).

Thus, the ability of circulating IgG, either complexed or not, to regulate RF-producing B cells appears to depend both on the nature of the antigen in the immune complex and the availability of T-cell help. This model explains the observation that the "physiologic" RF response is generally of the IgM class, of low affinity, and germline encoded. During infection or inflammation, immune complexes and T-cell help are transiently available, and RF production is stimulated. Under normal circumstances, once the Ag–Ab complexes have been cleared from the circulation and T-cell help is no longer available, high-affinity RF-producing B cells are deleted either by the high concentrations of circulating monomeric IgG or by cross-linking of the FcγRIIB receptor by immune complexes. The result of this regulatory mechanism is that high-affinity RFs do not enter the long-term B-cell compartment (119,130,141). In contrast, in patients with RA, the RF response is amplified and displays evidence of a T-dependent clonal expansion, including class switching to IgG and IgA isotypes, accumulation of somatic mutations, and epitope spreading to multiple Fc epitopes.

What Antigen Initiates the Rheumatoid Factor Response?

Although the studies of transgenic mice have shed light on the regulation of RF production under a variety of circumstances, the antigen or antigens responsible for the high titer RF response in RA remain unknown. One possibility is that the RF response arises incidentally in the course of an immune response to an unrelated antigen. From the studies of RF transgenic mice, it has become clear that there are at least four major factors that regulate RF-producing B cells. These are

1. The affinity of the particular RF for Fc
2. The amount of circulating Ig
3. The presence of Ig in the form of certain types of immune complexes
4. The availability of T-cell help and co-stimulation

Some investigators have postulated that the RF response in RA is due to chronic and persistent antigenic stimulation within the synovium. However, this hypothesis is not supported by studies showing that in long-term population surveys, RF seropositivity may precede the clinical onset of joint disease for several years. Alternatively, the antigen inducing the RF response in RA may be Ig itself in the form of immune complexes with any foreign antigen; in this case, RF production could be viewed more generally as a defect in immune tolerance to self. The latter hypothesis is supported by findings in the murine RF transgenic model in which clonal ignorance of the transgenic RF is replaced by activation and expansion of the autoreactive response if the mice are bred onto the autoimmune MRL/lpr background (136). Although this is an attractive hypothesis, there is, as yet, no evidence that patients with RA have a generalized defect in either B- or T-cell tolerance.

Loss of tolerance to self may also result from exposure to altered self-antigen. Although high-affinity autoreactive T cells are ordinarily deleted or rendered anergic in the course of immune development, T cells recognizing nonimmunodominant "cryptic" peptides may not be eliminated during immune development. This T-cell population may be expanded when increased amounts of the self-protein are produced or antigen presentation is increased or altered (143,144). The production of RF in RA patients may be similarly due to a breakdown in tolerization of T cells to Ig peptides.

One reason for alteration of self-peptides is posttranslational modification. It is, therefore, of interest that posttranslational modifications of Ig that could induce neoepitopes have been identified in RA patients. It is well established that the IgG in the peripheral blood of patients with RA is hypogalactosylated (145,146). An absence of galactose on the N-linked sugars attached to Asn 297 in the CH2 domain of IgG results in the formation of a truncated oligosaccharide (Fig. 17.5). As much as 70% of serum IgG in RA patients may bear agalactosyl structures, compared with 15% to 30% in healthy individuals (145). Levels of agalactosyl IgG in patients with RA vary with disease flares and remissions, and early agalactosylation is associated

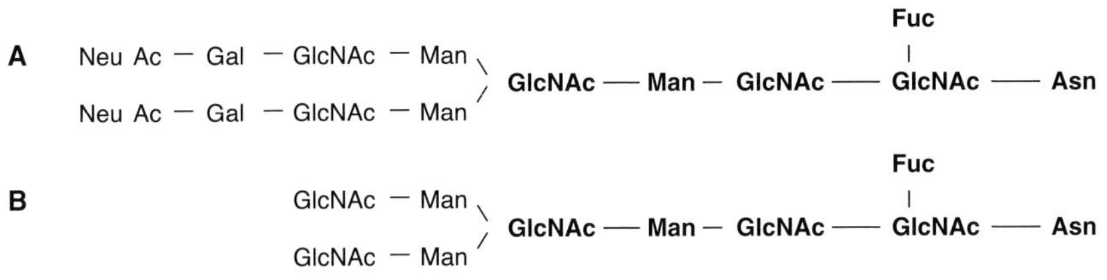

```
                                                       Fuc
                                                        |
A   Neu Ac — Gal — GlcNAc — Man \
                                 > GlcNAc — Man — GlcNAc — GlcNAc — Asn
    Neu Ac — Gal — GlcNAc — Man /

                                                       Fuc
                                                        |
B                  GlcNAc — Man \
                                 > GlcNAc — Man — GlcNAc — GlcNAc — Asn
                   GlcNAc — Man /
```

Figure 17.5. A: Structure of N-linked oligosaccharide attached to Asn 297 of immunoglobulin G (IgG)-CH2 domain. The core structure is shown in bold. Variant glycoforms arise from presence or absence of the sugars shown in plain type. **B:** Structure of the N-linked agalactosylated oligosaccharide found on circulating IgG of patients with rheumatoid arthritis.

with a more progressive disease course (145–147). Hypogalactosylation of serum IgG has been found in only a few conditions other than RA, notably in granulomatous T-cell–dependent diseases such as tuberculosis, Crohn's disease, and leprosy and in the mouse models of RA induced by pristane and type II collagen (148). The precise basis for the abnormal galactosylation found in RA patients is unknown. Galactosyl-transferase activity is decreased in the B cells of RA patients (148–150); however, because the RA glycosylation defect is reversible (145), it is unlikely that there is a mutation of the gene encoding either galactosyl-transferase or its kinases. Hypogalactosylation may be due to the action of interleukin-6, and, indeed, mice transgenic for interleukin-6 have high levels of circulating agalactosyl IgG (151).

Another abnormality that may occur in RA is the modification of Ig by advanced end glycation products (AGEs). This posttranslational modification can result from hyperglycemia or oxidative stress, or both. IgM antibodies against AGE-modified IgG (IgM anti-IgG-AGE) were found in three patients with aggressive RA and vasculitis (152). A larger number of patients with RA and other autoimmune diseases and a panel of healthy individuals were then tested for IgM and IgA anti-IgG-AGE by enzyme-linked immunoassay. Anti-AGE antibodies could be detected in 33% to 60% of RF-positive individuals but were not found in RF-negative individuals with RA or other rheumatic and autoimmune diseases. RF and IgM anti-IgG-AGE appeared to be a linked response.

Apart from possible effects related to breaking tolerance to Ig, posttranslational modifications of IgG might affect the function of the Ig itself, such as the ability to fix complement or bind Fc receptors, which could result in alterations in endocytosis of IgG-containing complexes. If endocytosis were decreased, this would result in prolonged exposure of cells to unprocessed complexes on the surface of APCs as is seen on FDCs in the GCs. If endocytosis were increased, this would result in rapid internalization of complexes and an increased load of processed antigenic peptides on the cell surface.

In conclusion, the reason for specific elicitation of high-titer RF in RA patients remains unclear. Possible stimuli for production of RF could include a defect in T- or B-cell tolerance to endogenous Ig, stimulation by a cross-reactive antigen, prolonged exposure to immune complexes, or exposure to neoepitopes generated from altered Ig.

Effect of Drugs and Disease Activity on Expression of Rheumatoid Factors

Several investigators have attempted to delineate the clinical significance of changes in RF levels in patients with RA. The interpretation of these studies has generally been complicated by accompanying changes in medication. Nonsteroidal antiinflammatory drugs were initially reported to directly suppress RF production *in vitro* and *in vivo* (153,154). More recent studies indicate that decreases in serum RF associated with nonsteroidal antiinflammatory drug administration correlate with improvement in disease activity (155). Treatment with methotrexate and, to a lesser extent, clinical improvement have been shown to correlate with a decrease of serum IgM-RF production in patients with RA (156). Suppression of spontaneous *in vitro* RF production by peripheral blood lymphocytes obtained from patients with RA after initiation of methotrexate therapy is also consistent with a direct effect of this agent on RF production (157). Treatment with other drugs, including tumor necrosis factor blockers (158), cyclophosphamide (159), and the B-cell–depleting anti-CD20 antibody (160), induces a decrease in RF titers. Taken together, these data indicate that RF levels in RA are likely influenced both by the clinical activity of the disease and the concomitant therapy.

Rheumatoid Factor and B-Cell Malignancies

It is of interest that, in malignancies of mature B cells, neoplastic transformation preferentially occurs in B cells with RF specificity. The reason why so many B-cell malignancies produce RF is unclear. Studies in humans have revealed that many of the antibodies produced by malignant B cells display autoreactivity apart from RF activity (161–163). It has, therefore, been postulated that two events might be necessary for malignant transformation to occur. One would be a gene alteration event that occurs randomly. The second would require cellular events that are a consequence of contact with antigen, such as gene rearrangement events. Contact with antigen would be more likely to occur for autoantigen than foreign antigen. Alternatively, potential carcinogens inside immune complexes, such as transforming viruses, are more likely to be engulfed by RF B cells. Finally, because RF B-cell precursors are common, and because they are constantly traversing the cell cycle, their likelihood of sustaining DNA damage that could lead to malignant transformation is increased (119).

FUNCTION AND PATHOGENICITY OF RHEUMATOID FACTOR AND RHEUMATOID FACTOR–PRODUCING B CELLS

Pathogenicity of Rheumatoid Factor

Plasma cells that secrete RF are abundant within the rheumatoid synovium, and the synovial fluid contains high titers of IgM and IgG RF. The high concentrations of IgG RF in the synovial fluid relative to the concentration of monomeric IgG can lead to self-association of RFs with formation of large aggregates (68). These aggregates are pathogenic because of their ability to further stimulate RF-producing B cells to proliferate as described above and because they are able to fix complement, thus triggering inflammatory cascades. Self-associating IgG RFs that escape into the serum usually dissociate into smaller complexes because of competition from circulating soluble IgG; however, when present in high titer, these complexes may not dissociate and are thought to be responsible for the vasculitis that complicates the course of some RA patients.

There is some evidence that the presence of agalactosyl IgG results in a more pathogenic immune complex. In collagen-induced arthritis, the agalactosyl forms of antibodies to type II collagen are more pathogenic than their fully glycosylated counterparts (164), perhaps because the vacant glycosylation sites on IgG create a lectin-like activity that promotes the self-association of IgG and enhances immune complex formation (147,164,165). Studies of agalactosyl IgG have suggested that complement activation may, in fact, be augmented through binding of agalactosyl IgG to the endogenous lectin mannose binding protein that activates complement through both classic and alternative pathways (148).

Pathogenicity of Rheumatoid Factor–Producing B Cells

It has become increasingly evident that B cells have multiple functions that are separate from their role as antibody-producing cells (166). These functions include the production of soluble molecules, such as cytokines, which can influence immune responses of T cells and APCs; release of chemokines that regulate organization of lymphoid structures; and, when activated, expression of co-stimulatory molecules, such as B7, that enhance antigen-presentation capability.

RF-producing B cells are ideally suited for some of these functions because they proliferate in response to immune complexes and T-cell help and because they are able to take up foreign antigens within immune complexes via their BCR. The ability of RF B cells to take up immune complexes confers markedly enhanced antigen-presenting function. Roosnek and Lanzavecchia (167) were the first to show that RF-positive B cells efficiently present antigen derived from Ag–Ab complexes and that RF-negative B cells do not, indicating that the uptake of immune complexes is much more effective via B-cell membrane Ig than via Fc receptors. These results were confirmed using the human-RF transgenic system. If the RF transgenic mice were immunized with tetanus toxoid, spleen cells from the mice were highly effective APCs of tetanus toxoid/human anti–tetanus toxoid immune complexes, indicating a role for RF-producing B cells as APCs *in vivo* (128). RF-producing B cells can effectively present antigen derived from immune complexes to T cells specific for that antigen; at the same time, those T cells augment the RF response. Under normal circumstances, the ability of RF B cells to present peptides derived from the antigen within the immune complex allows efficient amplification of the immune response to antigen to include epitopes of antigen that are only derived from B cells. The secreted RFs help clear the immune complexes, thus contributing to termination of the immune response.

Under pathologic circumstances, RF-producing B cells could greatly amplify abnormal immune responses by presenting cryptic epitopes of self-antigens present in immune complexes. Because abnormal lymphoid neogenesis occurs in the synovium, the large number of RF-producing B cells present locally could amplify self-reactive responses to other synovial antigens. The presence of large aggregates of self-associating IgG RFs and the availability of T-cell help in the lymphoid aggregates of the synovium help perpetuate the RF response. In addition, once plasma cells have been generated and are located within the synovial tissue or the bone marrow, they may no longer be responsive to any down-regulatory effects of the high concentration of circulating monomeric IgG that control the RF response under normal circumstances. Secretion of chemokines by synovial B cells may further perpetuate the continuing lymphoid infiltration of the joint. In particular, secretion of lymphotoxin alpha by B cells is important for recruitment of FDCs and organization of lymphoid follicular structures within the synovium (168,169).

In sum, these studies show that, although expression of RF in a nonautoimmune host is not sufficient to cause disease, in the setting of RA, both RFs and the B cells that produce them can play a pathogenic role by multiple mechanisms (Fig. 17.6). The recognition of a potential pathogenic role of RF-producing

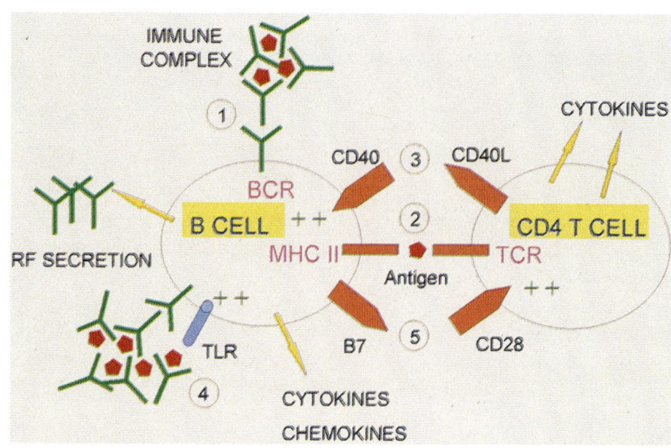

Figure 17.6. Multiple functions of rheumatoid factor (RF) B cells. RF–positive B cells recognize immune complexes via surface expression of B-cell receptor (BCR) (*1*) with RF specificity. Endocytosis of these complexes results in antigen presentation of the antigen within the immune complex to CD4$^+$ T cells via T-cell receptors (TCRs) (*2*), which recognize antigen in the context of class II major histocompatibility complex (MHC II). T cells co-stimulate (++) B cells through ligation of CD40 (*3*), resulting in secretion of soluble immunoglobulin. RF–positive B cells can also be stimulated to proliferate by immune complexes, possibly through co-ligation of Toll-like receptors (TLRs) (*4*). Activated B cells may secrete a variety of cytokines and chemokines important in organization of lymphoid tissue and may express B7 that co-stimulates T-cell activation and cytokine secretion through ligation of CD28 (*5*).

B cells in RA has led to the concept that B-cell depletion may be a beneficial therapeutic strategy.

TARGETING B CELLS IN RHEUMATOID ARTHRITIS

There is considerable rationale for the B lymphocyte as a target in RA, including the presence of RFs in synovial fluid and the presence of B lymphocytes in subsynovial inflammatory infiltrates. The recent availability of treatments to selectively deplete antibodies and B cells has provided a unique opportunity to clarify the role of B cells in the pathogenesis of RA.

Staphylococcal Protein A Immunoadsorption (Prosorba) Column

Apheresis using a SPA (Prosorba) column is among the currently approved treatments for RA. In a placebo-controlled trial of 91 patients with refractory disease, weekly treatments for 12 weeks were shown to be effective (170). Studies of the humoral effects of the Prosorba column were conducted in three RA patients in conjunction with this trial (171).

At the start of treatment, passage through the column reduces the plasma concentrations of IgG disproportionately compared to albumin, IgM, IgA, and IgM RF. After 15 minutes of treatment, only the concentration of IgM RF is decreased markedly by passage through the column. The IgM RF of one patient declined by 88%, but this patient was a nonresponder. All three patients tested had normal levels of CICs, and no quantitative changes in CIC concentration were noted after passage through the column. In conclusion, the Prosorba column reduced IgM RF levels in some patients but did not appear to improve disease activity through this mechanism.

Anti-CD20 Antibody (Rituximab)

Rituximab is a genetically engineered chimeric murine/human monoclonal antibody directed against the CD20 antigen found on the surface of most B lymphocytes, with the exception of plasma cells. This biologic agent is U.S. Food and Drug Administration–approved for the treatment of relapsed or refractory, low-grade or follicular, CD20-positive, B-cell non-Hodgkin's lymphoma (172). In an uncontrolled, unblinded pilot study of five RA patients, treatment with high-dose corticosteroids, intravenous cyclophosphamide, and anti-CD20 was found to be efficacious (173). Two of the five treated patients had return of normal numbers of circulating B cells but no flare in RA activity. It is unknown whether the B cells that repopulate the periphery after anti-CD20 therapy are different in maturity or specificity from those present before therapy. It is possible that prednisolone and cyclophosphamide initially induce significant clinical benefit, perhaps by depleting plasma cells, and that anti-CD20–associated B-cell depletion leads to continued control of disease activity.

Results of a larger placebo-controlled study of anti-CD20 in methotrexate partial responders have been reported (174). Patients were randomized to one of four groups: no additional drug (N = 30), anti-CD20 (N = 31), anti-CD20 plus cyclophosphamide (N = 31), and anti-CD20 plus methotrexate (N = 30). Percentages of patients achieving American College of Rheumatology 50 responses at 24 weeks were 10%, 32%, 45%, and 50% in groups 1 through 4, respectively. Decrease or normalization of serum C-reactive protein, anti–cyclic citrullinated peptide (CCP) antibodies, and RF levels were observed in subjects receiving anti-CD20 (175). Thus, anti-CD20 may have a therapeutic effect by depleting B lymphocytes, including those with autoreactive specificities, but these findings await confirmation.

Inhibitors of Co-Stimulation

As discussed in Regulation of Rheumatoid Factor Production, RF production is dependent on T-cell help and co-stimulation. Inhibitors of co-stimulatory molecules involved in T-cell activation have been recently investigated in the treatment of RA. In a study of MRL/lpr mice treated with CTLA4Ig, a soluble antagonist B7/CD28 co-stimulatory T-cell activation pathway (176), production of autoantibodies (anti–double-stranded DNA antibody and RF) was suppressed, as was organ damage. An investigational trial of CTLA4Ig in RA showed therapeutic benefit (177), although changes in RF levels were not reported.

Inhibition of other co-stimulatory receptor ligand pairs will undoubtedly be tested in future studies. One pathway of potential interest is the interaction of the lymphotoxin β receptor with its ligands, lymphotoxin $\alpha_1\beta_2$ and LIGHT. This interaction is responsible for up-regulating expression of the T-cell–attracting chemokine CCL21 and the B-cell–attracting chemokine CXCL13. High levels of lymphotoxin β and CXCL13 have been found in rheumatoid synovia and may be responsible for mediating lymphoid neogenesis (169). It is, therefore, of relevance to RA that soluble lymphotoxin-β receptor Ig-fusion protein can reverse lymphoid neogenesis in a mouse model of diabetes (178).

OTHER AUTOANTIBODIES FOUND IN RHEUMATOID ARTHRITIS

In addition to antibodies to the Fc region of IgG, multiple other autoantibodies have been reported in RA (Table 17.3). The identity of the cognate antigens for these antibodies may provide additional insight into the pathogenesis of RA.

Antibodies to Type II Collagen

Among the autoantigens that are potentially immunogenic in RA is type II collagen, a normal constituent of articular cartilage. It has been shown that immunization with type II collagen can cause an inflammatory arthritis that histologically resembles RA in rats, mice, and primates (179) and that this disease can be transferred by antibodies alone (180). Antibodies to type II collagen have been found frequently in synovia of RA patients compared to patients with other types of arthritis (181). They may also be seen in other rheumatic and infectious diseases (182). Anti–type II collagen antibodies early in the disease may predict more severe disease (183). Finally, studies of oral tolerance, in which type II collagen is administered orally to RA patients, reported a small but significant reduction in joint pain and swelling in treated patients compared to controls (184,185), although these results await confirmation in larger studies.

TABLE 17.3. Autoantibodies and Autoantigens in Rheumatoid Arthritis

Antibody	Antigen
Rheumatoid factor	Fc region of immunoglobulin G
Anti-collagen	Type II collagen
Anti–human cartilage gycoprotein-39	Human cartilage glycoprotein-39
Anti-aggrecan	Aggrecan
Anti–cartilage link protein	Cartilage link protein
Anti-perinuclear factor	(Pro)filaggrin
Anti-keratin	(Pro)filaggrin
Anti-filaggrin	Filaggrin
Anti–cyclic citrullinated peptides	Citrullinated peptides on multiple proteins
Anti-RA33	A2 protein of the heterogeneous nuclear ribonucleoprotein
Anti-Sa	? Citrullinated vimentin
Anti-calpastatin	Calpastatin
Anti-p68	Heavy chain binding protein
Anti–glucose-6-phosphate isomerase	Glucose-6-phosphate isomerase
Anti-enolase	Enolase

Antibodies to Human Cartilage gp-39

Human cartilage gp-39 (HC gp-39, also called *YKL-40*), glycoprotein expressed by articular chondrocytes and synoviocytes, has also received attention as a candidate autoantigen in RA (186). HC gp-39, a member of the chitinase protein family whose function is unknown, was originally isolated from RA synovial fluid and sera and described as a biochemical marker of joint injury (187). Immunization of BALB/c mice with HC gp-39 induces a chronic and relapsing arthritis; as in human RA, there is pannus production and degradation of cartilage. Plasma levels of HC gp-39 may be elevated in RA as well as in other inflammatory conditions, such as SLE and inflammatory bowel disease (188).

Antibodies to Aggrecan and Cartilage Link Protein

Cartilage proteoglycans, such as aggrecan, are autoantigens in some individuals with RA. Fragments of these molecules may be released from the cartilage and help to perpetuate the abnormal immune response in RA synovium. In RA, autoantibodies against proteoglycans are present as immune complexes or bound to the degraded, eroded cartilage surface. Antibodies against the G1 globular domain of aggrecan occur in a significant number of RA patients but only after keratan sulfate has been removed (189). BALB/c mice develop progressive polyarthritis similar to RA after immunization with deglycosylated core protein and with the G1 domain (190,191). Glycosylation of the proteoglycan and, perhaps, collagen and HC gp-39 molecules may influence antigen presentation and T-cell responses.

Anti-Perinuclear Factor and Anti-Keratin, Anti-Filaggrin, and Anti–Cyclic Citrullinated Peptide Antibodies

In 1964, Nienhuis and Mandema first reported the presence of antibodies directed against cytoplasmic granules in buccal mucosal cells in the serum of patients with RA, so-called anti-perinuclear factors (192). A naturally occurring antibody reactive against keratinized tissue of animal esophagus was first reported in 1979 (192a,193). Anti-keratin antibodies have been shown to be associated with RA (193–197). The antigenic target of these anti-keratin antibodies was subsequently identified as a neutral/acidic isoform of basic filaggrin, a cytokeratin filament–aggregating protein (198). Anti-perinuclear factors were found to bind an antigen related to human epidermal (pro)filaggrin (199). Anti-filaggrin antibodies are enriched in RA synovial membranes (200).

More recently, autoantibodies reactive with synthetic peptides containing citrulline, a posttranslationally modified (deiminated) arginine residue, have been described in RA (201). Citrullination of proteins is mediated by peptidylarginine deiminase, an enzyme that exists in at least five forms in humans and can occur during the process of apoptosis (Fig. 17.7). Activity of the enzyme is also influenced by estrogen. Many proteins can undergo citrullination, and it is yet to be determined whether a specific citrullinated protein is a specific autoantigen in RA (202). Antibodies to CCP may be responsible for the specificity of anti-perinuclear factors and anti-keratin antibodies. In addition, anti-filaggrin antibodies recognize citrulline-bearing epitopes present on various molecular forms of (pro)filaggrin (203,204). Anti-CCP antibodies appear to recognize several citrulline-containing proteins, including deiminated forms of the α and β chains of fibrin (203). Thus, deiminated forms of fibrin deposited in RA rheumatoid synovial membranes may represent the major target of anti-filaggrin antibodies. Anti-CCP antibodies have been found to be highly specific for RA (96%) compared to healthy controls (195), but conflicting reports have been published about their association with disease severity (195,205). Measurement of anti-CCP antibodies may have clinical utility in helping to establish a diagnosis of early RA or in RF-negative patients.

Anti-RA33 Antibodies

Autoantibodies to a nuclear antigen termed *RA33*, which were originally thought to be highly specific for RA, were first described in 1989 (206). The RA33 antigen was subsequently identified as the A2 protein of the heterogeneous nuclear ribonucleoprotein complex (207). Anti-RA33 antibodies are also found in SLE and in mixed connective tissue disease (197), so that it is unclear what information about the pathogenesis of RA can be gleaned from their presence.

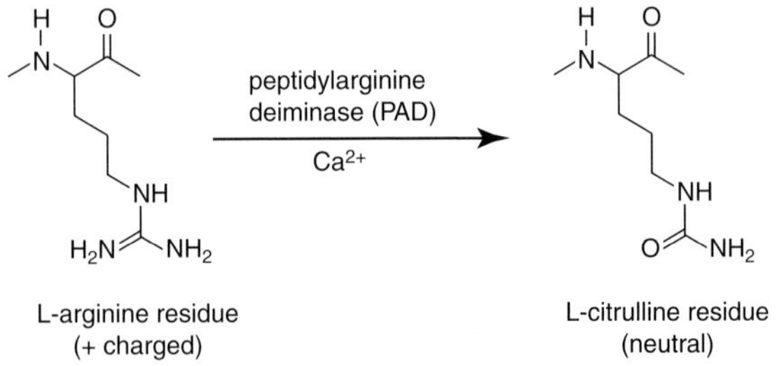

Figure 17.7. The enzymatic conversion of peptidyl-arginine to peptidyl-citrulline by peptidyl arginine deiminase. (From van Boekel MA, Vossenaar ER, van den Hoogen FH, et al. Autoantibody systems in rheumatoid arthritis: specificity, sensitivity and diagnostic value. *Arthritis Res* 2002;4:87–93, with permission.)

Anti-Sa Antibodies

Autoantibodies to a 50-kd protein present in healthy human spleen and placenta and in RA synovial tissue (anti-Sa antibodies) were first reported in 1994 (208). Anti-Sa antibodies were found to have a high specificity for RA (208–210) and were found to be distinct from RF, anti-filaggrin, and anti-calpastatin antibodies. In an analysis of patients with early arthritis, anti-Sa antibodies were found to identify a subset of predominantly male RA patients with severe, erosive disease (211). Identification of the cognate antigen of anti-Sa antibodies has proven to be quite difficult. Recent evidence suggests that the Sa antigen may be a citrullinated form of vimentin, a cytoskeletal intermediate filament protein (210).

In a study of 238 patients with early peripheral synovitis, sera were tested for RF and antibodies to Sa, RA33, (pro)filaggrin, CCP, calpastatin, and keratin (211). There was a high degree of correlation between anti-filaggrin, anti-keratin, anti-Sa, and anti-CCP antibodies. Of the 101 patients who were positive for at least one of these four autoantibodies, 57% were positive for only one. This modest degree of concordance between antibodies that likely recognize citrullinated antigens suggests that multiple antigens are responsible for these responses (211).

Anti-Calpastatin Antibodies

Calpastatin is a naturally occurring protein that serves as a specific inhibitor of calpains, calcium-dependent neutral cysteine proteinases. Although anti-calpastatin antibodies have been found in approximately 45% of RA sera (212,213), they have also been found in sera of patients with SLE, myositis, scleroderma, and in healthy sera (214).

Anti-p68 Antibodies

Antibodies to the p68 protein, recently identified as *heavy chain binding protein* (BiP), have been found in RA sera (215). The BiP protein is an antigen for both T and B cells in RA (216). BiP is a ubiquitously expressed chaperone protein expressed predominantly in the endoplasmic reticulum, but, with heat shock, it can localize to the cell nucleus (217). The major B-cell epitope on the BiP protein is an *N*-acetylglucosamine carbohydrate group (217). It has been speculated that the alteration in glycosylation pattern of BiP, along with its relocation to the nucleus, may induce anti-p68 antibodies in RA.

Antibodies to Enzymes of the Glycolytic Pathway

An enzyme of the glycolytic pathway, glucose-6-phosphate isomerase (GPI) has been found to be a B-cell autoantigen in a T-cell receptor transgenic mouse model (K/BxN) that spontaneously develops a disease that closely resembles RA in humans (218). Both B and T lymphocytes are required for development of arthritis in these mice (219), and there is evidence that the arthritis is a result of an adaptive immune response leading to an overexuberant innate immune response (220). Strikingly, once initiated, disease can be transferred with anti-GPI antibodies alone. GPI is a ubiquitous enzyme but appears to be expressed on the synovial lining, where it is available to bind Ig and complement. Inflammation may be joint specific because the articular cartilage surface lacks complement inhibitors (221).

It has been reported that up to 64% of RA patients, but not controls, have anti-GPI IgG in serum and synovial fluid and that the presence of these antibodies correlates with extraarticular manifestations and with Felty's syndrome (222,222a). The frequency of anti-GPI positivity and the specificity of anti-GPI antibodies for RA have been challenged, however, in a number of larger studies (223,224,224a). Antibodies to other enzymes, such as creatine kinase (224) and alpha-enolase (225), have also been reported in RA. The specificity of anti–alpha-enolase antibodies for RA is reportedly approximately 97% and may predict radiologic progression (225).

Other Autoantibodies

A variety of other autoantibodies have been described in RA, but these are often present in other inflammatory, autoimmune, or infectious diseases (182). Thus, their role in the pathogenesis of RA is unclear, and their presence may reflect the presence of inflammation or a normal immune response to antigens unrelated to the etiopathogenesis of RA. Such antibodies include those directed at fibronectin (226), nonhistone chromosomal proteins HMG1 and HMG2 (227), as well as antineutrophil cytoplasmic antibodies (228) and antiphospholipid antibodies (182).

REFERENCES

1. Waaler E. On the occurrence of a factor in human serum activating the specific agglutination of sheep blood corpuscles. *Acta Pathol Microbiol Scand* 1940;17:172–188.
2. Rose HM, Ragan C, Pearce E, et al. Differential agglutination of normal and sensitive sheep erythrocytes by sera of patients with rheumatoid arthritis. *Proc Soc Exp Biol Med* 1948;68:1–6.
3. Egeland T, Munthe E. The role of the laboratory in rheumatology. Rheumatoid factors. *Clin Rheum Dis* 1983;9:135–160.
4. Mageed RA, Børretzen M, Moyes SP, et al. Rheumatoid factor autoantibodies in health and disease. *Ann N Y Acad Sci* 1997;815:296–311.
5. Bridges SL Jr. Rheumatoid factor. In: Koopman WJ, ed. *Arthritis and allied conditions*, 14th ed. Baltimore: Williams and Wilkins, 2000:1223–1244.
6. Zvaifler NJ. Immunopathology of joint inflammation in rheumatoid arthritis. *Adv Immunol* 1973;16:265–336.
7. Möttönen T, Paimela L, Leirisalo-Repo M, et al. Only high disease activity and positive rheumatoid factor indicate poor prognosis in patients with early rheumatoid arthritis treated with "sawtooth" strategy. *Ann Rheum Dis* 1998;57:533–539.
8. Wolfe F, Sharp JT. Radiographic outcome of recent-onset rheumatoid arthritis: a 19-year study of radiographic progression. *Arthritis Rheum* 1998;41:1571–1582.
9. Jansen LM, van dH-B, I, van Schaardenburg D, et al. Predictors of radiographic joint damage in patients with early rheumatoid arthritis. *Ann Rheum Dis* 2001;60:924–927.
10. Combe B, Dougados M, Goupille P, et al. Prognostic factors for radiographic damage in early rheumatoid arthritis: a multiparameter prospective study. *Arthritis Rheum* 2001;44:1736–1743.
11. Mattey DL, Hassell AB, Dawes PT, et al. Independent association of rheumatoid factor and the HLA-DRB1 shared epitope with radiographic outcome in rheumatoid arthritis. *Arthritis Rheum* 2001;44:1529–1533.
12. van Zeben D, Hazes JM, Zwinderman AH, et al. Clinical significance of rheumatoid factors in early rheumatoid arthritis: results of a follow up study. *Ann Rheum Dis* 1992;51:1029–1035.
13. Jacobsson LT, Knowler WC, Pillemer S, et al. Rheumatoid arthritis and mortality. A longitudinal study in Pima Indians. *Arthritis Rheum* 1993;36:1045–1053.
14. van Schaardenburg D, Hazes JM, de Boer A, et al. Outcome of rheumatoid arthritis in relation to age and rheumatoid factor at diagnosis. *J Rheumatol* 1993;20:45–52.
15. Goodson NJ, Wiles NJ, Lunt M, et al. Mortality in early inflammatory polyarthritis: cardiovascular mortality is increased in seropositive patients. *Arthritis Rheum* 2002;46:2010–2019.
16. Ball J, Lawrence JS. The relationship of rheumatoid serum factor to rheumatoid arthritis: a 5-year follow up of a population sample. *Ann Rheum Dis* 1963;22:311–318.
17. Aho K, Palosuo T, Raunio V, et al. When does rheumatoid disease start? *Arthritis Rheum* 1985;28:485–489.
18. Del Puente A, Knowler WC, Pettitt DJ, et al. The incidence of rheumatoid arthritis is predicted by rheumatoid factor titer in a longitudinal population study. *Arthritis Rheum* 1988;31:1239–1244.
19. Halldorsdottir HD, Jonsson T, Thorsteinsson J, et al. A prospective study on the incidence of rheumatoid arthritis among people with persistent increase of rheumatoid factor. *Ann Rheum Dis* 2000;59:149–151.
20. Feldman D, Feldman D, Ginzler E, et al. Rheumatoid factor in patients with systemic lupus erythematosus. *J Rheumatol* 1989;16:618–622.
21. Pinillos RM, Sole JM, Roura X, et al. Rheumatoid factor in patients with systemic lupus erythematosus. *Ann Rheum Dis* 1987;46:877–878.
22. Richter Cohen M, Steiner G, Smolen JS, et al. Erosive arthritis in systemic lupus erythematosus: analysis of a distinct clinical and serological subset. *Br J Rheumatol* 1998;37:421–424.
23. Tarkowski A, Westberg G. Rheumatoid factor isotypes and renal disease in systemic lupus erythematosus. *Scand J Rheumatol* 1987;16:309–312.
24. Garcia-Carrasco M, Ramos-Casals M, Cervera R, et al. Cryoglobulinemia in systemic lupus erythematosus: prevalence and clinical characteristics in a series of 122 patients. *Semin Arthritis Rheum* 2001;30:366–373.
25. Meltzer M, Franklin EC, Elias K, et al. Cryoglobulinemia—a clinical and laboratory study. II. Cryoglobulins with rheumatoid factor activity. *Am J Med* 1966;40:837–856.
26. Murakami J, Shimizu Y, Kashii Y, et al. Functional B-cell response in intrahepatic lymphoid follicles in chronic hepatitis C. *Hepatology* 1999;30:143–150.
27. Tzioufas AG, Boumba DS, Skopouli FN, et al. Mixed monoclonal cryoglobulinemia and monoclonal rheumatoid factor cross-reactive idiotypes as predictive factors for the development of lymphoma in primary Sjögren's syndrome. *Arthritis Rheum* 1996;39:767–772.
28. Martin T, Weber JC, Levallois H, et al. Salivary gland lymphomas in patients with Sjögren's syndrome may frequently develop from rheumatoid factor B cells. *Arthritis Rheum* 2000;43:908–916.
29. Randen I, Pascual V, Victor K, et al. Synovial IgG rheumatoid factors show evidence of an antigen-driven immune response and a shift in the V gene repertoire compared to IgM rheumatoid factors. *Eur J Immunol* 1993;23:1220–1225.
30. Børretzen M, Randen I, Zdarsky E, et al. Control of autoantibody affinity by selection against amino acid replacements in the complementarity-determining regions. *Proc Natl Acad Sci U S A* 1994;91:12917–12921.
31. Artandi SE, Calame KL, Morrison SL, Bonagura VR. Monoclonal IgM rheumatoid factors bind IgG at a discontinuous epitope comprised of amino acid loops from heavy-chain constant-region domains 2 and 3. *Proc Natl Acad Sci U S A* 1992;89:94–98.
32. Bonagura VR, Artandi SE, Davidson A, et al. Mapping studies reveal unique epitopes on IgG recognized by rheumatoid arthritis-derived monoclonal rheumatoid factors. *J Immunol* 1993;151:3840–3852.
33. Bonagura VR, Agostino N, Børretzen M, et al. Mapping IgG epitopes bound by rheumatoid factors from immunized controls identifies disease-specific rheumatoid factors produced by patients with rheumatoid arthritis. *J Immunol* 1998;160:2496–2505.
34. Oppliger IR, Nardella FA, Stone GC, et al. Human rheumatoid factors bear the internal image of the Fc binding region of staphylococcal protein A. *J Exp Med* 1987;166:702–710.
35. Sasso EH, Barber CV, Nardella FA, et al. Antigenic specificities of human monoclonal and polyclonal IgM rheumatoid factors. The C gamma 2-C gamma 3 interface region contains the major determinants. *J Immunol* 1988;140:3098–3107.
36. Sutton B, Corper A, Bonagura V, et al. The structure and origin of rheumatoid factors. *Immunol Today* 2000;21:177–183.
37. Kunkel HG, Agnello V, Joslin FG, et al. Cross-idiotypic specificity among monoclonal IgM proteins with anti-gamma-globulin activity. *J Exp Med* 1973;137:331–342.
38. Chen PP, Fong S, Carson DA. Rheumatoid factor. *Rheum Dis Clin North Am* 1987;13:545–568.
39. Kunkel HG, Winchester RJ, Joslin FG, et al. Similarities in the light chains of anti-gamma-globulins showing cross-idiotypic specificities. *J Exp Med* 1974;139:128–136.
40. Agnello V. The etiology and pathophysiology of mixed cryoglobulinemia secondary to hepatitis C virus infection. *Springer Semin Immunopathol* 1997;19:111–129.
41. Carson DA, Chen PP, Kipps TJ, et al. Idiotypic and genetic studies of human rheumatoid factors. *Arthritis Rheum* 1987;30:1321–1325.
42. Koopman WJ, Schrohenloher RE, Carson DA. Dissociation of expression of two rheumatoid factor cross-reactive kappa L chain idiotopes in rheumatoid arthritis. *J Immunol* 1990;144:3468–3472.
43. Schrohenloher RE, Accavitti MA, Bhown AS, et al. Monoclonal antibody 6B6.6 define a cross-reactive kappa light chain idiotope on human monoclonal and polyclonal rheumatoid factors. *Arthritis Rheum* 1990;33:187–198.
44. Carson DA, Chen PP, Fox RI, et al. Rheumatoid factor and immune networks. *Annu Rev Immunol* 1987;5:109–126.
45. Lee SK, Bridges SL Jr., Koopman WJ, et al. The immunoglobulin kappa light chain repertoire expressed in the synovium of a patient with rheumatoid arthritis. *Arthritis Rheum* 1992;35:905–913.
46. Dobloug JH, Forre O, Natvig JB, et al. Demonstration of rheumatoid factor idiotypic antigens on peripheral blood B and T lymphocytes from patients with rheumatoid arthritis. *Scand J Immunol* 1979;9:273–279.
47. Gharavi AE, Patel BM, Hughes GR, et al. Common IgA and IgM rheumatoid factor idiotypes in autoimmune diseases. *Ann Rheum Dis* 1985;44:155–158.
48. Mageed RA, Dearlove M, Goodall DM, et al. Immunogenic and antigenic epitopes of immunoglobulins. XVII—Monoclonal antibodies reactive with common and restricted idiotopes to the heavy chain of human rheumatoid factors. *Rheumatol Int* 1986;6:179–183.
49. Ono M, Winearls CG, Amos N, et al. Monoclonal antibodies to restricted and cross-reactive idiotopes on monoclonal rheumatoid factors and their recognition of idiotope-positive cells. *Eur J Immunol* 1987;17:343–349.
50. Pasquali JL, Urlacher A, Storck D. A highly conserved determinant on human rheumatoid factor idiotypes defined by a mouse monoclonal antibody. *Eur J Immunol* 1983;13:197–201.
51. Davidson A, Lopez J, Sun D, et al. A monoclonal anti-idiotype specific for human polyclonal IgM rheumatoid factor. *J Immunol* 1992;148:3873–3878.

52. Shokri F, Mageed RA, Kitas GD, et al. Quantification of cross-reactive idiotype-positive rheumatoid factor produced in autoimmune rheumatic diseases. An indicator of clonality and B cell proliferative mechanisms. *Clin Exp Immunol* 1991;85:20–27.
53. Carson DA, Chen PP, Kipps TJ, et al. Regulation of rheumatoid factor synthesis. *Clin Exp Rheumatol* 1989;7[Suppl 3]:S69–S73.
54. Zhang M, Spey D, Ackerman S, et al. Rheumatoid factor idiotypic and antigenic specificity is strongly influenced by the light chain VJ junction. *J Immunol* 1996;156:3570–3575.
55. Sasso EH. Immunoglobulin V genes in rheumatoid arthritis. *Rheum Dis Clin North Am* 1992;18:809–836.
56. Silverman GJ, Schrohenloher RE, Accavitti MA, et al. Structural characterization of the second major cross-reactive idiotype group of human rheumatoid factors. Association with the VH4 gene family. *Arthritis Rheum* 1990;33:1347–1360.
57. Børretzen M, Chapman C, Natvig JB, et al. Differences in mutational patterns between rheumatoid factors in health and disease are related to variable heavy chain family and germ-line gene usage. *Eur J Immunol* 1997;27:735–741.
58. Victor KD, Randen I, Thompson K, et al. Rheumatoid factors isolated from patients with autoimmune disorders are derived from germline genes distinct from those encoding the Wa, Po, and Bla cross reactive idiotypes. *J Clin Invest* 1991;87:1603–1613.
59. Pascual V, Randen I, Thompson K, et al. The complete nucleotide sequences of the heavy chain variable regions of six monospecific rheumatoid factors derived from Epstein-Barr virus–transformed B cells isolated from the synovial tissue of patients with rheumatoid arthritis. *J Clin Invest* 1990;86:1320–1328.
60. Pascual V, Victor K, Randen I, et al. IgM rheumatoid factors in patients with rheumatoid arthritis derive from a diverse array of germline immunoglobulin genes and display little evidence of somatic variation. *J Rheumatol Suppl* 1992;32:50–53.
61. Randen I, Brown D, Thompson KM, et al. Clonally related IgM rheumatoid factors undergo affinity maturation in the rheumatoid synovial tissue. *J Immunol* 1992;148:3296–3301.
62. Carayannopoulos MO, Potter KN, Li Y, et al. Evidence that human immunoglobulin M rheumatoid factors can be derived from the natural autoantibody pool and undergo an antigen driven immune response in which somatically mutated rheumatoid factors have lower affinities for immunoglobulin G Fc than their germline counterparts. *Scand J Immunol* 2000;51:327–336.
63. Zhang M, Majid A, Bardwell P, et al. Rheumatoid factor specificity of a VH3-encoded antibody is dependent on the heavy chain CDR3 region and is independent of protein A binding. *J Immunol* 1998;161:2284–2289.
64. Crouzier R, Martin T, Pasquali J-L. Heavy chain variable region, light chain variable region, and heavy chain CDR3 influences on the mono- and polyreactivity and on the affinity of human monoclonal rheumatoid factors. *J Immunol* 1995;154:4526–4535.
65. Williams DG, Moyes SP, Mageed RA. Rheumatoid factor isotype switch and somatic mutation variants within rheumatoid arthritis synovium. *Immunology* 1999;98:123–136.
66. Corper AL, Sohi MK, Bonagura VR, et al. Structure of human IgM rheumatoid factor Fab bound to its autoantigen IgG Fc reveals a novel topology of antibody-antigen interaction. *Nat Struct Biol* 1997;4:374–381.
67. Breedveld FC, Otten HG, Daha MR. Rheumatoid factor production in the joint. *Scand J Rheumatol Suppl* 1995;101:183–185.
68. Munthe E, Natvig JB. Immunoglobulin classes, subclasses and complexes of IgG rheumatoid factor in rheumatoid plasma cells. *Clin Exp Immunol* 1972;12:55–70.
69. Smiley JD, Sachs C, Ziff M. In vitro synthesis of immunoglobulin by rheumatoid synovial membrane. *J Clin Invest* 1968;47:624–632.
70. Ziff M. Relation of cellular infiltration of rheumatoid synovial membrane to its immune response. *Arthritis Rheum* 1974;17:313–319.
71. Randen I, Mellbye OJ, Førre Ø, et al. The identification of germinal centres and follicular dendritic networks in rheumatoid synovial tissue. *Scand J Immunol* 1995;41:481–486.
72. Iguchi T, Ziff M. Electron microscopic study of rheumatoid synovial vasculature. Intimate relationship between tall endothelium and lymphoid aggregation. *J Clin Invest* 1986;77:355–361.
73. van Dinther-Janssen AC, Pals ST, Scheper R, et al. Dendritic cells and high endothelial venules in the rheumatoid synovial membrane. *J Rheumatol* 1990;17:11–17.
74. Thomas R, Davis LS, Lipsky PE. Rheumatoid synovium is enriched in mature antigen-presenting dendritic cells. *J Immunol* 1994;152:2613–2623.
75. Lindhout E, van Eijk M, van Pel M, et al. Fibroblast-like synoviocytes from rheumatoid arthritis patients have intrinsic properties of follicular dendritic cells. *J Immunol* 1999;162:5949–5956.
76. Kang YM, Zhang X, Wagner UG, et al. CD8 T cells are required for the formation of ectopic germinal centers in rheumatoid synovitis. *J Exp Med* 2002;195:1325–1336.
77. Kumon I. *In situ* characterization of mononuclear cell phenotype in intrahepatic lymphoid follicles in patients with chronic viral hepatitis. *Gastroenterol Jpn* 1992;27:638–645.
78. Freni MA, Artuso D, Gerken G, et al. Focal lymphocytic aggregates in chronic hepatitis C: occurrence, immunohistochemical characterization, and relation to markers of autoimmunity. *Hepatology* 1995;22:389–394.
79. Steere AC, Duray PH, Butcher EC. Spirochetal antigens and lymphoid cell surface markers in Lyme synovitis. Comparison with rheumatoid synovium and tonsillar lymphoid tissue. *Arthritis Rheum* 1988;31:487–495.
80. Berek C, Kim HJ. B-cell activation and development within chronically inflamed synovium in rheumatoid and reactive arthritis. *Semin Immunol* 1997;9:261–268.
81. Schroder AE, Sieper J, Berek C. Antigen-dependent B cell differentiation in the synovial tissue of a patient with reactive arthritis. *Mol Med* 1997;3:260–272.
82. Armengol MP, Juan M, Lucas-Martin A, et al. Thyroid autoimmune disease: demonstration of thyroid antigen-specific B cells and recombination-activating gene expression in chemokine-containing active intrathyroidal germinal centers. *Am J Pathol* 2001;159:861–873.
83. Bridges SL Jr. Frequent N addition and clonal relatedness among immunoglobulin lambda light chains expressed in rheumatoid arthritis synovia and PBL, and the influence of Vlambda gene segment utilization on CDR3 length. *Mol Med* 1998;4:525–553.
84. Weyand CM, Kurtin PJ, Goronzy JJ. Ectopic lymphoid organogenesis: a fast track for autoimmunity. *Am J Pathol* 2001;159:787–793.
85. Kim HJ, Krenn V, Steinhauser G, et al. Plasma cell development in synovial germinal centers in patients with rheumatoid and reactive arthritis. *J Immunol* 1999;162:3053–3062.
86. Kim HJ, Berek C. B cells in rheumatoid arthritis. *Arthritis Res* 2000;2:126–131.
87. Blades MC, Ingegnoli F, Wheller SK, et al. Stromal cell-derived factor 1 (CXCL12) induces monocyte migration into human synovium transplanted onto SCID mice. *Arthritis Rheum* 2002;46:824–836.
88. Nanki T, Hayashida K, El Gabalawy HS, et al. Stromal cell-derived factor-1-CXC chemokine receptor 4 interactions play a central role in CD4+ T cell accumulation in rheumatoid arthritis synovium. *J Immunol* 2000;165:6590–6598.
89. Calame KL. Plasma cells: finding new light at the end of B cell development. *Nat Immunol* 2001;2:1103–1108.
90. Bridges SL Jr., Lee SK, Johnson ML, et al. Somatic mutation and CDR3 lengths of immunoglobulin κ light chains expressed in patients with rheumatoid arthritis and normal individuals. *J Clin Invest* 1995;96:831–841.
91. Han S, Dillon SR, Zheng B, et al. V(D)J recombinase activity in a subset of germinal center B lymphocytes. *Science* 1997;278:301–305.
92. Papavasiliou F, Casellas R, Suh H, et al. V(D)J recombination in mature B cells: a mechanism for altering antibody responses. *Science* 1997;278:298–301.
93. Han S, Zheng B, Schatz DG, et al. Neoteny in lymphocytes: Rag1 and Rag2 expression in germinal center B cells. *Science* 1996;274:2094–2097.
94. Hikida M, Mori M, Takai T, et al. Reexpression of RAG-1 and RAG-2 genes in activated mature mouse B cells. *Science* 1996;274:2092–2094.
95. Prak EL, Weigert M. Light chain replacement: a new model for antibody gene rearrangement. *J Exp Med* 1995;182:541–548.
96. Chen C, Prak EL, Weigert M. Editing disease-associated autoantibodies. *Immunity* 1997;6:97–105.
97. Liu Y-J. Reuse of B lymphocytes in germinal centers. *Science* 1997;278:238–239.
98. Zhang Z, Bridges SL, Jr. Expression of RAG and TdT and evidence of receptor revision in synovial B lymphocytes in rheumatoid arthritis. *Scand J Immunol* 1999;50:101(abst).
99. Itoh K, Meffre E, Albesiano E, et al. Immunoglobulin heavy chain variable region gene replacement as a mechanism for receptor revision in rheumatoid arthritis synovial tissue B lymphocytes. *J Exp Med* 2000;192:1151–1164.
100. Zhang Z, Wu X, Limbaugh BH, et al. Expression of recombination-activating genes and terminal deoxynucleotidyl transferase and secondary rearrangement of immunoglobulin kappa light chains in rheumatoid arthritis synovial tissue. *Arthritis Rheum* 2001;44:2275–2284.
101. Meffre E, Davis E, Schiff C, et al. Circulating human B cells that express surrogate light chains and edited receptors. *Nat Immunol* 2000;1:207–214.
102. Meffre E, Chiorazzi M, Nussenzweig MC. Circulating human B cells that express surrogate light chains display a unique antibody repertoire. *J Immunol* 2001;167:2151–2156.
103. Stastny P. Association of the B-cell alloantigen DRw4 with rheumatoid arthritis. *N Engl J Med* 1978;298:869–871.
104. Alarcón GS, Koopman WJ, Acton RT, et al. Seronegative rheumatoid arthritis. A distinct immunogenetic disease? *Arthritis Rheum* 1982;25:502–507.
105. Dobloug JH, Førre Ø, Kass E, et al. HLA antigens and rheumatoid arthritis. Association between HLA-DRw4 positivity and IgM rheumatoid factor production. *Arthritis Rheum* 1980;23:309–313.
106. Olsen NJ, Callahan LF, Brooks RH, et al. Associations of HLA-DR4 with rheumatoid factor and radiographic severity in rheumatoid arthritis. *Am J Med* 1988;84:257–264.
107. Gregersen PK, Silver J, Winchester R. The shared epitope hypothesis: an approach to understanding the molecular genetics of susceptibility to rheumatoid arthritis. *Arthritis Rheum* 1987;30:1205–1213.
108. Gran JT, Husby G, Thorsby E. The prevalence of HLA-DR4 and HLA-DR3 in healthy persons with rheumatoid factor. *Scand J Rheumatol* 1985;14:79–82.
109. Silman AJ, Ollier B, Mageed RA. Rheumatoid factor detection in the unaffected first degree relatives in families with multicase rheumatoid arthritis. *J Rheumatol* 1991;18:512–515.
110. Perdriger A, Chales G, Semana G, et al. Role of HLA-DR-DR and DR-DQ associations in the expression of extraarticular manifestations and rheumatoid factor in rheumatoid arthritis. *J Rheumatol* 1997;24:1272–1276.
111. Calin A, Elswood J, Klouda PT. Destructive arthritis, rheumatoid factor, and HLA-DR4. Susceptibility versus severity, a case-control study. *Arthritis Rheum* 1989;32:1221–1225.
112. Nelson JL, Dugowson CE, Koepsell TD, et al. Rheumatoid factor, HLA-DR4, and allelic variants of DRB1 in women with recent-onset rheumatoid arthritis. *Arthritis Rheum* 1994;37:673–680.
113. Olsen NJ, Stastny P, Jasin HE. High levels of *in vitro* IgM rheumatoid factor synthesis correlate with HLA-DR4 in normal individuals. *Arthritis Rheum* 1987;30:841–848.

114. Garred P, Madsen HO, Petersen J, et al. CC chemokine receptor 5 polymorphism in rheumatoid arthritis. *J Rheumatol* 1998;25:1462–1465.
115. Jaraquemada D, Ollier W, Awad J, et al. HLA and rheumatoid arthritis: susceptibility or severity? *Dis Markers* 1986;4:43–53.
116. Walker DJ, Griffiths ID. HLA associations are with severe rheumatoid arthritis. *Dis Markers* 1986;4:121–132.
117. Weyand CM, Hicok KC, Conn DL, et al. The influence of HLA-DRB1 genes on disease severity in rheumatoid arthritis. *Ann Intern Med* 1992;117:801–806.
118. Pisetsky DS, Jelinek DF, McAnally LM, et al. *In vitro* autoantibody production by normal adult and cord blood B cells. *J Clin Invest* 1990;85:899–903.
119. Carson DA, Chen PP, Kipps TJ. New roles for rheumatoid factor. *J Clin Invest* 1991;87:379–383.
120. Frater JL, Hsi ED. Properties of the mantle cell and mantle cell lymphoma. *Curr Opin Hematol* 2002;9:56–62.
121. Pasquali JL, Fong S, Tsoukas CD, et al. Different populations of rheumatoid factor idiotypes induced by two polyclonal B cell activators, pokeweed mitogen and Epstein-Barr virus. *Clin Immunol Immunopathol* 1981;21:184–189.
122. Karsh J, Goldstein R, Lazarovits AI. *In vitro* IgM and IgM rheumatoid factor production in response to *Staphylococcus aureus* Cowan I and pokeweed mitogen: the contribution of CD5+ (Leu 1) B cells. *Clin Exp Immunol* 1989;77:179–183.
123. Burastero SE, Casali P, Wilder RL, et al. Monoreactive high affinity and polyreactive low affinity rheumatoid factors are produced by CD5+ B cells from patients with rheumatoid arthritis. *J Exp Med* 1988;168:1979–1992.
124. Tsoukas CD, Carson DA, Fong S, et al. Cellular requirements for pokeweed mitogen-induced autoantibody production rheumatoid arthritis. *J Immunol* 1980;125:1125–1129.
125. Tarkowski A, Czerkinsky C, Nilsson LA. Simultaneous induction of rheumatoid factor- and antigen-specific antibody-secreting cells during the secondary immune response in man. *Clin Exp Immunol* 1985;61:379–387.
126. Levinson AI, Tar L, Carafa C, et al. *Staphylococcus aureus* Cowan I. Potent stimulus of immunoglobulin M rheumatoid factor production. *J Clin Invest* 1986;78:612–617.
127. Nemazee DA. Immune complexes can trigger specific, T cell-dependent, autoanti-IgG antibody production in mice. *J Exp Med* 1985;161:242–256.
128. Tighe H, Chen PP, Tucker R, et al. Function of B cells expressing a human immunoglobulin M rheumatoid factor autoantibody in transgenic mice. *J Exp Med* 1993;177:109–118.
129. Tighe H, Heaphy P, Baird S, et al. Human immunoglobulin (IgG) induced deletion of IgM rheumatoid factor B cells in transgenic mice. *J Exp Med* 1995;181:599–606.
130. Tighe H, Warnatz K, Brinson D, et al. Peripheral deletion of rheumatoid factor B cells after abortive activation by IgG. *Proc Natl Acad Sci U S A* 1997;94:646–651.
131. Kyburz D, Corr M, Brinson DC, et al. Human rheumatoid factor production is dependent on CD40 signaling and autoantigen. *J Immunol* 1999;163:3116–3122.
132. Warnatz K, Kyburz D, Brinson DC, et al. Rheumatoid factor B cell tolerance via autonomous Fas/FasL-independent apoptosis. *Cell Immunol* 1999;191:69–73.
132a. Shlomchik MJ, Zharhary D, Saunders T, et al. A rheumatoid factor transgenic mouse model of autoantibody regulation. *Int Immunol* 1993;5:1329–1341.
133. Wang H, Shlomchik MJ. High affinity rheumatoid factor transgenic B cells are eliminated in normal mice. *J Immunol* 1997;159:1125–1134.
134. Wang H, Shlomchik MJ. Maternal Ig mediates neonatal tolerance in rheumatoid factor transgenic mice but tolerance breaks down in adult mice. *J Immunol* 1998;160:2263–2271.
135. Hannum LG, Ni D, Haberman AM, et al. A disease-related rheumatoid factor autoantibody is not tolerized in a normal mouse: implications for the origins of autoantibodies in autoimmune disease. *J Exp Med* 1996;184:1269–1278.
136. Wang H, Shlomchik MJ. Autoantigen-specific B cell activation in Fas-deficient rheumatoid factor immunoglobulin transgenic mice. *J Exp Med* 1999;190:639–649.
137. William J, Euler C, Christensen S, et al. Evolution of autoantibody responses via somatic hypermutation outside of germinal centers. *Science* 2002;297:2066–2070.
138. Ma J, Xu J, Madaio MP, et al. Autoimmune lpr/lpr mice deficient in CD40 ligand: spontaneous Ig class switching with dichotomy of autoantibody responses. *J Immunol* 1996;157:417–426.
139. Rifkin IR, Leadbetter EA, Beaudette BC, et al. Immune complexes present in the sera of autoimmune mice activate rheumatoid factor B cells. *J Immunol* 2000;165:1626–1633.
140. Mackay F, Woodcock SA, Lawton P, et al. Mice transgenic for BAFF develop lymphocytic disorders along with autoimmune manifestations. *J Exp Med* 1999;190:1697–1710.
141. Soulas P, Koenig-Marrony S, Julien S, et al. A role for membrane IgD in the tolerance of pathological human rheumatoid factor B cells. *Eur J Immunol* 2002;32:2623–2634.
142. Leadbetter EA, Rifkin IR, Hohlbaum AM, et al. Chromatin-IgG complexes activate B cells by dual engagement of IgM and Toll-like receptors. *Nature* 2002;416:603–607.
143. Moudgil KD, Sercarz EE. Dominant determinants in hen eggwhite lysozyme correspond to the cryptic determinants within its self-homologue, mouse lysozyme: implications in shaping of the T cell repertoire and autoimmunity. *J Exp Med* 1993;178:2131–2138.
144. Lin R-H, Mamula MJ, Hardin JA, et al. Induction of autoreactive B cells allows priming of autoreactive T cells. *J Exp Med* 1991;173:1433–1439.
145. Rudd PM, Leatherbarrow RJ, Rademacher TW, et al. Diversification of the IgG molecule by oligosaccharides. *Mol Immunol* 1991;28:1369–1378.
146. Young A, Sumar N, Bodman K, et al. Agalactosyl IgG: an aid to differential diagnosis in early synovitis. *Arthritis Rheum* 1991;34:1425–1429.
147. van Zeben D, Rook GA, Hazes JM, et al. Early agalactosylation of IgG is associated with a more progressive disease course in patients with rheumatoid arthritis: results of a follow-up study. *Br J Rheumatol* 1994;33:36–43.
148. Axford JS, Sumar N, Alavi A, et al. Changes in normal glycosylation mechanisms in autoimmune rheumatic disease. *J Clin Invest* 1992;89:1021–1031.
149. Furukawa K, Matsuta K, Takeuchi F, et al. Kinetic study of a galactosyltransferase in the B cells of patients with rheumatoid arthritis. *Int Immunol* 1990;2:105–112.
150. Wilson IB, Platt FM, Isenberg DA, et al. Aberrant control of galactosyltransferase in peripheral B lymphocytes and Epstein-Barr virus transformed B lymphoblasts from patients with rheumatoid arthritis. *J Rheumatol* 1993;20:1282–1287.
151. Rook G, Thompson S, Buckley M, et al. The role of oil and agalactosyl IgG in the induction of arthritis in rodent models. *Eur J Immunol* 1991;21:1027–1032.
152. Ligier S, Fortin PR, Newkirk MM. A new antibody in rheumatoid arthritis targeting glycated IgG: IgM anti-IgG-AGE. *Br J Rheumatol* 1998;37:1307–1314.
153. Ceuppens JL, Rodriguez MA, Goodwin JS. Non-steroidal anti-inflammatory agents inhibit the synthesis of IgM rheumatoid factor *in vitro*. *Lancet* 1982;1:528–530.
154. Goodwin JS, Ceuppens JL, Rodriguez MA. Administration of nonsteroidal anti-inflammatory agents in patients with rheumatoid arthritis. Effects on indexes of cellular immune status and serum rheumatoid factor levels. *JAMA* 1983;250:2485–2488.
155. Cush JJ, Lipsky PE, Postlethwaite AE, et al. Correlation of serologic indicators of inflammation with effectiveness of nonsteroidal antiinflammatory drug therapy in rheumatoid arthritis. *Arthritis Rheum* 1990;33:19–28.
156. Alarcón GS, Schrohenloher RE, Bartolucci AA, et al. Suppression of rheumatoid factor production by methotrexate in patients with rheumatoid arthritis: evidence for differential influences of therapy and clinical status on IgM and IgA rheumatoid factor expression. *Arthritis Rheum* 1990;33:1156–1161.
157. Olsen NJ, Callahan LF, Pincus T. Immunologic studies of rheumatoid arthritis patients treated with methotrexate. *Arthritis Rheum* 1987;30:481–488.
158. Camussi G, Lupia E. The future role of anti-tumour necrosis factor (TNF) products in the treatment of rheumatoid arthritis. *Drugs* 1998;55:613–620.
159. Townes AS, Sowa JM, Shulman LE. Controlled trial of cyclophosphamide in rheumatoid arthritis. *Arthritis Rheum* 1976;19:563–573.
160. De Vita S, Zaja F, Sacco S, et al. Efficacy of selective B cell blockade in the treatment of rheumatoid arthritis: evidence for a pathogenetic role of B cells. *Arthritis Rheum* 2002;46:2029–2033.
161. Davidson A, Preud'homme JL, Solomon A, et al. Idiotypic analysis of myeloma proteins: anti-DNA activity of monoclonal immunoglobulins bearing an SLE idiotype is more common in IgG than IgM antibodies. *J Immunol* 1987;138:1515–1518.
162. Watts RA, Williams W, Le Page S, et al. Analysis of autoantibody reactivity and common idiotype PR4 expression of myeloma proteins. *J Autoimmun* 1989;2:689–700.
163. Seligmann M, Brouet JC. Antibody activity of human myeloma globulins. *Semin Hematol* 1973;10:163–177.
164. Rademacher TW, Williams P, Dwek RA. Agalactosyl glycoforms of IgG autoantibodies are pathogenic. *Proc Natl Acad Sci U S A* 1994;91:6123–6127.
165. Malhotra R, Wormald MR, Rudd PM, et al. Glycosylation changes of IgG associated with rheumatoid arthritis can activate complement via the mannose-binding protein. *Nat Med* 1995;1:237–243.
166. Lipsky PE. Systemic lupus erythematosus: an autoimmune disease of B cell hyperactivity. *Nat Immunol* 2001;2:764–766.
167. Roosnek E, Lanzavecchia A. Efficient and selective presentation of antigen-antibody complexes by rheumatoid factor B cells. *J Exp Med* 1991;173:487–489.
168. Gause A, Berek C. Role of B cells in the pathogenesis of rheumatoid arthritis: potential implications for treatment. *BioDrugs* 2001;15:73–79.
169. Takemura S, Braun A, Crowson C, et al. Lymphoid neogenesis in rheumatoid synovitis. *J Immunol* 2001;167:1072–1080.
170. Felson DT, LaValley MP, Baldassare AR, et al. The Prosorba column for treatment of refractory rheumatoid arthritis: a randomized, double-blind, sham-controlled trial. *Arthritis Rheum* 1999;42:2153–2159.
171. Sasso EH, Merrill C, Furst TE. Immunoglobulin binding properties of the Prosorba immunadsorption column in treatment of rheumatoid arthritis. *Ther Apher* 2001;5:84–91.
172. Davis TA, Grillo-Lopez AJ, White CA, et al. Rituximab anti-CD20 monoclonal antibody therapy in non-Hodgkin's lymphoma: safety and efficacy of re-treatment. *J Clin Oncol* 2000;18:3135–3143.
173. Edwards JC, Cambridge G. Sustained improvement in rheumatoid arthritis following a protocol designed to deplete B lymphocytes. *Rheumatology (Oxford)* 2001;40:205–211.
174. Edwards JCW, Szczepanski L, Szechinski J, et al. Efficacy and safety of rituximab, a B-cell targeted chimeric monoclonal antibody: a randomized, placebo-controlled trial in patients with rheumatoid arthritis. *Arthritis Rheum* 2002;46:S197.
175. Cambridge G, Leandro MJ, Edwards JC, et al. Serologic changes following B lymphocyte depletion therapy for rheumatoid arthritis. *Arthritis Rheum* 2003;48:2146–2154.
176. Takiguchi M, Murakami M, Nakagawa I, et al. Blockade of CD28/CTLA4-B7 pathway prevented autoantibody-related diseases but not lung disease in MRL/lpr mice. *Lab Invest* 1999;79:317–326.
177. Moreland LW, Alten R, Van Den BF, et al. Costimulatory blockade in patients with rheumatoid arthritis: a pilot, dose-finding, double-blind, placebo-con-

trolled clinical trial evaluating CTLA-4Ig and LEA29Y eighty-five days after the first infusion. *Arthritis Rheum* 2002;46:1470–1479.
178. Wu Q, Salomon B, Chen M, et al. Reversal of spontaneous autoimmune insulitis in nonobese diabetic mice by soluble lymphotoxin receptor. *J Exp Med* 2001;193:1327–1332.
179. Cremer M. Type II collagen-induced arthritis in rats. In: Greenwald R, Diamond H, eds. *Handbook of animal models for the rheumatic diseases.* Boca Raton: CRC Press, 1988:17–27.
180. Terato K, Harper DS, Griffiths MM, et al. Collagen-induced arthritis in mice: synergistic effect of *E. coli* lipopolysaccharide bypasses epitope specificity in the induction of arthritis with monoclonal antibodies to type II collagen. *Autoimmunity* 1995;22:137–147.
181. Tarkowski A, Klareskog L, Carlsten H, et al. Secretion of antibodies to types I and II collagen by synovial tissue cells in patients with rheumatoid arthritis. *Arthritis Rheum* 1989;32:1087–1092.
182. van Boekel MA, Vossenaar ER, van den Hoogen FH, et al. Autoantibody systems in rheumatoid arthritis: specificity, sensitivity and diagnostic value. *Arthritis Res* 2002;4:87–93.
183. Cook AD, Rowley MJ, Mackay IR, et al. Antibodies to type II collagen in early rheumatoid arthritis. Correlation with disease progression. *Arthritis Rheum* 1996;39:1720–1727.
184. Trentham DE, Dynesius-Trentham RA, Orav EJ, et al. Effects of oral administration of type II collagen on rheumatoid arthritis. *Science* 1993;261:1727–1730.
185. Barnett ML, Kremer JM, St.Clair EW, et al. Treatment of rheumatoid arthritis with oral type II collagen. Results of a multicenter, double-blind, placebo-controlled trial. *Arthritis Rheum* 1998;41:290–297.
186. Verheijden GF, Rijnders AW, Bos E, et al. Human cartilage glycoprotein-39 as a candidate autoantigen in rheumatoid arthritis. *Arthritis Rheum* 1997;40:1115–1125.
187. Johansen JS, Jensen HS, Price PA. A new biochemical marker for joint injury. Analysis of YKL-40 in serum and synovial fluid. *Br J Rheumatol* 1993;32:949–955.
188. Vos K, Steenbakkers P, Miltenburg AM, et al. Raised human cartilage glycoprotein-39 plasma levels in patients with rheumatoid arthritis and other inflammatory conditions. *Ann Rheum Dis* 2000;59:544–548.
189. Guerassimov A, Zhang Y, Banerjee S, et al. Cellular immunity to the G1 domain of cartilage proteoglycan aggrecan is enhanced in patients with rheumatoid arthritis but only after removal of keratan sulfate. *Arthritis Rheum* 1998;41:1019–1025.
190. Zhang Y, Guerassimov A, Leroux JY, et al. Arthritis induced by proteoglycan aggrecan G1 domain in BALB/c mice. Evidence for T cell involvement and the immunosuppressive influence of keratan sulfate on recognition of T and B cell epitopes. *J Clin Invest* 1998;101:1678–1686.
191. Leroux JY, Guerassimov A, Cartman A, et al. Immunity to the G1 globular domain of the cartilage proteoglycan aggrecan can induce inflammatory erosive polyarthritis and spondylitis in BALB/c mice but immunity to G1 is inhibited by covalently bound keratan sulfate *in vitro* and *in vivo*. *J Clin Invest* 1996;97:621–632.
192. Nienhuis RL, Mandema E. A new serum factor in patients with rheumatoid arthritis: the antiperinuclear factor. *Ann Rheum Dis* 1964;23:302–305.
192a. Sondag-Tschroots IR, Aaij C, Smit JW, et al. The antiperinuclear factor. 1. The diagnostic significance of the antiperinuclear factor for rheumatoid arthritis. *Ann Rheum Dis* 1979;38:248–251.
193. Young BJ, Mallya RK, Leslie RD, et al. Anti-keratin antibodies in rheumatoid arthritis. *BMJ* 1979;2:97–99.
194. Saraux A, Berthelot JM, Chales G, et al. Value of laboratory tests in early prediction of rheumatoid arthritis. *Arthritis Rheum* 2002;47:155–165.
195. Bas S, Perneger TV, Seitz M, et al. Diagnostic tests for rheumatoid arthritis: comparison of anti-cyclic citrullinated peptide antibodies, anti-keratin antibodies and IgM rheumatoid factors. *Rheumatology (Oxford)* 2002;41:809–814.
196. Paimela L, Gripenberg M, Kurki P, et al. Antikeratin antibodies: diagnostic and prognostic markers for early rheumatoid arthritis. *Ann Rheum Dis* 1992;51:743–746.
197. Steiner G, Smolen J. Autoantibodies in rheumatoid arthritis and their clinical significance. *Arthritis Res* 2002;4[Suppl 2]:S1–S5.
198. Simon M, Girbal E, Sebbag M, et al. The cytokeratin filament-aggregating protein filaggrin is the target of the so-called "antikeratin antibodies," autoantibodies specific for rheumatoid arthritis. *J Clin Invest* 1993;92:1387–1393.
199. Sebbag M, Simon M, Vincent C, et al. The antiperinuclear factor and the so-called antikeratin antibodies are the same rheumatoid arthritis-specific autoantibodies. *J Clin Invest* 1995;95:2672–2679.
200. Masson-Bessiere C, Sebbag M, Durieux JJ, et al. In the rheumatoid pannus, anti-filaggrin autoantibodies are produced by local plasma cells and constitute a higher proportion of IgG than in synovial fluid and serum. *Clin Exp Immunol* 2000;119:544–552.
201. Schellekens GA, de Jong BA, van den Hoogen FH, et al. Citrulline is an essential constituent of antigenic determinants recognized by rheumatoid arthritis-specific autoantibodies. *J Clin Invest* 1998;101:273–281.
202. Smeets TJ, Vossenaar ER, van Venrooij WJ, et al. Is expression of intracellular citrullinated proteins in synovial tissue specific for rheumatoid arthritis? *Arthritis Rheum* 2002;46:2824–2826.
203. Masson-Bessiere C, Sebbag M, Girbal-Neuhauser E, et al. The major synovial targets of the rheumatoid arthritis-specific antifilaggrin autoantibodies are deiminated forms of the alpha- and beta-chains of fibrin. *J Immunol* 2001;166:4177–4184.
204. Union A, Meheus L, Humbel RL, et al. Identification of citrullinated rheumatoid arthritis-specific epitopes in natural filaggrin relevant for antifilaggrin autoantibody detection by line immunoassay. *Arthritis Rheum* 2002;46:1185–1195.
205. Kroot EJ, de Jong BA, van Leeuwen MA, et al. The prognostic value of anti-cyclic citrullinated peptide antibody in patients with recent-onset rheumatoid arthritis. *Arthritis Rheum* 2000;43:1831–1835.
206. Hassfeld W, Steiner G, Hartmuth K, et al. Demonstration of a new antinuclear antibody (anti-RA33) that is highly specific for rheumatoid arthritis. *Arthritis Rheum* 1989;32:1515–1520.
207. Steiner G, Hartmuth K, Skriner K, et al. Purification and partial sequencing of the nuclear autoantigen RA33 shows that it is indistinguishable from the A2 protein of the heterogeneous nuclear ribonucleoprotein complex. *J Clin Invest* 1992;90:1061–1066.
208. Despres N, Boire G, Lopez-Longo FJ, et al. The Sa system: a novel antigen-antibody system specific for rheumatoid arthritis. *J Rheumatol* 1994;21:1027–1033.
209. Tong CY, Hollingsworth RC, Williams H, et al. Effect of genotypes on the quantification of hepatitis C virus (HCV) RNA in clinical samples using the Amplicor HCV Monitor Test and the Quantiplex HCV RNA 2.0 assay (bDNA). *J Med Virol* 1998;55:191–196.
210. Menard HA, Lapointe E, Rochdi MD, et al. Insights into rheumatoid arthritis derived from the Sa immune system. *Arthritis Res* 2000;2:429–432.
211. Goldbach-Mansky R, Lee J, McCoy A, et al. Rheumatoid arthritis associated autoantibodies in patients with synovitis of recent onset. *Arthritis Res* 2000;2:236–243.
212. Despres N, Talbot G, Plouffe B, et al. Detection and expression of a cDNA clone that encodes a polypeptide containing two inhibitory domains of human calpastatin and its recognition by rheumatoid arthritis sera. *J Clin Invest* 1995;95:1891–1896.
213. Mimori T, Suganuma K, Tanami Y, et al. Autoantibodies to calpastatin (an endogenous inhibitor for calcium-dependent neutral protease, calpain) in systemic rheumatic diseases. *Proc Natl Acad Sci U S A* 1995;92:7267–7271.
214. Lackner KJ, Schlosser U, Lang B, et al. Autoantibodies against human calpastatin in rheumatoid arthritis: epitope mapping and analysis of patient sera. *Br J Rheumatol* 1998;37:1164–1171.
215. Blass S, Specker C, Lakomek HJ, et al. Novel 68 kDa autoantigen detected by rheumatoid arthritis specific antibodies. *Ann Rheum Dis* 1995;54:355–360.
216. Blass S, Union A, Raymackers J, et al. The stress protein BiP is overexpressed and is a major B and T cell target in rheumatoid arthritis. *Arthritis Rheum* 2001;44:761–771.
217. Blass S, Meier C, Vohr HW, et al. The p68 autoantigen characteristic of rheumatoid arthritis is reactive with carbohydrate epitope specific autoantibodies. *Ann Rheum Dis* 1998;57:220–225.
218. Korganow AS, Ji H, Mangialaio S, et al. From systemic T cell self-reactivity to organ-specific autoimmune disease via immunoglobulins. *Immunity* 1999;10:451–461.
219. Matsumoto I, Staub A, Benoist C, et al. Arthritis provoked by linked T and B cell recognition of a glycolytic enzyme. *Science* 1999;286:1732–1735.
220. Ji H, Ohmura K, Mahmood U, et al. Arthritis critically dependent on innate immune system players. *Immunity* 2002;16:157–168.
221. Matsumoto I, Maccioni M, Lee DM, et al. How antibodies to a ubiquitous cytoplasmic enzyme may provoke joint-specific autoimmune disease. *Nat Immunol* 2002;3:360–365.
222. Schaller M, Burton DR, Ditzel HJ. Autoantibodies to GPI in rheumatoid arthritis: linkage between an animal model and human disease. *Nat Immunol* 2001;2:746–753.
222a. Matsumoto I, Lee DM, Goldbach-Mansky R, et al. Low prevanlence of antibodies to glucose-6-phosphate isomerase in patients with rheumatoid arthritis and a spectrum of other chronic autoimmune disorders. *Arthritis Rheum* 2003;48:944–954.
223. Kassahn D, Kolb C, Solomon S, et al. Few human autoimmune sera detect GPI. *Nat Immunol* 2002;3:411–412.
224. Schubert D, Schmidt M, Zaiss D, et al. Autoantibodies to GPI and creatine kinase in RA. *Nat Immunol* 2002;3:411–413.
224a. Van Gaalen FA, Toes RE, Ditzel HJ, et al. Association of autoantibodies to glucose-6-phosphate isomerase with extraarticular complications in rheumatiod arthritis. *Arthritis Rheum* 2004;50:395–399.
225. Saulot V, Vittecoq O, Charlionet R, et al. Presence of autoantibodies to the glycolytic enzyme alpha-enolase in sera from patients with early rheumatoid arthritis. *Arthritis Rheum* 2002;46:1196–1201.
226. Atta MS, Lim KL, Ala'deen DA, et al. Investigation of the prevalence and clinical associations of antibodies to human fibronectin in systemic lupus erythematosus. *Ann Rheum Dis* 1995;54:117–124.
227. Uesugi H, Ozaki S, Sobajima J, et al. Prevalence and characterization of novel pANCA, antibodies to the high mobility group non-histone chromosomal proteins HMG1 and HMG2, in systemic rheumatic diseases. *J Rheumatol* 1998;25:703–709.
228. Mulder AH, Horst G, van Leeuwen MA, et al. Antineutrophil cytoplasmic antibodies in rheumatoid arthritis. Characterization and clinical correlations. *Arthritis Rheum* 1993;36:1054–1060.

CHAPTER 18

Immunosenescence and T-Cell Biology in Rheumatoid Arthritis

Cornelia M. Weyand and Jörg J. Goronzy

Paul Ehrlich is credited with the idea that immune responses cause harm when directed against the host. His concept of *horror autotoxicus* has had tremendous influence on studies investigating the mechanisms of autoimmune disease. Rheumatoid arthritis (RA) is a classic autoimmune syndrome that is characterized by the production of rheumatoid factors, antibodies that react against self (host) proteins (1,2). Cellular immune responses in patients with RA are aberrant and are sufficiently strong that standard means of immunosuppression cannot eradicate them but can only inhibit them. Our inability to eliminate the T cells and B cells that are responsible for anti–self-immunity can be explained by the power of immunologic memory. Once imprinted, the immune system will remember responses and react more swiftly and effectively when restimulated with the same antigen. However, if antigen-specific memory responses are the underlying immune abnormality in RA, then the disease should ebb with advancing age. Adaptive immune responses steadily deteriorate as the host ages (3,4). By the time individuals reach age 65, their ability to mount an immune response to a vaccine is severely impaired (5). Conversely, age is a strong risk factor for the development of RA—incidence rates increase with age and peak in 75- to 85-year-old individuals (6). It is difficult to envision how an aging immune system, compromised in its ability to generate antigen-specific immune responses, allows for the recognition of arthritogenic antigen.

Considering that RA is a disease of the middle-aged and elderly, it becomes important to integrate the principles of immunosenescence into disease models that attempt to dissect the underlying immunopathology. The immune system, of all organ systems, is particularly prone to age-dependent changes. Immune functions undergo profound alterations as individuals progress through the fourth, fifth, and sixth decades of life. Aging of the immune system starts almost immediately after birth, but it accelerates after age 40. It is now clear that immunosenescence is not a simple mechanism by which aging cells lose function. Cellular aging is also associated with *de novo* gene expression and the gain of functional capabilities. Unfortunately, these newly gained functions often have destructive potential. Because these changes occur late in life, they are not under evolutionary pressure. As such, it has been suggested that cellular senescence is an example of antagonistic pleiotropy (7,8). This hypothesis implies that changes that benefit young organisms have unselected deleterious consequences for older organisms. We will review how the concepts of immunosenescence apply to our understanding of the disease processes in RA and the possible consequences for our therapeutic approach to this chronic disorder.

CELLULAR SENESCENCE AND RHEUMATOID ARTHRITIS

Hematopoiesis, which includes the generation of lymphocytes, monocytes, and granulocytes, depends on the ability of precursor cells to proliferate. The sensitivity of hematopoietic cells to growth inhibition is exemplified in patients exposed to tumor therapy with DNA alkylating agents. Although this therapy hinders the expansion of malignant cells, bone marrow–derived cells are inevitably depleted, and the patient loses the ability to fight infections. Many immunocompetent cells, such as granulocytes, monocytes, and dendritic cells, can be replenished from hematopoietic stem cells that are not limited in their capacity for self-renewal. This rule does not hold for T cells because these highly sophisticated cells have additional hurdles to overcome before they are immunocompetent effector cells. T-cell replenishment is obviously affected by the functional capacity of the thymic gland, in which harmful T cells are eliminated and good T cells are selected. Once mature, T cells remain highly dependent on their ability to replicate. When challenged by antigen, individual T cells generate a population of sufficient size to find and promote removal of the antigen throughout the body.

Normal somatic cells have an intrinsic property that limits their proliferative potential (9). As cells age, their ability to proliferate declines until they reach replicative senescence. Cells sense the number of divisions they have completed, not their chronologic age. The number of cell cycles a cell can complete before it loses its ability to divide is genetically controlled (10,11) and depends on the cell type, the species, and the age of the donor.

Because RA is an autoimmune syndrome whose chronicity depends on the persistence and reinduction of pathogenic immune responses, it is important to understand how the biologic principle of cellular senescence impacts this disease. Incidence rates for RA increase steadily until age 84 (Fig. 18.1) (6). Issues of relevance include (a) the significance of an aging immune system for the induction and maintenance of active inflammatory infiltrates in the joints and (b) the implications for therapy of a syndrome that occurs preferentially in elderly hosts and that imposes profound replicative stress on the aged immune system.

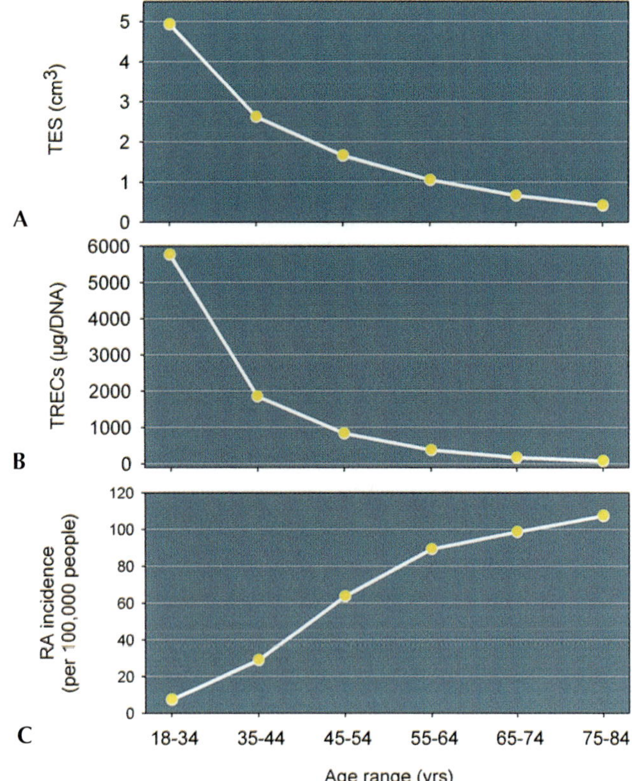

Figure 18.1. A–C: Age is a risk factor for rheumatoid arthritis (RA). The adaptive immune system, particularly the production of T cells, undergoes marked changes with progressive age. The component of the thymus involved in thymopoiesis, thymic epithelial space (TES), begins involution at the age of 1 year, compromising the output of T cells with advancing age (**A**, modified from Steinmann GG, Klaus B, Muller-Hermelink HK. The involution of the ageing human thymic epithelium is independent of puberty. A morphometric study. *Scand J Immunol* 1985;22:563–575). Accordingly, the number of recent thymic emigrants in the peripheral T-cell pool declines exponentially (**B**, modified from Koetz K, Bryl E, Spickschen K, et al. T cell homeostasis in patients with rheumatoid arthritis. *Proc Natl Acad Sci U S A* 2000;97:9203–9208). In parallel, the incidence rate of RA increases steeply and peaks in individuals 75 to 84 years of age (**C**, modified from Doran MF, Pond GR, Crowson CS, et al. Trends in incidence and mortality in rheumatoid arthritis in Rochester, Minnesota, over a forty-year period. *Arthritis Rheum* 2002;46: 625–631). TREC, T-cell receptor excision circles.

IMMUNOSENESCENCE—DEMANDS OF T-CELL HOMEOSTASIS

The size and composition of the T-cell population are under homeostatic control (12,13). Proliferation of progenitor cells must be in equilibrium with the death of T cells. Quantitative estimates of the total number of T cells predict that each person harbors ~2×10^{11} CD4$^+$ and ~1×10^{11} CD8$^+$ T cells (14,15). Half-lives of T cells have been measured *in vivo* by different methods. Estimates indicate that T cells live an average of 250 days. Survival times are estimated to be 1,250 days for naïve cells and 50 days for memory cells (16–18). From these data, daily production rates can be calculated. It has been estimated that approximately 1% of the total T-cell pool is replenished every day. As such, 2 to 3×10^9 new T cells must be generated each day.

The current model holds that thymopoiesis is the sole source of T cells in newborns and children. The functionally important part of the thymus, the epithelial space, begins to atrophy with the first year of age (19,20). The volume then shrinks by an estimated 3% per year through middle age; the involution slows to 1% per year later in life (21,22). It has been emphasized that some thymic epithelial tissue can be retained in individuals older than 60 years. However, thymopoietically active tissue comprises less than 20% of total space in donors 50 years and older.

Significant progress has been made in assessing thymic production rates in humans using a new method for the estimation of recent thymic emigrants (23–26). While undergoing T-cell receptor (TCR) rearrangement in the thymus, the excised DNA in thymocytes form episomes called *TCR excision circles* (TRECs). By virtue of expressing unique sequences, such TRECs can be traced. TRECs are not duplicated during cell division and are considered to be a marker of recent thymic emigrants. Quantification of TRECs in thymocytes has demonstrated stable levels per 100,000 cells through approximately age 50 (23,27,28). However, in the peripheral T-cell compartment, TREC concentrations decline with advancing age. Between the ages of 20 and 60 years, 90% to 95% of peripheral TREC$^+$CD4$^+$ T cells are lost (23,29). Low levels of TREC production or TREC survival continue into the seventh and eighth decades of life. Because TREC concentrations provide an upper estimate for thymic output, at best, only a small percentage of thymic function is maintained in adults.

In recent years, it has become clear that adults possess a second mechanism for generating new T cells. By driving peripheral T cells into division using a mechanism called *homeostatic expansion*, large numbers of T cells can be produced (12,30). With advancing age, homeostatic proliferation gains importance and contributes to the reconstitution of the peripheral T-cell pool (Fig. 18.2). The relative proportion of thymic production and peripheral proliferation is not known, but studies in patients undergoing chemotherapy have suggested that patients older than 18 years repopulate the compartment predominantly through expansion of memory T cells, not through the release of new naïve T cells (31,32).

It is obvious that proliferative expansion of postthymic T cells cannot occur without limits (Fig. 18.3). First, lymphocytes have a finite capacity for replication before they enter replicative senescence and can no longer respond to stimuli. Second, T-cell proliferation is associated with profound shifts in the cell-surface phenotype and functional competence of T cells. The best example of such a shift is the transition of naïve T cells into the memory state. Third, functionality of the T-cell pool is closely linked with extreme diversity of antigen-specific receptors. If selected T cells have a survival advantage during postthymic expansion, they could create size restraints by occupying space and preventing newly arriving T cells, either from outside or from within the pool, from entering the compartment. The consequence would be a sacrifice of diversity. Notably, the risk for development of RA is highest at an age when T-cell production can no longer depend on the influx of novel T cells from the thymus. During that period of life, the T-cell compartment is shaped by homeostatic proliferation (Fig. 18.1).

IMPAIRED T-CELL GENERATION IN PATIENTS WITH RHEUMATOID ARTHRITIS

Thymopoietic capacity has been measured in patients with RA by quantifying TRECs in CD4$^+$ T cells and in unseparated peripheral blood lymphocytes (29,33). These studies have demonstrated a reduction of TREC concentrations to approximately one-third of that in age-matched healthy controls (Fig. 18.4). Comparison of the relationship between age and TRECs in healthy controls and in patients with RA provides insights into the mechanism of premature loss of TREC$^+$ T cells. Reduced TREC concentrations are present in patients with RA at age 20, and these numbers decline during the next 3 decades at the same rate as in controls. Thus, the process of TREC dilution

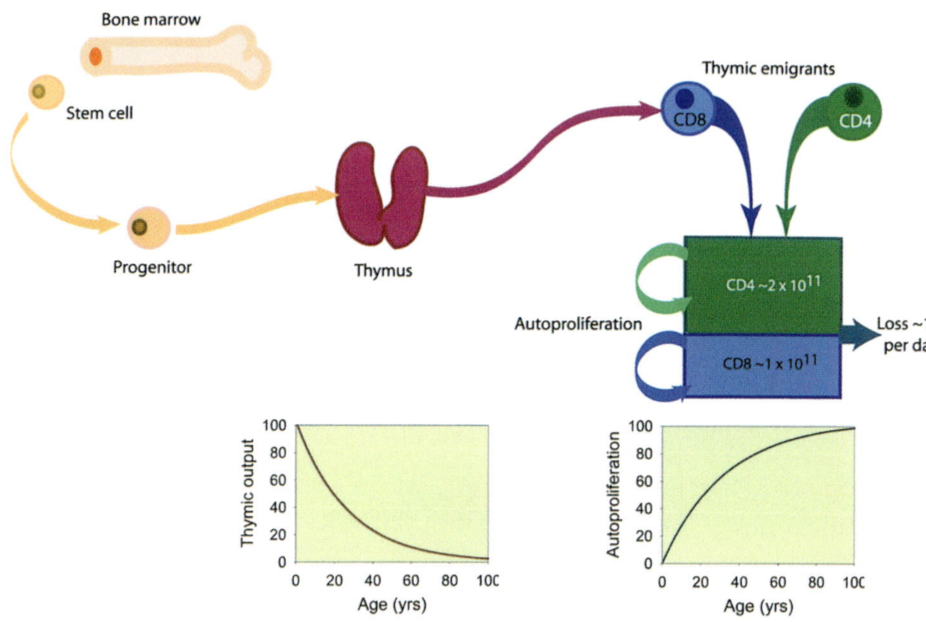

Figure 18.2. T-cell homeostasis. In humans, production of novel T cells is limited to the thymus. T-cell precursor cells derived from hematopoietic stem cells travel to the thymus and undergo T-cell receptor rearrangement. After a stringent selection process, mature CD4$^+$ and CD8$^+$ T cells are released into the periphery. Because the number of cells in the peripheral T-cell pool are homeostatically controlled and thymic output declines sharply with age, an alternate process of T-cell generation is necessary. This process has been named *autoproliferation* and involves replication of currently available mature T cells in the pool. Autoproliferation compensates for the decrease in T-cell input, but it can lead to fundamental changes in gene expression and function of replicated T cells.

over age, which is a consequence of TREC$^-$ cells expanding at the expense of recent thymic emigrants, is unchanged in patients. Instead, patients with RA start adult life with fewer TREC$^+$ cells in their circulating T-cell pool. The number of TREC$^+$ T cells in patients with RA is not dependent on disease duration. In other words, 20 to 30 years of active RA does not induce a progressive decline in thymic output, again suggesting that reduction in TREC$^+$ cells occurred before disease onset.

Although several mechanisms could account for reduced TREC concentrations among peripheral CD4$^+$ T cells in RA, the most likely explanation is reduced thymic activity. Redistribution of TREC$^+$ T cells away from the circulation appears to be unlikely. Rheumatoid tissue lesions are almost exclusively composed of memory CD4$^+$CD45RO$^+$ T cells that possess very low levels of TREC episomes, in line with their replicative history (34,35).

Also, low TREC concentrations in RA do not appear to be an epiphenomenon of a high T-cell turnover. Although TREC concentrations are negatively influenced by the rate of peripheral T-cell proliferation (25) and the abundance of proinflammatory cytokines in RA could increase T-cell proliferation, several findings are not compatible with a high turnover model. First, reduction in TRECs is most obvious in CD4$^+$CD45RO$^-$ T cells, suggesting that the reduced TREC content predominantly affects the naïve compartment. Relative proportions of CD4$^+$ T cells with naïve and memory phenotypes are not shifted in patients, indicating that memory T cells have not replaced those with a naïve phenotype. Finally, the proportion of CD4$^+$ T cells in the cell cycle is not increased but is, rather, reduced in patients with RA (*author's unpublished observation*).

A primary defect in thymopoiesis that is closely associated with disease in adults is not without precedence. Age-inappropriate reduction in thymic output has been described for myasthenia gravis and human immunodeficiency virus (HIV) infection (36,37). The true epithelial space in the thymus of patients with myasthenia gravis undergoes more rapid atrophy than in age-matched controls (15). With this accelerated loss of thymopoietically active tissue, TREC levels in peripheral CD4$^+$ and CD8$^+$ T-cell subsets are reduced (38). Severe functional consequences of insufficient thymic T-cell production have also been demonstrated in patients with HIV infection (15,39). Although T-cell homeostasis is modified through a combination of several mechanisms, there is agreement that induction of premature thymic atrophy is a hallmark of HIV infection. A combination of decreased T-cell survival in the periphery and exhaustion of compensatory mechanisms, mostly due to the failure to increase T-cell generation in the thymus, is considered to be the underlying cause of CD4$^+$ T-

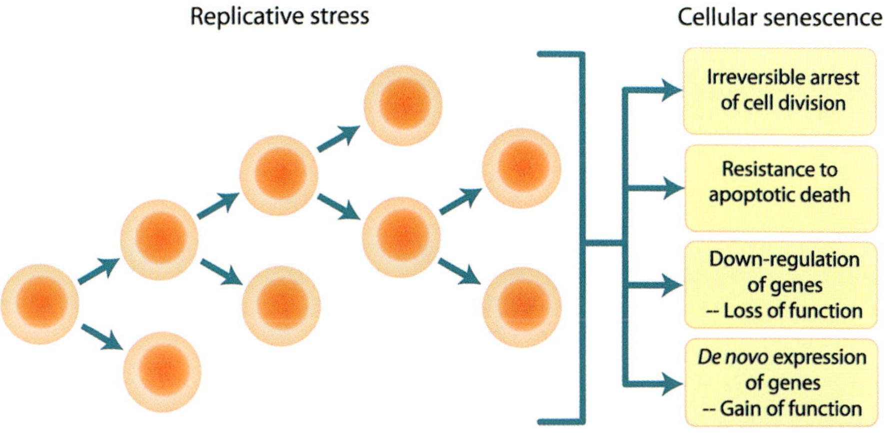

Figure 18.3. The process of cellular senescence. Lymphocytes are somatic cells, thereby limited in the number of replications they can experience. After a finite number of cell cycles, somatic cells reach cellular senescence. This is associated with profound changes in gene expression and function. Cellular senescence, although closely correlated with an arrest in cell division, is characterized by loss of function and also by *de novo* expression of genes.

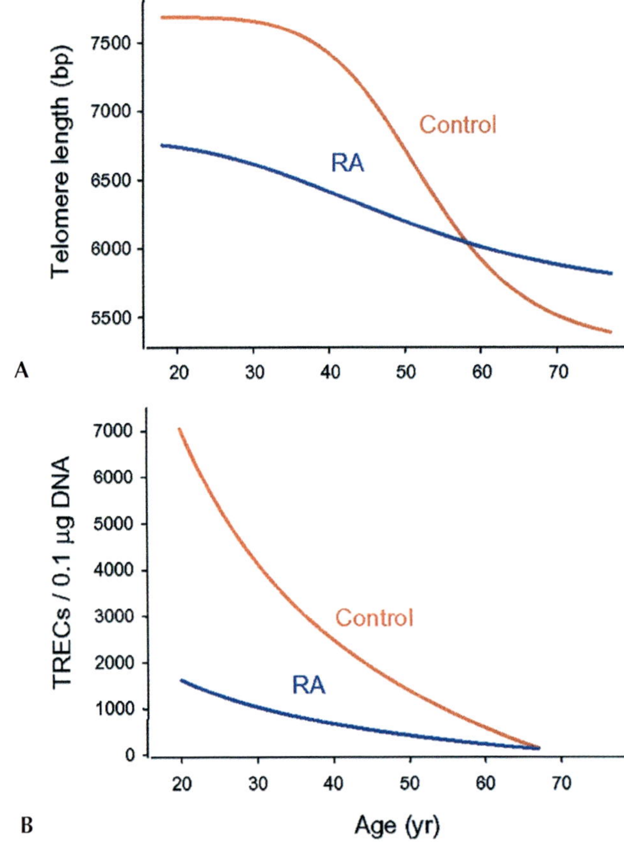

Figure 18.4. A,B: Premature immunosenescence in rheumatoid arthritis (RA). Telomeres are shortened with each cell division, making the length of telomeric sequences a surrogate marker for the replicative history of a cell population. TCR excision circles (TRECs) are episomes formed as a by-product of T-cell receptor rearrangement; TREC numbers in a cell population are proportional to the frequency of recent thymic emigrants. In healthy individuals, telomeres of lymphocytes decline with age. This process is accelerated in patients with RA **(A)**, with a minimal telomeric reserve already present in patients at age 20 years. As indicated by TREC measurements, thymic T-cell production in healthy individuals declines to a low level at 65 years of age. In patients with RA, TREC concentrations are severely reduced by age 20. Age-inappropriate loss of thymic T-cell production would necessitate compensatory T-cell proliferation, causing premature telomeric erosion. (From Goronzy JJ, Weyand CM. Thymic function and peripheral T-cell homeostasis in rheumatoid arthritis. *Trends Immunol* 2001;22:251–255, with permission.)

cell lymphopenia in HIV-infected individuals. Increases in circulating TREC$^+$ T cells after successful antiviral therapy have been interpreted as showing recovery of thymic function with suppression of viral infection (40,41).

In patients with RA, multiple mechanisms could contribute to premature failure of T-cell replenishment. Cytokines have been reported to play an important role in thymic atrophy. Overexpression of leukemia inhibitory factor and oncostatin M can cause severe thymocyte loss in experimental models (42–44). Physiologic degeneration of the human thymus has been associated with the accumulation of some cytokines [e.g., leukemia inhibitory factor, oncostatin M, and interleukin (IL)-6] and the decline of others (e.g., IL-2, IL-9, IL-10, IL-13, and IL-14) (28). An imbalance in the intrathymic cytokine milieu could result in age-inappropriate reduction of thymopoiesis. Alternatively, the process of thymocyte education and selection could be less efficient in individuals prone to develop RA. In terms of output, thymic selection is a highly inefficient process. Only 1% of T cells entering the organ survive and migrate into the periphery. Even minor shifts in efficacy of T-cell selection would translate into marked downstream effects. RA-associated HLA class II molecules, critically involved in the thymic selection process, have been implicated in altering T-cell repertoire formation. It has been proposed that the structural features of the ternary complex formed by TCRs, antigen, and RA-associated HLA class II molecules are unique and favor selection of certain T cells (45–48). It is, therefore, possible that the outcome of the thymic selection process is different in individuals predisposed to RA.

SENESCENT T CELLS IN RHEUMATOID ARTHRITIS

There are experimental data that T cells in patients with RA have molecular and functional characteristics of senescent cells (49). The causes of premature T-cell senescence in RA may be multiple, but it is conceivable that inappropriate postthymic expansion of T cells is the major component. Because the T-cell pool is homeostatically controlled, impairment of thymic T-cell generation will elicit homeostatic proliferation to regain and maintain stable size and numbers, despite insufficient T-cell influx. Given the fact that postthymic T cells are somatic cells with a finite potential for proliferation, such a response pattern could have profound consequences on the composition and functional competence of the T-cell pool.

Increased Replicative History of Postthymic T Cells in Rheumatoid Arthritis

Somatic cells vary in the number of cell cycles they can complete. One of the determinants that controls senescence and growth arrest is telomeres (50,51). Telomeres consist of repetitive DNA sequences that cap the ends of linear chromosomes. Telomeres prevent chromosome fusion and genomic instability. During cell division and DNA replication, 50 to 100 bases at the 3' end of the telomere remain unreplicated. Thus, as cells proliferate, telomeres shorten, and the loss of telomeric length can be used to estimate the number of cell cycles that have been completed. In the human germline, the average terminal telomeric restriction fragment amounts to approximately 15 to 20 kilobases (kb). Human cells proliferate until their average telomeric length is 5 to 7 kb. Once they have consumed their telomeres, the cells cease to divide and acquire a senescent phenotype. In contrast to the situation in rodent cells, in which telomeric length may not be a determinant of senescence, replicative growth arrest in human cells can be prevented by reversing telomeric shortening (52,53). It is believed that cells sense their replicative history through the length of telomeric ends.

Because they are highly dependent on proliferative burst, T cells are equipped with a mechanism that allows partial repair of their telomeres. On triggering of the T-cell antigen receptor and co-stimulatory molecules, T cells up-regulate telomerase (54,55). Telomerase is a ribonucleoprotein complex that can add telomeric repeats to chromosomes *de novo*. Thus, telomeric loss in T cells is always a minimal estimate of prior replicative stress.

To examine whether the impairment of thymic T-cell production in patients with RA is associated with an increased replicative history of postthymic T cells, telomeric restriction fragments have been measured in CD4$^+$ and CD8$^+$ T-cell populations (Fig. 18.4) (29,56). Both T-cell subsets showed age-inappropriate erosion of telomeres of 1 kb when compared with healthy 20- to 30-year-old individuals. Healthy individuals lose an average of 2 kb of telomeric repeats between the ages of 20 and 70. Thus, by age 20, the patients with RA had already used up half of their telomeric reserve. The premature erosion of telomeres suggests that

T cells in patients with RA have passed through an additional 20 to 40 cell cycles. This is comparable to another important benchmark of T-cell proliferation—namely, the number of T-cell doublings that occur in antigen-specific immune responses. It has been estimated that T cells replicate 10 to 15 times when mounting an antigen-specific immune response (57,58). The transition of naïve T cells into the memory compartment is associated with a rapid decline in telomeric lengths, indicating the high proliferative turnover of antigen-exposed T cells.

Telomeric shortening in lymphocytes has also been used to demonstrate the excessive replicative stress in individuals undergoing bone marrow transplantation (59,60). Comparative studies of telomeres in donors and recipients have revealed that the empty space in the T-cell compartment is filled by proliferative expansion of circulating cells. In summary, the postthymic T-cell pool of patients with RA has been exposed to marked replicative stress and has experienced multiple rounds of proliferation to the extent that the remaining replicative potential is compromised. Telomeric shortening in patients with RA preferentially affects cells with a naïve phenotype (29), strongly indicating that the stimulus for proliferation does not derive from antigen contact but from a signal that is driving homeostatic expansion.

Contraction of T-Cell Diversity in Rheumatoid Arthritis

A cardinal feature of the adaptive immune system is the enormous diversity of lymphocytes, each expressing a clonally distributed T-cell antigen receptor. The key to T-cell diversity lies in the thymus, where TCRs are randomly generated and then sorted for their suitability. A defect in thymic output, compensated by the expansion of postthymic T cells, should pose a threat to TCR diversity (61). Contraction of diversity could be further accelerated if peripheral T cells differ in their opportunity to divide. Nonrandomness of peripheral T-cell proliferation should lead to extensive remodeling of the T-cell repertoire.

An array of technical approaches has been developed to estimate the diversity in T-cell populations. Monoclonal reagents specific for the TCR α chain and β chain variable region gene segments can detect clonal expansion of T-cell populations. For detection with these reagents, however, such expansion must be gigantic, occupying several percent of the pool. T-cell clones that reach a size of 1×10^8 cells would only account for 0.1% of the T-cell compartment. Studies analyzing the representation of TCR β chain variable region–joining region combinations, an approach that evaluated population sizes of 0.1% of the T-cell pool, suggest that there are profound repertoire abnormalities in patients with RA, in comparison with healthy controls (45).

More sensitive techniques for analyzing T-cell populations involve TCR spectratyping. In this approach, TCR rearrangements are amplified by polymerase chain reaction and separated by size using gel electrophoresis. Because of junctional diversity between the TCR gene segments, TCR sequences differ in length. These length distributions are Gaussian, with most of the TCRs using an optimal length. Length separation of TCR rearrangements allows for the detection of T-cell subsets that account for 0.05% to 1% of the T-cell compartment. Considering the enormous number of T cells in the pool, these techniques are still insensitive. However, TCR spectratyping has been able to demonstrate clonal T-cell populations in the overall T-cell repertoire of patients with RA, and not only at the local inflammatory site (62–65). In these studies, most patients showed multiple T-cell clones. Although there was a trend for certain TCR β chain variable region gene segments to be overrepresented (66,67), no simple algorithm could explain the oligoclonality of the T-cell pool. Both the CD4$^+$ and the CD8$^+$ T-cell compartments contained clonally expanded cells, indicating a global defect in the maintenance of the T-cell repertoire. Clonally expanded CD4$^+$ T cells could be isolated from the patients' blood and synovial tissue (68), and these expanded clonotypes did not necessarily express a phenotype of cellular activation.

The most sensitive assessment of T-cell diversity involves tracing of individual T cells (56). This goal has been partially reached in studies that analyzed the frequencies of individual TCR β chains. TCR β chains were isolated by random cloning, probes specific for each TCR were generated, and the frequency of each individual TCR β chain was determined by limiting dilution. Control individuals harbored TCR β chains that were present at an average frequency of 1 in 2 to 3×10^7 T cells. TCRs expressed by naïve T cells were so infrequent that most of them could not be found again, even when a sensitivity threshold of 1 in 2×10^7 T cells was achieved. Conversely, patients with RA had a marked contraction in diversity. TCR β chains were detected at a median frequency of 1 in 2 to 3×10^6 T cells. The loss of diversity was most profound for the naïve CD4$^+$ T-cell subset. Such a repertoire contraction was not seen in chronic active viral infections, such as hepatitis C, suggesting that chronic, persistent, antigen-specific responses by themselves do not compromise T-cell diversity.

The finding that TCR diversity in RA was contracted to 10% of that of healthy controls implies that each T cell from a patient with RA must have expanded at least tenfold to fill the available space. An expansion by the factor of ten requires approximately three population doublings. Similar estimates are reached when extrapolating the number of rounds of division needed to compensate for a drop in thymic output to one-third of normal.

Together, these findings suggest that deficient generation of novel CD4$^+$ T cells necessitates expansion of remaining T cells, which leads to a contraction in diversity. Signals that control homeostatic expansions are incompletely known, and it is unclear how these signals shape the resulting T-cell repertoire. In lymphopenic animals, both naïve and memory T cells respond with proliferation (69,70). Depending on the lymphopenic host, the resulting T-cell phenotype and function differ. There is agreement that two major factors dictate how the T-cell pool repopulates when severely depleted. Most investigators believe that naïve peripheral T cells require recognition of self–major histocompatibility complex (MHC) molecules to undergo homeostatic proliferation (12). Interestingly, postthymic T cells may relive the selection process they have been exposed to in the thymic environment. T-cell survival as well as T-cell homeostatic expansion are dependent on the Src-family kinases, lck and fyn, supporting the view that TCR stimulation is necessary (71,72). If naïve peripheral T cells only enter the cell cycle after contacting relevant self-MHC ligands, the host's HLA genotype should modulate the outcome. Also, functional intactness of cell populations presenting MHC molecules to T cells could ultimately determine remodeling of the T-cell pool. These considerations are important because MHC class I–restricted CD8$^+$ T cells and MHC class II–restricted CD4$^+$ T cells would seek out distinct partners to receive a signal for homeostatic expansion.

The second factor determining T-cell survival and expansion is growth-promoting cytokines. Cytokines binding to receptors that contain a common γ chain are critical regulators of T-cell growth in the postthymic milieu (73–75). This group of cytokines includes IL-4, IL-7, IL-9, IL-15, and IL-21. A defect in Janus kinase 3, a kinase activated by all of these γ chain–containing receptors, leads to severe abnormalities in the T-cell compartment (76,77). IL-4, IL-7, and IL-15 form a core group of T-cell growth factors, with IL-7 having a nonredundant role in supporting the survival and expansion of both naïve CD4$^+$ and CD8$^+$ T cells *in vivo* (73,75). Although most of the currently available information is

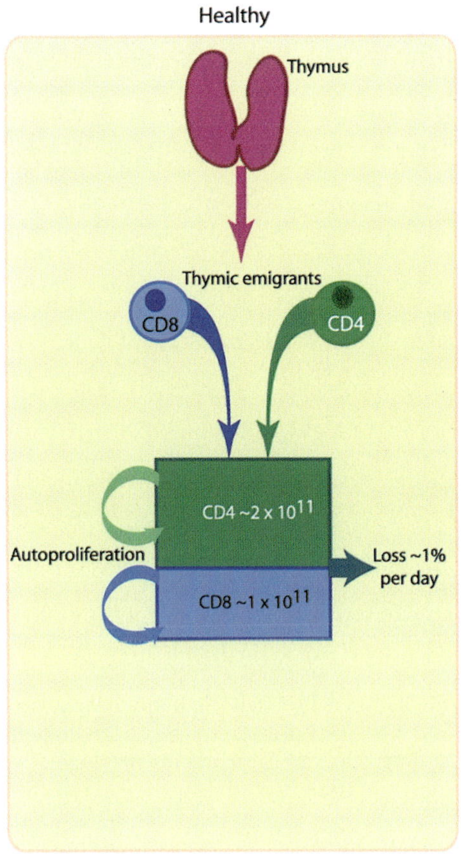

Figure 18.5. Abnormal T-cell homeostasis in rheumatoid arthritis. A comparative model of T-cell homeostasis is shown for healthy individuals and patients with rheumatoid arthritis. In healthy donors, thymic input into the peripheral T-cell pool declines with age. Autoproliferation of mature T cells helps maintain T-cell numbers, but it does not exhaust the replicative potential of lymphocytes. In patients with RA, premature loss of thymopoiesis forces the system to respond with accelerated autoproliferation. Replicative stress imposed on the peripheral T-cell pool has profound consequences, including exhaustion of the replicative reserve, remodeling of the repertoire due to nonrandom T-cell proliferation, and a survival advantage for senescent T cells.

based on experimental animal models, a unique role of IL-7 for T-cell homeostasis appears to exist in humans (74).

How patients with RA drive proliferative responses of post-thymic naïve T cells is currently not known. Of particular interest is the question of whether cytokines relevant in the disease process itself modulate homeostatic T-cell proliferation. Equally important, the functional outcome of homeostatic proliferation is determined by whether the patient can avoid the overgrowth of selected T cells. T cells with higher affinities for self-antigen are disproportionately favored during homeostatic expansion, leading to the selection of autoreactive T-cell populations. Also, T cells expressing receptors for ligands that are abundant should have an advantage and should compete successfully for space, and T cells with receptors that have very low affinity for self-derived antigens should have little chance to survive. Eventually, the risk for self-sustaining autoreactive immune responses would increase (78). Clonal populations that populate the circulating and the synovial tissue compartments in RA could be the result of such survival advantage. One important component in this breakdown in self-tolerance is the number of T cells with identical specificity. Once the clonal size of a self-reactive T cell surpasses a size threshold, autoreactivity may be unavoidable.

The model predicts that autoreactivity in a patient with RA is a dynamic process (Fig. 18.5). Dependent on the needs of T-cell homeostasis, T-cell clonotypes could expand and shrink, but, overall, the T-cell pool should become progressively more self-directed, providing fertile soil for autodestructive immunity.

T-Cell Senescence Program and Shifts in Functional Capacity

Senescence induces a complex phenotype in cells that cannot simply be described as a functional loss. Replicative senescence is an example of a broad cellular program developed to protect the organism from cells that have accumulated potentially oncogenic insults. Overall, three key features of the senescent phenotype have been defined (Fig. 18.3). Senescent cells display an essentially irreversible arrest of cell division. Quite unexpectedly, they acquire resistance to apoptotic death. Most importantly, they experience changes in cellular function that are associated with drastic alterations in their functional capabilities (7,8). Most intriguing is a shift toward secretory activity, including the potential to release large amounts of proinflammatory cytokines. There is overwhelming experimental evidence that patients with RA harbor senescent T cells with associated fundamental alterations in immunocompetence (Table 18.1, Fig. 18.5) (33,49).

Consistent with impaired cell cycle progression, $CD4^+CD45RO^-$ naïve T cells isolated from patients with RA displayed an aborted proliferative burst when stimulated through their TCR (29). Periph-

TABLE 18.1. $CD4^+$ T Cells in Rheumatoid Arthritis: Senescence-Induced Shift in Gene Expression

Gene expression down-regulated or lost
CD28
CD40 ligand
CD7
Gene expression up-regulated or gained
Killer immunoglobulin-like receptors (KIR2DL1, KIR2DL2, KIR2DS2)
C-type lectin receptor, CD161
Perforin
Granzyme
CD8α
Interleukin-12 receptor
Chemokine receptor, CCR5
Bcl-2

eral blood naïve CD4+ T cells from healthy individuals responded with 14 population doublings after TCR-mediated stimulation; a single CD4+ T cell gave rise to a progeny of 15,000 cells. Conversely, naïve CD4+ T cells from patients with RA were limited to nine population doublings and only grew to a clonal size of 1,200 T cells. The failure in clonal burst is sufficient to explain why patients with RA are prone to infectious complications (79). Impaired T-cell responsiveness has also been reported for T cells in the rheumatoid synovial lesion (80). Elegant studies have indicated that part of the T-cell nonresponsiveness is related to chronic exposure to tumor necrosis factor (TNF)-α (80–82). TNF-α down-regulates expression of the CD28 gene, thereby implicating this cytokine in the human T-cell senescence program (83).

In addition, TCR signaling is attenuated in synovial T cells. Again, this can be in part attributed to chronic TNF-α exposure (80). One of the key TCR signaling molecules that is down-regulated with chronic stimulation or TNF-α exposure is the TCR ζ chain. Depressed TCR ζ chain expression has been documented in several diseases, such as chronic infections, cancer, and RA (84,85), and it appears to be a feature of senescent T cells. A second mechanism of T cell low responsiveness involves the linker for activation of T cells adapter molecule. The action of linker for activation of T cells is dependent on its membrane localization, which is extremely sensitive to intracellular redox balance (86). Oxidative stress is known to be one of the most potent inducers of a cellular senescence program (87). Depletion of glutathione, as is the case with chronic oxidative stress, results in membrane replacement of linker for activation of T cells, which is in part responsible for the low responsiveness of synovial T cells (88).

Support for the accumulation of senescent T cells in RA has also come from studies that have shown resistance to apoptotic cell death in both synovial tissue–derived and in circulating T cells (89–91). Two distinct pathways underlying reduced susceptibility to apoptosis have been reported. In response to withdrawal of the growth factor IL-2, only a small fraction of patient-derived senescent CD4+ T cells entered apoptosis. Protection from cell death correlates with overexpression of the antiapoptotic molecule, bcl-2 (90). A different molecular mechanism has been linked to impaired Fas-induced apoptosis. Ineffectiveness of Fas-mediated apoptosis has been associated with impaired degradation of the antiapoptotic molecule, Fas-ligand IL-1–converting enzyme inhibitory protein (91). The outcome of both of these mechanisms is important for determining T-cell populations. Instead of allowing for appropriate clonal downsizing, the resistance to programmed cell death leads to accumulation of senescent T cells. Considering that space in the immune system is limited and that newly arriving cells can only be accepted if they can replace an old cell, insufficient removal of senescent T cells eventually causes profound shifts in the composition of the T-cell compartment.

Loss of Gene Expression in Senescent CD4+ T Cells: Emergence of CD28^{null} T Cells

An example of the functional loss with progressive T-cell senescence is the loss of the co-stimulatory molecule CD28. The CD28^{null} phenotype has been associated with T-cell populations that have undergone multiple rounds of division and have the characteristics of chronically stimulated lymphocytes (92,93). Especially in chronic viral infections, such as cytomegalovirus and HIV infection, replacement of CD28+ by CD28-deficient T cells has been described (94,95). In general, CD8+ T cells are more prone to lose surface expression of CD28 than are CD4+ T cells. This property may reflect differences in the homeostatic turnover of these two T-cell subpopulations.

Important insights into the mechanism of CD28 loss come from studies defining the transcriptional control of CD28. Expression of the CD28 gene, which is constitutive in T cells, is under the control of a transcriptional initiator complex (96–98). The assembly of the initiator complex is selectively lost with progressive age of CD4+ and CD8+ T cells. The molecular components of the initiator complex are partially known and include nucleolin and heterogeneous nuclear ribonucleoprotein D0-A as critical factors. Transcription of these two proteins is not affected by the senescence program, and posttranscriptional modification of these abundant nuclear proteins has been proposed as the underlying mechanism of CD28 loss (99).

CD28 expression can be modulated through three different interventions. Chronic cellular stimulation causes lack of initiator region binding proteins (96,97). Also, TNF-α can down-regulate CD28 in T cells (83). Prolonged exposure to excessive amounts of TNF-α accelerates the aging process of T cells, which is in part reversible, as documented by the increased T-cell responsiveness after TNF-α blockade *in vivo*. Cytokines can also enhance expression of CD28. Specifically, IL-12 reinduces CD28 in deficient T cells and restores its co-stimulatory function (100). These findings document that the cytokine environment plays an important modulatory role in T-cell senescence, a concept particularly relevant in RA.

Gene Induction in Senescent CD4+ T Cells: *De Novo* Expression of Killer Immunoglobulin-Like Receptors

Gene expression profiling has identified members of the killer immunoglobulin-like receptor (KIR) family as being preferentially transcribed in senescent CD4+ T cells (101,102). KIRs are type I transmembrane molecules with structural features of the immunoglobulin superfamily. They are present in primates but not in rodents and are part of the human leukocyte receptor complex located on chromosome 19. Because of their ability to recognize polymorphic HLA class I molecules, KIRs have critical immunoregulatory functions. KIRs were first identified in natural killer (NK) cells and have been implicated in controlling NK lytic and cytokine expression capacities. The KIR family includes inhibitory and activating receptors. Engagement of inhibitory KIRs by the appropriate HLA class I ligand activates kinases and leads to the phosphorylation of cytoplasmic immunoreceptor tyrosine-based inhibitory motifs. Phosphorylated immunoreceptor tyrosine-based inhibitory motifs act as recruitment points for cytosolic protein tyrosine phosphatases, resulting in the dephosphorylation of substrates critical in cellular activation. Activating KIRs lack immunoreceptor tyrosine-based inhibitory motifs but interact with the signal transduction adapter protein, DAP12. DAP12 activation leads to activation of the mitogen-activated protein kinase cascade, which ultimately induces degranulation of cytotoxic granules and production of cytokines. One of the important aspects of the KIR locus is its extreme polymorphism, generated by more than 15 genes. Haplotypes differ markedly in the number of genes and also contain allelic polymorphisms. It has been proposed that the KIR locus is under strong evolutionary pressure and is evolving in synergy with the polymorphic HLA class I locus (103,104).

Several KIRs have been found in CD4+ T cells from patients with RA (102,105). A unique role has been proposed for the stimulatory isoform, KIR2DS2. This receptor is specific for selected alleles of HLA-C. Cross-linking of KIR2DS2 has been demonstrated to provide a co-stimulatory signal, increasing cell proliferation and production of interferon γ (IFN-γ) (101). An interesting feature of KIR2DS2 expression in RA is the unopposed appearance of this stimulatory receptor (105). Whereas most NK cells express KIR isoforms that partially counteract each other, CD4$^+$ T cells from patients with RA are equipped with stimulatory variants only. An unanswered question is whether KIR2DS2-expressing CD4$^+$ T cells respond only to HLA class I ligands or whether alternative ligands are recognized. Recent studies have raised the possibility that murine stimulatory receptors bind viral proteins and, thus, possess a role in antiviral defenses (106).

The possibility that up-regulation of KIRs is only one aspect of a more complex senescence program has been suggested by the identification of a number of additional genes that also are overexpressed in CD4$^+$CD28^{null} T cells. A summary of genes preferentially expressed in senescent CD4$^+$ T cells is given in Table 18.1. Besides KIRs, this list also includes other receptors previously considered typical for NK cells. CD161 is a C-type lectin receptor that regulates the lytic function of NK cells; its physiologic ligand remains unidentified. CD161 has been implicated in the tissue migration of T cells and may function by regulating the trafficking pattern of senescent CD4$^+$ T cells. CD161 has been successfully used to trace CD4$^+$CD28^{null} T cells in synovial lesions (107). Accumulation of CD4$^+$CD161$^+$ T cells is typical for rheumatoid synovitis and is not a feature of the synovial infiltrates in patients with connective tissue disease.

Acquisition of HLA class I–binding receptors endows senescent CD4$^+$ T cells with new functional capabilities. Not only do these cells release large amounts of IFN-γ, they also sense HLA class I expression in an inflammatory microenvironment. In addition, many of the acquired genes are functionally linked with tissue destruction.

Destructive Phenotype of Senescent CD4$^+$ T Cells

Classic CD4$^+$ T cells are specialized in the release of cytokines, by which they control the function of other effector populations. Senescent CD4$^+$ T cells that accumulate in patients with RA are prone to secrete high concentrations of IFN-γ (105,108). Through IFN-γ, they stimulate the functional activity of tissue-infiltrating macrophages. This is not their only capability in mediating tissue injury. Senescent CD4$^+$ T cells express the pore-forming molecule, perforin, and the cytotoxic enzyme, granzyme B, and kill target cells after receiving a TCR-mediated signal (109). Cytolytic effector functions provided by CD4$^+$ T cells have not yet been explored in the synovium. Because CD4$^+$CD28^{null}KIR$^+$ T cells are able to initiate granule release, not only after sensing antigen through their TCR, but also after triggering of KIRs, these cells have a great potential for continuous tissue damage. In this sense, aberrant KIR expression is a mechanism of escaping tolerance. If signals derived from KIRs or other NK cell receptors can bypass the need for TCR triggering, then senescent CD4$^+$ T cells must be considered dangerous lymphocytes (Table 18.2).

Senescent CD4$^+$ T Cells and Vascular Injury: From Rheumatoid Arthritis to Acute Coronary Syndromes

The KIR gene region is highly polymorphic, raising the possibility that KIR genes function as disease-risk genes. Approximately 40% of the general population inherits a KIR2DS2-containing haplotype. Comparison of patients with RA who do and do not have a KIR2DS2-containing haplotype has demonstrated that this gene is associated with a special clinical phenotype of RA, rheumatoid vasculitis (105). Not only do almost all patients with vascular complications of RA express the KIR2DS2 gene, but the putative ligand HLA-Cw3 is also enriched. The co-occurrence of KIR2DS2 and HLA class I ligands suggests that susceptibility to rheumatoid vasculitis is conferred by gene complementation.

TABLE 18.2. Functional Consequences of T-Cell Senescence in Rheumatoid Arthritis

Impaired proliferative burst of naïve T cells in response to stimulation
Attenuated T-cell receptor signaling
Resistance of T cells to apoptosis
Clonal expansion of CD4$^+$ and CD8$^+$ T cells
Premature loss of telomeres
Loss of gene expression, including the co-stimulatory molecule, CD28
Excessive production of interferon γ
Acquisition of cytolytic capability in CD4$^+$ T cells
De novo expression of HLA class I–recognizing receptors (KIRs)
De novo expression of C-type lectin receptors (CD161)

Implicating senescent KIR2DS2-expressing CD4$^+$ T cells in the vascular injury of rheumatoid disease has opened a promising new line of research into the immunopathogenesis of acute coronary syndromes (ACS). Cardiovascular disease is recognized as one of the major reasons for premature mortality in patients with RA (110). This observation has fostered investigation of immune functions in patients who do not have RA but have ACS. Intriguing parallels have emerged from these studies, supporting the notion that pathogenic pathways of immune-mediated tissue injury are shared between RA and ACS (Table 18.3) (111).

Patients with RA are not the only individuals carrying clonal expansions of senescent CD4$^+$ T cells. Phenotypically and functionally equivalent T cells have also been isolated from patients with unstable angina (112). Senescent CD4$^+$ and CD8$^+$ T cells with abundant IFN-γ production can easily be demonstrated in the blood of patients with unstable angina (113). These IFN-γ–producing T cells distinguish patients with plaque instability from those with chronic, stable coronary atherosclerosis. Clonally expanded CD4$^+$ T-cell populations have been isolated from patients with plaque instability, and it has been demonstrated that these cells selectively infiltrate culprit plaque that has caused fatal myocardial infarction (114). The recruitment of senescent CD4$^+$ T cells to the ruptured plaque strongly supports a direct role of these cells in the process of plaque instability and disruption.

Sequence analysis of TCRs used by expanded clonotypes in patients with unstable angina has suggested diversity of antigenic stimuli, although a certain degree of nonrandomness in TCR sequences has been found. The TCR sequence analysis also demonstrates that senescent CD4$^+$ T cells are distinct from NK T cells that express canonical TCRs (114).

CD4$^+$CD28^{null} T cells facilitate tissue injury in the atherosclerotic plaque through one of several mechanisms. Endothelial cells are susceptible to the cytolytic attack of these cells, and it has been proposed that damage of the microvasculature in the plaque could cause structural instability (115). Activation of KIR2DS2 was sufficient to lyse endothelial cells, reemphasizing

TABLE 18.3. Rheumatoid Arthritis and Acute Coronary Syndromes: Shared Abnormalities in T-Cell Biology

Accumulation of CD4$^+$ T cells and macrophages in the disease-relevant lesion
Activation in circulating monocytes
Expansion of CD4$^+$ and CD8$^+$ T cells that have lost expression of CD28
Recruitment of CD4$^+$CD28^{null} T cells into the lesion
Contraction of the T-cell repertoire with emergence of large monoclonal T-cell populations
Production of excessive interferon γ by circulating T cells
De novo expression of granzyme and perforin and cytolytic capability by CD4$^+$ T cells
Acquisition of the C-type lectin receptor, CD161, by CD4$^+$ T cells

that specific antigen is not necessarily required to elicit the tissue-damaging properties of senescent CD4+ T cells. Increased cytotoxicity in the presence of the acute phase protein, C-reactive protein, has suggested an intriguing interaction between the innate and adaptive immune responses. C-reactive protein is a powerful biologic marker of risk for cardiovascular events. The molecular mechanism underlying the C-reactive protein–mediated enhancement of endothelial cell killing has not been revealed. Synergistic actions of innate and adaptive immune reactions in tissue damage would provide an elegant explanation for increasing cardiovascular risk with advancing age. Sharing of immune abnormalities in patients with RA and ACS would certainly support the notion that instability of the atherosclerotic plaque is one of the vascular complications of RA.

CONCLUSION

Incidence rates for RA increase steadily with age and peak in 75- to 85-year-old individuals, signifying age as major risk factor for this autoimmune syndrome. Due to the high demand for cellular proliferation, the immune system is particularly prone to senescence, a biologic program associated with profound changes in gene expression and function. The most age-dependent component of the immune system is thymopoiesis, the production of novel T cells in the thymus. On involution of the thymus, which starts at 1 year of age, the immune system must use alternative means of securing homeostasis, such as proliferative expansion of postthymic T cells. Patients with RA have markedly reduced numbers of recent thymic emigrants, in comparison with age-matched controls, suggesting premature deficiency of thymic T-cell production. In parallel, their peripheral T cells show signs of cellular senescence, such as age-inappropriate shortening of telomeres, loss of the co-stimulatory molecule CD28, and *de novo* expression of a number of gene products. Senescence-associated abnormalities in T cells of patients with RA generate a proinflammatory functional profile with high production of IFN-γ and the acquisition of cytotoxic capabilities. The accumulation of proinflammatory and tissue-destructive T cells is shared between patients with RA and those with ACS, providing a framework to explain the increased risk of patients with RA to develop complications of coronary atherosclerosis.

ACKNOWLEDGMENTS

Supported by grants from the National Institutes of Health (AR41974, AR42527, AG15043, and AI44142) and by the Mayo Foundation.

REFERENCES

1. Smith JB, Haynes MK. Rheumatoid arthritis—a molecular understanding. *Ann Intern Med* 2002;136:908–922.
2. Panayi GS, Corrigall VM, Pitzalis C. Pathogenesis of rheumatoid arthritis. The role of T cells and other beasts. *Rheum Dis Clin North Am* 2001;27:317–334.
3. Grubeck-Loebenstein B, Wick G. The aging of the immune system. *Adv Immunol* 2002;80:243–284.
4. Miller RA. The aging immune system: primer and prospectus. *Science* 1996;273:70–74.
5. Goronzy JJ, Fulbright JW, Crowson CS, et al. Value of immunological markers in predicting responsiveness to influenza vaccination in elderly individuals. *J Virol* 2001;75:12182–12187.
6. Doran MF, Pond GR, Crowson CS, et al. Trends in incidence and mortality in rheumatoid arthritis in Rochester, Minnesota, over a forty-year period. *Arthritis Rheum* 2002;46:625–631.
7. Campisi J. From cells to organisms: can we learn about aging from cells in culture? *Exp Gerontol* 2001;36:607–618.
8. Campisi J. Cellular senescence as a tumor-suppressor mechanism. *Trends Cell Biol* 2001;11:S27–S31.
9. Hayflick L, Moorehead PS. The serial cultivation of human diploid cell strains. *Exp Cell Res* 1961;25:585–621.
10. Campisi J. Replicative senescence: an old lives' tale? *Cell* 1996;84:497–500.
11. Stanulis-Praeger BM. Cellular senescence revisited: a review. *Mech Ageing Dev* 1987;38:1–48.
12. Jameson SC. Maintaining the norm: T-cell homeostasis. *Nat Rev Immunol* 2002;2:547–556.
13. Tuma RA, Pamer EG. Homeostasis of naive, effector and memory CD8 T cells. *Curr Opin Immunol* 2002;14:348–353.
14. Haase AT. Population biology of HIV-1 infection: viral and CD4+ T cell demographics and dynamics in lymphatic tissues. *Annu Rev Immunol* 1999;17:625–656.
15. Haynes BF, Markert ML, Sempowski GD, et al. The role of the thymus in immune reconstitution in aging, bone marrow transplantation, and HIV-1 infection. *Annu Rev Immunol* 2000;18:529–560.
16. Sachsenberg N, Perelson AS, Yerly S, et al. Turnover of CD4+ and CD8+ T lymphocytes in HIV-1 infection as measured by Ki-67 antigen. *J Exp Med* 1998;187:1295–1303.
17. McCune JM, Hanley MB, Cesar D, et al. Factors influencing T-cell turnover in HIV-1-seropositive patients. *J Clin Invest* 2000;105:R1–R8.
18. Hellerstein M, Hanley MB, Cesar D, et al. Directly measured kinetics of circulating T lymphocytes in normal and HIV-1-infected humans. *Nat Med* 1999;5:83–89.
19. Haynes BF, Sempowski GD, Wells AF, et al. The human thymus during aging. *Immunol Res* 2000;22:253–261.
20. Flores KG, Li J, Sempowski GD, et al. Analysis of the human thymic perivascular space during aging. *J Clin Invest* 1999;104:1031–1039.
21. Steinmann GG. Changes in the human thymus during aging. *Curr Top Pathol* 1986;75:43–88.
22. Steinmann GG, Klaus B, Muller-Hermelink HK. The involution of the ageing human thymic epithelium is independent of puberty. A morphometric study. *Scand J Immunol* 1985;22:563–575.
23. Douek DC, McFarland RD, Keiser PH, et al. Changes in thymic function with age and during the treatment of HIV infection. *Nature* 1998;396:690–695.
24. McFarland RD, Douek DC, Koup RA, et al. Identification of a human recent thymic emigrant phenotype. *Proc Natl Acad Sci U S A* 2000;97:4215–4220.
25. Ye P, Kirschner DE. Reevaluation of T cell receptor excision circles as a measure of human recent thymic emigrants. *J Immunol* 2002;168:4968–4979.
26. Okamoto Y, Douek DC, McFarland RD, et al. Effects of exogenous interleukin-7 on human thymus function. *Blood* 2002;99:2851–2858.
27. Jamieson BD, Douek DC, Killian S, et al. Generation of functional thymocytes in the human adult. *Immunity* 1999;10:569–575.
28. Sempowski GD, Hale LP, Sundy JS, et al. Leukemia inhibitory factor, oncostatin M, IL-6, and stem cell factor mRNA expression in human thymus increases with age and is associated with thymic atrophy. *J Immunol* 2000;164:2180–2187.
29. Koetz K, Bryl E, Spickschen K, et al. T cell homeostasis in patients with rheumatoid arthritis. *Proc Natl Acad Sci U S A* 2000;97:9203–9208.
30. Goldrath AW. Maintaining the status quo: T-cell homeostasis. *Microbes Infect* 2002;4:539–545.
31. Mackall CL, Fleisher TA, Brown MR, et al. Age, thymopoiesis, and CD4+ T-lymphocyte regeneration after intensive chemotherapy. *N Engl J Med* 1995;332:143–149.
32. Mackall CL, Fleisher TA, Brown MR, et al. Distinctions between CD8+ and CD4+ T-cell regenerative pathways result in prolonged T-cell subset imbalance after intensive chemotherapy. *Blood* 1997;89:3700–3707.
33. Weyand CM, Goronzy JJ. Premature immunosenescence in rheumatoid arthritis. *J Rheumatol* 2002;29:1141–1146.
34. Kohem CL, Brezinschek RI, Wisbey H, et al. Enrichment of differentiated CD45RBdim,CD27- memory T cells in the peripheral blood, synovial fluid, and synovial tissue of patients with rheumatoid arthritis. *Arthritis Rheum* 1996;39:844–854.
35. Matthews N, Emery P, Pilling D, et al. Subpopulations of primed T helper cells in rheumatoid arthritis. *Arthritis Rheum* 1993;36:603–607.
36. Bofill M, Janossy G, Willcox N, et al. Microenvironments in the normal thymus and the thymus in myasthenia gravis. *Am J Pathol* 1985;119:462–473.
37. Haynes BF, Hale LP. The human thymus. A chimeric organ comprised of central and peripheral lymphoid components. *Immunol Res* 1998;18:175–192.
38. Sempowski G, Thomasch J, Gooding M, et al. Effect of thymectomy on human peripheral blood T cell pools in myasthenia gravis. *J Immunol* 2001;166:2808–2817.
39. Haynes BF, Hale LP, Weinhold KJ, et al. Analysis of the adult thymus in reconstitution of T lymphocytes in HIV-1 infection. *J Clin Invest* 1999;103:453–460.
40. Sempowski GD, Haynes BF. Immune reconstitution in patients with HIV infection. *Annu Rev Med* 2002;53:269–284.
41. McCune JM. Thymic function in HIV-1 disease. *Semin Immunol* 1997;9:397–404.
42. Shen MM, Skoda RC, Cardiff RD, et al. Expression of LIF in transgenic mice results in altered thymic epithelium and apparent interconversion of thymic and lymph node morphologies. *EMBO J* 1994;13:1375–1385.
43. Malik N, Haugen HS, Modrell B, et al. Developmental abnormalities in mice transgenic for bovine oncostatin M. *Mol Cell Biol* 1995;15:2349–2358.
44. Metcalf D, Nicola NA, Gearing DP. Effects of injected leukemia inhibitory factor on hematopoietic and other tissues in mice. *Blood* 1990;76:50–56.
45. Walser-Kuntz DR, Weyand CM, Weaver AJ, et al. Mechanisms underlying the formation of the T cell receptor repertoire in rheumatoid arthritis. *Immunity* 1995;2:597–605.

46. Yang H, Rittner H, Weyand CM, et al. Aberrations in the primary T-cell receptor repertoire as a predisposition for synovial inflammation in rheumatoid arthritis. *J Investig Med* 1999;47:236–245.
47. Nepom GT. The role of the DR4 shared epitope in selection and commitment of autoreactive T cells in rheumatoid arthritis. *Rheum Dis Clin North Am* 2001;27:305–315.
48. Roudier J. Association of MHC and rheumatoid arthritis. Association of RA with HLA-DR4: the role of repertoire selection. *Arthritis Res* 2000;2:217–220.
49. Goronzy JJ, Weyand CM. Thymic function and peripheral T-cell homeostasis in rheumatoid arthritis. *Trends Immunol* 2001;22:251–255.
50. Chiu CP, Harley CB. Replicative senescence and cell immortality: the role of telomeres and telomerase. *Proc Soc Exp Biol Med* 1997;214:99–106.
51. Shiels PG, Kind AJ, Campbell KH, et al. Analysis of telomere lengths in cloned sheep. *Nature* 1999;399:316–317.
52. Bodnar AG, Ouellette M, Frolkis M, et al. Extension of life-span by introduction of telomerase into normal human cells. *Science* 1998;279:349–352.
53. Vaziri H, Benchimol S. Reconstitution of telomerase activity in normal human cells leads to elongation of telomeres and extended replicative life span. *Curr Biol* 1998;8:279–282.
54. Son NH, Murray S, Yanovski J, et al. Lineage-specific telomere shortening and unaltered capacity for telomerase expression in human T and B lymphocytes with age. *J Immunol* 2000;165:1191–1196.
55. Liu K, Schoonmaker MM, Levine BL, et al. Constitutive and regulated expression of telomerase reverse transcriptase (hTERT) in human lymphocytes. *Proc Natl Acad Sci U S A* 1999;96:5147–5152.
56. Wagner UG, Koetz K, Weyand CM, et al. Perturbation of the T cell repertoire in rheumatoid arthritis. *Proc Natl Acad Sci U S A* 1998;95:14447–14452.
57. Kaech SM, Wherry EJ, Ahmed R. Effector and memory T-cell differentiation: implications for vaccine development. *Nat Rev Immunol* 2002;2:251–262.
58. Blattman JN, Antia R, Sourdive DJ, et al. Estimating the precursor frequency of naive antigen-specific CD8 T cells. *J Exp Med* 2002;195:657–664.
59. Wynn RF, Cross MA, Hatton C, et al. Accelerated telomere shortening in young recipients of allogeneic bone-marrow transplants. *Lancet* 1998;351:178–181.
60. Mathioudakis G, Storb R, McSweeney PA, et al. Polyclonal hematopoiesis with variable telomere shortening in human long-term allogeneic marrow graft recipients. *Blood* 2000;96:3991–3994.
61. Mackall CL, Bare CV, Granger LA, et al. Thymic-independent T cell regeneration occurs via antigen-driven expansion of peripheral T cells resulting in a repertoire that is limited in diversity and prone to skewing. *J Immunol* 1996;156:4609–4616.
62. Jendro MC, Ganten T, Matteson EL, et al. Emergence of oligoclonal T cell populations following therapeutic T cell depletion in rheumatoid arthritis. *Arthritis Rheum* 1995;38:1242–1251.
63. Goronzy JJ, Bartz-Bazzanella P, Hu W, et al. Dominant clonotypes in the repertoire of peripheral $CD4^+$ T cells in rheumatoid arthritis. *J Clin Invest* 1994;94:2068–2076.
64. Schmidt D, Goronzy JJ, Weyand CM. $CD4^+$ $CD7^-$ $CD28^-$ T cells are expanded in rheumatoid arthritis and are characterized by autoreactivity. *J Clin Invest* 1996;97:2027–2037.
65. Fitzgerald JE, Ricalton NS, Meyer AC, et al. Analysis of clonal $CD8^+$ T cell expansions in normal individuals and patients with rheumatoid arthritis. *J Immunol* 1995;154:3538–3547.
66. Waase I, Kayser C, Carlson PJ, et al. Oligoclonal T cell proliferation in patients with rheumatoid arthritis and their unaffected siblings. *Arthritis Rheum* 1996;39:904–913.
67. Hingorani R, Monteiro J, Furie R, et al. Oligoclonality of V beta 3 TCR chains in the $CD8^+$ T cell population of rheumatoid arthritis patients. *J Immunol* 1996;156:852–858.
68. Rittner HL, Zettl A, Jendro MC, et al. Multiple mechanisms support oligoclonal T cell expansion in rheumatoid synovitis. *Mol Med* 1997;3:452–465.
69. Goldrath AW, Bevan MJ. Low-affinity ligands for the TCR drive proliferation of mature $CD8^+$ T cells in lymphopenic hosts. *Immunity* 1999;11:183–190.
70. Kieper WC, Jameson SC. Homeostatic expansion and phenotypic conversion of naive T cells in response to self peptide/MHC ligands. *Proc Natl Acad Sci U S A* 1999;96:13306–13311.
71. Seddon B, Legname G, Tomlinson P, et al. Long-term survival but impaired homeostatic proliferation of naive T cells in the absence of p56lck. *Science* 2000;290:127–131.
72. Seddon B, Zamoyska R. TCR signals mediated by Src family kinases are essential for the survival of naive T cells. *J Immunol* 2002;169:2997–3005.
73. Tan JT, Dudl E, LeRoy E, et al. IL-7 is critical for homeostatic proliferation and survival of naive T cells. *Proc Natl Acad Sci U S A* 2001;98:8732–8737.
74. Fry TJ, Mackall CL. Interleukin-7: master regulator of peripheral T-cell homeostasis? *Trends Immunol* 2001;22:564–571.
75. Goldrath AW, Sivakumar PV, Glaccum M, et al. Cytokine requirements for acute and basal homeostatic proliferation of naive and memory $CD8^+$ T cells. *J Exp Med* 2002;195:1515–1522.
76. Sohn SJ, Forbush KA, Nguyen N, et al. Requirement for Jak3 in mature T cells: its role in regulation of T cell homeostasis. *J Immunol* 1998;160:2130–2138.
77. Thomis DC, Berg LJ. Peripheral expression of Jak3 is required to maintain T lymphocyte function. *J Exp Med* 1997;185:197–206.
78. Goronzy JJ, Weyand CM. T cell homeostasis and autoreactivity in rheumatoid arthritis. *Curr Dir Autoimmun* 2001;3:112–132.
79. Doran MF, Crowson CS, Pond GR, et al. Predictors of infection in rheumatoid arthritis. *Arthritis Rheum* 2002;46:2294–2300.
80. Cope AP, Liblau RS, Yang XD, et al. Chronic tumor necrosis factor alters T cell responses by attenuating T cell receptor signaling. *J Exp Med* 1997;185:1573–1584.
81. Cope AP. Regulation of autoimmunity by proinflammatory cytokines. *Curr Opin Immunol* 1998;10:669–676.
82. Isomaki P, Panesar M, Annenkov A, et al. Prolonged exposure of T cells to TNF down-regulates TCR zeta and expression of the TCR/CD3 complex at the cell surface. *J Immunol* 2001;166:5495–5507.
83. Bryl E, Vallejo AN, Weyand CM, et al. Down-regulation of CD28 expression by TNF-alpha. *J Immunol* 2001;167:3231–3238.
84. Maurice MM, Lankester AC, Bezemer AC, et al. Defective TCR-mediated signaling in synovial T cells in rheumatoid arthritis. *J Immunol* 1997;159:2973–2978.
85. Nakagomi H, Petersson M, Magnusson I, et al. Decreased expression of the signal-transducing zeta chains in tumor-infiltrating T-cells and NK cells of patients with colorectal carcinoma. *Cancer Res* 1993;53:5610–5612.
86. Gringhuis SI, van der EA, Leow A, et al. Effect of redox balance alterations on cellular localization of LAT and downstream T-cell receptor signaling pathways. *Mol Cell Biol* 2002;22:400–411.
87. Sherr CJ, DePinho RA. Cellular senescence: mitotic clock or culture shock? *Cell* 2000;102:407–410.
88. Gringhuis SI, Leow A, van der EA, et al. Displacement of linker for activation of T cells from the plasma membrane due to redox balance alterations results in hyporesponsiveness of synovial fluid T lymphocytes in rheumatoid arthritis. *J Immunol* 2000;164:2170–2179.
89. Salmon M, Scheel-Toellner D, Huissoon AP, et al. Inhibition of T cell apoptosis in the rheumatoid synovium. *J Clin Invest* 1997;99:439–446.
90. Schirmer M, Vallejo AN, Weyand CM, et al. Resistance to apoptosis and elevated expression of Bcl-2 in clonally expanded $CD4^+CD28^-$ T cells from rheumatoid arthritis patients. *J Immunol* 1998;161:1018–1025.
91. Vallejo AN, Schirmer M, Weyand CM, et al. Clonality and longevity of $CD4^+$CD28null T cells are associated with defects in apoptotic pathways. *J Immunol* 2000;165:6301–6307.
92. Kern F, Ode-Hakim S, Vogt K, et al. The enigma of $CD57^+CD28^-$ T cell expansion—anergy or activation? *Clin Exp Immunol* 1996;104:180–184.
93. Hamann D, Kostense S, Wolthers KC, et al. Evidence that human $CD8^+CD45RA^+CD27^-$ cells are induced by antigen and evolve through extensive rounds of division. *Int Immunol* 1999;11:1027–1033.
94. Wang EC, Borysiewicz LK. The role of $CD8^+$, $CD57^+$ cells in human cytomegalovirus and other viral infections. *Scand J Infect Dis Suppl* 1995;99:69–77.
95. Evans TG, Kallas EG, Luque AE, et al. Expansion of the CD57 subset of CD8 T cells in HIV-1 infection is related to CMV serostatus. *AIDS* 1999;13:1139–1141.
96. Vallejo AN, Nestel AR, Schirmer M, et al. Aging-related deficiency of CD28 expression in $CD4^+$ T cells is associated with the loss of gene-specific nuclear factor binding activity. *J Biol Chem* 1998;273:8119–8129.
97. Vallejo AN, Brandes JC, Weyand CM, et al. Modulation of CD28 expression: distinct regulatory pathways during activation and replicative senescence. *J Immunol* 1999;162:6572–6579.
98. Vallejo AN, Weyand CM, Goronzy JJ. Functional disruption of the CD28 gene transcriptional initiator in senescent T cells. *J Biol Chem* 2001;276:2565–2570.
99. Vallejo AN, Bryl E, Klarskov K, et al. Molecular basis for the loss of CD28 expression in senescent T cells. *J Biol Chem* 2002;277:46940–46949.
100. Warrington KJ, Vallejo AN, Weyand CM, Goronzy JJ. CD28 loss in senescent $CD4^+$ T cells: reversal by interleukin-12 stimulation. *Blood* 2003;101(9):3543–3549.
101. Namekawa T, Snyder MR, Yen JH, et al. Killer cell activating receptors function as costimulatory molecules on $CD4^+$CD28null T cells clonally expanded in rheumatoid arthritis. *J Immunol* 2000;165:1138–1145.
102. Snyder MR, Muegge LO, Offord C, et al. Formation of the killer Ig-like receptor repertoire on $CD4^+$CD28null T cells. *J Immunol* 2002;168:3839–3846.
103. Valiante NM, Lienert K, Shilling HG, et al. Killer cell receptors: keeping pace with MHC class I evolution. *Immunol Rev* 1997;155:155–164.
104. Vilches C, Parham P. KIR: diverse, rapidly evolving receptors of innate and adaptive immunity. *Annu Rev Immunol* 2002;20:217–251.
105. Yen JH, Moore BE, Nakajima T, et al. Major histocompatibility complex class I-recognizing receptors are disease risk genes in rheumatoid arthritis. *J Exp Med* 2001;193:1159–1167.
106. Arase H, Mocarski ES, Campbell AE, et al. Direct recognition of cytomegalovirus by activating and inhibitory NK cell receptors. *Science* 2002;296:1323–1326.
107. Warrington KJ, Takemura S, Goronzy JJ, et al. $CD4^+$,$CD28^-$ T cells in rheumatoid arthritis patients combine features of the innate and adaptive immune systems. *Arthritis Rheum* 2001;44:13–20.
108. Park W, Weyand CM, Schmidt D, et al. Co-stimulatory pathways controlling activation and peripheral tolerance of human $CD4^+CD28^-$ T cells. *Eur J Immunol* 1997;27:1082–1090.
109. Namekawa T, Wagner UG, Goronzy JJ, et al. Functional subsets of CD4 T cells in rheumatoid synovitis. *Arthritis Rheum* 1998;41:2108–2116.
110. Turesson C, Jacobsson L, Bergstrom U. Extra-articular rheumatoid arthritis: prevalence and mortality. *Rheumatology (Oxford)* 1999;38:668–674.
111. Weyand CM, Goronzy JJ, Liuzzo G, et al. T-cell immunity in acute coronary syndromes. *Mayo Clin Proc* 2001;76:1011–1020.
112. Liuzzo G, Kopecky SL, Frye RL, et al. Perturbation of the T-cell repertoire in patients with unstable angina. *Circulation* 1999;100:2135–2139.
113. Liuzzo G, Vallejo AN, Kopecky SL, et al. Molecular fingerprint of interferon-gamma signaling in unstable angina. *Circulation* 2001;103:1509–1514.
114. Liuzzo G, Goronzy JJ, Yang H, et al. Monoclonal T-cell proliferation and plaque instability in acute coronary syndromes. *Circulation* 2000;101:2883–2888.
115. Nakajima T, Schulte S, Warrington KJ, et al. T-cell-mediated lysis of endothelial cells in acute coronary syndromes. *Circulation* 2002;105:570–575.

CHAPTER 19

Synovial Fibroblasts

Thomas Pap, Renate E. Gay, and Steffen Gay

Fibroblasts occur prominently in the synovium in rheumatoid arthritis (RA) and have activities that can promote inflammation and destruction. Appreciation of the role of these cells in the pathogenesis has come from evidence for their activation and capacity to serve as effector cells in progressive destruction of articular cartilage. Furthermore, there is accumulating evidence that RA synovial fibroblasts (RA-SF) contribute significantly to the initiation and perpetuation of disease. It has been demonstrated that RA-SF play an important role in the attraction of inflammatory cells to the synovium, and several studies have linked these cells to mechanisms that regulate the switch from acute to chronic inflammation (1). Importantly, it has been shown that the activation of RA-SF is accompanied by dramatic and long-lasting changes in their phenotype. These changes are seen particularly in the most superficial lining layer of the synovium, and it has been established that the phenotypic alterations of RA-SF are not purely a transient reaction to proinflammatory stimuli. These alterations are accompanied by changes in the function of RA-SF that are preserved in the absence of continuous inflammation (2). As a consequence, joint destruction may proceed, even when inflammation is well controlled. The use of molecular biology techniques, such as gene transfer, and novel *in vitro* and *in vivo* models of disease have resulted in a multitude of data expanding our knowledge on disease mechanisms. These data have not only changed the conception of RA pathology but have also complemented and linked previously conflicting observations. This chapter will review the role of fibroblast-like cells in synovial activation and summarize advances in understanding the role of RA-SF in the pathogenesis of RA.

SYNOVIAL ACTIVATION AND CHRONIC INFLAMMATION

In addition to synovial hyperplasia and altered immune phenomena, chronic inflammation is a hallmark of RA (3). This inflammatory process primarily affects the synovium and is characterized by the accumulation of macrophages, T and B lymphocytes. Inflammatory cells release a variety of cytokines that result in the stimulation of neighboring cells and contribute to the specific environment in the rheumatoid joint. Tumor necrosis factor α (TNF-α) and interleukin-1β (IL-1β) are the most prominent examples of proinflammatory cytokines that control synovial activation (4). Numerous data have shown the presence of these cytokines in the rheumatoid joint and demonstrated that stimulation of SF with TNF-α and IL-1 may up-regulate expression of adhesion molecules (5,6) and matrix-degrading enzymes (7–9). This strategy of stimulation of resident RA-SF by proinflammatory cytokines, therefore, appears to be an important element in the activation of RA-SF and contributes to the progressive destruction of inflamed joints. Consequently, novel therapeutic strategies have been developed that aim at inhibiting TNF-α and IL-1 (10,11). They are based on the delivery of recombinant antibodies, soluble receptors, or receptor antagonists and have been termed *biologics*. Biologics that block TNF-α and IL-1 have changed significantly the treatment of RA, and it has been demonstrated that their use inhibits synovial inflammation and may reduce joint destruction in RA (12–18).

Other cytokines, such as IL-15 and IL-18, have also been implicated in synovial inflammation (19). IL-15 is expressed at elevated levels in the RA synovium and is produced predominantly by synovial macrophages (20,21). Expression of IL-15 has also been found for RA-SF and for some endothelial cells (22). It appears that IL-15 has direct effects on T cells, particularly on the proliferation and maintenance of CD8$^+$ memory cells (23). In addition, IL-15 constitutes an important factor that promotes the ability of synovial T cells to stimulate the release of TNF-α by macrophages through cell-to-cell contact (24). Although the therapeutic potential of these findings remains to be established, data from animal models suggest that inhibition of IL-15 through delivery of its soluble receptor may suppress the development of antigen-induced arthritis (25). Recently, IL-18 has been detected in RA synovium, and both synovial macrophages and fibroblasts have been identified as source for this proinflammatory cytokine. It has been found that IL-18 acts on both lymphocytes and macrophages, but induction of TNF-α in macrophage-like cells could be a primary function of IL-18 (26).

The understanding that different cell types in the rheumatoid synovium create a cytokine network with complex interactions (Fig. 19.1) has largely replaced previous concepts positing that some cells in the synovium are active players, whereas others are just passive responders (27). It is now evident that the accumulation of inflammatory cells results in effects on SF and that, conversely, resident RA-SF cells mediate the accumulation and survival of these inflammatory cells. RA-SF overexpress various chemokines that mediate the recruitment of macrophages and lymphocytes to the joints (28). Proinflammatory cytokines, such as TNF-α and IL-1β, may stimulate RA-SF to produce monocyte chemoattractant protein-1 (MCP-1), a chemoattractant factor involved in the recruitment of mononu-

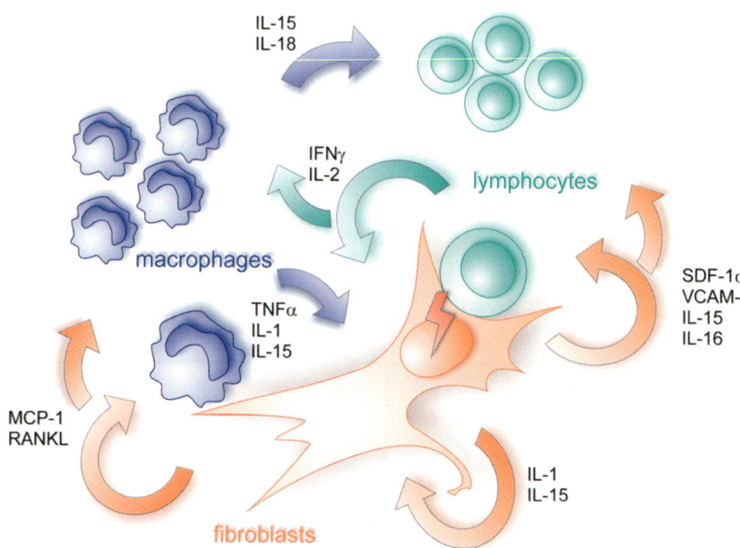

Figure 19.1. Cellular interactions in rheumatoid arthritis. IFN, interferon; IL, interleukin; MCP-1, monocyte chemoattractant protein-1; RANKL, receptor activator of nuclear factor–κB ligand; SDF, stromal cell–derived factor; TNF, tumor necrosis factor; VCAM-1, vascular cell adhesion molecule-1.

clear phagocytes during inflammation (29). In addition, Franz et al. demonstrated that IL-16, a cytokine that mediates the attraction of $CD4^+$ T cells, is expressed abundantly by RA-SF. The tissue distribution of IL-16 together with *in vitro* data (30) suggest that IL-16 contributes to the accumulation of T cells in the rheumatoid joint. Although the role of IL-16 in the pathogenesis of RA is uncertain, it appears that IL-16 produced by RA-SF may modulate the composition of the synovial T-cell repertoire.

Interactions between RA-SF and T cells appear to be of importance for the specific composition of the rheumatoid synovium. Using T cells at various stages of differentiation and activation, Haynes et al. found that human thymocytes and mitogen-activated peripheral blood T cells bind to RA-SF, whereas fresh peripheral blood T cells do not show this behavior. Of note, antibodies against CD2 and synovial cell lymphocyte function–associated antigen-3 inhibited this binding (31). There is now agreement that activated RA-SF are responsible for impaired apoptosis and anergy of synovial lymphocytes. Salmon et al. demonstrated first that RA-SF mediate the survival of T cells (32). After this observation, growing attention has focused on the mechanisms of fibroblast–lymphocyte interaction. It has been demonstrated that T and B cells are protected against apoptosis by the stromal cell–derived factor-1α (SDF-1α), a ligand of the chemokine receptor (CXCR)4. SDF-1α is produced by RA-SF and appears to inhibit T-cell apoptosis through the activation of phosphatidylinositol 3-kinase (PI 3-K) and mitogen-activated protein kinases pathways (33). Moreover, it has been shown that SDF-1α stimulates the migration of RA synovial T cells to the joints (33,34). RA-SF have been implicated in the attraction and accumulation of B lymphocytes that also are enriched in the inflamed joints of RA patients.

Lindhout et al. first showed that RA-SF may act as follicular dendritic cells and bind B cells (35). It appears that this function is intrinsic to RA-SF and quite specific for these cells when compared to non–RA-SF. B cells co-cultured with RA-SF show reduced apoptosis with an increase of mitochondrial apoptosis inhibitors, such as Bcl-X(L) (36). Hayashida et al. demonstrated that RA-SF promote the survival of B cells through the up-regulation of Bcl-X(L) expression and block their apoptosis through VLA-4 (CD49d/CD29)–vascular cell adhesion molecule (VCAM)-1 (CD106) interactions. Reparon-Schuijt et al. showed that B cells co-cultured with SF are protected from cell death in a cell contact– and VCAM-1–dependent mechanism (37), but the significance of these findings is less clear, as similar effects have been seen with SF from non-RA patients.

A variety of data support the notion that RA-SF play a significant role in the activation of macrophages and their differentiation into multinucleated, bone-resorbing cells. Specifically, the osteoclast differentiating factor, also called *receptor activator of nuclear factor–κB ligand*, has been identified as a major factor promoting osteoclastogenesis in the RA synovium. Shigeyama et al. demonstrated that RA-SF produce large amounts of receptor activator of nuclear factor–κB (NF-κB) ligand *in vivo* and that the levels of receptor activator of NF-κB ligand correlate with the ability of RA-SF cells to generate osteoclasts from peripheral blood mononuclear cells *in vitro* (38). It has been concluded that RA-SF contribute to the degradation of extracellular matrix not only directly, through the release of matrix-degrading enzymes, but also indirectly, through effecting the differentiation and activation of osteoclasts. This interaction of macrophages and fibroblasts in the RA synovium is highlighted further by a study of Hamann et al. (39). These investigators demonstrated that the cooperation of synovial macrophages and fibroblasts is mediated also through direct cell–cell interactions through ligation of CD55 on RA-SF with CD97 on macrophages. Interestingly, these interactions appear to take place predominantly in the synovial lining that mediates the progressive destruction of cartilage and bone.

WHAT IS UNIQUE ABOUT THE ACTIVATION OF RHEUMATOID ARTHRITIS SYNOVIAL FIBROBLASTS?

It has been widely accepted that RA-SF, particularly those of the most superficial lining layer, differ substantially from fibroblast-like synoviocytes of healthy individuals, as well as from SF of patients with other arthritic conditions, such as osteoarthritis (2,40,41). These RA-SF exhibit an altered morphology with a more round shape, a large pale nucleus, and multiple prominent nucleoli. The first description of this specific phenotype came from Fassbender in the 1980s (42). Subsequently, it has been shown that RA-SF not only have a different appearance but exhibit alterations of their behavior that are similar to that of tumors. Therefore, the phenotype of RA-SF has been termed *transformed appearing*, *tumor-like*, or—as will be used in

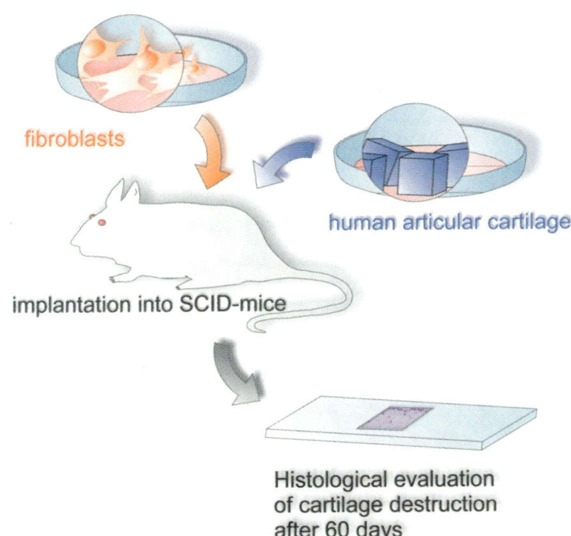

Figure 19.2. The severe combined immunodeficient (SCID) mouse model of rheumatoid arthritis (RA). In this model, RA synovial fibroblasts (RA-SF) are implanted together with normal human cartilage into SCID mice and kept for 60 days. After that time, the implants are removed, and the invasion of RA-SF into the cartilage is evaluated by histologic techniques.

this chapter—simply *activated*. Numerous data suggest that the activation of SF in RA is not merely a reaction to cytokine stimulation but, rather, is fixed in these cells and maintained, even when the fibroblasts are removed from their inflammatory environment. This notion is of importance because it helps to explain a number of findings that have demonstrated the progression of articular damage, even when inflammation is controlled through specific treatment (43).

In addition to clinical studies, histomorphologic analyses of RA-SF and studies of their growth characteristics, and cellular activation markers of RA-SF, the most convincing evidence for the stable activation of these cells has been derived from the severe combined immunodeficient (SCID) mouse model of cartilage destruction (44) (Fig. 19.2). In this model, RA-SF are co-implanted with normal human cartilage into SCID mice. Because they lack a functional immune system, SCID mice do not reject the implants and can be used to study the invasion of RA-SF into cartilage in the absence of human inflammatory cells. In this experimental setting, RA-SF maintain their specific phenotype and, unlike normal or osteoarthritis SF, progressively degrade the co-implanted cartilage. Therefore, this model has been used widely to study the specific characteristics of fibroblast activation in RA (45).

CYTOKINE-INDEPENDENT STIMULATION OF RHEUMATOID ARTHRITIS SYNOVIAL FIBROBLASTS

A major focus of research on RA-SF has been the search for exogenous and endogenous stimuli in the activation of SF in RA. Neidhart et al. have shown that endogenous retroviral L1 elements can be detected in synovial fluid, synovium, and synovial cells invading cartilage and bone in RA (46). In functional studies, it could be demonstrated that L1 induces the human stress-activated protein kinase-p38δ. p38δ can be detected in L1 transduced SF *in vitro*, but it has been also found expressed strongly at sites of synovial invasion into cartilage. Subsequent studies have shown that p38δ also induces matrix-degrading

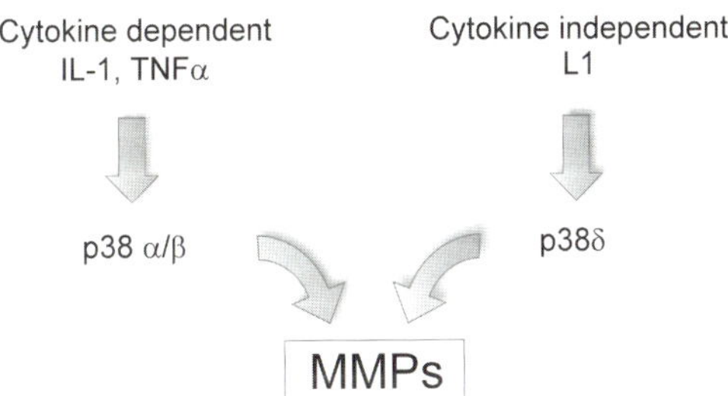

Figure 19.3. Regulation of matrix metalloproteinases by cytokine-dependent and cytokine-independent pathways. IL, interleukin; MMPs, matrix metalloproteinases; TNFα, tumor necrosis factor α.

enzymes, like collagenase-1 [matrix metalloproteinase-1 (MMP-1)] (47). These studies demonstrated that SF can be stimulated through T-cell/macrophage-independent pathways and may contribute, thereby, to joint destruction in the absence of inflammatory cytokines such as IL-1 and TNF-α. The L1-driven activation of p38δ appears independent of cytokines and may contribute to the progression of RA (Fig. 19.3). Future clinical trials designed to inhibit the L1-p38δ pathway may show the extent to which the process of synovial activation affects the therapeutic application of cytokine inhibitors.

It has also been demonstrated that SF appear to be major players in innate immunity. Kyburz et al. showed that bacterial peptidoglycans can stimulate SF to produce inflammatory cytokines, adhesion molecules (like VCAM-1 and ICAM-1), and a variety of matrix-degrading enzymes (48). This stimulation is mediated by the expression of Toll-like receptor-2 on SF, especially at sites of joint destruction in RA (49). This finding indicates that fibroblasts can participate in the innate immune system through the expression of pathogen pattern recognition receptors. These data further support the concept that SF may not only maintain the presence of inflammatory cells, but also initiate an inflammatory response in the synovium through the activation of NF-κB (49) and the production of chemokines and adhesion molecules (50).

UP-REGULATION OF PROTO-ONCOGENES AND TRANSCRIPTION FACTORS

A prominent feature of RA-SF is the activation of transcription factors and signaling pathways that ultimately result in altered apoptosis, up-regulation of adhesion molecules, and the expression of matrix-degrading enzymes (Fig. 19.4).

It has been demonstrated that early response genes, such as Egr-1, are expressed constitutively at high levels in RA-SF. Egr-1 is involved in cellular activation and is transcribed only transiently in normal cells (51). TNF-α may induce Egr-1 messenger RNA in fibroblast-like cells and mediate fibroblast proliferation, loss of growth inhibition by cell-to-cell contact, and altered cytokine expression pattern. Expression of Egr-1 in RA-SF is maintained over several passages *in vitro*, and Egr-1 binding sites are found in promoter regions of several genes that have been associated with stable activation of RA-SF (52). Thus, proto-oncogenes of the Egr family are involved in the activation of the cathepsin L gene (53), a matrix-degrading cysteine proteinase gene that is up-regulated in the RA synovium (54). Other data suggest that Egr-1 up-regulates naturally occurring antagonists of matrix-degrading enzymes, such as tissue metalloproteinases, as well as collagen production. Therefore, further studies are needed to elucidate the specific contribution of early response genes of the Egr family to synovial hyperplasia, joint destruction, and joint fibrosis in RA.

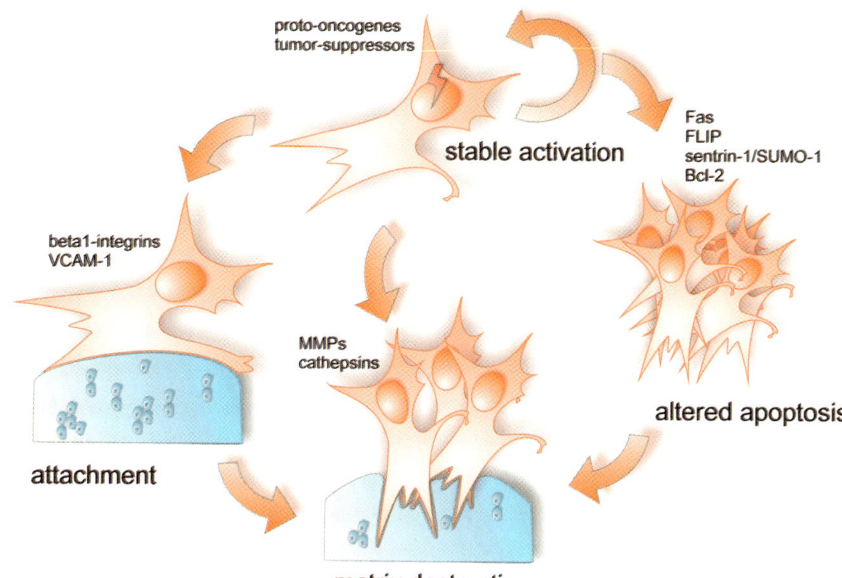

Figure 19.4. Activation of rheumatoid arthritis synovial fibroblasts (RA-SF). The stable activation of RA-SF results in the overexpression of adhesion molecules that mediate the attachment of RA-SF to the articular cartilage as well as alterations in apoptosis that are responsible for synovial hyperplasia. In addition, the activation of RA-SF leads to the up-regulation of cartilage-degrading enzymes that mediate the progressive destruction of cartilage and bone. FLIP, Fas-associated death domain–like interleukin-1–converting enzyme–like inhibitory protein; MMPs, matrix metalloproteinases; SUMO-1, small ubiquitin-like modifier-1; VCAM-1, vascular cell adhesion molecule-1.

Several other proto-oncogenes, such as *ras*, *raf*, *sis*, *myb*, and *myc*, have also been detected in RA synovium. They were found to be up-regulated predominantly in RA-SF attached to cartilage and bone (52), and binding sites for the aforementioned early response gene Egr-1 were identified in the promoters of the oncogenes *sis* and *ras*. There is evidence that some of these proto-oncogenes are involved in the up-regulation of MMPs contributing directly to cartilage destruction in RA. Specifically, c-Ras appears to play a role in the increased expression and proteolytic activation of MMPs in fibroblasts, and, through regulation of the Ras-Raf mitogen-activated protein kinases pathway, to contribute to the increased expression of disease-relevant MMPs in RA-SF. Consequently, inhibition of c-Raf through gene transfer of dominant negative mutants reduces the destructive potential of RA-SF in the SCID mouse model. Inhibition of c-Raf strongly induces apoptosis in RA-SF when blocked together with c-Myc (55). c-Myc is a downstream target of c-Raf that has been observed to be up-regulated in RA-SF, especially at sites of destruction in RA (56). Similar to the situation with c-Raf, blocking of c-Myc through dominant negative mutants reduced the invasion of RA-SF in the SCID mouse model. These findings complemented the observations by Hashiramoto et al., which showed a high-level inhibition of c-Myc through delivery of antisense oligodeoxynucleotides significantly reduced the proliferation of RA-SF and induced apoptosis through caspase signaling (57). Taken together, these data suggest that the pathologic expression of proto-oncogenes and the subsequent modulation of different signaling pathways constitute important steps in the activation of RA-SF. In addition, these data point to distinct, but overlapping, effects of different proto-oncogenes in RA.

Among the proto-oncogenes involved in the activation of RA-SF, c-fos has been assigned a special role. c-fos encodes a basic leucin zipper transcription factor and is part of the transcriptional activator AP-1 (jun/fos). Increased activity of c-fos has been found in RA-SF (56). Asahara et al. described a high DNA binding activity of AP-1 in the synovial tissues of RA patients, but negligible activity in osteoarthritis (OA) samples (58). AP-1 activity was detected predominantly in adherent cells and correlated with the *in situ* expression of c-fos and c-jun mRNA, as well as with disease activity. Morita et al. showed that the delivery of c-fos antisense oligonucleotides suppressed AP-1 activity and inhibited IL-1–mediated fibroblast proliferation (59). Of importance, the promoters of several MMP genes contain binding sites for the transcription factor AP-1. AP-1 sites have been proven to be involved in tissue-specific expression of MMPs. However, AP-1 sites do not appear to regulate transcription of MMPs alone. Rather, there are essential interactions with other cis-acting sequences in the promoters and with transcription factors that bind to these sequences (60). Thus, the up-regulation of *c-fos*, as well as of *fos*-related proto-oncogenes, appears to be important for cell activation via AP-1 formation and subsequent matrix degradation.

In addition to AP-1, NF-κB has been strongly implicated in synovial activation and in the up-regulation of matrix-degrading enzymes (61,62). NF-κB is a family of dimeric, regulatory DNA-binding proteins that is part of different signal cascades. NF-κB is bound to IκB in an inactive form in the cytoplasm. On phosphorylation by IκB kinase, IκB is released from NF-κB, which, in turn, is translocated to the nucleus. Binding sites for NF-κB have been found in a number of genes involved in the inflammatory response, and it has been demonstrated that NF-κB is highly activated in RA-SF (63). Specifically, NF-κB is involved in the regulation of inflammatory cytokines such as TNF-α, IL-1, IL-6, and IL-8 (64), as well as adhesion molecules (65) and matrix-degrading enzymes (66). As demonstrated by Han et al., NF-κB expression shows a better correlation with MMP expression than AP-1 (61). It has been suggested that the inflammation-dependent up-regulation of MMPs is mediated largely through NF-κB. Therefore, NF-κB appears to constitute an important link between synovial inflammation, hyperplasia, and matrix destruction (67).

ALTERATIONS IN TUMOR SUPPRESSORS

The role of known tumor suppressor genes in the cellular activation of RA-SF has been a topic of considerable interest in the pathogenesis of RA. Early studies by Firestein et al. found an increased expression of p53 in RA synovial tissues (68), and, together with data demonstrating somatic mutations of p53 in RA-SF (69–71), it was hypothesized that such mutations may contribute to the stable activation of RA-SF. This notion was challenged by the high variability of such mutations, as well as by data from other studies that

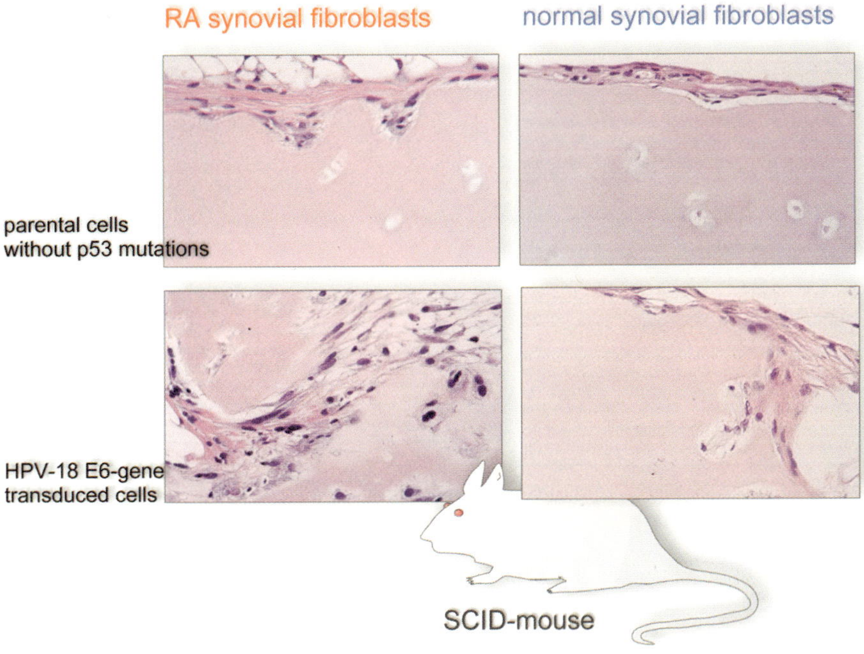

Figure 19.5. Effects of p53 inhibition on the invasiveness of rheumatoid arthritis synovial fibroblasts (RA-SF) in the severe combined immunodeficient (SCID) mouse model of RA. Gene transfer of the human papilloma virus (HPV)-18 E6 protein that inhibits p53 results in an increased invasiveness of RA-SF but also transforms normal SF to exhibit an RA-like invasive behavior. (Adapted from Pap T, Aupperle KR, Gay S, et al. Invasiveness of synovial fibroblasts is regulated by p53 in the SCID mouse in vivo model of cartilage invasion. *Arthritis Rheum* 2001;44:676–681.)

failed to detect p53 mutations in RA-SF (72). Based on these studies, Pap et al. analyzed whether mutations of p53 are required for the invasion of RA-SF into cartilage and found significant cartilage destruction in the SCID mouse model, even in the absence of p53 (73). However, inhibition of p53 through retroviral gene transfer of the human papilloma virus-18 E6 gene increased the invasion of RA-SF in the SCID mouse model (Fig. 19.5). Furthermore, inhibition of p53 induced an aggressive, RA-like phenotype also in normal SF, demonstrating clearly that inhibition of a single, disease-relevant signaling molecule may transform normal SF. Subsequent studies have revealed that p53 expression occurs during inflammation and counteracts local inflammatory responses (74). These data together have suggested that, although inhibition of p53 may induce normal synovial cells into an aggressive state, it constitutes only part of the cellular activation in RA. Initial events most likely do not include the inactivation of p53, but environmental factors may cause alteration in the function of p53 at later stages of disease. These may then enhance the activation of already altered RA-SF and transform normal cells.

Evidence that the tumor suppressor pentaerythritol tetranitrate (PTEN) is down-regulated in some RA-SF has contributed further to the concept that the activation of RA-SF involves a complex pattern of molecular alterations (75). PTEN is a tyrosine phosphatase that exhibits homology to the cytoskeletal proteins tensin and auxilin and has been found altered together with p53 in several cancers. Although no mutations of PTEN were found in studies by Pap et al. (75), it was an important observation that the expression of PTEN is lacking in the lining layer of RA synovium and in more than 50% of RA-SF *in vitro*. Studies in the SCID mouse model demonstrate further that RA-SF invading the cartilage show no expression of PTEN but at the same time produce disease-relevant MMPs (75).

Modulation of Apoptosis in Rheumatoid Arthritis Synovial Fibroblasts

Impaired apoptosis has been associated strongly with the stable activation of RA-SF. It has been understood that changes in the expression of apoptosis-regulating molecules affect internal, mitochondrial-dependent as well as external, death receptor–dependent pathways. Thus, members of the Bcl family, which are important regulators of mitochondrial pathways of apoptosis, have been shown to contribute to the pathogenesis of experimental arthritis (76). *In situ* analyses of human tissues have demonstrated expression of the antiapoptotic molecule Bcl-2 in RA-SF (77). Moreover, a correlation was found between the enhanced expression of the Bcl-2 and synovial lining thickening (78); elevated levels of Bcl-x(L) have also been detected in RA-SF (79). It was also shown that stimulation of RA-SF with the proinflammatory cytokine IL-15 suppressed Bcl-2 and Bcl-x(L) messenger RNA (79). It was found in this study that apoptosis can be increased when the autocrine stimulation of RA-SF with IL-15 is inhibited, which provides a link between cytokine-mediated stimulation of RA-SF and their resistance to cell death.

Apoptosis is triggered by cell-surface receptors that act through a death domain (80). Fas (CD-95/Apo-1) is the prominent member of the death domain family, and Fas–Fas ligand (FasL) interactions have been implicated most strongly in the modulation of apoptosis in RA-SF. There is growing evidence that RA-SF are relatively resistant to FasL-induced apoptosis, despite their high expression of Fas (77). The underlying mechanisms of this resistance to apoptosis are only incompletely understood, and it appears that several pathways are involved. As elevated levels of the soluble Fas (sFas) are found in the synovial fluids of patients with RA (81), it has been suggested that the increased expression of sFas in the joints may prevent Fas-induced apoptosis of synoviocytes. However, RA-SF maintain their resistance against FasL-induced apoptosis for extended periods of time *in vitro* (82,83). Therefore, intrinsic modulation of pathways downstream of the Fas receptor have been suggested to account for the resistance against Fas-induced apoptosis (Fig. 19.6). Aberrant expression of Fas-associated death domain–like IL-1–converting enzyme–like inhibitory protein (FLIP) has been one of the mechanisms implicated in the resistance of RA-SF to apoptosis. Perlman et al. demonstrated that activated RA macrophages are resistant to Fas-induced apoptosis, despite the expression of Fas, but, at the same time, show elevated levels of FLIP (84). The expression levels of FLIP were higher in RA than in OA synovium and correlated with lining thickening and inflammation. Schedel et al. found expression of FLIP mainly at sites of cartilage destruction (85). In a study of synovial tissues from patients with

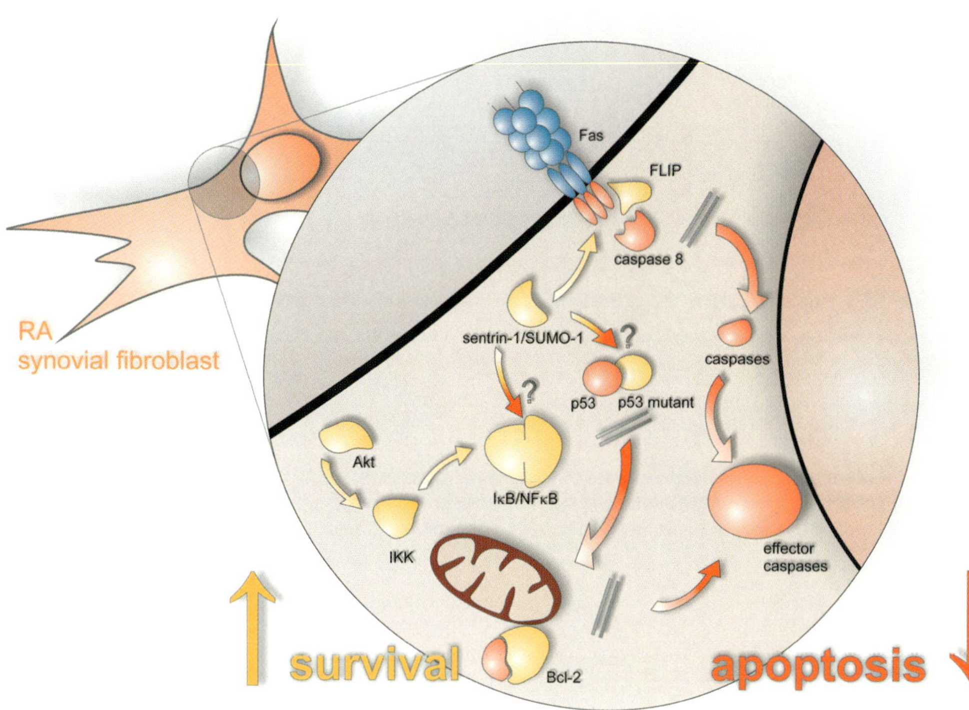

Figure 19.6. Regulation of apoptosis in rheumatoid arthritis–synovial fibroblasts. FLIP, Fas-associated death domain–like IL-1–converting enzyme–like inhibitory protein; IKK, IκB kinase; NF-κB, nuclear factor–κB; SUMO-1, small ubiquitin-like modifier-1.

RA, Catrina et al. suggested that the expression of FLIP depends on the stage of disease (86). In patients with long-term RA, increased levels of apoptosis were associated with low levels of FLIP, whereas patients with early RA showed decreased levels of apoptosis accompanied by high expression of FLIP. These data suggest that resistance of RA-SF to apoptosis occurs early in disease.

Another molecule that modulates downstream mechanisms of the Fas signaling is sentrin-1/small ubiquitin-like modifier-1 (SUMO-1). Sentrin-1/SUMO-1 is a small ubiquitin-like molecule found at very low levels in normal synovial tissues and synovial tissues of OA patients. In contrast, RA synovium shows marked expression of sentrin-1/SUMO-1 located predominantly in RA-SF of the lining layer and at sites of cartilage invasion (87). Moreover, RA-SF maintain their high expression of sentrin-1/SUMO-1 when analyzed in the SCID mouse model. Other data suggest that the levels of sentrin-1/SUMO-1 correlate directly with the resistance of RA-SF to Fas-induced apoptosis (82). Despite this strong association, functional data, including the inhibition of sentrin-1/SUMO-1, will be required to elucidate the specific effects of sentrinization in RA-SF. Specifically, it needs to be determined how the different, partly opposing effects of sentrin-1/SUMO-1 are balanced in RA-SF to mediate their resistance to apoptosis.

Among the different transcription factors that are involved in modulating apoptosis in RA-SF, NF-κB has been confirmed to be a key molecule (62). Inhibition of NF-κB through decoy oligonucleotides has been demonstrated to increase the apoptosis of RA-SF (88). NF-κB activity can be modulated by the serine-threonine protein kinase AKT, which is regulated by the PI 3-K (89,90). AKT is expressed at elevated levels in RA-SF (91) and mediates its antiapoptotic signaling through NF-κB. Conversely, blocking of PI 3-K/AKT leads to the proliferation of RA-SF (92).

DESTRUCTION OF ARTICULAR STRUCTURES BY MATRIX-DEGRADING ENZYMES

The progressive destruction of articular cartilage and bone in RA is mediated by the concerted action of different matrix-degrading enzymes, particularly cathepsins and MMPs. Cathepsins are classified by their catalytic mechanisms and cleave cartilage types II, IX, and XI, as well as proteoglycans. The cysteine proteases cathepsin B and L are up-regulated in RA synovium (54,93). In addition, cathepsin K expression by RA-SF and macrophages has been reported, especially at the site of synovial invasion into articular bone (94,95). As shown by Hou et al., cathepsin K mediates the intralysosomal hydrolysis of collagen fibrils in RA-SF (96). It was demonstrated that intracellular degradation of such fibrils is prevented by cathepsin K inhibitors but not by inhibitors of the cathepsins L and B. In addition, cathepsin K has aggrecan-degrading activity, and cleavage products of aggrecan appear to potentiate the collagenolytic activity of cathepsin K (96). In a similar fashion to MMPs, cathepsins are activated by proto-oncogenes. This notion is supported by the observation of combined *ras* and cathepsin L expression in the rheumatoid synovium (54). Cunanne et al. demonstrated the expression of cathepsins B and L very early in the course in disease (97). Several studies have also shown that proinflammatory cytokines, such as IL-1 and TNF-α, can stimulate the production of cathepsins by synovial fibroblast-like cells (95,98,99). Although Keyszer et al. found a more pronounced expression of MMPs messenger RNA, compared with the cathepsins B and L in RA, the elevated levels of these cysteine proteases in RA compared with OA suggest also a major role in matrix degradation in RA (100).

MMPs constitute the major group of enzymes involved in the progressive destruction of joints in RA and comprise a family of at least 20 zinc-containing endopeptidases that act extracellularly and are involved in the degradation and remodeling of extracellular matrix proteins. The expression of MMPs in the rheumatoid synovium has been studied extensively (101), and strong expression for a number of MMPs has been described in RA (102,103). Apart from MMP-2 and the membrane-type MMPs, which are expressed constitutively at significant levels, MMP expression is regulated strongly by proinflammatory cytokines, growth factors, and extracellular matrix molecules (101). In the past years, major steps of cartilage degradation by MMPs have been elucidated. It has been shown that MMP-1, -3, and -13 are involved most prominently in the cleavage of collagen type II, the major matrix constituent of hyaline cartilage. These enzymes also cleave collagen type IX, which provides a link between collagen type II fibrils and glucosaminoglycans (104). Rutkauskaite et al. demonstrated that the inhibition of MMP-1 in RA-SF by retroviral gene transfer of specific ribozymes significantly reduces the invasiveness of these cells in the SCID mouse model (105). Other studies have linked the expression of collagenases (MMP-1, MMP-13), gelantinases (MMP-2, MMP-9), and stromelysin (MMP-3) to the disease activity in RA (106–109) and have demonstrated that MMP-1, MMP-2, and MMP-3 together are sufficient to destroy the majority of structural proteins in the joints (110).

The role of MMPs in rheumatoid cartilage degradation is also highlighted by studies in transgenic mice. Thus, mice that are transgenic for MMP-13 develop severe cartilage damage, which may not necessarily resemble an RA-like disease (111). Knockout models of MMPs have also demonstrated the complexity of cartilage destruction by MMPs. These studies have challenged the role of MMP-3, an enzyme that has been implicated strongly in the destructive potential of RA-SF (112,113) and shown to be a key activator of other MMPs. MMP-3–deficient mice develop collagen-induced arthritis, and histologic analyses of the changes demonstrated no differences between wild-type and knockout mice (114). Observations in MT1-MMP knockout mice illustrate further that some MMPs may even have a key regulatory role, as MT1-MMP knockout mice develop arthritis (112,115). Unfortunately, there has been no precise assessment of the contribution of individual MMPs to the invasiveness of RA-SF. This lack of understanding has been an obstacle to developing specific strategies for the inhibition of MMPs in RA. In this context, the SCID mouse model offers the opportunity to selectively inhibit single MMPs or MMP activation pathways in human RA-SF and to assess their effects on the invasiveness of these cells. In this context, inhibition of plasmin—one major activator of MMPs—reduces the invasion of RA-SF by approximately 30% (116). Conversely, overexpression of tissue inhibitors of metalloproteinases in RA-SF through adenoviral gene transfer resulted in a nearly complete block of invasion compared to control fibroblasts (117). Other studies analyzing the role of individual MMPs in the SCID mouse model are under way and will provide more detailed insights into the concerted action of MMP family members in rheumatoid joint destruction.

CONCLUSION

RA-SF contribute significantly to the pathogenesis of RA. As part of a cellular network, these cells are involved in the regulation of inflammatory changes and play a major role in the progressive destruction of articular cartilage and bone. RA-SF display an activated phenotype that is preserved in the absence of continuous cytokine stimulation. Attachment to articular cartilage, production of matrix-degrading enzymes, and alterations in apoptosis are hallmarks of their stable activation. The fact that activated RA-SF express Toll-like receptor-2 and that Toll-like receptor-2 signaling results in the production of chemokines demonstrates that these cells participate also in the innate immune system through the expression of pathogen recognition receptors. Novel therapeutic strategies to inhibit joint destruction in RA will, therefore, have to include the specific targeting of activated RA-SF.

REFERENCES

1. Buckley CD, Pilling D, Lord JM, et al. Fibroblasts regulate the switch from acute resolving to chronic persistent inflammation. *Trends Immunol* 2001; 22:199–204.
2. Pap T, Muller-Ladner U, Gay RE, et al. Fibroblast biology. Role of synovial fibroblasts in the pathogenesis of rheumatoid arthritis. *Arthritis Res* 2000;2:361–367.
3. Pap T, Gay RE, Gay S. Rheumatoid arthritis. In: Theofilopoulos AN, Bona CA, eds. *The molecular pathology of autoimmune diseases*. New York: Taylor & Francis, 2002:376–401.
4. Dayer JM, Burger D. Interleukin-1, tumor necrosis factor and their specific inhibitors. *Eur Cytokine Netw* 1994;5:563–571.
5. Marlor CW, Webb DL, Bombara MP, et al. Expression of vascular cell adhesion molecule-1 in fibroblastlike synoviocytes after stimulation with tumor necrosis factor. *Am J Pathol* 1992;140:1055–1060.
6. Pirila L, Heino J. Altered integrin expression in rheumatoid synovial lining type B cells: in vitro cytokine regulation of alpha 1 beta 1, alpha 6 beta 1, and alpha v beta 5 integrins. *J Rheumatol* 1996;23:1691–1698.
7. Hanemaaijer R, Sorsa T, Konttinen YT, et al. Matrix metalloproteinase-8 is expressed in rheumatoid synovial fibroblasts and endothelial cells. Regulation by tumor necrosis factor-alpha and doxycycline. *J Biol Chem* 1997; 272:31504–31509.
8. Migita K, Eguchi K, Kawabe Y, et al. TNF-alpha-mediated expression of membrane-type matrix metalloproteinase in rheumatoid synovial fibroblasts. *Immunology* 1996;89:553–557.
9. Unemori EN, Hibbs MS, Amento EP. Constitutive expression of a 92-kD gelatinase (type V collagenase) by rheumatoid synovial fibroblasts and its induction in normal human fibroblasts by inflammatory cytokines. *J Clin Invest* 1991;88:1656–1662.
10. Arend WP, Dayer JM. Inhibition of the production and effects of interleukin-1 and tumor necrosis factor alpha in rheumatoid arthritis. *Arthritis Rheum* 1995;38:151–160.
11. Dayer JM. Interleukin 1 or tumor necrosis factor-alpha: which is the real target in rheumatoid arthritis? *J Rheumatol Suppl* 2002;65:10–15.
12. Elliott MJ, Maini RN, Feldmann M, et al. Randomised double-blind comparison of chimeric monoclonal antibody to tumour necrosis factor alpha (cA2) versus placebo in rheumatoid arthritis. *Lancet* 1994;344:1105–1110.
13. Maini R, St Clair EW, Breedveld F, et al. Infliximab (chimeric anti-tumour necrosis factor alpha monoclonal antibody) versus placebo in rheumatoid arthritis patients receiving concomitant methotrexate: a randomised phase III trial. ATTRACT Study Group. *Lancet* 1999;354:1932–1939.
14. Lipsky PE, van der Heijde DM, St Clair EW, et al. Infliximab and methotrexate in the treatment of rheumatoid arthritis. Anti-Tumor Necrosis Factor Trial in Rheumatoid Arthritis with Concomitant Therapy Study Group. *N Engl J Med* 2000;343:1594–1602.
15. Weinblatt ME, Kremer JM, Bankhurst AD, et al. A trial of etanercept, a recombinant tumor necrosis factor receptor:Fc fusion protein, in patients with rheumatoid arthritis receiving methotrexate. *N Engl J Med* 1999;340:253–259.
16. Dinarello CA. The role of the interleukin-1-receptor antagonist in blocking inflammation mediated by interleukin-1. *N Engl J Med* 2000;343:732–734.
17. Bresnihan B, Alvaro-Gracia JM, Cobby M, et al. Treatment of rheumatoid arthritis with recombinant human interleukin-1 receptor antagonist. *Arthritis Rheum* 1998;41:2196–2204.
18. Pisetsky DS. Tumor necrosis factor blockers in rheumatoid arthritis. *N Engl J Med* 2000;342:810–811.
19. Liew FY, McInnes IB. Role of interleukin 15 and interleukin 18 in inflammatory response. *Ann Rheum Dis* 2002;61(Suppl 2):ii100–ii102.
20. McInnes IB, al Mughales J, Field M, et al. The role of interleukin-15 in T-cell migration and activation in rheumatoid arthritis. *Nat Med* 1996;2:175–182.
21. McInnes IB, Liew FY. Interleukin 15: a proinflammatory role in rheumatoid arthritis synovitis. *Immunol Today* 1998;19:75–79.
22. Oppenheimer-Marks N, Brezinschek RI, Mohamadzadeh M, et al. Interleukin 15 is produced by endothelial cells and increases the transendothelial migration of T cells in vitro and in the SCID mouse-human rheumatoid arthritis model in vivo. *J Clin Invest* 1998;101:1261–1272.
23. Zhang X, Sun S, Hwang I, et al. Potent and selective stimulation of memory-phenotype CD8+ T cells in vivo by IL-15. *Immunity* 1998;8:591–599.
24. Vey E, Burger D, Dayer JM. Expression and cleavage of tumor necrosis factor-alpha and tumor necrosis factor receptors by human monocytic cell lines upon direct contact with stimulated T cells. *Eur J Immunol* 1996;26:2404–2409.
25. Ruchatz H, Leung BP, Wei XQ, et al. Soluble IL-15 receptor alpha-chain administration prevents murine collagen-induced arthritis: a role for IL-15 in development of antigen- induced immunopathology. *J Immunol* 1998;160:5654–5660.
26. McInnes IB, Gracie JA, Leung BP, et al. Interleukin 18: a pleiotropic participant in chronic inflammation. *Immunol Today* 2000;21:312–315.
27. Pap T, Franz JK, Gay RE, et al. Has research on lymphocytes hindered progress in rheumatoid arthritis? In: Bird H, Snaith M, eds. *Challenges in rheumatoid arthritis*. Oxford: Blackwell Science Ltd, 1999:61–77.
28. Hosaka S, Akahoshi T, Wada C, et al. Expression of the chemokine superfamily in rheumatoid arthritis. *Clin Exp Immunol* 1994;97:451–457.
29. Koch AE, Kunkel SL, Harlow LA, et al. Enhanced production of monocyte chemoattractant protein-1 in rheumatoid arthritis. *J Clin Invest* 1992;90:772–779.
30. Franz JK, Kolb SA, Hummel KM, et al. Interleukin-16, produced by synovial fibroblasts, mediates chemoattraction for $CD4^+$ T lymphocytes in rheumatoid arthritis. *Eur J Immunol* 1998;28:2661–2671.
31. Haynes BF, Grover BJ, Whichard LP, et al. Synovial microenvironment-T cell interactions. Human T cells bind to fibroblast-like synovial cells in vitro. *Arthritis Rheum* 1988;31:947–955.
32. Salmon M, Scheel Toellner D, Huissoon AP, et al. Inhibition of T cell apoptosis in the rheumatoid synovium. *J Clin Invest* 1997;99:439–446.

33. Nanki T, Hayashida K, El Gabalawy HS, et al. Stromal cell-derived factor-1-CXC chemokine receptor 4 interactions play a central role in CD4+ T cell accumulation in rheumatoid arthritis synovium. *J Immunol* 2000;165:6590–6598.
34. Suzuki Y, Rahman M, Mitsuya H. Diverse transcriptional response of CD4(+) T cells to stromal cell-derived factor (SDF)-1: cell survival promotion and priming effects of SDF-1 on CD4(+) T cells. *J Immunol* 2001;167:3064–3073.
35. Lindhout E, van Eijk M, van Pel M, et al. Fibroblast-like synoviocytes from rheumatoid arthritis patients have intrinsic properties of follicular dendritic cells. *J Immunol* 1999;162:5949–5956.
36. Hayashida K, Shimaoka Y, Ochi T, et al. Rheumatoid arthritis synovial stromal cells inhibit apoptosis and up-regulate Bcl-xL expression by B cells in a CD49/CD29-CD106-dependent mechanism. *J Immunol* 2000;164:1110–1116.
37. Reparon-Schuijt CC, van Esch WJ, van Kooten C, et al. Regulation of synovial B cell survival in rheumatoid arthritis by vascular cell adhesion molecule 1 (CD106) expressed on fibroblast-like synoviocytes. *Arthritis Rheum* 2000;43:1115–1121.
38. Shigeyama Y, Pap T, Kunzler P, et al. Expression of osteoclast differentiation factor in rheumatoid arthritis. *Arthritis Rheum* 2000;43:2523–2530.
39. Hamann J, Wishaupt JO, van Lier RA, et al. Expression of the activation antigen CD97 and its ligand CD55 in rheumatoid synovial tissue. *Arthritis Rheum* 1999;42:650–658.
40. Firestein GS. Invasive fibroblast-like synoviocytes in rheumatoid arthritis. Passive responders or transformed aggressors? *Arthritis Rheum* 1996;39:1781–1790.
41. Müller-Ladner U, Gay RE, Gay S. Cellular pathways of joint destruction. *Curr Opin Rheumatol* 1997;9:213–220.
42. Fassbender HG. Histomorphological basis of articular cartilage destruction in rheumatoid arthritis. *Coll Relat Res* 1983;3:141–155.
43. Mulherin D, Fitzgerald O, Bresnihan B. Clinical improvement and radiological deterioration in rheumatoid arthritis: evidence that the pathogenesis of synovial inflammation and articular erosion may differ. *Br J Rheumatol* 1996;35:1263–1268.
44. Müller-Ladner U, Kriegsmann J, Franklin BN, et al. Synovial fibroblasts of patients with rheumatoid arthritis attach to and invade normal human cartilage when engrafted into SCID mice. *Am J Pathol* 1996;149:1607–1615.
45. Pap T, Müller-Ladner U, Hummel KM, et al. Studies in the SCID mouse model. In: Evans CH, Robbins P, eds. *Gene therapy in inflammatory diseases*. Basel, Switzerland: Birkenhäuser, 1998.
46. Neidhart M, Rethage J, Kuchen S, et al. Retrotransposable L1 elements expressed in rheumatoid arthritis synovial tissue: association with genomic DNA hypomethylation and influence on gene expression. *Arthritis Rheum* 2000;43:2634–2647.
47. Kuchen S, Seemayer CA, Kuenzler P, et al. Cytokine-independent upregulation of matrix metalloproteinase 1 mRNA expression by the stress activated protein kinase 4. *Arthritis Rheum* 2002;44:S183.
48. Kyburz D, Rethage J, Seibl R, et al. Bacterial peptidoglycans but not CpG oligonucleotides activate synovial fibroblasts by Toll-like receptor signaling. *Arthritis Rheum* 2003;48:590–593.
49. Seibl R, Birchler T, Loeliger S, et al. Expression and regulation of Toll-like receptor 2 in rheumatoid arthritis synovium. *Am J Pathol* 2003;162:1221–1227.
50. Pierer M, Kyburz D, Rethage J, et al. TLR-2 dependent upregulation of chemokines in RA-SF. *Arthritis Rheum* 2003;46:S553.
51. Aicher WK, Heer AH, Trabandt A, et al. Overexpression of zinc-finger transcription factor Z-225/Egr-1 in synoviocytes from rheumatoid arthritis patients. *J Immunol* 1994;152:5940–5948.
52. Müller-Ladner U, Kriegsmann J, Gay RE, et al. Oncogenes in rheumatoid synovium. *Rheum Dis Clin North Am* 1995;21:675–690.
53. Ishidoh K, Taniguchi S, Kominami E. Egr family member proteins are involved in the activation of the cathepsin L gene in v-src-transformed cells. *Biochem Biophys Res Commun* 1997;238:665–669.
54. Trabandt A, Aicher WK, Gay RE, et al. Expression of the collagenolytic and Ras-induced cysteine proteinase cathepsin L and proliferation-associated oncogenes in synovial cells of MRL/L mice and patients with rheumatoid arthritis. *Matrix* 1990;10:349–361.
55. Nawrath M, Hummel KM, Pap T, et al. Effect of dominant negative mutants of raf-1 and c-myc on rheumatoid arthritis synovial fibroblasts in the SCID mouse model. *Arthritis Rheum* 1998;41:S95.
56. Xue C, Takahashi M, Hasunuma T, et al. Characterisation of fibroblast-like cells in pannus lesions of patients with rheumatoid arthritis sharing properties of fibroblasts and chondrocytes. *Ann Rheum Dis* 1997;56:262–267.
57. Hashiramoto A, Sano H, Maekawa T, et al. C-myc antisense oligodeoxynucleotides can induce apoptosis and down-regulate Fas expression in rheumatoid synoviocytes. *Arthritis Rheum* 1999;42:954–962.
58. Asahara H, Fujisawa K, Kobata T, et al. Direct evidence of high DNA binding activity of transcription factor AP-1 in rheumatoid arthritis synovium. *Arthritis Rheum* 1997;40:912–918.
59. Morita Y, Kashihara N, Yamamura M, et al. Antisense oligonucleotides targeting c-fos mRNA inhibit rheumatoid synovial fibroblast proliferation. *Ann Rheum Dis* 1998;57:122–124.
60. Benbow U, Brinckerhoff CE. The AP-1 site and MMP gene regulation: what is all the fuss about? *Matrix Biol* 1997;15:519–526.
61. Han Z, Boyle DL, Manning AM, et al. AP-1 and NF-kappaB regulation in rheumatoid arthritis and murine collagen-induced arthritis. *Autoimmunity* 1998;28:197–208.
62. Karin M, Lin A. NF-kappaB at the crossroads of life and death. *Nat Immunol* 2002;3:221–227.
63. Aupperle KR, Bennett BL, Boyle DL, et al. NF-kappa B regulation by I kappa B kinase in primary fibroblast-like synoviocytes. *J Immunol* 1999;163:427–433.
64. Georganas C, Liu H, Perlman H, et al. Regulation of IL-6 and IL-8 expression in rheumatoid arthritis synovial fibroblasts: the dominant role for NF-kappa B but not C/EBP beta or c- Jun. *J Immunol* 2000;165:7199–7206.
65. Li P, Sanz I, O'Keefe RJ, et al. NF-kappa B regulates VCAM-1 expression on fibroblast-like synoviocytes. *J Immunol* 2000;164:5990–5997.
66. Vincenti MP, Coon CI, Brinckerhoff CE. Nuclear factor kappaB/p50 activates an element in the distal matrix metalloproteinase 1 promoter in interleukin-1beta-stimulated synovial fibroblasts. *Arthritis Rheum* 1998;41:1987–1994.
67. Miagkov AV, Kovalenko DV, Brown CE, et al. NF-kappaB activation provides the potential link between inflammation and hyperplasia in the arthritic joint. *Proc Natl Acad Sci U S A* 1998;95:13859–13864.
68. Firestein GS, Nguyen K, Aupperle KR, et al. Apoptosis in rheumatoid arthritis: p53 overexpression in rheumatoid arthritis synovium. *Am J Pathol* 1996;149:2143–2151.
69. Firestein GS, Echeverri F, Yeo M, et al. Somatic mutations in the p53 tumor suppressor gene in rheumatoid arthritis synovium. *Proc Natl Acad Sci U S A* 1997;94:10895–10900.
70. Han Z, Boyle DL, Shi Y, et al. Dominant-negative p53 mutations in rheumatoid arthritis. *Arthritis Rheum* 1999;42:1088–1092.
71. Inazuka M, Tahira T, Horiuchi T, et al. Analysis of p53 tumour suppressor gene somatic mutations in rheumatoid arthritis synovium. *Rheumatology (Oxford)* 2000;39:262–266.
72. Kullmann F, Judex M, Neudecker I, et al. Analysis of the p53 tumor suppressor gene in rheumatoid arthritis synovial fibroblasts. *Arthritis Rheum* 1999;42:1594–1600.
73. Pap T, Aupperle KR, Gay S, et al. Invasiveness of synovial fibroblasts is regulated by p53 in the SCID mouse in vivo model of cartilage invasion. *Arthritis Rheum* 2001;44:676–681.
74. Yamanishi Y, Boyle DL, Pinkoski MJ, et al. Regulation of joint destruction and inflammation by p53 in collagen-induced arthritis. *Am J Pathol* 2002;160:123–130.
75. Pap T, Franz JK, Hummel KM, et al. Activation of synovial fibroblasts in rheumatoid arthritis: lack of expression of the tumour suppressor PTEN at sites of invasive growth and destruction. *Arthritis Res* 2000;2:59–65.
76. Perlman H, Liu H, Georganas C, et al. Differential expression pattern of the antiapoptotic proteins, Bcl-2 and FLIP, in experimental arthritis. *Arthritis Rheum* 2001;44:2899–2908.
77. Matsumoto S, Muller Ladner U, Gay RE, et al. Ultrastructural demonstration of apoptosis, Fas and Bcl-2 expression of rheumatoid synovial fibroblasts. *J Rheumatol* 1996;23:1345–1352.
78. Perlman H, Georganas C, Pagliari LJ, et al. Bcl-2 expression in synovial fibroblasts is essential for maintaining mitochondrial homeostasis and cell viability. *J Immunol* 2000;164:5227–5235.
79. Kurowska M, Rudnicka W, Kontny E, et al. Fibroblast-like synoviocytes from rheumatoid arthritis patients express functional IL-15 receptor complex: endogenous IL-15 in autocrine fashion enhances cell proliferation and expression of Bcl-x(L) and Bcl- 2. *J Immunol* 2002;169:1760–1767.
80. Itoh N, Nagata S. A novel protein domain required for apoptosis. Mutational analysis of human Fas antigen. *J Biol Chem* 1993;268:10932–10937.
81. Hasunuma T, Kayagaki N, Asahara H, et al. Accumulation of soluble Fas in inflamed joints of patients with rheumatoid arthritis. *Arthritis Rheum* 1997;40:80–86.
82. Baier A, Drynda A, Volkmer D, et al. Increased expression of Sentrin-1/SUMO-1 contributes to the resistance of rheumatoid arthritis synovial fibroblasts (RA-SF) to Fas-induced apoptosis versus osteoarthritis (OA)-SF. *Arthritis Rheum* 2002;46:S550.
83. Drynda A, van der Laan WH, Verheijen JH, et al. Induction of apoptosis in rheumatoid arthritis synovial fibroblasts (RA-SF) by adenoviral gene transfer with TIMP-3 is facilitated by TNF-alpha. *Ann Rheum Dis* 2002;61 (Suppl 1):73.
84. Perlman H, Pagliari LJ, Liu H, et al. Rheumatoid arthritis synovial macrophages express the Fas-associated death domain-like interleukin-1beta-converting enzyme-inhibitory protein and are refractory to Fas-mediated apoptosis. *Arthritis Rheum* 2001;44:21–30.
85. Schedel J, Gay RE, Kuenzler P, et al. FLICE-inhibitory protein expression in synovial fibroblasts and at sites of cartilage and bone erosion in rheumatoid arthritis. *Arthritis Rheum* 2002;46:1512–1518.
86. Catrina AI, Ulfgren AK, Lindblad S, et al. Low levels of apoptosis and high FLIP expression in early rheumatoid arthritis synovium. *Ann Rheum Dis* 2002;61:934–936.
87. Franz JK, Pap T, Hummel KM, et al. Expression of sentrin, a novel antiapoptotic molecule, at sites of synovial invasion in rheumatoid arthritis. *Arthritis Rheum* 2000;43:599–607.
88. Makarov SS. NF-kappaB in rheumatoid arthritis: a pivotal regulator of inflammation, hyperplasia, and tissue destruction. *Arthritis Res* 2001;3(4): 200–206.
89. Beraud C, Henzel WJ, Baeuerle PA. Involvement of regulatory and catalytic subunits of phosphoinositide 3-kinase in NF-kappaB activation. *Proc Natl Acad Sci U S A* 1999;96:429–434.
90. Ozes ON, Mayo LD, Gustin JA, et al. NF-kappaB activation by tumour necrosis factor requires the Akt serine-threonine kinase. *Nature* 1999;401:82–85.
91. Zhang HG, Wang Y, Xie JF, et al. Regulation of tumor necrosis factor alpha-mediated apoptosis of rheumatoid arthritis synovial fibroblasts by the protein kinase Akt. *Arthritis Rheum* 2001;44:1555–1567.

92. Kim G, Jun JB, Elkon KB. Necessary role of phosphatidylinositol 3-kinase in transforming growth factor beta-mediated activation of Akt in normal and rheumatoid arthritis synovial fibroblasts. *Arthritis Rheum* 2002;46:1504–1511.
93. Trabandt A, Gay RE, Fassbender HG, et al. Cathepsin B in synovial cells at the site of joint destruction in rheumatoid arthritis. *Arthritis Rheum* 1991;34:1444–1451.
94. Hummel KM, Petrow PK, Franz JK, et al. Cysteine proteinase cathepsin K mRNA is expressed in synovium of patients with rheumatoid arthritis and is detected at sites of synovial bone destruction. *J Rheumatol* 1998;25:1887–1894.
95. Hou WS, Li W, Keyszer G, et al. Comparison of cathepsins K and S expression within the rheumatoid and osteoarthritic synovium. *Arthritis Rheum* 2002;46:663–674.
96. Hou WS, Li Z, Gordon RE, et al. Cathepsin k is a critical protease in synovial fibroblast-mediated collagen degradation. *Am J Pathol* 2001;159:2167–2177.
97. Cunnane G, Fitzgerald O, Hummel KM, et al. Collagenase, cathepsin B and cathepsin L gene expression in the synovial membrane of patients with early inflammatory arthritis. *Rheumatology (Oxford)* 1999;38:34–42.
98. Lemaire R, Huet G, Zerimech F, et al. Selective induction of the secretion of cathepsins B and L by cytokines in synovial fibroblast-like cells. *Br J Rheumatol* 1997;36:735–743.
99. Huet G, Flipo RM, Colin C, et al. Stimulation of the secretion of latent cysteine proteinase activity by tumor necrosis factor alpha and interleukin-1. *Arthritis Rheum* 1993;36:772–780.
100. Keyszer G, Redlich A, Haupl T, et al. Differential expression of cathepsins B and L compared with matrix metalloproteinases and their respective inhibitors in rheumatoid arthritis and osteoarthritis: a parallel investigation by semiquantitative reverse transcriptase-polymerase chain reaction and immunohistochemistry. *Arthritis Rheum* 1998;41:1378–1387.
101. Pap T, Schett G, Gay S. Matrix metalloproteinases. In: Smolen J, Lipsky P. *Targeted therapies in rheumatology*. New York: Martin Dunitz Ltd, Taylor & Francis, 2003 (*in press*).
102. Konttinen YT, Ainola M, Valleala H, et al. Analysis of 16 different matrix metalloproteinases (MMP-1 to MMP-20) in the synovial membrane: different profiles in trauma and rheumatoid arthritis. *Ann Rheum Dis* 1999;58:691–697.
103. Pap T, Shigeyama Y, Kuchen S, et al. Differential expression pattern of membrane-type matrix metalloproteinases in rheumatoid arthritis. *Arthritis Rheum* 2000;43:1226–1232.
104. van Meurs JB, van Lent PL, Holthuysen AE, et al. Kinetics of aggrecanase- and metalloproteinase-induced neoepitopes in various stages of cartilage destruction in murine arthritis. *Arthritis Rheum* 1999;42:1128–1139.
105. Rutkauskaite E, Schedel J, Zacharias W, et al. Effects of retroviral gene transfer of specific ribozymes against MMP-1 on the production of MMP-1 and the invasiveness of synovial fibroblasts in the SCID mouse model of RA. *Arthritis Rheum* 2002;46:S587.
106. Ahrens D, Koch AE, Pope RM, et al. Expression of matrix metalloproteinase 9 (96-kd gelatinase B) in human rheumatoid arthritis. *Arthritis Rheum* 1996;39:1576–1587.
107. Ichikawa Y, Yamada C, Horiki T, et al. Serum matrix metalloproteinase-3 and fibrin degradation product levels correlate with clinical disease activity in rheumatoid arthritis. *Clin Exp Rheumatol* 1998;16:533–540.
108. Maeda S, Sawai T, Uzuki M, et al. Determination of interstitial collagenase (MMP-1) in patients with rheumatoid arthritis. *Ann Rheum Dis* 1995;54:970–975.
109. Yoshihara Y, Obata K, Fujimoto N, et al. Increased levels of stromelysin-1 and tissue inhibitor of metalloproteinases-1 in sera from patients with rheumatoid arthritis. *Arthritis Rheum* 1995;38:969–975.
110. Okada Y, Nagase H, Harris ED, Jr. Matrix metalloproteinases 1, 2, and 3 from rheumatoid synovial cells are sufficient to destroy joints. *J Rheumatol* 1987;(14)Spec No:41–42.
111. Neuhold LA, Killar L, Zhao W, et al. Postnatal expression in hyaline cartilage of constitutively active human collagenase-3 (MMP-13) induces osteoarthritis in mice. *J Clin Invest* 2001;107:35–44.
112. Okada Y, Takeuchi N, Tomita K, et al. Immunolocalization of matrix metalloproteinase 3 (stromelysin) in rheumatoid synovioblasts (B cells): correlation with rheumatoid arthritis. *Ann Rheum Dis* 1989;48:645–653.
113. Yamanaka H, Matsuda Y, Tanaka M, et al. Serum matrix metalloproteinase 3 as a predictor of the degree of joint destruction during the six months after measurement, in patients with early rheumatoid arthritis. *Arthritis Rheum* 2000;43:852–858.
114. Mudgett JS, Hutchinson NI, Chartrain NA, et al. Susceptibility of stromelysin 1-deficient mice to collagen-induced arthritis and cartilage destruction. *Arthritis Rheum* 1998;41:110–121.
115. Holmbeck K, Bianco P, Caterina J, et al. MT1-MMP-deficient mice develop dwarfism, osteopenia, arthritis, and connective tissue disease due to inadequate collagen turnover. *Cell* 1999;99:81–92.
116. van der Laan WH, Pap T, Ronday HK, et al. Cartilage degradation and invasion by rheumatoid synovial fibroblasts is inhibited by gene transfer of a cell surface-targeted plasmin inhibitor. *Arthritis Rheum* 2000;43:1710–1718.
117. van der Laan WH, Quax PH, Seemayer CA, et al. Cartilage degradation and invasion by rheumatoid synovial fibroblasts is inhibited by gene transfer of TIMP-1 and TIMP-3. *Gene Ther* 2003;10:234–242.

CHAPTER 20

Cartilage and Bone Degradation

Steven R. Goldring and Mary B. Goldring

The degradation of articular cartilage and erosion of juxtaarticular bone and resultant joint damage and deformity represent major factors in determining the long-term functional status of patients with rheumatoid arthritis (RA) (1–6). The introduction of techniques using magnetic resonance imaging have helped to establish that cartilage and bone loss occur early in the course of RA and that these changes tend to progress throughout the course of the illness (7,8). Such knowledge has led to a modification of the treatment strategy in RA in which aggressive intervention early in the course of the joint disease is advocated to prevent joint damage. Additional support for the use of early intervention has been provided by the results of several recent studies demonstrating that treatment with disease-modifying drugs can halt or retard the progression of joint destruction (9–13). Nevertheless, despite these encouraging results, many patients continue to show evidence of progressive joint damage and deterioration in functional status. For this reason, there remains the need to develop additional strategies for the treatment of RA. These strategies include therapies specifically targeted at preventing cartilage and bone degradation in parallel with approaches for suppressing synovitis and inflammation. An understanding of the cellular and molecular mechanism involved in cartilage and bone remodeling is essential for developing therapeutic approaches that specifically prevent cartilage and bone destruction.

Under physiologic conditions, the extracellular matrices of articular cartilage and periarticular bone do not exist in a static state but are remodeled to a variable degree through distinct cellular mechanisms that provide a system for degrading individual matrix components and restoring the integrity of the tissues through synthetic activities (Fig. 20.1). These remodeling processes are highly regulated to maintain the integrity and functional properties of the tissues. Although mechanical factors may contribute to the degradation of the articular cartilage and bone in inflammatory joint disorders, the principal mechanism by which these tissues are destroyed involves, directly or indirectly, dysregulated cellular activities. As discussed in the following section, the loss of cartilage and bone tissues in RA may result from either disequilibria in the activities of the cells that remodel these tissues under physiologic conditions or the adverse effects of inflammatory cells present within the inflamed rheumatoid synovium that have inappropriately gained access to the bone or cartilage microenvironment. This chapter focuses on the cellular, biochemical, and molecular mechanisms of physiologic cartilage and bone remodeling and compares and contrasts these processes to the events associated with pathologic remodeling in RA.

ARTICULAR CARTILAGE STRUCTURE AND REMODELING

The extracellular matrix of cartilage consists of highly cross-linked fibrils of type II collagen molecules associated with several cartilage-specific collagens, including types IX and XI, the large aggregating proteoglycan aggrecan, small proteoglycans (decorin, biglycan, fibromodulin, and lumican), and other collagens (VI, XII, and XIV), as well as noncollagenous matrix proteins (14). There are no blood vessels or lymphatics in cartilage, and the chondrocyte, which is the only cellular element, receives its nutrition via diffusion from the subchondral bone and the synovial fluid. The chondrocyte is responsible for remodeling the cartilage matrix. Under physiologic conditions, the degradative and synthetic activities that accompany the remodeling process are very low. For example, the turnover of type II collagen has been estimated to have a half-life of more than 100 years (15). The half-life of aggrecan subfractions has been estimated to be in the range of 3 to 24 years (16).

Histopathologic studies of joint tissues from patients with RA have demonstrated that the initial area of cartilage matrix degradation occurs in areas contiguous with the proliferating synovial pannus (17,18) (Fig. 20.2). In these regions, there is evidence of attachment of the synovial cells, including synovial fibroblasts and macrophages, to the cartilage surface. Both cell types have been implicated in the degradation of the adjacent cartilage matrix via release of proteinases capable of digesting the cartilage matrix components (19,20). Several authors have suggested a critical role for a distinctive fibroblast-like cell type, the so-called pannocyte, that is present within the inflamed RA-synovium (21–24). These cells exhibit anchorage-independent growth and, in contrast to synovial fibroblasts from normal or osteoarthritic tissue, demonstrate the capacity to invade cartilage in the absence of an inflammatory environment (25). In addition, there is evidence of loss of proteoglycan throughout the cartilage matrix, particularly in superficial zones that are in contact with the synovial fluid at sites that are not directly associated with the pannus–cartilage junction (19,20). These effects may be related to the release and activation of proteinases from polymorphonuclear leukocytes and other inflammatory cells present within the synovial fluid.

Numerous proteinases have been implicated in the pathogenesis of cartilage matrix degradation. Of the collagen-degrad-

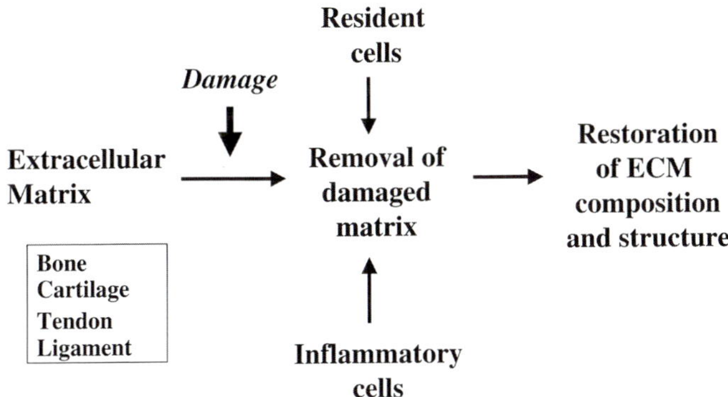

Figure 20.1. Proposed mechanisms of repair of extracellular matrices (ECMs) of joint structures. Injury to the matrices of bone, cartilage, tendons, or ligaments results in activation of resident cells that populate these tissues or in recruitment of inflammatory cells. These cells degrade or remove the damaged matrix components. Under physiologic conditions, synthetic activity of resident cells restores the integrity of the damaged matrices, leading to restoration of structural and functional integrity.

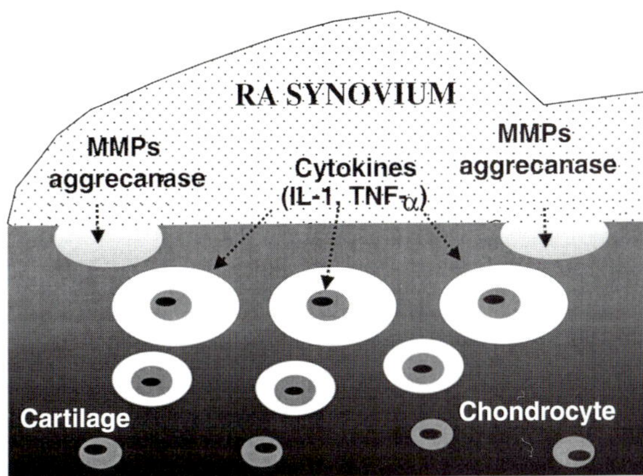

Figure 20.3. Dual mechanism of cartilage matrix degradation in rheumatoid arthritis (RA). Degradation of the cartilage matrix at the cartilage–pannus interface occurs by two principal mechanisms. Proteinases and related products released from the cells within the pannus are able to directly degrade the adjacent cartilage matrix. In addition, cytokines, such as interleukin (IL)-1 and tumor necrosis factor (TNF)-α derived from the inflamed synovium, act on chondrocytes at the cartilage–pannus interface and stimulate the chondrocytes to release proteinases and other products that degrade the pericellular cartilage matrix. MMPs, matrix metalloproteinases.

ing enzymes, collagenases-1, -2, and -3 [matrix metalloproteinase (MMP)-1, MMP-8, MMP-13] and membrane type I MMP (MMP-14) are believed to play the major roles based on their localization to regions of cartilage degradation and detection in synovial fluids from RA patients (26–29). Several of the MMPs, including MMP-3, MMP-8, and MMP-14, also have the capacity to degrade aggrecan. However, there is evidence that members of the reprolysin-related proteinases of the ADAM (a disintegrin and metalloproteinase) family, are the principal mediators of aggrecan degradation (30). Aggrecanase-1 and -2 have been cloned and are characterized as ADAMTS (ADAM with thrombospondin-1 domains)-4 and -5 (31–34). Other proteinases that may have roles in the degradation of various matrix components or participate in the proteinase activation cascade include plasminogen activator, the gelatinases, and MMP-2 and -9. Synovial fibroblasts express high levels of cathepsin K on the cartilage surface at the pannus–cartilage junction (35,36). Among the known cathepsins, cathepsin K has been shown to be the only protease that is capable of hydrolyzing types I and II collagens at multiple sites within their triple-helical region (37). Cells exhibiting a fibroblastic morphology appear to be the major source of this enzyme. Using *in vitro* cell culture techniques, mature cathepsin K has been shown to be secreted by primary cultures of synovial fibroblasts derived from RA synovium, and treatment of these cells with interleukin (IL)-1 or tumor necrosis factor (TNF)-α markedly up-regulates cathepsin K production. Cathepsin K requires an acidic pH to hydrolyze cartilage-associated collagens. pH values as low as 5.5 have been reported at the sites of cartilage degradation, and there is also evidence that synovial fibroblasts themselves are able to secrete acidic components that may provide the microenvironment suitable for the enzymatic activity of secreted active cathepsin K and for the autocatalytic activation of its secreted precursor form (38).

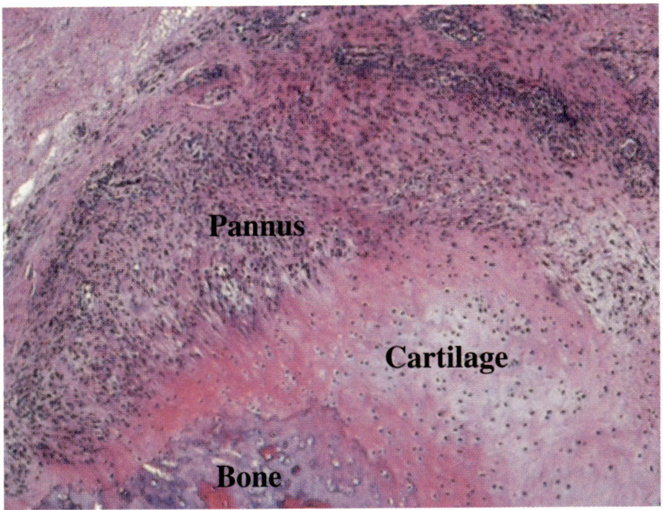

Figure 20.2. Degradation of the cartilage matrix at the pannus–cartilage junction in rheumatoid arthritis. Attachment of the inflamed synovial tissues to the articular cartilage surface leads to progressive destruction of the cartilage matrix.

In addition to the direct action of proteinases released from the pannus, the RA synovial tissues contribute to cartilage matrix degradation by releasing cytokines and other mediators that act on chondrocytes to inappropriately degrade their own pericellular matrix (Fig. 20.3). These proinflammatory cytokines and related products may also suppress chondrocyte synthetic function. The resultant disequilibria in remodeling likely contributes to the rapid loss of cartilage matrix components characteristic of the RA joint lesion. There is also evidence that the chondrocytes may participate in this destructive process not only by responding to the proinflammatory cytokines released from the synovium, but may themselves be the source of proinflammatory and catabolic cytokines that, via autocrine or paracrine mechanisms, contribute to cartilage matrix loss (39–42). The role of synovial- and cartilage-derived proinflammatory products on cartilage matrix degradation in RA is discussed in the following section.

The anatomic sites of cartilage matrix degradation associated with RA are

1. Pannus–cartilage junction
2. Synovial fluid–cartilage interface
3. Perichondrocytic zone
4. Cartilage adjacent to subchondral bone

The mechanisms associated with the pathogenesis of these changes are discussed above. In addition to these sites, a fourth region of the cartilage matrix is also susceptible to degradation by

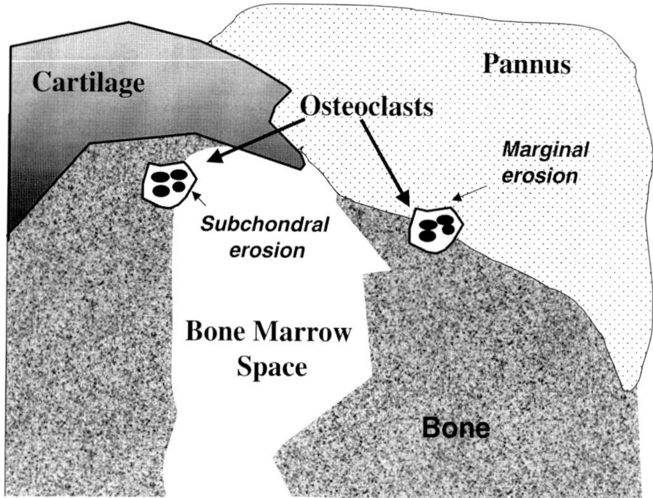

Figure 20.4. Bone erosions at the joint margins and at the subchondral bone surface are mediated by osteoclasts. Osteoclast-like cells derived from the rheumatoid arthritis synovium or the subchondral marrow resorb the bone at the joint margin and at the subchondral bone surface.

the inflammatory processes associated with RA (40,43–45). This site corresponds to the region of the deep zones of the cartilage matrix immediately adjacent to the subchondral bone (Fig. 20.4). Histopathologic examination of juxtaarticular bone from RA joints reveals that the synovial inflammation tends to invade the bone marrow space immediately beneath the subchondral bone. Similar changes are also detected in specimens from animal models of inflammatory arthritis. In these regions, there is replacement of the marrow elements by inflammatory cells, and numerous resorption lacunae containing multinucleated cells expressing osteoclast phenotypic markers can be seen lining the subchondral bone surface. This process eventually leads to degradation of the subchondral bone and exposure of the deeper zones of the articular cartilage to the advancing inflammatory cells. This inflammatory tissue, similar to the pannus associated with the articular cartilage surface, is a source of proteinases that can directly degrade the cartilage matrix. Cytokines produced by this tissue can also act on adjacent chondrocytes to stimulate these cells to elaborate proteinases that degrade their perichondrocytic matrix.

The importance of the subchondral mechanism of cartilage degradation is illustrated by the analysis of histopathologic changes observed in studies of inflammatory arthritis in animals in which the nuclear factor (NF)–κB ligand (RANKL) gene is deleted (43). Induction of inflammatory arthritis using a serum transfer model results in pannus formation and extensive periarticular joint inflammation. Because animals lack the capacity to generate osteoclasts, bone erosions at the pannus–bone interface fail to develop. The inflamed synovial tissue is able to invade the marrow space through existing vascular channels. However, despite extensive bone marrow inflammation adjacent to the subchondral bone, there is no evidence of bone resorption at this site. As a result, the deep zones of the articular cartilage in the RANKL knockout mice are protected from attack by the inflammatory tissue, and there is preservation of cartilage in this region.

PROINFLAMMATORY AND CATABOLIC CYTOKINES: ROLE IN CARTILAGE MATRIX DEGRADATION

Table 20.1 provides a summary of the proinflammatory cytokines implicated in cartilage matrix degradation in RA. Among these factors, IL-1 and TNF-α have received particular attention. These cytokines possess the capacity to induce synovial cells or chondrocytes to synthesize MMPs, aggrecanases, and other cartilage-degrading proteinases. They also stimulate the synthesis of several additional products implicated in joint inflammation and cartilage matrix degradation, including prostaglandin E_2; nitric oxide; soluble phospholipase A_2; other proinflammatory cytokines, such as IL-6, leukemia inhibitory factor, IL-17, and IL-18; and the chemokine IL-8 (42,46–50). Comparison of the relative potencies of IL-1 and TNF-α indicates that, with respect to effects on chondrocytes, IL-1 is 100- to 1,000-fold more potent on a molar basis, although strong synergies between these two cytokines can be demonstrated both *in vivo* and *in vitro* (51–53). For example, in animal models of inflammatory arthritis, TNF-α is sufficient to drive inflammation at the onset of arthritis. In contrast, IL-1 has a pivotal role in sustaining both inflammation and cartilage erosion (51).

TABLE 20.1. Cytokines That Regulate Cartilage Matrix Loss

IL-1
Tumor necrosis factor α
IL-17
IL-18
IL-6
Leukemia inhibitory factor
Oncostatin-M
IL-11
IL-8 (chemokine)

IL, interleukin.

Oncostatin M (OSM), which is a member of the IL-6 family of cytokines, is a product of macrophages and activated T cells. It is a potent stimulator of chondrocyte production of MMPs and aggrecanases and demonstrates a synergistic proinflammatory effect with IL-1 (54). Adenoviral overexpression of OSM in mouse knee joints results in induction of an inflammatory arthritis associated with synovial inflammation and cartilage damage (55). Furthermore, administration of neutralizing antibodies to OSM antibodies results in amelioration of collagen-induced or pristane-induced arthritis (56). Examination of the signaling pathways mediating OSM effects indicates that this cytokine stimulates MMP expression in chondrocytes via the JAK/STAT pathway. This contrasts with the results with IL-1 and TNF-α, indicating that these cytokines use the p38 and JNK pathways to regulate MMPs in chondrocytes (57).

IL-17 and IL-18 are potent inducers of catabolic responses in chondrocytes (58–62). IL-18 is a product of macrophages and belongs to the IL-1 family of cytokines. In addition to its effects on chondrocytes, IL-18 promotes T-cell differentiation and enhances inflammation in animal models of arthritis (63–65). IL-17 is a product of activated Th1 ($CD4^+$) lymphocytes. It acts via a unique receptor that is structurally unrelated to other cytokine receptor families. In contrast, the IL-18 receptor shares homology with the IL-1RI and possesses a Toll-family signaling domain. After receptor ligation, IL-17 and IL-18 activate NF-κB via interactions involving TRAF-6. Both cytokines have been shown to increase the expression of IL-1β, TNF-α, and IL-6 and to enhance cartilage breakdown by increasing stromelysin, nitric oxide synthase, and COX-2 expression in human articular chondrocytes (66,67). IL-17 also contributes to cartilage-matrix loss by suppressing chondrocyte synthetic activity and by enhancing aggrecanase-mediated proteoglycan degradation. These effects are independent of IL-1 (59,61,68–71). Overexpression of IL-17 with adenovirus infection in the context of collagen-induced arthritis produces major enhancement in the cartilage loss (70). IL-17 blockade suppresses bone and cartilage loss in collagen- and adjuvant-induced arthritis, but this treatment is most effective when used in concert with TNF blockade, suggesting that the proinflammatory effects of IL-17 require synergy with other cytokines (62,70,72). Blockade of IL-18 with IL-18–neutralizing antibody or IL-18–binding protein reduces inflammation and tissue destruction in animal models of inflammatory arthritis (56,60,73). However, this cytokine has been shown to play an important role in host defense against bacterial infection, and therapeutic targeting of this cytokine may carry a risk of infection.

ANTIINFLAMMATORY CYTOKINES: POTENTIAL ROLE IN CHONDROPROTECTION

IL-4, IL-10, IL-11, and IL-13 may be classified as inhibitory or antiinflammatory cytokines. It is not clearly established that these cytokines exert direct effects on chondrocytes. Their "chondroprotective" effects in models of inflammatory arthritis are most likely related to their capacity to decrease the production and/or activities of the proinflammatory cytokines and, via these effects, reduce cartilage damage in inflammatory arthritis (42,52,58). IL-1 receptor antagonist (IL-1Ra) has been included in this group of antiinflammatory cytokines. IL-1Ra is produced by the same cells that secrete IL-1 and exists as at least three isoforms, including an intracellular form. It exerts its antiinflammatory effects by competing with IL-1 for receptor occupancy (74–77). IL-4, IL-10, and IL-13 have been shown to increase IL-1Ra production and decrease the production and actions of proinflammatory cytokines (62,78). Intraarticular overexpression of IL-4 does not suppress inflammation but dramatically reduces cartilage and bone destruction. These effects appear to be related to suppression of IL-17 and inhibition of RANKL, which is a potent osteoclast-inducing and -activating factor (see Bone Loss in Rheumatoid Arthritis). In the severe combined immunodeficiency disease mouse model of tissue implantation, co-incubation of cartilage fragments with human synovial fibroblasts overexpressing IL-10 inhibits synovial invasion without affecting chondrocyte-mediated depletion of the cartilage matrix components (79).

CHEMOKINES: ROLE IN CARTILAGE DEGRADATION

In addition to their ability to produce proinflammatory cytokines, chondrocytes also possess the capacity, when activated by proinflammatory cytokines such as IL-1 or TNF-α, to produce chemokines. They also express chemokine receptors, including CCR1, CCR2, CCR3, CCR5, CXCR1, and CXCR2 (39,80,81). Borzi et al. (80,81) showed that interaction of these receptors with their corresponding ligands—monocyte chemoattractant protein-1; regulated on activation, normal T cell–expressed and –secreted (RANTES); and growth-related gene product-α (Gro-α)—results in up-regulation of MMP-3, and RANTES has been shown to induce expression of nitric oxide synthase, IL-6, and MMP-1 (82). There is also evidence that chemokines can influence the synthetic activity of chondrocytes. For example, Yuan et al. reported that monocyte chemoattractant protein-1 or RANTES inhibit proteoglycan synthesis and enhance proteoglycan release from the chondrocytes (83).

BIOMARKERS FOR MONITORING CARTILAGE MATRIX DEGRADATION

Assays have been developed for measuring various breakdown products derived from the degradation of cartilage matrix components, including aggrecan and type II collagen, collagen pyridinoline cross-links, cartilage oligomeric protein, and glycoprotein-39, also termed YKL-40. These products have been examined as molecular markers of the catabolic process in synovial fluids and sera (84,85). Fibronectin fragments that are found in increased levels in RA synovial fluids may enhance cartilage degradation by increasing MMP-13 via an IL-1–dependent mechanism (86).

BONE LOSS IN RHEUMATOID ARTHRITIS

The presence of focal marginal joint erosions is regarded as the radiologic hallmark of RA (39,40,45,87). However, additional skeletal sites may be affected by the focal synovitis and systemic inflammation that accompany the rheumatoid process. Four distinct patterns of bone loss have been described. These are focal joint margin erosions, subchondral bone erosions, juxtaarticular osteopenia, and systemic osteoporosis (87,88).

Focal Bone Erosions

Histopathologic examination of the sites of focal bone erosions reveals the presence of inflamed synovial tissue in direct contact with the bone surfaces (Fig. 20.5). The conclusion from these analyses is that the synovial tissue must, in some way, produce a local disorder in bone remodeling such that there is net loss of bone matrix. It has been challenging, however, to definitively establish the specific cell type responsible for degradation of the bone matrix because of the heterogeneity of the cells that line the bone surface at the bone–pannus interface. A general issue has been whether the resorption of bone at these sites is mediated by osteoclasts, which are the cells that mediate bone resorption under physiologic conditions, or whether other cells present within the inflamed synovium might be responsible for this process.

Initial observations indicating that osteoclasts were involved in the pathogenesis of focal bone erosions were provided by Bromley and Woolley (89,90), who noted the presence of multinucleated cells with phenotypic features of osteoclasts in resorption lacunae at the bone–pannus junction (89,90). They speculated that the interaction of the inflamed synovial tissues with the bone surface resulted in the recruitment and induction of osteoclasts that were responsible for digestion of the bone matrix. Leisen et al. (91), using electron microscopy to examine the bone–pannus

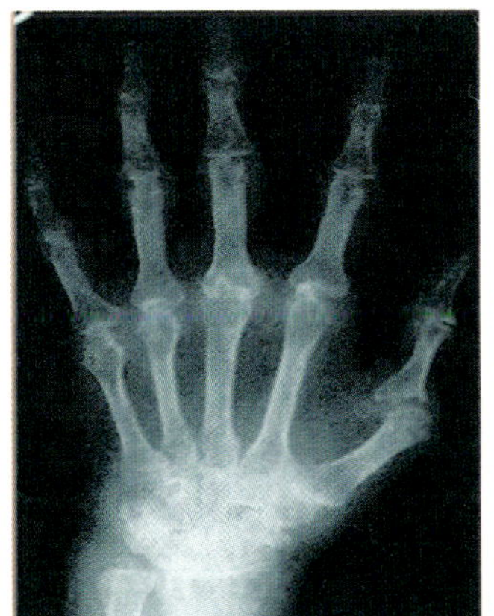

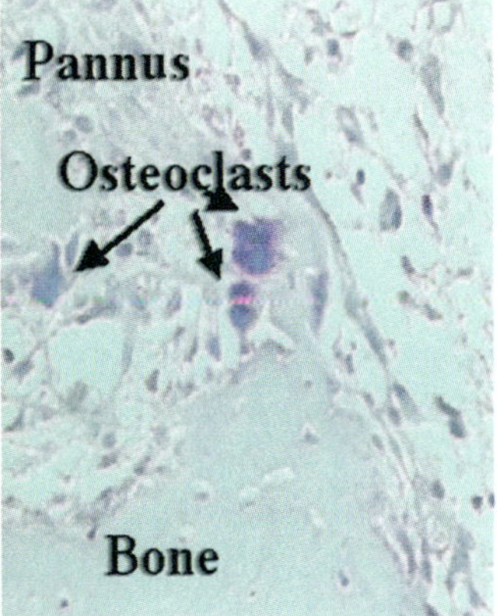

Figure 20.5. Radiographic and histopathologic features of bone erosions in rheumatoid arthritis (RA). Radiograph of the hand from a patient with RA demonstrating extensive marginal and subchondral bone erosions as well as joint-space narrowing. The histopathologic section demonstrates the presence of multinucleated osteoclast-like cells at the bone–pannus interface eroding the bone surface at the joint margin in a patient with RA.

interface, detected the presence of resorption bays typical of osteoclastic activity at the sites of pannus invasion into calcified cartilage and subchondral bone and also concluded that osteoclasts are involved in the resorptive process.

Osteoclasts are multinucleated cells that are derived from hematopoietic precursors of monocyte–macrophage lineage (92–95). During the process of differentiation and activation, they all acquire a number of distinctive phenotypic and functional activities that enable them to remove the mineralized bone matrix (95). Osteoclasts accomplish this by generating a local acidic environment at their site of attachment to the bone surface. They also develop membrane specializations consisting of a highly convoluted surface ("ruffled border") that creates a large surface area for digestion of the organic bone matrix through the action of acid proteases such as cathepsin K. In addition, osteoclasts express abundant receptors for the polypeptide hormone calcitonin. Binding of calcitonin to its surface receptor on osteoclasts inhibits osteoclast activity and induces osteoclast detachment from the bone surface (96). Studies by Gravallese et al. (44) and Haynes et al. (97) have used immunostaining and *in situ* hybridization techniques to examine the cells present at the bone–pannus junction for the expression of phenotypic features of osteoclasts. These studies reveal that the multinucleated (and some mononuclear cells) in resorption lacunae at the bone–pannus junction exhibit the full repertoire of osteoclast-specific phenotypic markers, including the expression of tartrate-resistant acid phosphatase activity, cathepsin K, and calcitonin receptors. These findings indicate that osteoclasts contribute to the pathogenesis of focal erosions in RA.

Despite the detection of cells with an osteoclast phenotype at the bone–pannus interface, in many areas, the cells lining this surface exhibit histologic features of synovial fibroblasts or macrophages. This finding has led some authors to speculate that these cells also contribute to the focal bone loss associated with marginal joint erosions (98). In support of this hypothesis, there is the evidence from *in vitro* studies that fibroblasts can produce cathepsin K (35,98) and that these cells, as well as activated macrophages, possess the capacity to resorb a mineralized bone matrix (99,100). In comparison to osteoclasts, however, the resorptive capacity of fibroblasts and activated macrophages is very restricted, suggesting that their contribution to the focal bone loss is likely to be limited.

Several different approaches using transgenic and knockout mice have helped to more definitively establish the primary role of osteoclasts in the pathogenesis of focal bone erosions. Inflammatory arthritis can be generated in mice lacking the gene for RANKL (43). As is discussed in the subsequent section, this cytokine is required for osteoclast differentiation and activation, and mice lacking this gene cannot generate osteoclasts (101). Inflammatory arthritis with features of RA can be induced in these animals using a serum transfer model of arthritis (43,102–104). Although wild-type and RANKL-deficient mice developed comparable levels of synovitis and joint inflammation, the RANKL knockout mice, which lack the ability to form osteoclasts, exhibit minimal evidence of bone erosions.

Redlich et al. (105) used a similar strategy to investigate the role of osteoclasts in the pathogenesis of focal erosions. In these studies, animals lacking the c-*fos* gene were back-crossed with TNF-α transgenic mice. C-*fos* is a transcription factor that is essential for osteoclastogenesis, and animals lacking this gene, similar to the RANKL knockout mice, are unable to generate osteoclasts (95). The TNF-α transgenic mice developed a form of spontaneous polyarthritis resembling RA. The back-crossed mice developed arthritis, but, similar to the findings with the RANKL knockout mice, the inability to form osteoclasts was associated with an absence of bone erosions. The observations from these two studies (43,105) provide further evidence that osteoclasts represent a necessary cellular pathway for bone resorption in inflammatory joint disease.

Given the strong evidence that osteoclasts mediate the focal bone loss associated with marginal joint erosions, there remains the question of the origin of these cells and the mechanisms involved in their recruitment, differentiation, and activation. To address the question of the origin of the osteoclasts associated with the focal bone erosions, several investigators have shown that macrophage lineage cells can be harvested from RA synovium or inflamed synovium from animal models of arthritis and, under appropriate culture conditions, can be induced to form multinucleated cells with phenotypic features of osteoclasts (106–110). An additional prerequisite for the formation of osteoclasts is the presence of a balance of cytokines and chemokines in the synovial tissues that have the capacity to recruit the osteoclast precursors to the bone–pannus interface and induce the differentiation of these precursors into fully functional bone-resorbing osteoclasts (39).

RA synovial tissue is a rich source of factors with the capacity to induce osteoclast differentiation and activation. These factors include IL-1, IL-6, IL-11, IL-15, IL-17, macrophage colony-stimulating factor (M-CSF), TNF-α, and parathyroid hormone–related peptide (the factor associated with humoral hypercalcemia of malignancy) (45,62,111–117) (Table 20.2). Included among these factors is RANKL, which, as discussed above, is an essential factor regulating osteoclast differentiation and activity (101,116,118–123). This factor, which is a member of the TNF-ligand family, was originally cloned and characterized as a product of activated T cells [TNF-related, activation-induced cytokine (TRANCE)] (124,125). RANKL exerts its actions by binding to its receptor, the receptor activator of NF-κB (RANK) that is a member of the TNF family of receptors. RANK is expressed on osteoclast precursors, osteoclasts, dendritic cells, and certain nonimmune cells, including chondrocytes and osteoblasts. RANKL–RANK signaling is essential for osteoclastogenesis, and deletion of either the ligand or its receptor results in the failure to form osteoclasts, which, in animal models, is manifested by an osteopetrotic phenotype (101,126). RANKL activity is regulated by an inhibitory molecule, osteoprotegerin (OPG), which is a member of the TNF-receptor family. OPG is a soluble protein that acts as a decoy receptor (127–129). Binding of OPG to RANKL prevents RANKL-RANK interaction and disrupts osteoclastogenesis. Many of the stimuli that up-regulate RANKL produce a reciprocal inhibition of OPG, thus enhancing osteoclastogenic activity. Similarly, agents that enhance OPG tend to inhibit RANKL production, resulting in a decrease in osteoclast formation and inhibition of bone resorption (130,131).

Evidence of a role for RANKL in the pathogenesis of focal bone erosions in inflammatory arthritis was first suggested by Kong et al. (101). They demonstrated the presence of RANKL in RA synovium. Using a rat model of adjuvant arthritis, they showed that treatment with OPG (the decoy receptor for RANKL that binds RANKL and inhibits its biologic activity) almost completely

TABLE 20.2. Osteoclast-Inducing and -Activating Factors Produced by the Rheumatoid Arthritis Synovium

RANKL
IL-1α and -1β
IL-6
IL-11
IL-15
IL-17
Macrophage colony-stimulating factor
Tumor necrosis factor α
Parathyroid hormone–related protein

IL, interleukin; RANKL, receptor activator of nuclear factor–κB ligand.

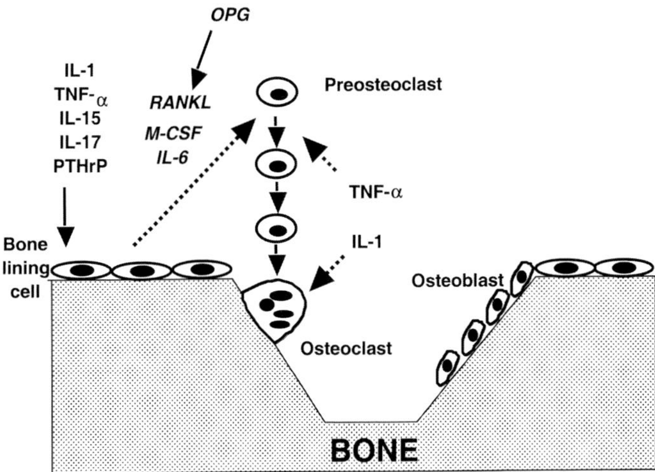

Figure 20.6. Proposed sites of action of cytokines on osteoclast differentiation and activation. Interleukin (IL)-1, tumor necrosis factor (TNF)-α, IL-15, IL-17, and parathyroid hormone–related peptide (PTHrP) enhance osteoclast formation by stimulating the production of osteoclast-inducing factors such as receptor activator of nuclear factor–κB ligand (RANKL), macrophage colony-stimulating factor (M-CSF), and IL-6. Osteoprotegerin (OPG) is a soluble decoy receptor that binds RANKL and inhibits its osteoclast-inducing activity. TNF-α also acts directly on osteoclast precursors to induce their differentiation into osteoclasts. IL-1 acts directly on osteoclasts to increase their resorbing activity.

TABLE 20.3. T-Cell–Derived Cytokines That Regulate Osteoclastogenesis

Stimulatory	Inhibitory
RANKL	Granulocyte-macrophage colony-stimulating factor
Tumor necrosis factor α	Interferon-γ
Macrophage colony-stimulating factor	Interferon-β
IL-6	IL-4
IL-7	IL-10
IL-15	IL-12
IL-17	IL-13
	IL-18

IL, interleukin; RANKL, receptor activator of nuclear factor–κB ligand .

blocked the development of joint erosions. Similar results demonstrating inhibition of bone erosions with OPG have been reported in the collagen-induced model of inflammatory arthritis (132) and in TNF-α transgenic animals with spontaneous arthritis (133). Further evidence implicating RANKL in the pathogenesis of erosions is provided by the demonstration of RANKL in RA synovial tissues (101,116,118,119). Expression is localized to both synovial fibroblasts and T cells, both of which have been shown to have the capacity to induce osteoclastogenesis *in vitro* (118,134,135). Recent studies by Weitzmann et al. (135,136) have demonstrated that treatment of co-cultures of activated T cells and osteoclast precursors with OPG did not completely block osteoclastogenesis, indicating that, in addition to RANKL, other products derived from T cells may have osteoclast-inducing activity.

As discussed above, RA synovial tissue is a source of multiple factors, in addition to RANKL, that have the capacity to enhance osteoclast formation and activity. These factors can be divided into those that (a) act indirectly by up-regulating the production of factors from the osteoblast-lineage bone-lining cells or cells in the bone marrow stroma adjacent to the remodeling surfaces and (b) those that act directly on the osteoclast or its precursors. Figure 20.6 is a schematic representation of the potential mechanism by which hormones or cytokines act indirectly via effects on bone-lining cells to up-regulate osteoclast differentiation. As shown in the figure, interaction of the lining cells with the inducing factor results in increased production by the lining cells of osteoclast-inducing factors such as RANKL, M-CSF, and IL-6. TNF-α and IL-1 are cytokines that have dual sites of action on osteoclast-mediated bone resorption. They can act indirectly via effects on bone lining cells to enhance RANKL and M-CSF production, but, in addition, TNF-α acts on osteoclast precursors to enhance differentiation into osteoclasts, and IL-1 acts directly on osteoclasts to increase their resorbing activity (92,95,137). Both IL-1 and TNF-α contribute further to bone loss in RA by impairing bone formation via induction of osteoblast apoptosis (138).

Several other proinflammatory products from RA synovium have effects on osteoclast-mediated bone resorption. IL-17 is a proinflammatory T-cell–derived cytokine implicated in both cartilage and bone loss (139). Elevated levels of IL-17 have been detected in synovial fluid from patients with RA, and it has been identified by immunostaining in T-cell–rich areas within RA synovial tissues (62,140). In experimental models, IL-17 stimulates osteoclast differentiation and induces bone resorption. The capacity of IL-17 to induce osteoclast differentiation and bone resorption *in vitro* is prostaglandin-dependent and appears to be mediated through the induction of RANKL on the surface of osteoblasts. This is supported by the observation that OPG inhibits IL-17–induced osteoclast differentiation (140). IL-15 is another T-cell product that possesses osteoclast-inducing activity (115). Similar to IL-17, its osteoclastogenic activity is probably not mediated via direct effects on osteoclast precursors. Although IL-15 is a potent inducer of TNF-α, its osteoclast-inducing activity appears to be independent of TNF stimulation (115,141,142). Several additional T-cell–derived cytokines have been shown to regulate osteoclast differentiation in a positive or negative manner; these are listed in Table 20.3.

Subchondral Bone Erosions

Although the initial bone loss associated with the RA synovial lesion occurs at the cortical bone surface adjacent to the synovial lining, as the disease progresses, the pannus invades through the bone cortex and into the marrow space below the subchondral bone. Erosion of subchondral bone by cells expressing an osteoclast phenotype can be detected in these regions of marrow invasion. Presumably, the osteoclast-like cells present in resorption lacunae are derived from macrophage lineage precursors within the bone marrow (43,44,116). Resorption of the subchondral bone provides additional access by the inflamed synovial tissues and cells to the cartilage, and it is likely that the destruction of the cartilage matrix occurs at this interface as well as in the regions within the joint where the pannus has attached to the cartilage surface. In our studies with the RANKL knockout mice with serum transfer arthritis and in the studies by Kong et al. (101) in animals with adjuvant arthritis treated with OPG, it is possible that preservation of the subchondral bone may be a factor in the reduced cartilage destruction seen in these models. It is interesting to speculate that these regions of marrow invasion by the synovium may correspond to the zones of marrow edema that have been detected adjacent to synovial inflammation using magnetic resonance imaging (7,8).

Generalized Bone Loss

There is evidence that patients with RA have increased generalized bone loss in the axial spine and appendicular skeleton

(143–150). Identification of the independent role of the systemic effects of RA on bone remodeling has been difficult because of multiple confounding factors, including reduced mobility, impaired nutrition, and the concomitant use of glucocorticoids and immunosuppressive therapies. In addition, epidemiologic studies examining the relationship between systemic bone loss and RA have been flawed by problems with study design, such as small numbers of subjects, variations in the stage of the disease and in the disease activity of the subjects, and inconsistent outcome measures. Despite these limitations, there is evidence indicating an increased incidence of fractures in patients with RA (147,151–155).

Conflicting findings are available concerning the mechanisms involved in the pathogenesis of generalized bone loss in RA. Histomorphometric analysis of bone biopsies from patients with RA have shown a decrease in bone-formation indices without findings indicative of an increase in bone resorption (156–158). In contrast, evaluation of bone remodeling based on analysis of biochemical markers of bone turnover indicate that there is an increase in bone-resorbing activity in patients with RA. The discrepancies in the results using these two approaches could reflect differences in the stages of the disease in which bone remodeling was being evaluated, as well as the confounding effects of corticosteroid treatment and disease activity in the patient populations. The bulk of the evidence suggests that increased bone resorption likely accounts for the increased incidence of generalized bone loss in RA, at least during the earlier stages of the disease.

Gough et al. (159) analyzed biochemical markers of bone turnover in 232 patients with RA in a longitudinal study over a 2-year period. He noted that the RA subjects demonstrated a significant increase in bone-resorption markers based on urinary pyridinoline and deoxypyridinoline excretion. He also observed a significantly greater rate of bone loss in the RA patients than in the controls (greater than 3% at the spine and greater than 5% at the hip). Of interest, the levels of bone-resorption markers were highly correlated with C-reactive protein levels, suggesting that increased disease activity was associated with enhanced bone resorption. There was no significant change in bone-formation markers as assessed by serum alkaline phosphatase and procollagen I carboxyterminal propeptide levels. The authors concluded that significant amounts of generalized bone loss occurred early in RA and that this loss was associated with the level of disease activity. Other investigators have also detected increases in urinary markers of bone resorption, particularly in patients with active disease who demonstrated rapid bone loss as determined by bone-mineral density (84,160). These findings are supported by the earlier studies of Sambrook et al. (161), who observed that joint count and C-reactive protein levels correlated with the magnitude of trabecular bone loss.

There is still controversy regarding the effects of corticosteroids on generalized bone loss in RA. In part, this situation is related to the tendency to use corticosteroids in patients with more severe disease who are already at greater risk for generalized bone loss related to confounding variables that can have independent adverse effects on bone remodeling. Michel et al. (154) analyzed data from five Arthritis, Rheumatism and Aging Medical Information System centers. They identified an association between fracture risk and the following: number of years taking prednisone, disability, age, lack of physical activity, female sex, disease duration, impaired grip strength, and low body mass. Similar findings have been reported by Haugeberg et al. (162) based on data from the Oslo County Rheumatoid Arthritis Registry. They found that older age, low body weight, lower functional status, and current use of corticosteroids were significant predictors of reduced bone mass.

Other investigators have suggested that the potentially adverse effects of corticosteroids on bone remodeling may be offset by providing a suppressive effect on inflammation and maintaining physical activity (150,163,164). In support of this, cross-sectional and longitudinal studies by Sambrook demonstrated no difference in the progression of bone loss in RA patients treated with or without low-dose glucocorticoids, although patients with RA had lower levels of bone-mineral density compared to that of normal controls (146,165). Similar findings have been reported by Lane et al. (166), who examined the association between corticosteroid use and bone-mineral density in a community-based sample of ambulatory white women of age 65 years and older with or without RA. Lane et al. found that women with RA who were current users of glucocorticoids had the lowest bone-density levels. Women with RA who had never used steroids also had a reduced bone density compared to that of the control population. They concluded that women with RA have lower appendicular and axial bone mass and that this decrease is not attributable to the use of steroids but rather to their lower functional status. Other studies, however, have suggested that even low-dose glucocorticoids may have a detrimental effect on bone density (167,168). For example, in a cross-sectional analysis using quantitative computed tomography, Laan et al. (168) demonstrated that low doses of glucocorticoids (mean dose, 6.8 mg prednisone per day) are associated with reduced bone density compared to non-steroid–treated patients with RA. In a case control analysis of 112 RA patients, Saag et al. (151) observed that long-term, low-dose glucocorticoid use is a significant predictor of adverse events, including fractures, gastrointestinal events, and infections.

Juxtaarticular Bone Loss

Juxtaarticular bone loss is among the earliest radiographic features of RA that characteristically occurs in joints affected by active synovitis and usually precedes the appearance of focal bone erosions. Histomorphometric examination of bone from the regions of juxtaarticular bone loss demonstrates evidence of increased bone remodeling, with a relative increase in resorption over formation (169). Increased numbers of cells with an osteoclast phenotype can be detected in resorption lacunae in these regions. Many of these zones of resorption are not in direct contact with the inflamed synovium and are distinct from the areas of bone loss associated with subchondral bone erosion described in the preceding section. Several mechanisms have been suggested for the enhanced bone-resorbing activity, including the effects of proinflammatory mediators released from the synovium and the effects of loss of joint loading and immobilization (170–175).

CONCLUSION

The characterization of the mechanisms associated with bone and cartilage loss in RA has revealed several potential therapeutic targets, such as RANKL, that act in tandem with IL-1 and TNF-α to produce joint destruction. Development of therapies that specifically target these cytokines, as well as other mediators and their signal pathways, represents a rational approach for more effective treatment of patients with RA.

REFERENCES

1. Scott D, Pugner K, Kaarela K, et al. The links between joint damage and disability. *Rheumatology* 2000;39:122–132.
2. van Zeben D, Hazes JMW, Zwinderman AH, et al. Factors predicting outcome of rheumatoid arthritis: results of a followup study. *J Rheumatol* 1993; 20:1288–1296.

3. Sharp JT, Wolfe F, Mitchell DM, et al. The progression of erosion and joint space narrowing scores in rheumatoid arthritis during the first twenty-five years of disease. *Arthritis Rheum* 1991;34:660–668.
4. Drossaers-Bakker KW, Zwinderman AH, Vlieland TP, et al. Long-term outcome in rheumatoid arthritis: a simple algorithm of baseline parameters can predict radiographic damage, disability, and disease course at 12-year followup. *Arthritis Rheum* 2002;47:383–390.
5. Drossaers-Bakker KW, Kroon HM, Zwinderman AH, et al. Radiographic damage of large joints in long-term rheumatoid arthritis and its relation to function. *Rheumatology (Oxford)* 2000;39:998–1003.
6. Drossaers-Bakker K, de Buck M, van Zeben D, et al. Long-term course and outcome of functional capacity in rheumatoid arthritis: the effect of disease activity and radiologic damage over time. *Arthritis Rheum* 1999;42:1854–1860.
7. McQueen FM, Stewart N, Crabbe J, et al. Magnetic resonance imaging of the wrist in early rheumatoid arthritis reveals a high prevalence of erosions at four months after symptom onset. *Ann Rheum Dis* 1998;57:350–356.
8. McGonagle D, Conaghan PG, O'Connor P, et al. The relationship between synovitis and bone changes in early untreated rheumatoid arthritis; a controlled magnetic resonance imaging study. *Arthritis Rheum* 1999;42:1706–1711.
9. Moreland LW, Schiff MH, Baumgartner SW, et al. Etanercept therapy in rheumatoid arthritis; a randomized, controlled trial. *Ann Intern Med* 1999;130:478–486.
10. Maini R, St. Clair EW, Breedveld FC, et al. Infliximab (chimeric anti-tumour necrosis factor alpha monoclonal antibody) versus placebo in rheumatoid arthritis patients receiving concomitant methotrexate: a randomized phase III trial. ATTRACT Study Group. *Lancet* 1999;354:1932–1939.
11. Strand V, Cohen S, Schiff M, et al. Treatment of active rheumatoid arthritis with leflunomide compared with placebo and methotrexate. *Arch Int Med* 1999;159:2542–2550.
12. Lipsky P, van der Hiejde D, St. Clair E, et al. Infliximab and methotrexate in the treatment of rheumatoid arthritis. Anti-tumor necrosis factor trial in rheumatoid arthritis with concomitant therapy study group. *N Engl J Med* 2000;343:1594–1602.
13. Bresnihan B, Alvaro-Gracia JM, Cobby M, et al. Treatment of rheumatoid arthritis with recombinant human interleukin-1 receptor antagonist. *Arthritis Rheum* 1998;41:2196–2204.
14. Poole AR, Kojima T, Yasuda T, et al. Composition and structure of articular cartilage: a template for tissue repair. *Clin Orthop* 2001;S26–33.
15. Verzijl N, DeGroot J, Thorpe SR, et al. Effect of collagen turnover on the accumulation of advanced glycation end products. *J Biol Chem* 2000;275:39027–39031.
16. Maroudas A, Bayliss MT, Uchitel-Kaushansky N, et al. Aggrecan turnover in human articular cartilage: use of aspartic acid racemization as a marker of molecular age. *Arch Biochem Biophys* 1998;350:61–71.
17. Kobayashi I, Ziff M. Electron microscopic studies of the cartilage-pannus junction in rheumatoid arthritis. *Arthritis Rheum* 1975;18:475–483.
18. Woolley DE, Crossley MJ, Evanson JM. Collagenase at sites of cartilage erosion in the rheumatoid joint. *Arthritis Rheum* 1977;20:1231–1239.
19. Dodge GR, Poole AR. Immunohistochemical detection and immunochemical analysis of type II collagen degradation in human normal, rheumatoid, and osteoarthritic articular cartilages and in explants of bovine articular cartilage cultured with interleukin 1. *J Clin Invest* 1989;83:647–661.
20. Kimura H, Tateishi HJ, Ziff M. Surface ultrastructure of rheumatoid articular cartilage. *Arthritis Rheum* 1977;20:1085–1098.
21. Zvaifler NJ, Tsai V, Alsalameh S, et al. Pannocytes: distinctive cells found in rheumatoid arthritis articular cartilage erosions. *Am J Pathol* 1997;150:1125–1138.
22. Zvaifler NJ, Firestein GS. Pannus and pannocytes. Alternative models of joint destruction in rheumatoid arthritis. *Arthritis Rheum* 1994;37:783–789.
23. Yamanishi Y, Firestein GS. Pathogenesis of rheumatoid arthritis: the role of synoviocytes. *Rheum Dis Clin North Am* 2001;27:355–371.
24. Firestein GS. Evolving concepts of rheumatoid arthritis. *Nature* 2003;423:356–361.
25. Muller-Ladner U, Kriegsmann J, Franklin BN, et al. Synovial fibroblasts of patients with rheumatoid arthritis attach to and invade normal human cartilage when engrafted into SCID mice. *Am J Pathol* 1996;149:1607–1615.
26. Tetlow LC, Adlam DJ, Woolley DE. Matrix metalloproteinase and proinflammatory cytokine production by chondrocytes of human osteoarthritic cartilage. *Arthritis Rheum* 2001;44:585–594.
27. Wu W, Billinghurst RC, Pidoux I, et al. Sites of collagenase cleavage and denaturation of type II collagen in aging and osteoarthritic articular cartilage and their relationship to the distribution of matrix metalloproteinase 1 and matrix metalloproteinase 13. *Arthritis Rheum* 2002;46:2087–2094.
28. Dahlberg L, Billinghurst RC, Manner P, et al. Selective enhancement of collagenase-mediated cleavage of resident type II collagen in cultured osteoarthritic cartilage and arrest with a synthetic inhibitor that spares collagenase 1 (matrix metalloproteinase 1). *Arthritis Rheum* 2000;43:673–682.
29. Cunnane G, Fitzgerald O, Beeton C, et al. Early joint erosions and serum levels of matrix metalloproteinase 1, matrix metalloproteinase 3, and tissue inhibitor of metalloproteinases 1 in rheumatoid arthritis. *Arthritis Rheum* 2001;44:2263–2274.
30. Arner EC. Aggrecanase-mediated cartilage degradation. *Curr Opin Pharmacol* 2002;2:322–329.
31. Tacchetti C, Quarto R, Nitsch L, et al. In vitro morphogenesis of chick embryo hypertrophic cartilage. *J Cell Biol* 1987;105:999–1006.
32. Tortorella MD, Burn TC, Pratta MA, et al. Purification and cloning of aggrecanase-1: a member of the ADAMTS family of proteins. *Science* 1999;284:1664–1666.
33. Abbaszade I, Liu RQ, Yang F, et al. Cloning and characterization of ADAMTS11, an aggrecanase from the ADAMTS family. *J Biol Chem* 1999;274:23443–23450.
34. Hurskainen TL, Hirohata S, Seldin MF, et al. ADAM-TS5, ADAM-TS6, and ADAM-TS7, novel members of a new family of zinc metalloproteases. General features and genomic distribution of the ADAM-TS family. *J Biol Chem* 1999;274:25555–25563.
35. Hou W, Li W, Keyszer G, et al. Comparison of cathepsins K and S expression within the rheumatoid and osteoarthritic synovium. *Arthritis Rheum* 2002;46:663–674.
36. Hou W, Li Z, Gordon R, et al. Cathepsin K is a critical protease in synovial-fibroblast mediated collagen degradation. *Am J Pathol* 2001;159:2167–2177.
37. Garnero P, Borel O, Byrjalsen I, et al. The collagenolytic activity of cathepsin K is unique among mammalian proteinases. *J Biol Chem* 1998;273:32347–32352.
38. Pap T, Claus A, Ohtsu S, et al. Osteoclast-independent bone resorption by fibroblast-like cells. *Arthritis Res* 2003;5:R163–173.
39. Goldring MB, Goldring SR. Role of cytokines and chemokines in cartilage and bone destruction in arthritis. *Curr Opin Orthopaed* 2002;13:351–362.
40. Goldring SR. Bone and joint destruction in rheumatoid arthritis: what is really happening? *J Rheumatol Suppl* 2002;65:44–48.
41. Goldring MB. The role of cytokines as inflammatory mediators in osteoarthritis: lessons from animal models. *Connect Tissue Res* 1999;40:1–11.
42. Goldring MB. Anticytokine therapy for osteoarthritis. *Expert Opin Biol Ther* 2001;1:817–829.
43. Pettit A, Hong J, von Stechow D, et al. TRANCE/RANKL knockout mice are protected from bone erosion in a serum transfer model of arthritis. *Am J Pathol* 2001;159:1689–1699.
44. Gravallese EM, Harada Y, Wang JT, et al. Identification of cell types responsible for bone resorption in rheumatoid arthritis and juvenile rheumatoid arthritis. *Am J Pathol* 1998;152:943–951.
45. Gravallese EM, Goldring SR. Cellular mechanisms and the role of cytokines in bone erosions in rheumatoid arthritis. *Arthritis Rheum* 2000;43:2143–2151.
46. Mengshol JA, Vincenti MP, Coon CI, et al. Interleukin-1 induction of collagenase 3 (matrix metalloproteinase 13) gene expression in chondrocytes requires p38, c-Jun N-terminal kinase, and nuclear factor κB. *Arthritis Rheum* 2000;43:801–811.
47. Feldmann M, Maini RN, Bondeson J, et al. Cytokine blockade in rheumatoid arthritis. *Adv Exp Med Biol* 2001;490:119–127.
48. Feldmann M, Brennan FM, Foxwell BM, et al. The role of TNF alpha and IL-1 in rheumatoid arthritis. *Curr Dir Autoimmun* 2001;3:188–199.
49. Feldmann M. Pathogenesis of arthritis: recent research progress. *Nat Immunol* 2001;2:771–773.
50. Evans CH, Ghivizzani SC, Herndon JH, et al. Clinical trials in the gene therapy of arthritis. *Clin Orthop* 2000;S300–307.
51. van den Berg WB. Uncoupling of inflammatory and destructive mechanisms in arthritis. *Semin Arthritis Rheum* 2001;30:7–16.
52. van den Berg WB. Anti-cytokine therapy in chronic destructive arthritis. *Arthritis Res* 2001;3:18–26.
53. van den Berg WB. The role of cytokines and growth factors in cartilage destruction in osteoarthritis and rheumatoid arthritis. *Zeitschrift fur Rheumatologie* 1999;58:136–141.
54. Koshy PJ, Lundy CJ, Rowan AD, et al. The modulation of matrix metalloproteinase and ADAM gene expression in human chondrocytes by interleukin-1 and oncostatin M: a time-course study using real-time quantitative reverse transcription-polymerase chain reaction. *Arthritis Rheum* 2002;46:961–967.
55. Langdon C, Kerr C, Hassen M, et al. Murine oncostatin M stimulates mouse synovial fibroblasts in vitro and induces inflammation and destruction in mouse joints in vivo. *Am J Pathol* 2000;157:1187–1196.
56. Plater-Zyberk C, Buckton J, Thompson S, et al. Amelioration of arthritis in two murine models using antibodies to oncostatin M. *Arthritis Rheum* 2001;44:2697–2702.
57. Li WQ, Dehnade F, Zafarullah M. Oncostatin M-induced matrix metalloproteinase and tissue inhibitor of metalloproteinase-3 genes expression in chondrocytes requires Janus kinase/STAT signaling pathway. *J Immunol* 2001;166:3491–3498.
58. Lubberts E, van den Berg WB. Cytokines in the pathogenesis of rheumatoid arthritis and collagen-induced arthritis. *Adv Exp Med Biol* 2003;520:194–202.
59. Lubberts E, van den Bersselaar L, Oppers-Walgreen B, et al. IL-17 promotes bone erosion in murine collagen-induced arthritis through loss of the receptor activator of NF-kappa B ligand/osteoprotegerin balance. *J Immunol* 2003;170:2655–2662.
60. Joosten LA, Radstake TR, Lubberts E, et al. Association of interleukin-18 expression with enhanced levels of both interleukin-1beta and tumor necrosis factor alpha in knee synovial tissue of patients with rheumatoid arthritis. *Arthritis Rheum* 2003;48:339–347.
61. Lubberts E, Joosten LA, van de Loo FA, et al. Overexpression of IL-17 in the knee joint of collagen type II immunized mice promotes collagen arthritis and aggravates joint destruction. *Inflamm Res* 2002;51:102–104.
62. Chabaud M, Lubberts E, Joosten L, et al. IL-17 derived from juxta-articular bone and synovium contributes to joint degradation in rheumatoid arthritis. *Arthritis Res* 2001;3:168–177.
63. Park CC, Morel JC, Amin MA, et al. Evidence of IL-18 as a novel angiogenic mediator. *J Immunol* 2001;167:1644–1653.
64. Nakanishi K, Yoshimoto T, Tsutsui H, et al. Interleukin-18 is a unique cytokine that stimulates both Th1 and Th2 responses depending on its cytokine milieu. *Cytokine Growth Factor Rev* 2001;12:53–72.

65. Leung BP, Culshaw S, Gracie JA, et al. A role for IL-18 in neutrophil activation. *J Immunol* 2001;167:2879–2886.
66. Olee T, Hashimoto S, Quach J, et al. IL-18 is produced by articular chondrocytes and induces proinflammatory and catabolic responses. *J Immunol* 1999;162:1096–1100.
67. Shalom-Barak T, Quach J, Lotz M. Interleukin-17-induced gene expression in articular chondrocytes is associated with activation of mitogen-activated protein kinases and NF-κB. *J Biol Chem* 1998;273:27467–27473.
68. Cai L, Yin JP, Starovasnik MA, et al. Pathways by which interleukin 17 induces articular cartilage breakdown in vitro and in vivo. *Cytokine* 2001;16:10–21.
69. Dudler J, Renggli-Zulliger N, Busso N, et al. Effect of interleukin 17 on proteoglycan degradation in murine knee joints. *Ann Rheum Dis* 2000;59:529–532.
70. Lubberts E, Joosten LA, Oppers B, et al. IL-1-independent role of IL-17 in synovial inflammation and joint destruction during collagen-induced arthritis. *J Immunol* 2001;167:1004–1013.
71. Lubberts E, Joosten LAB, van de Loo FAJ, et al. Reduction of interleukin-17-induced inhibition of chondrocyte proteoglycan synthesis in intact murine articular cartilage by interleukin-4. *Arthritis Rheum* 2000;43:1300–1306.
72. Bush KA, Farmer KM, Walker JS, et al. Reduction of joint inflammation and bone erosion in rat adjuvant arthritis by treatment with interleukin-17 receptor IgG1 Fc fusion protein. *Arthritis Rheum* 2002;46:802–805.
73. Wei XQ, Leung BP, Arthur HM, et al. Reduced incidence and severity of collagen-induced arthritis in mice lacking IL-18. *J Immunol* 2001;166:517–521.
74. Arend WP. The mode of action of cytokine inhibitors. *J Rheumatol Suppl* 2002;65:16–21.
75. Arend WP. Physiology of cytokine pathways in rheumatoid arthritis. *Arthritis Rheum* 2001;45:101–106.
76. Arend WP. Cytokines and cellular interactions in inflammatory synovitis. *J Clin Invest* 2001;107:1081–1082.
77. Arend WP. Cytokine imbalance in the pathogenesis of rheumatoid arthritis: the role of interleukin-1 receptor antagonist. *Semin Arthritis Rheum* 2001;30:1 6.
78. Woods JM, Katschke KJ, Jr., Tokuhira M, et al. Reduction of inflammatory cytokines and prostaglandin E2 by IL-13 gene therapy in rheumatoid arthritis synovium. *J Immunol* 2000;165:2755–2763.
79. Muller-Ladner U, Evans CH, Franklin BN, et al. Gene transfer of cytokine inhibitors into human synovial fibroblasts in the SCID mouse model. *Arthritis Rheum* 1999;42:490–497.
80. Borzi RM, Mazzetti I, Macor S, et al. Flow cytometric analysis of intracellular chemokines in chondrocytes in vivo: constitutive expression and enhancement in osteoarthritis and rheumatoid arthritis. *FEBS Lett* 1999;455:238–242.
81. Borzi RM, Mazzetti I, Cattini L, et al. Human chondrocytes express functional chemokine receptors and release matrix-degrading enzymes in response to C-X-C and C-C chemokines. *Arthritis Rheum* 2000;43:1734–1741.
82. Alaaeddine N, Olee T, Hashimoto S, et al. Production of the chemokine RANTES by articular chondrocytes and role in cartilage degradation. *Arthritis Rheum* 2001;44:1633–1643.
83. Yuan GH, Masuko-Hongo K, Sakata M, et al. The role of C-C chemokines and their receptors in osteoarthritis. *Arthritis Rheum* 2001;44:1056–1070.
84. Garnero P, Gineyts E, Christgau S, et al. Association of baseline levels of urinary glucosyl-galactosyl-pyridinoline and type II collagen C-telopeptide with progression of joint destruction in patients with early rheumatoid arthritis. *Arthritis Rheum* 2002;46:21–30.
85. Garnero P, Rousseau J-C, Delmas PD. Molecular basis and clinical use of biochemical markers of bone, cartilage and synovium in joint diseases. *Arthritis Rheum* 2000;43:953–968.
86. Yasuda T, Poole AR. A fibronectin fragment induces type II collagen degradation by collagenase through an interleukin-1-mediated pathway. *Arthritis Rheum* 2002;46:138–148.
87. Goldring SR, Gravallese EM. Mechanisms of bone loss in inflammatory arthritis: diagnosis and therapeutic implications. *Arthritis Res* 2000;2:33–37.
88. Goldring SR, Polisson RP. Bone disease in rheumatological disorders. In: Avioli L, Krane SM, eds. *Metabolic bone disease*, 2nd ed. San Diego: Academic Press, 1998: 621–635.
89. Bromley M, Woolley DE. Histopathology of the rheumatoid lesion; identification of cell types at sites of cartilage erosion. *Arthritis Rheum* 1984;27:857–863.
90. Bromley M, Woolley DE. Chondroclasts and osteoclasts at subchondral sites of erosions in the rheumatoid joint. *Arthritis Rheum* 1984;27:968–975.
91. Leisen JCC, Duncan H, Riddle JM, et al. The erosive front: a topographic study of the junction between the pannus and the subchondral plate in the macerated rheumatoid metacarpal head. *J Rheumatol* 1988;15:17–22.
92. Suda T, Takahashi N, Udagawa N, et al. Modulation of osteoclast differentiation and function by the new members of the tumor necrosis factor receptor and ligand families. *Endocr Rev* 1999;20:345–357.
93. Suda T, Udagawa N, Nakamura I, et al. Modulation of osteoclast differentiation by local factors. *Bone* 1995;17:87S–91S.
94. Suda T, Takahashi N, Martin TJ. Modulation of osteoclast differentiation. *Endocr Rev* 1992;13:66–80.
95. Teitelbaum S. Bone resorption by osteoclasts. *Science* 2000;289:1504–1508.
96. Galson DL, Goldring SR. *Structure and biology of the calcitonin receptor, principles of bone biology*. Bilezikian LR, Rodan G, eds. New York: Academic Press, 2002:603–617.
97. Haynes DR, Crotti TN, Loric M, et al. Osteoprotegerin and receptor activator of nuclear factor kappaB ligand (RANKL) regulate osteoclast formation by cells in the human rheumatoid arthritic joint. *Rheumatology (Oxford)* 2001;40:623–630.
98. Hummel KM, Petrow PK, Franz JK, et al. Cysteine proteinase cathepsin K mRNA is expressed in synovium of patients with rheumatoid arthritis and is detected at sites of synovial bone destruction. *J Rheumatol* 1998;25:1887–1894.
99. Hattersley G, Chambers TJ. Calcitonin receptors as markers for osteoclastic differentiation: correlation between generation of bone-resorptive cells and cells that express calcitonin receptors in mouse bone marrow cultures. *Endocrinology* 1989;125:1606–1612.
100. Chambers TJ, Horton MA. Failure of cells of the mononuclear phagocyte series to resorb bone. *Calcif Tissue Int* 1984;36:556–558.
101. Kong YY, Yoshida H, Sarosi I, et al. OPGL is a key regulator of osteoclastogenesis, lymphocyte development and lymph-node organogenesis. *Nature* 1999;397:315–323.
102. Matsumoto I, Maccioni M, Lee DM, et al. How antibodies to a ubiquitous cytoplasmic enzyme may provoke joint-specific autoimmune disease. *Nat Immunol* 2002;3:360–365.
103. Matsumoto I, Staub A, Benoist C, et al. Arthritis provoked by linked T and B cell recognition of a glycolytic enzyme. *Science* 1999;286:1732–1735.
104. Korganow A, Weber JC, Martin T. Animal models and autoimmune diseases. *Rev Med Interne* 1999;20:283–286.
105. Redlich K, Hayer S, Ricci R, et al. Osteoclasts are essential for TNF-alpha-mediated joint destruction. *J Clin Invest* 2002;110:1419–1427.
106. Fujikawa Y, Sabokbar A, Neale S, et al. Human osteoclast formation and bone resorption by monocytes and synovial macrophages in rheumatoid arthritis. *Ann Rheum Dis* 1996;55:816–822.
107. Suzuki Y, Tsutsumi Y, Nakagawa M, et al. Osteoclast-like cells in an in vitro model of bone destruction by rheumatoid synovium. *Rheumatology (Oxford)* 2001;40:673–682.
108. Romas E, Bakharevski O, Hards DK, et al. Expression of osteoclast differentiation factor at sites of bone erosion in collagen-induced arthritis. *Arthritis Rheum* 2000;43:821–826.
109. Kuratani T, Nagata K, Kukita T, et al. Induction of abundant osteoclast-like multinucleated giant cells in adjuvant arthritic rats with accompanying disordered high bone turnover. *Histol Histopathol* 1998;13:751–759.
110. Takayanagi H, Oda H, Yamamoto S, et al. A new mechanism of bone destruction in rheumatoid arthritis: synovial fibroblasts induce osteoclastogenesis. *Biochem Biophys Res Commun* 1997;240:279–286.
111. Feldmann M, Maini RN. The role of cytokines in the pathogenesis of rheumatoid arthritis. *Rheumatology* 1999;38:3–7.
112. Romas E, Martin TJ. Cytokines in the pathogenesis of osteoporosis. *Osteoporos Int* 1997;7:S47–S53.
113. Okano K, Tsukazaki T, Ohtsuru A, et al. Parathyroid hormone-related peptide in synovial fluid and disease activity of rheumatoid arthritis. *Br J Rheumatol* 1996;35:1056–1062.
114. Funk JL, Cordaro LA, Wei H, et al. Synovium as a source of increased amino-terminal parathyroid hormone-related protein expression in rheumatoid arthritis; a possible role for locally produced parathyroid hormone-related protein in the pathogenesis of rheumatoid arthritis. *J Clin Invest* 1998;101:1362–1371.
115. Ogata Y, Kukita A, Kukita T, et al. A novel role of IL-15 in the development of osteoclasts: inability to replace its activity with IL-2. *J Immunol* 1999;162:2754–2760.
116. Gravallese EM, Manning C, Tsay A, et al. Synovial tissue in rheumatoid arthritis is a source of osteoclast differentiation factor. *Arthritis Rheum* 2000;43:250–258.
117. Gravallese EM, Galson DL, Goldring SR, et al. The role of TNF-receptor family members and other TRAF-dependent receptors in bone resorption. *Arthritis Res* 2001;3:6–12.
118. Horwood NJ, Kartsogiannis V, Quinn JMW, et al. Activated T lymphocytes support osteoclast formation in vitro. *Biochem Biophys Res Commun* 1999;265:144–150.
119. Takayanagi H, Iizuka H, Juji T, et al. Involvement of receptor activator of nuclear factor kappa-B ligand/osteoclast differentiation factor in osteoclastogenesis from synoviocytes in rheumatoid arthritis. *Arthritis Rheum* 2000;43:259–269.
120. Lacey DL, Timms E, Tan HL, et al. Osteoprotegerin ligand is a cytokine that regulates osteoclast differentiation and activation. *Cell* 1998;93:165–176.
121. Lacey DL, Tan HL, Lu J, et al. Osteoprotegerin ligand modulates murine osteoclast survival in vitro and in vivo. *Am J Pathol* 2000;157:435–448.
122. Yasuda H, Shima N, Nakagawa N, et al. Osteoclast differentiation factor is a ligand for osteoprotegerin/osteoclastogenesis-inhibitory factor and is identical to TRANCE/RANKL. *Proc Natl Acad Sci U S A* 1998;95:3597–3602.
123. Yasuda H, Shima N, Nakagawa N, et al. Identity of osteoclastogenesis inhibitory factor (OCIF) and osteoprotegerin (OPG): a mechanism by which OPG/OCIF inhibits osteoclastogenesis in vitro. *Endocrinology* 1998;139:1329–1337.
124. Wong BR, Rho J, Arron J, et al. TRANCE is a novel ligand of the tumor necrosis factor receptor family that activates c-Jun N-terminal kinase in T cells. *J Biol Chem* 1997;272:25190–25194.
125. Wong BR, Josien R, Lee SY, et al. TRANCE (tumor necrosis factor [TNF]-related activation-induced cytokine), a new TNF family member predominantly expressed in T cells, is a dendritic cell-specific survival factor. *J Exp Med* 1997;186:2075–2080.
126. Dougall WC, Glaccum M, Charrier K, et al. RANK is essential for osteoclast and lymph node development. *Genes Dev* 1999;13:2412–2424.
127. Bucay N, Sarosi I, Dunstan CR, et al. Osteoprotegerin-deficient mice develop early onset osteoporosis and arterial calcification. *Genes Dev* 1998;12:1260–1268.

128. Emery JG, McDonnell P, Burke MB, et al. Osteoprotegerin is a receptor for the cytotoxic ligand TRAIL. *J Biol Chem* 1998;273:14363–14367.
129. Simonet WS, Lacey DL, Dunstan CR, et al. Osteoprotegerin: a novel secreted protein involved in the regulation of bone density. *Cell* 1997;89:309–319.
130. Hofbauer LC, Heufelder AE. Role of receptor activator of nuclear factor-kappa B ligand and osteoprotegerin in bone cell biology. *J Mol Med* 2001;79:243–253.
131. Hofbauer LC, Khosla S, Dunstan CR, et al. The roles of osteoprotegerin and osteoprotegerin ligand in the paracrine regulation of bone resorption. *J Bone Miner Res* 2000;15:2–12.
132. Romas E, Sims N, Hards D, et al. Osteoprotegerin reduces osteoclast numbers and prevents bone erosion in collagen-induced arthritis. *Am J Pathol* 2002;161:1419–1427.
133. Redlich K, Hayer S, Maier A, et al. Tumor necrosis factor-α-mediated joint destruction is inhibited by targeting osteoclasts with osteoprotegerin. *Arthritis Rheum* 2002;46:785–792.
134. Kotake S, Udagawa N, Hakoda M, et al. Activated human T cells directly induce osteoclastogenesis from human monocytes: possible role of T cells in bone destruction in rheumatoid arthritis patients. *Arthritis Rheum* 2001;44:1003–1012.
135. Weitzmann MN, Cenci S, Rifas L, et al. T cell activation induces human osteoclast formation via receptor activator of nuclear factor kappaB ligand-dependent and -independent mechanisms. *J Bone Miner Res* 2001;16:328–337.
136. Weitzmann MN, Cenci S, Rifas L, et al. Interleukin-7 stimulates osteoclast formation by up-regulating the T-cell production of soluble osteoclastogenic cytokines. *Blood* 2000;96:1873–1878.
137. Romas E, Gillespie M, Martin T. Involvement of receptor activator of NF-κB ligand and tumor necrosis factor-α in bone destruction in rheumatoid arthritis. *Bone* 2002;30:340–346.
138. Tsuboi M, Kawakami A, Nakashima T, et al. Tumor necrosis factor-alpha and interleukin-1beta increase the Fas-mediated apoptosis of human osteoblasts. *J Lab Clin Med* 1999;134:190–191.
139. Fossiez F, Djossou O, Chomarat P, et al. T cell interleukin-17 induces stromal cells to produce proinflammatory and hematopoietic cytokines. *J Exp Med* 1996;183:2593–2603.
140. Kotake S, Udagawa N, Takahashi N, et al. IL-17 in synovial fluids from patients with rheumatoid arthritis is a potent stimulator of osteoclastogenesis. *J Clin Invest* 1999;103:1345–1352.
141. McInnes I, Liew F. Interleukin 15: a proinflammatory role in rheumatoid synovitis. *Immunol Today* 1998;19:75–79.
142. McInnes IB, Leung BP, Sturrock RD, et al. Interleukin-15 mediates T cell-dependent regulation of tumour necrosis factor-alpha production in rheumatoid arthritis. *Nat Med* 1997;3:189–195.
143. Sambrook P, Nguyen T. Vertebral osteoporosis in rheumatoid arthritis. *Br J Rheum* 1992;31:573–574.
144. Sambrook P, Spector T, Seeman E, et al. Osteoporosis in rheumatoid arthritis: a monozygotic co-twin control study. *Arthritis Rheum* 1995;38:806–809.
145. Sambrook PN, Eisman A, Champion G, et al. Determinants of axial bone loss in rheumatoid arthritis. *Arthritis Rheum* 1987;30:721–728.
146. Sambrook P, Eisman J, Yeates M, et al. Osteoporosis in rheumatoid arthritis: safety of low-dose corticosteroids. *Ann Rheum Dis* 1986;45:950.
147. Peel NF, Eastell R, Russell RGG. Osteoporosis in rheumatoid arthritis—the laboratory perspective. *Br J Rheum* 1991;30:84–85.
148. Deodhar AA, Woolf AD. Bone mass measurement and bone metabolism in rheumatoid arthritis: a review. *Br J Rheumatol* 1996;35:309–322.
149. Woolf AD. Osteoporosis in rheumatoid arthritis—the clinical viewpoint. *Br J Rheum* 1991;30:82–84.
150. Gough AK, Lilley J, Eyre S, et al. Generalized bone loss in patients with rheumatoid arthritis. *Lancet* 1994;344:23–27.
151. Saag K, Rochelle K, Caldwell J, et al. Low dose longterm corticosteroid therapy in rheumatoid arthritis; an analysis of serious adverse events. *Am J Med* 1994;96:115–123.
152. Beat AM, Bloch DA, Fries JF. Predictors of fractures in early rheumatoid arthritis. *J Rheumatol* 1991;18:804–808.
153. Hooyman JR, Melton LJ, Nelson AM, et al. Fractures after rheumatoid arthritis; a population based study. *Arthritis Rheum* 1984;27:1353–1361.
154. Michel BA, Bloch DA, Wolfe F, et al. Fractures in rheumatoid arthritis: an evaluation of associated risk factors. *J Rheumatol* 1993;20:1666–1669.
155. Spector TD, Hall GM, McCloskey EV, et al. Risk of vertebral fracture in women with rheumatoid arthritis. *BMJ* 1993;306:558.
156. Compston JE, Vedi S, Croucher PI, et al. Bone turnover in non-steroid treated rheumatoid arthritis. *Ann Rheum Dis* 1994;53:163–166.
157. Kroger H, Arnala I, Alhava EM. Bone remodeling in osteoporosis associated with rheumatoid arthritis. *Calcif Tissue Int* 1991;49:S90.
158. Mellish RWE, O'Sullivan MM, Garrahan NJ, et al. Iliac crest trabecular bone mass and structure in patients with non-steroid treated rheumatoid arthritis. *Ann Rheum Dis* 1987;46:830–836.
159. Gough AK, Peel NF, Eastell R, et al. Excretion of pyridinium crosslinks correlates with disease activity and appendicular bone loss in early rheumatoid arthritis. *Ann Rheum Dis* 1994;53:14–17.
160. Iwamoto J, Takeda T, Ichimura S. Urinary cross-linked N-telopeptides of type I collagen levels in patients with rheumatoid arthritis. *Calcif Tissue Int* 2003;.72:491–497.
161. Sambrook P, Ansel B, Foster S, et al. Bone turnover in early rheumatoid arthritis; longitudinal bone density studies. *Ann Rheum Dis* 1985;44:580.
162. Haugeberg G, Orstavik RE, Uhlig T, et al. Bone loss in patients with rheumatoid arthritis: results from a population-based cohort of 366 patients followed up for two years. *Arthritis Rheum* 2002;46:1720–1728.
163. Kirwan JR. The effects of glucocorticoids on joint destruction in rheumatoid arthritis. *N Engl J Med* 1995;333:142–146.
164. Gough A, Sambrook P, Devlin J, et al. Osteoclastic activation is the principal mechanism leading to secondary osteoporosis in rheumatoid arthritis. *J Rheumatol* 1998;7:1282–1289.
165. Sambrook P, Cohen M, Eisman J, et al. Effects of low-dose corticosteroid on bone mass in rheumatoid arthritis: a longitudinal study. *Ann Rheum Dis* 1989;48:535.
166. Lane NE, Mroczkowski PJ, Hochberg MC. Prevention and management of glucocorticoid-induced osteoporosis. *Bull Rheum Dis* 1995;44:1–4.
167. Fries JF, Williams CA, Ramsey DR, et al. The relative toxicity of disease-modifying antirheumatic drugs. *Arthritis Rheum* 1993;44:406–411.
168. Laan R, van Riel P, van Erning L, et al. Vertebral osteoporosis in rheumatoid arthritis patients; effects of low-dose prednisone therapy. *Br J Rheumatol* 1992;31:91–96.
169. Shimizu S, Shiozawa S, Shiozawa K, et al. Quantitative histologic studies on the pathogenesis of periarticular osteoporosis in rheumatoid arthritis. *Arthritis Rheum* 1985;28:25–31.
170. Chu CQ, Field M, Allard S, et al. Detection of cytokines at the cartilage/pannus junction in patients with rheumatoid arthritis; implications for the role of cytokines in cartilage destruction and repair. *Br J Rheumatol* 1992;31:653–661.
171. Deleuran BW, Chu CQ, Field M, et al. Localization of interleukin-1 alpha, type 1 interleukin-1 receptor and interleukin-1 receptor antagonist in the synovial membrane and cartilage/pannus junction in rheumatoid arthritis. *Br J Rheumatol* 1992;31:801–809.
172. Chu CQ, Field M, Feldmann M, et al. Localization of tumor necrosis factor alpha in synovial tissues and at the cartilage-pannus junction in patients with rheumatoid arthritis. *Arthritis Rheum* 1991;34:1125–1132.
173. Firestein GS, Alcaro-Garcia JM, Maki R. Quantitative analysis of cytokine gene expression in rheumatoid arthritis. *J Immunol* 1990;144:3347–3353.
174. Harris EDJ. Rheumatoid arthritis. Pathophysiology and implications for therapy. *N Engl J Med* 1990;322:1277–1289.
175. Mazess RB, Whedon GD. Immobilization and bone. *Calcif Tissue Int* 1983; 32:265.

CHAPTER 21

Mechanisms of Joint Damage in Rheumatoid Arthritis

Beverley F. Fermor, J. Brice Weinberg, David S. Pisetsky, and Farshid Guilak

Rheumatoid arthritis (RA) is a chronic, debilitating arthropathy characterized by inflammation and proliferation of synovium that leads to joint destruction. In considering the pathogenesis of joint destruction, cartilage has usually been considered an "innocent bystander," with damage mediated by other cell types, including adjacent synoviocytes. Recent evidence suggests, however, that cartilage-degradation RA may also involve intrinsic disturbances that reflect an imbalance of the anabolic and catabolic activities of the articular chondrocytes themselves, as well as changes resulting from inflammation, synoviocyte activation, and changes in adjacent bone. Chondrocyte metabolic activity is influenced strongly by local microenvironmental factors that include soluble mediators (e.g., cytokines), extracellular matrix (ECM) components, and biophysical influences such as mechanical stress. In particular, biomechanical factors may play an important role in the onset and progression of osteoarthritic changes secondary to joint inflammation in RA.

The sequence of biomechanical and biochemical processes leading to joint destruction *in vivo* is unclear. The role of mechanical factors in disease pathogenesis is also relevant to treatment and to the role of physical therapy. Thus, there has long been debate over the role of joint use, including exercise and physical therapy, in RA treatment, as opposed to joint rest and even immobilization; studies indicate, however, that exercise can lead to decreased pain, increased mobility, and increased muscle strength. The effects of exercise (i.e., mechanical stress) on articular cartilage and other tissues in an inflamed RA joint remain unknown.

Recently introduced therapies for RA include inhibitors of inflammatory cytokines such as tumor necrosis factor (TNF)-α or interleukin (IL)-1. The action of these cytokines is associated with production of other proinflammatory mediators, such as nitric oxide (NO) and prostaglandins (PGs). Mechanical stress, an important factor in the physiology and pathophysiology of the synovial joint, can also induce production of these proinflammatory mediators in cell types such as chondrocytes, osteoblasts, osteocytes, and endothelial cells. This chapter reviews pathways for joint destruction in RA, focusing on the relationship between mechanical stress, the proinflammatory mediators NO and prostaglandin E_2 (PGE_2), and cytokines such as IL-1, TNF-α, and IL-17. Understanding the interaction between mechanical loading of the joint and production of inflammatory mediators could help identify new targets for RA treatment (Fig. 21.1).

STRUCTURE AND FUNCTION OF ARTICULAR CARTILAGE

Under normal conditions, articular cartilage in diarthrodial joints functions as a nearly frictionless surface that, for decades, can be exposed to loads of several times body weight. This remarkable function is attributed to the unique structure and composition of the cartilage ECM, which determine the mechanical properties (Fig. 21.2). The cartilage ECM is maintained by the metabolic activity of a sparse population of cells (chondrocytes) embedded within this tissue. The ECM of articular cartilage is primarily water, which comprises 60% to 85% of the wet weight of the tissue. The remaining solid matrix is composed of a cross-linked network of type II collagen (15–22% by wet weight), proteoglycan (4–7% by wet weight), and lesser amounts of other collagen types (e.g., VI, IX, X) and noncollagenous proteins (1). The aggregating proteoglycan, or aggrecan, in cartilage is composed of a hyaluronic-acid backbone to which numerous chondroitin and keratan sulfate chains are attached by a link protein.

The constituents of articular cartilage are organized in a stratified structure that confers the unique mechanical behavior of the ECM (2). Collagen fibers in the superficial-most zone of cartilage, which have a small diameter, are densely packed and oriented parallel to the articular surface. In the middle or transitional zone, the collagen fibers form an arcade-like structure on which is superimposed randomly arranged collagen fibers (3). In the deep zone, the collagen fibers are larger and form bundles, which are oriented perpendicular to the bone. In this tissue, chondrocytes are surrounded by a thin region of tissue termed the *pericellular matrix*, which is rich in proteoglycans and collagen types II, VI, and IX (4).

Mechanical leading of the joint, which occurs during normal activities of daily living, deforms the articular cartilage (5) and generates a combination of tensile, compressive, and shear stresses within the tissue (6). The properties of cartilage are highly specialized because of its unique composition and structural organization. Biomechanically, this tissue can be viewed as a fiber-reinforced, porous, and permeable composite matrix that is saturated with fluid (7). Because cartilage exhibits viscoelastic (i.e., time- or rate-sensitive) properties, loading is associated with shock

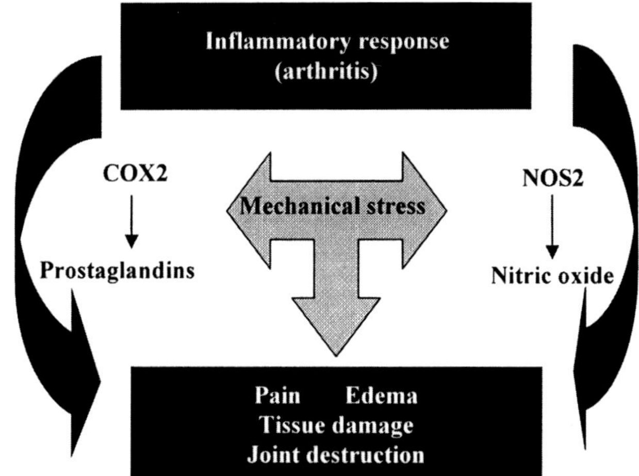

Figure 21.1. The inflammatory response in rheumatoid arthritis is associated with the production of nitric oxide and prostaglandins. Application of mechanical stress to articular cartilage also causes production of these two inflammatory mediators. There are also influences of the two pathways on each other and also with other inflammatory mediators. COX2, cyclooxygenase-2; NOS2, nitric oxide synthase.

absorption and energy dissipation (7). These viscoelastic behaviors arise from several mechanisms, including interstitial fluid flow through the porous-permeable solid matrix, and from physical interactions between the solid matrix constituents (e.g., collagen and proteoglycan). In a healthy joint, these characteristics contribute to normal load bearing, energy dissipation, and joint lubrication over the joint's lifetime. With injury or degeneration related to RA, cartilage undergoes a significant loss of mechanical function, as well as the potential to cause further degeneration of the joint.

ROLE OF BIOMECHANICAL FACTORS IN CARTILAGE PHYSIOLOGY

Many studies have shown that the mechanical-stress environment of the joint is an important factor, which, together with genetic factors and soluble mediators (e.g., growth factors and cytokines) (8), can modulate the activity of the chondrocytes *in vivo*. Mechanical stress is essential to maintain the components of the ECM in a state of slow turnover and to maintain a homeostatic balance between the catabolic and anabolic events of the chondrocytes. Alterations in the mechanical environment of the articular cartilage due to abnormal joint loading can lead to cellular and biochemical changes in the activity of the chondrocytes that are associated with cartilage degradation and the progression of degenerative joint disease (9–11). Alterations in joint loading may result from joint pain, immobilization, instability, or deformity and may be an important factor that modifies joint physiology after the onset of RA (Fig. 21.3). Furthermore, abnormal loading patterns may become more pronounced as the adjoining muscles weaken, a phenomenon often observed in progressive disease. For example, disuse of the joint, which occurs with casting or immobilization, results in a loss of proteoglycans, changes in proteoglycan sulfation patterns, a decrease in the compressive stiffness, increased hydration, and a decrease in cartilage thickness. These effects are partially reversible with remobilization (12,13). Exercise may cause site-specific changes in proteoglycan content and cartilage stiffness, although these changes are not deleterious (14) and may have a beneficial effect in the normal joint (15,16).

Mechanical loading of the joint *in vivo* exposes the articular cartilage to cyclic stresses, which have both static (i.e., constant) and dynamic (i.e., time-varying) components. Therefore, various investigations of the biophysical mechanisms of cellular response to stress have sought to separate "static" and "dynamic" loading conditions (8). To study the sequence of biomechanical and biochemical events involved in the transduction of mechanical stress to a cellular response in cartilage, *in vitro* explant models of mechanical loading have been used (Fig. 21.4). These model systems enable better control of the biomechanical and biochemical environments, as compared to the *in vivo* situation (17–20). Mechanical responses have been reported over a wide range of loading magnitudes and exhibit a stress-dose dependency (8). Excessive loading (e.g., high magnitude, long duration) seems to be deleterious, resulting in cell death, tissue disruption, and swelling (21,22). The majority of studies investigating cell death have used a mechanical regimen that involves a high-energy

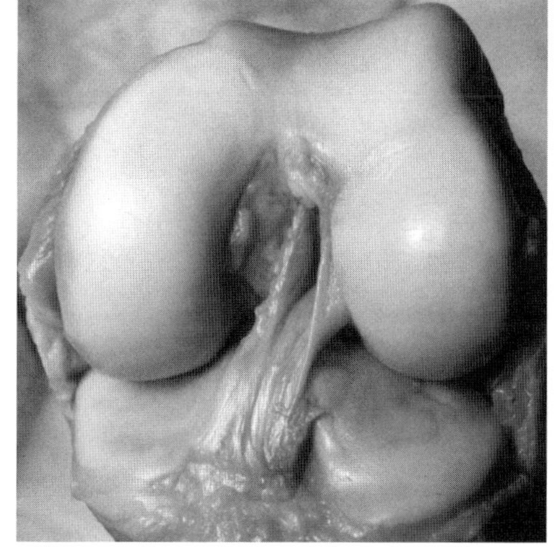

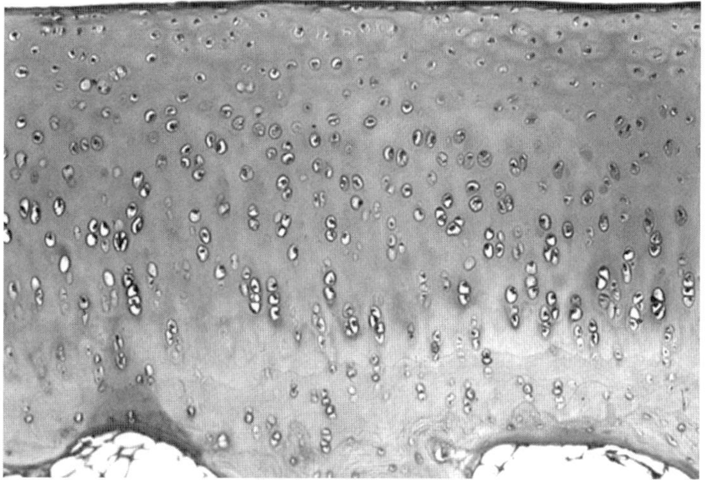

Figure 21.2. A: Articular cartilage of the knee joint. Cartilage is the thin layer of deformable, load-bearing material that lines the ends of bones in diarthrodial joints. Normal cartilage exhibits a smooth, white, translucent appearance. **B:** Histologic micrograph of adult articular cartilage. The extracellular matrix is composed primarily of water, making up 60% to 85% of the tissue's wet weight. The remaining solid matrix is composed of a cross-linked network of type II collagen (15–22% by wet weight), proteoglycan (4–7% by wet weight), and lesser amounts of other collagen types (e.g., VI, IX, X) and noncollagenous proteins. Chondrocytes are the only cell types in cartilage and make up 1% to 10% of the tissue volume in adult cartilage.

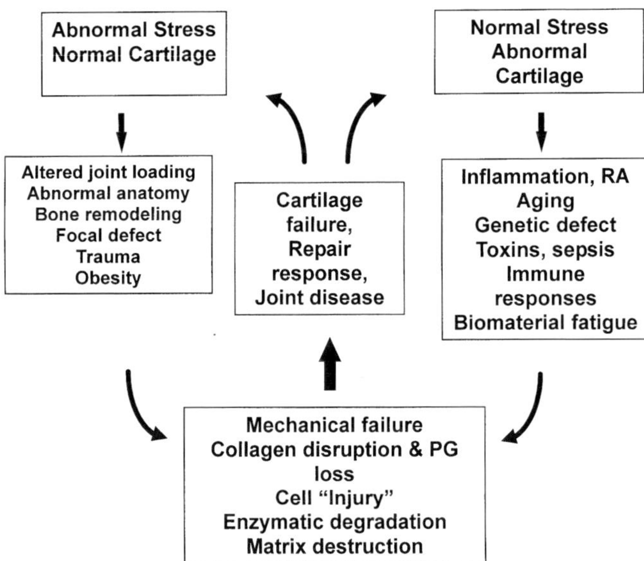

Figure 21.3. Biomechanical factors in joint degeneration. Biomechanical factors appear to play an important role in the pathways leading to progressive joint degeneration. The initiation and progression of cartilage degeneration in joint disease is due to a combination of abnormal biomechanical loading or abnormal physiology of the joint, or both. The outcome of these factors is an abnormal "remodeling" response of the chondrocytes that often results in increased matrix degradation and progressive degenerative changes. PG, prostaglandin; RA, rheumatoid arthritis.

impact load (23–27). Physiologic repetitive loading at 1 megapascal (MPa) can cause cell death in the superficial tangential zone only, and no apoptosis is detected (28,29).

Static compression of articular cartilage explants *in vitro* causes a stress-dependent decrease in proteoglycan and collagen synthesis rates (30–33). Under these loading conditions, exudation of the interstitial water leads to an increase in the solid volume fraction of the ECM, which, in turn, increases the density of matrix-associated negative charges or fixed-charge density. These effects alter the physicochemical and osmotic environment within the ECM and surrounding the cell. Conversely, dynamic compression at certain magnitudes and frequencies can lead to an increase in proteoglycan and collagen metabolism and gene expression (17–20). Dynamic compression exposes the chondrocytes to a diverse array of biophysical factors, such as fluid pressure, fluid flow, and resulting electrokinetic effects due to the movement of fluid and ions through the charged ECM.

EFFECTS OF INFLAMMATORY MEDIATORS ON CARTILAGE

Nitric Oxide

NO is a gaseous mediator that regulates diverse physiologic processes throughout the body. NO is synthesized by the heme-containing enzyme, NO synthase (NOS), from L-arginine in a reaction requiring nicotinamide-adenine dinucleotide phosphate, tetrahydrobiopterin, and molecular oxygen (O_2) as cofactors to produce L-citrulline and NO. Three isoforms of NOS have been identified (NOS-1, NOS-2, and NOS-3). NO has a half-life of several seconds and, therefore, cannot diffuse long distances. Thus, to regulate the functioning of diarthrodial joints, NO must be synthesized locally. NOS-1 and NOS-3 are expressed constitutively and generate NO for cell-signaling purposes. NOS-2 produces NO in larger quantities during inflammation and host defense and can promote tissue damage. Potential sources of NO in the joint in response to inflammatory mediators include the endothelial cells lining the synovial capillaries, infiltrating leukocytes, and the resident mesenchymal cells of the joint (34), synoviocytes (35), articular chondrocytes (36), and bone (37).

Normal cartilage produces low levels of NO (38). Production of high levels of NO requires the presence of arthritis or stimulation by cytokines (IL-1, TNF-α, and IL-17), endotoxin, or immune complexes. Increased NO production and NOS-2 expression occur in several animal models of RA, including MRL/lpr mice (39), streptococcal cell-wall fragment model (40), adjuvant-induced arthritis (41), and collagen-induced arthritis (42). Elevated NO production has been observed in human RA (43–46).

Studies on bovine and human articular cartilage show that the superficial cells produce more NO per cell in response to IL-1 than do deep cells (36,47). Also, superficial cells are more respon-

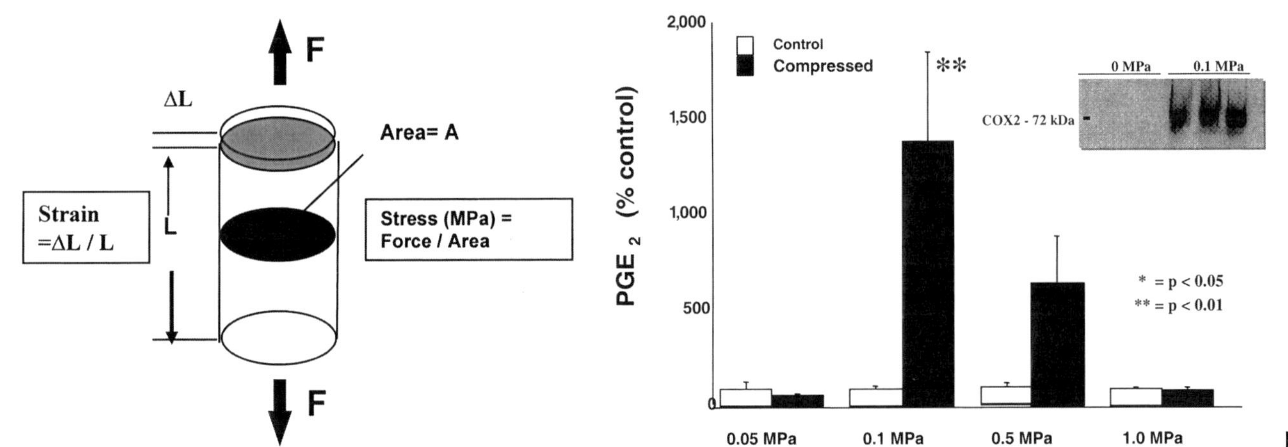

Figure 21.4. **A:** The relationship between stress and strain in a tissue. The units of megapascal (MPa) are used to measure the magnitude of stress applied when articular cartilage is compressed. **B:** Using *in vitro* models, increasing the magnitude of stress applied to porcine articular cartilage explants is associated with increased prostaglandin E_2 (PGE_2) production, which is associated with increased cyclocoxygenase-2 (COX-2) protein. This graph represents a range of stress magnitudes at constant frequency (0.5 Hz) and duration (24 hours) of loading. F, force; L, length.

sive to IL-1, possibly because they contain more type 1 IL-1 receptors. Increased NO production at the interface of cartilage and synovial fluid may play an important role in the modulation of cartilage damage in inflammatory arthritis. NO may be involved as an endogenous modulator of cartilage matrix turnover to different degrees in different zones of the cartilage.

NO can have pleiotropic effects on articular cartilage depending on the environment and concentration. NO can inhibit adhesion-modulating signal transduction and modulate cytokine expression, suppress matrix collagen and proteoglycan synthesis, activate matrix metalloproteinases (MMPs), or suppress proliferation and promotion of chondrocyte apoptosis (35,48,49).

NO can also decrease cartilage degradation and increase bone formation. Likewise, NO can have a protective effect on matrix catabolism, measured by release of $^{35}SO_4$ into the medium from slices of bovine (50) and lapine (51) articular cartilage, as well as alginate cultures of human articular chondrocytes (47). This protection may be mediated by inhibition of MMPs. The NOS-2 nonselective inhibitor N^G-monomethyl-L-arginine (L-NMA) partially reduces IL-1–induced bovine-chondrocyte MMP-1 messenger RNA (mRNA) expression (52) and IL-1–stimulated MMP-9 mRNA expression in rabbit articular chondrocytes (53).

The most direct effect of NO on chondrocytes appears to be the suppression of energy metabolism as manifested by decreased adenosine triphosphate (ATP) production (54,55), decreased O_2 consumption (55), decreased matrix synthesis (49), and heightened matrix calcification (54). Insufficient mitochondrial ATP generation may be one of the factors contributing to "metabolic failure" in articular cartilage (56); in this situation, matrix synthesis cannot keep pace with the heightened matrix degradation triggered by biomechanical or other factors (57,58).

Although many of the physiologic actions of NO are mediated through the activation of soluble guanylate cyclase, the mechanisms by which NO exerts its cytostatic/cytotoxic or tissue-damaging effects are unclear (59). NO nitrosylates the iron in the heme of cytochrome oxidase, the terminal enzyme in the mitochondrial electron transport chain. This nitrosylation inhibits the enzyme activity. Nanomolar concentrations of NO inhibit cytochrome oxidase reversibly and competitively with molecular O_2 and lead to diminished ATP and cell death. NO is linked to energy generation in the mitochondrion and the control of cell death in certain cell types (59,60). ATP levels are proposed as an important determinant of cell death, either by apoptosis or necrosis (61). For a cell to survive, a certain ATP level is required. When ATP falls below this level, apoptosis occurs if sufficient ATP is available for the energy-requiring apoptotic processes such as enzymatic hydrolysis of macromolecules, nuclear condensation, and bleb formation. With a severe drop in ATP levels, cellular-controlled cell death ceases and necrosis occurs (61). Decreased cellular ATP is characteristic of cell death, but it is unclear whether the decrease is the cause or consequence of cell death.

The effects of NO may be mediated by peroxynitrite. Many cell types produce both NO and superoxide and, consequently, peroxynitrite, a molecule that may lead to tissue injury due to its strong oxidatory capacity and long half-life. Superoxide can limit the effects of NO by diverting it to peroxynitrite. Alternatively, NO can be a scavenger of superoxide anion and could provide a chemical barrier to cytotoxic O_2 free radicals. Some of the conflicting findings on the role of NO or peroxynitrite in cell death can be attributed to the type of NO donor used for *in vitro* experiments. To understand the responses to exogenous NO, it is important to know the precise reactive species that is generated by the NO donor used, either directly by the NO donor compound itself or indirectly as a consequence of a secondary reaction with an additional reactive O_2 species (62).

Prostaglandins

Inflammation in RA has been attributed in part to the actions of prostanoids such as PGE_2, which can regulate the expression of many target genes. PGE_2 production is mediated by the enzyme cyclooxygenase (COX), and inhibitors of this enzyme inhibit pain and inflammation (63). Although the role of PGE_2 in disease pathogenesis is not fully understood (64), its involvement in mechanotransduction in articular cartilage suggests a mechanism by which joint use can lead to inflammation and damage. COX is a membrane-bound heme protein that is localized to both the endoplasmic reticulum and the nuclear membrane (65). COX-1 is constitutively expressed by many cells, whereas COX-2 expression is induced by a range of stimuli, including cytokines, mitogens, hormones, and serum (65). Increased PGE_2 synthesis from COX-2 in articular cartilage is a cellular response to activation by proinflammatory stimuli (66) and an important component in disease pathogenesis (67). Osteoarthritic cartilage produces more PGE_2 than nonarthritic cartilage (68,69), and antiinflammatory cytokines and glucocorticoids decrease prostanoid production. New COX-2–selective inhibitors are rapidly replacing COX nonselective, nonsteroidal antiinflammatory drugs for the treatment of both RA and osteoarthritis (OA) (64,70). These highly selective COX-2 inhibitors exhibit potent antiinflammatory effects with significantly reduced gastric toxicity (71).

PG receptors are comprised of eight genes encoding transmembrane G protein–coupled receptors (72). The receptors are classified on the basis of the selective affinities for naturally occurring prostanoids. There are at least four different receptors for PGE, EP_1, EP_2, EP_3, and EP_4, and there are multiple subtypes of each (Table 21.1) (73). Each receptor is associated with a unique G protein and second messenger system. EP_2 and EP_4 lead to the activation of adenylate cyclase via G_s and increased cyclic adenosine monophosphate (cAMP) concentration. EP_1 is coupled to the mobilization of Ca^{2+} via an unknown species of G protein and phosphatidylinositol turnover. EP_3 generally activates G_i but, due to its alternate splicing forms, it can induce a range of effects, and there is considerable species specificity (74,75). Stimulation of different EP receptors can have different consequences. EP_1 receptors are related to proliferation and inhibition of differentiation, and EP_4/EP_2 receptors to growth inhibition and differentiation promotion (73). Mice with a genetically disrupted EP_2 receptor exhibit a

TABLE 21.1. Classification of Prostaglandin E Receptors

Prostaglandin E Receptor	G Protein	Pathway	Biologic Effect
EP_1	Unknown	Mobilization of Ca^{2+} via phosphatidylinositol turnover	Increased proliferation Inhibition of differentiation
EP_2	G_s	Activates adenylate cyclase Increased cyclic adenosine monophosphate	Growth inhibition Promotion of differentiation
EP_3	G_i	—	Alternate splicing leads to range of effects
EP_4	G_s	Activates adenylate cyclase, Increased cyclic adenosine monophosphate	Growth inhibition Promotion of differentiation

weaker skeleton in terms of biomechanical properties compared with similar wild-type mice (76). It has been suggested that articular chondrocytes preferentially express EP_1 and EP_2 and, to a lesser extent, EP_3, whereas others suggest only EP_4 receptors are present (77). Antagonists of specific PG receptors may have the potential to provide selective therapeutic benefit. However, progress in this area of research has been hampered by the lack of specificity of the receptor antagonists available.

INHIBITION OF INFLAMMATORY MEDIATORS AS THERAPEUTIC TARGETS

The severity of arthritis in animal models is decreased by NOS inhibitors, suggesting that NO could play an important role in the onset and progression of arthritis. N^6-(1-iminoethyl)-L-lysine, dihydrochloride, an inhibitor of NOS-2, inhibits the progression of OA in the canine meniscectomy model (78). Streptococcal wall–induced arthritis in rats is inhibited by arginine analogues, such as the nonspecific inhibitors of NOS-2, L-NMMA N^G-monomethyl-L-arginine, monoacetate salt (40), L-NMA (41), and L-N^G-nitroarginine methyl ester (hydrochloride) (79) and also by N^6-(1-iminoethyl)-L-lysine, dihydrochloride (80). Streptococcal wall–induced arthritis is not inhibited by aminoguanidine in rats (81), and murine collagen–induced arthritis is resistant to NOS inhibitors, as well as to disruption of the NOS gene (82).

There is also evidence, however, that NOS-2 selective inhibitors can exacerbate the inflammation. Nonselective NOS inhibitors have more antiarthritic properties than selective NOS-2 inhibitors, particularly with respect to reduction of synovitis. These findings suggest that NOS-2 potentially exhibits a protective effect in the joint (83). There is evidence that NOS-2 is the isoform of NOS responsible for excessive and autotoxic levels of NO in chronic pathogenic inflammatory lesions (38,84). NO has previously been shown to have a protective role in cartilage *in vitro*. Administration of NOS-2 inhibitors can also be proinflammatory in the carrageenin-induced pleurisy model, perhaps due to increased production of leukotriene B_4 (LTB_4) (85).

Nonsteroidal antiinflammatory drugs have been used for many years in the treatment of arthritis (86). However, development of the selective COX-2 inhibitors has proven beneficial due to the reduction in gastrointestinal side effects associated with nonsteroidal antiinflammatory drugs. PGE_2 can also exert anticatabolic and antiinflammatory effects by reducing the expression and synthesis of IL-1 and TNF-α, as well as NOS-2 and MMP-1 and MMP-3 (87–89). Surprisingly, there is relatively little known about the effects of PGs on articular cartilage.

The catabolic effects of proinflammatory cytokines are believed to play a role in arthritis. A major cytokine involved in the arthritic process is IL-1, and both local and systemic levels of IL-1 reflect disease activity (90). IL-1 has profound catabolic effects on articular cartilage explants from numerous species (91). Elevated levels of IL-1 present in the synovial fluids of inflamed joints implicate it as a major etiologic agent in arthritis. Also, intraarticular injection of IL-1 induces arthritis in experimental animals (92). IL-1 decreases ECM synthesis and increases metalloproteinase synthesis via production of NO in chondrocytes (93). IL-1 receptor antagonist is an effective therapeutic agent in animal models of RA and human RA (94). Difference in potency has not been shown between the two isoforms of IL-1 (α and β). Some investigators believe that IL-1α is a major cytokine in the early stages of inflammation, whereas IL-1β is the more dominant cytokine in advanced disease (95). The increased synthesis of NO by IL-1β–activated chondrocytes is due to increased expression of NOS-2. Inhibition of NOS-2 and NO production prevents IL-1β–mediated suppression of proteoglycan and type II collagen synthesis and increased expression of metalloproteinases in chondrocytes, demonstrating that NO acts as an endogenous mediator of the catabolic actions of IL-1β.

Production of inflammatory mediators in response to catabolic cytokines is affected by O_2 tension, and O_2 tension can also alter the effect of one inflammatory pathway on another (96–98). O_2 tension is particularly relevant to cartilage physiology because of its avascular structure. As a result, articular cartilage functions at a lower O_2 tension than do most tissues (99). O_2 and other nutrients must diffuse into the tissue from the synovial fluid surrounding the joint, and an O_2 gradient is created in cartilage. The superficial zones of the tissue exist at approximately 6% O_2 (45.6 mm Hg) and the deep zones at nearly 0% O_2 (99). At rest, the synovial joint is a relatively hypoxic environment, and joint tissues become even more hypoxic during stress due to inflammation or mechanical loading (54). Articular chondrocytes are highly glycolytic but also show mitochondrial respiration/oxidative phosphorylation *in vitro* (54,100,101).

INTERACTION BETWEEN MECHANICAL STRESS AND INFLAMMATORY CYTOKINES

The interplay of mechanical stimuli, cytokines, NO production, and matrix synthesis remains an important issue in disease pathogenesis. NO is produced in response to IL-1 in cartilage. IL-1 is associated with a decrease in synthesis and an increase in degradation of the proteoglycans and collagens (102). Transforming growth factor β (TGF-β) stimulates synthesis of collagens and proteoglycans in chondrocytes and acts to reduce the activity of IL-1, thus opposing the inhibitory and catabolic effects of IL-1. NO does not reduce TGF-β production by lapine chondrocytes but, in the presence of L-NMA, IL-1β can increase TGF-β production by rabbit chondrocyte slices (103).

Cyclic tension is proposed as an antagonist of IL-1β actions in chondrocyte and fibrochondrocyte monolayers. Cyclic tension exerts its effects via transcriptional regulation of IL-1β response elements together with inhibition of NOS-2 and NO production, as well as COX-2 and MMP-1 (104–106). Conversely, cyclic tension can suppress collagen degradation by abrogating IL-1β–induced inhibition of tissue inhibitor of metalloproteinase-II and collagen type II expression. Cyclic tension also counteracts IL-1β–dependent inhibition of aggrecan mRNA expression through hyper-induction of aggrecan, a prominent component of cartilage proteoglycans. Other studies suggest that cyclic tension inhibits DNA and matrix synthesis in monolayers of chondrocytes with increased IL-1, MMP-2, and MMP-9 mRNA (107). However, it is important to note that these studies have been done using monolayers of articular chondrocytes, a system with two potential limitations: (a) chondrocytes can readily de-differentiate to a fibroblastic phenotype, and (b) mechanical stimuli are applied in the absence of the natural cartilage ECM.

In other cartilaginous tissues, such as the knee meniscus, mechanical stress may regulate, at least in part, the metabolic activity of meniscal fibrochondrocytes *in vivo*. Mechanical stress and IL-1 have interacting effects on the metabolic activity of fibrochondrocytes, potentially through NOS-2–mediated production of NO. The biosynthetic response to dynamic compression with IL-1 is restored by inhibition of NOS-2, suggesting that the inhibitory influence of IL-1 on mechanically induced biosynthesis requires NO production and NOS-2 activation (108). Dynamic compression can also increase proteoglycan degradation, which is further increased by IL-1. These findings suggest that the actions of IL-1 on mechanically stimulated biosynthesis may involve a separate mechanism as compared to mechanically induced proteoglycan breakdown.

Endogenous synthesis of NO does not affect the synthesis of noncollagenous proteins in cartilage, and NO fails to reduce the abundance of Col2Al mRNA (102). Blocking the induction of NO by chondrocytes treated by IL-1 restores translational/post-translational processes but fails to increase mRNA abundance (102). These findings suggest that the alterations in collagen synthesis rates may occur without significantly affecting levels of mRNAs encoding the various collagen α chains. This finding is consistent with a report showing that 24 hours of dynamic compression does not alter collagen I gene mRNA levels (109).

BIOMECHANICAL REGULATION OF INFLAMMATORY MEDIATORS IN CARTILAGE

Mechanical Stress Causes Increased Nitric Oxide Production in Articular Cartilage

Physiologic magnitudes and frequencies of either static or dynamic mechanical compression can lead to increased production of inflammatory mediators, such as NO, by articular cartilage (110). Fluid shear stress can also increase NO production and proteoglycan synthesis in bovine articular chondrocytes (111). Bovine chondrocytes embedded in agarose, however, exhibit decreased NO production when subjected to 15% nominal strain at frequencies of 0.3, 1.0, or 3.0 Hz (112). In this system, using isolated bovine articular chondrocytes embedded in an agarose gel, mechanical compression was performed in the absence of the natural ECM (112). In this regard, the mechanical "environment" of chondrocytes embedded in agarose differs significantly from that of chondrocytes in cartilage explants. Interactions between cell-surface receptors, such as integrins (113) and ECM molecules, can play an important role in mechanotransduction in cartilage (114) and would be expected to differ significantly in the two systems.

NO is an important mediator of the synthesis and breakdown of various macromolecular components of the cartilage ECM. The question of whether NO is catabolic or anabolic to the cartilage remains unclear. Findings that NO production is increased by either static or dynamic compression may reflect the dual role of NO in the suppression of proteoglycan synthesis and breakdown in this loading configuration. Conversely, increased NO production in response to shear stress on single-cell suspension of chondrocytes is associated with increased proteoglycan synthesis (111). There is agreement that endogenously produced NO inhibits incorporation of ^{35}S-sulphate into proteoglycans in explants of articular chondrocytes derived from rabbits, rats, or humans (115–117). Bovine articular chondrocytes lack this response, however (118).

Mechanical Stress Increases Production of Prostaglandins in Articular Cartilage

Mechanical compression of articular cartilage can significantly increase COX-2 protein expression and PGE_2 (119), which may regulate chondrocyte metabolism in physiologic and pathologic settings. In an explant culture system, the frequencies and magnitudes of mechanical stress used were representative of a physiologic range and were generally associated with increased proteoglycan synthesis in cartilage explants (22,120). Thus, increased production of PGE_2 may act anabolically. Such anabolic effects of PGE_2 on cartilage have previously been identified *in vitro* by demonstration of increased proteoglycan, DNA, and collagen synthesis (121,122). PGE_2 causes a biphasic response, with low concentrations of PGE_2 increasing and high doses decreasing collagen synthesis (123). This biphasic effect has also been attributed to the ability of PGE_2 to activate both the cAMP–protein kinase A and the Ca^{2+} and protein kinase C second messenger systems (122).

These second messenger systems also modulate the response of chondrocytes to mechanical stress (8,124). One of the earliest events in the response of chondrocytes to mechanical stress may be an increase in the intracellular concentration of calcium ion as a result of cell deformation initiated through mechanosensitive ion channels (125). The increased Ca^{2+} may be responsible for the activation of phospholipase A_2, an enzyme required for the release of arachidonic acid from the cell membrane to form PGE_2 (126).

Activation of COX-2 could also play an antiinflammatory role, as COX-2 mediates the synthesis of cyclopentenone PGs such as 15d-PGJ_2 (127). These lipid mediators may exert antiinflammatory activity through activation of peroxisome proliferator–activated receptor γ (PPARγ) (128,129). The activation of the PPARγ pathway inhibits mouse and human osteoclast differentiation, blocking the effects of macrophage colony-stimulating factor (M-CSF) and osteoprotegerin (OPG) ligand–induced osteoclast formation and activity (130).

BIOMECHANICAL REGULATION OF INFLAMMATORY MEDIATORS IN BONE

Bone contains three major cell types. Osteoblasts are associated with bone formation, osteoclasts with bone resorption, and osteocytes with mechanotransduction. Osteocytes are considered the primary mechanosensors. These cells are located in the bone matrix and can convey strain-related information and influence bone remodeling (131–133). Osteocytes are found embedded deep within the bone in small osteocytic lacunae (25,000 per mm^3 of bone). Osteocytes differentiate from osteoblasts and become trapped in the bone matrix produced by the osteocytes that later becomes calcified. Osteocytes have numerous long processes that are rich in microfilaments. These cells contact processes from other osteocytes (and show numerous gap junctions) or contact cells lining the bone surfaces (osteoblasts or flat lining cells in the endosteum or periosteum). These processes, which are organized during the formation of the matrix before its calcification, form a network of thin canaliculi permeating the entire bone matrix. This is evidence that fluid flow is an important stimulus in mechanotransduction in bone.

Both NO and PGs have been implicated in the mechanical loading response in bone. Although studies have not been done particularly with respect to RA, production of inflammatory mediators by osteoblasts and osteocytes are also of interest because pathologic changes in bone in inflammatory RA lead to osteoporosis (37). An excellent review of the effects of mechanical strain on bone has been written by Ehrlich and Lanyon (134).

With respect to NO and PGs, physiologic levels of pulsating fluid flow cause significantly more PGE_2 and PGI_2 production by osteocytes than by osteoblasts (135,136). *In vivo* inhibition of PG production by the administration of indomethacin prevents bone adaptation to mechanical strain (137–139). *In vivo,* the selective COX-2 inhibitor NS398 inhibits the bone formation that occurs in response to mechanical loading (140). PGE_2 can be anabolic to bone by recruiting osteoblast precursor cells and increasing osteoblast proliferation, alkaline phosphatase activity, and collagen synthesis (132,141,142). *In vivo* administration of PGE_2 enhances bone formation in response to four-point bending (143), a maneuver causing a physiologic level of mechanical stress. Fluid shear stress and mechanical stretching likewise increases cAMP in a manner that is PGE_2 dependent (144,145).

NO can also be a mediator of mechanically induced bone formation. Both NO and prostanoid production are increased after exposure to physiologic levels of mechanical strain induced by axial loading or fluid flow in organ and cell cultures of calvarial and long-bone osteocytes and osteoblasts (146–152). Mechanically induced formation of NO appears to result from activation of endothelial NOS (NOS-3) in bone cells (153,154). *In vivo* inhibition of NO also inhibits mechanically induced bone formation in rats (155–157). Pharmacologic NO donors can increase bone mass in experimental animals, and preliminary evidence suggests that these agents may also influence bone turnover in humans (37).

Osteoclasts are specialized multinucleated cells found in bone that mediate bone resorption (158–160). These form from circulating hematopoietic cells of bone marrow origin (158,161). Because of their morphologic similarity to inflammatory multinucleated giant cells, investigators have postulated an origin from emigrated blood monocytes (158,159,161). Blood monocytes and peritoneal macrophages can degrade bone *in vitro* (162,163). In murine systems, bone degrading ability relates to the degree of macrophage multinuclearity (162). In osteopetrosis, there is an inability to produce M-CSF, with a resultant defect in osteoclast function (164–166). Some studies have provided evidence that osteoclasts may be derived from a hematopoietic cell that is different from monocytes and macrophages (167). Osteoclasts, but not mononuclear phagocytes, respond to calcitonin (168); isolated osteoclasts do not express most antigens characteristic of mononuclear phagocytes (169); osteoclasts do not have the macrophage antigen F4/80 (161); and monoclonal anti-osteoclast antibodies do not react with mononuclear phagocytes (170). Nevertheless, it is likely that the osteoclast represents a highly differentiated mononuclear phagocyte despite some phenotypic differences.

Although osteoclasts lack certain surface molecules usually found on macrophages (e.g., Fc and C3 receptors), they express high levels of tartrate-resistant acid phosphatase, the vitronectin receptor, and calcitonin receptors (171). Several factors have been discovered that enhance osteoclast formation *in vitro*. These factors include 1,25 dihydroxyvitamin D_3, PGE_2, IL-1, IL-11, TNF, and glucocorticoids. These factors work through induction of OPG ligand (OPGL), which is identical to TNF-related activation-induced cytokine, in osteoblasts. OPGL, in turn, binds to a molecule called *receptor activator of nuclear factor (NF)-κB* on osteoclast precursors, and, in the presence of M-CSF, the osteoclast precursors develop into mature osteoclasts. OPG is a soluble decoy receptor for OPGL that can inhibit osteoclast formation and differentiation (171,172). TGF-β increases the proportion of precursors that become osteoclasts, and it is an essential co-stimulator of osteoclast formation. Research using mice with disruption of various genes has been very helpful in understanding the control of osteoclast formation and function and bone resorption. Mice with disruptions of M-CSF, C-src, C-fos, NF-κB, OPGL, and receptor activator of NF-κB have osteopetrosis, whereas those with disrupted OPG have osteoporosis (171).

BIOMECHANICAL REGULATION OF INFLAMMATORY MEDIATORS IN MENISCUS AND SYNOVIUM

Alterations in the distribution and magnitude of stress in the menisci may have important consequences on joint physiology and function. Studies suggest that the meniscus may also serve as an important target for pharmacologic or biophysical therapies for RA. Studies on the relationship of mechanical stress and its effect on the menisci are limited. For example, exercise increases collagen and proteoglycan content in rat menisci (173), whereas joint immobilization decreases aggrecan gene expression in intact menisci (174) and inhibits collagen accumulation in healing menisci (175). Furthermore, injury or loss of the meniscus can initiate pathologic changes in the articular cartilage of the knee (176–181) that are associated with alterations in the stress–strain environment in the joint (182–184).

In explant compression models, mechanical stress can increase NO production through a NOS-2–dependent mechanism in porcine meniscus (185) that is associated with increased matrix synthesis (108). There is increased total protein synthesis in bovine meniscal explants exposed to similar magnitudes of oscillatory compression (186). Some studies show that dynamic compression stimulates proteoglycan synthesis (108), whereas others show no influence of dynamic stress on proteoglycan synthesis (186). Static compression on meniscal explants decreases mRNA levels of type I collagen and decorin and up-regulate MMP-1 (109).

Although synovial inflammation is a key feature of RA (187–192), little is known about the effects of mechanical stress on synoviocytes, although human MH7A cells originating from an RA patient show down-regulation of MMP-13 with mechanical loading and up-regulation with mechanical unloading (193). In this study, gentle oscillatory motion was applied using a reciprocal shaker so that flow was applied to the cells. Another study showed that application of hydrostatic pressure to bovine synovial cells caused increased hsp70 mRNA (194).

INTERACTIONS BETWEEN INFLAMMATORY MEDIATORS

Effects of the Nitric Oxide Synthase Pathway on the Cyclooxygenase Pathway

Inflammation in RA involves a complex relationship between the pathways of NOS and COX. Induction of NO can inhibit or stimulate PGE_2 production in many different cell types. Inhibition of NO production by the NOS inhibitor L-NMMA leads to a twofold increase in PGE_2 production in OA cartilage explants (195), RAW.274 macrophages (196), lapine meniscal cells (197), and human OA meniscus explants (198). The presence of NO may decrease PGs in arthritis, which, in turn, may diminish the extent of the inflammatory response.

Mechanically induced NO production can also affect the activity of the COX pathway. The NOS-2–selective inhibitor (1400W) enhances PGE_2 production in response to mechanical stress. Likewise, inhibition of NO enhances PGE_2 production in human osteoarthritic articular cartilage and lipopolysaccharide-stimulated macrophages (195,199). These findings have important implications concerning the possible use of NOS-2 inhibitors to treat joint disease (200); inhibition of NOS-2 could potentially increase the inflammatory response of the chondrocytes due to a "superinduction" of PGE_2. Although the mechanism of this interaction is not fully understood, inhibition of PGE_2 production by NO may be due to decreased expression and nitration of the tyrosine residue (Tyr^{385}) of COX-2 (63). NO can also inhibit the translocation of COX-2 to a cytosolic compartment that favors enzyme activity (201).

In contrast, inhibition of NOS in bone may inhibit COX. Inhibition of bone NOS activity prevents PGE_2 production in response to fluid flow (149). In addition, the nonselective COX inhibitor, indomethacin, and the selective prostacyclin synthase inhibitor, 15-hydroperoxyeicosatetraenoic acid, inhibit loading-induced NO production in bone (148,202). Cytochrome P450 may be the level of interaction of the two pathways (203) because in bone, cytochrome P450 activity is responsible for the release of PGI_2 and P450 reductase activity is responsible for the production of NO.

A better understanding of the interactions between the NOS and COX pathways may provide insights into the potentially "protective" role of NO in arthritis. The selective NOS-2 inhibitor N[6]-(iminoethyl)-L-lysine can exacerbate joint disease in streptococcal cell wall–induced arthritis in rats, whereas L-NMMA N[G]-monomethyl-L-arginine, monoacetate salt, a nonselective inhibitor of both constitutive and inducible forms of NOS, prevents intraarticular accumulation of leukocytes, joint swelling, and bone erosion (83). The site of NO production may influence the acute inflammatory response *in vivo* because local production of NO may have a protective role, whereas systemically produced NO may be destructive (85). In other studies, NOS inhibitors decreased PGE_2 production (204) or had no effect on the COX pathway (205).

Effects of the Nitric Oxide Synthase Pathway on the Lipoxygenase Pathway

Leukotrienes are potent inflammatory mediators derived from arachidonic acid and, like other prostanoids, have been implicated as mediators in arthritis. Lipoxygenase (LOX) is the rate-limiting enzyme in leukotriene production. Production of LTB_4 induces a complex cascade of molecular and cellular events that ultimately recruits cells from the immune system to the sites of inflammation.

Mice deficient in 5-LOX–activating protein (and, as a consequence, in LTB_4 synthesis) are protected from developing collagen-induced arthritis (206). LTB_4 in synovial fluids from patients with active RA is fivefold higher than that from patients with OA (207,208). LTB_4 is a potent chemoattractant of neutrophils (209) and also promotes adhesion of neutrophils to vascular endothelium (210). Neutrophils are found in large numbers in synovial fluids and are postulated to be involved in cartilage and bone erosion in RA (211,212). LTB_4-receptor antagonists can inhibit collagen-induced arthritis in mice (213).

Many cell types associated with joint inflammation can produce leukotrienes (207,214,215). There is limited evidence, however, that articular chondrocytes produce leukotrienes. Articular cartilage can express mRNA for 5-LOX and 12-LOX in response to fatty acids and IL-1 (216) and LTB_4 at a barely detectable level in response to IL-1 (217). If mechanical compression is applied to articular cartilage explants in the presence of the NOS-2–inhibitor 1400W, LTB_4 is produced in sufficient quantity to elicit a chemotactic response (218). LOX protein, but not LTB_4, is detected in response to mechanical compression without a NOS-2 inhibitor. This finding suggests that NO may regulate the enzymatic activity of preformed LOX and, thus, diminish LTB_4 production. This effect of NO on LOX and LTB_4 production would be antiinflammatory and would have a protective role in arthritis.

Reports of failure of NOS-2 selective inhibitors to improve experimental models of arthritis (83) could be due to the enhanced production of the prostanoids LTB_4 or PGE_2 secondary to a release of the NO-mediated block of COX and LOX activity. NOS-2 is the isoform of NOS thought to be responsible for excessive and autotoxic levels of NO in chronic inflammatory lesions (38,84). However, it is now becoming evident that NOS-2–produced NO is protective or that NOS-1/NOS-3 are also involved in tissue injury, or both (83). Administration of NOS-2 inhibitors can be proinflammatory in the carrageenin-induced pleurisy model, partially due to increased production of LTB_4 (85). Similarly, models of experimental allergic encephalitis (multiple sclerosis) in NOS-2 knockout mice show disease worsening (219).

A potential mechanism for the interplay between the NOS, COX, and LOX pathways is the formation of the cyclopentenone prostanoids that are among the endogenous activators of a class of nuclear receptors, the peroxisome proliferator-activated gamma receptors (PPARγ) (220,221). PPARγ can modulate transcription of genes that regulate lipid metabolism, as well as genes involved in inflammation (128). Mice with PPARα disruption have a prolonged response to inflammation induced by LTB_4 (221). However, activation of PPARγ can also be antiinflammatory (127–129).

CONCLUSION

The joint functions in a dynamic environment, with a critical level and pattern of mechanical stress required to maintain the balance of cartilage synthesis and breakdown. With RA, this balance may be disrupted because of the effects of proinflammatory mediators, as well as because of altered biomechanics from damage of articular structures. Better understanding of the interactions between the mechanical environment and inflammatory response may lead to new approaches for treatment and prevention.

ACKNOWLEDGMENTS

Supported by Veterans' Administration Medical Research and National Institutes of Health grants AR48182, AR47920, AR50245, and AG15768.

REFERENCES

1. Heinegard D, Oldberg A. Structure and biology of cartilage and bone noncollagenous macromolecules. *FASEB J* 1989;3:2042–2051.
2. Mow VC, Ratcliffe A, Poole AR. Cartilage and diathrodial joints as paradigms for hierarchical materials and structures. *Biomaterials* 1992;13:67–97.
3. Hunziker EB, Michel M, Studer D. Ultrastructure of adult human articular cartilage matrix after cryotechnical processing. *Microsc Res Tech* 1997;37:271–284.
4. Poole AR, Flint MH, Beaumont BW. Chondrons extracted from canine tibial cartilage: preliminary report on their isolation and structure. *J Orthop Res* 1988;6:408–419.
5. Armstrong CG, Bahrani AS, Gardner DL. In vitro measurement of articular cartilage deformations in the intact human hip joint under load. *J Bone Joint Surg* 1979;61:744–755.
6. Ateshian GA, Lai WM, Zhu WB, et al. An asymptotic solution for the contact of two biphasic cartilage layers. *J Biomech* 1994;27:1347–1360.
7. Mow VC, Kuei SC, Lai WM, et al. Biphasic creep and stress relaxation of articular cartilage in compression: theory and experiments. *J Biomech Eng* 1980;102:73–84.
8. Guilak F, Sah R, Setton LA. Physical regulation of cartilage metabolism. In: Mow VC, Hayes WC, eds. *Basic orthopaedic biomechanics*. Philadelphia: Lippincott–Raven, 1997:179–208.
9. Minor MA. Exercise in the treatment of osteoarthritis. *Osteoarthritis* 1999;25:397–415.
10. Helminen HJ, Jurvelin J, Kiviranta I, et al. Joint loading effects on articular cartilage: a historical review. In: Helminen HJ, Kiviranta I, Tammi M, et al., eds. *Joint loading: biology and health of articular structures*. Bristol: Wright and Sons, 1987:1–46.
11. Howell DS, Treadwell BV, Trippel SB. Etiopathogenesis of osteoarthritis. In: Moskowitz RW, Howell DS, Goldberg VM, et al., eds. *Osteoarthritis, diagnosis and medical/surgical management*. Philadelphia: WB Saunders, 1992:233–252.
12. Akeson W, Amiel D, Abel M, et al. Effects of immobilization on joints. *Clin Orthop* 1987;219:28–37.
13. Palmoski M, Perricone E, Brandt K. Development and reversal of a proteoglycan aggregation defect in normal canine knee cartilage after immobilization. *Arthritis Rheum* 1979;22:508–517.
14. Lammi MJ, Hakkinen TP, Parkkinen JJ, et al. Adaptation of canine femoral head articular cartilage to long distance running exercise in young beagles. *Ann Rheum Dis* 1993;52:369–377.
15. Kraus VB. Pathogenesis and treatment of osteoarthritis. *Med Clin North Am* 1997;81:85–112.
16. Lane N, Buckwalter J. Exercise: a cause of osteoarthritis? *Rheum Dis Clin North Am* 1993;19:617–633.
17. Bachrach NM, Valhmu WB, Stazzone E, et al. Changes in proteoglycan synthesis of chondrocytes in articular cartilage are associated with the time-dependent changes in their mechanical environment. *J Biomech* 1995;28:1561–1569.
18. Buschmann MD, Gluzband YA, Grodzinsky AJ, et al. Mechanical compression modulates matrix biosynthesis in chondrocyte/agarose culture. *J Cell Sci* 1995;108:1497–1508.

19. Sah RL, Grodzinsky AJ, Plaas AH, et al. Effects of tissue compression on the hyaluronate-binding properties of newly synthesized proteoglycans in cartilage explants. *Biochem J* 1990;267:803–808.
20. Torzilli PA, Grigiene R. Continuous cyclic load reduces proteoglycan release from articular cartilage. *Osteoarthritis Cartilage* 1998;6:260–268.
21. Farquhar T, Todhunter RJ, Fubini SL, et al. Effect of methylprednisolone and mechanical loading on canine articular cartilage in explant culture. *Osteoarthritis Cartilage* 1996;4:55–62.
22. Guilak F, Meyer BC, Ratcliffe A, et al. The effects of matrix compression on proteoglycan metabolism in articular cartilage explants. *Osteoarthritis Cartilage* 1994;2:91–101.
23. Jeffrey JE, Gregory DW, Aspden RM. Matrix damage and chondrocyte viability following a single impact load on articular cartilage. *Arch Biochem Biophys* 1995;322:87–96.
24. Repo RU, Finlay JB. Survival of articular cartilage after controlled impact. *J Bone Joint Surg* 1977;59:1068–1076.
25. Borrelli J, Torzilli PA, Grigiene R, et al. Effect of impact load on articular cartilage: development of an intra-articular fracture model. *J Orthop Trauma* 1997;11:319–326.
26. Torzilli PA, Grigiene R, Borrelli J, et al. Effect of impact load on articular cartilage: cell metabolism and viability, and matrix water content. *J Biomech Eng* 1999;121:433–441.
27. Loening AM, James IE, Levenston ME, et al. Injurious mechanical compression of bovine articular cartilage induces chondrocyte apoptosis. *Arch Biochem Biophys* 2000;381:205–212.
28. Steinmeyer J, Knue S. The proteoglycan metabolism of mature bovine articular cartilage explants superimposed to continuously applied cyclic mechanical loading. *Biochem Biophys Res Commun* 1997;240:216–221.
29. Lucchinetti E, Adams CS, Horton WEJ, et al. Cartilage viability after repetitive loading: a preliminary report. *Osteoarthritis Cartilage* 2002;10:71–81.
30. Gray ML, Pizzanelli AM, Lee RC, et al. Kinetics of the chondrocyte biosynthetic response to compressive load and release. *Biochim Biophys Acta* 1989;991:415–425.
31. Kim YJ, Sah RL, Grodzinsky AJ, et al. Mechanical regulation of cartilage biosynthetic behavior: physical stimuli. *Arch Biochem Biophys* 1994;311:1–12.
32. Schneiderman R, Keret D, Maroudas A. Effects of mechanical and osmotic pressure on the rate of glycosaminoglycan synthesis in the human adult femoral head cartilage: an in vitro study. *J Orthop Res* 1986;4:393–408.
33. Guilak F, Ratcliffe A, Lane N, et al. Mechanical and biochemical changes in the superficial zone of articular cartilage in canine experimental osteoarthritis. *J Orthop Res* 1994;12:474–484.
34. Evans CH, Watkins SC, Stefanovic-Racic M. Nitric oxide and cartilage metabolism. *Methods Enzymol* 1996;269:75–88.
35. Lotz M. The role of nitric oxide in articular cartilage damage. *Rheum Dis Clin North Am* 1999;25:269–282.
36. Hayashi T, Abe E, Yamate T, et al. Nitric oxide production by superficial and deep articular chondrocytes. *Arthritis Rheum* 1997;40:261–269.
37. Van't Hof RJ, Ralston SH. Nitric oxide and bone. *Immunology* 2001;103:255–261.
38. Clancy RM, Amin AR, Abramson SB. The role of nitric oxide in inflammation and immunity. *Arthritis Rheum* 1998;41:1141–1151.
39. Weinberg JB, Granger DL, Pisetsky DS, et al. The role of nitric oxide in the pathogenesis of spontaneous murine autoimmune disease: increased nitric oxide production and nitric oxide synthase expression in MRL-lpr/lpr mice, and reduction of spontaneous glomerulonephritis and arthritis by orally administered NG-monomethyl-L-arginine. *J Exp Med* 1994;179:651–660.
40. McCartney-Francis N, Allen JB, Mizel DE, et al. Suppression of arthritis by an inhibitor of nitric oxide synthase. *J Exp Med* 1993;178:749–754.
41. Stefanovic-Racic N, Meyers K, Meschter C, et al. N-Monomethyl arginine, an inhibitor of nitric oxide synthase, suppresses the development of adjuvant induced arthritis in rats. *Arthritis Rheum* 1994;7:1062–1069.
42. Cannon GW, Openshaw SJ, Hibbs JB, et al. Nitric oxide production during adjuvant-induced and collagen-induced arthritis. *Arthritis Rheum* 1996;39:1677–1684.
43. Ueki Y, Miyake S, Tominaga Y, et al. Increased nitric oxide levels in patients with rheumatoid arthritis. *J Rheumatol* 1996;23:230–236.
44. Grabowski PS, England AJ, Dykhuizen R, et al. Elevated nitric oxide production in rheumatoid arthritis. Detection using the fasting urinary nitrate: creatinine ratio. *Arthritis Rheum* 1996;39:643–647.
45. McInnes IB, Leung BP, Field M, et al. Production of nitric oxide in the synovial membrane of rheumatoid and osteoarthritis patients. *J Exp Med* 1996;184:1519–1524.
46. St Clair EW, Wilkinson WE, Lang T, et al. Increased expression of blood mononuclear cell nitric oxide synthase type 2 in rheumatoid arthritis patients. *J Exp Med* 1996;39:1173–1178.
47. Hauselmann HJ, Stefanovic-Racic M, Michel BA, et al. Differences in nitric oxide production by superficial and deep human articular chondrocytes: implications for proteoglycan turnover in inflammatory joint diseases. *J Immunol* 1998;160:1444–1448.
48. Pelletier JP, Jovanovic D, Fernandes JC, et al. Reduction in the structural changes of experimental osteoarthritis by a nitric oxide inhibitor. *Osteoarthritis Cartilage* 1999;7:416–418.
49. Studer RK, Levicoff E, Georgesc H, et al. Nitric oxide inhibits chondrocyte response to IGF1: inhibition of IGF-1Rbeta tyrosine phosphorylation. *Am J Physiol* 2000;279:C961–C969.
50. Stefanovic-Racic M, Morales TI, Taskiran D, et al. The role of nitric oxide in proteoglycan turnover by bovine articular cartilage organ cultures. *J Immunol* 1996;156:1213–1220.
51. Stefanovic-Racic M, Mollers MO, Miller LA, et al. Nitric oxide and proteoglycan turnover in rabbit articular cartilage. *J Orthop Res* 1997;15:442–449.
52. Lo YYC, Conquer JA, Grinstein S, et al. Interleukin-1-beta induction of *C-fos* and collagenase expression in articular chondrocytes—involvement of reactive oxygen species. *J Cell Biochem* 1998;69:19–29.
53. Sasaki K, Hattori T, Fujisawa T, et al. Nitric oxide mediates interleukin-1-induced gene expression of matrix metalloproteinases and basic fibroblast growth factor in cultured rabbit articular chondrocytes. *J Biochem* 1998;123:431–439.
54. Johnson K, Jung A, Murphy A, et al. Mitochondrial oxidative phosphorylation is a downstream regulator of nitric oxide effects on chondrocyte matrix synthesis and mineralization. *Arthritis Rheum* 2000;43:1560–1570.
55. Tomita M, Sato EF, Nishikawa M, et al. Nitric oxide regulates mitochondrial respiration and functions of articular chondrocytes. *Arthritis Rheum* 2001;44:96–104.
56. Terkeltaub R, Johnson K, Murphy A, et al. Invited review: the mitochondrion in osteoarthritis [Review]. *Mitochondrion* 2002;1:301–319.
57. Nuki G. Osteoarthritis: a problem of joint failure. *Zeitschrift fur Rheumatologie* 1999;58:142–147.
58. Sandell LJ, Aigner T. Articular cartilage and changes in arthritis. An introduction: cell biology of osteoarthritis. *Arthritis Res* 2001;3:107–113.
59. Moncada S, Erusalimsky JD. Does nitric oxide modulate mitochondrial energy generation and apoptosis? *Nat Rev Mol Cell Biol* 2002;3:214–220.
60. Granger DL, Lehninger AL, Hibbs JB Jr. Aberrant oxygen metabolism in neoplastic cells injured by cytotoxic macrophages. *Adv Exp Med Biol* 1985;184:51–63.
61. Richter C, Schweizer M, Cossarizza, A, et al. Control of apoptosis by cellular ATP levels. *FEBS Lett* 1996;378:107–110.
62. Del Carlo M Jr., Loeser RF. Nitric oxide-mediated chondrocyte cell death requires the generation of additional reactive oxygen species. *Arthritis Rheum* 2002;46:394–403.
63. Clancy RM, Varenika B, Huang W, et al. Nitric oxide synthase/COX cross-talk: nitric oxide activates COX-1 but inhibits COX-2–derived prostaglandin production. *J Immunol* 2000;165:1582–1587.
64. Vane JR, Mitchell JA, Appleton I, et al. Inducible isoforms of cyclooxygenase and nitric-oxide synthase in inflammation. *Proc Natl Acad Sci U S A* 1994;91:2046–2050.
65. O'Banion M. Cyclooxygenase-2: molecular biology, pharmacology, and neurobiology. *Crit Rev Neurobiol* 1999;13:45–82.
66. Vane JR, Botting RM. Mechanism of action of antiinflammatory drugs. *Int J Tissue React* 1998;20:3–15.
67. Harris E. Rheumatoid arthritis: pathophysiology and implications for therapy. *N Engl J Med* 1990;322:1277.
68. Crofford LJ, Wilder RL, Ristimaki AP, et al. Cyclooxygenase-1 and -2 expression in rheumatoid synovial tissues: effects of interleukin-1beta, phorbol ester, and corticosteroids. *J Clin Invest* 1994;93:1095–1101.
69. Abramson SB. The role of COX-2 produced by cartilage in arthritis. *Osteoarthritis Cartilage* 1999;7:380–381.
70. Anderson GD, Hauser SD, McGarity KL, et al. Selective inhibition of cyclooxygenase (COX)-2 reverses inflammation and expression of COX-2 and interleukin-6 in rat adjuvant arthritis. *J Clin Invest* 1996;97:2672–2679.
71. Penning TD, Talley JJ, Bertenshaw SR, et al. Synthesis and biological evaluation of the 1,5–diarylpyrazole class of cyclooxygenase-2 inhibitors: identification of 4–[5–(4–methylphenyl)-3–(trifluoromethyl)-1H-pyrazol-1–yl]benzenesulfonamide (SC-58635, celecoxib). *J Med Chem* 1997;40:1347–1365.
72. Coleman R, Kennedy I, Humphrey P, et al. Prostanoids and their receptors. In: Comprehensive medicinal chemistry. Membranes and receptors. Oxford: Pergamon Press, 1990:643–714.
73. Coleman R, Smith W, Narumiya S. Classification of prostanoid receptors: properties, distribution, and structure of the receptors and their subtypes. *Pharmacol Rev* 1994;46:205–229.
74. Narumiya S, Sugimoto Y, Ushikubi F. Prostanoid receptors: structures, properties, and functions. *Physiol Rev* 1999;79:1193–1226.
75. Versteeg H, van Bergen en Henegouwen P, van Deventer S, et al. Cyclooxygenase-dependent signalling: molecular events and consequences. *FEBS Lett* 1999;445:1–5.
76. Akhter M, Cullen D, Gong G, et al. Biomechanical properties of bone in prostaglandin EP2 knockout mice. *Trans Orthop Res Soc* 2000:743.
77. de Brum-Fernandes AJ, Morisset S, Bkaily G, et al. Characterization of the PGE_2 receptor subtype in bovine chondrocytes in culture. *Br J Pharmacol* 1996;118:1597–1604.
78. Pelletier JP, Jovanovic D, Fernandes JC, et al. Reduced progression of experimental osteoarthritis *in vivo* by selective inhibition of inducible nitric oxide synthase. *Arthritis Rheum* 1998;41:1275–1286.
79. Ialenti A, Moncada S, DiRosa M. Modulation of adjuvant arthritis by endogenous nitric oxide. *Br J Pharmacol* 1993;110:701–706.
80. Connor JR, Manning PT, Settle SL, et al. Suppression of adjuvant-induced arthritis by selective inhibition of inducible nitric oxide synthase. *Eur J Pharmacol* 1995;273:15–24.
81. Stefanovic-Racic M, Meyers K, Meschter C, et al. Comparison of the nitric oxide synthase inhibitors methylarginine and aminoguanidine as prophylactic and therapeutic agents in rat adjuvant arthritis. *J Rheumatol* 1995;22:1922–1928.
82. Visco DM, Fletcher DS, Orevillo CJ, et al. NOS-2 deficient mice are susceptible to collagen-induced arthritis. *Trans Orthop Res Soc* 1997;22:416.

83. McCartney-Francis NL, Song X, Mizel DE, et al. Selective inhibition of inducible nitric oxide synthase exacerbates erosive joint disease. *J Immunol* 2001;166:2734–2740.
84. Bogdan C. The multiplex function of nitric oxide in (auto)immunity. *J Exp Med* 1998;187:1361–1365.
85. Paul-Clark MJ, Gilroy DW, Willis D, et al. Nitric oxide synthase inhibitors have opposite effects on acute inflammation depending on their route of administration. *J Immunol* 2001;166:1169–1177.
86. Willoughby DA, Colville-Nash PR, Seed MP. Inflammation, prostaglandins, and loss of function. *J Lipid Mediat* 1993;6:287–293.
87. Blanco FJ, Lotz M. IL-1–induced nitric oxide inhibits chondrocyte proliferation via PGE_2. *Exp Cell Res* 1995;218:319–325.
88. Di Battista JA, Martel-Pelletier J, Fujimoto N, et al. Prostaglandins E_2 and E_1 inhibit cytokine-induced metalloprotease expression in human synovial fibroblasts. Mediation by cyclic-AMP signalling pathway. *Lab Invest* 1994;71:270–278.
89. Milano S, Arcoleo F, Dieli M, et al. Prostaglandin E_2 regulates inducible nitric oxide synthase in the murine macrophage cell line J774. *Prostaglandins* 1995;49:105–115.
90. van den Berg WB and Bresnihan B. Pathogenesis of joint damage in rheumatoid arthritis: evidence of a dominant role for interleukin-1. *Baillieres Best Pract Res Clin Rheumatol* 1999;13:577–597.
91. Dingle J, Page Thomas D, Hazelman B. The role of cytokines in arthritic diseases: in vitro and in vivo measurements of cartilage degradation. *Int J Tissue React* 1987;9:349–354.
92. van den Berg WB. Lessons for joint destruction from animal models. *Curr Opin Rheumatol* 1997;9:221–228.
93. Pelletier JP, DiBattista JA, Roughley P, et al. Cytokines and inflammation in cartilage degradation. *Rheum Dis Clin North Am* 1993;19:545–568.
94. Evans CH, Ghivizzani SC, Robbins PD. Blocking cytokines with genes. *J Leukoc Biol* 1998;64:55–61.
95. van den Berg WB. The role of cytokines and growth factors in cartilage destruction in osteoarthritis and rheumatoid arthritis. *Z Rheumatol* 1999;58: 1136–1341.
96. Cernanec J, Guilak F, Weinberg JB, et al. Influence of hypoxia and reoxygenation on cytokine-induced production of proinflammatory mediators in articular cartilage. *Arthritis Rheum* 2002;46:968–975.
97. Dudhia J, Wheeler-Jones C, Bayliss M. Transient activation of P42/ P44MAPK by IL-1alpha is enhanced by a low oxygen tension in human articular cartilage. *Trans Orthop Res Soc* 2000:0943.
98. Grimshaw MJ, Mason RM. Bovine articular chondrocyte function in vitro depends upon oxygen tension. *Osteoarthritis Cartilage* 2000;8:386–392.
99. Silver IA. Measurement of pH and ionic composition of pericellular sites. *Philos Trans R Soc Lond B Biol Sci* 1975;271:261–272.
100. Bywaters EGL. The metabolism of joint tissues. *J Pathol Bact* 1937;44:247–268.
101. Stefanovic-Racic M, Stadler J, Georgescu HI, et al. Nitric oxide and energy production in articular chondrocytes. *J Cell Physiol* 1994;159:274–280.
102. Cao M, Westerhausen-Larson A, Niyibizi C, et al. Nitric oxide inhibits the synthesis of type-II collagen without altering Col2A1 mRNA abundance: prolyl hydroxylase as a possible target. *Biochem J* 1997;324:305–310.
103. Studer RK, Georgescu HI, Miller LA, et al. Inhibition of transforming growth factor beta production by nitric oxide-treated chondrocytes—implications for matrix synthesis. *Arthritis Rheum* 1999;42:248–257.
104. Gassner R, Buckley M, Georgescu R, et al. Cyclic tensile stress exerts antiinflammatory actions on chondrocytes by inhibiting inducible nitric oxide synthase. *J Immunol* 1999;163:2187.
105. Xu Z, Buckley M, Evans C, et al. Cyclic tensile strain acts as an antagonist of IL1beta actions in chondrocytes. *J Immunol* 2000;165:453–460.
106. Agarwal S, Long P, Gassner R, et al. Cyclic tensile strain suppresses catabolic effects of interleukin-1beta in fibrochondrocytes from the temporomandibular joint. *Arthritis Rheum* 2001;44:608–617.
107. Fujisawa T, Hattori T, Takahashi K, et al. Cyclic mechanical stress induces extracellular matrix degradation in cultured chondrocytes via gene expression of matrix metalloproteinases and interleukin-1. *J Biochem* 1999;125:966–975.
108. Shin SJ, Fermor B, Weinberg JB, et al. Regulation of matrix turnover in meniscal explants: the role of mechanical stress, interleukin 1 and nitric oxide. *J Appl Physiol* 2003;95:308–313.
109. Upton ML, Chen J, Guilak F, et al. Differential effects of static and dynamic compression on meniscal cell gene expression. *J Orthop Res* 2003;21:963–969.
110. Fermor B, Weinberg JB, Pisetsky DS, et al. The effects of static and intermittent compression on nitric oxide production in articular cartilage explants. *J Orthop Res* 2001;19:72–80.
111. Das P, Schurman DJ, Smith RL. Nitric oxide and G proteins mediate the response of bovine articular chondrocytes to fluid-induced shear. *J Orthop Res* 1997;15:87–93.
112. Lee DA, Frean SP, Lees P, et al. Dynamic mechanical compression influences nitric oxide production by articular chondrocytes seeded in agarose. *Biochem Biophys Res Commun* 1998;251:580–585.
113. Millward-Sadler S, Wright M, Lee H, et al. Integrin-regulated secretion of interleukin 4: a novel pathway of mechanotransduction in human articular chondrocytes. *J Cell Biol* 1999;145:183–189.
114. Clancy RM, Rediske J, Tang X, et al. Outside-in signaling in the chondrocyte. Nitric oxide disrupts fibronectin-induced assembly of a subplasmalemmal actin/rho A/focal adhesion kinase signaling complex. *J Clin Invest* 1997;100: 1789–1796.
115. Taskirin D, Stefanovic-Racic M, Georgescu HI, et al. Nitric oxide mediates suppression of cartilage proteoglycan synthesis by interleukin-1. *Biochem Biophys Res Commun* 1994;200:142–148.
116. Jarvinen T, Moilanen T, Jarvinen T, et al. Nitric oxide mediates interleukin-1 induced inhibition of glycosaminoglycan synthesis in rat articular cartilage. *Med Inflamm* 1995;4:107–111.
117. Hauselmann H, Oppliger L, Michel B, et al. Nitric oxide and proteoglycan biosynthesis by human articular chondrocytes in alginate culture. *FEBS Lett* 1994;352:361–364.
118. Stefanovic-Racic M, Watkins SC, Kang R, et al. Identification of inducible nitric oxide synthase in human osteoarthritic cartilage. *Trans Ortho Res Soc* 1996;21:534.
119. Fermor B, Weinberg JB, Pisetsky DS, et al. Induction of cyclooxygenase-2 by mechanical stress through a nitric oxide-regulated pathway. *Osteoarthritis Cartilage* 2002;10:792–798.
120. Sah RL, Kim YJ, Doong JY, et al. Biosynthetic response of cartilage explants to dynamic compression. *J Orthop Res* 1989;7:619–636.
121. Dingle J. Cartilage maintenance in osteoarthritis: interaction of cytokines, NSAID and prostaglandins in articular cartilage damage and repair. *J Rheumatol Suppl* 1991;28:30.
122. Lowe GN, Fu YH, McDougall S, et al. Effects of prostaglandins on deoxyribonucleic acid and aggrecan synthesis in the RCJ 3.1C5.18 chondrocyte cell line: role of second messengers. *Endocrinology* 1996;137:2208–2216.
123. Di Battista JA, Dore S, Martel-Pelletier J, et al. Prostaglandin E_2 stimulates incorporation of proline into collagenase digestible proteins in human articular chondrocytes: identification of an effector autocrine loop involving insulin-like growth factor I. *Mol Cell Endocrinol* 1996;123:27–35.
124. Stockwell RA. Structure and function of the chondrocyte under mechanical stress. In: Helminen HJ, Kiviranta I, Tammi M, eds. *Joint loading: biology and health of articular structures*. Bristol: John Wright & Sons, 1987:126–148.
125. Guilak F, Zell RA, Erickson GR, et al. Mechanically induced calcium waves in articular chondrocytes are inhibited by gadolinium and amiloride. *J Orthop Res* 1999;17:421–429.
126. Gijon MA, Leslie CC. Regulation of arachidonic acid release and cytosolic phospholipase A_2 activation. *J Leukoc Biol* 1999;65:330–336.
127. Rossi A, Kapahi P, Natoli G, et al. Antiinflammatory cyclopentenone prostaglandins are direct inhibitors of IkappaB kinase. *Nature* 2000;403:103–108.
128. Ricote M, Li AC, Willson TM, et al. The peroxisome proliferator-activated receptor-gamma is a negative regulator of macrophage activation. *Nature* 1998;391:79–82.
129. Jiang C, Ting AT, Seed B. PPAR-gamma agonists inhibit production of monocyte inflammatory cytokines. *Nature* 1998;391:82–86.
130. Mbalaviele G, Abu-Amer Y, Meng A, et al. Activation of peroxisome proliferator-activated receptor-gamma pathway inhibits osteoclast differentiation. *J Biol Chem* 2000;275:14388–14393.
131. Burger EH, Klein-Nulend J. Mechanotransduction in bone—role of the lacuno-canalicular network. *FASEB J* 1999;13:S101–S112.
132. Duncan RL, Turner CH. Mechanotransduction and the functional response of bone to strain. *Calcif Tissue Int* 1995;57:344–358.
133. Lanyon LE. Osteocytes, strain detection, bone modeling and remodeling. *Calcif Tissue Int* 1993;53:102–107.
134. Ehrlich PJ, Lanyon LE. Mechanical strain and bone cell function: a review. *Osteoporos Int* 2002;13:688–700.
135. Ajubi NE, Klein-Nulend J, Nijweide PJ, et al. Pulsating fluid flow increases prostaglandin production by cultured chicken osteocytes—a cytoskeleton-dependent process. *Biochem Biophys Res Commun* 1996;225:62–68.
136. Klein-Nulend J, Burger EH, Semeins CM, et al. Pulsating fluid flow stimulates prostaglandin release and inducible prostaglandin G/H synthase mRNA expression in primary mouse bone cells. *J Bone Miner Res* 1997;12:45–51.
137. Forwood MR, Owan I, Takano Y, et al. Increased bone formation in rat tibiae after a single short period of dynamic loading in vivo. *Am J Physiol Endocrinol Metab* 1996;270:E419–E423.
138. Pead MJ, Lanyon LE. Indomethacin modulation of load-related stimulation of new bone formation in vivo. *Calcif Tissue Int* 1989;45:34–40.
139. Chow JWM, Chambers TJ. Indomethacin has distinct early and late actions on bone formation induced by mechanical stimulation. *Am J Physiol Endocrinol Metab* 1994;267:E287–E292.
140. Forwood M. Inducible cyclo-oxygenase (COX-2) mediates the induction of bone formation by mechanical loading in vivo. *J Bone Miner Res* 1996;11:1688–1693.
141. Cui L, Ma YF, Yao W. Cancellous bone of aged rats maintains its capacity to respond vigorously to the anabolic effects of prostaglandin E_2 by modeling-dependent bone gain. *J Bone Miner Metab* 2001;19:29–37.
142. Yao W, Jee WS, Zhou H. Anabolic effect of prostaglandin E_2 on cortical bone of aged male rats comes mainly from modeling-dependent bone gain. *Bone* 1999;25:697–702.
143. Tang LY, Cullen DM, Yee JA, et al. Prostaglandin E_2 increases the skeletal responses to mechanical loading. *J Bone Miner Res* 1997;12:276–282.
144. Reich KM, Gay CV, Frangos JA. Fluid shear stress as a mediator of osteoblast cyclic adenosine monophosphate production. *J Cell Physiol* 1990;143:100–104.
145. Binderman I, Zor U, Kaye AM, et al. The transduction of mechanical force into biochemical events in bone cells may involve activation of phospholipase A_2. *Calcif Tissue Int* 1988;42:261–266.
146. Fermor B, Gundle R, Evans M, et al. Primary human osteoblast proliferation and PGE_2 release in response to mechanical strain in vitro. *Bone* 1998;22:637–643.
147. Rawlinson SC, el-Haj AJ, Minter SL, et al. Loading-related increases in prostaglandin production in cores of adult canine cancellous bone in vitro: a role for prostacyclin in adaptive bone remodeling? *J Bone Miner Res* 1991;6:1345–1351.
148. Pitsillides AA, Rawlinson SCF, Suswillo FL, et al. Mechanical strain-induced

NO production by bone cells: a possible role in adaptive bone (re)modelling. *FASEB J* 1995;9:1614–1622.
149. Klein-Nulend J, Semeins CM, Ajubi NE, et al. Pulsating fluid flow increases nitric oxide (NO) synthesis by osteocytes but not periosteal fibroblasts—correlation with prostaglandin upregulation. *Biochem Biophys Res Commun* 1995;217:640–648.
150. Harrell A, Dekel S, Binderman I. Biochemical effect of mechanical stress on cultured bone cells. *Calcif Tissue Res* 1977;22:202–207.
151. Johnson DL, McAllister TN, Frangos JA. Fluid flow stimulates rapid and continuous release of nitric oxide in osteoblasts. *Am J Physiol* 1996;271:E205–E208.
152. McAllister TN, Frangos JA. Steady and transient fluid shear stress stimulate NO release in osteoblasts through distinct biochemical pathways. *J Bone Miner Res* 1999;14:930–936.
153. Klein-Nulend J, Helfrich MH, Sterck JG, et al. Nitric oxide response to shear stress by human bone cell cultures is endothelial nitric oxide synthase dependent. *Biochem Biophys Res Commun* 1998;250:108–114.
154. Zaman G, Pitsillides AA, Rawlinson SC, et al. Mechanical strain stimulates nitric oxide production by rapid activation of endothelial nitric oxide synthase in osteocytes. *J Bone Miner Res* 1999;14:1123–1131.
155. Turner CH, Takano Y, Owan I, et al. Nitric oxide inhibitor L-NAME suppresses mechanically induced bone formation in rats. *Am J Physiol* 1996;270:E634–E639.
156. Chow JW, Fox SW, Lean JM, et al. Role of nitric oxide and prostaglandins in mechanically induced bone formation. *J Bone Miner Res* 1998;13:1039–1044.
157. Chambers TJ, Fox S, Jagger CJ, et al. The role of prostaglandins and nitric oxide in the response of bone to mechanical forces. *Osteoarthritis Cartilage* 1999;7:422–423.
158. Bonucci E. New knowledge on the origin, function, and fate of osteoclasts. *Clin Orthop* 1981;158:252.
159. Mundy GR. Monocyte-macrophage system and bone resorption. *Lab Invest* 1983;49:119.
160. Hall TJ, Chambers TJ. Molecular aspects of osteoclast function. *Inflamm Res* 1996;l45:1.
161. Hume DA, Loutit JF, Gordon S. The mononuclear phagocyte system of the mouse defined by immunohistochemical localization of antigen f4/80: macrophages of bone and associated connective tissue. *J Cell Sci* 1984;66:189.
162. Fallon MD, Teitelbaum SL, Kahn AJ. Multinucleation enhances macrophage-mediated bone resorption. *Lab Invest* 1983;49:159.
163. Teitelbaum SL, Kahn AJ. Mononuclear phagocytes, osteoclasts and bone resorption. *Mineral Electrolyte Metabolism* 1980;3:2.
164. Wiktor JW, Bartocci A, Ferrante AWJ, et al. Total absence of colony stimulating factor 1 in the macrophage-deficient osteopetrotic (op/op) mouse. *Proc Natl Acad Sci U S A* 1990;87:4328.
165. Witmer-Pack MD, Hughes DA, Schuler G, et al. Identification of macrophages and dendritic cells in the osteopetrotic (op/op) mouse. *J Cell Sci* 1993;104:1021.
166. Marks SCJ, Seifert MF. The development and structure of osteoclasts in osteopetrosis. In: Butler ED, ed. *The chemistry and biology of mineralized tissues.* Birmingham: Ebsco Media, 1984.
167. Loutit JF, Nisbet NW. The origin of the osteoclast. *Immunobiology* 1982;161:193.
168. Chambers TJ, Magnus CJ. Calcitonin alters behaviour of isolated osteoclasts. *J Pathol* 1982;136:27.
169. Horton MA, Lewis D, McNulty K. Human fetal osteoclasts fail to express macrophage integrins. *Br J Exp Pathol* 1985;66:103.
170. Horton MA, Pringle JAS, Chambers TJ. Identification of human osteoclasts with monoclonal antibodies. *N Engl J Med* 1985;312:923.
171. Chambers TJ. Regulation of the differentiation and function of osteoclasts. *J Pathol* 2000;192:4.
172. Yasuda H, Shima N, Nakagawa N, et al. A novel molecular mechanism modulating osteoclast differentiation and function. *Bone* 1999;25:109.
173. Vailas AC, Zernicke RF, Matsuda J, et al. Adaptation of rat knee meniscus to prolonged exercise. *J Appl Physiol* 1986;60:1031–1104.
174. Djurasovic M, Aldridge JW, Grumbles R, et al. Knee joint immobilization decreases aggrecan gene expression in the meniscus. *Am J Sports Med* 1998;26:460–466.
175. Dowdy PA, Miniaci A, Arnoczky SP, et al. The effect of cast immobilization on meniscal healing. An experimental study in the dog. *Am J Sports Med* 1995;23:721–728.
176. Arnoczky SP, Warren RF, Kaplan N. Meniscal remodeling following partial meniscectomy—an experimental study in the dog. *Arthroscopy* 1985;1:247–252.
177. Carlson CS, Guilak F, Vail TP, et al. Articular cartilage damage following medial meniscectomy in dogs is predicted by synovial fluid biomarker levels. *J Orthop Res* 2002;20:92–100.
178. Elliott DM, Guilak F, Vail TP, et al. Tensile properties of articular cartilage are altered by meniscectomy in a canine model of osteoarthritis. *J Orthop Res* 2002;20:996–1002.
179. Fairbank TJ. Knee joint changes after meniscectomy. *J Bone Joint Surg* 1948;30B:664–670.
180. Moskowitz RW, Davis W, Sammarco J. Experimentally induced degenerative joint lesions following partial menisectomy in the rabbit. *Arthritis Rheum* 1973;16:397–405.
181. Roos H, Lauren M, Adalberth T, et al. Knee osteoarthritis after meniscectomy: prevalence of radiographic changes after twenty-one years, compared with matched controls. *Arthritis Rheum* 1998;41:687–693.
182. LeRoux MA, Arokoski J, Vail TP, et al. Simultaneous changes in the mechanical properties, quantitative collagen organization, and proteoglycan concentration of articular cartilage following canine meniscectomy. *J Orthop Res* 2000;18:383–392.
183. Levy IM, Torzilli PA, Warren RF. The effect of medial meniscectomy on anterior-posterior motion of the knee. *J Bone Joint Surg Am* 1982;64:883–888.
184. Setton LA, Guilak F, Hsu EW, et al. Biomechanical factors in tissue engineered meniscal repair. *Clin Orthop* 1999;367[Suppl]:S254–S272.
185. Fink C, Fermor B, Weinberg JB, et al. The effect of dynamic mechanical compression on nitric oxide production in the meniscus. *Osteoarthritis Cartilage* 2001;9:481–487.
186. Imler SM, Vanderploeg EJ, Hunter CJ, et al. Static and oscillatory compression modulate protein and proteoglycan synthesis by meniscal fibrochondrocytes. *Trans Orthop Res Soc* 2001;26:552.
187. Edwards JCW. The origin of type a synovial cells. *Immunobiology* 1982; 161:227.
188. Harris EDJ. Rheumatoid arthritis. Pathophysiology and implications for therapy. *N Engl J Med* 1990;322:1277.
189. Mulherin D, Fitzgerald O, Bresnihan B. Synovial tissue macrophage populations and articular damage in rheumatoid arthritis. *Arthritis Rheum* 1996;39:115.
190. Hirohata S, Yanagida T, Itoh K, et al. Accelerated generation of $CD14^+$ monocyte-lineage cells from the bone marrow of rheumatoid arthritis patients. *Arthritis Rheum* 1996;39:836.
191. Kinne RW, Schmidt-Weber CB, Hoppe R, et al. Long term amelioration of rat adjuvant arthritis following systemic elimination of macrophages by clodronate-containing liposomes. *Arthritis Rheum* 1995;38:1777.
192. Sakurai H, Kohsaka H, Liu MF. Nitric oxide production and inducible nitric oxide synthase expression in inflammatory arthritides. *J Clin Invest* 1995; 96:2357–2363.
193. Sun HB, Yokota H. Altered mRNA level of matrix metalloproteinase-13 in MH7A synovial cells under mechanical loading and unloading. *Bone* 2001; 28:399–403.
194. Kaarniranta K, Elo M, Sironen R, et al. Hsp70 Accumulation in chondrocytic cells exposed to high continuous hydrostatic pressure coincides with mRNA stabilization rather than transcriptional activation. *Proc Natl Acad Sci U S A* 1998;95:2319–2324.
195. Amin AR, Attur M, Patel RN, et al. Superinduction of cyclooxygenase-2 activity in human osteoarthritis-affected cartilage. Influence of nitric oxide. *J Clin Invest* 1997;99:1231–1237.
196. Weinberg JB. Nitric oxide synthase 2 and cyclooxygenase 2 interactions in inflammation. *Immunol Res* 2001;22:319–341.
197. Cao M, Stefanovic-Racic M, Georgescu HI, et al. Generation of nitric oxide by lapine meniscal cells and its effect on matrix metabolism: stimulation of collagen production by arginine. *J Orthop Res* 1998;16:104–111.
198. LeGrand A, Fermor B, Fink C, et al. IL1, TNFalpha, and IL17 synergistically upregulate nitric oxide and prostaglandin E_2 production in explants of human osteoarthritic cartilage knee menisci. *Arthritis Rheum* 2001;44:2078–2083.
199. Henrotin YE, Zheng SX, Deby GP, et al. Nitric oxide downregulates interleukin 1–beta (Il-1–beta) stimulated Il-6, Il-8, and prostaglandin E-2 production by human chondrocytes. *J Rheum* 1998;25:1595–1601.
200. Pelletier JP, Jovanovic D, Fernandes JC, et al. Reduced progression of experimental osteoarthritis in vivo by selective inhibition of inducible nitric oxide synthase. *Arthritis Rheum* 1998;41:1275–1286.
201. Patel R, Attur MG, Dave M, et al. Regulation of cytosolic COX-2 and prostaglandin E_2 production by nitric oxide in activated murine macrophages. *J Immunol* 1999;162:4191–4197.
202. Rawlinson SCF, Pitsillides AA, Lanyon LE. The prostacyclin synthetase inhibitor, 15–HPETE blocks strain-related increases in osteocytic G6PD activity and reduces nitric oxide release. *Bone* 1996;17:571.
203. Rawlinson SC. *Early loading-related responses of resident cells in mammalian bone organ explants.* Doctoral dissertation: University of London, 1999.
204. Manfield L, Jang D, Murrell GA. Nitric oxide enhances cyclooxygenase activity in articular cartilage. *Inflamm Res* 1996;45:254–258.
205. Jarvinen TA, Moilanen T, Jarvinen TL, et al. Endogenous nitric oxide and prostaglandin E_2 do not regulate the synthesis of each other in interleukin-1 beta-stimulated rat articular cartilage. *Inflammation* 1996;20:683–692.
206. Griffiths R, Smith MA, Roach ML, et al. Collagen-induced arthritis is reduced in 5–lipoxygenase-activating protein-deficient mice. *J Exp Med* 1997; 185:1123–1129.
207. Davidson EM, Rae SA, Smith MJ. Leukotriene B_4, a mediator of inflammation present in synovial fluid in rheumatoid arthritis. *Ann Rheum Dis* 1983;42:677–679.
208. Ahmadzadeh N, Shingu M, Nobunaga M, et al. Relationship between leukotriene B_4 and immunological parameters in rheumatoid synovial fluid. *Inflammation* 1991;15:497–503.
209. Ford-Hutchinson AW, Bray MA, Doig MV, et al. Leukotriene B_4, a potent chemokinetic and aggregating substance released from polymorphonuclear leukocytes. *Nature* 1980;286:264–265.
210. Gimbrone MA, Brock AF, Schafer AI. Leukotriene B_4 stimulates polymorphonuclear leukocyte adhesion to cultured vascular endothelial cells. *J Clin Invest* 1984;74:1552–1555.
211. Pillinger MH, Abraham SN. The neutrophil in rheumatoid arthritis. *Rheum Dis Clin North Am* 1995;21:691–714.
212. Jones AK, Al-Janabi MA, Solanki K, et al. In vivo leukocyte migration in arthritis. *Arthritis Rheum* 1991;34:270–275.
213. Griffiths RJ, Pettipher ER, Koch K, et al. Leukotriene B_4 plays a critical role in the progression of collagen-induced arthritis. *Proc Natl Acad Sci U S A* 1995; 92:517–521.

214. Borgeat P, Samuelsson B. Arachidonic acid metabolism in polymorphonuclear leukocytes: unstable intermediate in formation of dihydroxy acids. *Proc Natl Acad Sci U S A* 1979;76:3213–3217.
215. Atik OS. Leukotriene B_4 and prostaglandin E_2 like activity in synovial fluid in osteoarthritis. *Prostaglandins Leukot Essent Fatty Acids* 1990;39:253–254.
216. Curtis C, Flannery C, Harwood J, et al. Effect of fatty acids on the expression of lipoxygenases (LOX) in chondrocytes. *Trans Orthop Res Soc* 2001;26:378.
217. Tawara T, Shingu M, Nobunaga M, et al. Effects of recombinant human IL-1 beta on production of prostaglandin E_2, leukotriene B_4, NAG, and superoxide by human synovial cells and chondrocytes. *Inflammation* 1991;15:145–157.
218. Fermor B, Haribabu B, Weinberg JB, et al. Mechanical stress and nitric oxide influence leukotriene production in cartilage. *Biochem Biophys Res Commun* 2001;285:806–810.
219. Koprowski H, Zheng YM, Heber-Katz E, et al. In vivo expression of inducible nitric oxide synthase in experimentally induced neurologic diseases. *Proc Natl Acad Sci U S A* 1993;90:3024–3027.
220. Colville-Nash PR, Qureshi SS, Willis D, et al. Inhibition of inducible nitric oxide synthase by peroxisome proliferator-activated receptor agonists: correlation with induction of heme oxygenase 1. *J Immunol* 1998;161:978–984.
221. Devchand PR, Keller H, Peters JM, et al. The PPAR alpha leukotriene B4 pathway to inflammation control. *Nature* 1996;384:39.

CHAPTER 22

Animal Models

Wim B. van den Berg

Much of the pathogenesis of chronic arthritis and concomitant joint destruction remains to be elucidated. In addition, treatments have to be developed that selectively inhibit progression of destructive arthritis, yet leave host defense mechanisms virtually intact. This requires critical understanding of cells and mediators involved in destruction and initiation, maintenance, and remission of the arthritic process. Studies in human arthritis are hampered by the fact that the precise time of onset is unknown, whereas lesional tissue is often obtained from end-stage disease at the moment of joint replacement. The latter holds, in particular, for cartilage specimens, because it is widely accepted that this tissue has a limited capacity for repair. Moreover, specimens come from patients who have been receiving various drugs, and the shortage of control tissue is obvious. Numerous arthritis units recently have started early arthritis clinics, in which biopsies are taken in early stages of the disease process by blind needle technologies or miniarthroscopy, and this will enhance our knowledge of the disease process. Another focused approach is the use of experimental animal models of arthritis.

Although not ideal in terms of precise mimicry of human arthritic disease, experimental models of arthritis do reflect key aspects of their human counterparts. Their established time course, the easy access to tissue samples, and the ease of experimental therapeutic manipulation offer a useful approach to further understanding of the pathogenesis of arthritis. Models also provide valuable tools to obtain insight in biologic approaches and advanced arthritis therapy. Potential therapies then need to be evaluated in human disease, indirectly approving the predictive value of findings in particular models. It must be accepted that no single animal model of arthritis truly represents the human disease. In fact, the wide variety of agents that can induce an experimental arthritis with clinical and histopathologic features close to those of human arthritis supports the hypothesis that rheumatoid arthritis (RA) may have a variety of causes and that characteristic features reflect common end points. Analysis of aspects peculiar to an individual model are of value, but emphasis should be on general validity and common concepts in various models. In the following sections, models most widely used in the study of RA will be summarized, and their value will be illustrated with some research findings. Because the questions answered in models arise from elements of human disease, current concepts will be briefly addressed first.

GENERAL CONCEPTS AND FEATURES OF ARTHRITIS

RA is characterized by chronic inflammation in multiple joints and progressive destruction of bone and cartilage. Its pathogenesis is unknown, but the disease is generally considered an autoimmune process. The articular cartilage is an intriguing tissue, because it is the victim of the disease, but it may also function as the trigger, by releasing potential autoantigens and trapping exogenous antigens. Chronic synovial inflammation can result from direct activation of the synovial cells by nonantigenic triggers, including continuous stimulation by bacterial or viral triggers; often, RA synovial macrophages and fibroblasts show deranged behavior and tumor-like growth. In addition, the process can be driven and amplified by persistent T- and B-cell stimulation by as-yet-unknown (auto)antigens. T cells will drive macrophage activation through cytokines, such as interferon γ (IFN-γ) and interleukin-17 (IL-17), whereas antibodies will trigger the process by immune-complex formation and interaction through complement and Fc receptors on synovial cells. Either way, the end effect of multiple pathways is enhanced production of degradative enzymes and destructive cytokines such as tumor necrosis factor (TNF), IL-1, and IL-17. These mediators cause cartilage destruction and, indirectly, through activation of osteoclasts, bone erosion (Fig. 22.1). Destruction of articular cartilage is prominent at sites of pannus formation, where inflamed synovial tissue overgrows the edges of the cartilage surface, providing direct contact and uninhibited extrusion of mediators.

Characteristic histopathologic features in the RA joint include immune complexes in the articular cartilage layers and variable amounts of macrophages, T cells, and plasma cells in the synovium, often accompanied by fibrosis and synovial hyperplasia (see Chapter 11). Autoantibody formation, including rheumatoid factor and anticitrulline antibodies, is prominent, making B cells and a contribution of immune complex–mediated cellular activation processes a likely event. The antigens trapped in immune complexes in the cartilage surface layers are still poorly defined and, although candidates for a role in synovitis, may even reflect an epiphenomenon of immune-complex deposition and retention in damaged areas. Increasing attention is currently focused on the role of cytokines, with TNF and IL-1 being seen as master cytokines, orchestrating the synovial inflammation and concomitant tissue destruction. Considerable variation is found in relative cytokine levels and immune elements between RA patients and at various stages in one patient. This makes it impossible to define critical criteria for the best animal model. As suggested above, the analysis of different animal models reflecting various specific aspects have their value and will contribute to our overall understanding of key elements of the arthritic process.

The simplified process depicted in Figure 22.1 illustrates various levels of potential therapeutic interference, which can be studied in models ranging from antigen presentation by dendritic cells to T cells, control by regulatory T cells, production of

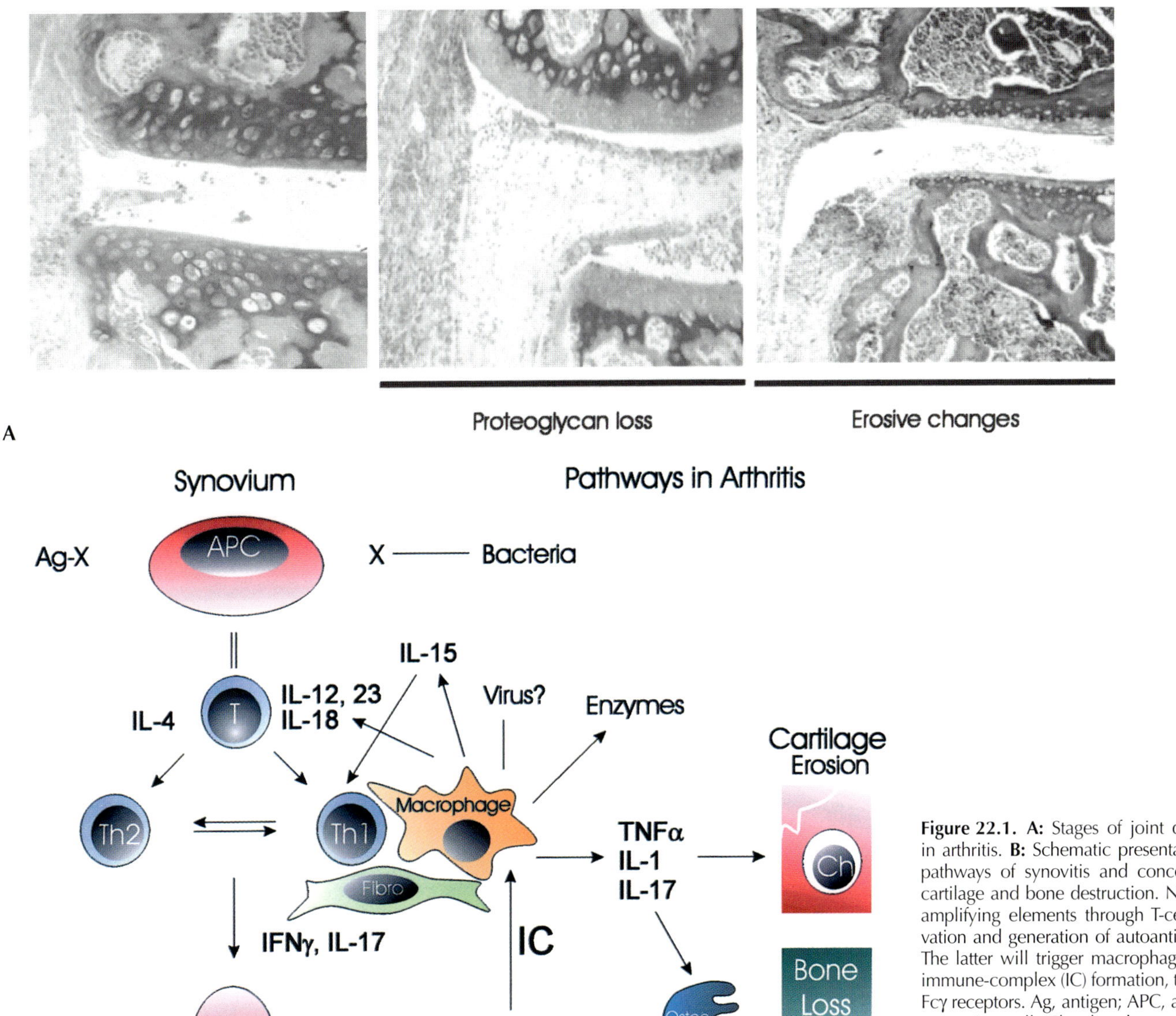

Figure 22.1. **A:** Stages of joint damage in arthritis. **B:** Schematic presentation of pathways of synovitis and concomitant cartilage and bone destruction. Note the amplifying elements through T-cell activation and generation of autoantibodies. The latter will trigger macrophages after immune-complex (IC) formation, through Fcγ receptors. Ag, antigen; APC, antigen-presenting cell; Ch, chondrocyte; Fibro, fibroblast; IFN, interferon; IL, interleukin; Th1, T helper 1; Th2, T helper 2; TNF, tumor necrosis factor.

autoantibodies, activation of synovial cells, and release of inflammatory and destructive mediators, to blockade of its interaction with cartilage and bone. It is, of course, attractive to target research in animal models at the level of specific arthritogens and immune triggering. However, in the absence of an established RA antigen, and given the likelihood that human RA probably is not driven by one particular antigen, it seems equally valuable to seek further understanding of effector mechanisms characteristic of joint inflammation and destruction.

MODELS OF ARTHRITIS

Historically, models of arthritis have been used to understand the stimuli provoking chronic arthritis and the mechanisms regulating chronicity and tissue destruction. When a model is established, the potential of a given stimulus is proven. The next step would be to obtain evidence that such reactions do occur in human arthritis, for instance, T-cell reactivity against a cartilage antigen. If this is the case, it still has to be proved that this reactivity is of pathogenetic importance and not an epiphenomenon, for example, by showing that antigen-specific immunomodulation affects the course of the human disease. Up until now, such research has not yielded a clue about dominant pathogenic triggers for RA. Present studies can be categorized into those that attempt further understanding of principles in established models and those that are still looking for new, putative triggers and novel models and concepts.

In line with historical concepts in RA, the models most widely studied in the past decades were those of adjuvant arthritis, collagen-induced arthritis, antigen-induced arthritis, and streptococcal cell-wall (SCW) arthritis (1). T cells play a dominant part in all of these models (Table 22.1). The second common principle is the presence of a chronic stimulus, either in the form of a persistent antigen or an autoantigen akin to joint structures. Examples of persisting antigens are nondegradable bacterial cell walls in the synovial tissue or antigen trapped in collagenous reservoirs, such as ligaments and articular cartilage (a feature of antigen-induced arthritis). Both conditions reflect escape from proper clearance by the phagocytic system. A second category of persistent stimuli is formed by autoantigens from the articular cartilage, such as collagen type II (CII) and proteoglycans. In adjuvant and SCW arthritis, the cartilage could as well function as an autoantigen, related to structural

TABLE 22.1. Models of Arthritis

Model	Abbreviation	Species[a]	Feature	IC	T cell
Adjuvant arthritis	AA	Lewis rat	AI	–	+
Streptococcal cell-wall arthritis	SCW-A	Lewis rat	Persistent bacteria, AI	–	+
Collagen-induced arthritis	CIA	DBA mouse	CII, AI	+	+
Proteoglycan arthritis	PG-A	BALB/c mouse	PG,AI	+	+
Antigen-induced arthritis	AIA	Rabbit, mouse	Persistent antigen	+	+
KRN arthritis	KRN	K/BxN mouse	GPI-AI	+	+
TNF transgenic arthritis	TNFtg	Mouse	TNF overexpression	–	–
IL-1 transgenic arthritis	IL-1tg	Mouse	IL-1 overexpression	–	–
IL-1ra transgenic arthritis	IL-1ra–/–	BALB/c mouse	IL-1ra deficiency	?	+
Oil-induced arthritis	OIA	DA rat	AI	–	+
Pristane-induced arthritis	PIA	DA rat	AI	–	+
MRL–lpr/lpr	MRL	Mouse	Fas defect	–	–
HTLV-induced arthritis	HTLV	Mouse	Viral, transgenic	–	+

AI, autoimmune; CII, collagen type II; DA, dark agouti; GPI, glucose-6-phosphate isomerase; HTLV, human T-cell lymphotropic virus; IC, immune complex; IL, interleukin; TNF, tumor necrosis factor.
[a]Mostly used.

mimicry between bacterial peptidoglycans and cartilage proteoglycans. However, ultimate proof that these cross-reactive responses really contribute has still to be provided. Of interest, destructive forms of RA tend to decline at the time that the cartilage is fully destroyed. Moreover, total joint replacement often results in a complete remission of arthritis in that particular joint, without the need for concomitant synovectomy. These are possible arguments for a direct role of cartilage antigens in the pathogenesis or an indirect role of cartilage components in the maintenance of the inflammatory process in the joint. The latter receives recent attention, because it is shown that degraded fragments of cartilage components can directly stimulate synoviocytes to release inflammatory cytokines.

Adjuvant Arthritis

Adjuvant arthritis is the first and historically the most extensively studied model of polyarthritis, discovered in 1954 (2). It is induced by intradermal injection of Freund's complete adjuvant, containing heat-killed mycobacteria, and arthritis develops within 2 weeks in susceptible rat strains. In general, the model is induced in Lewis rats. The volume, type of oil, and composition of the suspension are critical variables that determine incidence and severity of the arthritis. The active component in bacteria is the cell-wall peptidoglycan, and the disease can be induced with various bacteria.

The histopathologic features of adjuvant arthritis mainly reflect a periarthritis, with marked periostitis instead of a synovitis, and massive inflammation in the bone marrow. Immune-complex deposition in the cartilage is not a characteristic feature, and cartilage destruction is limited in early disease. Adjuvant arthritis is a plain T-cell model, and the strongest argument for an autoimmune process is the induction of arthritis by passive transfer of T cells from diseased animals. The joint inflammation may reflect the generation of a T-cell reaction to bacterial epitopes cross-reacting with endogenous bacterial fragments continuously present in synovial tissues or with cartilaginous antigens. It may also be based on nonspecific immunomodulation, reflecting the adjuvant properties of the bacterium in oil preparations and the generation of a dysregulated expression of autoimmunity to whatever autoimmune epitope. The fact that nonantigenic adjuvants, such as the oil preparation avridine (CP 20961) and other mineral oils, can induce an arthritis indistinguishable from adjuvant arthritis underlines the potential existence of such a pathway.

In classic adjuvant arthritis, a bacterium-specific pathogenesis remains most likely because conventionally bred rats are generally resistant to adjuvant arthritis, whereas germ-free Fisher or Wistar rats are susceptible (3,4). The germ-free rats lack early contact with bacteria and are, therefore, not tolerized; colonization with bacteria before the induction of adjuvant arthritis prevented susceptibility (5).

The most striking observation in the model of adjuvant arthritis is the occurrence of spontaneous remission and the lack of susceptibility to reinduction. This resistance is antigen specific and makes the model highly suitable for studies in regulation of T-cell tolerance. T-cell lines and clones were isolated that can induce disease, but, when attenuated, can also induce protective responses (6,7). The identification of epitopes on bacterial heat-shock proteins and the recognition of cross-reactive, highly conserved, endogenous heat-shock proteins in eukaryotes has implicated these proteins as potential target antigens in adjuvant arthritis (8,9).

Studies on cytokine involvement identified a role of both TNF-α and IL-1, and the most optimal blockade of inflammation and tissue destruction was obtained with a combination therapy (10). Intriguingly, when treated with osteoprotegerin (OPG), which neutralizes the osteoclast-activating mediator receptor activator of nuclear factor–κB ligand (RANKL), the model shows persistent inflammation, but bone erosion is fully absent (11). In adjuvant arthritis, most of the cartilage damage is indirect, after major loss of underlying bone, and this might explain protection of cartilage erosion seen with OPG.

In the pharmaceutical industry, adjuvant arthritis is often the model of first choice for screening novel therapeutic agents for antiarthritic efficacy. This choice is based mainly on its ease of induction and simple macroscopic observation of arthritis in the paws. Potentially, its merits rely on the pure T-cell–driven pathogenesis. However, the fact that nonsteroidal antiinflammatory drugs are effective inhibitors of cartilage and bone destruction in this model warrants care with interpretation of therapeutic effects of novel compounds.

Streptococcal Cell-Wall Arthritis

This model was originally described by Cromartie, Craddock, and Schwab (12). It is induced in Lewis rats by the systemic injection of cell-wall fragments of group A streptococci, which are highly resistant to biodegradation. A similar disease can be induced with cell-wall fragments from other bacteria, such as *Lactobacillus casei* or *Eubacterium aerofaciens*. The common principle resides in the poor degradability of the fragments, thereby creating a persistent stimulus. The lactobacillus and eubacterial models are of particular interest for human disease, because these bacteria are part of the normal gastrointestinal flora (13,14). It implies that an enormous load of potential arthritogenic stimuli is continuously present in the normal gastrointestinal tract and may spread to other tissues.

Within 24 hours of administration of cell-wall fragments, acute inflammation develops in peripheral joints, coincident with dissemination of cell-wall fragments in blood vessels of the synovium and subchondral bone marrow. Acute, complement-dependent inflammation subsides over the next week and is followed within 2 weeks by a chronic, erosive polyarthritis, involving mainly peripheral joints. In contrast with the acute phase, chronic joint inflammation develops only in susceptible strains, with the highest incidence in Lewis rats. The chronic phase shows waxing and waning of arthritis, bringing it close to human RA.

Although macrophages become stimulated by persistent bacterial fragments, cogent evidence now exists that the chronic phase is dependent on specific T cells, with limited involvement of antibodies. It was not inducible in nude Lewis rats (no T cells), and cyclosporin A effectively inhibited this phase. SCW-specific T-cell responses were found in arthritis-susceptible Lewis rats, whereas resistant Fisher rats did not mount this immune reaction. In addition, germ-free Fisher rats were susceptible and did show SCW-specific T-cell reactivity. This suggests that chronic arthritis is driven by this SCW-specific T-cell reaction to persistent bacteria. Most rat strains are strongly tolerant of threatening arthritogenic reactions to bacterial cell walls, whereas Lewis rats display weak tolerance and easily lose tolerogenic control. Mice strains studied so far are not susceptible to the single intraperitoneal injection model. Female rats show a more severe arthritis than male rats. It is tempting to speculate that similar loss of tolerance may occur in RA patients and sustain arthritis.

In addition to SCW-specific T-cell reactions, cross-reactive autoimmunity to cartilage proteoglycans may contribute to chronicity. However, it is unlikely that this is a major factor at onset. In fact, the early histopathologic appearance of the joint is that of a strong, mononuclear synovitis, with a sparse exudate in the joint space and limited loss of proteoglycan from the articular cartilage. Only at later stages were marked pannus formation and severe erosions of underlying cartilage and bone frequently observed (Fig. 22.2).

In line with involvement of growth factors and tumor-like behavior of synovial cells in patients with RA, similar characteristics have been found in synoviocytes from SCW arthritic rats. Probably because of persistent bacterial stimuli, synovial cells do show continued proliferation *ex vivo*, with apparent paracrine and autocrine regulation by growth factors (15). This observation suggests that sustained macrophage–fibroblast activation may be a perpetuating principle, but, *in vivo*, the T cell is still a critical, driving factor.

Studies on involvement of cytokines showed a combined role of TNF-α and IL-1, as found in adjuvant arthritis (10). In mice, a chronic relapsing SCW model can be induced by repeated

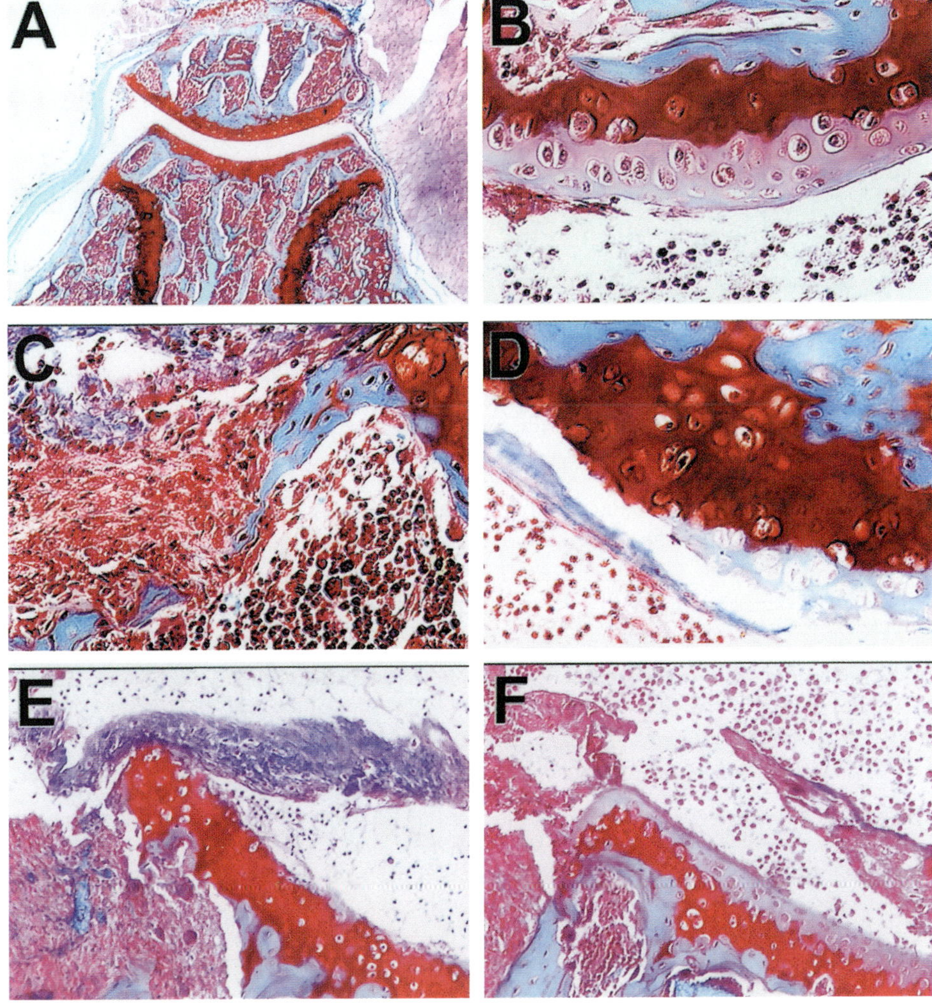

Figure 22.2. **A–F:** Histology sections of murine knee joints at various stages of arthritis: **(A)** control, **(B)** cartilage proteoglycan loss, **(C)** erosive ingrowth and bone loss, **(D)** loss of cartilage surface, **(E)** aggressive murine collagen arthritis with cartilage surface loss and bone erosion. **F:** Local overexpression of interleukin-4 prevents surface erosion and bone loss, as compared to **(E)**.

weekly injection of SCW fragments directly into the knee joint. Further details are discussed in the section Flares of Arthritis.

The rat SCW model has not been frequently used for drug studies. Cyclosporin A shows efficacy, and steroids are suppressive as well, whereas methotrexate showed moderate activity. The main reason for limited studies in this model is the difficulty of preparing proper arthritogenic bacterial cell-wall fragments.

CpG ARTHRITIS

As an extension of involvement of bacteria in arthritis, it was recently identified that bacterial DNA could induce arthritis. In particular, the CpG motifs in bacterial DNA are arthritogenic, and substantial amounts can be found in joint tissues (16). Macrophages play a major role in this arthritis through TNF production. However, in comparison to cell-wall fragments, the cytokine-inducing capacity is weak. Normal joints of individuals contain both bacterial fragments and bacterial CpG motifs, and it is conceivable that both principles contribute to arthritis.

Collagen-Induced Arthritis

The model of collagen arthritis in rats was first described in 1977 by Trentham et al. (17). It was found accidentally, after immunization with purified collagen preparations. The initial observation indicated that arthritis was confined to sensitization with native CII, a major component of articular cartilage. Denatured CII or collagen type I was not arthritogenic. Later, it was identified that minor collagen types from articular cartilage may also function as arthritogens, for instance, collagen types IX and XI (18).

The crucial element in this arthritis is the induction of immunity to foreign CII, subsequently cross-reacting with homologous CII. Plain immunization with homologous CII can also be used, but then much stronger immunization regimens are needed to override natural tolerance. The disease can easily be induced in rats, with full-blown expression within 14 days, whereas expression in mice follows more tight genetic restriction (19). Moreover, disease expression in mice is gradual, starting after 3 to 4 weeks in some, whereas a 100% incidence commonly takes 8 to 10 weeks. Of interest, collagen arthritis can be induced in nonhuman primates. Most rhesus monkeys were susceptible. Instead of a susceptibility gene, linkage studies on the major histocompatibility complex revealed the presence of a gene-regulating resistance.

Unlike adjuvant arthritis, collagen arthritis is less systemic as an illness but involves mainly the peripheral joints and spares the spine. Ears may be affected. This feature is mainly found at late stages in rats and can be used to study polychondritis. In murine collagen-induced arthritis, marked expression of arthritis was also found in knee joints, in addition to the paws, ankles, and wrists. Histopathology of collagen arthritis shows a distinct, acute synovitis with numerous granulocytes and bone erosions, as well as periosteal new bone formation. Involvement of the bone marrow is limited in early disease. A characteristic feature is the direct erosive attack by granulocytes at the cartilage surface. In contrast to findings in other models, a complete loss of articular cartilage is often seen within a few weeks (Fig. 22.2E). The arthritis ends up in ankylosis, with limited inflammation. The lack of sustaining antigen is probably the main reason for remission of arthritis.

The mechanism of arthritis expression is based on two principles: anticollagen antibodies and anti-CII T-cell immunity. Although antibodies alone are able to induce arthritis after passive administration to naïve recipient animals, high concentrations and repeated dosing are needed to obtain persistent arthritis. Passive transfer with bulk T cells or clones alone yielded poor disease expression. Probably, antibodies are needed to bind to the cartilage surface and to release further collagen epitopes, on complement fixation and the attraction of leukocytes, including granulocytes and lymphocytes. Influx of anti-CII–specific T cells will then further drive the arthritic process, as substantiated by blocking activity of anti-CD40 antibodies (20).

Arthritis expression can be enhanced by immune boosting with IL-12 and IL-18 or addition of extra anti-CII antibodies. Around the time of onset, nonspecific inflammatory stimuli, such as lipopolysaccharide or yeast particles (zymosan), or the addition of single inflammatory mediators, IL-1, TNF-α, or transforming growth factor β (TGF-β), will enhance expression (21). This principle can be used to synchronize expression at a given day in all mice and multiple joints. It proves an intriguing principle that quiescent autoimmune arthritis comes to a full expression with a combination of potentiating elements, which may include bacterial infections and IL-12–IL-18 release (22). Recent studies not only implicate potentiating cytokines but also the control by modulators, such as IL-4 and IL-10 (23). In terms of genetics, it turns out that both the relative levels of potentiating, as well as inhibitory cytokines, determine the susceptibility of a particular mouse strain (24). In addition, variations in stimulatory and inhibitory Fcγ receptor expression levels on macrophages, linked to immune complex–mediated activation, are a crucial element in severity and chronicity (25,26).

In the murine model, anti–IL-1 and anti-TNF have been used before onset, shortly after onset, and in the established phase. TNF plays an important part in the onset of collagen-induced arthritis (27,28) but is less dominant in late arthritis. In contrast, IL-1 is a pivotal mediator in both early and established collagen-induced arthritis (Fig. 22.3). The elimination of IL-1 greatly suppressed the arthritis and yielded marked protection against cartilage destruction (29,30). The protection could be demonstrated using either neutralizing antibodies or IL-1 receptor antagonist, provided that large amounts (1 mg per day per mouse) of the antagonist were continuously supplied in osmotic minipumps.

Apart from the abundant cytokine-related studies, much research has been focused on oral and nasal tolerance induction with CII fragments. It is now accepted that the route of administration and the local cytokine milieu, rather than the existence of tolerizing or arthritogenic epitopes on fragments, determine the impact on arthritis (24,31). Collagen-induced arthritis, using a defined autoantigen, is also a suitable model for investigating whether usage of T-cell receptors (TCR) is restricted and the possibility of suppressing arthritis by blocking a particular receptor. A major problem is epitope spreading during progression of autoimmune arthritis. Although challenging scientifically, therapeutic applicability of TCR blockade in RA patients remains a remote possibility. Significant T-cell reactivity to CII cannot easily be detected in patients with RA, making it difficult to analyze efficacy of specific immunomodulation. Recent immunomodulation approaches include the principle of bystander suppression, where oral or nasal administration of a nonrelated antigen is used to generate the production of suppressive cytokines (IL-4, IL-10, TGF-β). These mediators will then, by way of bystander activity, suppress anti-CII immunity and, indirectly, collagen arthritis (32,33). If variable antigen usage is accepted as a likely condition reflecting heterogeneity in various RA patients, such a nonspecific therapeutic approach might prove more useful.

A worrisome finding in terms of comparison with human arthritis is the highly destructive character of collagen arthritis and the marked sensitivity to nonsteroidal antiinflammatory drugs. Indomethacin is a very potent suppressor of both the inflammation and the joint destruction; steroids are also highly effective. The latter complicates experimental studies, because stress influences can profoundly affect the expression of arthri-

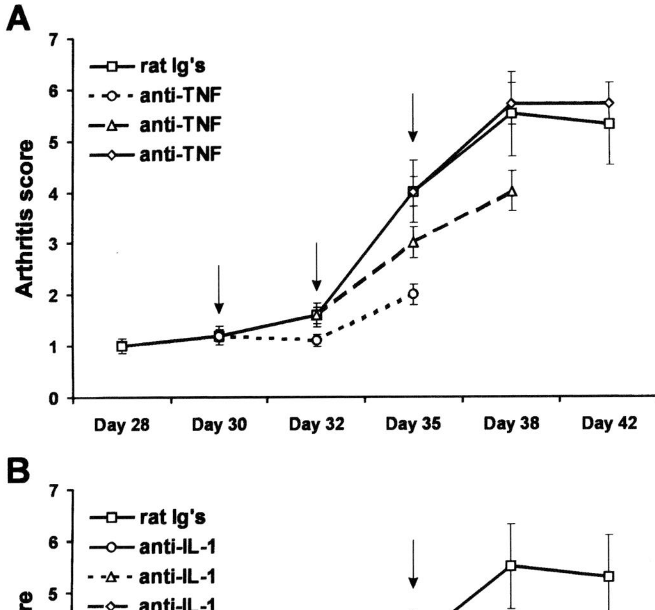

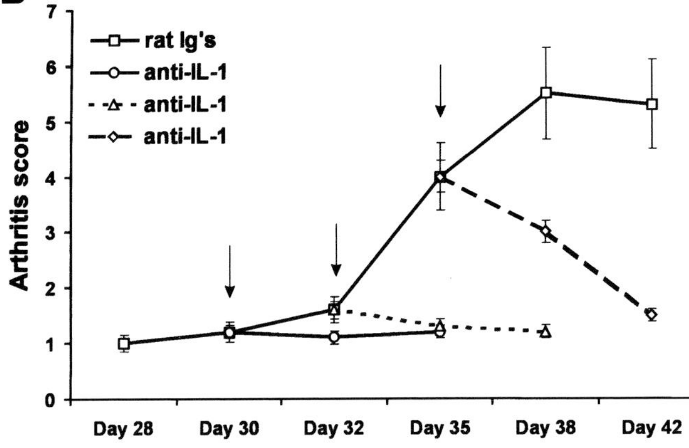

Figure 22.3. Impact of anticytokine treatment on murine collagen arthritis. Treatment with anti–tumor necrosis factor (TNF) **(A)** or anti–interleukin (IL)-1ab antibodies **(B)** was started at various time points. Note that anti-TNF treatment is only effective when started early, whereas anti–IL-1 is still effective in established disease. Ig, immunoglobulin.

tis. In contrast to the female preponderance in RA, male rodents are more susceptible to collagen arthritis.

Proteoglycan Arthritis

The proteoglycan arthritis model is a logical extension of collagen arthritis, because both CII and proteoglycan are major components of articular cartilage. Yet, again, the discovery of the model was coincidental, after the immunization of mice to prepare antibodies. Repeated boosting was needed to induce consistent arthritis after 8 weeks, implicating poor antigenicity or strong tolerance. Arthritis was noticed in inbred female BALB/c mice on immunization with human fetal articular proteoglycan, stripped of chondroitin sulphate (34,35). The arthritogenic epitope resides in the core protein. The mechanism of induction of arthritis is probably quite similar to that in collagen-induced arthritis: the induction of immunity to fetal human proteoglycan, subsequently cross-reacting with murine proteoglycans.

The proteoglycan model shows a polyarthritis, with severe cartilage erosion and marked ankylosis. In addition, involvement of the lumbar spine and disc regions was found, making it a model for spondylitis, also. Like collagen arthritis, the most severe expression of proteoglycan arthritis is found in the presence of both antibodies and antiproteoglycan T-cell immunity. In general, cytokine involvement follows the observations in collagen arthritis, with the striking exception that, although both models are considered to be driven by T helper 1 (Th1), IFN-γ deficiency makes BALB/c mice susceptible to collagen-induced arthritis, whereas it prevents proteoglycan arthritis. Detailed analysis of shifts in subclasses of antibodies produced may shed some light on these observations (36). Of interest, antiproteoglycan antibodies on their own were capable of causing marked loss of proteoglycan from the cartilage in the absence of distinct synovitis. The genetics of this model is extensively studied by the group of Glant, using crosses of susceptible and resistant mice (37,38).

Screening for the occurrence of antiproteoglycan immunity in patients with RA did not yield unequivocal data in support of a role in human arthritis so far. Further characterization of proteoglycan subtypes and epitopes is warranted.

Antigen-Induced Arthritis

In support of an immunologically mediated disease process in RA, a clean mechanistic model, based on local antigenic challenge in a primed host, appeared logical at the time. Such a model was first developed by Dumonde and Glynn in rabbits (39). In principle, it can be induced in any species, provided that proper immunity to a particular antigen can be mounted, and extensions have since been developed in mice, rats, and guinea pigs. In contrast to the polyarthritis models described so far, this type of arthritis remains confined to the injected joint, enabling comparison with a contralateral control joint of the same animal.

Commonly used antigens were ovalbumin, bovine serum albumin, and fibrin. Preimmunization is performed with antigen in complete Freund's adjuvant to induce strong humoral as well as cell-mediated immunity. Arthritis is usually induced 3 weeks later by a local injection in the knee joint of a large amount of antigen. Initially, an immune complex type of reaction dominates, followed by a T-cell–mediated chronic inflammation. In the rabbit, chronicity may last for years. Histopathology shows a granulocyte-rich exudate in the joint space, thickening of the synovial lining layer, and, at later stages, a predominantly mononuclear infiltrate in the synovium, which later includes numerous T cells and clusters of plasma cells. Interestingly, a large proportion (50%) of these plasma cells are still making antibodies to the inciting antigen, suggesting that retained antigen still is a driving force in chronic arthritis. Intense immune-complex formation is seen in superficial layers of the articular cartilage, which may contribute to localized cartilage destruction. Early loss of proteoglycan, followed by pannus formation and cartilage and bone erosion, is a common finding. Of the models described so far, these characteristics are the closest to those found in human RA.

Two important principles emerged: First, chronicity is only found in the presence of sufficient antigen retention in joint tissues, in combination with proper T-cell–mediated delayed hypersensitivity; second, joints contain numerous non- or avascular collagenous tissues, such as cartilage, ligaments, and tendons, which allow for prolonged antigen retention by antibody-mediated trapping and charge-mediated binding (40,41). A key finding was the observation that antigen injected in the skin produced transient inflammation, whereas a similar dose in the joints caused chronic inflammation.

The chronicity of arthritis is caused by the generation of local hyperreactivity (Table 22.2). Antigen initially trapped in collagenous tissues will be slowly released in time to sustain low-grade chronic arthritis. As a consequence, the local T-cell infiltrate will gain specificity, because retention of specific T cells is shaped by homologous antigen. This identified that small amounts of antigen are sufficient to sustain arthritis, whereas relatively large amounts were needed to induce its onset. This condition forms the basis for exacerbations (flares) of arthritis with low doses of antigen, described below.

TABLE 22.2. Features of Classic Arthritis Models

Features	AA	SCW-A	CIA	AIA
Impact of bacterial flora[a]	+	+	–	–
Stimulus	?	Persistent bacteria	CII	Planted Ag
Self-limiting arthritis	+	–	±	–
Flares	Refractory	Spontaneous	Inducible	Inducible
Chronic synovitis	±	++	+	++
Bone marrow inflammation[b]	++	+	±	±
Main site of expression	Ankle	Ankle	Peripheral	Chosen[c]
Bone erosion	++	+	++	+
Cartilage erosion	±	±	++	++
Dominant feature	Periostitis	Fibrosis	Destructive	Local hyperreactivity

AA, adjuvant arthritis; AIA, antigen-induced arthritis; CII, collagen type II; CIA, collagen-induced arthritis; SCW-A, streptococcal cell-wall arthritis.
[a]Impact on susceptibility of strains.
[b]As an early feature.
[c]Chosen by intraarticular injection.

In rabbits, antibody responses are generally high and allow for sufficient immune complex–mediated trapping of antigen in the joint. Cationic antigens are proper arthritogens in the murine model, owing to their ability to stick to the negatively charged collagenous structures of the joint and to accumulate immune complexes at the surface (41). Of interest, this principle appears of importance in the more recently developed KRN model of arthritis, in which anti–glucose-6-phosphate isomerase (GPI) antibodies stick to GPI antigen trapped at cartilage surfaces and contribute to chronicity and destruction (see below).

In antigen-induced arthritis in the rabbit and the mouse, elimination of TNF-α and IL-1 was poorly effective in suppressing joint inflammation, pointing to substantial overkill by other mediators in this severe onset of arthritis (42–44). However, elimination of IL-1 did yield impressive protection against cartilage destruction (43,45). This was even more striking in the antigen-induced flare, when induced 4 weeks after first onset of arthritis (46).

The model of antigen-induced arthritis is most suited to studies into the mechanism of cartilage destruction, as induced by a mix of immune complexes and T-cell reactivity. It is facilitated by knowledge of the exact time of onset, accessibility of the knee joint (as compared with ankles), and the presence of a contralateral control joint. Moreover, the model can be adequately used to evaluate the regulation of local T-cell hyperreactivity against a retained foreign antigen, in comparison with similar events against autoimmune antigens in progressing collagen arthritis.

Antigen-induced arthritis is insensitive to nonsteroidal anti-inflammatory drugs (47,48), although steroids are highly effective, cytotoxic drugs are potent suppressants, and gold compounds were shown to be effective in the rabbit model.

Flares of Arthritis

In comparison to the chronic process of human RA, a general shortcoming of most models is the relatively short duration of a severe and rapidly destructive inflammation. In that respect, models of repeated flares of arthritis, with slower development of lesions, provide a valuable extension.

An arthritic joint bearing retained antigen and a chronic antigen-specific T-cell infiltrate display a state of local hyperreactivity. This is not restricted to retained antigen but also applies to new antigen entering the sensitized joint from the circulation. Flares of smoldering arthritis can be induced with as little as 10 ng of antigen and are highly T-cell dependent (49). Flares can be induced by local, intravenous, or even oral rechallenge. Higher dosages are, of course, needed for intravenous or oral challenges, and access to the joint is dependent on systemic antibodies and physicochemical properties of the antigen. A model of repeated flares is more akin to the human state than is a model showing severe inflammation for some weeks, followed by rapid waning of arthritis. In a considerable proportion of patients with RA, the disease course is characterized by exacerbations and remissions.

An important extension of the flare model is formed by exacerbations induced by cytokines. Joints bearing a chronic infiltrate, compared to naïve joints, are more sensitive to IL-1, and this reactivity seems to reside in the macrophage infiltrate. Most importantly, IL-1–induced flares are more destructive to the articular cartilage than initial IL-1 insults.

In addition to flare models based on protein antigen, similar models have been developed in rats and mice using bacterial cell-wall constituents. In contrast to small protein antigens, which are only inflammatory in the context of an immune response, bacterial fragments may function as an antigen as well as a phlogistic irritant; ensuing reactions are a mixture of T-cell– and macrophage-driven processes. The generation of local hyperreactivity asks for large, persistent bacterial peptidoglycan–polysaccharide components, but the recurrence may happen with a variety of components, ranging from cell-wall fragments, lipopolysaccharide, CpG motifs, to cytokines such as IL-1. The strongest flares occur in the presence of T-cell immunity, and a correlation was found between the potential of fragments to induce an exacerbation and to elicit cell-wall–specific T-cell proliferation (50). In the mouse system, strong tolerance exists, and flares result from a mixture of macrophage and T-cell reactivity. Separate roles of TNF and IL-1 were found in swelling and erosion (51). TNF dependency of the swelling response was seen for every flare, but IL-1 became involved at later stages and was dominant in the chronic erosive process (Fig. 22.4). Histology showed that erosion was completely absent in IL-1–deficient mice, but did occur in TNF-deficient mice (Fig. 22.5). Of note, the model is more severe and erosive in DBA mice, compared to C57Bl mice; erosion is absent in T- and B-cell–deficient RAG mice; and IL-12 and IL-18 promote an erosive phenotype (22).

Of note, considerable cross-reactivity occurs between cell walls of different bacterial origins, and flares may result from homologous as well as heterologous fragments. This may extend to cross-reactive autoantigens from cartilage, which underlines the idea that arthritis can start against a particular antigen but may spread to other antigens, including autoantigens. Recently, Toll receptors were identified as recognition sites for bacteria, cross-reacting with numerous fragments of damaged connective tissue components.

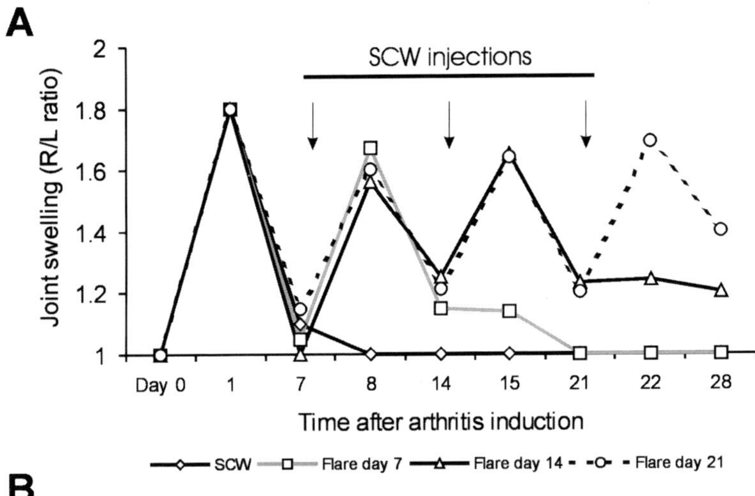

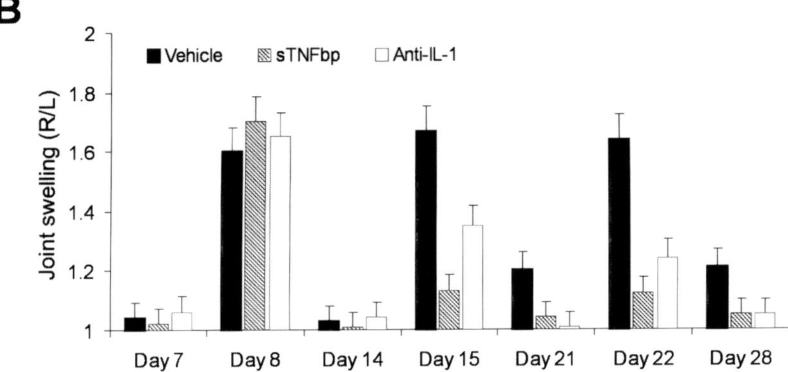

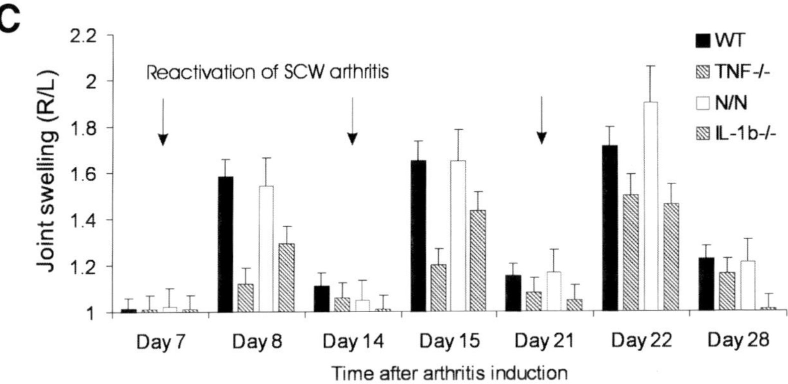

Figure 22.4. Repeated flares after consecutive injection of streptococcal cell wall (SCW) fragments in the murine knee joint **(A)**. Using this model, two approaches were followed: **(B)** treatment with tumor necrosis factor (TNF)bp or interleukin (IL)-1 antibodies, given shortly before each flare and starting treatment at day 14, and **(C)** comparisons in TNF- and IL-1b–deficient mice with their respective wild-type (WT) controls. Note the TNF dependence of joint swelling of every flare, but increasing IL-1 dependence with time. The waning of TNF involvement is more pronounced in the knockout animals, suggesting adverse effects of complete TNF neutralization. N/N, control strain, normal background to IL-1b–/–; R/L, right to left.

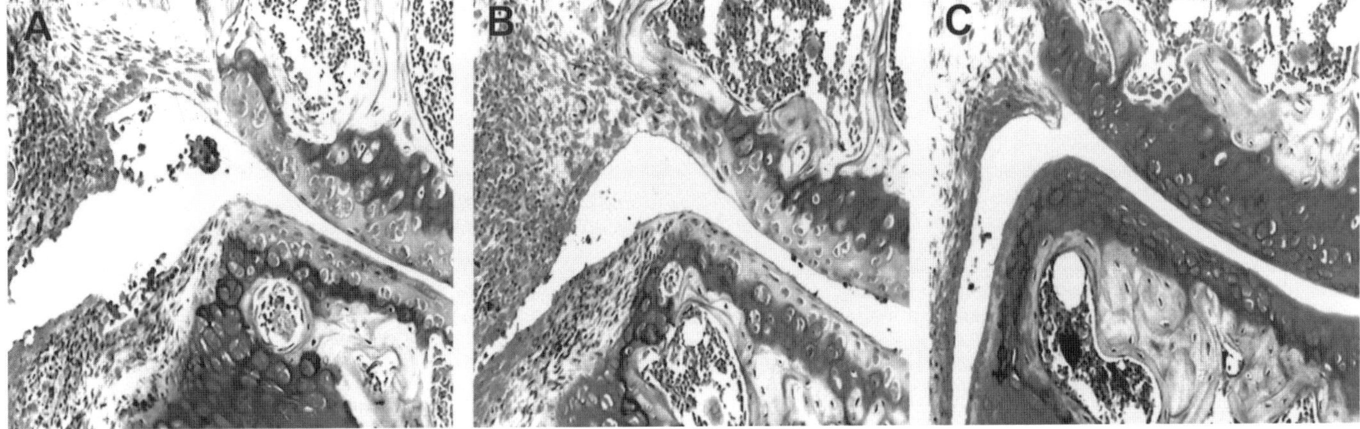

Figure 22.5. Histology at day 28 of repeated streptococcal cell-wall challenge in wild-type control **(A)**, tumor necrosis factor (TNF)–/– **(B)** and interleukin (IL)-1b–deficient **(C)** mice. Note sustained inflammatory infiltrate and joint damage in the TNF knockout and absence of damage in the IL-1b knockout mouse.

Their presence on dendritic cells and role in regulation of autoimmune responses is intriguing. These principles open up a wide range of putative stimuli involved in exacerbations, simultaneously complicating the search for the driving antigen in humans. Fortunately, flares can be efficiently blocked with a combination of antibodies to TNF and IL-1, as already mentioned.

Immune-Complex Arthritis

Autoantibodies are a key feature of RA. In some of the models discussed above, such as collagen-, proteoglycan-, and antigen-induced arthritis, immune-complex formation at joint tissues is a major element (Table 22.1). Although there is no doubt that excessive immune-complex formation can cause destructive arthritis, common observations indicate that chronicity is limited and, in fact, only seen in the presence of T cells. The latter may be linked to the need of T cells to sustain antibody production or may point to the greater potential of T-cell–macrophage interaction to sustain joint pathology. Minute amounts of antigen suffice to stimulate T cells, whereas considerable amounts of immune complexes are needed to stimulate inflammatory mediator release from phagocytes. Either way, immune-complex models mimic part of the RA pathology.

There is growing interest in the use of passive immune-complex models, along with availability of a range of transgenic knockouts, to identify crucial pathways of inflammation and tissue destruction. In general, the advantage of passive systems is the lower dependence of genetic background, herein avoiding excessive backcrossing to create transgenics in suitable susceptible mouse strains. Passive transfer of collagen arthritis can be done with a critical mixture of a number of anti-CII monoclonal antibodies, including complement-binding immunoglobulin G (IgG)2a. Sets are now commercially available, routinely recommending DBA mice as sensitive recipients. Accepted concepts of inflammation pathways include immune complex–mediated complement and Fcγ receptor activation on phagocytes.

Proteoglycan antibodies from the proteoglycan arthritis model can induce transient arthritis on transfer, with concomitant proteoglycan loss from the cartilage, but no erosive damage. IgG1 seems the critical subclass, but the limited destructive potential is yet unclear.

An immune-complex model emerging from the murine antigen–induced arthritis model and using the principle of cationic retention is the passive transfer of antilysozyme antibodies to mice, which are locally injected in one knee joint with poly-L-lysine–lysozyme. Poly-L-lysine–coupled lysozyme is highly cationic and sufficiently large to be retained in the joint for prolonged periods of time. Both association with synovial tissue and heavy sticking to cartilage surfaces contributes to chronicity and cartilage destruction. An intriguing observation was the more chronic and destructive nature of this arthritis in DBA/1j mice (Table 22.3), which seems related to high sustained levels of activating Fc receptors on macrophages of this mouse strain (52). The model shows strong dependence of IL-1, whereas TNF blockade was ineffective (53).

TABLE 22.3. Passive Immune-Complex Arthritis Models in Mice

Antigen	Antibodies	Destructive	Sensitive Strains
PLL-lysozyme	Rabbit Ig	++	DBA>B10RIII>BALB/c
Collagen II	IgG2	++	DBA
Proteoglycan	IgG1	±	BALB/c
GPI	IgG1	++	BALB/c>DBA>129/Sv

GPI, glucose-6-phophate isomerase; Ig, immunoglobulin; PLL, poly-L-lysine.

A final model to be mentioned here is the passive GPI model, which will be addressed in the next section. Differences between the various immune-complex models reside mainly in the subclasses of antibodies (Table 22.3) and related complement-binding activity or Fcγ receptor–mediated activation of granulocytes, macrophages, and mast cells.

KRN Arthritis

An intriguing novel arthritis model emerged from the elegant series of experiments in transgenic mice overexpressing a self-reactive TCR. The cross of K/BxN mice developed arthritis (54). In principle, many insults or adjuvants, which will skew regulation of T-cell tolerance, have the potential to create autoimmune pathology, including joint inflammation. This holds for adjuvant arthritis and also for the oil-induced models described below. The major breakthrough and the beauty of the KRN model was the elucidation of the driving antigen and the identification that the passive transfer with antibodies induced a protracted arthritis. It was found that the TCR recognized the ubiquitous self-antigen GPI and provoked through B-cell differentiation and proliferation high levels of anti-GPI antibodies. These antibodies are directly pathogenic on transfer and appear to recognize endogenous GPI, which seems to associate preferentially with the cartilage surface (55). The latter may underlie the dominance of joint pathology in these mice, although GPI is also abundant at other sites in the body. IgG1 antibodies are the major subclass and cause a sustained erosive arthritis after continued transfer. This pathology brings the model close to passive collagen-induced arthritis or immune-complex arthritis, with planted cartilage associated antigen, all having immune-complex formation at the cartilage surface. Differences relate to IgG subclasses.

As mentioned above, for passive immune-complex models, in general, the severity is dependent on complement factors and Fcγ receptors. Activation of complement through the alternative pathway appeared crucial, in line with dominance of IgG1. Because activity of complement and the level of expression of Fcγ receptors on phagocytes is variable in various mouse strains, this determines to a great extent the variable susceptibility. BALB/c mice are hyperreactive, whereas DBA/1 and C57Bl6 were less susceptible, and minor responsiveness was seen in 129/Sv mice (56,57). Similar antibodies are found in RA patients, but certainly not in all, and levels are moderate. Its role in RA remains to be identified (58). The involvement of IL-1 and TNF follows roughly earlier observations in similar models. IL-1 is really obligatory, with no arthritis in IL-1–deficient mice. TNF was also essential, although less critically than IL-1, because a proportion of TNF-deficient mice developed robust arthritis (59). When compared to the passive arthritis induced with antibodies to the cationic antigen poly-L-lysine–lysozyme, a higher TNF sensitivity was obvious, as well as a dependence of mast cells. This all fits with a role of environmental initiating elements. Probably, onset of mild GPI arthritis is facilitated by local TNF generation and mast-cell–dependent histamine release, whereas a model with a planted cationic antigen in the joint generates sufficient nonspecific inflammation to set arthritis in motion without the need of additional facilitating mediators, such as TNF. Once affected, the role of TNF is limited, also in GPI arthritis.

TUMOR NECROSIS FACTOR TRANSGENIC MICE

In an elegant series of experiments, the group of George Kollias provided great insight into the possible role of TNF in arthritis induction. By the introduction in mice of a modified human TNF transgene lacking a TNF 3' untranslated region involved in translational repression of TNF, it was shown that pronounced TNF overexpression results in chronic polyarthritis with a 100% incidence (60). Hyperplasia of the synovium, inflammatory infiltrates in the joint space, pannus formation, and cartilage destruction were observed. Intriguingly, a similar form of arthritis also developed in targeted mutant mice lacking the 3' adenylate uridylate–rich elements, confirming the role of these elements in the maintenance of a physiologic TNF response in the joint (61). A proposed mechanism is the inability of natural antiinflammatory signals, such as IL-10, to suppress TNF production under these conditions. These exciting findings stimulated a major search for functional mutations around TNF production in RA patients. However, so far, no clear indications have been found.

The model is of great interest for identifying pathways of TNF-induced arthritis and screening efficacy of various TNF-directed therapies. It comes as no surprise that anti-TNF treatment blocks the pathology, but it was a remarkable observation that antibodies to the IL-1 receptor also prevented arthritis, indirectly identifying that this arthritis runs through induction of IL-1 (62). The model does not need T or B cells, because arthritis is undisturbed in TNF transgenics backcrossed to RAG mice, and the pathology can be transferred with selected TNF-producing fibroblasts. Further identification of TNF receptor involvement showed a crucial role of the p55 type I receptor in mediating the TNF pathology and a suppressive role of the p75 type II receptor.

Apparently, the type II receptor does not have a clear suppressive role in inflammatory bowel disease, which is a pathology also found in TNF transgenic mice. The latter is a T- and B-cell–dependent disease. It is known that the cytotoxic anti-TNF and the TNF- and lymphotoxin-scavenging TNF-soluble receptor treatments have different efficacy in human RA, compared to Crohn's disease, but the reason for this is not fully understood. Recent studies substantiate a dualistic proinflammatory and immunosuppressive role of TNF and heterogeneity of TNF receptor usage in autoimmune suppression versus inflammatory tissue damage (63,64). This provides a rationale for future treatment of RA with selective anti-TNF receptor, instead of anti-TNF. However, full understanding is complicated by the finding of cooperative activity of p55 and p75 TNF receptor in arthritis induced with membrane-bound TNF, in line with the identification of preferential binding of transmembrane, compared to soluble, TNF to the p75 receptor. It remains to be elucidated to what extent human RA is driven by soluble, or membrane TNF. Of note, soluble TNF is hard to detect in RA synovial fluid, and models with dominant overexpression of soluble TNF hamper proper identification of the role of p75 TNF receptor.

IL-1α TRANSGENIC MICE AND IL-1RA–/– MICE

Recently, transgenic IL-1α overexpression was also shown to induce chronic, destructive arthritis (65). Transgenic mice expressing human IL-1α had high serum levels of IL-1 and developed a severe polyarthritis within 4 weeks of age. Hyperplasia of the synovial lining, pannus formation, and, ultimately, cartilage destruction were evident. T and B cells were scant, but active granulocytes were abundant.

The opposite approach, elimination of IL-1 control by gene targeting of the endogenous IL-1 receptor antagonist (IL-1ra), also yielded a model of arthritis. IL-1ra deficiency in a BALB/ca background resulted in pronounced arthritis at the age of 8 weeks (66). Marked synovial and periarticular inflammation was noted, with invasion of granulation tissue and articular erosion. Moreover, elevated levels of antibodies against IgGs, CII and double-stranded DNA were found, suggestive of autoimmune responses. Intriguingly, IL-1ra deficiency in a C57Bl/6j background did not yield arthritis but, instead, showed arteritis (67). This genetic variation, although not well understood, underscores an immunologic pathogenetic pathway. Overexpression of a range of cytokines, including IL-1β, TNF, and IL-6, was observed in the joints before onset of arthritis. Interestingly, autoantibody levels did not correlate with disease severity, which may imply that it reflects a reaction to damaged joint tissue.

In sharp contrast to the TNF transgenic model, the arthritis in IL-1ra–/– mice seems dependent on T cells, in line with the strong genetic restriction. It is consistent with the view that IL-1 is a crucial regulator of T-cell function. Undisturbed IL-1 action, in the absence of IL-1ra, probably permits activation of T cells directed against exogenous triggers or endogenous autoantigens. Impaired T-cell activation is found in IL-1–deficient mice, linked to low levels of CD40 ligand and OX40 expression on T cells, and underlies the suppression of collagen arthritis in these mice (20). Moreover, altered susceptibility to collagen arthritis is found in transgenic mice with aberrant expression of IL-1ra, with earlier onset and more severe arthritis in IL-1ra–deficient mice and reduced arthritis in IL-1ra transgenics (68).

OTHER MODELS

Adjuvant Oils and Pristane

Adjuvant oils can induce a symmetric destructive polyarthritis when injected intradermally in dark agouti rats (69). Expression of arthritis occurs between days 11 and 14, is found in 100% of rats, and lasts for 6 weeks. As in classic adjuvant arthritis, readministration of oil to rats that had recovered from oil-induced arthritis fails to induce arthritis a second time. This points to an immunologic background and, indeed, the arthritis could be transferred with concanavalin A–activated T cells from arthritic rats to irradiated recipients. The model runs in germ-free dark agouti rats. A seemingly similar disease could be induced with adjuvant oil in certain strains of mice and was termed *pristane arthritis* (70,71). The pristane disease in mice, however, has proved difficult to characterize because of late onset, variable penetrance, and difficulty of transfer. In late disease, numerous types of autoantibodies were noted, including rheumatoid factor, which may contribute to the propagation of arthritis and make this model less clearly T-cell driven. In marked contrast to findings in oil, classic adjuvant, and SCW arthritis in rats, pristane arthritis was suppressed in germ-free mice, implying a bacterium-specific pathogenesis.

The pristane model can easily be induced in most rat strains, shows a chronic relapsing disease course, and is extensively used by Holmdahl et al. to identify genes that control onset, severity, and chronicity of the disease (72,73). There is no indication of B-cell involvement at onset. Using crosses of highly susceptible dark agouti rats and resistant E3 strains, different loci were identified that control in a complex way the various stages of the disease. Similar studies have been done in other arthritis models, including collagen arthritis, by Joe et al., and some recent studies are suggested for further reading (74,75).

MRL/lpr Mice

Spontaneous arthritis is also described in MRL–lpr/lpr mice (76–78). These animals develop a severe autoimmune disease, characterized by massive lymphadenopathy, arteritis, immune complex–mediated glomerulonephritis, and chronic arthritis. The serologic abnormalities in these animals include antibodies against native DNA, rheumatoid factors, and circulating immune complexes. This strain of mice may thus be regarded as a model of both systemic lupus erythematosus and RA. The presence of rheumatoid factors, which is lacking in most of the induced models, makes this model of potential interest. However, the incidence of arthritis is much lower than the incidence of the systemic lupus–like syndrome and is much more variable in presentation. Moreover, on standard breeding, it is often noted that the incidence of arthritis is further diminished, due to preferential breeding of the more healthy individuals. The arthritis is characterized by early synovial and mesenchymal cell hyperplasia, late T-cell infiltration, and preceding cartilage destruction. The first signs are synovial cells with a transformed appearance and invasion of these cells into cartilage and bone, resulting in an RA-like pannus. Significant arthritis occurs only in aged mice, and signs are mild or absent before the age of 5 months. These mice display prolonged cell survival because of defective FAS-mediated apoptosis. The potential involvement of retroviral antigens in chronic arthritis, which was claimed earlier on in MRL mice, was underlined by the occurrence of arthritis after 2 to 3 months in mice transgenic for human T-cell leukemia virus (79,80).

Severe Combined Immunodeficiency Disease Mice

The immunocompromised severe combined immunodeficiency disease (SCID) mouse allows for *in vivo* study of the pathologic potential of cells from animal models or patients with RA. For this purpose, cells or pieces of synovial tissue are transferred to the SCID mouse and behavior and pathologic changes analyzed (81). An interesting design is the combination of cells or tissue with cartilage as a target tissue, to obtain further insight into mechanisms of cartilage destruction (82). Using the latter approach, it was found that RA synovial fibroblasts, without the need of T cells, can display invasive behavior and cause cartilage destruction. This destruction is promoted by IL-1 (83).

CYTOKINES IN ARTHRITIS SUSCEPTIBILITY AND JOINT DESTRUCTION

Major findings on TNF and IL-1 involvement have already been addressed under the headings of the various models. Instead of going through all the details in the common models, recent findings are summarized in Table 22.4, and relative importance of TNF and IL-1 in various pathways of cell activation is shown in Figure 22.6. Reviews are suggested for further reading (84–87). TNF is a major mediator in early stages of joint inflammation in every model. Although IL-1 is not a dominant inflammatory cytokine in all models, it is certainly the pivotal cytokine in the inhibition of chondrocyte proteoglycan synthesis in all models studied so far, and the blocking of IL-1 has a great beneficial impact on net cartilage destruction. In line with this, chronic destructive arthritis could not be induced in IL-1–deficient mice using any of the standard models mentioned above. In contrast, TNF deficiency reduced incidence of autoimmune arthritis expression, but, once joints become afflicted, full progression to erosive arthritis did occur (86,88). The novel T-cell cytokine IL-17 provides an additional target apart from TNF and IL-1. Local overexpression showed that it can accelerate inflammation and tissue destruction in collagen-induced arthritis, independent of IL-1 (89). In addition, the macrophage-derived cytokines IL-12, IL-15, and IL-18 are abundant in RA synovia, can contribute to Th1 maturation and activation, and were shown to promote collagen arthritis (90,91).

Regulation of Arthritis Susceptibility

Apart from the cytokines TNF-α and IL-1, modulatory cytokines, such as IL-4, IL-10, IL-12, and TGF-β, and specific endogenous inhibitors, such as shed receptors or IL-1ra, are of prime importance in the pathogenesis of arthritis. Although it has long been thought that susceptibility or resistance of a particular mouse strain to induction of collagen arthritis was entirely related to different epitope recognition, it is now clear that the cytokine milieu and the different production and sensitivity to regulatory cytokines has a major impact. In general, endogenous T helper 2 cytokines IL-4 and IL-10 are protective. Enhanced incidence of models like collagen-induced arthritis and proteoglycan arthritis is seen in IL-4– and IL-10–deficient mice, and treatment with IL-4/IL-10 suppresses arthritis (23,92). In addition, IL-12 and IL-18 promote such diseases, through enhancement of Th1 reactivity, and strong immunization with high or repeated adjuvant exposure makes seemingly resistant mouse strains susceptible (21,22,93). Enhanced expression of autoimmune arthritis can be induced with a single lipopolysaccharide or bacterial fragment injection shortly before expected onset, through generation of IL-12 and promotion of TNF and IL-1 production. It reflects the potential impact of environmental bacterial pressure, and variability in suscepti-

TABLE 22.4. Cytokine Involvement in Various Murine Arthritis Models

		Acute Inflammation		Mononuclear Infiltrate		Cartilage Destruction	
Model	References	TNF	IL-1	TNF	IL-1	TNF[a]	IL-1
SCW	51	++	–	+	++	–	+
SCW flares	84,85	+	+	–	++	–	++
CIA	27–30	++	+++	±	++	+	++
AIA	43–45	±	±	–	+	–	++
AIA flare	46	+	+	–	+	–	++
ICA[b]	53	±	++	–	++	±	++
GPI-A[c]	59	+	++	+	++	+	++

AIA, antigen-induced arthritis; CIA, collagen-induced arthritis; GPI, glucose-6-phophate isomerase arthritis; ICA, immune-complex arthritis; IL, interleukin; SCW-A, streptococcal cell-wall arthritis; TNF, tumor necrosis factor.
[a]The role of TNF in destruction is mainly indirect, by preventing onset of the arthritic process.
[b]ICA, passive immune-complex arthritis with poly-L-lysine lysozyme as antigen.
[c]Passive arthritis induced with antibodies from the K/BxN arthritic mice.

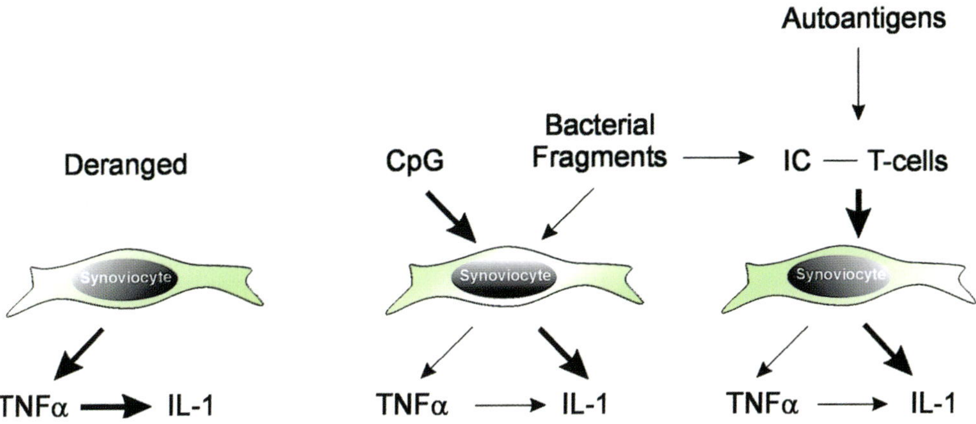

Figure 22.6. Various pathways of tumor necrosis factor (TNF) and interleukin (IL)-1 triggering. When there is defective TNF production (mimicking the TNF transgenic mice), IL-1 production is fully dependent of TNF. With inflammatory stimuli and immune-driven activation, in particular, TNF-independent IL-1 production is pronounced. In most induced animal models, late disease includes immune elements, which might explain skewed IL-1 sensitivity. IC, immune complex.

bility probably is dependent on marked variation of Toll receptor levels observed in various mouse strains.

Cartilage and Bone Destruction

Animal models are excellent tools to characterize destructive pathways. Cartilage damage observed in different models ranges from a selective loss of cartilage, underlying pannus tissue, to an overall loss of matrix, starting with proteoglycan release and progressing to collagen damage. Killing of chondrocytes and complete loss of the superficial and middle cartilage layer are noted in severe forms (Fig. 22.2). This underlines that arthritic processes can be more or less destructive, depending on the underlying process and cytokines mixture. Enhanced degradation of matrix and inhibited synthesis of proteoglycans by the chondrocyte are general findings in all models. Aggressive overall cartilage loss is only noted in the presence of immune-complex deposition, whereas milder, more gradual forms of damage are noted in models driven by macrophage or T-cell activation. Large variation in progressive destruction is also noted in populations of patients with RA, which may indicate separate pathogenic pathways.

The contribution of neutrophils to cartilage destruction is still unclear. Although enzymes from neutrophils, such as elastase, can be highly destructive *in vitro*, neutrophils also contain TGF-β and IL-1ra and can be protective as well. Normally, neutrophils do not attach to the cartilage surface, and released enzymes will be scavenged by enzyme inhibitors of the synovial fluid. Depletion of neutrophils in antigen-induced arthritis did not influence cartilage destruction, and damage was similar in elastase-deficient mice. However, in the presence of dense immune complexes in the superficial cartilage layers, marked sticking of neutrophils is found in antigen- and collagen-induced arthritis, in particular. This attachment is increased by immobilization of the joint. The ruffled cartilage surface under those conditions indicates direct destruction by attached cells (94,95).

Although neutrophils may be destructive under certain conditions, these cells are not essential to the destruction, and neither are lymphocytes. Observations in MRL–lpr/lpr mice and the H_2-c-*fos* transgenic mice bearing cells with enhanced levels of metalloproteinases indicate that macrophage-rich infiltrates can be highly destructive without the presence of neutrophils and lymphocytes. Plain overexpression of c-*fos* in synovial cells did not lead to arthritis. However, the eliciting of antigen-induced or collagen arthritis in these c-*fos* mice yielded more severe and more destructive arthritis. Remarkably, the cellular infiltrate in these mice contained hardly any lymphocytes, yet, marked cartilage destruction was found, stressing the role of mesenchymal cells in that damage (96).

Similarly, macrophage, but not lymphocyte, numbers in rheumatoid synovial tissue correlate with the radiologic progression of joint destruction (97). The critical enzymes involved in destruction in arthritis models and human RA are still far from understood and warrant further study in animal models.

A general lesson that may be deduced from observations in various models is that continuing irreversible destruction can occur under conditions that will hardly be considered inflamma-

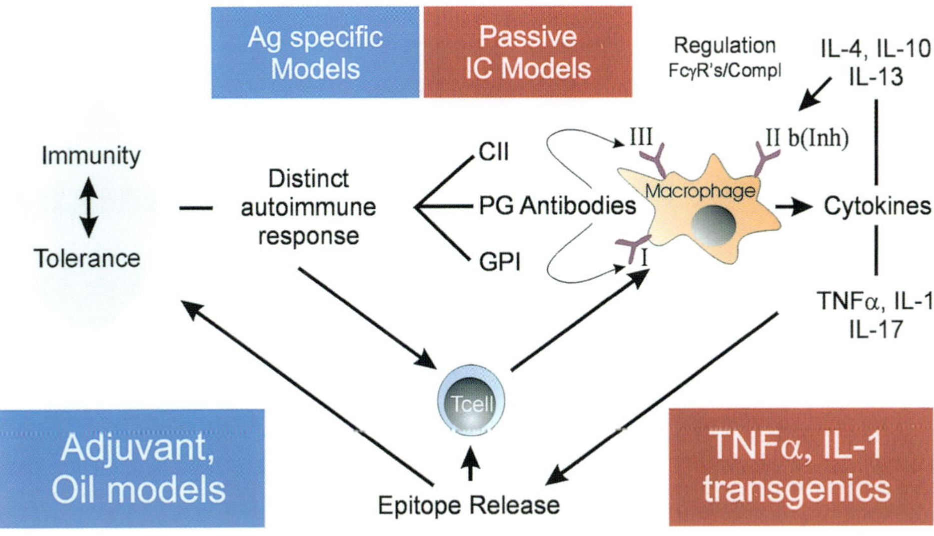

Figure 22.7. Apart from the continued interest in regulation of tolerance, various elements of the arthritis process are shown, which can be explored with the respective animal models. At present, much interest is focused on the role of autoantibodies and immune complex (IC)–mediated triggering of Fcγ receptors (FcγR) on macrophages. In the mouse, FcγR I and III are activating, whereas IIb is inhibitory (Inh). Sensitivity of various mouse strains to immune-complex arthritis is dependent on genetic differences in relative levels and skewing of receptor expression by the cytokine milieu. Distinct destructive pathways are explored in cytokine-specific transgenics. Ag, antigen; CII, collagen type II; GPI, glucose-6-phosphate isomerase; IL, interleukin; PG, proteoglycan; TNF, tumor necrosis factor.

tory, whereas the opposite occurs as well. Symptomatic relief by antiinflammatory therapy is promising, but the main challenge remains to interrupt joint destruction. As an example, local gene transfer with IL-4 did not suppress local inflammation, yet, markedly reduced cartilage and bone destruction in collagen-induced arthritis (98). It has recently been identified that RANKL is the crucial activating cytokine of the bone-resorbing osteoclasts. In the absence of RANKL, joint inflammation continues in the passive GPI immune-complex arthritis, but bone erosion is prevented (99). Similarly, when TNF transgenic mice were crossed with *c-fos*–deficient mice, joint inflammation continued, yet bone erosion was fully absent. *C-fos* mice lack functional osteoclasts, and this study identifies that TNF-driven bone erosion is osteoclast dependent, and the absence of osteoclasts alters TNF-mediated arthritis from a destructive to a nondestructive phenotype. In line with this, treatment with OPG, which is the natural inhibitor of RANKL, does not reduce inflammation in adjuvant arthritis and TNF transgenic mice, yet, bone erosion was reduced (11,100,101), and similar findings were obtained with local OPG treatment of the joints of mice collagen arthritis (*author's personal observation*). These promising results reveal that animal models will yield further insight in inflammatory versus destructive mechanisms. A brief summary scheme of some research areas in models is depicted in Figure 22.7. Careful monitoring of both joint inflammation and destructive features is warranted in clinical trials with novel therapeutics.

REFERENCES

1. Wooley PH. Animal models of rheumatoid arthritis. *Curr Opin Rheumatol* 1991;3:407–420.
2. Pearson CM. Development of arthritis, periarthritis and periostitis in rats given adjuvants. *Proc Soc Exp Biol (New York)* 1956;91:95–101.
3. Van de Langerijt AGM, Kingston AE, van Lent PLEM, et al. Cross-reactivity to proteoglycans in bacterial arthritis: lack of evidence for in vivo role in induction of disease. *Clin Immunol Immunopathol* 1994;71:273–280.
4. Van de Langerijt AGM, van Lent PLEM, Hermus ARMM, et al. Susceptibility to adjuvant arthritis: relative importance of adrenal activity and bacterial flora. *Clin Exp Immunol* 1994;97:33–38.
5. Kohashi O, Kohashi Y, Takahashi T, et al. Suppressive effect of *Escherichia coli* on adjuvant-induced arthritis in germ-free rats. *Arthritis Rheum* 1986;29:547–553.
6. Holoshitz J, Naparstek Y, Ben-Num A, et al. Lines of T lymphocytes induce or vaccinate against autoimmune arthritis. *Science* 1983;219:56–58.
7. Billingham MEJ. Monoclonal antibody therapy of experimental arthritis: comparison with cyclosporin A for elucidating cellular and molecular disease mechanisms. In: Davies ME, Dingle JT, eds. *Immunopharmacology of joints and connective tissue.* New York: Academic Press, 1994:65–86.
8. Van Eden W. Heatshock proteins as immunogenic bacterial antigens with the potential to induce and regulate autoimmune arthritis. *Immunol Rev* 1991;121:5–28.
9. Van Eden W. Heat shock proteins in rheumatoid arthritis. *Stress Proteins* 1999;136:329–346.
10. Bendele AM, Chlipala ES, Scherrer J, et al. Combination benefit of treatment with the cytokine inhibitors IL-1ra and PEGylated soluble TNF receptor type I in animal models of RA. *Arthritis Rheum* 2000;43:2648–2659.
11. Kong YY, Feige U, Sarosi I, et al. Activated T cells regulate bone loss and joint destruction in adjuvant arthritis through osteoprotegerin ligand. *Nature* 1999;402:304–309.
12. Cromartie WJ, Craddock JG, Schwab JH, et al. Arthritis in rats after systemic injection of streptococcal cell walls. *J Exp Med* 1977;146:1585–1602.
13. Stimpson SA, Brown RR, Anderle SK, et al. Arthropathic properties of peptidoglycan-polysaccharide polymers from normal flora bacteria. *Infect Immun* 1986;51:240–249.
14. Hazenberg MP, Klasen IS, Kool J, et al. Are intestinal bacteria involved in the etiology of rheumatoid arthritis? *APMIS* 1992;100:1–9.
15. Lafyatis R, Thompson NL, Remmers EF, et al. Transforming growth factor-β production by synovial tissues from rheumatoid patients and streptococcal cell wall arthritic rats. *J Immunol* 1989;143:1142–1148.
16. Deng GM, Tarkowski A. Synovial cytokine mRNA expression during arthritis triggered by CpG motifs of bacterial DNA. *Arthritis Res* 2001;3:48–53.
17. Trentham DE, Townes AS, Kang AH. Autoimmunity to type II collagen: an experimental model of arthritis. *J Exp Med* 1977;146:857–868.
18. Holmdahl R, Malmstrom V, Vuorio E. Autoimmune recognition of cartilage collagens. *Ann Med* 1993;25:251–264.
19. Wooley PH, Luthra HS, Stuart JM, et al. Type II collagen-induced arthritis in mice. I. MHC (I-region) linkage and antibody correlates. *J Exp Med* 1981;154: 688–700.
20. Saijo S, Asano M, Horai R, et al. Suppression of autoimmune arthritis in IL-1 deficient mice in which T cell activation is impaired due to low levels of CD40 ligand and OX40 expression on T cells. *Arthritis Rheum* 2002;46:553–544.
21. Joosten LAB, Helsen MMA, van den Berg WB. Accelerated onset of collagen-induced arthritis by remote inflammation. *Clin Exp Immunol* 1994;97:204–211.
22. Joosten LAB, Heuvelmans-Jacobs M, Lubberts E, et al. Local IL-12 gene transfer promotes conversion of an acute arthritis to a chronic destructive arthritis. *Arthritis Rheum* 2002;46:1379–1389.
23. Joosten LAB, Lubberts E, Durez P, et al. Role of IL-4 and IL-10 in murine collagen-induced arthritis: protective effect of IL-4 and IL-10 treatment on cartilage destruction. *Arthritis Rheum* 1997;40:249–260.
24. Ortman RA, Shevach EM. Susceptibility to collagen-induced arthritis: cytokine-mediated regulation. *Clin Immunol* 2001;98:109–118.
25. Ravetch JV, Bolland S. IgG Fc receptors. *Annu Rev Immunol* 2001;19:275–290.
26. Van Lent PLEM, Nabbe K, Blom AB, et al. Role of activatory Fcγ RI and Fcγ RIII and inhibitory Fcγ RII in inflammation and cartilage destruction during experimental antigen-induced arthritis. *Am J Pathol* 2001;159:2309–2320.
27. Williams RO, Feldmann M, Maini RN. Anti-tumor necrosis factor ameliorates joint disease in murine collagen-induced arthritis. *Proc Natl Acad Sci U S A* 1992a;89:9784–9788.
28. Wooley PH, Dutcher J, Widmer MB, et al. Influence of a recombinant human soluble tumor necrosis factor receptor FC fusion protein on type II collagen-induced arthritis in mice. *J Immunol* 1993;151:6602–6607.
29. Van den Berg WB, Joosten LAB, Helsen M, et al. Amelioration of established murine collagen-induced arthritis with anti-IL-1 treatment. *Clin Exp Immunol* 1994;95:237–243.
30. Joosten LAB, Helsen MMA, van de Loo FAJ, et al. Anticytokine treatment of established type II collagen-induced arthritis in DBA/1 mice: a comparative study using anti-TNFα, anti-IL-1α/β and IL-1ra. *Arthritis Rheum* 1996;39:797–809.
31. Brand DD, Myers LK, Whittington KB, et al. Detection of early changes in autoimmune T cell phenotype and function following intravenous administration of type II collagen induced TCR-transgenic model. *J Immunol* 2002;168:490–498.
32. Miossec P, van den Berg WB. Th1/Th2 cytokine balance in arthritis. *Arthritis Rheum* 1997;40:2105–2115.
33. Joosten LAB, Coenen-de Roo CJJ, Helsen MMA, et al. Induction of tolerance with intranasal administration of human cartilage gp39 in DBA/1 mice. Amelioration of clinical, histologic, and radiologic signs of type II collagen-induced arthritis. *Arthritis Rheum* 2000;43:645–655.
34. Mikecz K, Glant TT, Buzas E, et al. Proteoglycan induced polyarthritis and spondylitis adoptively transferred to naive BALB/C mice. *Arthritis Rheum* 1990;33:866–876.
35. Finnegan A, Mikecz K, Tao P, et al. Proteoglycan (aggrecan)-induced arthritis in BALB/c mice is a Th1-type disease regulated by Th2 cytokines. *J Immunol* 1999;163:5383–5390.
36. Rosloniec EF, Latham K, Guedez YB. Paradoxical roles of IFN-gamma in models of Th1-mediated autoimmunity. *Arthritis Res* 2003;4:333–336.
37. Adarichev VA, Bardos T, Christodoulou S, et al. Major histocompatibility complex controls susceptibility and dominant inheritance, but not the severity of the disease in mouse models of RA. *Immunogenetics* 2002;54:184–192.
38. Otto JM, Chandrasekeran R, Vermes C, et al. A genome scan using a novel genetic cross identifies new susceptibility loci and traits in a mouse model of RA. *J Immunol* 2000;165:5278–5286.
39. Dumonde DC, Glynn LE. The production of arthritis in rabbits by an immunological reaction to fibrin. *Br J Exp Pathol* 1962;43:373–383.
40. Cooke TDV, Hird ER, Ziff M, et al. The pathogenesis of chronic inflammation in experimental antigen induced arthritis. *J Exp Med* 1972;135:323–338.
41. Van den Berg WB, van de Putte LBA, Zwarts WA, et al. Electrical charge of the antigen determines intraarticular antigen handling and chronicity of arthritis in mice. *J Clin Invest* 1984;74:1850–1859.
42. Lewthwaite J, Blake SM, Hardingham TE, et al. The effect of recombinant human IL-1 receptor antagonist on the induction phase of antigen induced arthritis in the rabbit. *J Rheumatol* 1994;21:467–472.
43. Van de Loo AAJ, Arntz OJ, Otterness IG, et al. Protection against cartilage proteoglycan synthesis inhibition by anti-interleukin 1 antibodies in experimental arthritis. *J Rheumatol* 1992;19:348–356.
44. Henderson B, Blake S. Therapeutic potential of cytokine manipulation. *Trends Pharmacol Sci* 1992;13:145–152.
45. Van Meurs JBJ, van Lent PLEM, Singer II, et al. IL-1ra prevents expression of the metalloproteinase-generated neoepitope VDIPEN in antigen-induced arthritis. *Arthritis Rheum* 1998;41:647–656.
46. Van de Loo AAJ, Arntz OJ, Bakker AC, et al. Role of interleukin-1 in antigen-induced exacerbations of murine arthritis. *Am J Pathol* 1995;146:239–249.
47. De Vries BJ, van den Berg WB. Impact of NSAIDs on murine antigen induced arthritis. I. An investigation of antiinflammatory and chondroprotective effects. *J Rheumatol* 1989;18[Suppl16]:10–18.
48. Hunneyball IM, Billingham MEJ, Rainsford KD. Animal models of arthritic disease: influence of novel compared with classical antirheumatic agents. In: Rainsford KD, ed. *New developments in antirheumatic therapy*. Kluwer: Dordrecht, 1989:93–132.
49. Lens JW, van den Berg WB, van de Putte LBA. Flare-up of antigen-induced arthritis in mice after challenge with intravenous antigen. Studies on the characteristics of and mechanisms involved in the reaction. *Clin Exp Immunol* 1984;55:287–294.

50. Van den Broek MF, van den Berg WB, van de Putte LBA, et al. Streptococcal cell wall induced arthritis and flare-up reactions in mice induced by homologous and heterologous cell walls. *Am J Pathol* 1988;133:139–149.
51. Kuiper S, Joosten LAB, Bendele AM, et al. Different roles of TNFα and IL-1 in murine streptococcal cell wall arthritis. *Cytokine* 1998;10:690–702.
52. Blom AB, van Lent PLEM, van Vuuren H et al. FcgammaR expression on macrophages is related to severity and chronicity of synovial inflammation and cartilage destruction during experimental immune-complex-mediated arthritis (ICA). *Arthritis Res* 2000;2:489–503.
53. Van Lent PLEM, van de Loo FAJ, Holthuysen AEM, et al. Major role for IL-1 but not for TNF in early cartilage damage in immune complex arthritis in mice. *J Rheumatol* 1995;22:2250–2258.
54. Korganow AS, Ji H, Mangialaio S, et al. From systemic T cell self-reactivity to organ-specific autoimmune disease via immunoglobulins. *Immunity* 1999;10: 451–461.
55. Maccioni M, Zeder-Lutz G, Huang H, et al. Arthritogenic monoclonal antibodies from K/BxN mice. *J Exp Med* 2002;195:1071–1077.
56. Ji H, Gauguier D, Ohmura K, et al. Genetic influences on the end stage effector phase of arthritis. *J Exp Med* 2001;194:321–330.
57. Ji H, Ohmura K, Mahmood U, et al. Arthritis critically dependent on innate immune system players. *Immunity* 2002;16:157–168.
58. Matsumoto I, Maccioni M, Lee DM, et al. How antibodies to a ubiquitous cytoplasmic enzyme may provoke joint-specific autoimmune disease. *Nat Immunol* 2002;3:360–365.
59. Ji H, Pettit A, Ohmura K, et al. Critical roles for IL-1 and TNFα in antibody-induced arthritis. *J Exp Med* 2002;196:77–85.
60. Keffer J, Probert L, Cazlaris H, et al. Transgenic mice expressing human tumor necrosis factor: a predictive genetic model of arthritis. *EMBO J* 1991;13:4025–4031.
61. Kontoyiannis D, Pasparakis M, Pizarro TT, et al. Impaired on/off regulation of TNF biosynthesis in mice lacking TNF AU-rich elements: implications for joint and gut-associated immunopathologies. *Immunity* 1999;10:387–398.
62. Kollias G, Douni E, Kassiotis G, et al. On the role of TNF and receptors in models of multiorgan failure, RA, multiple sclerosis and inflammatory bowel disease. *Immunol Rev* 1999;169:175–194.
63. Kassiotis G, Kollias G. Uncoupling the proinflammatory from the immunosuppressive properties of TNF at the p55 TNF receptor level: implications for pathogenesis and therapy of autoimmune demyelination. *J Exp Med* 2001;193:427–434.
64. Douni E, Kollias G. A critical role of the p75 TNF-R in organ inflammation independent of TNF, lymphotoxin α, or the p55TNF-R. *J Exp Med* 1998; 188:1343–1352.
65. Niki Y, Yamada H, Seki S, et al. Macrophage- and neutrophil-dominant arthritis in human IL-1 alpha transgenic mice. *J Clin Invest* 2001;107:1127–1135.
66. Horai R, Saijo S, Tanioka H, et al. Development of chronic inflammatory arthropathy resembling RA in IL-1ra-deficient mice. *J Exp Med* 2000;191:313–320.
67. Nicklin MJ, Hughs DE, Barton JL, et al. Arterial inflammation in mice lacking the IL-1ra gene. *J Exp Med* 2000;191:303–312.
68. Ma Y, Thornton S, Boivin GP, et al. Altered susceptibility to collagen-induced arthritis in transgenic mice with aberrant expression of IL-1ra. *Arthritis Rheum* 1998;41:1798–1805.
69. Kleinau S, Erlandsson H, Holmdahl R, et al. Adjuvant oils induce arthritis in the DA rat. I. Characterization of the disease and evidence for an immunological involvement. *J Autoimmune* 1991;4:871–880.
70. Wooley PH, Seibold JR, Whalen JD, et al. Pristane induced arthritis. The immunologic and genetic features of an experimental murine model of autoimmune disease. *Arthritis Rheum* 1989;32:1022–1030.
71. Thompson SJ, Elson CJ. Susceptibility to pristane-induced arthritis is altered with changes in bowel flora. *Immunol Lett* 1993;36:227–232.
72. Holmdahl R, Lorentzen JC, Lu S, et al. Arthritis induced in rats with nonimmunogenic adjuvants as models for RA. *Immunol Rev* 2001;184:184–202.
73. Lu S, Nordquist N, Holmberg J, et al. Both common and unique susceptibility genes in different rat strains with pristane-induced arthritis. *Eur J Hum Genet* 2002;10:475–483.
74. Joe B, Cannon GW, Griffiths MM, et al. Evaluation of quantitative trait loci regulation severity of mycobacterial adjuvant induced arthritis in monocongenic and polycongenic rats: identification of a new regulatory locus on rat chromosome 10 and evidence of overlap with RA susceptibility loci. *Arthritis Rheum* 2002;46:1075–1085.
75. Remmers EF, Joe B, Griffiths MM, et al. Modulation of multiple experimental arthritis models by collagen-induced arthritis quantitative trait loci isolated in congenic rat lines: different effects of non-major histocompatibility complex quantitative trait loci in males and females. *Arthritis Rheum* 2002;46: 2225–2234.
76. Hang L, Theofilopoulos AN, Dixon FJ. A spontaneous rheumatoid arthritis-like disease in MRL/1 mice. *J Exp Med* 1982;155:1690–1701.
77. Koopman WJ, Gay S. The MRL-lpr/lpr mouse. A model for the study of rheumatoid arthritis. *Scand J Rheumatol* 1988;75[Suppl]:284–289.
78. Bartlett RR, Popovic S, Raiss RX. Development of autoimmunity in MRL/lpr mice and the effects of drugs on this murine disease. *Scand J Rheumatol* 1988;75[Suppl]:290–299.
79. Iwakura Y, Tosu M, Yoshida E, et al. Induction of inflammatory arthropathy resembling rheumatoid arthritis in mice transgenic for HTLV-I. *Science* 1991;253:1026–1028.
80. Yamamoto H, Sekiguchi T, Itagaki K, et al. Inflammatory polyarthritis in mice transgenic for human T cell leukemia virus type I. *Arthritis Rheum* 1993;36:1612–1620.
81. Williams RO, Plater-Zyberk C, Williams DG, et al. Successful transfer of collagen-induced arthritis to severe combined immunodeficient (SCID) mice. *Clin Exp Immunol* 1992b;88:455–460.
82. Müller-Ladner U, Kriegsmann J, Franklin BN, et al. Synovial fibroblasts of patients with RA attach to and invade normal human cartilage when engrafted into SCID mice. *Am J Pathol* 1996;149:1607–1615.
83. Neumann E, Judex M, Kullmann F, et al. Inhibition of cartilage destruction by double gene transfer of IL-1ra and IL-10 involves the activin pathway. *Gene Ther* 2002;9:1508–1519.
84. Van den Berg WB, Bresnihan B. Pathogenesis of joint damage in RA: evidence of a dominant role for IL-1. *Baillieres Clin Rheumatol* 1999;13:577–597.
85. Van den Berg WB. What we learn from arthritis models to benefit arthritis patients. *Baillieres Clin Rheumatol* 2000;14:599–616.
86. Van den Berg WB. Uncoupling of inflammatory and destructive mechanisms in arthritis. *Semin Arthritis Rheum* 2001;30[Suppl2]:7–16.
87. Van den Berg WB. Lessons from animal models of arthritis. *Curr Rheumatol Rep* 2002;4:232–239.
88. Campbell IK, O'Donnell K, Lawlor KE, et al. Severe inflammatory arthritis and lymphadenopathy in the absence of TNF. *J Clin Invest* 2001;107:1519–1527.
89. Lubberts E, Joosten LAB, Oppers B, et al. IL-1 independent role of IL-17 in synovial inflammation and joint destruction during collagen induced arthritis. *J Immunol* 2001;167:1004–1013.
90. Gracie JA, Forsey RJ, Chan WL, et al. A proinflammatory role for IL-18 in rheumatoid arthritis. *J Clin Invest* 1999;104:1393–1401.
91. McInnes IB, Liew FY. Interleukin-15: a proinflammatory role in rheumatoid arthritis synovitis. *Immunol Today* 1998;19:75–79.
92. Finnegan A, Grusby MJ, Kaplan CD, et al. IL-4 and IL-12 regulate proteoglycan-induced arthritis through Stat dependent mechanisms. *J Immunol* 2002;169:3345–3352.
93. Campbell IK, Hamilton JA, Wicks IP. Collagen-induced arthritis in C57Bl/6 (H-2b) mice: new insights into an import disease model of rheumatoid arthritis. *Eur J Immunol* 2000;30:1568–1575.
94. Van Lent PLEM, van den Bersselaar L, van de Putte LBA, et al. Immobilization aggravates cartilage damage during antigen-induced arthritis in mice. Attachment of polymorphonuclear leucocytes to articular cartilage. *Am J Pathol* 1990;136:1407–1416.
95. Van Lent PLEM, Blom A, Holthuysen AEM, et al. Monocytes/macrophages rather than PMN are involved in early cartilage degradation in cationic immune complex arthritis in mice. *J Leukoc Biol* 1997;61:267–278.
96. Shiozawa S, Tanka Y, Fujita T, et al. Destructive arthritis without lymphocyte infiltration in H_2-c-*fos* transgenic mice. *J Immunol* 1992;148:3100–3104.
97. Bresnihan B. Pathogenesis of joint damage in RA. *J Rheumatol* 1999;26:717–719.
98. Lubberts E, Joosten LAB, Chabaud M, et al. IL-4 gene therapy for collagen arthritis suppresses synovial IL-17 and osteoprotegerin ligand and prevents bone erosion. *J Clin Invest* 2000;105:1697–1710.
99. Pettit AR, Ji H, von Stechow D, et al. TRANCE/RANKL knockout mice are protected from bone erosion in a serum transfer model of arthritis. *Am J Pathol* 2001;159:1689–1699.
100. Redlich K, Hayer S, Ricci R, et al. Osteoclasts are essential for TNFα-mediated joint destruction. *J Clin Invest* 2002;110:1419–1427.
101. Redlich K, Hayer S, Maier A, et al. TNFα-mediated joint destruction is inhibited by targeting osteoclasts with osteoprotegerin. *Arthritis Rheum* 2002; 46:785–792.

CHAPTER 23

Nonsteroidal Antiinflammatory Drugs and Analgesics

Leslie J. Crofford

Inflammation is a key clinical feature of rheumatoid arthritis (RA). Agents that inhibit symptoms of inflammation have been used for more than a century in the treatment of RA. Even in the era of biologic therapies, antiinflammatory drugs continue to be an important part of the therapeutic armamentarium. It was established in 1971 that nonsteroidal antiinflammatory drugs (NSAIDs) act to block the production of prostaglandins (PGs), lipid mediators important in normal physiology, as well as in inflammation. PG production occurs by the action of at least three enzymes, including the cyclooxygenase (COX) enzymes, whose metabolic activity is blocked by NSAIDs. Inhibiting PG production has both therapeutic and adverse effects that must be understood in order to use NSAIDs safely.

In recent years, important progress has been made toward understanding the clinical effects of NSAIDs by clarifying the biology of PG production. This advance came with the discovery of COX-2, the isoform whose expression is increased during inflammation. Specific inhibition of COX-2 blocks PG production at sites of inflammation while preserving production in certain other tissues, most importantly, platelets and the gastroduodenal mucosa. The relative roles of nonspecific NSAIDs compared with specific COX-2 inhibitors in treatment of RA continue to evolve.

The simple analgesic acetaminophen can be a useful alternative for management of pain, but it lacks any appreciable effect on inflammation. In patients unable to tolerate nonspecific or COX-2–specific NSAIDs or in those with contraindications to their use, acetaminophen and other analgesics may be useful treatments. This chapter will review biology of COX enzymes and the mechanism of action and clinical pharmacology of aspirin and salicylates, nonspecific and COX-2–specific NSAIDs, and acetaminophen. The comparative safety and efficacy of nonspecific and COX-2–specific NSAIDs in the treatment of RA will be discussed. Finally, a brief guide to the selection of an NSAID and clinical situations where a non-NSAID analgesic agent may be preferred will be presented.

CYCLOOXYGENASE BIOLOGY

Background

The diversity of PG function is achieved by cell- and tissue-specific generation of different stable PGs, multiple PG receptors linked to different intracellular signaling pathways, and PG production pathways involving enzymes that are induced to dramatically increase local PG production (Fig. 23.1). PGs are members of a family of lipid mediators derived from the 20 carbon-containing polyunsaturated fatty acid, arachidonic acid, and termed *eicosanoids* (eicosa meaning *twenty*). Eicosanoids were first recognized in the 1930s as the substance in semen that caused contraction of smooth muscle, hence the name *prostaglandin*. The structures of the PGs were identified 30 years later, and the biosynthetic pathways were described shortly thereafter (1). An important evolution in the understanding of the PG biosynthetic pathways has developed since 1990 with molecular cloning of multiple synthetic enzymes, study of their expression and regulation, and solving the crystal structures.

Prostaglandin Biosynthetic Pathway

Biosynthesis of PGs involves a three-step sequence: hydrolysis of arachidonic acid from glycerophospholipid membranes, oxygenation of arachidonate to the endoperoxide PGH_2, and conversion of PGH_2 to the biologically active end products via specific synthases (2). The first step in PG synthesis is mediated by a phospholipase A_2 (PLA_2) (3). The principal secreted PLA_2 participating in inflammatory processes is type IIA–secreted PLA_2 (4). Very high concentrations of type IIA–secreted PLA_2 are found in synovial fluid of patients with RA (5). The type IV cytosolic PLA_2 has a preference for phospholipids containing arachidonate and is likely to be importantly involved in regulating generation of lipid mediators during inflammation (6,7). Although the synthesis of PGs is regulated acutely by activation of phospholipases and release of arachidonate, the net level of prostanoid production is determined by expression of enzymes distal in the metabolic pathway (8).

The first committed step for prostanoid biosynthesis is the two-step formation of PGH_2 by the bifunctional enzyme, PGH synthase, or COX. There are two isoforms of the enzyme, COX-1 and COX-2, the genes for which are found on human chromosomes 9 and 1, respectively. After biosynthesis of PGH_2 by COX, this endoperoxide is converted to one of several possible prostanoids by a terminal synthase. In general, this process is cell specific, with differentiated cells producing only one PG in abundance (3). The most important stable prostanoids are PGD_2, PGE_2, $PGF_2\alpha$, prostacyclin, and thromboxane A_2.

PGE_2 is an important mediator of inflammation in RA and other inflammatory arthritides (9). There are several forms of PGE synthase enzymes, including the microsomal PGE syn-

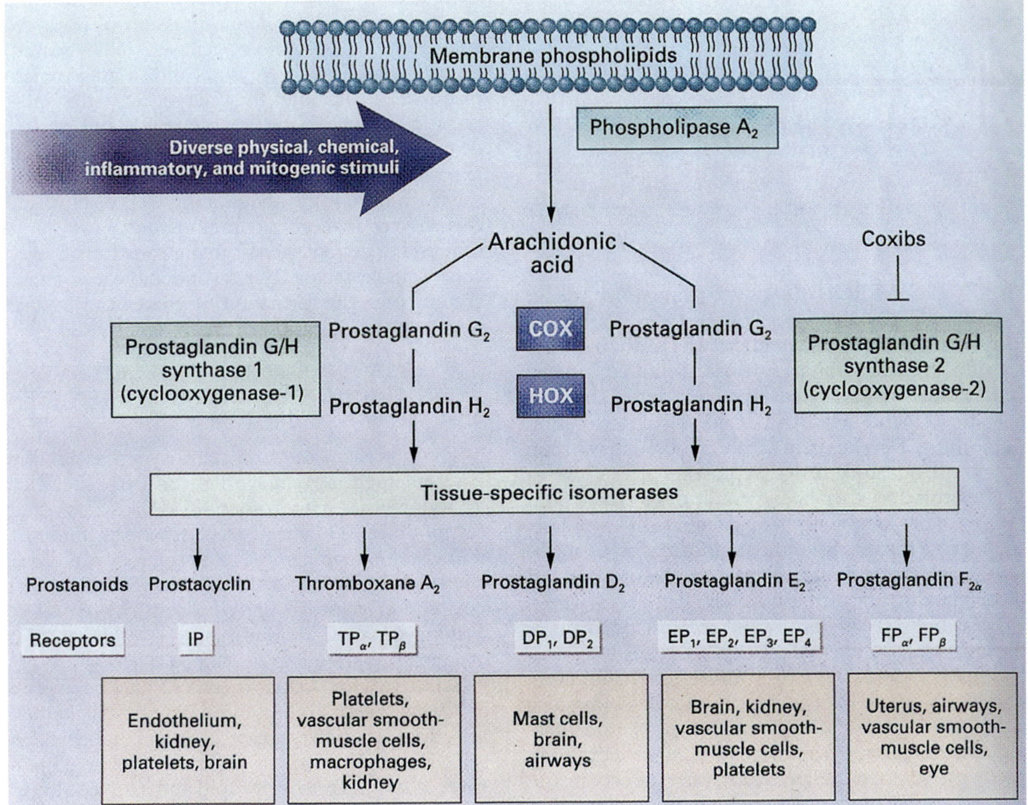

Figure 23.1. Biosynthesis and actions of prostaglandins (PGs). Many diverse stimuli trigger release of arachidonic acid from membrane phospholipids by phospholipase A_2. Arachidonate is metabolized by PG G/H synthase [PGHS or cyclooxygenase (COX-1)] or COX-2, which have both COX and hydroperoxidase (HOX) activity, to the unstable intermediate PG, PGH_2. Nonspecific nonsteroidal antiinflammatory drugs inhibit both COX-1 and COX-2, whereas specific COX-2 inhibitors block the activity of only that isoform. PGH_2 is further metabolized by tissue-specific isomerases or synthases, some constitutive and some inducible, to form the stable prostanoids. These PGs act on G-protein–coupled cell-surface receptors located on target tissues to generate diverse biologic effects. (From FitzGerald GA, Patrono C. The coxibs, selective inhibitors of cyclooxygenase-2. *N Engl J Med* 2001;345:433–442, with permission.)

thase-1 (PGES-1), which is expressed in arthritic tissues and is regulated by proinflammatory cytokines (9–11). It is likely that microsomal PGES-1 acts in concert with COX-2 to generate high levels of PGE_2 (12).

Biochemistry

COX-1 and COX-2 are bifunctional enzymes that mediate a COX reaction whereby arachidonate plus two molecules of O_2 are converted to PGG_2, followed by a hydroperoxidase reaction in which PGG_2 undergoes a two-electron reduction to PGH_2 (2). These two reactions occur at distinct but structurally and functionally interconnected sites. The peroxidase activity occurs at a heme-containing active site located near the protein surface whereas the COX reaction occurs in a hydrophobic channel in the core of the enzyme. The COX reaction is peroxide dependent and requires that the heme group at the peroxidase site undergo a two-electron oxidation. A tyrosine residue (Tyr385), located at the COX active site, is involved as a reaction intermediate (2). The physiological heme oxidant *in vivo* is not known, but it has been shown that the COX activity of COX-2 can be activated at tenfold lower concentrations of hydroperoxide than COX-1 (2).

Structural Biology

COX enzymes are integral membrane proteins that sit within the inner leaflet of the lipid bilayer of intracellular phospholipid membranes of the nuclear envelope and endoplasmic reticulum (13,14). The crystal structure of both COX isoforms has been determined, and they have essentially identical domain structures (Fig. 23.2) (15,16). Both COX-1 and COX-2 are homodimers, and each monomer consists of three structural domains. Both enzymes also contain sequences that target the endoplasmic reticulum and the associated nuclear envelope (2). The epidermal growth factor–like domain located at the N-terminus is likely to be involved in dimerization. The membrane-binding domain consists of four amphipathic α-helices that are inserted into one-half of the lipid bilayer. These α-helices are arranged to form an entrance to the hydrophobic channel in the center of the large, globular catalytic domain that contains the COX active site. This structure allows the entrance of arachidonate and O_2 directly from the lipid bilayer (2). NSAID binding occurs in the upper half of the hydrophobic channel and overlaps with the COX active site.

Most of the amino acids that form the hydrophobic channel of the COX-1 and COX-2 molecules are identical, with the exception of the substitution of the small amino acid valine in COX-2 for the isoleucine with a bulky side chain in COX-1 at position 523. This substitution opens a side pocket to the hydrophobic channel in COX-2 that was found to be critical for the development of pharmaceutical compounds that specifically inhibit COX-2 (16). The interaction of arachidonate with COX-1 and COX-2 may be different, as evidenced by differing effects of amino acid substitutions for the arginine (Arg120) located at the mouth of the hydrophobic channel in both enzymes. It is likely that an ionic bond with arachidonate is formed by COX-1, whereas a hydrogen bond is formed by COX-2 (17). Overall, COX-2 has a wider and somewhat more flexible interior channel, which has been exploited for the development of specific inhibitors (18).

Molecular Biology

The most striking difference between the COX isoforms is at the level of expression and regulation of messenger RNA (mRNA) and protein levels (19). These differences in expression and regulation are reflected in their differing biologic roles (Table 23.1). The promoter region of COX-1 has the characteristics of a housekeeping gene, a gene that is continuously transcribed and stably expressed. COX-1 mRNA and protein are expressed in most tissues under basal conditions as a result of these molecu-

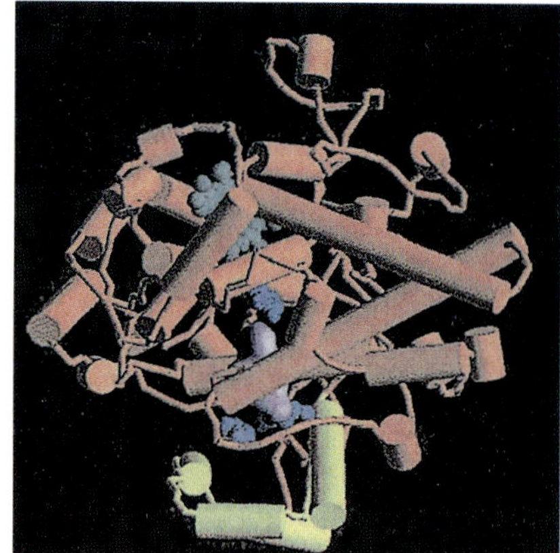

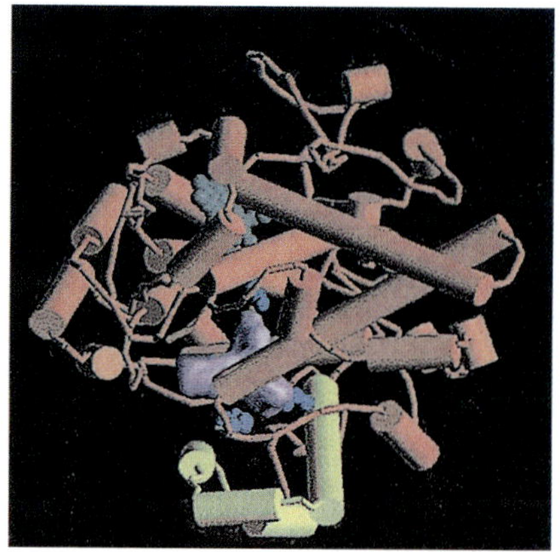

Figure 23.2. Crystal structures of cyclooxygenase (COX)-1 and COX-2. The domain structures of both COX enzymes are essentially identical. In this representation of the COX-1 **(A)** and COX-2 **(B)** monomers, the α-helices that insert into one-half of the lipid bilayer are depicted in yellow. The globular catalytic domain is represented in red. The epidermal growth factor–like domain is located on the right side face of each globular domain. The hydrophobic channels are occupied by a flurbiprofen for COX-1 and a celecoxib-related inhibitor for COX-2, both shown in purple. Note that the celecoxib-like drug has a large side chain that fills the side pocket of the hydrophobic channel. The side chains in blue represent important amino acid contacts. The heme critical for hydroperoxidase activity is shown in gray. (Modified from Picot D, Loll PJ, Garavito M. The X-ray crystal structure of the membrane protein prostaglandin H2 synthase-1. *Nature* 1994;367:243–249 and Kurumbail RA, Stevens AM, Gierse JK, et al. Structural basis for selective inhibition of cyclooxygenase-2 by antiinflammatory agents. *Nature* 1996;384:644–648.)

lar characteristics of the promoter (20). mRNA and protein levels do not vary greatly in response to external stimuli in differentiated tissues. COX-1 is available to increase PG production acutely when an abrupt increase in arachidonate substrate occurs, whereas COX-2 generally must be induced over a period of hours (12,21). COX-1 is the only isoform expressed in mature platelets and is the dominant isoform in normal gastric mucosa (22).

The COX-2 gene has the structure typical of highly regulated gene products (22). The promoter region has binding sites for transcription factors that act to increase gene transcription immediately in response to external stimuli (22,23). Increased levels of mRNA are seen as early as 15 to 30 minutes after a stimulus, and protein levels increase in 1 to 2 hours, reaching maximal levels by 4 hours after stimulation in most cell types and tissues (24). As anticipated from the promoter structure, COX-2 expression is highly induced by a number of cytokines, including interleukin-1, tumor necrosis factor α, and other stimuli associated with inflammation and growth (22,24,25). It has been confirmed that COX-2 expression is inhibited by glucocorticoids in all cells and tissues studied to date (22). Both COX-1 and COX-2 are expressed in synovial tissues of patients with arthritis. COX-1 is localized at the synovial lining layer, and there is no difference in the level of expression in inflammatory versus noninflammatory arthritides (26). COX-2 is localized to the sublining layers, particularly the vascular endothelial cells, infiltrating mononuclear inflammatory cells, and fibroblast-like synoviocytes. COX-2 expression is increased in inflammatory forms of arthritis (26,27).

Although COX-2 is clearly induced after stimulation by inflammatory stimuli in many tissues, COX-2 is also expressed under basal conditions in some tissues and induced by physiologic stimuli in others. The most important sites of basal COX-2 expression are the brain and kidney (28,29), and COX-2 has an important role in reproductive, cardiovascular, and skeletal physiology (22,30–32). It appears that, in some tissues, such as the vasculature and the kidney, PGs derived from the different COX isoforms may have antagonistic physiologic roles (33). The biologic roles of COX-1 and COX-2 help predict the adverse effects associated with nonspecific and COX-2–specific NSAIDs.

TABLE 23.1. Selected Biologic Roles of Cyclooxygenase (COX)-1 and COX-2

Organ/System	COX-1	COX-2
Inflammation, tissue damage, and repair	—	Induced. Mediates inflammatory symptoms, role in resolution, and repair in normal physiology.
Gastrointestinal tract	Constitutive. Cytoprotection of normal gastroduodenal mucosa.	Induced. Increased by inflammation and injury, especially important for mucosal defense in the colon.
Kidney	Constitutive. Expressed in vasculature, glomerulus, medullary collecting ducts. Role in GFR and solute homeostasis.	Constitutive. Expressed in vasculature, macula densa, medullary interstitium. Role in GFR, renin secretion, and solute homeostasis. Induced. In glomerulus during inflammation and in macula densa with salt or water deprivation.
Cardiovascular	Constitutive. Platelet thromboxane production, activation, hemostasis or thrombosis, vasoconstriction.	Constitutive. Prostacyclin production in normal arteries, inhibits platelet activation, vasodilation. Induced. In atherosclerosis, vasculitis.
Reproductive	—	Induced. Acute increase during ovulation, implantation, parturition.
Skeleton	—	Constitutive/induced. Osteoclastogenesis, endochondral bone formation.
Pulmonary	Constitutive. Counterbalances leukotriene synthesis in aspirin-exacerbated respiratory disease.	—

GFR, glomerular filtration rate.

MECHANISM OF ACTION

Cyclooxygenase Inhibition

The most important mechanism of NSAID action is to inhibit production of PGs by competing with arachidonic acid for binding in the COX catalytic site. NSAIDs have little effect on peroxidase activity (34). NSAIDs may exhibit different kinetic modes of inhibition, including (a) rapid, reversible binding (e.g., ibuprofen), (b) rapid, lower-affinity reversible binding followed by time-dependent, higher-affinity, slowly reversible binding, or (c) rapid, reversible binding followed by covalent modification (e.g., aspirin) (2). Time-dependent inhibition of COX enzymes appears to depend on the arginine (Arg120) near the entrance to the hydrophobic channel, which serves as the counterion for the carboxylate group of many NSAIDs. Many NSAIDs are optical isomers or enantiomers whereby the S-enantiomer, but not the R-enantiomer, are active COX inhibitors. The tyrosine (Tyr355) at the closed end of the hydrophobic channel governs the stereospecificity of NSAIDs (2,34). Time-dependent inhibition of COX-2 by specific inhibitors appears to depends on an arginine (Arg513) in the side pocket (35).

Cyclooxygenase-2 Specificity

From a clinical perspective, it is important to characterize NSAIDs according to specificity for inhibition of COX-1 or COX-2 (Table 23.2) (36–38). All NSAIDs currently in clinical use that inhibit COX-1 also inhibit COX-2 at therapeutic concentrations. All currently available COX-2–specific inhibitors exhibit time-dependent, slowly reversible inhibition of COX-2. The specificity for COX-2 is based on the structural difference between the hydrophobic channels resulting in an NSAID binding site approximately 20% larger than COX-1 and including the side pocket, with currently available specific COX-2 inhibitors containing a bulky sulfa-containing side chain (Fig. 23.3). Mutagenesis of COX-2 to eliminate access to the side pocket completely abrogates the differential sensitivity of COX-2 to specific inhibitors (16).

Although specific COX-2 inhibitors are selective in *in vitro* assays, the large number of variables makes *in vitro* assays suggestive at best (36). The most widely accepted definition of a specific COX-2 inhibitor is based on the *ex vivo* whole blood assay (38). Whole blood is collected from human subjects after a single dose of an NSAID or after several days of dosing to achieve steady state. The magnitude of COX-1 inhibition is measured by determining the degree of inhibition of platelet thromboxane production or aggregation of stimulated platelets. In the same blood sample, inhibition of COX-2 activity in peripheral blood mononuclear cells after stimulation with lipopolysaccharide is determined (39). Specific COX-2 inhibitors are characterized by lack of inhibitory effect on COX-1 activity at doses at or above those that maximally inhibit COX-2 (Fig. 23.4) (36,38).

TABLE 23.2. Cyclooxygenase-2 (COX-2) Selectivity of Nonsteroidal Antiinflammatory Drugs by Whole Blood Assay

Highly COX-2 Selective[a]	Somewhat COX-2 Selective[a]	Nonselective
Etoricoxib	Diclofenac	Ibuprofen
Rofecoxib	Meloxicam	Naproxen
Valdecoxib	Nimesulide	Indomethacin
Parecoxib		
Celecoxib		

[a]More selective from left to right.

Adapted from Riendeau D, Percival MD, Brideau C, et al. Etoricoxib (MK-0663): preclinical profile and comparison with other agents that selectively inhibit cyclooxygenase-2. *J Pharmacol Exp Ther* 2000;296:558–566 and FitzGerald GA, Patrono C. The coxibs, selective inhibitors of cyclooxygenase-2. *N Engl J Med* 2001;345:433–442.

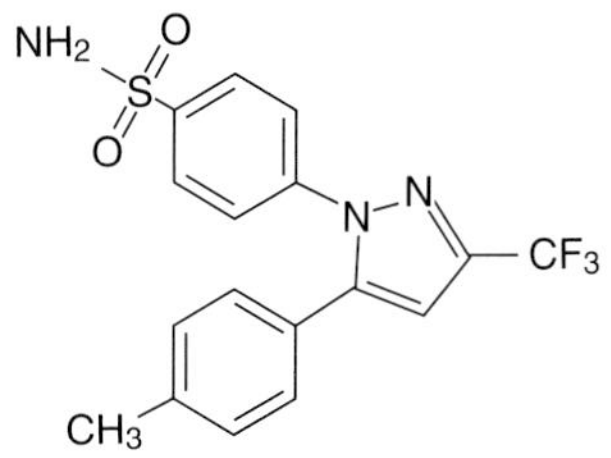

Celecoxib (sulfonamide)

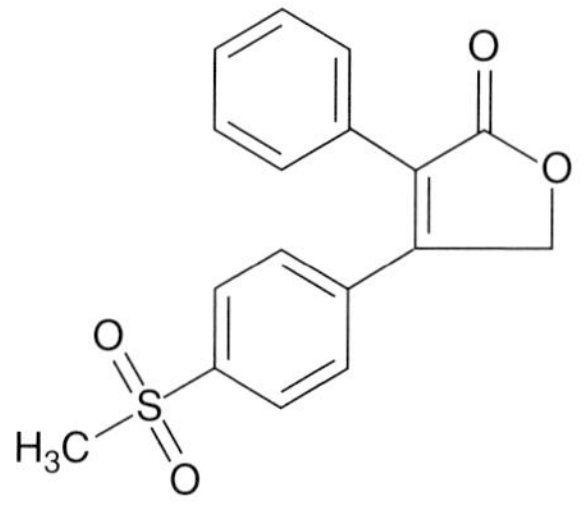

Rofecoxib (methyl sulfone)

Figure 23.3. Chemical structures of two cyclooxygenase-2 (COX-2)–specific nonsteroidal antiinflammatory drugs. Celecoxib and rofecoxib share structural features that promote specificity for the COX-2 isoform. Both agents, as well as other COX-2–specific NSAIDs, such as valdecoxib, contain bulky sulfa-containing side chains that insert into the side pocket of the hydrophobic channel.

Aspirin

Aspirin remains unique among NSAIDs as an irreversible inhibitor of the COX enzymes by virtue of the covalent acetylation of a serine (Ser529) located near the apex of the hydrophobic channel (34). Aspirin has an important therapeutic use as an agent for prophylaxis against cardiovascular thrombosis (40). Platelets provide a unique target for irreversible inhibition of COX-1, the only isoform in mature platelets, as they lack a nucleus and, therefore, the ability to resynthesize the enzyme. Aspirin, but not other NSAIDs, provides the complete and long-lasting inhibition of platelet COX-1 that is required to translate antiplatelet activity into clinical benefit (41). Some, but not all, NSAIDs may interfere with the antiplatelet effect of aspirin, presumably by blocking access to the COX-1 hydrophobic channel during the brief aspirin half-life (42).

Acetaminophen

Although most investigators believe that the most important mechanism for the antipyretic and analgesic activity of acetaminophen is inhibition of COX in the central nervous system, the exact mechanism remains unclear. At therapeutic doses, acetaminophen does not inhibit COX in peripheral tissues, which could explain its very weak antiinflammatory activity (43). The observations that inhibition of recombinant COX-1 and COX-2 by acetaminophen is dependent on hydroperoxide concentrations suggest a mechanism by which it acts to reduce the active oxidized form of COX to the inactive form (43,44). Inhibition of COX would, therefore, be more effective under conditions of low peroxide concentration, consistent with activity in the central nervous system, but not at inflammatory sites (43,44). Others have argued that alternatively spliced

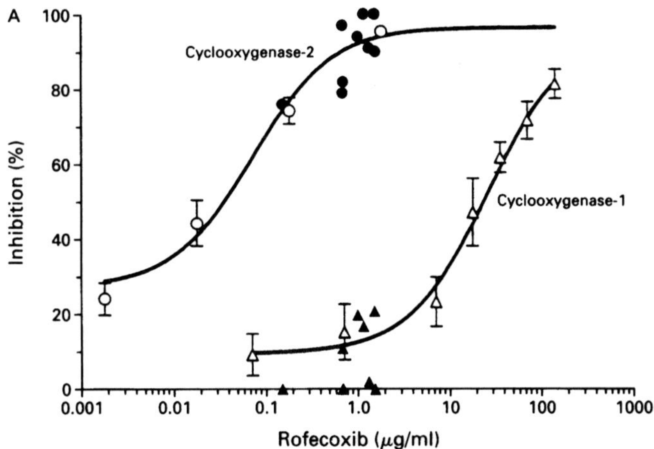

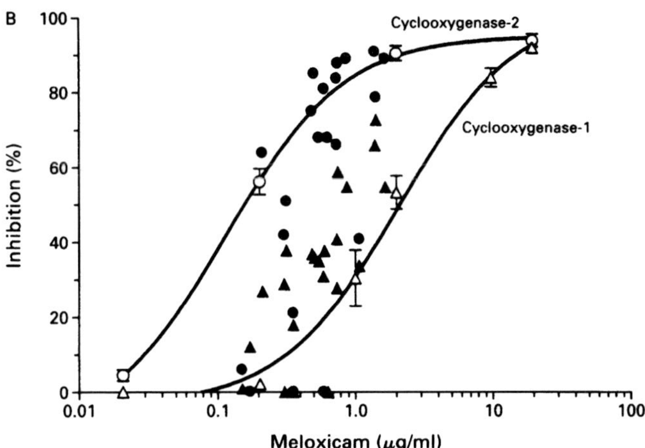

Figure 23.4. Representative examples of the whole blood assay for cyclooxygenase-2 (COX-2) specificity. The open symbols represent concentration–effect curves for the degree of inhibition of COX-1 (*triangles*) and COX-2 (*circles*) from *in vitro* whole blood experiments. In these experiments, increasing concentrations of rofecoxib **(A)** or meloxicam **(B)** were added to 1 mL of heparin-treated whole blood in the presence of lipopolysaccharide for 24 hours, and plasma prostaglandin E_2 was measured as an index of COX-2 activity. To determine COX-1 activity, increasing concentrations of rofecoxib or meloxicam were added to 1 mL whole blood and allowed to clot for 60 minutes, and serum thromboxane was measured. Superimposed on theses curves are data from *ex vivo* whole blood assays. The closed triangles represent the degree of inhibition of COX-1, and the closed circles represent the degree of inhibition of COX-2. In **(A)**, nine patients with rheumatoid arthritis were given 50 mg of rofecoxib daily for 7 days, and in **(B)**, 21 normal subjects received 7.5 or 15 mg of meloxicam once daily for 7 days. Blood was drawn 4 hours after the last dose of rofecoxib and 24 hours after the last dose of meloxicam, then COX-1 and COX-2 activity was determined, as described for the *in vitro* assay. (From FitzGerald GA, Patrono C. The coxibs, selective inhibitors of cyclooxygenase-2. *N Engl J Med* 2001;345:433–442, with permission.)

forms of COX-1 and COX-2 may be more sensitive to inhibition by acetaminophen and that tissue specificity is dictated by the presence of these COX variants (45,46).

Cyclooxygenase-Independent Actions of Salicylates and Nonsteroidal Antiinflammatory Drugs

Very high doses of NSAIDs have been shown to have COX-independent activities that could contribute to some of their actions. The practical importance of these mechanisms is unknown. Sodium salicylate and aspirin were shown to inhibit activation of the transcription factor nuclear factor–κB (NF-κB), suggesting a potentially important antiinflammatory mechanism (47). However, in mice genetically deficient for the p105 subunit of NF-κB, salicylates retain their antiinflammatory activity (48). Other NSAIDs, including inactive enantiomers of flurbiprofen, were also found to inhibit NF-κB (49). Other cell signaling molecules, such as mitogen-activated protein kinases and the transcription factor AP-1, may also be modulated by salicylates and NSAIDs (49). Some NSAIDs bind to and activate members of the peroxisome proliferator-activated receptor family and other intracellular receptors (49). Another potential mechanism of action is induction of endogenous antiinflammatory mechanisms. It was shown that the antiinflammatory effect of salicylate can be inhibited by an adenosine A_2 receptor antagonist in a murine model of inflammation, suggesting that salicylate may stimulate adenosine release (48). Specific COX-2 inhibitors may have unique structural features that promote COX-independent apoptosis and angiogenesis (50).

CLINICAL PHARMACOLOGY

Nonspecific and Cyclooxygenase-2–Specific Nonsteroidal Antiinflammatory Drugs

For a complete discussion of the clinical pharmacology of each nonspecific and COX-2–specific NSAID, the reader is directed to the package insert of the specific agent. The chemical class of selected nonspecific NSAIDs is shown in Table 23.3. Most NSAIDs are completely absorbed from the gastrointestinal (GI) tract. Once absorbed, NSAIDs are highly bound to plasma proteins, and the amount of free drug is relatively small. The relationship between the free and bound drug is stable for most NSAIDs, but some have dose-dependent protein binding and, consequently, the unbound concentration increases proportionally with dose (51). A relationship between plasma concentration of NSAIDs (e.g., naproxen) and therapeutic efficacy has been demonstrated (52). It has been shown that a higher dose of a single NSAID or NSAID combination can increase toxicity (53–55).

The nonspecific and COX-2–specific NSAIDs can be divided into those with longer and shorter plasma half-lives. Those drugs with a longer half-life take a longer time to reach steady-state concentrations. This can have consequences for the time to reach full therapeutic effect. The clearance of nonspecific and COX-2–specific NSAIDs is usually by hepatic metabolism with production of inactive metabolites that are excreted in the bile and urine. Most NSAIDs are metabolized through the microsomal cytochrome P450–containing mixed-function oxidase system (56). NSAIDs are most often metabolized by CYP3A (e.g., diclofenac, etoricoxib), CYP2C9 (e.g., naproxen, celecoxib), or both (e.g., valdecoxib). Other NSAIDs use completely different metabolic pathways; for example, rofecoxib is reduced by cytosolic enzymes. Because approximately 60% of drug interactions occur through CYP3A, drugs metabolized through this pathway are expected to have drug interactions. Those metabolized by CYP2C9 may have interactions with phenytoin and warfarin. Furthermore, there is genetic variation in enzyme activity, such that some individuals and ethnic groups may metabolize drugs more slowly. For example, Asians are frequently slow metabolizers through the CYP2C9 pathway. The pharmacokinetics of some NSAIDs can be affected by liver disease, renal disease, or old age (57).

Aspirin and Salicylates

Salicylates are acetylated (e.g., aspirin) or nonacetylated (e.g., sodium salicylate, choline salicylate, choline magnesium trisalicylate, salicylsalicylic acid) (58). Although the nonacetylated salicylates are only weak inhibitors of COX *in vitro*, they are able to reduce inflammation *in vivo*. Aspirin and salicylates are readily absorbed in the acidic or neutralized stomach and intestine. The formulation of these agents affects the absorption properties but not bioavailabil-

TABLE 23.3. Chemical Class of Nonspecific Nonsteroidal Antiinflammatory Drugs

Carboxylic Acids						Enolic Acids		Nonacidic Compounds
Salicylic Acids, Esters	Acetic Acids		Propionic Acids	Fenamic Acids		Pyrazolones	Oxicams	
	Phenylacetic Acids	Carbo- and Heterocyclic Acids						
Aspirin Diflunisal	Diclofenac	Etodolac Indomethacin Sulindac Tolmetin	Flurbiprofen Ketoprofen Oxaprozin Ibuprofen Naproxen	Meclofenamic		Phenylbutazone	Piroxicam Meloxicam	Nabumetone

Adapted from Brooks PM. NSAIDs. In: Klippel JH, Dieppe PA, eds. *Rheumatology*. London: Mosby, 1998:3.5.1–3.5.6.

ity. Buffered aspirin tablets contain antacids that increase the pH of the microenvironment, whereas enteric coating slows absorption. The bioavailability of rectal aspirin suppositories increases with retention time (56). Aspirin is rapidly deacetylated to salicylate either spontaneously or enzymatically. Albumin is the dominant protein to which salicylates bind, and in conditions in which albumin concentrations are low, such as active RA, the pharmacologic and toxic effects of an increment in dose are more pronounced. Salicylates diffuse into most body fluids, including synovial fluid, fairly rapidly. Salicylate is metabolized principally by the liver and excreted primarily by the kidney. The major metabolite is the glycine conjugate, and there are two glucuronide conjugates. The metabolites appear to be excreted as soon as they reach the kidney. In the kidney, salicylate and its metabolites are freely filtered by the glomerulus, then reabsorbed and secreted by the tubules (58).

The serum levels of salicylate bear only a modest relationship to the dose ingested, and a small increment in dose may lead to a profound increment in serum level. The rate of disappearance of serum salicylate varies with serum level. The major determinants of serum salicylate levels are urinary pH and the activity of the enzyme that conjugates glycine to salicylate. Urinary pH profoundly affects clearance of salicylate. Below pH 6.0, salicylate clearance is approximately one-tenth of creatinine clearance. Above pH 7.0, salicylate clearance rises steeply and may reach almost twice creatinine clearance at a slightly alkaline pH. The activity of metabolic enzymes is under genetic control, and continued ingestion of salicylate can induce enzyme expression several fold (58).

Acetaminophen

The absorption of therapeutic doses of acetaminophen is usually rapid and complete (59). The systemic bioavailability is approximately 75%, and the plasma half-life is 1.5 to 2.5 hours. Acetaminophen is metabolized in the liver by glucuronidation and sulfation. These conjugates are eliminated from the liver and blood mainly via urine and bile. A small amount of acetaminophen given in therapeutic doses is oxidized by the microsomal cytochrome P450–containing mixed-function oxidase system. The P450-catalyzed oxidative biotransformation of acetaminophen may produce the species responsible for acute and fulminant liver toxicity when very high doses are ingested (59).

THERAPEUTIC ACTIONS

Preclinical Studies

NSAIDs have antipyretic, analgesic, and antiinflammatory properties. The majority of evidence suggests that most of these properties are mediated by inhibition of COX-2 (22). Fever occurs in response to inflammation and induction of cytokines that function as endogenous pyrogens. PGs have long been known to mediate the fever response. COX-2 expression is induced in the brain vasculature with temporal correlation to the development of fever (60). Moreover, mice with targeted COX-2 gene disruption fail to develop fever in response to inflammatory stimuli (61).

In virtually all models studied, COX-2 expression increases in response to inflammatory stimuli and other types of tissue damage. Animal models of inflammation and pain have been used to address the relative roles of COX-1 and COX-2. These studies demonstrate that peripheral PG production can be a function of both COX-1 and COX-2 in different types of models (62). Markedly increased COX-2 expression has been observed in animal models of inflammatory arthritis and the rat carrageenan- or lipopolysaccharide-stimulated air pouch models that parallel increased PG production. Pharmacologic compounds that specifically inhibit COX-2 reversed inflammation in both these models (63,64). In the air pouch models, a specific inhibitor of COX-1 had no effect on PGE_2 production (62).

It has long been known that PGs are produced at the site of inflammation in the periphery where they sensitize peripheral nociceptors (65). In peripheral tissues, PGs prolong proinflammatory actions of bradykinin, histamine, nitric oxide, and other mediators. Recent studies have also demonstrated a role for PGs in central sensitization at the spinal level, resulting in induction of hyperalgesia and allodynia. In the dorsal horn of the spinal cord, COX-2 is constitutively expressed, although it can be up-regulated during inflammation (66–68). The antiinflammatory and analgesic activity of specific COX-2 inhibition is correlated with decreased cerebrospinal fluid PG levels (62). Intrathecal and systemic administration of a specific COX-2 inhibitor can block the initiation of thermal hyperalgesia (68,69). Inhibition of COX-2, but not COX-1, reduces spinal PG production after an inflammatory stimulus (68). These data suggest that constitutive and induced expression of COX-2 in the spinal cord may contribute to inflammatory hyperalgesia. Therefore, inhibition of spinal COX-2 may play a role in the therapeutic efficacy of NSAIDs and specific COX-2 inhibitors to control pain symptoms in inflammatory states.

Clinical Trials of Nonspecific and Cyclooxygenase-2–Specific Nonsteroidal Antiinflammatory Drugs in Rheumatoid Arthritis

The antiinflammatory effects of NSAIDs are well documented in patients with RA, as well as in other arthritides such as osteoarthritis, seronegative spondyloarthropathies, and crystal arthritis. The most recent clinical trials in RA patients have compared the efficacy of nonspecific NSAIDs, specific COX-2 inhibitors, or placebo (70–77). Clinical trials of NSAID efficacy in RA often, but not always, use a design whereby the current NSAID is discontinued and the patient must have an increase in symptoms or flare to enter the study. Although there is some variation in primary outcome measures, most include parameters that make up the American College of Rheumatology-20 (see Appendix B), such as tender joints, swollen joints, morning stiffness, patient assessment of arthritis pain, patient global assessment of disease activity, patient assessment of physical function, and acute phase reactants. Despite improvement in pain and stiffness with NSAIDs, these agents do not usually reduce erythrocyte sedimentation rate or C-reactive protein levels. Furthermore, there are no data to suggest that NSAIDs modify disease as measured by radiographs.

Clinical trials indicate that NSAIDs and COX-2 inhibitors are superior to placebo for control of RA symptoms, and data from these studies demonstrate that therapeutic efficacy is not different among nonspecific and COX-2–specific NSAIDs (70–77). There have been clinical observations to suggest that individual patients may respond differently to different drugs. In comparing fixed doses of different NSAIDs, minor differences in mean responses do not preclude marked variations in individual response and preference for a particular drug (78). The data suggest that the beneficial effects of NSAIDs in RA are sustained over time.

Other Therapeutic Applications

ACUTE PAIN

In addition to use in arthritis (RA and osteoarthritis), many NSAIDs are approved for use in acute pain based on efficacy in such clinical models as dysmenorrhea and dental pain. Indications specific to each drug can be found in the package inserts. Specific COX-2 inhibitors have also been shown to be effective in acute pain models, including dysmenorrhea, dental pain, and postoperative pain (79,80).

CARDIOPROPHYLAXIS

Aspirin is indicated for secondary prevention of cardiovascular disease (81). The role of aspirin in preventing cardiovascular events in patients without a prior history of cardiovascular disease is less clear. However, recent recommendations from the U.S. Preventive Services Task Force suggest that those patients with an increased (3% to 5%) risk for coronary heart disease events over 5 years may receive greater benefit than harm from aspirin chemoprophylaxis (82,83). There is no consensus that any NSAID other than aspirin is effective for prophylaxis of cardiovascular thrombotic events.

CANCER CHEMOPREVENTION

The possibility that inhibiting PG production prevents carcinogenesis or slows the growth of some cancers, particularly colon cancer, grew out of epidemiological studies (29). Subsequently, clinical trials demonstrated that NSAIDs (e.g., sulindac) could cause regression of polyps in patients with familial adenomatous polyposis (84). It was demonstrated that human colorectal cancers overexpress COX-2 and that inhibitors of COX-2, or genetic deficiency of COX-2, were associated with a marked reduction in tumor burden in animal models of familial adenomatous polyposis (29). Because of the potential for improved safety of specific COX-2 inhibitors, there is renewed interest in the potential for these drugs as chemopreventive agents. Celecoxib has been approved for reduction of polyps in patients with familial adenomatous polyposis (85). Studies are ongoing in many different forms of cancer to determine if COX inhibitors, either as single agents or in combination, may be useful chemopreventive agents (86). Chemopreventive activity of these drugs, particularly celecoxib, may be COX dependent and COX independent (50,87).

ADVERSE EFFECTS

Gastrointestinal

EPIDEMIOLOGY

Injury to the upper GI tract in the form of ulcers and their complications is the most important toxicity associated with aspirin and nonspecific NSAIDs (Table 23.4). Millions of individuals regularly use salicylates and nonspecific NSAIDs, magnifying the overall importance of NSAID gastroenteropathy from a public health standpoint. The expectation of reduced gastroduodenal injury drove development of specific COX-2 inhibitors. The data supporting their reduced GI toxicity is a major reason that specific COX-2 inhibitors are among the most frequently prescribed of all drugs, despite their increased cost.

Prospective data derived from the Arthritis, Rheumatism, and Aging Medical Information System showed that 13 of every 1,000 patients with RA taking nonspecific NSAIDs for 1 year have a serious GI complication (88). Although the rate of NSAID-related serious GI complications has decreased, in part due to use of protective strategies and COX-2–specific NSAIDs, no protective strategy has eliminated the risk of NSAID use (89). Unfortunately, despite a number of strategies available for risk reduction, a study suggested that there was a high level of failure to adequately protect patients using NSAIDs (90). The mortality rate among patients who are hospitalized for NSAID-

TABLE 23.4. Adverse Effects of Nonspecific and Cyclooxygenase-2 (COX-2)–Specific Nonsteroidal Antiinflammatory Drugs (NSAIDs)

Organ System	Nonspecific NSAIDs	Differences with COX-2–Specific NSAIDs
Gastrointestinal	Dyspepsia Gastroduodenal ulceration Bleeding (all levels) Colitis	Decreased UGI ulceration Decreased bleeding
Renal	Hypertension Edema Acute renal failure Interstitial nephritis Papillary necrosis	—
Hepatic	Elevated transaminases Rare severe hepatic reactions	—
Asthma	Exacerbation of AERD	No cross-reactivity in AERD
Allergic reactions	Hypersensitivity reactions	Celecoxib and valdecoxib contraindicated in patients with sulfonamide allergies
Cardiovascular	Platelet dysfunction	Possible risk of arterial thrombosis in high-risk patients with high-dose, highly specific inhibitors
Central nervous system	Dizziness Somnolence Cognitive dysfunction Aseptic meningitis	—

AERD, aspirin-exacerbated respiratory disease; UGI, upper gastrointestinal tract.

induced upper GI bleeding is 5% to 10% (89). Bleeding is by far the most common ulcer complication, but obstruction and perforation may also occur.

Epidemiological studies have shown that the use of nonspecific NSAIDs increases the risk of ulcer complications by a factor of 4 compared with nonusers, and low-dose aspirin (less than or equal to 325 mg) doubles the risk of bleeding ulcers (53,91,92). The absolute risk of serious GI complications (bleeding, perforation, or obstruction) in a patient with no other risk factors is approximately 0.5% per year, and the risk in RA patients is approximately 2% to 4% per year (88). It is of interest that recent data have suggested that acetaminophen at high doses (≥2 grams daily) is also associated with an increased relative risk of upper GI bleeding (91).

In addition to injury of the gastroduodenal mucosa, NSAID use is associated with symptoms of dyspepsia and damage to other regions of the GI tract. At least 10% to 20% of patients taking NSAIDs experience dyspepsia (89). Symptoms are not good predictors of NSAID-related GI complications because only a minority of patients with serious GI events report antecedent dyspepsia (88). Other adverse GI events include pill esophagitis, small-bowel ulceration, small-bowel strictures, colonic strictures, diverticular disease, and exacerbation of inflammatory bowel disease (89). Patients admitted to the hospital with large- or small-bowel perforations or bleeding are twice as likely to be taking NSAIDs (93). In an autopsy series of more than 700 patients, 8% of patients taking NSAIDs or low-dose aspirin, compared with 0.6% of those not taking NSAIDs, revealed small intestinal ulceration (94). In this study, 24% of NSAID users had gastroduodenal ulcers. COX-2 expression is higher in the colon than in more proximal portions of the GI tract under basal conditions and increases markedly if colonic inflammation is present (95). COX-2 inhibition or genetic deficiency markedly exacerbates experimental colitis, suggesting that COX-2–derived PGs may be a protective mechanism for mucosal defense (95).

MECHANISMS OF INJURY

Mucosal damage associated with inhibiting PG synthesis is associated with a decrease in epithelial mucus, secretion of bicarbonate, mucosal blood flow, epithelial proliferation, and mucosal resistance to injury (89). Impaired mucosal resistance permits injury by endogenous factors (e.g., acid, pepsin, and bile salts) and exogenous factors (e.g., NSAIDs), thereby amplifying bleeding risk by causing new mucosal lesions. Topical mucosal injury is initiated by the acidic properties of aspirin and many other NSAIDs. In addition, topical injury may occur as a result of indirect mechanisms, mediated through the biliary excretion and subsequent duodenogastric reflux of active NSAID metabolites (e.g., sulindac) (89). Inhibition of PGs, however, is the principal mechanism underlying development of gastroduodenal ulceration, as graphically illustrated by the fact that enteric coating and parenteral or rectal administration fails to reduce ulcer risk (89). In addition, platelet dysfunction can increase the risk of bleeding associated with damaged GI mucosa (96).

In the normal gastroduodenal mucosa and in platelets, COX-1 is the isoform responsible for PG production. Cytoprotective mechanisms other than PGs are also likely to be present, however, because it has been shown that mice genetically deficient in COX-1 do not develop spontaneous mucosal ulcers (97). In addition, inhibition of COX-2 may contribute to ulcer risk in situations where damage is present. During injury of the GI tract, as in other tissues, COX-2 is induced (98). PGs derived from COX-2 would normally exert suppressive effects on inflammatory cells, notably neutrophils, that contribute to damage (99,100). NSAID-induced injury occurs in association with enhanced adherence of neutrophils to the gastric vascular endothelium, which causes injury through release of reactive oxygen species, a process that may be enhanced if COX-2 is inhibited (100).

TABLE 23.5. Risk Factors for Nonsteroidal Antiinflammatory Drug (NSAID)–Induced Upper Gastrointestinal Ulcers

Established risk factors
Advanced age (linear increase in risk, substantial risk after age 65)
History of complicated or uncomplicated ulcer
Concomitant use of anticoagulants
Concomitant use of glucocorticoids
Serious systemic disorder
Higher-dose or multiple NSAIDs (including low-dose aspirin)
Possible risk factors
Cigarette smoking
Alcohol consumption
Concomitant infection with *Helicobacter pylori*

Adapted from Wolfe MM, Lichtenstein DR, Singh G. Gastrointestinal toxicity of nonsteroidal antiinflammatory drugs. *N Engl J Med* 1999;340:1888–1899.

RISK FACTORS FOR NONSTEROIDAL ANTIINFLAMMATORY DRUG GASTROPATHY

Patients differ in their risk for NSAID-related GI bleeding. Factors consistently associated with increased risk for developing NSAID-associated gastroduodenal ulcers are shown in Table 23.5 (89). These risk factors can be identified in prospective clinical trials of gastroprotective strategies, and risk reduction is higher in those at greatest risk (101,102).

SPECIFIC CYCLOOXYGENASE-2 INHIBITION

It has been demonstrated that the most important COX isoform responsible for gastroduodenal cytoprotection is COX-1 and that specific COX-2 inhibitors do not reduce gastric PG production (103,104). The clinical data suggest that specific COX-2 inhibitors reduce the relative risk for endoscopic ulcers, clinically significant ulcers, and ulcer complications (70,72,105–108). Two reports reviewed annualized incidence of ulcer complications in pooled data from randomized controlled trials of rofecoxib and celecoxib (105,106). There were significantly fewer patients with upper GI complications in patients treated with specific COX-2 inhibitors.

Two large randomized, controlled clinical trials were performed to evaluate the occurrence of clinically significant ulcers and ulcer complications in patients treated with specific COX-2 inhibitors compared to nonspecific NSAIDs (Table 23.6) (109). The Vioxx GI Outcome Research (VIGOR) study enrolled 8,076 patients with RA and randomized subjects to receive rofecoxib, 50 mg per day, or naproxen, 500 mg twice daily (72). An intent-to-treat analysis was performed, with the primary outcome measure being confirmed clinical upper GI events, including symptomatic gastroduodenal ulcer, upper GI bleeding, perforation, or obstruction. Patients were not allowed to use low-dose aspirin. There was a highly significant reduction of clinical GI events (2.1 per 100 patient-years vs. 4.5 per 100 patient-years, $p = .001$) (Fig. 23.5). This difference translates into a relative risk of 0.46 [95% confidence interval (CI): 0.33–0.64] for rofecoxib with a calculation that 41 patients would need to be treated to prevent one clinical GI event. An analysis of VIGOR revealed that previously identified risk factors for clinical ulcer and ulcer complications were also risks for those events with specific COX-2 inhibitors (102). However, the higher the risk, the greater the absolute risk reduction associated with use of the rofecoxib.

The Celecoxib Long-Term Safety Study (CLASS) was a combination of two randomized, controlled trials that enrolled 7,968 patients with osteoarthritis (72%) or RA (28%) to receive treatment

TABLE 23.6. Comparison of the Vioxx GI Outcome Research (VIGOR) Study and the Celecoxib Long-Term Safety Study (CLASS)

Variable	VIGOR (N = 8,076)	CLASS (N = 7,968)
Patient population	RA	OA (72%) and RA (28%)
Drug or dosage	Rofecoxib 50 mg/day	Celecoxib 400 mg b.i.d.
Active comparator	Naproxen 500 mg b.i.d.	Ibuprofen 800 mg t.i.d. or diclofenac 75 mg b.i.d.
Aspirin co-therapy	No	Yes, ≤325 mg/day (22%)
GI drugs	Antacids, OTC H_2-blockers	Antacids
Duration	Median 9 mo, maximum 13 mo	Initial report 6 mo, median 9 mo, maximum 13 mo
Primary end point	Clinical upper GI events (PUB)	Complicated upper GI events (POB)
Secondary end point	Complicated upper GI events (POB)	Clinical upper GI events (PUB)

GI, gastrointestinal; OA, osteoarthritis; OTC, over the counter; POB, perforation, obstruction, or GI bleeding; PUB, perforation, symptomatic gastroduodenal ulcer, or GI bleeding; RA, rheumatoid arthritis.
Modified from Simon LS, Smolen JS, Abramson SB, et al. Controversies in COX-2 selective inhibition. *J Rheumatol* 2002;29:1501–1510.

with celecoxib, 400 mg twice daily, or ibuprofen, 800 mg three times daily, in one trial and celecoxib, 400 mg twice daily, or diclofenac, 75 mg twice daily, in the other. The randomization scheme was for one of these two comparisons, but the intent-to-treat analysis from the originally published data compared the patients receiving celecoxib to the patients who received either ibuprofen or diclofenac, termed the *NSAID group* (107). Low-dose aspirin (≤325 mg per day) was allowed in CLASS and used by 22% of the enrolled patients. The primary outcome measure in CLASS was complicated ulcer (perforations, obstructions, or bleeding) with the secondary outcome that included symptomatic ulcers. Planned subanalyses of patients using aspirin were also reported. After 6 months of treatment, the annualized incidence of ulcer complications was 0.76% in the celecoxib-treated patients and 1.45% in the ibuprofen/diclofenac groups (p = .09) (Fig. 23.6). For the entire cohort over the entire study period (median follow-up of

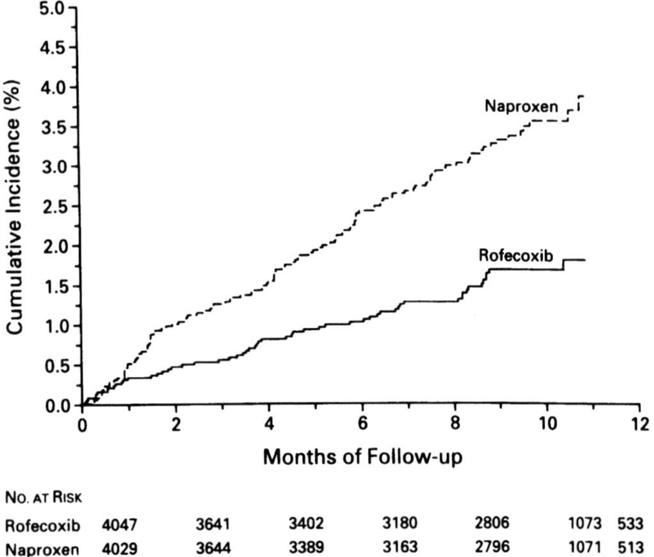

Figure 23.5. Clinical upper gastrointestinal events in the Vioxx Gastrointestinal Outcomes Research (VIGOR) trial. These curves represent the cumulative incidence of confirmed clinical upper gastrointestinal events in patients taking naproxen, 500 mg twice daily (*dotted line*), or rofecoxib, 50 mg once daily (*solid line*), for all randomized patients in the VIGOR trial. The number of patients at risk is shown. The median duration of treatment was 9 months. (From Bombardier C, Laine L, Reicin A, et al. Comparison of upper gastrointestinal toxicity of rofecoxib and naproxen in patients with rheumatoid arthritis. *N Engl J Med* 2000;343:1520–1528, with permission.)

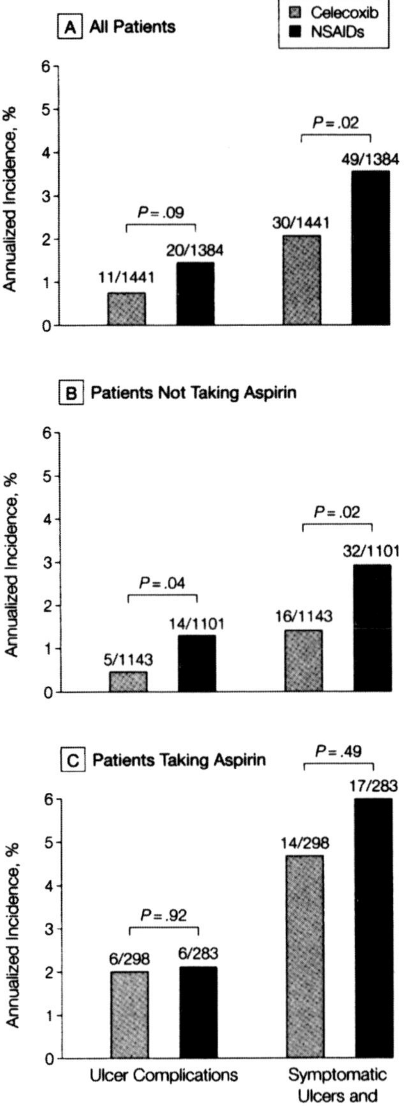

Figure 23.6. Annualized incidence of upper gastrointestinal (GI) tract ulcer complications and clinical upper gastrointestinal events in Celecoxib Long-Term Safety Study (CLASS). These bars represent GI events from the CLASS. Events were defined as occurring 48 hours after the first dose day or before 14 days after the last known dose and within the 6-month period. The data are expressed as annualized incidence rates (number of events per 100 patient-years exposure) for patients taking celecoxib, 400 mg twice daily (*light bars*), and ibuprofen, 800 mg three times daily, or diclofenac, 75 mg twice daily (*dark bars*). The numbers above the bars indicate events per patient-years of exposure. **A:** Data for all patients. **B,C:** Data for patients not taking aspirin and taking concomitant low-dose (≤325 mg daily) aspirin, respectively. NSAIDs, nonsteroidal antiinflammatory drugs. (From Silverstein FE, Faich G, Goldstein JL, et al. Gastrointestinal toxicity with celecoxib vs nonsteroidal antiinflammatory drugs for osteoarthritis and rheumatoid arthritis. The CLASS study: a randomized controlled trial. *JAMA* 2000;284:1247–1255, with permission.)

9 months, maximum follow-up of 13 months), celecoxib was associated with a significant reduction in the secondary end point of symptomatic ulcers plus ulcer complications versus ibuprofen (1.85% vs. 4.31%; $p = .005$) but not diclofenac (109). There was no significant difference in the primary end point of complicated ulcers comparing celecoxib with either ibuprofen of diclofenac (110). In the aspirin-treated group, there was no reduction in the incidence of complicated ulcers (107).

In addition to these randomized controlled clinical trials, a recent observational study was performed in elderly (at least 66 years old) Canadian patients receiving their first prescription of nonspecific or COX-2–specific NSAID. The relative risk of upper GI hemorrhage was determined for patients taking nonselective NSAIDs (4.0; 95% CI: 2.3–6.9), diclofenac plus misoprol (3.0; 95% CI: 1.7–5.6), rofecoxib (1.9; 95% CI: 1.2–2.8), and celecoxib (1.0; 95% CI: 0.7–1.6) (111). Specific COX-2 inhibitors were significantly less likely to develop upper GI bleeding than those taking nonspecific NSAIDs, and the risk with celecoxib was significantly lower than for rofecoxib. Covariates included all well-known risk factors, but the authors were unable to control for smoking or alcohol consumption. It should be noted that the frequency of gastroprotective agent use was higher in those patients taking specific COX-2 inhibitors, but differences in upper GI hemorrhage were present comparing nonspecific and COX-2–specific drugs, regardless of whether patients received GI drugs. In fact, patients using GI protective agents had a higher rate of GI bleeding in all groups.

ULCER PREVENTION

The only way to completely prevent NSAID-associated GI injury is not to use them (112). Using the lowest effective dose of an NSAID can reduce risk, compared with a higher dose (91). Changing from an NSAID to acetaminophen at a dose of less than or equal to 2 g daily or other analgesics will also reduce overall risk (91). There are several other strategies available to reduce the risks of upper GI complications due to aspirin and NSAID use. As previously noted, use of specific COX-2 inhibitors can reduce the risk of ulcers and ulcer complications in clinical trials and in observational studies (72,107,111). The utility of changing to a specific COX-2 inhibitor in patients who also use low-dose aspirin is not known, but the effectiveness of this strategy may be reduced or eliminated in aspirin-treated patients (107).

Another strategy proven effective is replacement of PGs with misoprostol, a stable analogue of PGE_1. Misoprostol at a dose of 200 mg four times daily was shown to reduce serious GI complications by 40% (odds ratio, 0.598; 95% CI: 0.36–0.98) compared with placebo in RA patients taking nonspecific NSAIDs (113). Misoprostol is often poorly tolerated at high doses, with the most important side effect being diarrhea (113,114). A combination agent consisting of diclofenac plus misoprostol, 200 mg given twice daily, is available. Although misoprostol given twice daily is less effective than three or four times daily, it is more effective than placebo in preventing GI ulceration (115). In observational studies, this combination agent is less effective than specific COX-2 inhibitors in preventing upper GI bleeding (111).

There are endoscopic studies that suggest proton pump inhibitors (PPIs) may be effective in healing of gastroduodenal ulcers and reducing recurrence of gastroduodenal ulcers in patients taking NSAIDs (114,116,117). An epidemiologic study also suggested a 40% risk reduction for NSAID-associated GI bleeding associated with use of antisecretory agents, although these studies are inconsistent (92,111,118). In patients continuing to use aspirin or NSAIDs after ulcers due to *Helicobacter pylori*, the PPI omeprazole was superior to the eradication of *H. pylori* in preventing recurrent bleeding in patients on NSAIDs (119). In patients taking NSAIDs and with a recent history of ulcer bleeding, the risk of recurrent ulcer bleeding was similar in patients receiving celecoxib (4.9%; 95% CI: 3.1–6.7) and diclofenac plus omeprazole (6.4%; 95% CI: 4.3–8.4) (120). There are no data that use of H_2-blockers or antacids prevents serious GI complications (88).

Renal

NONSPECIFIC AND CYCLOOXYGENASE-2–SPECIFIC NONSTEROIDAL ANTIINFLAMMATORY DRUGS

Renal PGs are important for salt and water homeostasis and maintaining renal blood flow. Potential adverse effects of NSAIDs on renal function include fluid and electrolyte disturbances, acute deterioration of renal function, interstitial nephritis, and papillary necrosis (109). The most common effects are hypertension and edema associated with altered solute homeostasis. Acute renal failure is more likely in those patients with decreased effective circulating volume and, in particular, those with congestive heart failure, cirrhosis, and renal insufficiency. An increased risk for worsening chronic renal failure is seen in patients with preexisting renal disease who regularly use aspirin (121).

Both COX-1 and COX-2 are constitutively expressed in the kidney; however, their distribution is somewhat different (28). Both COX-1 and COX-2 are expressed in the renal vasculature and glomerulus. COX-2 is expressed in the macula densa and is critical for basal and up-regulated secretion of renin (122–124). In the medulla, COX-1 is expressed primarily in the medullary collecting ducts and COX-2 in the interstitial cells (125). In COX null mice and mice treated with specific inhibitors, COX-1 and COX-2 exert opposite effects on systemic blood pressure and renal function (125). COX-2 inhibitors reduce renal medullary blood flow, decrease urine flow, and enhance the pressor effect of angiotensin II. In contrast, the pressor effect of angiotensin II is blunted by specific COX-1 inhibition by either pharmacologic or genetic means.

Studies of renal physiology demonstrate that specific COX-2 inhibitors have similar effects on renal function as nonspecific inhibitors (126–129). In clinical trials, renal effects of specific COX-2 inhibitors are similar to nonspecific inhibitors (72,107,109,130). Acute papillary necrosis and acute renal failure have been reported in patients taking specific COX-2 inhibitors (131). Therefore, similar to nonselective NSAIDs, patients taking specific COX-2 inhibitors should be monitored for blood pressure and development of edema (109). Furthermore, in patients with moderate to severe renal insufficiency or other risk factors for acute renal failure, both nonspecific and COX-2–specific NSAIDs should be avoided or used with great caution.

ACETAMINOPHEN

Analgesics, including acetaminophen, have been associated with a nephropathy leading to chronic renal failure (121,132,133). A large case control study demonstrated that subjects taking high doses of acetaminophen (≥1.4 g per day) had an increased risk of developing chronic renal failure (odds ratio, 5.3; 95% CI: 1.8–15.1) (121). However, preexisting renal or systemic disease was a necessary precursor to analgesic-associated chronic renal failure, and those without preexisting renal disease had only a small risk of end-stage renal disease (121,134).

Hepatic

NONSPECIFIC AND CYCLOOXYGENASE-2–SPECIFIC NONSTEROIDAL ANTIINFLAMMATORY DRUGS

Small elevations of one or more liver tests may occur in up to 15% of patients taking NSAIDs, and notable elevations of alanine aminotransferase or aspartate aminotransferase (approximately three or more times the upper limit of normal) have been reported in approximately 1% of patients in clinical trials with NSAIDs. These laboratory abnormalities may progress, may remain unchanged, or may be transient with continuing therapy. Rare cases of severe hepatic reactions, including jaundice and fatal fulminant hepatitis, liver necrosis, and hepatic failure (some with fatal outcome) have been reported with NSAIDs. Those NSAIDs that appear most likely to be associated with hepatic adverse events are diclofenac and sulindac (56). In children with viral illnesses, hepatocellular failure and fatty degeneration (Reye's syndrome) is associated with aspirin ingestion (135).

ACETAMINOPHEN

At therapeutic doses, acetaminophen is unlikely to cause hepatic abnormalities (136). In large doses, the usually small portion of acetaminophen is metabolized by the P450 CYP2E1 increases, dramatically leading to formation of an electrophilic metabolite, *N*-acetyl-*p*-benzoquinoneimine. Normally, *N*-acetyl-*p*-benzoquinoneimine would be detoxified by intracellular glutathione, but, in overdose, the detoxification system can be overwhelmed, leading to fulminant hepatic injury (59).

Asthma and Allergic Reactions

Up to 10% to 20% of the general asthmatic population have hypersensitivity to aspirin and nonspecific NSAIDs leading to severe exacerbation of asthma and nasoocular reactions (137,138). Formerly termed *aspirin-sensitive asthma*, these patients are now characterized as having aspirin-exacerbated respiratory disease (AERD) because they have chronic upper and lower respiratory mucosal inflammation, sinusitis, nasal polyposis, and asthma independent of their hypersensitivity reactions (139). A number of studies have now been reported that demonstrate the safety of the specific COX-2 inhibitors, rofecoxib and celecoxib, in patients with AERD (139–142). Although these studies were performed as challenge tests rather than long-term placebo-controlled trials, they are convincing.

The fact that specific COX-2 inhibitors appear safe in AERD does not imply that other hypersensitivity reactions do not occur. Aspirin and all NSAIDs, nonspecific and COX-2–specific, can cause hypersensitivity reactions, such as skin rash (including toxic epidermal necrolysis and Stevens-Johnson syndrome), urticaria/angioedema, cutaneous vasculitis, and anaphylactoid or anaphylactic reaction (143). Celecoxib and valdecoxib contain a sulfonamide group and should not be given to patients who report allergy to sulfa-containing drugs. Celecoxib and valdecoxib have been associated with numerous reports of severe allergic reactions, some of which have been fatal (144–147). It is suggested that these agents not be administered to patients with a known history of allergic reactions to aspirin or other NSAIDs. Although it was initially speculated that cutaneous allergic reactions may be reduced with specific COX-2 inhibitor rofecoxib, cases of angioedema have been reported (148–150).

Cardiovascular

Consideration of the cardiovascular effects of COX inhibition has accompanied the development and widespread use of specific COX-2 inhibitors. The reason behind this scrutiny is the observation that vascular PGI_2 production is mediated predominantly by COX-2 (38,151). PGI_2 is functionally antagonistic to thromboxane A_2 in the vasculature, inhibiting platelet activation and acting as an important mediation of vasodilation (31). Nevertheless, it is now clear that inhibition of PG formation by either nonspecific or COX-2–specific NSAIDs is not likely to be associated with adverse vascular events in otherwise healthy, low-risk patients (152,153). However, in patients with a high risk for thrombosis, inhibition of COX-2–derived PGI_2 without concomitant inhibition of platelet thromboxane A_2 represents a theoretical hazard (33,154). Two studies suggest that this hazard may be associated most strongly with high doses of rofecoxib. In the VIGOR trial, patients with RA taking rofecoxib, 50 mg daily, were five times more likely to have a myocardial infarction than those taking naproxen, 500 mg twice daily (72). This result has been speculated to be the result of chance or of a lower risk attributable to naproxen (152,155). However, a retrospective case control study reported an increased risk for serious coronary heart disease (acute myocardial infarction or death) in patients using more than 25 mg daily of rofecoxib. The risk for new users of this high dose of rofecoxib had a relative risk of 1.93 (95% CI: 1.09–3.42) compared with non-NSAID users (55). It should be noted that, in this study, there was no excess risk for users on nonspecific NSAIDs, celecoxib at any dose, or doses of rofecoxib less than or equal to 25 mg daily.

Central Nervous System

Minor central nervous system symptoms, including dizziness, headache, hypersomnolence, and insomnia, are commonly reported with NSAIDs. Elderly patients may be particularly susceptible to developing cognitive dysfunction and other central nervous system effects. Some agents (e.g., ibuprofen, naproxen) have been associated with aseptic meningitis, particularly in female patients with systemic lupus or other connective tissue diseases. It has been reported that rofecoxib can also be associated with aseptic meningitis (156).

Salicylate Intoxication

The new appearance of tachypnea, confusion, ataxia, oliguria, or a rising blood urea nitrogen/creatinine ratio in a patient, particularly an elderly patient, taking aspirin or salicylates should suggest the possibility of salicylate intoxication (157,158). In adults, metabolic acidosis is masked by hyperventilation, with stimulation of respiratory centers a direct effect of salicylates. Sudden rises in salicylate levels can occur, even if there is no change in dose, in patients who develop dehydration or acidosis from any cause and in patients who ingest other drugs that displace salicylate from protein-binding sites. Therapy consists of removing residual drug from the GI tract; forced diuresis, maintaining the urinary pH in the alkaline range and with potassium replacement; hemodialysis, if diuresis is unsatisfactory; and other supportive measures. Vitamin K has been recommended because large doses of salicylate may interfere with the synthesis of the vitamin K–dependent clotting factors.

SELECTED DRUG INTERACTIONS

Salicylate and Nonsteroidal Antiinflammatory Drug Interactions

Salicylates and NSAIDs compete with one another for protein binding sites, and there may be metabolic interactions as well. This competition can result in either increased (e.g., indomethacin) or decreased (e.g., ibuprofen, naproxen) NSAID concentrations. It has also been shown that chronic dosing of certain NSAIDs (e.g., ibuprofen, but not diclofenac) can prevent aspirin from blocking platelet COX-1 and inhibiting the antiplatelet effect of aspirin (42).

Antihypertensives

NSAIDs reduce the response to diuretics, particularly loop diuretics. This effect is due to inhibition of PG synthesis, as opposed to a pharmacokinetic interaction. NSAIDs also inhibit the effectiveness of angiotensin-converting enzyme inhibitors, perhaps due to increased sodium retention (159).

Anticoagulants

Clinically significant increases in prothrombin times can be seen in patients taking virtually any NSAID with warfarin. This can occur either due to protein binding displacement or due to altered metabolism of warfarin. Because patients taking warfarin are at increased risk of GI bleeding and may be more likely to receive COX-2–specific NSAIDs, it is noteworthy that prothrombin time should be monitored more closely than usual in patients taking specific COX-2 inhibitors. Celecoxib did not alter prothrombin time in a clinical trial, but, in postmarketing experience, bleeding has occurred, predominantly in the elderly. Rofecoxib and valdecoxib also have been shown to increase prothrombin time.

Methotrexate

Aspirin reduces clearance of methotrexate, and this effect is shared by some other NSAIDs (56). Neither celecoxib nor rofecoxib altered methotrexate pharmacokinetics in patients with RA (160,161).

PRACTICAL ASPECTS OF CHOOSING AN ANTIINFLAMMATORY ANALGESIC AGENT

Nonspecific versus Cyclooxygenase-2–Specific Nonsteroidal Antiinflammatory Drugs

Because there are no data to suggest that nonspecific and COX-2–specific NSAIDs differ in clinical efficacy for the treatment of RA, the choice of agent is driven primarily by safety issues and cost (162,163). GI toxicity with nonspecific NSAIDs in RA patients is common and associated with significant mortality (88). In addition to other risk factors, corticosteroid use is more common in RA than in other disorders for which NSAIDs are indicated. It is clear that patients with RA at risk for GI events should have a protective strategy considered. The choice of strategy could include a specific COX-2 inhibitor, misoprostol three or four times daily, or a PPI. Combinations of these strategies (e.g., specific COX-2 inhibitor plus PPI) have not been tested in prospective clinical trials.

Specific COX-2 inhibitors may be associated with reduced downstream costs, particularly in patients at very high risk for GI toxicity, despite the fact that they are more expensive (102,164). It remains unclear if these cost analyses hold true for patients requiring aspirin for cardioprophylaxis (107). Understanding the economic implications of GI and cardiovascular risks may be a very important consideration in RA patients who are at increased risk of myocardial infarction, particularly because these patients may have an increased risk of serious cardiovascular events if treated with high doses of specific COX-2 inhibitors, as seen in VIGOR (72).

To summarize recommendations taking into account GI and cardiovascular comorbidities, for patients with RA and low risk for GI toxicity, nonspecific NSAIDs are acceptable. In patients with higher GI risk and no indication for prophylactic aspirin, specific COX-2 inhibitors are suggested. In high-risk patients requiring low-dose aspirin for cardioprophylaxis, in addition to an NSAID, misoprostol or a PPI should be used. Prospective data are not yet available to determine if a specific COX-2 inhibitor combined with other protective strategies will prove most effective in preventing serious upper GI toxicity.

There are no differences in the renal adverse events comparing nonspecific and COX-2–specific NSAIDs. Patients should be monitored for aggravated hypertension, and in those patients with preexisting renal disease, renal function should be monitored. Specific COX-2 inhibitors may be used cautiously in those patients with a history of AERD, but they should be avoided in patients with a history of other types of hypersensitivity reactions to NSAIDs. Celecoxib and valdecoxib should not be used in patients with a history of sulfa allergy.

Nonsteroidal Antiinflammatory Drugs versus Analgesics

Acetaminophen is an effective analgesic and may be useful for treatment of mild pain in RA patients on effective disease-modifying agents. However, because RA is an inflammatory disease, it is expected that patients may derive more benefit from NSAIDs than acetaminophen. However, in patients in whom NSAIDs are contraindicated (e.g., allergy) or not tolerated (e.g., dyspepsia), acetaminophen may provide useful analgesia. In patients with severe renal disease, caution is advised with NSAIDs and acetaminophen. In those patients, addition of other analgesics, such as tramadol and opioids, may be required to maintain adequate pain control (165).

REFERENCES

1. Crofford LJ. Prostaglandin biology. *Gastroenterol Clin North Am* 2001;30:863–876.
2. Smith WL, DeWitt DL, Garavito RM. Cyclooxygenases: structural, cellular, and molecular biology. *Annu Rev Biochem* 2000;69:145–182.
3. Smith WL. Prostanoid biosynthesis and mechanisms of action. *Am J Physiol* 1992;263:F181–F191.
4. Murakami M, Nakatani Y, Atsumi G-I, et al. Regulatory functions of phospholipase A_2. *Crit Rev Immunol* 1997;17:225–283.
5. Wery J-P, Schevitz RW, Clawson DK, et al. Structure of recombinant human rheumatoid arthritic synovial fluid phospholipase A_2 at 2.2 A resolution. *Nature* 1991;352:79–82.
6. Murakami M, Kuwata H, Amakasu Y, et al. Prostaglandin E2 amplifies cytosolic phospholipase A_2- and cyclooxygenase-2-dependent delayed prostaglandin E2 generation in mouse osteoblastic cells. Enhancement by secretory phospholipase A_2. *J Biol Chem* 1997;272:19891–19897.
7. Leslie CC. Properties and regulation of cytosolic phospholipase A_2. *J Biol Chem* 1997;272:16709–16712.
8. DeWitt DL. Prostaglandin endoperoxide synthase: regulation of enzyme expression. *Biochim Biophys Acta* 1991;1083:121–134.
9. Stichtenoth DO, Thoren S, Bian H, et al. Microsomal prostaglandin E synthase is regulated by pro-inflammatory cytokines and glucocorticoids in primary rheumatoid synovial cells. *J Immunol* 2001;167:469–474.
10. Kojima F, Naraba H, Sasaki Y, et al. Coexpression of microsomal prostaglandin E synthase with cyclooxygenase-2 in human rheumatoid synovial cells. *J Rheumatol* 2002;29:1836–1842.
11. Mancini JA, Blood K, Guay J, et al. Cloning, expression, and up-regulation of inducible rat prostaglandin E synthase during lipopolysaccharide-induced pyresis and adjuvant-induced arthritis. *J Biol Chem* 2001;276:4469–4475.
12. Ueno N, Murakami M, Tanioka T, et al. Coupling between cyclooxygenase, terminal prostanoid synthase, and phospholipase A_2. *J Biol Chem* 2001;276:34918–34927.
13. Morita I, Schindler M, Regier MK, et al. Different intracellular locations for prostaglandin endoperoxide H synthase-1 and -2. *J Biol Chem* 1995;270:10902–10908.
14. Spencer AG, Woods JW, Arakawa T, et al. Subcellular localization of prostaglandin endoperoxide H synthases-1 and -2 by immunoelectron microscopy. *J Biol Chem* 1998;273:9886–9893.
15. Picot D, Loll PJ, Garavito M. The X-ray crystal structure of the membrane protein prostaglandin H2 synthase-1. *Nature* 1994;367:243–249.
16. Kurumbail RA, Stevens AM, Gierse JK, et al. Structural basis for selective inhibition of cyclooxygenase-2 by antiinflammatory agents. *Nature* 1996;384:644–648.
17. Reike CJ, Mulichak AM, Garavito RM, et al. The role of arginine 120 of human prostaglandin endoperoxide H synthase-2 in the interaction with fatty acid substrates and inhibitors. *J Biol Chem* 1999;274:17109–17114.
18. Luong C, Miller A, Barnett J, et al. Flexibility of the NSAID binding site in the structure of human cyclooxygenase-2. *Nat Struct Biol* 1996;3:927–933.
19. Crofford LJ. COX-1 and COX-2 tissue expression: implications and predictions. *J Rheumatol* 1997;24(Suppl 49):15–19.
20. Wang LH, Hajibeigi A, Xu XM, et al. Characterization of the promoter of human prostaglandin H synthase-1 gene. *Biochem Biophys Res Commun* 1993;190:406–411.

21. Morham SG, Langenbach R, Loftin CD, et al. Prostaglandin synthase 2 gene disruption causes severe renal pathology in the mouse. *Cell* 1995;83:473–482.
22. Crofford LJ, Lipsky PE, Brooks P, et al. Basic biology and clinical application of specific COX-2 inhibitors. *Arthritis Rheum* 2000;43:4–13.
23. Yamamoto K, Arakawa T, Ueda N, et al. Transcriptional roles of nuclear factor κB and nuclear factor-interleukin-6 in the tumor necrosis factor-dependent induction of cyclooxygenase-2 in MC3T3-E1 cells. *J Biol Chem* 1995;270:31315–31320.
24. Crofford LJ, Tan B, McCarthy CJ, et al. NF-κB is involved in the regulation of cyclooxygenase-2 expression by interleukin-1β in rheumatoid synoviocytes. *Arthritis Rheum* 1997;40:226–236.
25. Crofford LJ, Wilder RL, Ristimaki AP, et al. Cyclooxygenase-1 and -2 expression in rheumatoid synovial tissues: effects of interleukin-1β, phorbol ester, and corticosteroids. *J Clin Invest* 1994;93:1095–1101.
26. Siegle I, Klein T, Backman JT, et al. Expression of cyclooxygenase 1 and cyclooxygenase 2 in human synovial tissue. Differential elevation of cyclooxygenase 2 in inflammatory joint diseases. *Arthritis Rheum* 1998;41:122–129.
27. Sano H, Hla T, Maier JAM, et al. In vivo cyclooxygenase expression in synovial tissues of patients with rheumatoid arthritis and osteoarthritis and rats with adjuvant and streptococcal cell wall arthritis. *J Clin Invest* 1992;89:97–108.
28. Brater DC, Harris C, Redfern JS, et al. Renal effects of COX-2 selective inhibitors. *Am J Nephrol* 2001;21:1–15.
29. DuBois RN, Abramson SB, Crofford L, et al. Cyclooxygenase in biology and disease. *FASEB J* 1998;12:1063–1073.
30. Catella-Lawson F, Crofford LJ. Cyclooxygenase inhibition and thrombogenicity. *Am J Med* 2001;110:28S–32S.
31. Cheng Y, Austin SC, Rocca B, et al. Role of prostacyclin in the cardiovascular response to thromboxane A_2. *Science* 2002;296:539–541.
32. Simon AM, Manigrasso MB, O'Connor JP. Cyclo-oxygenase 2 function is essential for bone fracture healing. *J Bone Miner Res* 2002;17:963–976.
33. FitzGerald GA. The choreography of cyclooxygenases in the kidney. *J Clin Invest* 2002;110:33–34.
34. Smith WL, Garavito RM, DeWitt DL. Prostaglandin endoperoxide H synthases (cyclooxygenases)-1 and -2. *J Biol Chem* 1996;271:33157–33160.
35. Wong E, Bayly C, Waterman HL, et al. Conversion of prostaglandin G/H synthase-1 into an enzyme sensitive to PGHS-2-selective inhibitors by a double His513 → Arg and Ile523 → val mutation. *J Biol Chem* 1997;271:9280–9286.
36. Lipsky PE, Abramson SB, Crofford L, et al. The classification of cyclooxygenase inhibitors. *J Rheumatol* 1998;25:2298–2303.
37. Riendeau D, Percival MD, Brideau C, et al. Etoricoxib (MK-0663): preclinical profile and comparison with other agents that selectively inhibit cyclooxygenase-2. *J Pharmacol Exp Ther* 2000;296:558–566.
38. FitzGerald GA, Patrono C. The coxibs, selective inhibitors of cyclooxygenase-2. *N Engl J Med* 2001;345:433–442.
39. Patrignani P, Panara MR, Greco A. Biochemical and pharmacological characterization of the cyclooxygenase activity of human blood prostaglandin endoperoxide synthases. *J Pharmacol Exp Ther* 1994;271:1705–1712.
40. Patrono C. Aspirin as an antiplatelet drug. *N Engl J Med* 1994;330:1287–1294.
41. Patrono C, Coller B, Dalen JE, et al. Platelet-active drugs: the relationships among dose effectiveness and side effects. *Chest* 2001;119:39S–63S.
42. Catella-Lawson F, Reilly M, Kapoor SC, et al. Cyclooxygenase inhibitors and the antiplatelet effects of aspirin. *New Engl J Med* 2001;345:1809–1817.
43. Ouellet M, Percival MD. Mechanism of acetaminophen inhibition of cyclooxygenase isoforms. *Arch Biochem Biophys* 2001;387:273–280.
44. Boutaud O, Aronoff DM, Richardson JH, et al. Determinants of the cellular specificity of acetaminophen as an inhibitor of prostaglandin H2 synthases. *Proc Natl Acad Sci U S A* 2002;99:7130–7135.
45. Botting R. Paracetamol-inhibitable COX-2. *J Physiol Pharmacol* 2000;51:609–618.
46. Chandrasekharan NV, Dai H, Roos KLT, et al. COX-3, a cyclooxygenase-1 variant inhibited by acetaminophen and other analgesic/antipyretic drugs: cloning, structure, and expression. *Proc Natl Acad Sci U S A* 2002;99:13926–13931.
47. Kopp E, Gosh S. Inhibition of NF-kappa B by sodium salicylate and aspirin. *Science* 1994;265:956–959.
48. Cronstein BN, Montesinos MC, Weissmann G. Salicylates and sulfasalazine, but not glucocorticoids, inhibit leukocyte accumulation by an adenosine-dependent mechanism that is independent of inhibition of prostaglandin synthesis and p105 of NFkappaB. *Proc Natl Acad Sci U S A* 1999;96:6377–6381.
49. Tegeder I, Pfeilschifter J, Geisslinger G. Cyclooxygenase-independent actions of cyclooxygenase inhibitors. *FASEB J* 2001;15:2057–2072.
50. Zhu J, Song X, Lin HP, et al. Using cyclooxygenase-2 inhibitors as molecular platforms to develop a new class of apoptosis-inducing agents. *J Natl Cancer Inst* 2002;94:1745–1757.
51. Brooks PM. NSAIDs. In: Klippel JH, Dieppe PA, eds. *Rheumatology*. London: Mosby, 1998:3.5.1–3.5.6.
52. Tonkin AL, Wing LMH. Interactions of non-steroidal antiinflammatory drugs. *Bailliere's Clin Rheumatol* 1988;2:455–483.
53. Garcia Rodriguez LA, Jick H. Risk of upper gastrointestinal bleeding and perforation associated with individual non-steroidal antiinflammatory drugs. *Lancet* 1994;343:769–772.
54. Gutthann SP, Garcia-Rodrigues LA, Raiford DS. Individual nonsteroidal antiinflammatory drugs and other risk factors for upper gastrointestinal bleeding and perforation. *Epidemiology* 1997;8:18–24.
55. Ray WA, Stein CM, Daugherty JR, et al. COX-2 selective non-steroidal antiinflammatory drugs and risk of serious coronary heart disease. *Lancet* 2002; 360:1071–1073.
56. Furst DE, Hillson J. Aspirin and other nonsteroidal antiinflammatory drugs. In: Koopman WJ, ed. *Arthritis and allied conditions*. Philadelphia: Lippincott Williams & Wilkins, 2001:665–716.
57. Verbeek RK. Pathophysiologic factors affecting the pharmacokinetics on non-steroidal antiinflammatory drugs. *J Rheumatol* 1988;15:44–57.
58. Kimberly RP, Plotz PH. Salicylates including aspirin and sulfasalazine. In: Kelley WN, Harris ED, Ruddy S, et al., eds. *Textbook of rheumatology*, 3rd ed. Philadelphia: W.B. Saunders Company, 1989:739–764.
59. Bessems JGM, Vermeulen NPE. Paracetamol (acetaminophen)-induced toxicity: molecular and biochemical mechanisms, analogues and protective approaches. *Crit Rev Toxicol* 2001;31:55–138.
60. Cao C, Matsumura K, Yamagata K, et al. Induction by lipopolysaccharide of cyclooxygenase-2 mRNA in rat brain; its possible role in the febrile response. *Brain Res* 1995;697:187–196.
61. Li S, Wang Y, Matsumura K, et al. The febrile response to lipopolysaccharide is blocked in cyclooxygenase-2(−/−), but not in cyclooxygenase-1(−/−) mice. *Brain Res* 1999;825:86–94.
62. Smith CJ, Zhang Y, Koboldt CM, et al. Pharmacological analysis of cyclooxygenase-1 in inflammation. *Proc Natl Acad Sci U S A* 1998;95:13313–13318.
63. Anderson GD, Hauser SD, Bremer ME, et al. Selective inhibition of cyclooxygenase-2 reverses inflammation and expression of COX-2 and IL-6 in rat adjuvant arthritis. *J Clin Invest* 1996;97:2672–2679.
64. Seibert K, Zhang Y, Leahy K, et al. Pharmacological and biochemical demonstration of the role of cyclooxygenase 2 in inflammation and pain. *Proc Natl Acad Sci U S A* 1994;91:12013–12017.
65. Ito S, Okuda-Ashitaka E, Minami T. Central and peripheral roles of prostaglandins in pain and their interactions with novel neuropeptides nociceptin and nocistatin. *Neurosci Res* 2001;41:299–332.
66. Beiche F, Scheuerer S, Brune K, et al. Up-regulation of cyclooxygenase-2 mRNA in the rat spinal cord following peripheral inflammation. *FEBS Lett* 1996;390:165–169.
67. Samad TA, Moore KA, Sapirstein A, et al. Interleukin-1beta-mediated induction of COX-2 in the CNS contributes to inflammatory pain hypersensitivity. *Nature* 2001;410:471–475.
68. Yaksh TL, Dirig DM, Conway CM, et al. The acute antihyperalgesic action of nonsteroidal, antiinflammatory drugs and release of spinal prostaglandin E2 is mediated by inhibition of constitutive spinal cyclooxygenase-2 (COX-2) but not COX-1. *J Neurosci* 2001;21:5847–5853.
69. Dirig DM, Isakson PC, Yaksh TL. Effect of COX-1 and COX-2 inhibition on induction and maintenance of carrageenan-evoked thermal hyperalgesia. *J Pharmacol Exp Ther* 1998;285:1031–1038.
70. Simon LS, Lanza FL, Lipsky PE, et al. Preliminary study of the safety and efficacy of SC-58635, a novel cyclooxygenase 2 inhibitor: efficacy and safety in two placebo-controlled trials in osteoarthritis and rheumatoid arthritis, and studies of gastrointestinal and platelet effects. *Arthritis Rheum* 1998;41:1591–1602.
71. Emery P, Zeidler H, Kvien TK, et al. Celecoxib versus diclofenac in long-term management of rheumatoid arthritis: randomised double-blind comparison. *Lancet* 1999;354:2106–2111.
72. Bombardier C, Laine L, Reicin A, et al. Comparison of upper gastrointestinal toxicity of rofecoxib and naproxen in patients with rheumatoid arthritis. *N Engl J Med* 2000;343:1520–1528.
73. Furst DE, Kolba KS, Fleischmann R, et al. Dose response and safety study of meloxicam up to 22.5 mg daily in rheumatoid arthritis: a 12 week multicenter, double blind, dose response study versus placebo and diclofenac. *J Rheumatol* 2002;29:436–446.
74. Geusens PP, Truitt K, Sfaikakis P, et al. A placebo and active comparator-controlled trial of rofecoxib for the treatment of rheumatoid arthritis. *Scand J Rheumatol* 2002;31:230–238.
75. Matsumoto AK, Melian A, Mandel DR, et al. Randomized, controlled, clinical trial of etoricoxib in the treatment of rheumatoid arthritis. *J Rheumatol* 2002;29:1623–1630.
76. Bensen W, Weaver A, Espinoza L, et al. Efficacy and safety of valdecoxib in treating the signs and symptoms of rheumatoid arthritis: a randomized, controlled comparison with placebo and naproxen. *Rheumatology* 2002;41:1008–1016.
77. Collantes E, Curtis SP, Lee KW, et al. A multinational randomized, controlled, clinical trial of etoricoxib in the treatment of rheumatoid arthritis. *BMC Fam Pract* 2002;3:10–20.
78. Brooks PM, Day RO. Non-steroidal antiinflammatory drugs: differences and similarities. *New Engl J Med* 1991;324:1716–1725.
79. Daniels SE, Talwalker S, Torri S, et al. Valdecoxib, a cyclooxygenase-2-specific inhibitor, is effective in treating primary dysmenorrhea. *Obstet Gynecol* 2002;100:350–358.
80. Barton SF, Langeland FF, Snabes MC, et al. Efficacy and safety of intravenous parecoxib sodium in relieving acute postoperative pain following gynecologic laparotomy surgery. *Anesthesiology* 2002;97:306–314.
81. Antiplatelet Trialists' Group. Collaborative meta-analysis of randomised trials of antiplatelet therapy for prevention of death, myocardial infarction, and stroke in high risk patients. *BMJ* 2002;324:71–86.
82. Hayden M, Pignone M, Phillips C, et al. Aspirin for the primary prevention of cardiovascular events: a summary of the evidence for the U.S. Preventive Services Task Force. *Ann Intern Med* 2002;136:161–172.

83. Force USPST. Aspirin for the primary prevention of cardiovascular events: recommendation and rationale. *Ann Intern Med* 2002;136:157–160.
84. Giardeillo FM, Offerhaus GJA, DuBios RN. The role of nonsteroidal antiinflammatory drugs in colorectal cancer prevention. *Eur J Cancer* 1995;31A:1071–1076.
85. Phillips RK, Wallace MH, Lynch PM, et al. A randomised, double blind, placebo controlled study of celecoxib, a selective cyclooxygenase 2 inhibitor, on duodenal polyposis in familial adenomatous polyposis. *Gut* 2002;50:857–860.
86. Hawk ET, Viner JL, Dannenberg A, et al. COX-2 in cancer—a player that's defining the rules. *J Natl Cancer Inst* 2002;94:545–546.
87. Hwang DH, Fung V, Dannenberg AJ. National Cancer Institute workshop on chemopreventive properties of nonsteroidal antiinflammatory drugs: role of COX-dependent and -independent mechanisms. *Neoplasia* 2002;4:91–97.
88. Singh G, Ramey DR, Morfeld D, et al. Gastrointestinal tract complications of nonsteroidal antiinflammatory drug treatment in rheumatoid arthritis: a prospective observational cohort study. *Arch Intern Med* 1996;156:1530–1536.
89. Wolfe MM, Lichtenstein DR, Singh G. Gastrointestinal toxicity of nonsteroidal antiinflammatory drugs. *N Engl J Med* 1999;340:1888–1899.
90. Bakowsky VS, Hanly JG. Complications of nonsteroidal antiinflammatory drug gastropathy and use of gastric cytoprotection: experience at a tertiary care health center. *J Rheumatol* 1999;26:1557–1563.
91. Garcia Rodriguez LA, Hernandez-Diaz S. Relative risk of upper gastrointestinal complications among users of acetaminophen and nonsteroidal antiinflammatory drugs. *Epidemiology* 2001;12:570–576.
92. Lanas A, Bajador E, Serrano P, et al. Nitrovasodilators, low-dose aspirin, other nonsteroidal antiinflammatory drugs, and the risk of upper gastrointestinal bleeding. *N Engl J Med* 2000;343:834–839.
93. Houchen CW. Clinical implications of prostaglandin inhibition in the small bowel. *Gastroenterol Clin North Am* 2001;30:953–969.
94. Allison MC, Howatson AG, Torrance CJ, et al. Gastrointestinal damage associated with the use of nonsteroidal antiinflammatory drugs. *N Engl J Med* 1992;327:749–754.
95. Wallace JL. Prostaglandin biology in inflammatory bowel disease. *Gastroenterol Clin North Am* 2001;30:971–980.
96. Patrono C, Patrignani P, Garcia-Rodrigues LA. Cyclooxygenase-selective inhibition of prostanoid formation: transducing biochemical selectivity into clinical read-outs. *J Clin Invest* 2002;108:7–13.
97. Langenbach R, Morham SG, Tiano HF, et al. Prostaglandin synthase 1 gene disruption in mice reduces arachidonic acid-induced inflammation and indomethacin-induced gastric ulceration. *Cell* 1995;83:483–492.
98. McCarthy CJ, Crofford LJ, Greensom J, et al. Cyclooxygenase-2 expression in gastric antral mucosa before and after eradication of *Helicobacter pylori* infection. *Am J Gastroenterol* 1999;94:1218–1223.
99. Wallace JL, Keenan CM, Granger DN. Gastric ulceration induced by nonsteroidal anti-inflammatory drugs is a neutrophil-dependent process. *Am J Physiol* 1990;259:G462–G467.
100. Wallace JL. Nonsteroidal antiinflammatory drugs and gastroenteropathy: the second hundred years. *Gastroenterology* 1997;112:1000–1016.
101. Simon LS, Hatoum HT, Bittman RM, et al. Risk factors for serious nonsteroidal-induced gastrointestinal complications: regression analysis of the MUCOSA trial. *Fam Med* 1996;28:404–410.
102. Laine L, Bombardier C, Hawkey CJ, et al. Stratifying the risk of NSAID-related upper gastrointestinal clinical events: results of a double-blind outcomes study in patients with rheumatoid arthritis. *Gastroenterology* 2002;123:1006–1012.
103. Cryer B. Mucosal defense and repair. Role of prostaglandins in the stomach and duodenum. *Gastroenterol Clin North Am* 2001;30:877–894.
104. Cryer B, Feldman M. Cyclooxygenase-1 and cyclooxygenase-2 selectivity of widely used nonsteroidal antiinflammatory drugs. *Am J Med* 1998;104:413–421.
105. Langman MJ, Jensen DM, Watson DJ, et al. Adverse upper gastrointestinal effects of rofecoxib compared with NSAIDs. *JAMA* 2000;282:1929–1933.
106. Goldstein JL, Silverstein FE, Agrawal NM, et al. Reduced risk of upper gastrointestinal ulcer complications with celecoxib, a novel COX-2 inhibitor. *Am J Gastroenterol* 2000;95:1681–1690.
107. Silverstein FE, Faich G, Goldstein JL, et al. Gastrointestinal toxicity with celecoxib vs nonsteroidal antiinflammatory drugs for osteoarthritis and rheumatoid arthritis. The CLASS study: a randomized controlled trial. *JAMA* 2000;284:1247–1255.
108. Sikes DH, Agrawal NM, Zhao WW, et al. Incidence of gastroduodenal ulcers associated with valdecoxib compared with that of ibuprofen and diclofenac in patients with osteoarthritis. *Eur J Gastroenterol Hepatol* 2002;14:1101–1111.
109. Simon LS, Smolen JS, Abramson SB, et al. Controversies in COX-2 selective inhibition. *J Rheumatol* 2002;29:1501–1510.
110. Juni P, Rutjes AWS, Dieppe PA. Are selective COX-2 inhibitors superior to traditional non steroidal antiinflammatory drugs? *BMJ* 2002;324:1287–1288.
111. Mamdani M, Rochon PA, Juurlink DN, et al. Observational study of upper gastrointestinal haemorrhage in elderly patients given selective cyclo-oxygenase-2 inhibitors or conventional non-steroidal antiinflammatory drugs. *BMJ* 2002;325:624–629.
112. Lichenstein DR, Syngal S, Wolfe MM. Nonsteroidal antiinflammatory drugs and the gastrointestinal tract. The double-edged sword. *Arthritis Rheum* 1995;38:5–18.
113. Silverstein FE, Graham DY, Senior JR, et al. Misoprostol reduces serious gastrointestinal complications in patients with rheumatoid arthritis receiving nonsteroidal antiinflammatory drugs. *Ann Intern Med* 1995;123:241–249.
114. Graham DY, Agrawal NM, Campbell DR, et al. Ulcer prevention in long-term users of nonsteroidal antiinflammatory drugs. *Arch Intern Med* 2002;162:169–175.
115. Bocanegra TS, Weaver AL, Tindall EA, et al. Diclofenac/misoprostol compared with diclofenac in the treatment of osteoarthritis of the knee or hip: a randomized, placebo controlled trial. *J Rheumatol* 1998;25:1602–1611.
116. Hawkey CJ, Karrasch JA, Szczepanski L, et al. Omeprazole compared with misoprostol for ulcers associated with nonsteroidal antiinflammatory drugs. *N Engl J Med* 1998;338:727–734.
117. Yeomans ND, Tulassay Z, Juhasz L, et al. A comparison of omeprazole with ranitidine for ulcers associated with nonsteroidal antiinflammatory drugs. *N Engl J Med* 1998;338:719–726.
118. Wolfe F, Anderson J, Burke TA, et al. Gastroprotective therapy and risk of gastrointestinal ulcers: risk reduction by COX-2 therapy. *J Rheumatol* 2002;29:467–473.
119. Chan FKL, Chung SCS, Suen BY, et al. Preventing recurrent upper gastrointestinal bleeding in patients with *Helicobacter pylori* infection who are taking low-dose aspirin or naproxen. *N Engl J Med* 2001;344:967–973.
120. Chan FKL, Hung LCT, Suen BY, et al. Celecoxib versus diclofenac and omeprazole in reducing the risk of recurrent ulcer bleeding in patients with arthritis. *N Engl J Med* 2002;347:2104–2110.
121. Fored CM, Ejerblad E, Lindblad P, et al. Acetaminophen, aspirin, and chronic renal failure: a nationwide case-control study in Sweden. *N Engl J Med* 2001;345:1801–1808.
122. Harris RC, McKanna JA, Aiai Y, et al. Cyclooxygenase-2 is associated with the macula densa of rat kidney and increases with salt restriction. *J Clin Invest* 1994;94:2504–2510.
123. Traynor TR, Smart A, Briggs JP, et al. Inhibition of macula densa-stimulated renin secretion by pharmacological blockade of cyclooxygenase-2. *Am J Physiol* 1999;277:F706–F710.
124. Yang T, Endo Y, Huang YG, et al. Renin expression in COX-2-knockout mice on normal or low-salt diets. *Am J Physiol* 2000;279:F819–F825.
125. Qi Z, Hao C-M, Langenbach RI, et al. Opposite effects of cyclooxygenase-1 and -2 activity on the pressor response to angiotensin II. *J Clin Invest* 2002;110:61–69.
126. Swan SK, Rudy DW, Lasseter KC, et al. Effects of cyclooxygenase-2 inhibition on renal function in elderly persons receiving a low-salt diet. *Ann Intern Med* 2000;133:1–9.
127. McAdam BF, Catella-Lawson F, Mardini IA, et al. Systemic biosynthesis of prostacyclin by cyclooxygenase (COX)-2: the human pharmacology of a selective inhibitor of COX-2. *Proc Natl Acad Sci U S A* 1999;96:272–277.
128. Catella-Lawson F, McAdam B, Morrison BW, et al. Effects of specific inhibition of cyclooxygenase-2 on sodium balance, hemodynamics and vasoactive eicosanoids. *J Pharmacol Exp Ther* 1999;298:735–741.
129. Rossat J, Maillard M, Nussberger J, et al. Renal effects of selective cyclooxygenase-2 inhibition in normotensive salt-depleted subjects. *Clin Pharmacol Ther* 1999;66:76–84.
130. Whelton A, Maurath CJ, Vergurg KM, et al. Renal safety and tolerability of celecoxib, a novel cyclooxygenase inhibitor. *Am J Ther* 2000;7:159–174.
131. Akhund L, Quinet RJ, Ishaq S. Celecoxib-related renal papillary necrosis. *Arch Intern Med* 2003;163:114–115.
132. Segasothy M, Suleiman AB, Puvaneswary M, et al. Paracetamol: a cause for analgesic nephropathy and end-stage renal disease. *Nephron* 1988;50:50–54.
133. Pernager TV, Whelton PK, Klag MJ. Risk of kidney failure associated with the use of acetaminophen, aspirin, and nonsteroidal antiinflammatory drugs. *N Engl J Med* 1994;331:1675–1679.
134. Rexrode KM, Buring JE, Glynn RJ, et al. Analgesic use and renal function in men. *JAMA* 2001;286:315–321.
135. Belay ED, Bresee JS, Holman RC, et al. Reye's syndrome in the United States from 1981 through 1997. *N Engl J Med* 1999;340:1377–1382.
136. Prescott LF. Paracetamol: past, present, and future. *Am J Ther* 2000;7:143–147.
137. Szczeklik A, Nizankowska E, Duplaga M, et al. Natural history of aspirin-induced asthma. *Eur Respir J* 2000;16:432–436.
138. Hedman J, Kaprio J, Poussa T, et al. Prevalence of asthma, aspirin intolerance, nasal polyposis and chronic obstructive pulmonary disease in a population-based study. *Int J Epidemiol* 1999;28:717–722.
139. Woessner KM, Simon RA, Stevenson DD. The safety of celecoxib in patients with aspirin-sensitive asthma. *Arthritis Rheum* 2002;46:2201–2206.
140. Szczeklik A, Nizankowska E, Bochenek G, et al. Safety of a specific COX-2 inhibitor in aspirin-induced asthma. *Clin Exp Allergy* 2000;31:219–225.
141. Dahlen B, Szczeklik A, Murray JJ. Celecoxib in patients with asthma and aspirin intolerance. *N Engl J Med* 2001;344:142.
142. Stevenson DD, Simon RA. Lack of cross-reactivity between rofecoxib and aspirin in aspirin-sensitive patients with asthma. *J Allergy Clin Immunol* 2001;108:47–51.
143. Stevenson DD, Sanchez-Borges M, Szczeklik A. Classification of allergic and pseudoallergic reactions to drugs that inhibit cyclooxygenase enzymes. *Ann Allergy Asthma Immunol* 2001;87:177–180.
144. Grob M, Scheidegger P, Wuthrich B. Allergic skin reaction to celecoxib. *Dermatology* 2000;201:383.
145. Skowron F, Berard F, Bernard N, et al. Cutaneous vasculitis related to celecoxib. *Dermatology* 2002;204:305.
146. Schneider F, Meziani F, Chartier C, et al. Fatal allergic vasculitis associated with celecoxib. *Lancet* 2002;359:852–853.
147. Ernst EJ, Egge JA. Celecoxib-induced erythema multiforme with glyburide cross-reactivity. *Pharmacotherapy* 2002;22:637–640.

148. Quiralte J, Saenz de San Pedro B, Florido JJ. Safety of selective cyclooxygenase-2 inhibitor rofecoxib in patients with NSAID-induced cutaneous reactions. *Ann Allergy Asthma Immunol* 2002;89:63–66.
149. Pacor ML, Di Lorenzo G, Biasi D, et al. Safety of rofecoxib in subjects with a history of adverse cutaneous reactions to aspirin and/or non-steroidal anti-inflammatory drugs. *Clin Exp Allergy* 2002;32:397–400.
150. Kumar NP, Wild G, Ramasamy KA, et al. Fatal haemorrhagic pulmonary oedema and associated angioedema after the ingestion of rofecoxib. *Postgrad Med J* 2002;78:439–440.
151. Hennan JK, Huang J, Barrett TC, et al. Effects of selective cyclooxygenase-2 inhibition on vascular responses and thrombosis in canine coronary arteries. *Circulation* 2001;104:820–825.
152. Konstam MA, Weir MR, Reicin A, et al. Cardiovascular thrombotic events in controlled, clinical trials of rofecoxib. *Circulation* 2001;104:2280–2288.
153. Strand V, Hochberg MC. The risk of cardiovascular thrombotic events with selective cyclooxygenase-2 inhibitors. *Arthritis Care Res* 2002;47:349–355.
154. Crofford LJ, Oates JC, McCune WJ, et al. Thrombosis in patients with connective tissue diseases treated with specific COX-2 inhibitors: a report of four cases. *Arthritis Rheum* 2000;43:1891–1896.
155. Dalen JE. Selective COX-2 inhibitors, NSAIDs, aspirin, and myocardial infarction. *Arch Intern Med* 2002;162:1091–1092.
156. Bonnel RA, Villalba ML, Karwoski CB, et al. Aseptic meningitis associated with rofecoxib. *Arch Intern Med* 2002;162:713–715.
157. Hill JB. Salicylate intoxication. *N Engl J Med* 1973;288:1110–1113.
158. Durnas C, Cusack BJ. Salicylate intoxication in the elderly. Recognition and recommendations on how to prevent it. *Drugs Aging* 1992;2:20–34.
159. Brater DC. Effects of nonsteroidal antiinflammatory drugs on renal function: focus on cyclooxygenase-2-selective inhibition. *Am J Med* 1999;107:65S–71S.
160. Schwartz JI, Agrawal NG, Wong PH, et al. Lack of pharmacokinetic interaction between rofecoxib and methotrexate in rheumatoid arthritis patients. *J Clin Pharmacol* 2001;41:1120–1130.
161. Karim A, Tolbert DS, Hunt TL, et al. Celecoxib, a specific COX-2 inhibitor, has no significant effect on methotrexate pharmacokinetics in patients with rheumatoid arthritis. *J Rheumatol* 1999;26:2539–2543.
162. Fendrick AM, Bandekar RR, Chernew ME, et al. Role of initial NSAID choice and patient risk factors in the prevention of NSAID gastropathy: a decision analysis. *Arthritis Rheum* 2002;47:36–43.
163. Crofford LJ. Is there a place for non-selective NSAIDs in the treatment of arthritis? *Joint Bone Spine* 2002;69:4–7.
164. Cantor SB. Pharmacoeconomics of coxib therapy. *J Pain Symptom Manage* 2002;24:S28–S37.
165. Portenoy RK. Opioid therapy for chronic nonmalignant pain: a review of the critical issues. *J Pain Symptom Manage* 1996;11:203–217.

CHAPTER 24

Corticosteroids

Dinesh Khanna and Harold E. Paulus

Philip Hench (1) introduced glucocorticoids (GCs) in clinical practice after successfully treating a patient with rheumatoid arthritis (RA). He received a Nobel Prize, along with Kendall and Reichstein, in 1950 for this discovery. Since then, for more than half a century, GCs have been used for treatment of RA. No other treatment in RA has generated so much excitement and controversy as use of GCs. This chapter focuses on the therapeutic use of GCs in RA and briefly reviews GC pharmacology and mechanism of action. Published reports of clinical trials in RA are evaluated with emphasis on clinical manifestations, radiographic progression, and major side effects.

Cortisol (hydrocortisone) is the main endogenous GC and is secreted primarily in response to adrenocorticotropic hormone (ACTH). Estimates of GC excretion are approximately 5 mg per m^2 per day of cortisol (approximately 20–30 mg per day of hydrocortisone or 5–7 mg per day of prednisone) (2,3). GC levels have diurnal variation, with peak level between 4 A.M. and 8 A.M. (2). Synthetic GCs, more potent and with fewer side effects, have been developed (Fig. 24.1). Examples and their relative GC and mineralocorticoid potency are described in Table 24.1 (4).

PHARMACOLOGY

Pharmacokinetics

ABSORPTION

Natural and synthetic GCs are commonly used in RA for suppression of inflammation. The different preparations of GCs have largely the same rate of absorption (5). Prednisone is 80% to 90% absorbed whether on an empty or full stomach, both in normal volunteers and in various patient populations (6). The absorption probably occurs in the upper jejunum. The systemic bioavailability of prednisone and prednisolone are similar. GC bioavailability does not appear to be affected by pregnancy (7).

DISTRIBUTION

Cortisol, the endogenously produced GC (Fig. 24.2), is 80% bound to cortisol-binding globulin (CBG; transcortin), but the synthetic GCs bind less to CBG (5). Prednisone has approximately 60%; prednisolone, 5%; and other preparations, less than 1% of the affinity of cortisol for CBG. The remainder is bound to albumin, which binds with a low affinity and high capacity (5). CBG- and albumin-bound GCs are inactive during transport in the plasma. The unbound concentrations of prednisolone are biologically active, and free fraction ranges from less than 0.1% to 0.5% (8).

METABOLISM

Cortisol is reduced and hydroxylated in the liver, made water soluble by conjugation with sulfate or glucuronic acid, and excreted in urine. 6-Beta hydroxylation by the cytochrome P450 microsomal enzyme CYP3A4 also enhances water solubility and urinary excretion of GCs (9). Exogenous GCs are subject to the same metabolic reactions as cortisol. Cortisone and prednisone are rapidly reduced to the active forms, cortisol and prednisolone (10).

CLEARANCE

The clearance of prednisone from the circulation is 210 mL per minute per 1.73 m^2, with an elimination half-life of approximately 3 hours. Corticosteroids exhibit dose-dependent kinetics; higher doses are cleared more rapidly, perhaps due to concentration-dependent increases in the unbound free fraction in plasma. Dose-dependent pharmacokinetics partly explain the clinical observation that alternate-day prednisone dosing yields fewer biologic effects than equivalent daily dosing (8), as shown by a decrease in efficacy (11) and side effects (12). Clearance of both prednisone and methylprednisolone is lower by 18% to 28% in the morning than evening (13,14). This, along with the disruption of the usual diurnal rhythm of cortisol production, may result in variations in efficacy when steroids are administered at different times of the day. Prednisolone clearance is slower in blacks than whites and in women than men (15). However, these differences may not have any clinical implications, and dose adjustments are not required. There is an inverse correlation between prednisolone clearance and age (8,16).

DISTRIBUTION IN BREAST MILK

GCs are excreted in small amounts in human milk. One study found approximately 0.23% of a 5-mg prednisolone dose in breast milk (17).

Pharmacodynamics

The half-life of a GC in the circulation (pharmacokinetics) is not directly related to the duration of its intracellular effects (pharmacodynamics), which have been estimated by measuring the duration of suppression of ACTH activity after a dose of GC (Table 24.2). Short-acting GCs (e.g., cortisone, cortisol, prednisone, prednisolone, methylprednisolone) suppress ACTH activity for 24 to 30 hours, intermediate-acting GCs (e.g., triamcinolone) for 48 hours,

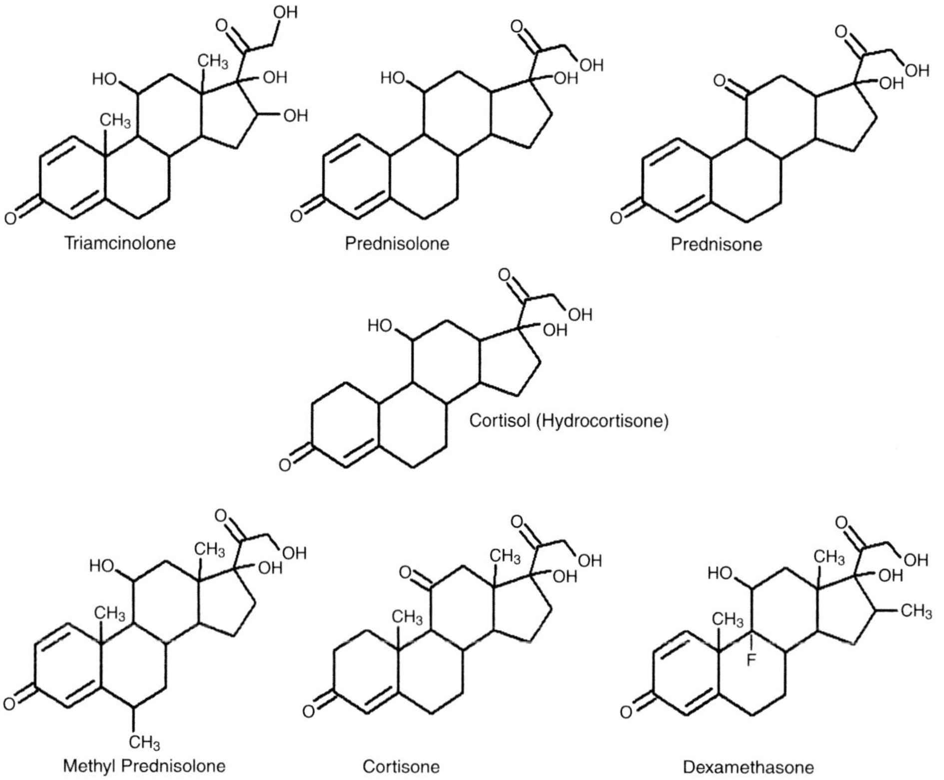

Triamcinolone Prednisolone Prednisone

Cortisol (Hydrocortisone)

Methyl Prednisolone Cortisone Dexamethasone

Figure 24.1. Chemical structures of some commonly used endogenous (cortisol) and synthetic corticosteroids.

and long-acting GCs (e.g., dexamethasone and betamethasone) for more than 48 hours (18,19). Thus, alternate-day administration of a short-acting GC allows normal ACTH production for 12 to 24 hours out of each 48-hour dosing interval.

MECHANISM OF ACTION

An understanding of the mechanism of action of GCs in humans and, especially, on cells lagged behind clinical observations of the effects in RA. In active, untreated RA, secretion of cortisol is impaired despite intact ACTH response, consistent with relative adrenal GC insufficiency and probably related to the effects of proinflammatory cytokines (23). Since the 1980s, the cellular mechanisms of action of GCs have been better defined (4).

Molecular Mechanisms of Glucocorticoid Action

Unbound GC passes through the cell membrane into cytoplasm (Fig. 24.2) and activates the cytoplasmic GC receptor (GR). GRs are cytoplasmic proteins that operate as hormone-activated transcriptional regulators (24). Two members of the receptor family bind GCs with high affinity. The type 1 receptor, the mineralocorticoid receptor, binds certain GCs and mediates aldosterone-like effects. The type 2 receptor is the more widely expressed GR. After activation by GC, the GR dissociates from complexed heat shock proteins and other factors (25,26). The activated ligand-bound GR is then able to dimerize and translocate into the nucleus. In the nucleus, the activated GR binds to palindromic DNA sequences in the promoter regions of several genes referred to as *GC response elements*. GR binding to GC response elements modulates transcriptional activity of the respective genes. Both endogenous and exogenous GCs mediate their effects mostly by the same transcription factor—the GR.

These findings lead to the question of whether the control of inflammation and autoimmunity by GCs may be affected by changes at the level of the GR. Investigations of the density of GR in RA showed a diminished number of GR molecules (27). Further analysis in rheumatic disease has shown that this GR down-

TABLE 24.1. Relative Potencies of Various Glucocorticoids

Glucocorticoid	Relative Antiinflammatory Potency	Equivalent Dose (mg)	Relative Mineralocorticoid Activity	Half-Life (min)	Biologic Half-Life (h)
Cortisol	1	20	1	60	8–12
Cortisone	0.8	25	0.8	60	8–12
Prednisone	4	5	0.8	180	12–36
Prednisolone	4	5	0.8	180	12–36
Methylprednisolone	5	4	0.5	180	12–36
Triamcinolone	5	4	0	180	12–36
Dexamethasone	20–30	0.75	0	220	36–72

From Kirou KA, Boumpas DT. Systemic glucocorticoid therapy in systemic lupus erythematosus. In: Wallace DJ, Hahn BH, eds. *Dubois' lupus erythematosus*, 6th ed. Philadelphia: Lippincott Williams & Wilkins, 2001:1173–1194, with permission.

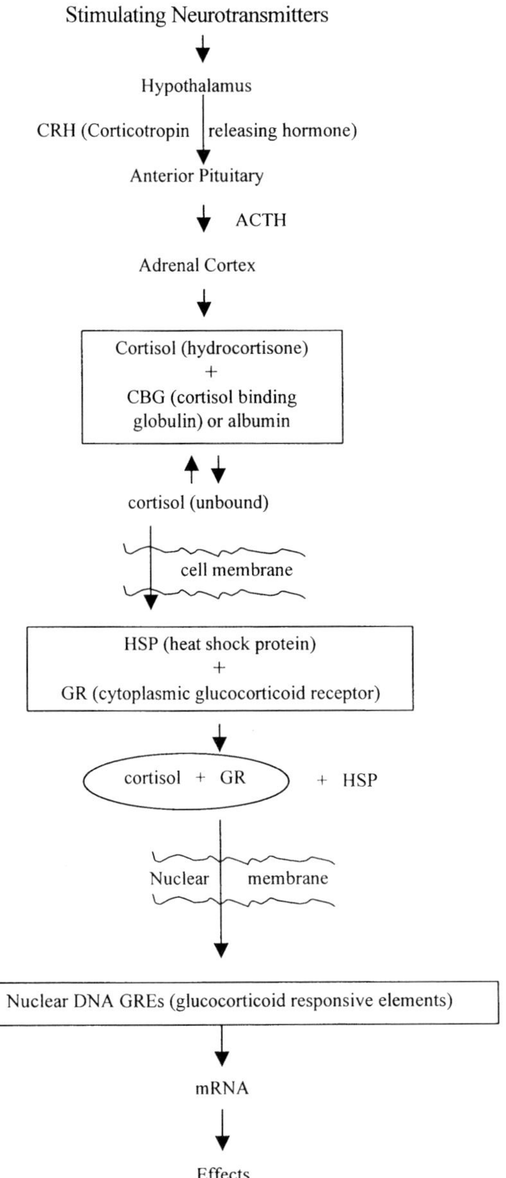

Figure 24.2. Induction of endogenous corticosteroid production, distribution, intracellular transport, and effects. ACTH, adrenocorticotropic hormone; mRNA, messenger RNA.

regulation may be due to the GC therapy and that the decrease in number of GRs is dose dependent (28). A recent study assessed the changes in GR numbers during treatment of RA for a period of 2 years, with either 10 mg prednisone or placebo (29). At the initiation of the study, the number of GRs was lower in the RA group than in healthy controls, but a steady increase in the GR numbers, independent of GC treatment, was seen reaching levels of healthy controls after 2 years. These findings suggest that up-regulation of GR may reflect a recovery or a compensatory response to ongoing inflammation; however, this might not be enough to efficiently control the inflammatory situation.

The transcription factors nuclear factor–κB (NF-κB) and activating protein 1 play an important role in the pathogenesis of RA (30,31). In most cell types, NF-κB in the cytoplasm is an inactive complex bound to its inhibitor protein, IκB. On activation, IκB is rapidly degraded, and free NF-κB dimers translocate to the nucleus and activate target genes. Asahara et al. (30) reported a markedly high DNA-binding affinity of NF-κB in nuclear extracts derived from synovial membranes of RA patients. NF-κB is involved in the regulation of several genes that are up-regulated in RA, such as the cyclooxygenase-2 gene, matrix metalloproteinase-1, and interleukin (IL)-1, -2, and -6. The GR antagonizes proinflammatory gene expression through transcriptional interference of NF-κB and activating protein 1 (32). This inhibition is achieved by inducing gene transcription and protein synthesis of NF-κB inhibitor, IκB (33). Activated GR also antagonizes NF-κB activity through direct complexing with, and inhibition of, NF-κB binding to DNA (34) or association with NF-κB bound to κB DNA sites (35). This competitive inhibition prevents induction of gene expression of a number of proinflammatory proteins. The proteins inhibited by GCs through this mechanism include IL-1, -2, -6, and -18; tumor necrosis factor (TNF); and interferon-γ, metalloproteinase-1, and cyclooxygenase-2 enzymes (33).

TABLE 24.2. Clinical Implications of Corticosteroid Pharmacokinetics, Pharmacodynamics, and Drug Interactions

- In liver failure, there is a decrease in conversion of prednisone to prednisolone, which is overcompensated for by reduced clearance of unbound prednisolone. Therefore, there is no need to replace prednisone with an inherently active GC agent (e.g., prednisolone, cortisol) in these patients.
- Hypoproteinemia per se does not cause increased unbound concentrations of prednisolone *in vivo* and, therefore, no dose adjustments are necessary (8).
- Patients with Crohn's disease have unpredictably reduced concentrations due to malabsorption.
- Patients with liver failure, renal failure, and renal transplant have an increased unbound fraction of prednisolone, depending on the residual hepatic or renal function.
- Drugs that induce hepatic microsomal enzymes (especially CYP3A4), such as phenobarbital, phenytoin, rifampicin, and carbamazepine, increase GC elimination (20).
- Drugs that inhibit CYP3A4, such as ketoconazole, erythromycin, cimetidine, and ethynyl estradiol, can increase GC activity (20).
- Doses of aluminum/magnesium hydroxide antacids do not decrease prednisone bioavailability (21).
- Patients with hyperthyroidism need higher doses of prednisone to achieve the same immunosuppressive effects as those in euthyroid states. This probably is due to a combination of enhanced nonrenal clearance and decreased intestinal absorption of prednisone (8).
- Some evidence suggests that indomethacin and naproxen increase GC concentrations (22). Additional studies are required to determine the clinical significance of this interaction.

GC, glucocorticoid.

Immunosuppressive Effects

The biologic effects of GCs are multiple and are essential for body homeostasis during normal or stress conditions. Although GCs are used as drugs to suppress inflammation and pathologic immune responses, a growing number of studies show a "paradoxical" immune-enhancing effect of GCs (36,37). Endogenous GCs have an important overall regulatory role in modulating immune responses that develop during infection or stress. Higher (pharmacologic) levels, such as those occurring after the initiation of stress, are, in general, immunosuppressive, whereas low physiologic levels of GC present before stress may enhance immune responses (4). Notably, acute stresses or short exposure to GCs enhances immune responses, whereas chronic exposure to stress or GCs has the opposite effect (36).

In peripheral blood, GCs induce neutrophilia, but the numbers of basophils, eosinophils, monocytes, and lymphocytes decrease on brief exposure to GCs (38). Lymphopenia is attributed to redirection of lymphocytes to bone marrow and spleen

(39,40), as well as to skin and regional lymph nodes of the inflammatory sites (36). Oral administration of prednisolone to healthy volunteers in various doses ranging from 10 to 60 mg affects the T lymphocytes in the blood more than B lymphocytes and CD4 T cells more than CD8 T cells (41). Inhibition of various stages of T-cell activation, including calcineurin-dependent pathways (42), calcium/calmodulin-dependent protein kinase II (43), and early tyrosine phosphorylation events, mediate GC immunosuppression. GC also inhibits IL-2 and its signaling, which is critical for T-cell proliferation (44). GCs indirectly also affect T-cell function by inhibiting the expression of major histocompatibility complex–class 2 molecules (38). B-cell function and immunoglobulin synthesis are relatively less affected by GCs. GCs also have an effect on mature helper T cells (Th) (45). Although GCs inhibit the acute production of both Th1 and Th2 cytokines, their presence may, nevertheless, promote the differentiation to the Th2 phenotype. This Th2 bias occurs with inhibition of IL-2 production (which favors Th1 development) by GC, whereas IL-10 production (favoring Th2 development) is relatively resistant to suppression (46,47). This action may explain its beneficial effect in the treatment of diseases characterized by Th1-type cytokine predominance, such as RA.

GCs induce apoptosis of thymocytes (45) and activated T cells (48). These mechanisms may be important in the regulation of immune responses and in prevention of autoimmunity.

Antiinflammatory Effects

The antiinflammatory effects of GCs are mediated via their GRs and correlate with dose and duration of GC treatment (4).

INHIBITION OF NEUTROPHIL MIGRATION TO PERIPHERY

GCs primarily affect neutrophils in their ability to migrate to inflammatory sites by inhibiting chemokine synthesis (49), adhesion molecule expression (50), and induction of lipocortin-1 (51). In RA, inhibition of neutrophil ingress into inflamed joints occurs as early as 90 minutes after pulse GC (methylprednisolone, 1,000 mg) and is associated with rapid modulation of adhesion molecules and inflammatory mediators (IL-8 and TNF-α levels) within the joints (52,53).

INHIBITION OF SYNTHESIS OF INFLAMMATORY MEDIATORS

Eicosanoid generation is inhibited by GC through induction of transcription of lipocortin-1 (54) and inhibition of IL-1β–mediated cyclooxygenase-2 induction (55). Additionally, there is down-regulation of destructive enzymes such as collagenase (56,57).

ALTERATION OF CYTOKINE BALANCE

Inhibition of cytokine generation constitutes another important antiinflammatory effect, for example, synthesis and action of TNF-α; IL-1β, -2, -3, -4, -5, -6, -8, -10, and -13; and granulocyte-macrophage colony-stimulating factor (49,58). Where mechanisms have been explored, cytokine inhibition is due to interference with gene expression. GCs appear to interfere with the binding and function of critical transcription factors, probably by direct protein–protein interactions and direct inhibition by the GR. On the other hand, synthesis of the antiinflammatory cytokines IL-10 and transforming growth factor β is either not affected or is induced by GCs (46,59).

INHIBITION OF BLOOD VESSEL DILATATION AND PERMEABILITY

GC inhibits vasodilatation and vascular permeability, thus limiting erythema and swelling. The inhibitory effect of GC on inducible nitric oxide synthase and, therefore, on nitric oxide synthesis, may contribute to this effect (60).

Cortisol Production by Healthy Adults

GC excretion is approximately 5 to 10 mg per m^2 per day of cortisol (equivalent to approximately 20–30 mg per day of hydrocortisone or 5–7 mg per day of prednisone) (2,3,61). Synthesis of cortisol may increase five- to tenfold under conditions of severe stress, to a maximal level of approximately 100 mg per m^2 per day (2,61). During surgical procedures, serum cortisol levels rise rapidly but usually return to baseline values within 24 to 48 hours. The magnitude of this increase is positively correlated with the extent of the surgery and anesthesia. In adults, cortisol secretion is approximately 50 mg per 24 hours during minor surgery and 75 to 150 mg per 24 hours during major surgeries, seldom exceeding 200 to 300 mg. This suggests that, in critically ill patients, these doses of hydrocortisone should be administered, preferably in a continuous infusion (61).

CLINICAL EFFICACY IN RHEUMATOID ARTHRITIS

Placebo Trials, Relative Efficacy, and Combination Use

SHORT- AND MEDIUM-TERM USE OF GLUCOCORTICOIDS

Short- and medium-term oral GCs have been used mainly for symptomatic relief of acute exacerbations of RA and as "bridge therapy" before disease-modifying antirheumatic agents (DMARDs) have taken effect. A metaanalysis conducted for the Cochrane database on short-term use (1 week) of low-dose GCs (62) (Table 24.3) confirmed the efficacy of prednisolone (15 mg or less) over placebo in terms of joint tenderness [standardized effect size (SES), 1.31], pain (SES, 1.75), and grip strength (SES, 0.41). In the individual studies, SES is the mean change of an outcome measure divided by the pooled baseline standard deviation of that measure. SES provides a unitless estimate of the relative magnitude of change (improvement or worsening) of an outcome measure during a clinical trial and is used in metaanalysis to compare effects across trials that may have used similar, but not identical, outcome measures. Standardized mean difference (SMD) is similar but divides the mean change in a measure by the standard deviation of the change. Similar results were obtained with comparison to nonsteroidal antiinflammatory drugs (NSAIDs). A previous Cochrane Library review (63) and a metaanalysis (64) were conducted to evaluate the effect of moderate-term use (approximately 7 months) of low-dose prednisone (defined as ≤15 mg) (Table 24.3). Four placebo-controlled trials were evaluated by Saag et al. (64) and an additional one by the Cochrane database (63). The results of the Cochrane analysis showed marked improvement in joint tenderness (SMD, –0.37), swelling (SMD, –0.41), pain (SMD, –0.43), and functional status (SMD, –0.57) over placebo, and the Saag et al. (64) analysis showed improvement in joint tenderness and erythrocyte sedimentation rate (ESR) over placebo; due to small sample sizes, however, the confidence intervals are wide and include 0. Prednisone was also found to be as effective as deflazacort (64) and chloroquine (65).

LONG-TERM USE OF GLUCOCORTICOIDS

Long-term studies have provided less evidence of extended symptomatic relief (Table 24.3). The initial study published in 1959 and 1960 by the Medical Research Council and Nuffield Foundation (66,67) compared prednisolone (mean dosage, 12 mg per day for 1 year and then 10 mg per day for the next year) with aspirin and found marked improvement in the prednisolone group for the initial weeks. However, a 12-month follow-up showed dissipation of

TABLE 24.3. Clinical Benefit in Rheumatoid Arthritis: Summary of Pivotal Trials

	Author (Reference)	Type of Study	Mean Dosage/d	Number of Patients Completing Study	Duration of Study (mo)	Tender Joints or Articular Index	Swollen Joints	Pain Visual Analog Scale (0–10)	Health Assessment Questionnaire–Disability Index Score (0–3)	Patient Global Severity Score (0–3)	Acute Phase Reactants (Erythrocyte Sedimentation Rate in mm/h)
Short-term studies	Gotzsche 2002 (62) (meta-analysis)	Prednisone vs. placebo	15 mg	NA	1	1.31[a]	NR	1.75[a]	NR	NR	NR
Moderate-term studies	Saag 1996 (64) (metaanalysis)	Prednisone vs. placebo	15 mg	NA	7	0.90[a]	1.05[a]	NR	NR	NR	1.20[a]
Long-term studies in rheumatoid arthritis	Medical Research Council 1959–1960 (66,67)	Prednisolone vs.	12 mg/first yr; 10 mg/second yr	41	24	NS[b]	NS[d]	ND	—	ND	−16
		Aspirin or phenbutazone	6 g or 400 mg	26	—	—	—	—	—	—	−7
	van Schaardenburg 1993 (65)	Prednisone vs.	7.1 mg	24	24	0	−3	ND	−0.50	ND	−22
		Chloroquine	200 mg[c]	13	—	−4	−3.5	—	−0.52	—	−17
	Kirwan 1995 (72)	Prednisolone vs.	7.5 mg	106	24	−133[e]	ND	−0.42	−0.30	—	NS
		Placebo	—	—	—	−109[e]	—	0.45	−0.24	—	—
	van Everdingen 2002 (71)	Prednisolone vs.	10 mg	37	24	−2	−2	−5	0.1	−1	−1[f]
		Placebo	—	34	—	0	−1	1	0.0	0	0[f]

NA, not applicable; ND, not done; NR, not reported; NS, not significant.
[a]Standardized effect size = means of each outcome in a study divided by its baseline pooled SD.
[b]Chi square test = 0.49.
[c]Loading dose of chloroquine at 100 mg p.o. t.i.d. for first month, followed by 100 mg p.o. b.i.d. during the second month.
[d]Chi square test = 0.16.
[e]Thompson's articular index of tender and swollen joints (maximum score = 534).
[f]C-reactive protein.

the beneficial effect on the acute phase response and clinical efficacy. A case control study evaluated the effect of prednisone (mean dosage, 8 mg per day) on RA outcomes in a cohort of 893 patients (68). Five and 10 years after the initiation of prednisone, Health Assessment Questionnaire (HAQ) scores were similar between the two groups, although there was a worsening of physician global assessment at 10 years in the prednisone group. This finding may be due to selection bias, as patients on prednisone used significantly more DMARDs than controls, suggesting more severe disease. In this cohort, there was no definitive advantage of low-dose prednisone. In 1999, an open-label study randomized 102 patients with active RA to either DMARDs or a combination of DMARDs and prednisolone for 1 year (69). Prednisolone was given in a dose regimen adapted to the disease activity of the patient, with a mean dose of 6 mg and cumulative dose of 2,160 mg. Within 2 weeks, there was clinically significant improvement in number of swollen joints, acute phase reactant, HAQ score, and grip strength in the prednisone group, although, at 6 months, no difference was seen in terms of swollen joints and C-reactive protein. However, a positive effect on the HAQ score and grip strength persisted.

With marked short-term beneficial effect on clinical parameters, there has been interest in using prednisone as a bridge therapy before slow-acting DMARDs have taken effect. This possibility was evaluated in 40 RA patients starting intramuscular gold who were randomized to receive either prednisone or placebo for 18 weeks (70). The disease duration was 21.5 months in the prednisone group and 29.5 months in placebo patients. The prednisone group was assigned to 10 mg per day for the first 12 weeks, followed by tapering over the next 6 weeks. Patients were tracked for 44 weeks. In the first 12 weeks, Disease Activity Score improved from a baseline value of 4.88 to 3.62 with prednisone, as compared to 4.97 to 4.58 with placebo ($p = .0001$). After tapering prednisone, rebound deterioration was observed at week 24 in 58% of the responders. No significant differences in radiographic progression were found between the two groups. The rebound deterioration led the authors to not recommend prednisone as bridge therapy.

Use in Early Rheumatoid Arthritis

Increased understanding of the pathogenesis of RA has led to the hypothesis that aggressive treatment of early RA is critical in controlling long-term sequelae such as radiographic progression and functional disability. Studies have been conducted to evaluate the clinical efficacy of low-dose GC (prednisone or prednisolone) in early RA.

In a prospective trial, 81 DMARDs-naïve patients with early RA (disease duration <1 year) were assigned to receive either 10 mg of prednisone per day or placebo for a period of 2 years (71). Most of the clinical response in terms of joint-count score, acute phase reactants, and grip strength was seen during the initial 6 months of the study. As in previous trials, the clinical efficacy of prednisone waned with time; however, grip strength and joint-tenderness count at the end of 24 months were better in the prednisone group ($p = .05$ and .01, respectively). Moreover, the patients taking prednisone required fewer intraarticular steroid injections and physiotherapy sessions during the first 6 months.

Many studies in the 1990s evaluated the role of corticosteroids in conjunction with baseline DMARD therapy. In 1995, a prospective, randomized clinical trial was conducted with 128 patients with early RA (symptoms <2 years) comparing the effect of prednisolone, 7.5 mg per day, to placebo (72). The study duration was 2 years, and background NSAIDs and DMARDs were comparable. At 3 months, there was statistically significant improvement in the prednisolone group in terms of pain, articular index, and HAQ score, as compared to placebo. However, the antiinflammatory effect of prednisolone declined considerably after 1 year. There was no difference between treatment groups in acute phase response by 6 months, in articular index by 9 months, and in HAQ score after 15 months. Taken together, these clinical trials and observational studies do not support the use of long-term prednisone to control the symptomatic disease activity in early RA.

Another prospective study in early RA that used prednisolone as a bridge therapy compared the combination therapy [sulfasalazine, 2 g per day; methotrexate (MTX), 7.5 mg per week; and initial prednisolone dosage, 60 mg per day, lowered over 6 weeks to 7.5 mg per day] to sulfasalazine alone in early RA (median duration of disease, 4 months) (73). Prednisolone and MTX were completely withdrawn by 28 and 40 weeks, respectively. The efficacy was assessed by a pooled index of five measures (mean change divided by pooled standard deviation; range = 0–5): tender joint count, physician global assessment, grip strength, ESR, and McMaster Toronto arthritis questionnaire. At week 28 (primary end point), the improvement in pooled index for combination therapy (1.4) was significant when compared to sulfasalazine alone (0.8) ($p < .0001$), but, at week 56, after prednisolone was withdrawn, there was no difference between the two groups in the pooled index (1.1 vs. 0.9) or individual variables. This result and those of other trials have failed to show significant rebound deterioration in clinical symptoms after prednisolone has been tapered off (71,73,74) (Table 24.4).

PULSE CORTICOSTEROID

A double-blind crossover pilot study evaluated ten patients with RA unresponsive to conventional treatment randomized to either receive 1 g of methylprednisolone or placebo, intravenously, once a month for 6 months (75). During the study, compared to placebo, patients receiving methylprednisolone "pulses" showed significantly better mean tender-joint counts and grip strength ($p < .05$), when measured 30 days after the previous pulse. Studies conducted in the early 1990s evaluated the role of GC as a DMARD pulse intervention. A prospective trial compared monthly intravenous methylprednisolone (15 mg per kg) to normal saline for 6 months in the background of a single DMARD (mostly D-penicillamine) (76). Ninety-seven RA patients (mean duration, 9 years) were followed for 1 year. At the end of the 1-year study, there were no differences between groups in swollen and tender-joint counts, patient and physician global assessment, morning stiffness and acute phase reactants, and radiographic progression.

In contrast to these results, a prospective study showed a short-term advantage of intramuscular depot methylprednisolone acetate over placebo to control disease flares (77). Fifty-nine patients commencing intramuscular gold therapy were randomized to receive 120-mg intramuscular depot methylprednisolone acetate or matching placebo at weeks 0, 4, and 8. The group receiving methylprednisolone injections had more rapid disease improvement. This advantage persisted for up to 12 weeks, although, by 24 weeks, both groups exhibited similar benefits due to continued improvement in the group treated with gold alone. Two studies have shown similar clinical efficacy when 1,000-mg doses of pulse methylprednisolone were compared to 100- to 320-mg doses (78,79) or when intravenous versus intramuscular routes of administration were compared (79).

INTRAARTICULAR STEROIDS

In RA, intraarticular steroids are used to reduce local inflammation and swelling, provide symptomatic relief, and prevent incipient contractures. A prospective study compared intraarticular treatment of RA knee-joint effusion with triamcinolone hexacetonide versus sodium morrhuate, a sclerosing agent (80).

TABLE 24.4. Dosage and Administration of Corticosteroids

Oral corticosteroids
- For active RA, ≤10 mg prednisone, given with breakfast every day.
- Use 1-mg tablets. Taper by 1 mg at a time until <5 mg, at which point, taper by 0.5 mg at a time. Usually taper every 2–4 wk or as soon as the post-taper RA flare subsides.
- Bridge therapy should last no longer than 12 mo.
- Long-term, low-dose GC as a substitute for DMARDs is not recommended.
- Monitor for opportunistic infections, diabetes, cataracts, glaucoma, hypertension, myopathy, osteoporosis, psychosis, and atherosclerosis.
- Patient should receive adequate calcium and vitamin D supplementation and antiresorptive agent, if indicated, to prevent osteoporosis. Consider statins to prevent atherosclerosis.
- Give stress doses of corticosteroids for general anesthesia, major trauma, surgeries, or severe illnesses.

Intravenous or intramuscular corticosteroid pulse
- Intravenous pulse therapy with methylprednisolone at 500–1,000 mg/d for 1–3 d reserved for extremely active RA or severe extraarticular disease, such as vasculitis, until DMARDs take effect.
- Pulse therapy should be given as an infusion over 45–60 min to avoid abrupt potassium and fluid shifts.
- Intramuscular pulse with 80–100 mg depot methylprednisolone can be used as bridge therapy for active RA.
- Intravenous or intramuscular pulses may be repeated every 3–4 wk until DMARDs take effect.
- There is a theoretic risk of causing adrenal suppression with this regimen; however, this complication has not been shown.

Alternate-day corticosteroid
- Alternate-day corticosteroid can be used in patients with serious side effects with daily regimen and also may be helpful with steroid taper, but is often unsuccessful because the RA flares on the day without steroids.
- Alternate-day steroid administration involves the same total prednisone dose, but it is given as one morning dosage every 48 h with breakfast.

Intraarticular corticosteroids
- For one to two active RA joints, use intraarticular glucocorticoid injection to control the disease flare.
- Limit to three injections per joint per year.
- Use either triamcinolone acetonide or methylprednisolone (depot form).
- Dose: for large joints (e.g., knees), 40–60 mg; medium joints (e.g., wrists, ankles), 20–30 mg; small joints (e.g., metacarpophalangeal, interphalangeal, or tendon sheaths), 10 mg.
- Mix with 1% lidocaine for tendon sheath injections (optional for intraarticular injections).
- Use careful sterile technique to minimize risk of introducing infection.

DMARDs, disease-modifying antirheumatic agents; GC, glucocorticoid; RA, rheumatoid arthritis.

Triamcinolone hexacetonide was more effective than sodium morrhuate in controlling disease flares in the affected joints over a 1-year period. A retrospective chart review of 140 RA patients found that approximately 75% who had triamcinolone hexacetonide joint injections (followed by bed rest) maintained remission during a 7-year mean follow-up (81). These patients received concomitant DMARD therapy for their disease, which may have influenced the results. Nevertheless, intraarticular steroid injections are an attractive option to control mono- and oligoarticular flares in RA. Intraarticular injection of GC, apart from its antiinflammatory effect, causes an increase in synovial hyaluronan concentrations to normal levels and restores the barrier to hyaluronan flux across the synovium (82).

RADIOGRAPHIC PROGRESSION AND GLUCOCORTICOIDS

The Joint Committee of the Medical Research Council of Great Britain reported on a randomized controlled trial of 3-year duration in 1959 and 1960 (66,67) (Table 24.5). The cohort studied consisted of patients with early RA (disease duration of less than 2 years). Forty-five patients were treated with 20 mg per day of prednisolone once a day, with slow taper to 10 mg per day over 1 year; and 39 patients were assigned to aspirin and other analgesics. At 1, 2, and 3 years, detailed analysis of hands and feet radiographs showed decreased bony changes in the prednisolone group as compared to the analgesic group, especially in the first year. West published the analysis of those patients who were followed for 4 years or longer (83). Thirty-nine patients from the initial cohort were treated with a mean dose of 11 mg of prednisolone daily for 4 years, 19 of whom continued at a lower dosage for an average of 3 additional years. Among the 19 patients, there was a total of 169 new erosions or 8.5 erosions per person, as compared to patients in an analgesic group (mean follow-up of 5 years), 32 of whom had 553 erosions or 17.3 erosions per patient ($p < .001$) (84).

Some further studies attempted to relate radiologic progression to corticosteroid use, but they contained important weaknesses that limited their contribution, such as small sample size, inadequate follow-up time, or the fact that they were not controlled trials. In a small, double-blind, placebo-controlled study, 5 mg per day of prednisone was added to DMARDs in 18 patients with active RA, as compared to 16 patients receiving DMARDs and placebo (85). After 6 months, erosions were reported in 4 of 16 controls versus 1 of 18 prednisone patients ($p = .057$). A retrospective comparison of 183 GC-treated RA patients with 205 patients either taking gold or analgesics reported similar radiographic deterioration in both groups (86); however, GC doses were uncertain. As mentioned previously, an open-labeled study randomized 102 patients with active RA to either DMARDs or a combination of DMARDs and prednisolone for 1 year (69) (mean dose of 6 mg and a cumulative dose of 2,160 mg). There was a nonsignificant trend toward reduction in radiographic progression among those randomized to the prednisolone group ($p < .07$). When treatment with monthly intravenous methylprednisolone (15 mg per kg) was compared to normal saline for 6 months in the background of a single DMARD (mostly D-penicillamine) (76), there was no difference in the radiologic scores between the methylprednisolone and placebo group at the end of 12 months.

After the initial trial by the Joint Committee of the Medical Research Council of Great Britain in 1995 (66,67) involving patients with less than 2 years of RA, a long period of uncertainty and confusion concerning the role of GCs in RA radiographic progression remained. In 1995, a prospective, randomized, clinical trial was conducted involving 128 patients with early RA (symptoms <2 years), comparing the effect of prednisolone, 7.5 mg per day, to placebo (72) (Table 24.5). Both groups had comparable NSAID and DMARD use. After 2 years, the Larsen score increased by a mean of 0.72 U (indicating very little change) in the prednisolone group and by 5.37 U (indicating substantial joint damage) in the placebo group ($p = .004$). This trial was the first modern study to show a substantial reduction in radiographic progression of RA with low-dose prednisolone. The results of this study were questioned due to the chance occurrence of more severe radiographic disease with high baseline Larsen scores in three of the patients in the placebo group and due to the statistical analysis of the radiographic assessment (87). No information was provided about these three patients, but erosive disease and high radiographic scores are the best predictors of further radiographic progression. Another disadvantage of the study was that the use and dosage of DMARDs was not standardized. Subsequently, a variety of statistical analyses excluding the two highest-scoring patients in the placebo group produced the same results (88). Follow-up of the majority of these prednisolone-treated patients, after discontinuation of prednisolone, showed that joint destruction resumed at a rate comparable to the placebo group, supporting the role of GCs as "true" DMARDs (74).

TABLE 24.5. Effects of Corticosteroids on Radiographic Progression in Early Rheumatoid Arthritis: Major Clinical Trials

Author (Reference)	Type of Study	Duration of Study	Mean Duration Rheumatoid Arthritis in Prednisolone Group	Dosage of Prednisolone/d	Number of Patients Treated with Prednisolone	Baseline Score in Prednisolone Group (Mean)	Baseline Score in Placebo/Disease-Modifying Antirheumatic Agent (Mean)	Change[a] in Score Prednisolone (Mean)	Change[a] in Score Placebo (Mean)	p Value
Medical Research Council, 1959–1960 (66,67)	Nonsteroidal antiinflammatory drugs vs. prednisolone. Initial blind observer for 2 yr with observational follow-up.	5.6 yr	<2 yr	11 mg	41	ND	ND	8.5/patient[b]	17.3/patient[b]	<.001
Kirwan, 1995 (72)	Blind observer vs. placebo with disease-modifying antirheumatic agent background.	104 wk	1.28 yr	7.5 mg	61	2.65[c]	6.23[c]	0.72[c]	5.37[c]	.004
Boers, 1997 (73)	Blind observer; comparison of combination[d] vs. SSZ.	80 wk	4 mo (median)	7.5 mg[d]	77	3[e]	5[e]	4[e]	12[e]	.01
Landewe, 2002 (90)	Open; extension of Boers trial[f].	4–5 yr	4 mo (median)	NR	74	6.5[e]	17[e]	23.4/ or 5.6/yr[e]	43.4/ or 8.6/yr[e]	.001
van Everdingen, 2002 (71)	Blind observer vs. placebo.	104 wk	<1 yr	10 mg[g]	40[g]	11[e]	15[e]	16[e]	29[e]	.007

ND, not done; NR, not reported. Protocol specified discontinuation of prednisolone by week 28; SSZ, sulfasalazine.
[a]Change in the radiographic score during the study.
[b]New erosions/patient with a mean of 5.6 years follow-up in prednisolone group and 5.0 years in analgesics group.
[c]Larsen score.
[d]Prednisolone at 60 mg/d with rapid taper to 7.5 mg/d by week 7 and to 0 after 28 weeks, in combination with methotrexate 7.5 mg/wk (tapered to zero at week 40) and SSZ, 2 g/day, compared to SSZ, 2 g/d alone.
[e]Modified total Sharp score.
[f]Patients initially randomized to combination therapy compared to those originally assigned to SSZ, although both groups were treated the same (SSZ, 2 g/d) after week 40.
[g]Prednisone.

Preliminary results from another randomized study of low-dose prednisolone treatment were published in 2000 (89). This 24-month study explored the concept of "bridging" treatment with low-dose prednisolone for 6 to 12 months until the full DMARD effect is reached. One hundred ninety-two DMARD-naïve RA patients with a mean disease duration of 9 months were randomized to receive either 5 mg of prednisolone or a placebo in a double-blind fashion, starting at the same time as a DMARD (MTX in 38% of patients or parenteral gold in 62%). Radiographic progression, as measured by the Sharp score, was rapidly inhibited with prednisolone (plus MTX or gold) treatment and remained suppressed thereafter (24-month change in Sharp erosion score with prednisolone +1.9 and with placebo +7.9). In the placebo group (placebo plus MTX or gold), progression was significantly greater during the first half year (+5.1 over 6 months) but decreased significantly during the second half year (2.0 over the next 6–12 months) and was nearly equal to the prednisolone group during the second year (+0.4 over the next 12 months) of DMARD therapy. These results are from a subset of patients, as analysis of the whole study has not yet been presented. However, this study supports the concept of "bridge therapy" for both efficacy and retardation of radiographic progression for 6 to 12 months until DMARDs are effective, at which time the prednisone may be tapered off. In another prospective trial, 81 DMARD-naïve early-RA patients (disease duration of <1 year) were randomly assigned to either 10 mg of oral prednisone per day or to placebo for a period of 2 years (71). After 12- and 24-month periods, radiologic scores showed significantly less progression in the prednisone group than in the placebo group ($p < .008$ and .007, respectively).

In addition, Boers et al. (73) evaluated the response of combination therapy (sulfasalazine, 2 g per day; MTX, 7.5 mg per week; and prednisone at an initial dosage of 60 mg per day, tapered over 6 weeks to 7.5 mg per day, and completely withdrawn by week 28) to sulfasalazine alone in early RA. Compared to sulfasalazine alone, the radiographic benefits due to the combination therapy were significant at weeks 28, 56, and 80. At follow-up 5 years after the baseline, the patients initially allocated to combination therapy had sustained the advantage in regard to radiographic joint-disease progression, as compared to the sulfasalazine treatment arm ($p = .033$), independent of subsequent DMARD therapy (90). This study has provided the most convincing evidence thus far for using the step-down approach for the treatment of RA and its role in retardation of radiographic progression even 4 years after the end of the study. In contrast to results seen in Kirwan (72,74), in which the radiographic progression resumed after low-dose prednisolone was discontinued, the Boers et al. trial (73) showed that the group randomized to initial high-dose GC with rapid taper and discontinuation continued to retard radiographic progression for nearly 5 years after discontinuing GC (90). This trial also used low-dose MTX for the initial 40 weeks, along with sulfasalazine in the combination group, so all of the credit cannot be given to GC for the sustained benefit seen on the radiographic retardation.

It is not clear whether there is a minimum GC dose that is effective in retarding radiographic progression. In a 3-year prospective study of NSAID-treated patients, patients continuing pre-study 5 mg of prednisone daily did not have less radiographic progression than those who did not take prednisone (91).

CHRONIC LOW-DOSE STEROIDS

There is a substantial use of chronic, low-dose prednisone (defined as less than or equal to 10 mg per day of prednisone) in rheumatology clinical practices. Pincus et al. (92) examined treatment preferences of seven private rheumatology practices in the United States. More than 50% of patients were treated with prednisone for longer than 60 months. Wolfe et al. (93) also surveyed 3,200 U.S. rheumatologists regarding their short- and long-term preferences according to prednisone and DMARDs' effectiveness. Approximately 65% found prednisone to be an effective treatment at the end of 1 year, and 50% still considered it effective after 4 years, second only to MTX and combination therapy (93).

The initial use of low-dose prednisone in RA is due to its rapid control of the signs and symptoms of active disease. This can be achieved within days to weeks. Some rheumatologists believe that GCs are more effective and are also safer, especially from a gastrointestinal standpoint, than NSAIDs. Evidence presented above also suggests a favorable effect on radiographic retardation. With chronic use of GCs, there is an inability to taper the dose or discontinue GCs because of the withdrawal symptoms. Steroid withdrawal syndrome is defined as a symptom complex resembling true adrenal insufficiency, with non-specific symptoms such as weakness, nausea, and arthralgias occurring in patients experiencing recent GC-dose reduction and normal hypothalamic-pituitary-adrenal (HPA)-axis testing (3). Unlike true adrenal insufficiency, withdrawal-associated flares of synovitis and joint pain can develop even if the reduced dosage remains supraphysiologic (3,94). Slower steroid taper and NSAIDs may be helpful.

TAPERING OF DAILY GLUCOCORTICOIDS

The decision to reduce daily low-dose GC in RA is made when (a) the disease is under control, (b) the GCs have been used as a bridge therapy and DMARDs have had enough time to act, or (c) serious side effects necessitate the reduction of the dose. Before taper is considered, risks of HPA-axis suppression should be considered.

Risks factors for HPA-axis suppression include the antiinflammatory potency and biologic effect of the chosen GC preparation. Dexamethasone has the greatest and hydrocortisone has the least suppression of the HPA axis (95). A second risk factor is the amount of time that the patient has been taking GC. Literature suggests blunting of the HPA axis with a short course of high-dose GC for 5 or more days, but, usually, at least 3 weeks of daily therapy is needed to cause clinical suppression of the axis (96). A third risk factor is the dose of GC. Dose was the best predictor of HPA-axis suppression in a retrospective chart review of patients receiving chronic low-dose prednisone. Patients receiving less than 5 mg of prednisone daily had a normal HPA-axis response, whereas those receiving 5 mg or more had widely varied responses on ACTH-stimulation testing (97).

Different authors have suggested different regimens of GC taper (3,96). The goal of tapering is to use a rate of change that will prevent both flare of RA and symptoms of adrenal insufficiency due to HPA suppression. These recommendations are not based on evidence-based medicine but on the experience of the authors (96,98). We and others generally aim at a decrement of 1 mg per day every 3 to 4 weeks at prednisone doses between 5 and 10 mg per day. If this is successful, prednisone is usually tapered every 2 to 3 weeks by 0.5 mg per day, for doses between 1 and 5 mg per day.

If this method of tapering is not successful and the patient has a minor flare or withdrawal symptoms, especially if this dose is below the physiologic replacement range, there is a difference of opinion between authors. One possibility is to treat the patient with a slight increase in the GC dosage (96), whereas others recommend testing to evaluate for HPA suppression, along with increasing the dose of the GC (3). In difficult cases, it is reasonable to convert patients from their low-dose prednisone to equipotent doses of hydrocortisone (99). The hydrocortisone dose can be tapered until the patient is taking only a single morning dose of 10 mg. Patients may remain on this until HPA-axis recovery, which may take up to 1 year. Although not proven, hydrocortisone's shorter duration of action may speed recovery of the HPA axis (3).

ARE GLUCOCORTICOIDS DISEASE-MODIFYING AGENTS?

The term *disease-modifying antirheumatic agents* was coined to describe medications that provided additional symptomatic benefit in RA patients who were receiving NSAIDs and/or low-dose GC; these agents often also reduced the acute phase reactants. Another feature of the disease-modifying agents is their delayed onset of benefit, usually taking weeks to months before their full efficacy is noted; these drugs are also referred to as *slow-acting antirheumatic drugs* (100). In 1993, a new classification was proposed by Edmonds et al. (101,102), introducing the term *disease-controlling antirheumatic therapy* (DC-ART). They defined a *DC-ART* as an agent that, for a minimum period of 1 year or more, (a) improves and sustains function in association with decreased inflammatory synovitis and (b) prevents or significantly decreases the rate of progression of structural joint damage. The review of clinical trials of GC in RA, as described in previous sections, supports their role in decreasing inflammation, as measured by joint counts and acute phase reactants and improvement of functional capacity (a few months to 1–2 years). However, a step-up increase in GC dosage may be necessary to successfully control the inflammatory synovitis. Long-term observational studies of up to 10 years have not shown sustained improvement or maintenance of functional capacity, as measured by disability and HAQ. Clinical trials have defined the role of GC in retarding radiographic damage over a period ranging from 2 years (71,72) to 5.6 years (83). The study by Boers et al. (73), which used initial high doses of prednisone with a rapid taper, showed a retardation in radiographic progression, as compared to sulfasalazine alone, and the initial radiographic benefit persisted at 5 years of follow-up. However, the patients in the combination group also received MTX, which makes the precise role of prednisone in this group difficult to determine.

Currently, GCs appear to qualify as a DC-ART, improving function and inflammatory synovitis and exhibiting a beneficial effect on radiographic progression for at least 1 year. Whether the beneficial effect of a short course of bridge GC persists for years is still unknown. Also unknown is whether the effect on radiographic progression, as that on inflammatory synovitis and acute phase reactants, wanes with time.

TABLE 24.6. Major Side Effects of Glucocorticoids (GCs)

Adverse Effect	Intervention and Monitoring
Bone	
Osteoporosis	Lifestyle modifications, adequate calcium and vitamin D, antiresorptive (bisphosphonates or hormone replacement therapy) for high-risk patients (>7.5 mg/d prednisone for >1 mo), bone mineral density at baseline for long-term therapy (>6 mo) and annually thereafter
Avascular necrosis	Avoidance of weightbearing; surgery
Cardiovascular	
Hypertension	Dietary modifications, treatment with antihypertensives
Premature atherosclerosis	Dietary modifications, treatment with lipid-lowering agents
Dermatologic	
Skin thinning and purpura	Patient awareness
Acne and hirsutism	Treatment with topical/oral acne medications
Alopecia	Awareness and cosmetic
Cushingoid appearance	Reassurance and decrease the dose or every other day steroids
Endocrine	
Diabetes mellitus	Aggressive monitoring of fasting blood sugars, treatment as necessary with oral hypoglycemics/insulin
Hypothalamic-pituitary-adrenal insufficiency	Lower-dose steroids or every other day regimen, stress-dose steroids, medical-alert bracelet
Gastrointestinal	
Peptic ulcer disease	Avoid use with nonsteroidal antiinflammatory drugs. Add proton pump inhibitor
Visceral perforation	Patient awareness and very careful monitoring
Pancreatitis	Patient awareness and treatment
Infections	
Increased risk of atypical and opportunistic infections	Patient education and awareness, purified protein derivative skin test before initiation of long-term GCs and, if positive, chemoprophylaxis with antitubercular medications
Increased risk of bacterial infections	Patient education and prompt treatment of minor infections
Muscle	
Proximal myopathy	Awareness and decrease or discontinuation of GC
Acute necrotizing myopathy	Physician awareness and discontinuation of GC
Neuropsychiatric	
Euphoria	Reduction in the dosage of GC
Depression	Reduction in the dosage of GC and antidepressants if necessary
Mania/psychosis	Reduction in the dosage and antipsychotics
Pseudotumor cerebri	Carbonic anhydrase inhibitors and acute treatment with high-dose GC
Ophthalmologic	
Glaucoma	Awareness and regular ophthalmology visit
Posterior subcapsular cataract	Awareness and regular ophthalmology visit

SIDE EFFECTS

Overshadowing questions about efficacy, the major concern with long-term GC use is the potential for numerous serious toxicities (103) (Table 24.6). This section reviews the common and serious side effects of GCs, especially those related to long-term use of low-dose prednisone.

Mortality, Hospitalizations, Serious Adverse Effects, and Dose Relationships

Many studies of various historic cohorts evaluated the effect of prednisone on morbidity and mortality in RA patients. Wolfe et al. (104), using a large Arthritis and Rheumatism and Aging Medical Information System (ARAMIS) constituting four different databases, showed a standarized mortality ratio ranging between 1.60 and 3.36 in GC-treated patients compared to controls, but did not provide the dosage or duration of prednisone usage. Another study, evaluating the mortality of RA in 75 patients over 15 years (105), found an increased mortality in patients on prednisone (N = 59), as compared to controls (N = 15). This increase was attributed to more severe disease in the former group ($p = .05$ after 9 years and $p = .15$ after 15 years). In another ARAMIS study, prednisone, 6.9 mg per day, resulted in a high frequency of hospitalizations, especially due to vertebral fractures and cataracts (106). A cohort

TABLE 24.7. Relative Contraindications to Corticosteroids

Oral corticosteroids
- Active infection
- Pulmonary granulomatous disease
- Uncontrolled hypertension
- Uncontrolled diabetes
- Severe osteoporosis with fractures

Acute high-dose corticosteroid pulses (intravenous, intramuscular, or oral)
- Active infection, occult abscesses
- Electrolyte imbalance, especially hypokalemia
- Uncontrolled hypertension
- Uncontrolled diabetes
- Bipolar, mania, or severe depression requiring treatment

study by Saag et al. (103) explored the serious side effects of prednisone doses of less than 15 mg per day for greater than 1 year in 112 RA patients; the mean dosage of this group is 6.1 mg per day for 6.2 years. Patients taking prednisone had more severe disease, characterized by presence of more extraarticular disease, higher ESR and use of a greater number of DMARDs; 92 serious adverse events were noted in the prednisone group, as compared to 31 in the control group. Prednisone doses between 0 and 5 mg per day, 5 and 10 mg per day, and 10 and 15 mg per day were associated with odds ratios of 1.9, 4.5, and 32.3, respectively, for a first serious adverse event. The prednisone-treated patients could occasionally receive intraarticular, parenteral, or pulse GC, not exceeding the equivalent of 900 mg of prednisone per year, and the control group could receive up to 300 mg of intermittent prednisone per year. There was no subanalysis of patients without the influence of the pulse GC.

Relative contraindications to GC therapy are presented in Table 24.7.

Osteoporosis

MECHANISM

Soon after use of GCs in RA was begun, it was realized that prolonged high-dose therapy had many side effects, of which osteoporosis was the most debilitating (107). GCs cause osteoporosis by reducing bone formation and increasing bone resorption (108). The bone formation is affected by a direct inhibitory effect on osteoblasts (109), inhibition of production of insulin-like growth factor-1 (108) and testosterone (110), and an increase in osteoblast and osteocyte apoptosis (111). There is also stimulation of osteoclast proliferation by suppressing synthesis of osteoprotegerin, an inhibitor of osteoclast differentiation from hemopoietic cells (112,113).

The bone reabsorption induced by GC is mediated by a direct effect on the activity of osteoclast-like cells (114), inhibition of sex hormones (110), and increased secretion of parathyroid hormone (PTH) by inhibition of intestinal calcium absorption (115). GCs also increase renal calcium excretion by decreasing renal calcium reabsorption (116).

GC inhibition of bone formation and increased bone resorption can lead to rapid bone loss. A prospective, longitudinal study found that the patients beginning prednisone (mean dose, 21 mg per day) on average lost 27% of their lumbar spine bone density during the first year of therapy (117). However, bone loss slows substantially thereafter, to an estimated rate of 3% per year (109,118). Even a single intraarticular GC injection can cause transient decreases in serum osteocalcin, a marker for bone formation (119).

IMPACT OF RHEUMATOID ARTHRITIS ON BONE LOSS

Active RA may, itself, lead to bone loss. In a longitudinal trial to evaluate the effect of early RA on bone density, dual-energy x-ray absorptiometry (DEXA) studies of 148 early RA patients before treatment were compared with 730 healthy controls. For patients with at least 2 years of active disease, mean loss of mineral density at the lumbar spine and greater trochanter was 5.5% and 10%, respectively ($p < .01$ compared to patients with inactive disease). Suppression of disease activity stabilized this bone loss (120). Similar results were seen in another cohort of 76 patients with mean disease duration of 2.35 years (118). RA patients had lower bone mineral density (BMD) compared with the reference values. For this study, repeat measurements were performed at 8.9 years. Between the two measurements there was a small decrease in BMD of –0.28% per year, showing that the bone loss slows down with time. HAQ was not a predictor of change in BMD in this study. A systematic review of published studies between 1966 and 1995 showed lumbar bone mass change of –0.6% per year and femoral neck change of –0.7% per year in RA patients treated without GCs (121). Most bone was lost in the first half year and in early or uncontrolled disease, especially in the femur.

LOW-DOSE PREDNISONE AND BONE LOSS

The debate about use of low-dose prednisone (<10 mg per day) and its effect on bone density has been satisfactorily answered with recent trials. A prospective study randomized 40 patients with active RA receiving intramuscular gold salts to receive either prednisone (initial dose, 10 mg per day, which was tapered between weeks 12 and 20) or placebo (122). Despite favorable effects on disease activity, trabecular BMD in the lumbar spine decreased in the prednisone-treated patients between baseline and week 20 (mean change, –8.2%); little change was found in the placebo-treated patients. After discontinuation of prednisone at week 20, an increase was found in trabecular BMD between weeks 20 and 44 (mean change, +5.3%). There was no significant loss of cortical bone in the spine. In contrast, a longitudinal study of a Japanese-American cohort taking 5 mg per day of prednisone found a decrease in both trabecular and cortical bone during a mean follow-up of 2 years (123). Another placebo-controlled trial in elderly early RA patients compared chloroquine to prednisone (mean, 15 mg per day) for 1 year (65). The disease duration was 11 months, and mean age in the prednisone group was 69 years. There was a 3.3% loss in the prednisone group, as compared to 0.1% loss of bone density in the placebo group at 6 months; at 1 year, the difference had decreased to 1.8% and was not significant during second-year follow-up.

A cross-sectional study of BMD, as measured by DEXA, was performed in 139 RA patients to assess the effect of low doses of GC on bone BMD (124). Patients receiving daily doses of prednisone between 1 and 4 mg per day had BMD similar to control patients who were not receiving GC, but patients taking 5 to 9 mg per day and those taking more than 10 mg per day had significantly lower BMD of the lumbar spine (84.3% and 80.5% of controls, respectively) than patients who received 1 to 4 mg per day (99.2% of controls). Alternate-day steroid dosing also has been shown to cause osteoporosis (125).

IMPACT ON FRACTURES

In a cohort of 395 early RA patients (mean age, 49 years) with a mean follow-up of 6.7 years, the 5-year probability of having a first fracture of any bone was 34% for 46 females taking 5 mg or more (average, 8.6 ± 0.8 mg per day) of prednisone (126) compared to 7% for 304 patients taking less than 5 mg (average, 0.2 mg) daily. In a recent 2-year randomized prospective trial evaluating the effects of alendronate on bone density in patients on chronic GC (mean, 17.4 mg daily of prednisone or equivalent daily), the placebo group (taking calcium and vitamin D) had 6.8% new vertebral fractures, as compared to 0.7% in those taking alendronate ($p = .026$) (127).

In aggregate, the data suggest that most disease-related bone loss occurs early in RA and is dependent on uncontrolled or aggressive disease. Low-dose prednisone (5–10 mg per day) has an adverse effect on BMD, but, probably, 1 to 4 mg per day has little or no effect.

TREATMENT OF GLUCOCORTICOID-INDUCED OSTEOPOROSIS

In 2001, an American College of Rheumatology committee published guidelines for the prevention and treatment of GC-induced osteoporosis (128). The committee recommended obtaining a baseline measurement of BMD at the lumbar spine or hip, or both, in patients who had begun long-term (i.e., more than 6 months) GC therapy, with annual follow-up measurements (Table 24.8).

Calcium and Vitamin D. Adequate calcium and vitamin D supplementation is essential. In a 2-year trial in RA patients who were receiving chronic GC (mean dose, 5.6 mg per day), subjects were randomized to 1,000 mg of calcium carbonate with 500 IU of vitamin D or matching placebo (129). Patients who received placebo lost bone at a rate of 2.0% and 0.9% per year in the lumbar spine and greater trochanter, respectively, whereas patients who received 1,000 mg of calcium carbonate and 500 IU of vitamin D daily gained bone at a rate of 0.7% and 0.9%, respectively. Placebo control groups in several randomized clinical trials of bisphosphonates received supplementation with calcium at 800 to 1,000 mg per day and vitamin D at 250 to 500 mg per day. In one study of patients receiving GC (median prednisone dosage, 11 mg per day), bone mass at the lumbar spine was maintained in the calcium-and-vitamin D–treated placebo patients (130). Similar results were noted in placebo-treated patients taking prednisone at a mean dosage of 15 mg per day who received 1,000 mg of calcium and 400 IU vitamin D daily during a randomized controlled trial of risedronate in patients receiving long-term GC treatment (131). These patients had stable BMD at both the lumbar spine and the greater trochanter after 48 weeks of treatment.

TABLE 24.8. Recommendations for the Prevention and Treatment of Glucocorticoid-Induced Osteoporosis

Patient beginning therapy with glucocorticoid (prednisone equivalent of ≥5 mg/d) with plans for treatment duration of ≥3 mo:
- Modify lifestyle risk factors for osteoporosis.
  - Smoking cessation or avoidance.
  - Reduction of alcohol consumption if excessive.
- Instruct in weightbearing physical exercise.
- Initiate calcium supplementation.
- Initiate supplementation with vitamin D (plain or activated form).
- Prescribe bisphosphonate (use with caution in premenopausal women).

Patient receiving long-term glucocorticoid therapy (prednisone equivalent of ≥5 mg/d):
- Modify lifestyle risk factors for osteoporosis.
  - Smoking cessation or avoidance.
  - Reduction of alcohol consumption if excessive.
- Instruct in weightbearing physical exercise.
- Initiate calcium supplementation.
- Initiate supplementation with vitamin D (plain or activated form).
- Prescribe treatment to replace gonadal sex hormones if deficient or otherwise clinically indicated.
- Measure BMD at lumbar spine and/or hip.
- If BMD is not normal (i.e., T score below –1), then
  - Prescribe bisphosphonate (use with caution in premenopausal women).
  - Consider calcitonin as second-line agent if patient has contraindication to or does not tolerate bisphosphonate therapy.
- If BMD is normal, follow up and repeat BMD measurement either annually or biannually.

BMD, bone mineral density.
From American College of Rheumatology Ad Hoc Committee on Glucocorticoid-Induced Osteoporosis. Recommendations for the prevention and treatment of glucocorticoid-induced osteoporosis: 2001 update. *Arthritis Rheum* 2001;44:1496–1503, with permission.

A Cochrane Database metaanalysis evaluated five randomized controlled trials to assess the effects of calcium and vitamin D compared to calcium alone or placebo in the prevention of bone loss in patients taking systemic corticosteroids. The metaanalysis was performed after 2 years of treatment (132), when there was a significant weighted mean difference between treatment and control groups in lumbar spine bone mass. The other outcome measures (femoral neck bone mass, fracture incidence, biochemical markers of bone resorption) were not significantly different. However, calcium alone does not prevent bone loss in patients receiving GC therapy. In a randomized prospective study in patients starting on chronic GC therapy, patients on calcium alone (1,000 mg daily) lost 4.3 percent of lumbar spine mineral density at the end of 1 year and another 2.3 percent at the end of 2 years (133). The active treatment group who also received calcitriol did not lose any bone mass.

It should be noted that if activated forms of vitamin D are used, patients should be carefully monitored for the development of hypercalcemia and hypercalciuria; if these adverse events develop, the dosage of the activated vitamin D supplement should be reduced.

Hormone Replacement Therapy. The effect of hormone replacement therapy (HRT) on bone mass in RA patients treated with chronic GC (mean, 7 mg per day) was evaluated in 200 postmenopausal women with RA who were randomly allocated to receive transdermal estradiol (50 μg daily) or calcium (400 mg daily) for 2 years (134). In the HRT group, lumbar spine BMD increased by 3.75%, whereas in patients taking calcium, BMD decreased by 0.85% at the end of 2 years. In the Women's Health Initiative Trial, 16,608 postmenopausal women were randomized to a combination of estrogen and progesterone (0.625 and 2.50 mg, respectively) or placebo (135). No information was provided regarding background calcium and vitamin D supplementation. The rate of osteoporotic fractures was decreased with HRT [hazard ratio, 0.77; confidence interval (CI): 0.63–0.94], as compared to placebo over a mean follow-up of 5 years (135).

Another prospective study examined the effect of HRT alone and in combination with human PTH 1-34 in postmenopausal patients who had taken a mean GC dose of 9.4 mg per day for an average of 14.9 years (136). The 1-year trial showed maintenance of bone mass in the HRT-alone group with a mean change of +0.01% in the lumbar spine by DEXA scan and a significant increase of +11% in the combination group. Trabecular bone is more susceptible to GC-induced bone loss because of its high turnover rate. PTH has a major effect on the trabecular bone.

Currently, there are no published reports regarding the efficacy of HRT in preventing bone loss at the initiation of GC treatment or of the protective effect of HRT when moderate-to-high doses of GCs are used for long-term treatment (129).

Bisphosphonates. Five randomized, placebo-controlled trials using bisphosphonates for prevention and treatment of GC-induced osteoporosis have been published (Table 24.9). Two of these trials included patients beginning more than 7.5 mg per day of prednisone (137,138). One publication compared 228 patients taking less than 3 months of GCs with another group of 290 patients receiving more than 6 months of GCs (139). Two other studies evaluated the role of bisphosphonates in patients taking more than 3 to 4 months of GC therapy (131,140). Approximately one-half of the patients in these studies were postmenopausal women, and baseline prednisone dosage was between 15 and 22 mg per day. Significant increases in BMD

TABLE 24.9. Comparison of Five Large, Randomized, Controlled Trials Assessing Bisphosphonates in the Treatment and Prevention of Glucocorticoid-Induced Osteoporosis

Characteristic or Outcome Measure	Authors (Reference)				
	Adachi et al. (140) (N = 141)	Roux et al. (137) (N = 117)	Saag et al. (130) (N = 477)	Cohen et al. (138) (N = 228)	Reid et al. (131) (N = 290)
	Etidronate	Etidronate	Alendronate	Risedronate	Risedronate
Sex and menopausal status (%)					
Postmenopausal women	50	49	49	46	53
Premenopausal women	12	15	22	20	9
Men	38	36	29	34	38
Baseline vertebral fractures (%)					
Treatment group	45	3.4	15	30	33
Placebo group	49	1.7	17	29	37
Baseline osteoporosis defined by bone mineral density criteria (%)	NA	24.5	32	NA	23
Mean daily prednisone dosage (mg)					
Baseline	22	NA	18	21	15
End of study	11	11	9	11	13
Supplements provided during study					
Calcium (mg/d)	500	500	800–1,000	500	1,000
Vitamin D (IU/d)	None	None	250–500	None	400
Bone mineral density increase (%)[a]					
Lumbar spine					
From baseline	0.6	0.3	2.9[b]	0.6[b]	2.9[b]
From placebo	3.7	3.1	3.3[b]	3.4[b]	2.5[b]
Trochanter					
From baseline	1.5	NA	2.7[b]	1.4[b]	2.4[b]
From placebo	4.1	NA	3.4[b]	4.4[b]	1.4[b]
Femoral neck					
From baseline	0.2	NA	1.0[b]	0.8[b]	1.8[b]
From placebo	1.9	NA	2.2[b]	3.8[b]	2.1[b]
Vertebral fracture reduction (%)					
Overall	40 (*p* NS)	NA	38 (*p* NS)[c]	67 (*p* NS)[b]	67[b]
Postmenopausal women	85 ($p = .05$)	NA	51 (*p* NS)[c]	60 (*p* NS)[b]	NA

NA, information not available; NS, not significant.
[a]Only 1-year values that were significant at the $p < .05$ level are shown.
[b]For alendronate at 10 mg/day and risedronate at 5 mg/day.
[c]Results shown are for the primary fracture outcome measured using vertebral morphometry among pooled alendronate users (both 5-mg/day and 10-mg/day dosages).
From American College of Rheumatology Ad Hoc Committee on Glucocorticoid-Induced Osteoporosis. Recommendations for the prevention and treatment of glucocorticoid-induced osteoporosis: 2001 update. *Arthritis Rheum* 2001;44:1496–1503, with permission.

occurred with bisphosphonate treatment and was most consistently observed in the lumbar spine. This increase was observed in patients with many different GC-treated disorders, most often RA and polymyalgia rheumatica, and generally occurred regardless of patient age, sex, and menopausal status. All of these bisphosphonate trials showed fracture risk reduction in postmenopausal women. In addition, the trial by Wallach et al. (139) showed a statistically significant reduction of 70% in the relative risk of incident radiographic vertebral fractures after 1 year of treatment with risedronate. A similar significant reduction in the risk of incident radiographic vertebral fractures (0.7% with alendronate vs. 6.8% with placebo; $p < .05$) was seen in alendronate-treated patients who completed 2 years (1-year study and 1-year extension) of a study of alendronate in the prevention and treatment of GC-induced osteoporosis (127).

Skin and Soft Tissues

The most frequent toxicities attributable to GC are skin thinning and purpura. Five ARAMIS patient populations from different data sets showed the incidence of purpura as 32 per 1,000 patient-years (106). Other skin adverse events include acne, alopecia (6%, from ARAMIS data set), hypertrichosis, and striae. A population-based case control study evaluated the risk of nonmelanoma skin cancer with use of GC for longer than 1 month (141). The risk of squamous cell carcinoma was increased among users of oral GC (adjusted odds ratio = 2.31) and risk of basal cell carcinoma was elevated modestly (adjusted odds ratio = 1.49). The patients in this study were not questioned about the dose of the GC, although most of the use of GC was for respiratory and musculoskeletal problems. This risk of skin cancer has not been confirmed independently.

The development of cushingoid features is troublesome for patients (142). This side effect usually occurs with more than 7.5 mg per day of prednisone or equivalent. In one trial, moon facies developed in 13% of patients taking 4 to 12 mg per day of triamcinolone for fewer than 60 days (143). Facial changes usually regress quickly after decreasing the dose or using an alternate-day steroid regimen.

Cataracts and Glaucoma

Visual symptoms are common complaints of patients taking GC. The ARAMIS analysis by Fries et al. (106) showed an incidence of blurred vision at 7 events per 1,000 patient-years. Posterior subcapsular cataracts (PSCs) are a common complication of prolonged use of GC. Cataracts are often bilateral; they develop slowly and may stabilize if the steroid dose is reduced (144). The incidence of PSCs associated with steroid use increases with cumulative dosage of GCs, but there is considerable interindividual variation in susceptibility (145,146). Although PSCs have been reported to develop after as little as 5 mg of oral prednisone per day for as short as 2 months, the usual time until onset is at least 1 year with dosage equivalent to 10 mg per day of oral prednisone (145,147). The incidence of corticosteroid-induced cataracts in several randomized, controlled trials ranged from 6.4% to 38.7% with oral GC use (148,149). Inhalation steroids have also been implicated in PSCs (150); however, this effect has not been definitively established. A retrospective observational cohort study showed the incidence rate of cataract (1.0 per 1,000 person-years) among users of intranasal GC to be similar to that of the general population (151). However, oral GC users were at higher risk of cataract (2.2 per 1,000 person-years). Multiple epidural steroid injections have been associated with development of PSCs (152).

Glaucomatous changes have been noted with various routes of corticosteroid administration, including systemic (oral and intravenous), topical (ocular and cutaneous), injected (periocular and subcutaneous), as well as inhalation and nasal administration (153–155).

Physicians should be careful and vigilant about these ophthalmologic complications, and patients should be examined periodically by ophthalmologists for early detection.

TABLE 24.10. Guidelines for Adrenal Supplementation Therapy[a]

Medical or Surgical Stress	Corticosteroid Dosage
Minor	
Inguinal hernia repair Colonoscopy Mild febrile illness Mild-moderate nausea/vomiting Gastroenteritis	25 mg of hydrocortisone or 5 mg of methylprednisolone i.v. on day of procedure only
Moderate	
Open cholecystectomy Hemicolectomy Significant febrile illness Pneumonia Severe gastroenteritis	50–70 mg of hydrocortisone or 10–15 mg of methylprednisolone i.v. on day of procedure; taper quickly over 1–2 d to usual dose
Severe	
Major cardiothoracic surgery Whipple procedure Liver resection Pancreatitis	100–150 mg of hydrocortisone or 20–30 mg of methylprednisolone i.v. on day of procedure; rapid taper to usual dose over next 1–2 d
Critically ill	
Sepsis-induced hypotension or shock	50–100 mg of hydrocortisone i.v. every 6–8 h or 0.18 mg/kg/h as a continuous infusion, plus 50 μg/d of fludrocortisone until shock resolved—may take several days to a week or more—then gradually taper, following vital signs and serum sodium

[a]Data are based on extrapolation from the literature, expert opinion, and clinical experience. Patients receiving ≤5 mg/d prednisone should receive their normal daily replacement but do not require supplementation. Patients who receive >5 mg/day prednisone should receive the above therapy in addition to their maintenance therapy. From Coursin DB, Wood KE. Corticosteroid supplementation for adrenal insufficiency. *JAMA* 2002;287(2):236–240, with permission.

Hypothalamic-Pituitary-Adrenal Insufficiency

RA itself may be associated with subtle dysfunction of the HPA axis (156). GC-induced HPA insufficiency appears to be both dose- and duration-specific. High-dose oral GC can result in transient suppression of ACTH release in as few as 5 days (157). Even a single large dose of intravenous methylprednisolone can cause transient HPA suppression, with function returning to normal in 5 days (158). "Steroid burst therapy" with 40 mg per day prednisone for 3 days followed by rapid taper did not cause HPA suppression when analyzed 1 week later (159). Subphysiologic doses (<7.5 mg per day) for long periods may lead to HPA blunting (160). It is believed that divided daily doses of prednisone increase HPA suppression. However, in a prospective trial in patients with active giant-cell arteritis, prednisone three times a day and once a day had similar HPA suppression (11). Alternate-day dosing with a short-acting GC produces less HPA suppression (161). Recovery of the HPA axis after discontinuation of the GC may take up to 1 year (61).

Patients on chronic GCs require an extra boost of steroids in time of stress, such as medical illnesses or surgeries. Normally, stress induces the activation of the HPA axis, resulting in increased corticotropin-releasing hormone, ACTH, and cortisol production. During GC-induced HPA suppression or blunting, supplemental therapy, in addition to the daily GC doses, is required to prevent adrenal insufficiency (2). The recommendations for adrenal supplementation therapy are provided in Table 24.10.

Gastrointestinal Tract

GC has little or no effect on peptic ulcer disease. In a nested case control study, the estimated relative risk of development of peptic ulcer disease in patients taking GCs was 1.1 (CI: 0.5–2.1); however, addition of traditional NSAIDs increased the estimated relative risk significantly, to 4.4 (CI: 2.0–9.7) (162). There are reports of visceral rupture (163), pancreatitis (164), and fatty liver (165) with use of GCs.

Myopathy

Myopathy is an infrequent complication of GC therapy. Myopathy usually occurs with high doses of GC (>30 mg of prednisone or equivalent) given for more than a few weeks (166), although there is considerable variability (167). Patients usually present with progressive, painless, proximal muscle weakness. Electromyography may be normal or show myopathic changes; type 2 muscle fiber atrophy is the most frequent finding on muscle biopsy. The myopathy is usually reversible within 3 to 4 weeks after reduction in the GC doses. Activation of the GR appears to be involved, because myopathy can be prevented in the rat by a GR antagonist (168).

An acute, severe myopathy, "acute necrotizing myopathy of intensive-care patients," can occur within days of initiation of high-dose intravenous GC therapy (169). The trigger for this condition could be immobility, underlying disease, or neuromuscular blockade. Immobility sensitizes skeletal muscle to the catabolic effect of steroids (170). In a case series of four patients with this disorder (169), all patients were on mechanical ventilators for various reasons and presented with inability to wean and sudden onset of flaccid quadriplegia. Patients had high muscle enzymes, and needle electromyography identified abnormal spontaneous activity. Motor unit potentials were polyphasic of low amplitude and short duration, characteristic of a myopathic process. Muscle biopsy demonstrated a prominent acute necrotizing myopathy with a loss of thick filaments in all four patients. These findings also can be seen in association with critical-care polyneuropathy, which is a separate entity (169).

Central Nervous System

GC effects on the central nervous system are relatively common. Most patients taking GCs experience a feeling of well-being independent of any improvement in their underlying disease. In a prospective, uncontrolled trial, 50 patients who were beginning to take high-dose GC (methylprednisolone, 119 mg mean dose) participated in neuropsychological testing (171).

During 8 days, no overt mania or delirium occurred. However, a significant proportion of patients experienced an organic mood disorder, 26% to 34% experienced a hypomanic syndrome, and 10% to 12% experienced a depressive syndrome. To evaluate the neurochemical effects of GC, prednisone (80 mg per day orally for 5 days) was given to 12 healthy volunteers in a double-blind manner (172). Prednisone administration was associated with decreases in cerebrospinal fluid levels of corticotropin, norepinephrine, beta-endorphin, beta-lipotropin, and somatostatin-like immunoreactivity, and 75% had associated alterations in behavior and mood.

The affective symptoms usually occur in the first week of GC treatment (173) and rarely may start within the first day (174). Later reactions are exceedingly rare. Women are at higher risk of developing a GC-induced psychiatric syndrome (173). It is well known that high-dose GC (greater than 40 mg of prednisone or equivalent) can cause psychosis (175), but neither dosage nor duration of treatment seems to affect the time of onset, duration, severity, or type of mental disturbances (176). In general, the psychiatric disorder responds to dose reduction or discontinuation of the medication (176).

GCs can also interfere with rapid eye movement sleep, especially if given in divided doses. Benign intracranial hypertension (pseudotumor cerebri) can occur occasionally.

Effects on Metabolism of Glucose, Lipids, and Protein

Glucose intolerance and diabetes mellitus from GCs are primarily mediated through increased gluconeogenesis in the liver and decreased peripheral utilization of glucose (177).

GCs have an important impact on lipid metabolism by activating lipolysis in adipose tissue and inducing a centripetal body fat distribution. Several studies have compared serum levels of lipids from RA patients with controls. Total and low-density lipoprotein cholesterol levels were elevated in some studies (178) and reduced in others (179). A more consistent finding has been decreased levels of high-density lipoprotein cholesterol in active or untreated RA in both men and women, which is an unfavorable profile with regard to cardiovascular risk. Lipoprotein(a), a cholesterol-rich modified form of low-density lipoprotein identified as an independent risk factor for coronary heart disease, has been found to be elevated in RA patients with both active and treated disease (180,181).

Administration of 0.35 mg per kg per day of prednisone for 14 days in healthy volunteers induces a significant increase in levels of very-low-density lipoprotein, high-density lipoprotein-cholesterol apolipoprotein A-I and apolipoprotein E (182). All values return to normal within 2 weeks after discontinuation of the prednisone. In systemic lupus erythematosus (SLE), patients already have baseline dyslipoproteinemia, but a prednisone dose of 10 mg daily is associated with a 7.5-mg per dL increase in cholesterol level (183). In the same study, hydroxychloroquine lowered serum cholesterol (–8.9 mg %). A 10-mg increase in prednisone dose was associated with a mean weight gain of 5.5 lb.

Cardiovascular Effects

The mortality in patients with RA is increased compared to that of the general population (181). A pooled analysis of various studies found a mean standardized mortality ratio of 1.7 (184). In epidemiologic studies, 34% to 40% of mortality in RA has been attributed to cardiovascular disease (105,185). In addition to traditional risk factors, chronic inflammation is considered to be a risk factor for the development of atherosclerosis. However, long-term epidemiologic studies have not shown any mortality benefit with GCs, possibly due to more severe disease in these patients (104,105,186).

In addition to its effect on lipids, GC has atherogenic effects that may be due to increased cholesterol esterification in human macrophages, resulting from an increase in the activity and expression of acyl coenzyme A cholesterol: acyl transferase (187). This effect is antagonized by progesterone, partly explaining the low prevalence of atherogenic disease in premenopausal women (188).

GC promotes fluid retention because of its permissive effects on the vasoactive substance and its inhibition of prostaglandin E_2. Fluid retention is not a problem in patients with normal renal function due to compensating mineralocorticoid escape. In 264 patients with SLE, a 10-mg change in prednisone dose led to a change in mean arterial blood pressure of 1.1 mm Hg after adjustment for age, weight, and antihypertensive drug use (183).

Avascular Necrosis

Avascular necrosis (osteonecrosis) is a well-known side effect of GC therapy. GCs induce osteoporosis by an increase in osteoblast and osteocyte apoptosis (112). Weinstein and Manolagas (189) evaluated the prevalence of osteocyte apoptosis in femoral heads with GC osteonecrosis. Cancellous bone in femurs from the patients taking GC was lined with apoptotic osteocytes and cells. In contrast, apoptotic bone cells were absent from specimens taken from patients with trauma or sickle cell disease and were rare with alcohol abuse.

Avascular necrosis most often affects the subchondral bone of the femoral head, but the knees, shoulders, and the other bones may be affected. It usually is associated with high-dose GC therapy, but may develop even in patients receiving physiologic doses for adrenal insufficiency (142,190). Intraarticular steroids have also been implicated in developing avascular necrosis (191). Most studies have found the risk to be low (<3%) in patients taking less than 15 to 20 mg per day of prednisone (103,192).

Infection

Patients treated with prednisone are at risk for serious infections. The major mechanism of infectious complications appears to be due to immunosuppression resulting from inhibition of NF-κB by activation of its inhibitor IκB (32). NF-κB is involved in the regulation of several cytokine genes and is a mediator of the proinflammatory action of TNF (142). NF-κB inhibition by GC may also lead to a reduction in the inflammatory and febrile response to bacterial infection, obscuring the diagnosis.

A metaanalysis of 71 controlled clinical trials using GC (193) showed an overall rate of infectious complications of 12.7%, with a relative risk of 1.6. The rate was not increased in patients given a daily dose of less than 10 mg or a cumulative dose of less than 700 mg of prednisone. A prospective analysis of the clinical course in SLE patients found a 1.5-fold increase in infections, with an average dose of prednisone of less than 10 mg per day; this study also showed a more than eightfold increase of infections in patients taking more than 40 mg per day (194). The frequency of all infections, and of bacterial and opportunistic infections specifically, increased progressively with dose.

The risk of infections with atypical or opportunistic organisms is increased in patients taking GC (7). One study found the rate to be 40 times that of patients who had not received GC (195), but the risk was significantly decreased if GC was used every other day. Pulmonary tuberculosis is a well-documented complication of GC therapy (196). In patients who have recieved GC therapy

TABLE 24.11. Use of Corticosteroids in Pregnancy, in Renal/Hepatic Disease, and with Other Comorbid Conditions

Pregnancy
- Category B.[a]
- No risk of teratogenesis.
- Excreted in breast milk (at approximately <10% of serum concentration).
- American Academy of Pediatrics guidelines—compatible with breast feeding.

Renal/hepatic diseases
- No adjustment required in mild to moderate hepatic/renal impairment.
- Patients with liver and renal failure may have increased unbound prednisolone, so dose adjustment may be necessary.

Other comorbid conditions
- Patients with hyperthyroidism need higher doses due to a combination of enhanced nonrenal clearance and decreased intestinal absorption of prednisone.

[a]Category B = no evidence of risk in humans.

for 1 month or longer at more than 15 mg per day, a purified protein derivative skin reaction of greater than 5 mm is considered positive and calls for preventive therapy (197).

Patients on chronic GC therapy should receive vaccinations with influenza (killed), pneumococcus, and tetanus at regular intervals (198). They can generate an adequate antibody response to killed influenza virus vaccine (199).

In summary, GC therapy is associated with varying complications, ranging from troublesome bruising to life-threatening infections. The risk of complications increases with increases in the dosage and duration of treatment. Some of the side effects are preventable with careful monitoring and preventive therapies.

USE OF CORTICOSTEROIDS IN PREGNANCY AND LACTATION

In pregnant rodents, exposure to GCs can result in cleft palate in offspring (200). However, controlled trials in humans have failed to show an increased risk of congenital malformations from GC therapy (201) (Table 24.11). GCs may be associated with a high incidence of premature ruptured membranes and preterm delivery (202). Gestational hypertension or diabetes mellitus is not uncommon (202).

Prednisone and prednisolone are considered safe in breast-feeding mothers, as less than 10% of active drug is secreted in milk (203). If a lactating mother is taking a high dose of GC, a wait of at least 4 hours after a dose has been suggested before resuming breast-feeding (203,204). No wait is required at maternal prednisolone doses of 20 mg once or twice daily (205).

ROLE OF CORTICOSTEROIDS IN THE MANAGEMENT OF RHEUMATOID ARTHRITIS

The mechanisms of action and clinical efficacy of corticosteroids almost seem to have been designed to treat RA. Indeed, for the past 50 years, discovery of a new mediator or mechanism of inflammation has been accompanied by the discovery that it could be moderated or ablated by corticosteroids. The rapid symptomatic relief and marked improvement in function with GC therapy produced grateful patients and satisfied physicians but rapidly led to overuse during the euphoria of the early 1950s. This enthusiasm was lost when many potentially serious and sometimes lethal adjuncts of corticosteroid use were recognized. In addition, most patients needed increasing doses to maintain the initial improvement, and attempts to taper and discontinue corticosteroids frequently were unsuccessful because they were accompanied by intolerable exacerbations of disease activity and physical dysfunction. The enthusiasm of the early 1950s was replaced with pessimism in the 1960s and 1970s, but corticosteroids remained a mainstay of many rheumatology practices because the available DMARDs were either too toxic or insufficiently effective to displace "bridge" corticosteroids.

Since the 1980s, effective methods to prevent steroid-induced osteoporosis, accompanied by more effective use of new DMARDs, combinations of DMARDs, and more effective "biologic" DMARDs have enabled many rheumatologists to use corticosteroids as true bridge therapy, during the induction of a DMARD response and to manage acute flares of RA, followed by successful tapering and discontinuation of the corticosteroid before serious steroid-induced adverse events occur. In the long-term observational study of early seropositive RA by the Western Consortium of Practicing Rheumatologists (Paulus HE, Khanna D, *personal communication*, 2002), 68% of 320 patients entered within 12 months of symptom onset were treated with low-dose daily corticosteroids at some time during the first 5 years; 33% of them were able to discontinue the corticosteroid within 1 year of its initiation—as one would expect with successful "bridge" therapy. An additional 7% received joint injections or brief pulses of intravenous, intramuscular, or oral corticosteroids. Only 24% did not receive any corticosteroid during the period of observation. Thus, the management of 45% of these early RA patients by rheumatologists included chronic low-dose corticosteroids. The remaining 55% were managed either without steroids, with occasional joint injections or systemic pulses, or with bridge therapy of less than 12 months' duration.

The clinical trials by Kirwan (72) and others (71,89,90) demonstrating retardation of radiographic evidence of joint damage by corticosteroids has led to debate among rheumatologists about whether chronic low-dose corticosteroids are indicated in the treatment of RA (206,207). The long experience of rheumatologists who have watched joints deteriorate progressively while serious adverse events accumulated during years of chronic oral corticosteroid therapy tempers enthusiasm for this approach. However, intermittent administration and withdrawal of low-dose corticosteroids by expert rheumatologists with well-informed and motivated patients now seems to be possible in approximately one-third of patients and, along with brief steroid pulses and joint injections when needed, may help to maintain a reasonably functional life for patients who are also being treated vigorously with DMARDs.

ACKNOWLEDGMENTS

We gratefully acknowledge Marlene Rosensweig for word processing and Ali Farrokh for technical assistance with the figures. This chapter was supported by grants from the National Institutes of Health P60 AR 36834, the Oregon Chapter Arthritis Foundation, the Charlotte Mundt Trust, and the Centocor Health Outcome in Rheumatic Diseases Fellowship.

REFERENCES

1. Hench PS, Kendall E, Slocumb CH, et al. The effect of a hormone of the adrenal cortex (17-hydroxy-11-dehydrocorticosterone: compound E) and the pituitary adrenocorticotropic hormone on rheumatoid arthritis. Preliminary report. *Proceedings of the Staff Meeting of the Mayo Clinic* 1949;24:181–197.
2. Coursin DB, Wood KE. Corticosteroid supplementation for adrenal insufficiency. *JAMA* 2002;287:236–240.
3. Krasner AS. Glucocorticoid-induced adrenal insufficiency. *JAMA* 1999;282:671–676.
4. Kirou KA, Boumpas DT. Systemic glucocorticoid therapy in systemic lupus

erythematosus. In: Wallace DJ, Hahn BH, eds. *Dubois' lupus erythematosus*, 6th ed. Philadelphia: Lippincott Williams & Wilkins, 2001:1173–1194.

5. Furst DE, Saag KG. Determinants of corticosteroid dosing. In: Rose BD, ed. *UptoDate*, computer software. Wellesley, MA: UptoDate, 2002.
6. Frey FJ, Frey BM. Altered plasma protein-binding of prednisolone in patients with the nephrotic syndrome. *Am J Kidney Dis* 1984;3:339–348.
7. Egerman RS, Pierce WF 4th, Andersen RN, et al. A comparison of the bioavailability of oral and intramuscular dexamethasone in women in late pregnancy. *Obstet Gynecol* 1997;89:276–280.
8. Frey BM, Frey FJ. Clinical pharmacokinetics of prednisone and prednisolone. *Clin Pharmacokinet* 1990;19:126–146.
9. Orth DN, Kovacs WJ. The adrenal cortex. In: Wilson D, Foster DW, Kronenberg HM, et al., eds. *Williams' textbook of endocrinology*, 9th ed. Philadelphia: WB Saunders, 1998:517–664.
10. Hale VG, Aizawa K, Sheiner LB, et al. Disposition of prednisone and prednisolone in the perfused rabbit liver: modeling hepatic metabolic processes. *J Pharmacokinet Biopharm* 1991;19:597–614.
11. Hunder GG, Sheps SG, Allen GL, et al. Daily and alternate-day corticosteroid treatment of giant cell arteritis. *Ann Intern Med* 1975;82:613–618.
12. Curtis JJ, Galla JH, Woodford SY, Saykaly RJ, Luke RG. Comparison of daily and alternate-day prednisone during chronic maintenance therapy: a controlled crossover study. *Am J Kidney Dis* 1981;1:166–171.
13. Meffin PJ, Wing LM, Sallustio BC, et al. Alterations in prednisolone disposition as a result of oral contraceptive use and dose. *Br J Clin Pharmacol* 1984;17:655–664.
14. Fisher LE, Ludwig EA, Wald JA, et al. Pharmacokinetics and pharmacodynamics of methylprednisolone when administered at 8 am versus 4 pm. *Clin Pharmacol Ther* 1992;51:677–688.
15. Magee MH, Blum RA, Lates CD, et al. Prednisolone pharmacokinetics and pharmacodynamics in relation to sex and race. *J Clin Pharmacol* 2001;41:1180–1194.
16. Tornatore KM, Logue G, Venuto RC, et al. Pharmacokinetics of methylprednisolone in elderly and young healthy males. *J Am Geriatr Soc* 1994;42:1118–1122.
17. Brooks PM, Needs CJ. The use of antirheumatic medication during pregnancy and in the puerperium. *Rheum Dis Clin North Am* 1989;15:789–806.
18. Harter JG, Reddy WI, Thorn GW. Studies on an intermittent corticosteroid dosage regimen. *N Engl J Med* 1963;269:591–596.
19. Axelrod L. Glucocorticoids. In: Kelly WM, Harris ED Jr., Reddy S, Sledge CB, eds. *Textbook of rheumatology*, 4th ed. Philadelphia: Saunders, 1993:779–796.
20. Feldweg AM, Leddy JP. Drug interactions affecting the efficacy of corticosteroid therapy. A brief review with illustrative case. *J Clin Rheumatol* 1999;5:143–150.
21. Tanner AR, Caffin JA, Halliday JW, et al. Concurrent administration of antacids and prednisone: effect on serum levels of prednisolone. *Br J Clin Pharmacol* 1979;7:397–400.
22. Rae SA, Williams IA, English J, et al. Alteration of plasma prednisolone levels by indomethacin and naproxen. *Br J Clin Pharmacol* 1982;14:459–461.
23. Gudbjornsson B, Skogseid B, Oberg K, et al. Intact adrenocorticotropic hormone secretion but impaired cortisol response in patients with active rheumatoid arthritis. Effect of glucocorticoids. *J Rheumatol* 1996;23:596–602.
24. Manglesdorf DJ, Thummel C, Beato M, et al. The nuclear receptor superfamily: the second decade. *Cell* 1995;83:835.
25. Pratt WB, Toft DO. Steroid receptor interactions with heat shock protein and immunophilin chaperones. *Endocrinology* 1997;18:306–310.
26. Dittmar KD, Banach M, Galigniana MD, et al. The role of DnaJ-like proteins in glucocorticoid receptor.hsp90 heterocomplex assembly by the reconstituted hsp90.p60.hsp70 foldosome complex. *J Biol Chem* 1998;273:7358–7736.
27. Schlaghecke R, Beuscher D, Kornely E, et al. Effects of glucocorticoids in rheumatoid arthritis. Diminished glucocorticoid receptors do not result in glucocorticoid resistance. *Arthritis Rheum* 1994;37:1127–1131.
28. Sanden S, Tripmacher R, Weltrich R, et al. Glucocorticoid dose dependent downregulation of glucocorticoid receptors in patients with rheumatic diseases. *J Rheumatol* 2000;27:1265–1270.
29. Huisman MA, van Everdingen AA, Wenting MJG, et al. Glucocorticoid receptor up-regulation in early rheumatoid arthritis upon low-dose prednisone and placebo. *Arthritis Rheum* 2002;46[Suppl]:S341.
30. Asahara T, Bauters C, Zheng LP et al. Synergistic effect of vascular endothelial growth factor and basic fibroblast growth factor on angiogenesis in vivo. *Circulation* 1995;92:11365–11371.
31. Asahara H, Fujisawa K, Kobata T, et al. Direct evidence of high DNA binding activity of transcription factor AP-1 in rheumatoid arthritis synovium. *Arthritis Rheum* 1997;40:912–918.
32. Scheinman RI, Cogswell PC, Lofquist AK, et al. Role of transcriptional activation of IκBa in mediation of immunosuppression by glucocorticoids. *Science* 1995;23:596–602.
33. Auphan N, DiDonato JA, Rosette C, et al. Immunosuppression by glucocorticoids: inhibition of NF-κB activity through induction of IκB synthesis. *Science* 1995;270:283–286.
34. Adcock IM, Brown CR, Gelder CM, et al. Effects of glucocorticoids on transcription factor activation in human peripheral blood mononuclear cells. *Am J Physiol* 1995;268:C331–C338.
35. Freedman LP. Increasing the complexity of coactivation in nuclear receptor signaling. *Cell* 1999;97:5–8.
36. Dhabhar FS, McEwen BS. Enhancing versus suppressive effects of stress hormones on skin immune function. *Proc Natl Acad Sci U S A* 1999;96:1059–1064.
37. Wiegers GJ, Labeur MS, Stec IE, et al. Glucocorticoids accelerate anti-T cell receptor-induced T cell growth. *J Immunol* 1995;155:1893–1902.
38. Boumpas DT, Chrousos GP, Wilder RL, Cupps TR, Balow JE. Glucocorticoid therapy for immune-mediated diseases: basic and clinical correlates. *Ann Intern Med* 1993;119:1198–1208.
39. Fauci AS, Dale DC. The effect of hydrocortisone on the kinetics of normal human lymphocytes. *Blood* 1975;46:235–243A.
40. Fauci AS. Mechanisms of corticosteroid action on lymphocyte subpopulations. I. Redistribution of circulating T and B lymphocytes to the bone marrow. *Immunology* 1975;28:669–680.
41. ten Berge RJ, Sauerwein HP, Yong SL, et al. Administration of prednisolone in vivo affects the ratio of OKT4/OKT8 and the LDH-isoenzyme pattern of human T lymphocytes. *Clin Immunol Immunopathol* 1984;30:91–103.
42. Paliogianni F, Boumpas DT. Glucocorticoids regulate calcineurin-dependent trans-activating pathways for interleukin-2 gene transcription in human T lymphocytes. *Transplantation* 1995;59:1333–1339.
43. Paliogianni F, Hama N, Balow JE, et al. Glucocorticoid-mediated regulation of protein phosphorylation in primary human T cells. Evidence for induction of phosphatase activity. *J Immunol* 1995;155:1809–1817.
44. Paliogianni F, Ahuja SS, Balow JP, et al. Novel mechanism for inhibition of human T cells by glucocorticoids. Glucocorticoids inhibit signal transduction through IL-2 receptor. *J Immunol* 1993;151:4081–4089.
45. Ashwell JD, Lu FW, Vacchio MS. Glucocorticoids in T cell development and function. *Annu Rev Immunol* 2000;18:309–345.
46. Visser J, van Boxel-Dezaire A, Methorst D, et al. Differential regulation of interleukin-10 (IL-10) and IL-12 by glucocorticoids in vitro. *Blood* 1998;91:4255–4264.
47. DeKruyff RH, Fang Y, Umetsu DT. Corticosteroids enhance the capacity of macrophages to induce Th2 cytokine synthesis in CD4+ lymphocytes by inhibiting IL-12 production. *J Immunol* 1998;160:2231–2237.
48. Kirsch AH, Mahmood AA, Endres J, et al. Apoptosis of human T-cells: induction by glucocorticoids or surface receptor ligation in vitro and ex vivo. *J Biol Regul Homeost Agents* 1999;13:80–89.
49. Mukaida N, Morita M, Ishikawa Y, et al. Novel mechanism of glucocorticoid-mediated gene repression. Nuclear factor-kappa B is target for glucocorticoid-mediated interleukin 8 gene repression. *J Biol Chem* 1994;269:13289–13295.
50. Cronstein BN, Kimmel SC, Levin RI, et al. A mechanism for the antiinflammatory effects of corticosteroids: the glucocorticoid receptor regulates leukocyte adhesion to endothelial cells and expression of endothelial-leukocyte adhesion molecule 1 and intercellular adhesion molecule 1. *Proc Natl Acad Sci U S A* 1992;89:9991–9995.
51. Lim LH, Solito E, Russo-Marie F, et al. Promoting detachment of neutrophils adherent to murine postcapillary venules to control inflammation: effect of lipocortin 1. *Proc Natl Acad Sci U S A* 1998;95:14535–14539.
52. Youssef PP, Triantafillou S, Parker A, et al. Effects of pulse methylprednisolone on cell adhesion molecules in the synovial membrane in rheumatoid arthritis. Reduced E-selectin and intercellular adhesion molecule 1 expression. *Arthritis Rheum* 1996;39:1970–1979.
53. Youssef PP, Haynes DR, Triantafillou S, et al. Effects of pulse methylprednisolone on inflammatory mediators in peripheral blood, synovial fluid, and synovial membrane in rheumatoid arthritis. *Arthritis Rheum* 1997;40:1400–1408.
54. Goulding NJ, Godolphin JL, Sharland PR, et al. Anti-inflammatory lipocortin 1 production by peripheral blood leucocytes in response to hydrocortisone. *Lancet* 1990;335:1416–1418.
55. O'Banion MK, Winn VD, Young DA. cDNA cloning and functional activity of a glucocorticoid-regulated inflammatory cyclooxygenase. *Proc Natl Acad Sci U S A* 1992;89:4888–4892.
56. Jonat C, Rahmsdorf HJ, Park KK, et al. Antitumor promotion and antiinflammation: down-modulation of AP-1 (Fos/Jun) activity by glucocorticoid hormone. *Cell* 1990;62:1189–1204.
57. Yang-Yen HF, Chambard JC, Sun YL, et al. Transcriptional interference between c-Jun and the glucocorticoid receptor: mutual inhibition of DNA binding due to direct protein-protein interaction. *Cell* 1990;62:1205–1215.
58. Waage A, Bakke O. Glucocorticoids suppress the production of tumour necrosis factor by lipopolysaccharide-stimulated human monocytes. *Immunology* 1988;63:299–302.
59. Batuman AO, Ferrero AP, Diaz A, et al. Regulation of transforming factor B1 gene expression by glucocorticoids in normal human T lymphocytes. *J Clin Invest* 1991;88:1574–1580.
60. Geller DA, Nussler AK, Di Silvio M, et al. Cytokines, endotoxin, and glucocorticoids regulate the expression of inducible nitric oxide synthase in hepatocytes. *Proc Natl Acad Sci U S A* 1993;90:522–526.
61. Lamberts SW, Bruining HA, de Jong FH. Corticosteroid therapy in severe illness. *N Engl J Med* 1997;337:1285–1292.
62. Gotzsche PC, Johansen HK. Short-term low-dose corticosteroids vs placebo and nonsteroidal antiinflammatory drugs in rheumatoid arthritis (Cochrane Review). *Cochrane Database Syst Rev* 2002;CD000189.
63. Criswell LA, Saag KG, Sems KM, et al. Moderate-term, low-dose corticosteroids for rheumatoid arthritis. *Cochrane Database Syst Rev* 2000;CD001158.
64. Saag KG, Criswell LA, Sems KM, et al. Low-dose corticosteroids in rheumatoid arthritis. A meta-analysis of their moderate-term effectiveness. *Arthritis Rheum* 1996;39:1818–1825.
65. van Schaardenburg D, Valkema R, Dijkmans BA, et al. Prednisone treatment of elderly-onset rheumatoid arthritis. Disease activity and bone mass in comparison with chloroquine treatment. *Arthritis Rheum* 1995;38:334–342.

66. Report by Joint Committee of the Medical Research Council and Nuffield Foundation on Clinical Trials of Cortisone, ACTH, and Other Therapeutic Measures in Chronic Rheumatic Diseases. A comparison of prednisolone with aspirin or other analgesics (first report). *Ann Rheum Dis* 1959;18:173–187.
67. Report by Joint Committee of the Medical Research Council and Nuffield Foundation on Clinical Trials of Cortisone, ACTH, and Other Therapeutic Measures in Chronic Rheumatic Diseases. A comparison of prednisolone with aspirin or other analgesics (second report). *Ann Rheum Dis* 1960;19:331–337.
68. McDougall R, Sibley J, Haga M, et al. Outcome in patients with rheumatoid arthritis receiving prednisone compared to matched controls. *J Rheumatol* 1994;21:1207–1213.
69. Hansen M, Podenphant J, Florescu A, et al. A randomised trial of differentiated prednisolone treatment in active rheumatoid arthritis. Clinical benefits and skeletal side effects. *Ann Rheum Dis* 1999;58:713–718.
70. van Gestel AM, Laan RF, Haagsma CJ, et al. Oral steroids as bridge therapy in rheumatoid arthritis patients starting with parenteral gold. A randomized double-blind placebo-controlled trial. *Br J Rheumatol* 1995;34:347–351.
71. van Everdingen AA, Jacobs JW, Siewertsz Van Reesema DR, et al. Low-dose prednisone therapy for patients with early active rheumatoid arthritis: clinical efficacy, disease-modifying properties, and side effects: a randomized, double blind, placebo-controlled clinical trial. *Ann Intern Med* 2002;136:1–12.
72. Kirwan JR. The effect of glucocorticoids on joint destruction in rheumatoid arthritis. The Arthritis and Rheumatism Council Low-Dose Glucocorticoid Study Group. *N Engl J Med* 1995;333:142–146.
73. Boers M, Verhoeven AC, Markusse HM, et al. Randomised comparison of combined step-down prednisolone, methotrexate and sulphasalazine with sulphasalazine alone in early rheumatoid arthritis. *Lancet* 1997;350: 309–318.
74. Hickling P, Jacoby RK, Kirwan JR. Joint destruction after glucocorticoids are withdrawn in early rheumatoid arthritis. Arthritis and Rheumatism Council Low Dose Glucocorticoid Study Group. *Br J Rheumatol* 1998;37:930–936.
75. Liebling MR, Lieb E, McLaughlin K, et al. A double-blind cross-over trial of pulse methylprednisolone in rheumatoid arthritis. *Ann Intern Med* 1981; 94:21–26.
76. Hansen TM, Kryger P, Elling H, et al. Double blind placebo controlled trial of pulse treatment with methylprednisolone combined with disease modifying drugs in rheumatoid arthritis. *BMJ* 1990;301:268–270.
77. Corkill MM, Kirkham BW, Chikanza IC, et al. Intramuscular depot methylprednisolone induction of chrysotherapy in rheumatoid arthritis: a 24–week randomized controlled trial. *Br J Rheumatol* 1990;29:274–279.
78. Iglehart IW 3rd, Sutton JD, Bender JC, et al. Intravenous pulsed steroids in rheumatoid arthritis: a comparative dose study. *J Rheumatol* 1990;17:159–162.
79. Radia M, Furst DE. Comparison of three pulse methylprednisolone regimens in the treatment of rheumatoid arthritis. *J Rheumatol* 1988;15:242–246.
80. Menninger H, Reinhardt S, Sondgen W. Intra-articular treatment of rheumatoid knee-joint effusion with triamcinolone hexacetonide versus sodium morrhuate. A prospective study. *Scand J Rheumatol* 1994;23:249–254.
81. McCarty DJ, Harman JG, Grassanovich JL, et al. Treatment of rheumatoid joint inflammation with intrasynovial triamcinolone hexacetonide. *J Rheumatol* 1995;22:1631–1635.
82. Pitsillides AA, Will RK, Bayliss MT, et al. Circulating and synovial fluid hyaluronan levels. Effects of intraarticular corticosteroid on the concentration and the rate of turnover. *Arthritis Rheum* 1994;37:1030–1038.
83. West HF. Rheumatoid arthritis: the relevance of clinical knowledge to research activities. *Abstracts World Med* 1967;41:401–417.
84. Masi AT. Low dose glucocorticoid therapy in rheumatoid arthritis (RA): transitional or selected add-on therapy? *J Rheumatol* 1983;10:675–678.
85. Harris ED Jr., Emkey RD, Nichols JE, et al. Low dose prednisone therapy in rheumatoid arthritis: a double blind study. *J Rheumatol* 1983;10:713–721.
86. Berntsen CA, Freyberg RH. Rheumatoid patients after five or more years of corticosteroid treatment: a comparative analysis of 183 patients. *Ann Intern Med* 1961;54:938–953.
87. Porter D. Glucocorticoids and joint destruction in rheumatoid arthritis. *N Engl J Med* 1995;333:1569.
88. Kirwan JR. Glucocorticoids and joint destruction in rheumatoid arthritis. *N Engl J Med* 1995;333:1569.
89. Rau R, Wassenberg S, Zeidler H, LDPT-Study Group. Low dose prednisolone therapy (LDPT) retards radiographically detectable destruction in early rheumatoid arthritis—preliminary results of a multicenter, randomized, parallel, double blind study. *Zeitschrift für Rheumatologie* 2000;59[Suppl 2]:II/90–96.
90. Landewe RB, Boers M, Verhoeven AC, et al. COBRA combination therapy in patients with early rheumatoid arthritis: long-term structural benefits of a brief intervention. *Arthritis Rheum* 2002;46:347–356.
91. Paulus HE, Di Primeo D, Sanda M, et al. Progression of radiographic joint erosion during low dose corticosteroid treatment of rheumatoid arthritis. *J Rheumatol* 2000;27:1632–1637.
92. Pincus T, Marcum SB, Callahan LF. Long term drug therapy for rheumatoid arthritis in seven rheumatology private practices: II. Second line drugs and prednisone. *J Rheumatol* 1992;19:1885–1894.
93. Wolfe F, Albert D, Pincus T. A survey of United States rheumatologists concerning effectiveness of disease-modifying antirheumatic drugs and prednisone in the treatment of rheumatoid arthritis. *Arthritis Care Res* 1998;373–381.
94. Dixon RB, Christy NP. On the various forms of corticosteroid withdrawal syndrome. *Am J Med* 1980;68:224–230.
95. Axelrod L. Glucocorticoid therapy. *Medicine* (Baltimore) 1976;55:39–65.
96. Furst DE, Saag KG, Glucocorticoid withdrawal regimen. In: Rose BD, ed. *UptoDate*, computer software. Wellesley, MA: UptoDate, 2002.
97. LaRochelle GE Jr., LaRochelle AG, Ratner RE, Borenstein DG. Recovery of the hypothalamic-pituitary-adrenal (HPA) axis in patients with rheumatic diseases receiving low-dose prednisone *Am J Med* 1993;95:258–264.
98. Garber ED, Targoff C, Paulus HE. Corticosteroids in the rheumatic diseases: chronic low doses, chronic high doses, "pulses," intra-articular. In: Paulus HE, Furst DE, Dromgoole SH, eds. *Drugs for rheumatic disease*. New York: Churchill Livingstone, 1987:443–476.
99. Byyny RL. Withdrawal from glucocorticoid therapy. *N Engl J Med* 1976;295: 30–32.
100. Cash JM, Klippel JH. Second-line drug therapy for rheumatoid arthritis. *N Engl J Med* 1994;330:1368–1375.
101. Edmonds JP, Scott DL, Furst DE, et al. New classification of antirheumatic drugs. The evolution of a concept. *J Rheumatol* 1993;20:585–587.
102. Edmonds JP, Scott DL, Furst DE, et al. Antirheumatic drugs: a proposed new classification. *Arthritis Rheum* 1993;36:336–339.
103. Saag KG, Koehnke R, Caldwell JR, et al. Low dose long-term corticosteroid therapy in rheumatoid arthritis: an analysis of serious adverse events. *Am J Med* 1994;96:115–123.
104. Wolfe F, Mitchell DM, Sibley JT, et al. The mortality of rheumatoid arthritis. *Arthritis Rheum* 1994;37:481–494.
105. Pincus T, Brooks RH, Callahan LF. Prediction of long-term mortality in patients with rheumatoid arthritis according to simple questionnaire and joint count measures. *Ann Intern Med* 1994;120:26–34.
106. Fries JF, Williams CA, Ramey D, Bloch DA. The relative toxicity of disease-modifying antirheumatic drugs. *Arthritis Rheum* 1993;36:297–306.
107. Curtis PH, Clark WS. Vertebral fractures resulting from prolonged cortisone and corticotropin therapy. *JAMA* 1954;156:467.
108. Canalis E. Mechanisms of glucocorticoid action in bone: implications to glucocorticoid-induced osteoporosis. *J Clin Endocrinol Metab* 1996;81:3441–3447.
109. Lukert BP, Raisz LG. Glucocorticoid-induced osteoporosis: pathogenesis and management. *Ann Intern Med* 1990;112:352–364.
110. Pearce G, Tabensky DA, Delmas PD, et al. Corticosteroid-induced bone loss in men. *J Clin Endocrinol Metab* 1998;83:801–806.
111. Manolagas SC, Weinstein RS. New developments in the pathogenesis and treatment of steroid-induced osteoporosis. *J Bone Miner Res* 1999;14:1061–1066.
112. Manolagas SC. Birth and death of bone cells: basic regulatory mechanisms and implications for the pathogenesis and treatment of osteoporosis. *Endocrincol Rev* 2000;21:115–137.
113. Orth DN. Glucocorticoid effects on bone, muscle, and connective tissue. In: Rose BD, ed. *UptoDate*, computer software. Wellesley, MA: UptoDate, 2002.
114. Kaji H, Sugimoto T, Kanatani M, et al. Dexamethasone stimulates osteoclast-like cell formation by directly acting on hemopoietic blast cells and enhances osteoclast-like cell formation stimulated by parathyroid hormone and prostaglandin E_2. *J Bone Miner Res* 1997;12:734–741.
115. Fucik RF, Kukreja SC, Hargis GK, et al. Effect of glucocorticoids on function of the parathyroid glands in man. *J Clin Endocrinol Metab* 1975;40:152–155.
116. Suzuki Y, Ichikawa Y, Saito E, et al. Importance of increased urinary calcium excretion in the development of secondary hyperparathyroidism of patients under glucocorticoid therapy. *Metabolism* 1983;32:151–156.
117. Reid IR, Heap SW. Determinants of vertebral mineral density in patients receiving long-term glucocorticoid therapy. *Arch Intern Med* 1990;150:2545–2548.
118. Kroot EJ, Nieuwenhuizen MG, de Waal Malefijt MC, et al. Change in bone mineral density in patients with rheumatoid arthritis during the first decade of the disease. *Arthritis Rheum* 2001;44:1254–1260.
119. Emkey RD, Lindsay R, Lyssy J, et al. The systemic effect of intraarticular administration of corticosteroid on markers of bone formation and bone resorption in patients with rheumatoid arthritis. *Arthritis Rheum* 1996;39:277–282.
120. Gough AK, Lilley J, Eyre S, et al. Generalised bone loss in patients with early rheumatoid arthritis. *Lancet* 1994;344:23–27.
121. Verhoeven AC, Boers M. Limited bone loss due to corticosteroids; a systematic review of prospective studies in rheumatoid arthritis and other diseases. *J Rheumatol* 1997;24:1495–1503.
122. Laan RF, van Riel PL, van de Putte LB, et al. Low-dose prednisone induces rapid reversible axial bone loss in patients with rheumatoid arthritis. A randomized, controlled study. *Ann Intern Med* 1993;119:963–968.
123. Saito JK, Davis JW, Wasnich RD, et al. Users of low-dose glucocorticoids have increased bone loss rates: a longitudinal study. *Calcif Tissue Int* 1995;57:115–119.
124. Buckley LM, Leib ES, Cartularo KS, et al. Effects of low dose corticosteroids on the bone mineral density of patients with rheumatoid arthritis. *J Rheumatol* 1995;22:1055–1059.
125. Gluck OS, Murphy WA, Hahn TJ, Hahn B. Bone loss in adults receiving alternate day glucocorticoid therapy. A comparison with daily therapy. *Arthritis Rheum* 1981;24:892–898.
126. Michel BA, Bloch DA, Fries JF. Predictors of fractures in early rheumatoid arthritis. *J Rheumatol* 1991;18:804–808.
127. Adachi JD, Saag KG, Delmas PD, et al. Two-year effects of alendronate on bone mineral density and vertebral fracture in patients receiving glucocorticoids: a randomized, double-blind, placebo-controlled extension trial. *Arthritis Rheum* 2001;44:202–211.
128. American College of Rheumatology Ad Hoc Committee on Glucocorticoid-Induced Osteoporosis. Recommendations for the prevention and treatment of

glucocorticoid-induced osteoporosis: 2001 update. *Arthritis Rheum* 2001;44: 1496–1503.

129. Buckley LM, Leib ES, Cartularo KS, et al. Calcium and vitamin D3 supplementation prevents bone loss in the spine secondary to low-dose corticosteroids in patients with rheumatoid arthritis. A randomized, double-blind, placebo-controlled trial. *Ann Intern Med* 1996;125:961–968.
130. Saag KG, Emkey R, Schnitzer TJ, et al. Alendronate for the prevention and treatment of glucocorticoid-induced osteoporosis. Glucocorticoid-Induced Osteoporosis Intervention Study Group. *N Engl J Med* 1998;339:292–299.
131. Reid DM, Hughes RA, Laan RF, et al. Efficacy and safety of daily risedronate in the treatment of corticosteroid-induced osteoporosis in men and women: a randomized trial. *J Bone Miner Res* 2000;2:15:1006–1020.
132. Homik J, Suarez-Almazor ME, Shea B, et al. Calcium and vitamin D for corticosteroid-induced osteoporosis. *Cochrane Database Syst Rev* 2000;2:CD000952.
133. Sambrook P, Birmingham J, Kelly P, et al. Prevention of corticosteroid osteoporosis. A comparison of calcium, calcitriol, and calcitonin. *N Engl J Med* 1993;328:1747–1752.
134. Hall GM, Daniels M, Doyle DV, et al. Effect of hormone replacement therapy on bone mass in rheumatoid arthritis patients treated with and without steroids. *Arthritis Rheum* 1994;37:1499–1505.
135. Women's Health Initiative Trial. Risks and benefits of estrogen plus progestin in healthy postmenopausal women. Principal results from the Women's Health Initiative randomized controlled trial. *JAMA* 2002;3:321–333.
136. Lane NE, Sanchez S, Modin GW, et al. Parathyroid hormone treatment can reverse corticosteroid-induced osteoporosis. Results of a randomized controlled clinical trial. *J Clin Invest* 1998;102:1627–1633.
137. Roux C, Oriente P, Laan R, et al. Randomized trial of effect of cyclical etidronate in the prevention of corticosteroid-induced bone loss. Ciblos Study Group. *J Clin Endocrinol Metab* 1998;83:1128–1133.
138. Cohen S, Levy RM, Keller M, et al. Risedronate therapy prevents glucocorticoid-induced bone loss: a twelve-month, multicenter, randomized, double-blind, placebo-controlled, parallel-group study. *Arthritis Rheum* 1999;42:2309–2318.
139. Wallach S, Cohen S, Reid DM, et al. Effects of risedronate treatment on bone density and vertebral fracture in patients on corticosteroid therapy. *Calcif Tissue Int* 2000;67:277–285.
140. Adachi JD, Bensen WG, Brown J, et al. Intermittent etidronate therapy to prevent corticosteroid-induced osteoporosis. *N Engl J Med* 1997;377:382–387.
141. Karagas MR, Cushing GL Jr, Greenberg ER, et al. Non-melanoma skin cancers and glucocorticoid therapy. *Br J Cancer* 2001;85:683–686.
142. Saag KG, Furst D. Major side effects of corticosteroids. In: Rose BD, ed. *UptoDate*, computer software. Wellesley, MA: UptoDate, 2002.
143. Shubin H. Long term (five or more years) administration of corticosteroids in pulmonary diseases. *Dis Chest* 1965;48:287–290.
144. Carnahan MC, Goldstein DA. Ocular complications of topical, peri-ocular, and systemic corticosteroids. *Curr Opin Ophthalmol* 2000;11:478–483.
145. Black RL, Oglesby RB, von Sallman L, et al. Posterior subcapsular cataracts induced by corticosteroids in patients with rheumatoid arthritis. *JAMA* 1960,174:166–171.
146. Hanania NA, Chapman KR, Kesten S. Adverse effects of inhaled corticosteroids. *Am J Med* 1995;98:196–208.
147. Urban RC Jr., Cotlier E. Corticosteroid-induced cataracts. *Surv Ophthalmol* 1986;31:102–110.
148. Tarantino A, Aroldi A, Stucchi L, et al. A randomized prospective trial comparing cyclosporine monotherapy with triple drug therapy in renal transplantation. *Transplantation* 1991;52:53–57.
149. Ponticelli S, Pisani F, Montagnino G, et al. A randomized study comparing cyclosporine alone versus double and triple therapy in renal transplants. Italian Multicenter Study Group for Renal Transplantation (SIMTRe). *Transplant Proc* 1997;29:290–291.
150. Cumming RG, Mitchell P, Leeder SR. Use of inhaled corticosteroids and the risk of cataracts. *N Engl J Med* 1997;337:8–14.
151. Ozturk F, Yuceturk AV, Kurt E, et al. Evaluation of intraocular pressure and cataract formation following the long-term use of nasal corticosteroids. *Ear Nose Throat J* 1998;77:846–848:850–851.
152. Chen YC, Gajraj NM, Clavo A, et al. Posterior subcapsular cataract formation associated with multiple lumbar epidural corticosteroid injections. *Anesth Analg* 1998,86:1054–1055.
153. Skuta GL, Morgan RK. Corticosteroid-induced glaucoma. In: Ritch R, Shields MB, Krupin T, eds. *The glaucomas*, 2nd ed. St. Louis: Mosby, 1996:1177–1188.
154. Garbe E, LeLoner J, Boivin JF, et al. Inhaled and nasal glucocorticoids and the risks of ocular hypertension or open angle glaucoma. *JAMA* 1997,277:722–727.
155. Akduman L, Kolker AE, Black DL, et al. Treatment of persistent glaucoma secondary to periocular corticosteroids. *Am J Ophthalmol* 1996;122:275–277.
156. Gutierrez MA, Garcia ME, Rodriguez JA, et al. Hypothalamic-pituitary-adrenal axis function in patients with active rheumatoid arthritis: a controlled study using insulin hypoglycemia stress test and prolactin stimulation. *J Rheumatol* 1999;26:277–281.
157. Streck WF, Lockwood DH. Pituitary adrenal recovery following short-term suppression with corticosteroids. *Am J Med* 1979;66:910–914.
158. Wenning GK, Wietholter H, Schnauder G, et al. Recovery of the hypothalamic-pituitary-adrenal axis from suppression by short-term, high-dose intravenous prednisolone therapy in patients with MS. *Acta Neurol Scand* 1994;89:270–273.
159. Carella MJ, Srivastava LS, Gossain VV, et al. Hypothalamic-pituitary-adrenal function one week after a short burst of steroid therapy. *J Clin Endocrinol Metab* 1993;76:1188–1191.
160. Daly JR, Myles AB, Bacon PA, et al. Pituitary adrenal function during corticosteroid withdrawal in rheumatoid arthritis. *Ann Rheum Dis* 1967;26:18–25.
161. Martin MM, Gaboardi F, Podolsky S, et al. Intermittent steroid therapy. Its effect on hypothalamic-pituitary-adrenal function and the response of plasma growth hormone and insulin to stimulation. *N Engl J Med* 1968;279:273–278.
162. Piper JM, Ray WA, Daugherty JR, et al. Corticosteroid use and peptic ulcer disease: role of nonsteroidal anti-inflammatory drugs. *Ann Intern Med* 1991;114:735–740.
163. Sterioff S, Orringer MB, Cameron JL. Colon perforations associated with steroid therapy. *Surgery* 1974;75:56–58.
164. Carone F, Liebon A. Acute pancreatic lesion in patients treated with ACTH and adrenal corticosteroids. *N Engl J Med* 1957;257:690.
165. Hill RB. Fatal fat embolism from steroid-induced fatty liver. *N Engl J Med* 1961;273:1453.
166. Bowyer SL, LaMothe MP, Hollister JR. Steroid myopathy: incidence and detection in a population with asthma. *J Allergy Clin Immunol* 1985;76:234–242.
167. Batchelor TT, Taylor LP, Thaler HT, et al. Steroid myopathy in cancer patients. *Neurology* 1997;48:1234–1238.
168. Konagaya M, Bernard PA, Max SR. Blockade of glucocorticoid receptor binding and inhibition of dexamethasone-induced muscle atrophy in the rat by RU38486, a potent glucocorticoid antagonist. *Endocrinology* 1986;119:375–380.
169. Hanson P, Dive A, Brucher JM, et al. Acute corticosteroid myopathy in intensive care patients. *Muscle Nerve* 1997;20:1371–1380.
170. Ferrando AA, Stuart CA, Sheffield-Moore M, et al. Inactivity amplifies the catabolic response of skeletal muscle to cortisol. *J Clin Endocrinol Metab* 1999;84:3515–3521.
171. Naber D, Sand P, Heigl B. Psychopathological and neuropsychological effects of 8–days' corticosteroid treatment. A prospective study. *Psychoneuroendocrinology* 1996;21:25–31.
172. Wolkowitz OM, Rubinow D, Doran AR, et al. Prednisone effects on neurochemistry and behavior. Preliminary findings. *Arch Gen Psychiatry* 1990;47:963–968.
173. Lewis DA, Smith RE. Steroid-induced psychiatric syndromes. A report of 14 cases and a review of the literature. *J Affect Disord* 1983;5:319–332.
174. Greeves JA. Rapid-onset steroid psychosis with very low dosage of prednisolone. *Lancet* 1984;1:1119–1120.
175. Boston Collaborative Drug Surveillance Program. Acute adverse effects reactions to prednisone in relation to dosage. *Clin Pharmacol Ther* 1972;13:694–698.
176. Ling MH, Perry PJ, Tsuang MT. Side effects of corticosteroid therapy. Psychiatric aspects. *Arch Gen Psychiatry* 1981;38:471–477.
177. Orth DN. Glucocorticoid effects on carbohydrate and lipid metabolism. In: Rose BD, ed. *UptoDate*, computer software. Wellesley, MA: UptoDate, 2002.
178. Lakatos J, Harsagyi A. Serum total, HDL, LDL cholesterol, and triglyceride levels in patients with rheumatoid arthritis. *Clin Biochem* 1988;21:93–96.
179. Lazarevic MB, Vitic J, Mladenovic V, et al. Dyslipoproteinemia in the course of active rheumatoid arthritis. *Semin Arthritis Rheum* 1992;22:172–178.
180. Lee YH, Choi SJ, Ji JD, et al. Lipoprotein(a) and lipids in relation to inflammation in rheumatoid arthritis. *Clin Rheumatol* 2000;19:324–325.
181. Van Doornum S, McColl G, Wicks IP. Accelerated atherosclerosis: an extraarticular feature of rheumatoid arthritis? *Arthritis Rheum* 2002;46:862–873.
182. Ettinger WH Jr, Hazzard WR. Prednisone increases very low density lipoprotein and high density lipoprotein in healthy men. *Metabolism* 1988;37:1055–1058.
183. Petri M, Lakatta C, Magder L, et al. Effect of prednisone and hydroxychloroquine on coronary artery disease risk factors in systemic lupus erythematosus: a longitudinal data analysis. *Am J Med* 1994;96:254–259.
184. Ward MM. Recent improvements in survival in patients with rheumatoid arthritis: better outcomes or different study designs? *Arthritis Rheum* 2001;44:1467–1469.
185. Symmons DP, Jones MA, Scott DL, et al. Long term mortality outcome in patients with rheumatoid arthritis: early presenters continue to do well. *J Rheumatol* 1998;25:1072–1077.
186. Mitchell DM, Spitz PW, Young DY, et al. Survival, prognosis, and causes of death in rheumatoid arthritis. *Arthritis Rheum* 1986;29:706–714.
187. Cheng W, Kvilekval KV, Abumrad NA. Dexamethasone enhances accumulation of cholesteryl esters by human macrophages. *Am J Physiol* 1995;269:E642–E648.
188. Cheng W, Lau OD, Abumrad NA. Two antiatherogenic effects of progesterone on human macrophages; inhibition of cholesteryl ester synthesis and block of its enhancement by glucocorticoids. *J Clin Endocrinol Metab* 1999;84:265–271.
189. Weinstein RS, Manolagas SC. Apoptosis and osteoporosis. *Am J Med* 2000;108:153–164.
190. Vreden SG, Hermus AR, van Liessum PA, et al. Aseptic bone necrosis in patients on glucocorticoid replacement therapy. *Neth J Med* 1991;39:153–157.
191. Laroche M, Arlet J, Mazieres B. Osteonecrosis of the femoral and humeral heads after intraarticular corticosteroid injections. *J Rheumatol* 1990;17:549–551.
192. Zizic TM, Marcoux C, Hungerford DS, et al. Corticosteroid therapy associated with ischemic necrosis of bone in systemic lupus erythematosus. *Am J Med* 1985;79:596–604.
193. Stuck AE, Minder CE, Frey FJ. Risk of infectious complications in patients taking glucocorticosteroids. *Rev Infect Dis* 1989;11:954–963.

194. Ginzler E, Diamond H, Kaplan D, et al. Computer analysis of factors influencing frequency of infection in systemic lupus erythematosus. *Arthritis Rheum* 1978;21:37–44.
195. Fauci AS, Dale DC, Balow JE. Glucocorticosteroid therapy: mechanisms of action and clinical considerations. *Ann Intern Med* 1976;84:304–315.
196. Dursun AB, Kalac N, Ozkan B, et al. Pulmonary tuberculosis in patients with rheumatoid arthritis (four case reports). *Rheumatol Int* 2002;21:153–157.
197. American Thoracic Society. Targeted tuberculin testing and treatment of latent tuberculosis infection. *MMWR Morb Mortal Wkly Rep* 2000;49:1–51.
198. Singer NG, McCune WJ. Prevention of infectious complications in rheumatic disease patients: immunization, *Pneumocystis carinii* prophylaxis, and screening for latent infections. *Curr Opin Rheumatol* 1999;11:173–178.
199. Kubiet MA, Gonzalez-Rothi RJ, Cottey R, et al. Serum antibody response to influenza vaccine in pulmonary patients receiving corticosteroids. *Chest* 1996;110:367–370.
200. Pinsky L, DiGeorge AM. Cleft palate in the mouse: a teratogenic index of glucocorticoid potency. *Science* 1965;147:402.
201. Schatz M, Patterson R, Zeitz S, et al. Corticosteroid therapy for the pregnant asthmatic patient. *JAMA* 1975;233:804–807.
202. Cowchock FS, Reece EA, Balaban D, et al. Repeated fetal losses associated with antiphospholipid antibodies: a collaborative randomized trial comparing prednisone with low-dose heparin treatment. *Am J Obstet Gynecol* 1992;166:1318–1323.
203. Bermas BL, Hill JA. Effects of immunosuppressive drugs during pregnancy. *Arthritis Rheum* 1995;38:1722–1732.
204. American Academy of Pediatrics Committee on Drugs: Transfer of drugs and other chemicals into human milk. *Pediatrics* 1989;84:924–936.
205. Ost L, Wettrell G, Bjorkhem I, Rane A. Prednisolone excretion in human milk. *J Pediatr* 1985;106:1008–1011.
206. Conn DL. Resolved: low-dose prednisone is indicated as a standard treatment in patients with rheumatoid arthritis. *Arthritis Rheum* 2001;45:462–467.
207. Saag KG. Resolved: low-dose glucocorticoids are neither safe nor effective for the long-term treatment of rheumatoid arthritis. *Arthritis Rheum* 2001;45:468–471.

CHAPTER 25

Methotrexate and Azathioprine

David M. Lee and Michael E. Weinblatt

METHOTREXATE

History

The development of methotrexate (MTX) and other folic acid antagonists occurred soon after the identification of folic acid as the active compound in liver extract that allowed regeneration of red blood cells for certain macrocytic anemias. Knowing that folic acid compounds were active in formation of blood cells and that administration of these compounds could accelerate childhood leukemias, Farber and colleagues (1) successfully administered the folate antagonist aminopterin (the parent compound of MTX) to children with leukemia in 1948. During the early 1950s, Gubner and colleagues (2) hypothesized that there may be a therapeutic role for antimetabolite therapy in inflammatory disease because the joint tissues in inflammatory arthritis appeared to be metabolically highly active. This hypothesis, combined with a shortage of cortisone, prompted the initial clinical use of aminopterin in a series of patients with inflammatory arthritis and psoriasis. In this series, seven of eight patients noted a decrease in their inflammatory arthritis after administration of aminopterin.

Structure

The structure of MTX (amethopterin) is similar to the physiologic folate cofactors and demonstrates three structural components: (a) a multi-ring pteridine group, (b) a paraaminobenzoic acid moiety, and (c) a glutamate residue (Fig. 25.1). Compared to folic acid, MTX has an amino substitution at the 4 position of the pteridine group and an addition of a methyl group at the 10 position of the paraaminobenzoic acid moiety. On entry into cells, enzymatic polyglutamation occurs with addition of up to five glutamate residues.

Pharmacology

PHARMACOKINETICS

MTX in rheumatoid arthritis (RA) is used exclusively as a weekly low-dose administration via oral or parenteral (subcutaneous or intramuscular) routes. Oral administration at low dosage generally demonstrates high bioavailability (mean = 70%), although there exists significant patient variability in efficiency of absorption (range, 40–100%) (3,4). Gastrointestinal (GI) absorption is rapid, with peak serum values achieved after 1 to 2 hours (5,6) and an elimination half-life of 3 to 10 hours (3,5,6). Bioavailability of the tablet form and the parenteral (liquid) forms of MTX is identical at the low doses used to treat RA (7,8), thus allowing for significant cost savings with the parenteral formulation taken orally. Bioavailability is not affected by food intake (9,10). At higher doses, absorption becomes more variable, and bioavailability from parenteral administration may be superior to oral administration (8,11). Parenteral administration, generally well tolerated and equivalent via subcutaneous or intramuscular routes (8,12), results in complete absorption, with peak serum concentrations achieved within 2 hours (13).

MTX distributes in fluid and tissues with a volume of distribution of 22.2 L per m^2 (3). Binding to plasma proteins occurs with approximately 50% of the drug protein bound (5). Although increased serum concentrations of free MTX have been documented due to protein displacement by other medications used in RA (such as salicylates, nonsteroidal antiinflammatory drugs, and sulfonamides), these interactions are of limited significance in RA therapy given its low dose.

Excretion of MTX is predominantly via the renal system through glomerular filtration and active tubular secretion of unmetabolized medication (14,15). A small fraction of the drug is excreted in bile and feces, with evidence of enterohepatic recirculation (16). There are a number of medications that decrease renal clearance of MTX, either by competition for excretion or by decreasing renal function. These medications include some antibiotics (penicillins, tetracycline) (17), probenecid (via competition for excretion) (18), and the nonsteroidal antiinflammatory drugs (14,19). Although the clinical relevance of these drug interactions is limited for low-dose MTX administered with antibiotics and nonsteroidal antiinflammatory drugs, the decreased clearance associated with probenecid can result in toxicity. Because decreased renal clearance, either from drug interaction or from renal insufficiency, has been associated with substantial increases in toxicity (20), monitoring of renal function is mandated. It should be noted that MTX is excreted in the milk of lactating mothers; thus, administration is contraindicated while breast-feeding postpartum.

PHARMACODYNAMICS

The majority of MTX is excreted unchanged via the kidneys; no additional metabolism is required for excretion or for dihydrofolate reductase (DHFR) inhibition (21). A small fraction of MTX is metabolized to an active metabolite, 7-hydroxy-MTX, by the enzyme aldehyde oxidase (21,22). Both MTX and 7-hydroxy-MTX exert their influence after uptake into the cell by active transport (23). Both molecules undergo subsequent modification by the addition of glutamate, which broadens their

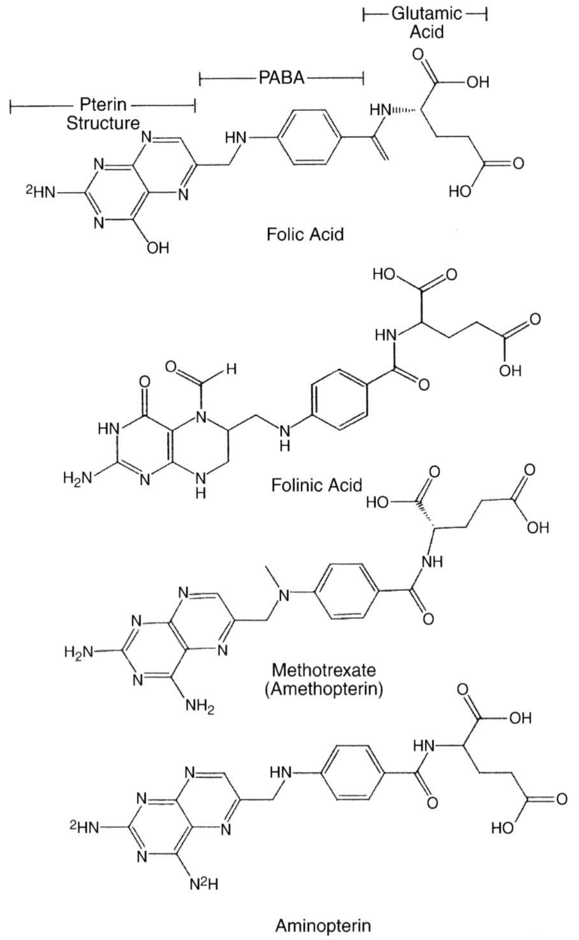

Figure 25.1. Chemical structures of folic acid, folinic acid, methotrexate, and aminopterin. PABA, paraaminobenzoic acid.

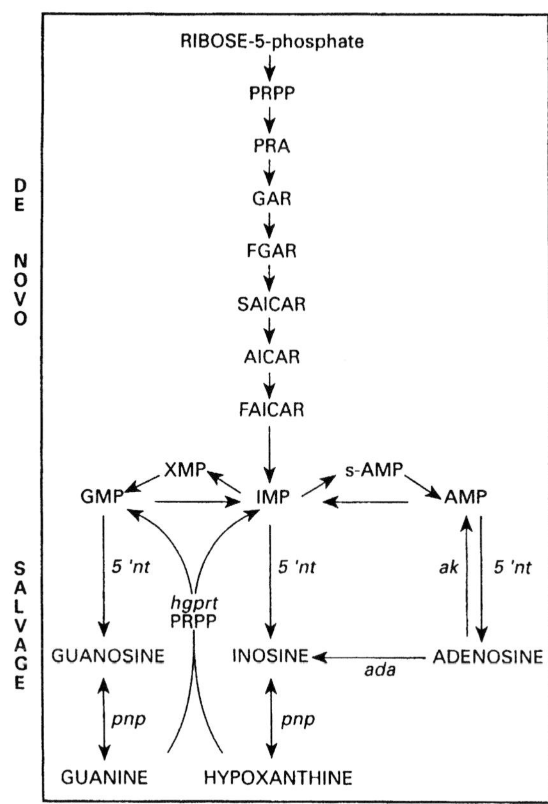

Figure 25.2. Methotrexate mechanism of actions. Pathways in purine metabolism, which is composed of a *de novo* synthesis (upper part of figure) and a salvage route (lower part of figure). ada, adenosine deaminase; AICAR, amino-imidazolcarboxamide ribosyl-5-phosphate; AK, adenosine kinase; AMP, adenosine monophosphate; FCAIR, form AICAR; FGAR, form GAR; GAR, glycinamide ribosyl-5-phosphate; GMP, guanosine monophosphate; hgprt, hypoxanthine-guanine phosphoribosyl; IMP, inosine monophosphate; 5'nt, purine-5'nucleotidase; pnp, purine nucleoside phosphorylase; PRA, phosphoribosylamine; PRPP, 5-phosphoribosyl-1-pyophosphate; SAICAR, succinyl amino-imidazolcarboxamide ribosyl-5-phosphate; s-AMP, succinyl-AMP; XMP, xanthine monophosphate. (From van Ede AE, Laan RF, Blom HJ, et al. Methotrexate in rheumatoid arthritis: an update with focus on mechanisms involved in toxicity. *Semin Arthritis Rheum* 1998;27:277.)

pharmacologic activity to other enzymes in the nucleic acid metabolic pathways (see Mechanism of Action).

Mechanism of Action

MTX, an analogue of folic acid, was originally designed as a specific competitive inhibitor of the enzyme DHFR that catalyzes the conversion of dihydrofolate to tetrahydrofolate. Tetrahydrofolate is a methyl donor required for the generation of the pyrimidine bases in DNA. Lack of sufficient substrate for formation of DNA halts the growth of dividing cells. At the high doses of MTX used for cancer chemotherapy, inhibition of DHFR is likely its major activity. However, in the low-dose weekly regimen used in RA therapy, there is little evidence to support an effect mediated solely by DHFR inhibition. Supplementation of folic acid, which competes with MTX for DHFR activity, does not generally result in reduced efficacy in RA (24,25). Folate supplementation does diminish the stomatitis and bone marrow suppression that result from decreased cellular proliferation due to DHFR inhibition. Furthermore, MTX therapy in the context of folate supplementation does not inhibit lymphocyte proliferation in RA. In contrast, clinical studies found stable or increased lymphocyte numbers in RA patients on MTX (26,27). Taken together, these observations suggest other mechanisms of action of MTX in RA.

MTX and its active metabolite, 7-hydroxy-MTX, are actively transported into cells (23), where they are modified by the addition of up to five glutamate moieties by the enzyme folylpolyglutamyl synthetase (28,29). The addition of glutamates traps MTX within the cell (30). Varying degrees of polyglutamation ensure that the concentration of the monoglutamated form remains low, allowing continued active transport into the cell and continued enzymatic conversion of each polyglutamated species while accumulating large quantities of total intracellular MTX. Furthermore, polyglutamated forms of MTX have significantly increased inhibitor activity for several key metabolic enzymes. Specifically, polyglutamated MTX demonstrates inhibitory activity for enzymes involved in both purine (glycinamide ribonucleotide transformylase) (29) and 5-aminoimidazole-4-carboxamide ribonucleotide transformylase (AICAR T'ase) (31,32) and pyrimidine (thymidylate synthetase) nucleic acid synthesis (33). Because the pentaglutamate form of MTX has tenfold more activity against AICAR T'ase than thymidylate synthetase, and 2,500-fold more activity than the monoglutamate form (31,33), it is likely that the effects of MTX on the purine biosynthetic pathway are substantially greater than its effects on the pyrimidine synthetic pathway (Fig. 25.2).

Given the lack of evidence for direct suppression of leukocyte proliferation, many studies have focused on other antiinflammatory effects of MTX in RA. These analyses have suggested that MTX inhibits production of inflammatory cytokines and increases production of antiinflammatory cytokines. Decreased levels of tumor necrosis factor α after MTX therapy have been documented in humans and in animal models of inflammatory arthritis (34). Similar analyses suggest both decreased interleukin (IL)-1 production and decreased cellular responses to IL-1 (35,36). RA patients treated with MTX demonstrate decreased serum levels of IL-6 (34,37), erythrocyte sedimentation rate, C-reactive protein (38), and rheumatoid factor (39), and *ex vivo* studies of mononuclear cells from RA patients show decreased production of IL-8 and leukotrienes (40) as well as immunoglobulin M rheumatoid factor (39,41). In contrast, serum levels of the antiinflammatory cytokine IL-10 in RA patients increase after treatment with MTX (42).

Although the exact mechanism of action of MTX in RA remains unknown, there are several animal models that suggest a prominent role for the adenosine pathway (43,44). In these models, treatment with MTX leads to increased extracellular concentration of adenosine (45), which has antiinflammatory properties. This accumulation of adenosine results from increased intracellular levels of both adenosine and adenosine monophosphate, which, in turn, result from AICAR T'ase inhibition and accumulation of AICAR (32) (Fig. 25.2). Intracellular adenosine monophosphate diffuses to the extracellular space in which conversion to adenosine can occur (45–47). The antiinflammatory effects of adenosine are similar to those noted for MTX. Many inflammatory leukocyte populations express G-protein–coupled adenosine A_2 receptors whose ligation leads to inhibition of production of inflammatory cytokines and decreased inflammatory cellular trafficking (48). In addition, engagement of A_2 receptors increase the production of antiinflammatory cytokines. Furthermore, blockade of the A_2 receptors in animal models abrogates the therapeutic effect of MTX (48).

Pivotal Trial Results

EARLY STUDIES

The earliest published use of the DHFR antagonist aminopterin (the predecessor to MTX) for arthritis was a series of eight patients reported in 1951 (2). Improvement was noted in short-term aminopterin usage in seven of the eight patients with subsequent increased disease activity after drug discontinuation. The observation that antifolates could be effective in RA was lost to the rheumatology community. Part of this was attributable to the enthusiasm for corticosteroids and concerns about the toxicity of MTX. Almost 30 years later, results from the first long-term use in 78 patients treated for up to 15 years were published in 1983 (49). In this series, 58% of patients experienced "marked" improvement. Other noncontrolled series published through 1985 reported similar positive results (50–53). Although encouraging, these studies were open, non–placebo controlled, and lacked the instruments such as the American College of Rheumatology (ACR) 20% or Disease Activity Score for accurate, validated outcomes measurement. These results did, however, provide impetus for further study.

MONOTHERAPY

Four initial double-blind trials, published in 1984 to 1985, compared MTX therapy with placebo for patients who had failed previous treatment with other disease-modifying antirheumatic drugs (DMARDs) (gold or D-penicillamine) (27,54–56). These studies, of 12 to 24 weeks in duration, used MTX dosages from 7.5 to 25.0 mg per week and followed indices similar to the current ACR 20% response. Although no durable remissions were reported, these and other clinical trials of MTX document a consistent 50% to 80% clinical response relative to baseline (57,58), with long-term stabilization of functional status (58–61). Improvement in clinical scores was noted as early as 3 weeks after initiation of therapy, and flare of disease activity was often noted within 3 weeks after MTX discontinuation in those trials that featured crossover arms (27,55). More recent trials have used slightly higher dosing regimens (15–20 mg per week) than early trials (7.5–15.0 mg per week); this higher dosing regimen is well tolerated with better efficacy than historic trials. In addition to assessing inflammatory indices and the functional status of patients, recent trials with MTX have measured radiographic progression of joint destruction. In these analyses, MTX has been shown to slow radiographic joint destruction and improve quality of life (61–63). Furthermore, low-dose weekly MTX monotherapy demonstrates high rates of long-term compliance, with 60% to 71% of patients continuing use at 5 years, and 34% to 38% continuing use at longer than 10 years (58–60,64–66).

The efficacy of MTX has been compared to other disease-modifying agents in head-to-head trials (Table 25.1). In particular, MTX has been compared to sulfasalazine (67,68), hydroxychloroquine (68), leflunomide (69–71), azathioprine (72–76), gold (27,57,58,77–81), and etanercept (82–84). To date, no other medication has been distinctly superior to MTX in terms of ACR criteria for improvement. In patients with recent onset of disease, etanercept and MTX therapy showed similar clinical efficacy after 12 months, as measured by the ACR 20% response (etanercept = 72%, MTX = 65%, $p = .16$) (83). Patients treated with etanercept demonstrated slightly less radiographic erosion compared to those treated with MTX (Δ Sharp score, 0.47 vs. 1.03, respectively; $p = .002$) (Table 25.1); however, the rate of

TABLE 25.1. Active Comparator Trials with Methotrexate and Other Delayed Mechanism of Action Antirheumatic Drugs

Comparison	Design	ACR% (DAS) Response (MTX vs. Comparator)	Δ Sharp Score[a] (U) (MTX vs. Comparator)	Reference
MTX vs. etanercept	Early RA (<3 yr); 1-yr RCT	ACR 20%: 65% vs. 72%	1.03 vs. 0.47	83
MTX vs. leflunomide	Established RA; 1-yr RCT	ACR 20%: 46% vs. 52% ACR 50%: 23% vs. 34% ACR 70%: 9% vs. 20%	0.88 vs. 0.53	85
MTX vs. azathioprine	Established RA; 48-wk RCT	ACR or DAS: not done Other: MTX, 45%; AZA, 26%	Not done	89
MTX vs. sulfasalazine	Early RA (<1 yr); 1-yr RCT	ACR 20%: 59% vs. 59% DAS: –0.87 vs. –1.15	Not done "Damage score": 4.50 vs. 4.64	197
MTX vs. auranofin	Established RA; 36-wk RCT	ACR or DAS: not done Other: MTX, 70%; AUR, 41% Post hoc analysis: ACR 20%: 68% vs. 30%	Not done	57

ACR, American College of Rheumatology; AUR, auranofin; AZA, azathioprine; DAS, Disease Activity Score; MTX, methotrexate; RA, rheumatoid arthritis; RCT, randomized controlled trial.
[a]Sharp score is an aggregate score of joint space narrowing and erosions (198).

radiographic change during the second 6 months of therapy was similar for etanercept and MTX (83). MTX has been compared to leflunomide over 12 months of therapy in patients with established disease. In this trial, MTX demonstrated an ACR 20% response rate of 46% (vs. leflunomide, 52%) and a Δ radiographic Sharp score of 0.88 (vs. leflunomide Δ Sharp score of 0.53) (85). Trials data demonstrate similar efficacy for MTX and other DMARDs (with ACR response rates similar to those quoted earlier), but, with the exception of etanercept, other DMARDs frequently displayed the same or higher rates of toxicity than MTX. MTX has demonstrated superior results in retarding progression of joint erosions relative to both gold and azathioprine therapy (62,72,86–88). Given its superior tolerability and efficacy, MTX has become a benchmark agent to which other agents are compared in clinical trials. Furthermore, MTX is the "anchor" agent in combination therapeutic approaches.

COMBINATION THERAPY

Using therapeutic concepts successfully applied to hypertension and cancer, wherein multiple agents of differing classes are used in combination to achieve a therapeutic goal, recent trials in RA have assessed the efficacy of combination DMARD therapy. The goals of these trials have been to decrease inflammatory symptoms, maintain functional status, and retard joint destruction relative to monotherapy. Balancing these end points is the goal of maintaining a tolerable toxicity profile. Initial randomized controlled trials of combination DMARD therapy have shown conflicting results, with some suggesting no benefit or worse outcomes (81,89–92). Potential explanations of those results include the generally short duration of study, use of surrogate markers of disease as end points, and choice of therapeutic agents.

A number of trials centering around MTX have shown a clear benefit from combination therapy with tolerable toxicity profiles. These studies have evaluated MTX plus cyclosporine (93–95), MTX plus infliximab (96–98), MTX plus etanercept (99), MTX plus leflunomide (100), MTX plus sulfasalazine plus hydroxychloroquine (68), MTX plus sulfasalazine plus prednisolone (101), and MTX plus sulfasalazine plus hydroxychloroquine plus prednisolone (102). Therapeutic benefits were established both in patients with new onset of symptoms, as well as in patients who had disease of several years' duration and who had failed previous DMARD therapy. Recent trials also support slowing of joint erosions with MTX in combination therapy (98,101,102). From a disease-management standpoint, the results of these trials validate the concurrent use of MTX with multiple other DMARD agents in the therapy of RA. Furthermore, these results suggest that patients in many stages of disease progression can benefit from more aggressive therapy.

In addition to data regarding the benefit of using MTX to treat articular symptoms and reduce joint destruction, evidence has emerged that treatment with MTX may confer a long-term mortality benefit as well. Epidemiology studies have documented a decreased life expectancy in patients with RA (103–105). There exists evidence that people with RA may have increased rates of heart disease, infection, and certain cancers, which contribute to this historic risk of decreased life expectancy in RA patients. Multiple analyses have demonstrated a survival benefit for RA patients treated with MTX (106–108). In the largest series, 1,240 patients were followed during the period from 1981 to 1999 (106). Approximately one-half of these patients (N = 588) were treated with MTX. The MTX-treated patients tended to have more severe disease activity. Analysis of life expectancy demonstrated a significant impact from treatment with MTX: The MTX-treated patients displayed a 60% reduction in mortality after adjusting for disease severity. Cardiovascular deaths were reduced by 70% in the MTX group. This survival increase was specific for MTX and was not seen in patients treated with other medications used in the study (sulfasalazine, penicillamine, hydroxychloroquine, and gold). These data highlight an emerging long-term consideration in RA therapy—namely, mortality benefit—and demonstrate a therapeutic benefit of MTX in this regard.

Toxicity

The most common adverse events associated with MTX use are GI related and include stomatitis, nausea, diarrhea, and anorexia (27,49,56,109–112). Headache and fatigue are also frequent complaints. GI toxicities tend to correlate with dosage level and may be responsive to concomitant folate or folinic acid administration, dosage reduction, and divided dosing on a cycled regimen (113,114). Antiemetics can also be used for isolated nausea. These side effects tend to diminish with chronic use. Less common but more serious organ-system toxicities include those in the hematologic, hepatic, and pulmonary systems. Rare adverse events are also reported for many other organ systems.

Bone Marrow Suppression

Bone marrow suppression can present with involvement of any of the hematopoietic lineages (lymphopenia, leukopenia, megaloblastic anemia, thrombocytopenia, pancytopenia) (115). Although idiosyncratic cases have been reported, marrow suppression often occurs in the context of dietary folate insufficiency or antifolate medications such as trimethoprim-sulfamethoxazole. MTX overdosing, either from inappropriate administration (accidental daily dosing, wrong dosage administered) or from decreased renal clearance (including use in dialysis) (115,116), can also manifest with bone marrow suppression. Intrinsic renal insufficiency and administration of medications that affect renal clearance of MTX are important considerations when treating with MTX (117). Although MTX tends to elevate the erythrocyte mean corpuscular volume in a large number of patients, a marked elevation in mean corpuscular volume has been reported to predict hematologic toxicity (116,118). Acute infections with organisms, such as parvovirus, have also been associated with marrow toxicity during MTX therapy (119).

Hepatic Toxicity

Hepatic toxicity from MTX therapy was reported soon after its introduction as a therapeutic agent. There is a spectrum of histopathologic changes associated with MTX usage. The changes include fatty infiltration, necrosis, portal tract inflammation, and varying degrees of fibrosis, to the point of cirrhosis (120,121). Risk factors for hepatotoxicity with weekly administration include renal insufficiency, alcohol consumption, insulin-dependent diabetes mellitus, morbid obesity, increased age, length of MTX use, and cumulative MTX dosage (122–124). Many of these risk factors were identified in patients with psoriasis taking MTX, as frequent use of MTX for this indication preceded its use in RA. In RA, MTX therapy has been associated with a low incidence of cirrhosis (125). This finding may be due, in part, to lower dosing regimens and frequent laboratory monitoring by rheumatologists. Analysis of eight studies representing a cohort of 295 RA patients taking MTX who underwent liver biopsy before initiation of therapy demonstrated one case of cirrhosis (0.3%) and 11 incidents of mild fibrosis (4%) (125). In another series of 23 patients receiving MTX therapy for more than 10 years, there were no cases of cirrhosis (126). An analysis

TABLE 25.2. Methotrexate Use: Dosage, Contraindications, Adverse Events, and Monitoring for Methotrexate Therapy

Methotrexate Dosing	Contraindications	Common Adverse Events	Rare Adverse Events	Suggested Monitoring
Initial dose: 7.5–10.0 mg/wk Dose escalation: every 4 wk Maximal dose: 20–25 mg/wk Concomitant folic or folinic acid	Renal insufficiency Dialysis Preexisting active liver disease Underlying pulmonary disease Alcohol consumption Lack of contraception Folate deficiency Serious concomitant illness Chronic viral hepatitis (suggested)	Hepatic transaminase elevation Gastrointestinal intolerance: stomatitis, nausea, diarrhea Alopecia Weight loss Fatigue Headache	Pulmonary toxicity Lymphoma Oligospermia Opportunistic infection Bone marrow suppression Hepatic fibrosis	Baseline Complete blood cell count Creatinine Hepatic transaminases Serum albumin Alkaline phosphatase Viral hepatitis serologies Consider chest radiograph Serially Complete blood cell count Creatinine Hepatic transaminases Serum albumin Alkaline phosphatase

From American College of Rheumatology Subcommittee on Rheumatoid Arthritis, G2002. Guidelines for the management of rheumatoid arthritis: update. *Arthritis Rheum* 2002;46:328, with permission.

of 719 patients who underwent biopsy after 1.3 to 3.0 g of cumulative MTX showed that 14% had mild fibrosis, 6% had moderate fibrosis, and 2% had cirrhosis (125). Other studies have placed the 5-year risk of serious liver disease at less than 0.1% (122). Adherence to ACR laboratory monitoring guidelines (Table 25.2), restriction of alcohol consumption, and judicious use of liver biopsies (Table 25.3) in patients with persistent elevations in hepatic transaminases greatly diminish the risk of severe hepatic damage.

Pulmonary Toxicity

A hypersensitivity pneumonitis is associated with the use of MTX in RA; the incidence of this reaction appears to be higher in RA than in other illnesses treated with MTX. This toxicity usually occurs early in the course of therapy (mean time, 79 weeks in one study) and can be seen with any dose of MTX (127). Histologically, biopsies of involved lung demonstrate varying degrees of inflammatory infiltrates consisting of mononuclear cells, giant cells with granuloma formation, as well as bronchiolitis and fibrosis (127,128). These findings are indistinguishable from those of rheumatoid lung disease (129). The pathogenic mechanisms leading to toxicity remain poorly understood and complicated due to the difficulty of distinguishing MTX lung disease from rheumatoid lung disease. Risk factors for acute lung toxicity identified in one study were increased age, diabetes mellitus, hypoalbuminemia, and presence of underlying rheumatoid lung disease (130,131).

These analyses suggest that the presenting symptoms of pulmonary toxicity can be subtle and nonspecific (130). In 29 patients, the presenting symptom was dyspnea persisting for 3 weeks before diagnosis (130). Headaches, malaise, nonproductive cough, and fever also occurred in a subset of these patients (132,133). Chest radiographs may initially be normal, with development of bilateral interstitial infiltrates typical later in the course (132,134). Other radiographic findings include diffuse nodular infiltrates, alveolar infiltrates, hilar adenopathy, or pleural effusions. Treatment includes evaluation for infection, cessation of MTX, administration of corticosteroid therapy, and ventilatory support as needed. Of note, treatment with folic acid or folinic acid appears to have no benefit for treatment of acute pulmonary toxicity. Poor outcomes, including death, chronic dyspnea, and progression to chronic interstitial lung disease, are not infrequent. One analysis of 29 patients reported a pulmonary toxicity mortality of 17% (127). Severe underlying lung disease is a contraindication to MTX therapy in RA.

Rare Toxicities

Several organ systems affected by rare toxicities have been the subject of case reports. Skin toxicities have included alopecia, reactivation of ultraviolet light–induced erythema, and cutaneous vasculitis (135–138). Osteoporosis and fractures of bone have been reported (139), although results of trials assessing osteoporosis risk have yielded equivocal results. Reactivation of chronic viral hepatitis after MTX discontinuation has been observed (140). High-dose MTX therapy can lead to drug precipitation in the renal tubule with concomitant renal failure (141). Although this is generally not seen at doses used for RA therapy, there are reports of declines in glomerular filtration rate with MTX therapy (142). Although absent in some analyses, central nervous system toxicities, including headache, fatigue, mood alteration, dizziness, and depression, have been reported. Rarely, opportunistic infections with *Nocardia* or *Pneumocystis carinii*, fungal infections with *Cryptococcus*, and viral infections with herpes zoster have also been reported with MTX use (143–147). In addition, general systemic complaints of fever, myalgias, and polyarthralgias have been seen with MTX therapy (148).

Fertility and Pregnancy

MTX is absolutely contraindicated in pregnancy. MTX at high doses is an abortifacient (149) and, at low doses, as with other folate antagonists, is a known teratogen. Specific fetal abnormalities, including skeletal defects, hydrocephalus, cleft palate, ear malformation, and anencephaly, are teratogenic features of an entity known as *aminopterin syndrome* (150,151). Thus, extensive discussion of teratogenic risks, plans for effective contraception, and absence of pregnancy should be guaranteed before initiation of therapy in women of childbearing age. Although MTX does not appear to damage ovarian function (152), it may cause reversible defects in spermatogenesis and lead to impaired fertility in males (153,154). In planning for pregnancy, women should discontinue MTX one menstrual cycle before attempting conception to avoid teratogenesis.

TABLE 25.3. Management of Hepatic Transaminase Elevation and Liver Biopsy: Recommendations for Monitoring for Hepatic Safety in Rheumatoid Arthritis Patients Receiving Methotrexate (MTX)

A. Baseline
  1. Tests for all patients
    a. Liver blood tests [aspartate aminotransferase (AST), alanine aminotransferase, alkaline phosphatase, albumin, bilirubin], hepatitis B and C serologic studies
    b. Other standard tests, including complete blood cell count and serum creatinine
  2. Pretreatment liver biopsy (Menghini suction-type needle) only for patients with
    a. Prior excessive alcohol consumption
    b. Persistently abnormal baseline AST values
    c. Chronic hepatitis B or C infection
B. Monitor AST, alanine aminotransferase, albumin at 4- to 8-wk intervals
C. Perform liver biopsy if
  1. Five of nine determinations of AST within a given 12-mo interval (6 of 12 if tests are performed monthly) are abnormal (defined as an elevation above the upper limit of normal)
  2. There is a decrease in serum albumin below the normal range (in the setting of well-controlled rheumatoid arthritis)
D. If results of liver biopsy are
  1. Roenigk grade I, II, or IIIA, resume MTX and monitor as in B, C1, and C2
  2. Roenigk grade IIIB or IV, discontinue MTX
E. Discontinue MTX in patients with persistent liver test abnormalities, as defined in C1 and C2, who refuse liver biopsy

From Kremer JM, Alarcón GS, Lightfoot RW Jr., et al. Methotrexate for rheumatoid arthritis: suggested guidelines for monitoring liver toxicity. *Arthritis Rheum* 1994;37:316, with permission.

Lymphoma

There are no clear data implicating MTX in carcinogenesis; however, there are reports of patients developing lymphoma while taking MTX. A study of a large French cohort of approximately 30,000 RA patients on MTX noted the development of 25 cases of lymphoma (18 non-Hodgkin's and seven Hodgkin's) over a 3-year period (155). This number of lymphoma cases represented no increase over what was expected in the healthy population for non-Hodgkin's lymphoma and a slight increase relative to the healthy population for Hodgkin's disease. Another large series of 16,263 patients seen over 16 years at the Mayo Clinic noted no increased rate of malignancy in RA patients treated with MTX relative to patients treated with other DMARD medications (156). One confounding fact that must be considered in interpretation of studies assessing risk of malignancy from RA therapy is the increased rate of cancer in RA patients not on DMARD therapy (157). In none of these large studies assessing MTX-associated risk of malignancy was there control for the incidence of lymphoma in RA patients not on therapy. Although there does not appear to be an increase in the rate of malignancy with MTX therapy in RA, there has been observed an unusual type of lymphoma with MTX therapy. These lymphomas are similar to those seen with cyclosporine and azathioprine, the occurrence of which has been termed the *posttransplant lymphoproliferative syndrome* (158).

Some atypical features of the lymphomas seen with MTX include extranodal location and a high rate of Epstein-Barr virus infection in the tumor cells (155). For a significant subset of these tumors, withdrawal of MTX was sufficient to cause tumor regression (155,159,160). Whether this tumor regression represents a direct oncogenic effect of MTX or an indirect effect due to immunosuppression or another undetermined cause remains unknown. Clinically, physicians need to be aware of the possibility of lymphoma development. On diagnosis of lymphoma, documentation of tumor Epstein-Barr virus status should be performed and, if positive for Epstein-Barr virus, consideration given for delaying lymphoma-directed therapy for a period of up to 6 weeks to allow for potential spontaneous regression.

Clinical Use

Although the selection of DMARD therapy for RA should be individualized, MTX therapy should be considered for any patient with active RA—even late in the disease process. Initial low dosing in the range of 7.5 to 10.0 mg per week is recommended with subsequent dose escalation as tolerated to maximal efficacy up to a dose of 15 to 25 mg per week (average maximal dose, 20 mg per week). After escalation to maximal dosing, at least 6 weeks must elapse before final therapeutic benefit can be assessed. In patients with active disease, the dose is usually started at 7.5 mg per week at our institution, increased at week 4 (if no adverse events) to 15 mg per week, and increased at week 8 to 20 mg per week. This way, it is known within 3 months whether MTX will be effective or whether another agent should be tried or added to MTX. To prevent the onset of toxicity and reduce adverse events, concomitant administration of folic acid at a dosage of 1 mg per day should be initiated coincident with MTX; the addition of folic acid appears to have no effect on efficacy (25,113,114,161). If side effects develop or persist, increasing the dose of folate to 2 to 5 mg per day or switching to weekly administration of folinic acid (starting dose, 5 mg), 8 to 12 hours after administration of MTX, is recommended. Contraindications to MTX therapy include renal insufficiency, dialysis, active liver disease, inability to cease alcohol consumption, untreated folate deficiency, serious concomitant medical illness, planned conception or lack of adequate contraception, and noncompliance. There exists controversy regarding dosing of MTX during the surgical period. At our institution, we suspend MTX dosing the week of surgery and 1 week postoperatively and resume when the patient is medically stable.

The safety of MTX use in patients with chronic viral hepatitis remains unknown. Although case reports of fulminant hepatitis on cessation of MTX therapy in patients with chronic viral hepatitis (B or C) infections have been published (140,162), there exist no large clinical trials addressing this issue. Thus, the use of MTX therapy in patients with chronic hepatitis B or hepatitis C infection remains a relative contraindication, with differing opinions about usage among experts. We do not use MTX in this setting, but other rheumatologists do—in which case, consultation with a gastroenterologist for consideration of pretreatment liver biopsy in patients with persistent antigenemia for either hepatitis B or C is recommended (125). Detailed explanation to the patient regarding potential side effects, the rationale for laboratory screening, and securing a commitment to regular laboratory tests and physician evaluation is highly recommended.

ACR guidelines for laboratory evaluation before initiation of MTX therapy includes baseline hepatic transaminases (alanine aminotransferase, aspartate aminotransferase), alkaline phosphatase, serum albumin, hepatitis B and C serologies, complete blood cell count (CBC), and serum creatinine (4). A baseline chest radiograph within the previous 12 months should be considered, particularly in patients with underlying lung disease. After initiation of therapy, monthly screening laboratories including CBC, creatinine, and liver function tests (alanine aminotransferase, aspartate aminotransferase, alkaline phosphatase, and albumin) are mandated for the first 6 months and then every 4 to 8 weeks thereafter. Guidelines for management of transaminase elevations have also been published by the ACR (Tables 25.2 and 25.3) (125,163).

AZATHIOPRINE

Structure

Azathioprine [6-(1-methyl-4-nitroimidazol-5-yl)thio] is a prodrug with an imidazole ring attached to its active metabolite 6-mercaptopurine (6-MP) (Fig. 25.3).

Pharmacology

PHARMACOKINETICS AND PHARMACODYNAMICS

Azathioprine is variably absorbed after oral ingestion (164), with an average bioavailability of 47%. This variable absorption may account for much of the interindividual variability in efficacy and toxicity seen in therapy. After absorption, the drug is rapidly distributed into a volume of 4 to 8 L. Plasma levels peak within 2 hours, with a serum half-life of 3 hours and a biologic half-life of 24 hours (165). Protein binding occurs at a level of 30% (165). Azathioprine is extensively metabolized with urinary excretion of less than 2% unmetabolized drug (166). The majority of azathioprine is excreted renally in the form of various metabolites (166). Because the biologic half-lives of the active intracellular metabolites of azathioprine are approximately 2 weeks, with little change in concentration during a 24-hour dosing interval, monitoring of serum levels is not effective (167–169).

METABOLISM

Azathioprine first undergoes chemical (not enzymatic) nucleophilic attack at the 5 position of the nitroimidazole ring by sulfhydryl containing compounds (166) to an active metabolite, 6-MP. This conversion occurs in the blood due to glutathione activity in red blood cells. Further metabolism of 6-MP is extensive (Figs. 25.3 and 25.4). 6-MP is taken up into cells where it undergoes enzymatic conversion to one of three metabolites: (a) 6-methylmercaptopurine via the enzyme thiopurine methyltransferase (TPMT), (b) 6-methylthiouric acid via the enzyme xanthine oxidase, or (c) 6-thiopurine nucleotides via the enzyme hypoxanthine-guanine phosphoribosyltransferase (164,170) (Fig. 25.3). Of these metabolites, only the 6-thiopurine nucleotides are thought to mediate biologic activity in RA (171). There exist genetic polymorphisms in the TPMT enzyme that can dramatically affect metabolism, and, thus, toxicity, of azathioprine (172–174). Population analysis has suggested that 90% of individuals have high TPMT activity, 10% have intermediate activity, and 0.3% have low or no activity (175). These findings have led some authorities to suggest measuring TPMT levels before initiation of azathioprine therapy (172). The inhibition of xanthine oxidase by allopurinol can also dramatically decrease rates of metabolism of azathioprine, leading to severe toxicities. This drug interaction arises frequently when caring for patients with solid organ transplants and coexistent gout. The coadministration of allopurinol and azathioprine should be avoided if possible. If there exist no other therapeutic options, reduction of azathioprine dosage and extreme care in follow-up laboratory monitoring must accompany initiation of allopurinol therapy in a patient taking azathioprine.

Mechanism of Action

The exact mechanism of action of azathioprine remains unclear. The immunosuppressive effects are probably mediated by the 6-thiopurine metabolites (171). 6-thioinosinic acid (6-IMP) blocks the synthesis of the purine bases and prevents the metabolic interconversion of purine bases, particularly inosinic to guanylic acid. Furthermore, by mimicking IMP, 6-IMP acts as a negative feedback regulator of purine synthesis. A separate pathway of action of azathioprine is the conversion of 6-MP to 6-thioguanine (176). Thioguanine, when incorporated into RNA or DNA, acts as a

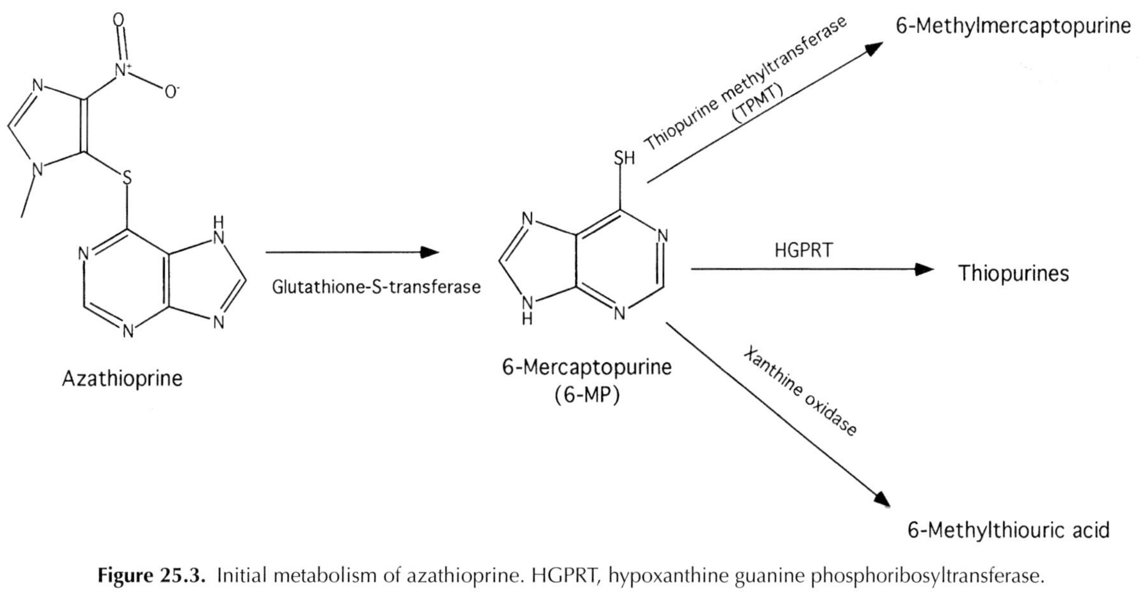

Figure 25.3. Initial metabolism of azathioprine. HGPRT, hypoxanthine guanine phosphoribosyltransferase.

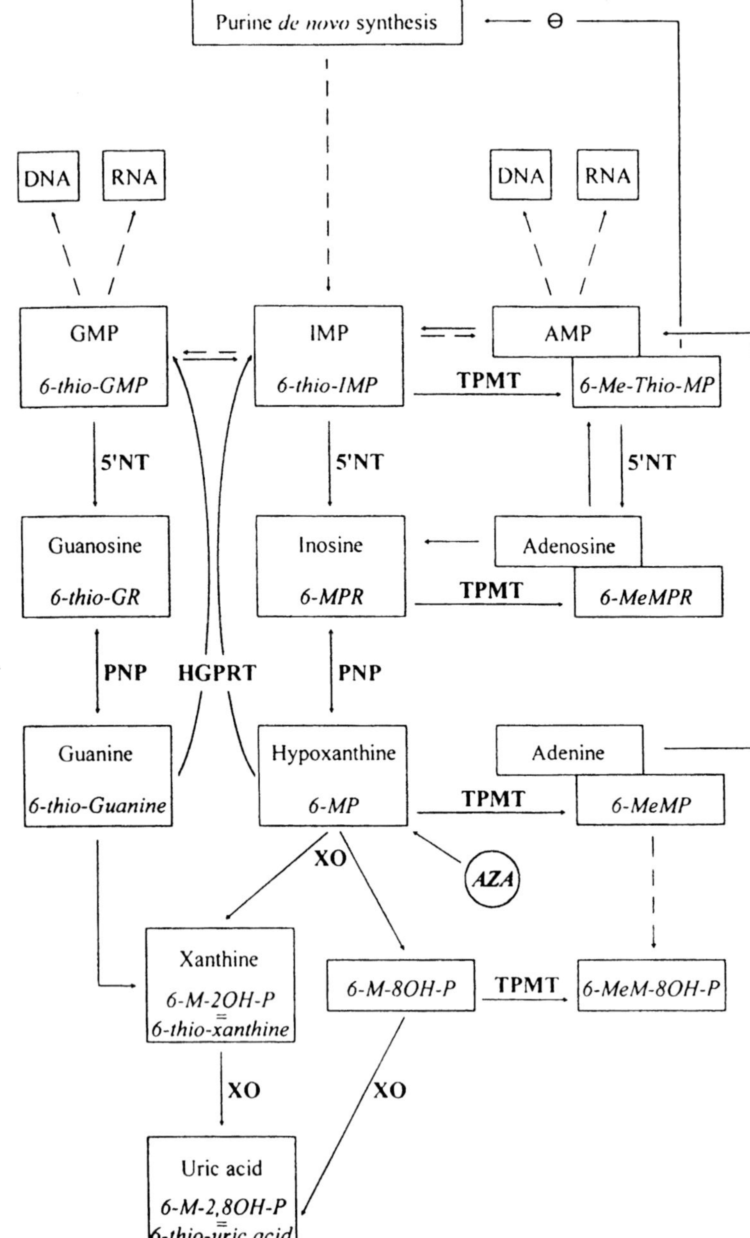

Figure 25.4. Azathioprine (AZA) and purine metabolism and mechanism of action. AMP, adenosine monophosphate; GMP, guanosine monophosphate; HGPRT, hypoxanthine guanine phosphoribosyltransferase; IMP, inosine monophosphate; 6-MeMPR, 6-methyl-mercaptopurine ribonucleoside; 6-MeM-8OH-P, 6-methylmercapto-8-hydroxy-purine; 6-Me-Thio-MP, 6-methyl-thio-mercaptopurine; 6-M-2OH-P, 6-mercapto-2-hydroxy-purine; 6-M-2,8OH-P, 6-mercapto-2, 8-dihydroxy-purine; 6-M-8OH-P, 6-mercapto-8-hydroxy-purine; 6-MPR, 6-mercaptopurine ribonucleoside; 5'NT, 5'-nucleotidase; PNP, purine nucleoside phosphorylase; 6-thio-GR, 6-thio-guanosine ribonucleoside; TPMT, thiopurine methyltransferase; XO, xanthine. (From Stolk JN, Boerbooms AM, de Abreu RA, et al. Reduced thiopurine methyltransferase activity and development of side effects of azathioprine treatment in patients with rheumatoid arthritis. *Arthritis Rheum* 1998;41: 1858, with permission.)

potent immunosuppressive (177). Some of the bone marrow toxicity of azathioprine has also been attributed to thioguanine (178).

Pivotal Trial Results

Monotherapy with azathioprine demonstrates clear efficacy relative to placebo (88,179–183). In general, these treatment responses are inferior to MTX, with greater incidence of toxic side effects (72–74,76). Response rates are similar to those seen with cyclosporine, cyclophosphamide, gold, D-penicillamine, and chloroquine, although most of these studies are limited by small sample sizes (182,184–186).

The use of azathioprine in combination therapy with other DMARDs has been studied only with MTX (89,90). The results of these trials suggest no benefit over monotherapy with MTX alone.

Toxicity

Poor tolerance of azathioprine therapy is one of the main reasons for its lack of use as a therapy for RA. Up to 30% of patients discontinue use of azathioprine within the first 6 months of therapy (187–189), with higher rates of discontinuation over longer time frames (182,185,187). The most common toxicity is GI intolerance with prominent nausea, vomiting, and diarrhea (190). Hepatic toxicity, including cholestasis and transaminase elevations, can occur in 5% to 10% of patients (191,192). Hypersensitivity reactions have been documented (192). Bone marrow suppression, most frequently leukopenia, is common and often dose limiting (190,192,193). Data for the risk of neoplasm are conflicting; the risk of neoplasm in treatment of rheumatic conditions remains unclear. Reversible lymphoma has been documented during treatment for Crohn's disease (194). However, a study of 755 patients with inflammatory bowel disease treated with azathioprine failed to show an increase in neoplasms (195).

As noted earlier, coadministration of allopurinol, and, less prominently, of sulfasalazine, can increase toxicities from azathioprine dramatically and should be avoided if possible.

Clinical Use

Presently, azathioprine is used infrequently in the treatment of RA (196) and is generally reserved for those patients who are intolerant of other first-line agents. Azathioprine dosing generally begins at 50 mg daily, with increasing dose as tolerated to 2.0 to 2.5 mg per kg (150 mg) daily. The onset of action occurs over 4 months. Consideration should be given for evaluation of TPMT enzyme activity before initiation of therapy. If TPMT activity is abnormal, azathioprine use should be avoided. Laboratory monitoring of hepatic transaminases, creatinine, and CBC are mandated. Blood counts should be monitored frequently (weekly to bimonthly) while increasing the dose. CBC monitoring can be extended to monthly and other laboratory tests to every 3 months once dosing is stabilized (196).

REFERENCES

1. Farber S, Diamond LK, Mercer RD, et al. Temporary remissions in acute leukemia in children produced by folic acid antagonist, 4-aminopteroylglutamic acid (aminopterin). *N Engl J Med* 1948;238:787.
2. Gubner R, August S, Ginsberg V. Therapeutic suppression of tissue reactivity II: effect of aminopterin in rheumatoid arthritis and psoriasis. *Am J Med Sci* 1951;22:176.
3. Herman RA, Veng-Pedersen P, Hoffman J, et al. Pharmacokinetics of low-dose methotrexate in rheumatoid arthritis patients *J Pharm Sci* 1989;78:165.
4. American College of Rheumatology Subcommittee on Rheumatoid Arthritis, G2002. Guidelines for the management of rheumatoid arthritis: update. *Arthritis Rheum* 2002;46:328.
5. Edno L, Bressolle F, Gomeni R, et al. Total and free methotrexate pharmacokinetics in rheumatoid arthritis patients. *Ther Drug Monit* 1996;18:128.
6. Sinnett MJ, Groff GD, Raddatz DA, et al. Methotrexate pharmacokinetics in patients with rheumatoid arthritis. *J Rheumatol* 1989;16:745.
7. Marshall PS, Gertner E. Oral administration of an easily prepared solution of injectable methotrexate diluted in water: a comparison of serum concentrations vs. methotrexate tablets and clinical utility. *J Rheumatol* 1996;23:455.
8. Jundt JW, Browne BA, Fiocco GP, et al. A comparison of low dose methotrexate bioavailability: oral solution, oral tablet, subcutaneous and intramuscular dosing. *J Rheumatol* 1993;20:1845.
9. Kozlowski GD, DeVito JM, Kisicki JC, Johnson JB. The effect of food on the absorption of methotrexate sodium tablets in healthy volunteers. *Arthritis Rheum* 1992;35:761.
10. Hamilton RA, Kremer JM. The effects of food on methotrexate absorption *J Rheumatol* 1995;22:630.
11. Campbell MA, Perrier DG, Dorr RT, et al. Methotrexate: bioavailability and pharmacokinetics. *Cancer Treat Rep* 1985;69:833.
12. Brooks PJ, Spruill WJ, Parish RC, Birchmore DA. Pharmacokinetics of methotrexate administered by intramuscular and subcutaneous injections in patients with rheumatoid arthritis. *Arthritis Rheum* 1990;33:91.
13. Edelman J, Biggs DF, Jamali F, Russell AS. Low-dose methotrexate kinetics in arthritis. *Clin Pharmacol Ther* 1984;35:382.
14. Liegler DG, Henderson ES, Hahn MA, Oliverio VT. The effect of organic acids on renal clearance of methotrexate in man. *Clin Pharmacol Ther* 1969;10:849.
15. Huffman DH, Wan SH, Azarnoff DL, Hogstraten B. Pharmacokinetics of methotrexate. *Clin Pharmacol Ther* 1973;14:572.
16. Nuernberg B, Koehnke R, Solsky M, et al. Biliary elimination of low-dose methotrexate in humans. *Arthritis Rheum* 1990;33:898.
17. Yamamoto K, Sawada Y, Matsushita Y, et al. Delayed elimination of methotrexate associated with piperacillin administration. *Ann Pharmacother* 1997;31:1261.
18. Bourke RS, Chheda G, Bremer A, et al. Inhibition of renal tubular transport of methotrexate by probenecid. *Cancer Res* 1975;35:110.
19. Thyss A, Milano G, Kubar J, et al. Clinical and pharmacokinetic evidence of a life-threatening interaction between methotrexate and ketoprofen. *Lancet* 1986;1:256.
20. Anonymous. The effect of age and renal function on the efficacy and toxicity of methotrexate in rheumatoid arthritis. Rheumatoid Arthritis Clinical Trial Archive Group. *J Rheumatol* 1995;22:218.
21. Bleyer WA. The clinical pharmacology of methotrexate: new applications of an old drug. *Cancer* 1978;41:36.
22. Jacobs SA, Stoller RG, Chabner BA, Johns DG. 7-Hydroxymethotrexate as a urinary metabolite in human subjects and rhesus monkeys receiving high dose methotrexate. *J Clin Invest* 1976;57:534.
23. Goldman ID. The characteristics of the membrane transport of amethopterin and the naturally occurring folates. *Ann N Y Acad Sci* 1971;186:400.
24. Morgan SL, Baggott JE, Vaughn WH, et al. The effect of folic acid supplementation on the toxicity of low-dose methotrexate in patients with rheumatoid arthritis. *Arthritis Rheum* 1990;33:9.
25. Morgan SL, Baggott JE, Vaughn WH, et al. Supplementation with folic acid during methotrexate therapy for rheumatoid arthritis. A double-blind, placebo-controlled trial. *Ann Intern Med* 1994;121:833.
26. Schuerwegh AJ, Fvan Offel J, Bridts CH, et al. Influence of longterm therapy with methotrexate and low dose corticosteroids on type 1 and type 2 cytokine production in CD4+ and CD8+ T lymphocytes of patients with rheumatoid arthritis. *J Rheumatol* 2001;28:1793.
27. Weinblatt ME, Coblyn JS, Fox DA, et al. Efficacy of low-dose methotrexate in rheumatoid arthritis. *N Engl J Med* 1985;312:818.
28. McGuire JJ, Bertino JR. Enzymatic synthesis and function of folylpolyglutamates. *Mol Cell Biochem* 1981;38:19.
29. Chabner BA, Allegra CJ, Curt GA, et al. Polyglutamation of methotrexate. Is methotrexate a prodrug? *J Clin Invest* 1985;76:907.
30. Jolivet J, Chabner BA. Intracellular pharmacokinetics of methotrexate polyglutamates in human breast cancer cells. Selective retention and less dissociable binding of 4-NH2-10-CH3-pteroylglutamate4 and 4-NH2-10-CH3-pteroylglutamate5 to dihydrofolate reductase. *J Clin Invest* 1983;72:773.
31. Allegra CJ, Drake JC, Jolivet J, Chabner BA. Inhibition of phosphoribosylaminoimidazolecarboxamide transformylase by methotrexate and dihydrofolic acid polyglutamates. *Proc Natl Acad Sci U S A* 1985;82:4881.
32. Baggott JE, Vaughn WH, Hudson BB. Inhibition of 5-aminoimidazole-4-carboxamide ribotide transformylase, adenosine deaminase and 5'-adenylate deaminase by polyglutamates of methotrexate and oxidized folates and by 5-aminoimidazole-4-carboxamide riboside and ribotide. *Biochem J* 1986;236:193.
33. Allegra CJ, Chabner BA, Drake JC, et al. Enhanced inhibition of thymidylate synthase by methotrexate polyglutamates. *J Biol Chem* 1985;260:9720.
34. Barrera P, Boerbooms AM, Janssen EM, et al. Circulating soluble tumor necrosis factor receptors, interleukin-2 receptors, tumor necrosis factor alpha, and interleukin-6 levels in rheumatoid arthritis. Longitudinal evaluation during methotrexate and azathioprine therapy. *Arthritis Rheum* 1993;36:1070.
35. Thomas R, Carroll GJ. Reduction of leukocyte and interleukin-1 beta concentrations in the synovial fluid of rheumatoid arthritis patients treated with methotrexate. *Arthritis Rheum* 1993;36:1244.
36. Segal R, Mozes E, Yaron M, Tartakovsky B. The effects of methotrexate on the production and activity of interleukin-1. *Arthritis Rheum* 1989;32:370.
37. Crilly A, McInness IB, McDonald AG, et al. Interleukin 6 (IL-6) and soluble IL-2 receptor levels in patients with rheumatoid arthritis treated with low dose oral methotrexate. *J Rheumatol* 1995;22:224.
38. Segal R, Caspi D, Tishler M, et al. Short term effects of low dose methotrexate on the acute phase reaction in patients with rheumatoid arthritis. *J Rheumatol* 1989;16:914.
39. Alarcon GS, Schrohenloher RE, Bartolucci AA, et al. Suppression of rheumatoid factor production by methotrexate in patients with rheumatoid arthritis. Evidence for differential influences of therapy and clinical status on IgM and IgA rheumatoid factor expression. *Arthritis Rheum* 1990;33:1156.
40. Sperling R, Benincaso AI, Austen KF, et al. Effects of methotrexate therapy on 5-lipoxygenase pathway metabolism of arachidonic acid in rheumatoid arthritis. *Arthritis Rheum* 1990;33:S38.
41. Olsen NJ, Callahan LF, Pincus T. Immunologic studies of rheumatoid arthritis patients treated with methotrexate. *Arthritis Rheum* 1987;30:481.
42. Constantin A, Loubet-Lescoulié P, Lambert N, et al. Antiinflammatory and immunoregulatory action of methotrexate in the treatment of rheumatoid arthritis—evidence of increased interleukin-4 and interleukin-10 gene expression demonstrated in vitro by competitive reverse transcriptase polymerase chain reaction. *Arthritis Rheum* 1998;41:48.
43. Cronstein BN. Molecular therapeutics. Methotrexate and its mechanism of action. *Arthritis Rheum* 1996;39:1951.
44. Kremer JM. Methotrexate and leflunomide: biochemical basis for combination therapy in the treatment of rheumatoid arthritis. *Semin Arthritis Rheum* 1999;29:14.
45. Gruber HE, Hoffer ME, McAllister DR, et al. Increased adenosine concentration in blood from ischemic myocardium by AICA riboside. Effects on flow, granulocytes, and injury. *Circulation* 1989;80:1400.
46. Cronstein BN, Eberle MA, Gruber HE, Levin RI. Methotrexate inhibits neutrophil function by stimulating adenosine release from connective tissue cells. *Proc Natl Acad Sci U S A* 1991;88:2441.
47. Morabito L, Montesinos MC, Schreibman DM, et al. Methotrexate and sulfasalazine promote adenosine release by a mechanism that requires ecto-5'-nucleotidase-mediated conversion of adenine nucleotides. *J Clin Invest* 1998;101:295.
48. Cronstein BN, Naime D, Ostad E. The antiinflammatory mechanism of methotrexate. Increased adenosine release at inflamed sites diminishes leukocyte accumulation in an in vivo model of inflammation. *J Clin Invest* 1993;92:2675.
49. Hoffmeister RT. Methotrexate therapy in rheumatoid arthritis: 15 years experience. *Am J Med* 1983;75:69.
50. Michaels RM, Nashel DJ, Leonard A, et al. Weekly intravenous methotrexate in the treatment of rheumatoid arthritis. *Arthritis Rheum* 1982;25:339.
51. Steinsson K, Weinstein A, Korn J, Abeles M. Low dose methotrexate in rheumatoid arthritis. *J Rheumatol* 1982;9:860.
52. Willkens RF, Watson MA, Paxson CS. Low dose pulse methotrexate therapy in rheumatoid arthritis. *J Rheumatol* 1980;7:501.

53. Groff GD, Shenberger KN, Wilke WS, Taylor TH. Low dose oral methotrexate in rheumatoid arthritis: an uncontrolled trial and review of the literature. *Semin Arthritis Rheum* 1983;12:333.
54. Williams HJ, Willkens RF, Samuelson CO Jr., et al. Comparison of low-dose oral pulse methotrexate and placebo in the treatment of rheumatoid arthritis. A controlled clinical trial. *Arthritis Rheum* 1985;28:721.
55. Andersen PA, West SG, O'Dell JR, et al. Weekly pulse methotrexate in rheumatoid arthritis. Clinical and immunologic effects in a randomized, double-blind study. *Ann Intern Med* 1985;103:489.
56. Thompson RN, Watts C, Edelman J, et al. A controlled two-centre trial of parenteral methotrexate therapy for refractory rheumatoid arthritis. *J Rheumatol* 1984;11:760.
57. Weinblatt ME, Kaplan H, Germain BF, et al. Low-dose methotrexate compared with auranofin in adult rheumatoid arthritis. A thirty-six-week, double-blind trial. *Arthritis Rheum* 1990;33:330.
58. Weinblatt ME, Kaplan H, Germain BF, et al. Methotrexate in rheumatoid arthritis: a five year prospective multicenter trial. *Arthritis Rheum* 1994;37:1492.
59. Weinblatt ME, Maier AL, Fraser PA, Coblyn JS. Longterm prospective study of methotrexate in rheumatoid arthritis: conclusion after 132 months of therapy. *J Rheumatol* 1998;25:238.
60. Kremer JM. Safety, efficacy, and mortality in a long-term cohort of patients with rheumatoid arthritis taking methotrexate: followup after a mean of 13.3 years. *Arthritis Rheum* 1997;40:984.
61. Tugwell P, Wells G, Strand V, et al. Clinical improvement as reflected in measures of function and health-related quality of life following treatment with leflunomide compared with methotrexate in patients with rheumatoid arthritis—sensitivity and relative efficiency to detect a treatment effect in a twelve-month, placebo-controlled trial. *Arthritis Rheum* 2000;43:506.
62. Weinblatt ME, Polisson R, Blotner SD, et al. The effects of drug therapy on radiographic progression of rheumatoid arthritis: results of a 36-week randomized trial comparing methotrexate and auranofin. *Arthritis Rheum* 1993;36:613.
63. Sharp JT, Strand V, Leung H, et al. Treatment with leflunomide slows radiographic progression of rheumatoid arthritis—results from three randomized controlled trials of leflunomide in patients with active rheumatoid arthritis. *Arthritis Rheum* 2000;43:495.
64. Wluka A, Buchbinder R, Mylvaganam A, et al. Longterm methotrexate use in rheumatoid arthritis: 12 year followup of 460 patients treated in community practice. *J Rheumatol* 2000;27:1864.
65. Rau R, Schleusser B, Herborn G, Karger T. Longterm treatment of destructive rheumatoid arthritis with methotrexate. *J Rheumatol* 1997;24:1881.
66. Weinstein A, Marlowe S, Korn J, Farouhar R. Low dose methotrexate treatment of rheumatoid arthritis: long term observations. *Am J Med* 1985;79:331.
67. Haagsma CJ, Lvan Riel P, de Jong AJ, van de Putte LB. Combination of sulphasalazine and methotrexate versus the single components in early rheumatoid arthritis: a randomized, controlled, double-blind, 52 week clinical trial. *Br J Rheumatol* 1997;36:1082.
68. O'Dell JR, Haire CE, Erikson N, et al. Treatment of rheumatoid arthritis with methotrexate alone, sulfasalazine and hydroxychloroquine, or a combination of all three medications. *N Engl J Med* 1996;334:1287.
69. Cohen S, Cannon GW, Schiff M, et al. Two-year, blinded, randomized, controlled trial of treatment of active rheumatoid arthritis with leflunomide compared with methotrexate. *Arthritis Rheum* 2001;44:1984.
70. Emery P, Breedveld FC, Lemmel EM, et al. A comparison of the efficacy and safety of leflunomide and methotrexate for the treatment of rheumatoid arthritis. *Rheumatology* 2000;39:655.
71. Strand V, Cohen S, Schiff M, et al. Treatment of active rheumatoid arthritis with leflunomide compared with placebo and methotrexate. Leflunomide Rheumatoid Arthritis Investigators Group. *Arch Int Med* 1999;159:2542.
72. Kerstens PJ, Boerbooms AM, Jeurissen ME, et al. Radiological and clinical results of longterm treatment of rheumatoid arthritis with methotrexate and azathioprine. *J Rheumatol* 2000;27:1148.
73. Kerstens PJ, Stolk JN, Ade Abreu R, et al. Azathioprine-related bone marrow toxicity and low activities of purine enzymes in patients with rheumatoid arthritis. *Arthritis Rheum* 1995;38:142.
74. Hamdy H, McKendry RJ, Mierins E, Liver JA. Low-dose methotrexate compared with azathioprine in the treatment of rheumatoid arthritis. A twenty-four-week controlled clinical trial. *Arthritis Rheum* 1987;30:361.
75. Arnold MH, O'Callaghan J, McCredie M, et al. Comparative controlled trial of low-dose weekly methotrexate versus azathioprine in rheumatoid arthritis: 3-year prospective study. *Br J Rheumatol* 1990;29:120.
76. Jeurissen ME, Boerbooms AM, van de Putte LB, et al. Methotrexate versus azathioprine in the treatment of rheumatoid arthritis. A forty-eight-week randomized, double-blind trial. *Arthritis Rheum* 1991;34:961.
77. Rau R, Herborn G, Menninger H, Blechschmidt J. Comparison of intramuscular methotrexate and gold sodium thiomalate in the treatment of early erosive rheumatoid arthritis: 12 month data of a double-blind parallel study of 174 patients. *Br J Rheumatol* 1997;36:345.
78. Morassut P, Goldstein R, Cyr M, et al. Gold sodium thiomalate compared to low dose methotrexate in the treatment of rheumatoid arthritis—a randomized, double blind 26-week trial. *J Rheumatol* 1989;16:302.
79. Suarez-Almazor ME, Fitzgerald A, Grace M, Russell AS. A randomized controlled trial of parenteral methotrexate compared with sodium aurothiomalate (Myochrysine) in the treatment of rheumatoid arthritis. *J Rheumatol* 1988;15:753.
80. Rau R, Herborn G, Karger T, et al. A double blind randomized parallel trial of intramuscular methotrexate and gold sodium thiomalate in early erosive rheumatoid arthritis. *J Rheumatol* 1991;18:328.
81. Williams HJ, Ward JR, Reading JC, et al. Comparison of auranofin, methotrexate, and the combination of both in the treatment of rheumatoid arthritis: a controlled clinical trial. *Arthritis Rheum* 1992;35:259.
82. Finck BK, Martin R, Fleischmann R, et al. A phase III trial of etanercept vs. methotrexate in early rheumatoid arthritis (Enbrel ERA trial). *Arthritis Rheum* 1999;42[Suppl]:S117.
83. Bathon JM, Martin RW, Fleischmann RM, et al. A comparison of etanercept and methotrexate in patients with early rheumatoid arthritis. *N Engl J Med* 2000;343:1586.
84. Genovese MC, Bathon J, Martin RW, et al. Etancercept versus methotrexate in patients with early rheumatoid arthritis. *Arthritis Rheum* 2002;46:1443.
85. Strand V, Cohen S, Schiff M, et al. Treatment of active rheumatoid arthritis with leflunomide compared with placebo and methotrexate. *Arch Int Med* 1999;159:2542.
86. Rau R, Herborn G, Karger T, Werdier D. Retardation of radiologic progression in rheumatoid arthritis with methotrexate therapy. A controlled study. *Arthritis Rheum* 1991;34:1236.
87. López-Méndez A, Daniel WW, Reading JC, et al. Radiographic assessment of disease progression in rheumatoid arthritis patients enrolled in the cooperative systematic studies of the rheumatic diseases program randomized clinical trial of methotrexate, auranofin, or a combination of the two. *Arthritis Rheum* 1993;36:1364.
88. Jeurissen ME, Boerbooms AM, van de Putte LB, et al. Influence of methotrexate and azathioprine on radiologic progression in rheumatoid arthritis. A randomized, double-blind study [see comments]. *Ann Intern Med* 1991;114:999.
89. Willkens RF, Sharp JT, Stablein D, et al. Comparison of azathioprine, methotrexate, and the combination of the two in the treatment of rheumatoid arthritis. A forty-eight-week controlled clinical trial with radiologic outcome assessment [see comments]. *Arthritis Rheum* 1995;38:1799.
90. Willkens RF, Urowitz MB, Stablein DM, et al. Comparison of azathioprine, methotrexate, and the combination of both in the treatment of rheumatoid arthritis. A controlled clinical trial [see comments]. *Arthritis Rheum* 1992;35:849.
91. Faarvang KL, Egsmose C, Kryger P, et al. Hydroxychloroquine and sulphasalazine alone and in combination in rheumatoid arthritis: a randomised double blind trial. *Ann Rheum Dis* 1993;52:711.
92. Porter DR, Capell HA, Hunter J. Combination therapy in rheumatoid arthritis—no benefit of addition of hydroxychloroquine to patients with a suboptimal response to intramuscular gold therapy. *J Rheumatol* 1993;20:645.
93. Bensen W, Tugwell P, Roberts RM, et al. Combination therapy of cyclosporine with methotrexate and gold in rheumatoid arthritis (2 pilot studies). *J Rheumatol* 1994;21:2034.
94. Tugwell P, Pincus T, Yocum D, et al. Combination therapy with cyclosporine and methotrexate in severe rheumatoid arthritis/ The Methotrexate-Cyclosporine Combination Study Group. *N Engl J Med* 1995;333:137.
95. Stein CM, Pincus T, Yocum D, et al. Combination treatment of severe rheumatoid arthritis with cyclosporine and methotrexate for forty-eight weeks: an open-label extension study. The Methotrexate-Cyclosporine Combination Study Group [see comments]. *Arthritis Rheum* 1997;40:1843.
96. Maini RN, Breedveld FC, Kalden JR, et al. Therapeutic efficacy of multiple intravenous infusions of anti-tumor necrosis factor α monoclonal antibody combined with low-dose weekly methotrexate in rheumatoid arthritis. *Arthritis Rheum* 1998;41:1552.
97. Maini R, St. Clair EW, Breedveld F, et al. Infliximab (chimeric anti-tumour necrosis factor alpha monoclonal antibody) versus placebo in rheumatoid arthritis patients receiving concomitant methotrexate: a randomised phase III trial. ATTRACT Study Group. *Lancet* 1999;354:1932.
98. Lipsky PE, Mvan der Heijde D, St. Clair EW, et al. Infliximab and methotrexate in the treatment of rheumatoid arthritis. *N Engl J Med* 2000;343:1594.
99. Weinblatt ME, Kremer JM, Bankhurst AD, et al. A trial of etanercept, a recombinant tumor necrosis factor receptor:Fc fusion protein, in patients with rheumatoid arthritis receiving methotrexate. *N Engl J Med* 1999;340:253.
100. Weinblatt ME, Kremer JM, Coblyn JS, et al. Pharmacokinetics, safety, and efficacy of combination treatment with methotrexate and leflunomide in patients with active rheumatoid arthritis. *Arthritis Rheum* 1999;42:1322.
101. Boers M, Verhoeven AC, Markusse HM, et al. Randomised comparison of combined step-down prednisolone, methotrexate and sulphasalazine with sulphasalazine alone in early rheumatoid arthritis. *Lancet* 1997;350:309.
102. Möttönen T, Hannonen P, Leirisalo-Repo M, et al. Comparison of combination therapy with single-drug therapy in early rheumatoid arthritis: a randomised trial. *Lancet* 1999;353:1568.
103. Wolfe F, Mitchell DM, Sibley JT, et al. The mortality of rheumatoid arthritis. *Arthritis Rheum* 1994;37:481.
104. Prior P, Symmons DP, Scott DL, et al. Cause of death in rheumatoid arthritis. *Br J Rheumatol* 1984;23:92.
105. Erhardt CC, Mumford PA, Venables PJ, Maini RN. Factors predicting a poor life prognosis in rheumatoid arthritis: an eight year prospective study. *Ann Rheum Dis* 1989;48:7.
106. Choi HK, Hernan MA, Seeger JD, et al. Methotrexate and mortality in patients with rheumatoid arthritis: a prospective study. *Lancet* 2002;359:1173.
107. Landewe RB, Evan den Borne B, Breedveld FC, Dijkmans BA. Methotrexate effects in patients with rheumatoid arthritis with cardiovascular comorbidity. *Lancet* 2000;355:1616.
108. Krause D, Schleusser B, Herborn G, Rau R. Response to methotrexate treatment is associated with reduced mortality in patients with severe rheumatoid arthritis. *Arthritis Rheum* 2000;43:14.

109. Furst DE, Erikson N, Clute L, Koehnke R, et al. Adverse experience with methotrexate during 176 weeks of a longterm prospective trial in patients with rheumatoid arthritis. *J Rheumatol* 1990;17:1628.
110. Weinblatt ME. Toxicity of low dose methotrexate in rheumatoid arthritis. *J Rheumatol* 1985;12:35.
111. McKendry RJ, Cyr M. Toxicity of methotrexate compared with azathioprine in the treatment of rheumatoid arthritis. A case-control study of 131 patients. *Arch Intern Med* 1989;149:685.
112. Gispen JG, Alarcon GS, Johnson JJ, et al. Toxicity of methotrexate in rheumatoid arthritis. *J Rheumatol* 1987;14:74.
113. Ortiz Z, Shea B, Suarez-Almazor ME, et al. The efficacy of folic acid and folinic acid in reducing methotrexate gastrointestinal toxicity in rheumatoid arthritis. A metaanalysis of randomized controlled trials. *J Rheumatol* 1998;25:36.
114. Shiroky JB, Neville C, Esdaile JM, et al. Low-dose methotrexate with leucovorin (folinic acid) in the management of rheumatoid arthritis. Results of a multicenter randomized, double-blind, placebo-controlled trial. *Arthritis Rheum* 1993;36:795.
115. Gutierrez-Urena S, Molina JF, Garcia CO, et al. Pancytopenia secondary to methotrexate therapy in rheumatoid arthritis. *Arthritis Rheum* 1996;39:272.
116. al-Awadhi A, Dale P, McKendry RJ. Pancytopenia associated with low dose methotrexate therapy. A regional survey. *J Rheumatol* 1993;20:1121.
117. Ellman MH, Ginsberg D. Low-dose methotrexate and severe neutropenia in patients undergoing renal dialysis. *Arthritis Rheum* 1990;33:1060.
118. Weinblatt ME, Fraser P. Elevated mean corpuscular volume as a predictor of hematologic toxicity due to methotrexate therapy. *Arthritis Rheum* 1989;32:1592.
119. Naides SJ. Acute parvovirus B19-induced pancytopenia in the setting of methotrexate therapy for rheumatoid arthritis. *Arthritis Rheum* 1995;38:1023.
120. Roenigk HH Jr, Auerbach R, Maibach HI, Weinstein GD. Methotrexate guidelines—revised. *J Am Acad Dermatol* 1982;6:145.
121. Kremer JM, Lee RG, Tolman KG. Liver histology in rheumatoid arthritis patients receiving long-term methotrexate therapy. A prospective study with baseline and sequential biopsy samples. *Arthritis Rheum* 1989;32:121.
122. Walker AM, Funch D, Dreyer NA, et al. Determinants of serious liver disease among patients receiving low-dose methotrexate for rheumatoid arthritis. *Arthritis Rheum* 1993;36:329.
123. Roenigk HH Jr, Maibach HI, Weinstein GD. Use of methotrexate in psoriasis. *Arch Dermatol* 1972;105:363.
124. Whiting-O'Keefe QE, Fye KH, Sack KD. Methotrexate and histologic hepatic abnormalities: a meta-analysis. *Am J Med* 1991;90:711.
125. Kremer JM, Alarcón GS, Lightfoot RW Jr., et al. Methotrexate for rheumatoid arthritis: suggested guidelines for monitoring liver toxicity. *Arthritis Rheum* 1994;37:316.
126. Aponte J, Petrelli M. Histopathologic findings in the liver of rheumatoid arthritis patients treated with long-term bolus methotrexate. *Arthritis Rheum* 1988;31:1457.
127. Kremer JM, Alarcon GS, Weinblatt ME, et al. Clinical, laboratory, radiographic, and histopathologic features of methotrexate-associated lung injury in patients with rheumatoid arthritis: a multicenter study with literature review. *Arthritis Rheum* 1997;40:1829.
128. Smith GJ. The histopathology of pulmonary reactions to drugs. *Clin Chest Med* 1990;11:95.
129. Yousem SA, Colby TV, Carrington CB. Lung biopsy in rheumatoid arthritis. *Am Rev Resp Dis* 1985;131:770.
130. Alarcon GS, Kremer JM, Macaluso M, et al. Risk factors for methotrexate-induced lung injury in patients with rheumatoid arthritis. A multicenter, case-control study. Methotrexate-Lung Study Group. *Ann Intern Med* 1997; 127:356.
131. Ohosone Y, Okano Y, Kameda H, et al. Clinical characteristics of patients with rheumatoid arthritis and methotrexate induced pneumonitis. *J Rheumatol* 1997;24:2299.
132. Sostman HD, Matthay RA, Putman CE, Smith GJ. Methotrexate-induced pneumonitis. *Medicine* 1976;55:371.
133. Carson CW, Cannon GW, Egger MJ, et al. Pulmonary disease during the treatment of rheumatoid arthritis with low dose pulse methotrexate. *Semin Arthritis Rheum* 1987;16:186.
134. Cannon GW, Ward JR, Clegg DO, et al. Acute lung disease associated with low-dose pulse methotrexate therapy in patients with rheumatoid arthritis. *Arthritis Rheum* 1983;26:1269.
135. Armstrong RB, Poh-Fitzpatrick MB. Methotrexate and ultraviolet radiation. *Arch Dermatol* 1982;118:177.
136. Marks CR, Willkens RF, Wilske KR, Brown PB. Small-vessel vasculitis and methotrexate. *Ann Intern Med* 1984;100:916.
137. Navarro M, Pedragosa R, Lafuerza A, et al. Leukocytoclastic vasculitis after high-dose methotrexate. *Ann Intern Med* 1986;105:471.
138. Weinblatt ME. Toxicity of low dose methotrexate in rheumatoid arthritis. *J Rheumatol* 1985;12 [Suppl]:35.
139. Maenaut K, Westhovens R, Dequeker J. Methotrexate osteopathy, does it exist? *J Rheumatol* 1996;23:2156.
140. Ito S, Nakazono K, Murasawa A, et al. Development of fulminant hepatitis B (precore variant mutant type) after the discontinuation of low-dose methotrexate therapy in a rheumatoid arthritis patient. *Arthritis Rheum* 2001;44:339.
141. Perazella MA. Crystal-induced acute renal failure. *Am J Med* 1999;106:459.
142. Kremer JM, Petrillo GF, Hamilton RA. Pharmacokinetics and renal function in patients with rheumatoid arthritis receiving a standard dose of oral weekly methotrexate: association with significant decreases in creatinine clearance and renal clearance of the drug after 6 months of therapy. *J Rheumatol* 1995;22:38.
143. Keegan JM, Byrd JW. Nocardiosis associated with low dose methotrexate for rheumatoid arthritis. *J Rheumatol* 1988;15:1585.
144. Perruquet JL, Harrington TM, Davis DE. *Pneumocystis carinii* pneumonia following methotrexate therapy for rheumatoid arthritis. *Arthritis Rheum* 1983;26:1291.
145. Altz-Smith M, Kendall LG Jr., Stamm AM. Cryptococcosis associated with low-dose methotrexate for arthritis. *Am J Med* 1987;83:179.
146. Ching DW. Severe, disseminated, life threatening herpes zoster infection in a patient with rheumatoid arthritis treated with methotrexate. *Ann Rheum Dis* 1995;54:155.
147. Lyon CC, Thompson D. Herpes zoster encephalomyelitis associated with low dose methotrexate for rheumatoid arthritis. *J Rheumatol* 1997;24:589.
148. Halla JT, Hardin JG. Underrecognized postdosing reactions to methotrexate in patients with rheumatoid arthritis. *J Rheumatol* 1994;21:1224.
149. Hausknecht RU. Methotrexate and misoprostol to terminate early pregnancy. *N Engl J Med* 1995;333:537.
150. Buckley LM, Bullaboy CA, Leichtman L, Marquez M. Multiple congenital anomalies associated with weekly low-dose methotrexate treatment of the mother. *Arthritis Rheum* 1997;40:971.
151. Feldkamp M, Carey JC. Clinical teratology counseling and consultation case report: low dose methotrexate exposure in the early weeks of pregnancy. *Teratology* 1993;47:533.
152. Roubenoff R, Hoyt J, Petri M, et al. Effects of antiinflammatory and immunosuppressive drugs on pregnancy and fertility. *Semin Arthritis Rheum* 1988;18:88.
153. Sussman A, Leonard JM. Psoriasis, methotrexate, and oligospermia. *Arch Dermatol* 1980;116:215.
154. Sherins RJ, DeVita VT Jr. Effect of drug treatment for lymphoma on male reproductive capacity. Studies of men in remission after therapy. *Ann Intern Med* 1973;79:216.
155. Mariette X, Cazals-Hatem D, Warszawki J, et al. Lymphomas in rheumatoid arthritis patients treated with methotrexate: a 3-year prospective study in France. *Blood* 2002;99:3909.
156. Moder KG, Tefferi A, Cohen MD, et al. Hematologic malignancies and the use of methotrexate in rheumatoid arthritis: a retrospective study. *Am J Med* 1995;99:276.
157. Symmons DP. Neoplasms of the immune system in rheumatoid arthritis. *Am J Med* 1985;78:22.
158. Kinlen LJ. Incidence of cancer in rheumatoid arthritis and other disorders after immunosuppressive treatment. *Am J Med* 1985;78:44.
159. Kamel OW, Van de Rijn M, Weiss LM, et al. Reversible lymphomas associated with Epstein-Barr virus occurring during methotrexate therapy for rheumatoid arthritis and dermatomyositis. *N Engl J Med* 1993;328:1317.
160. Salloum E, Cooper DL, Howe G, et al. Spontaneous regression of lymphoproliferative disorders in patients treated with methotrexate for rheumatoid arthritis and other rheumatic diseases. *J Clin Oncol* 1996;14:1943.
161. Weinblatt ME, Maier AL, Coblyn JS. Low dose leucovorin does not interfere with the efficacy of methotrexate in rheumatoid arthritis: an 8 week randomized placebo controlled trial. *J Rheumatol* 1993;20:950.
162. Flowers MA, Heathcote J, Wanless IR, et al. Fulminant hepatitis as a consequence of reactivation of hepatitis B virus infection after discontinuation of low-dose methotrexate therapy. *Ann Intern Med* 1990;112:381.
163. Erickson AR, Reddy V, Vogelgesang SA, West SG. Usefulness of the American College of Rheumatology recommendations for liver biopsy in methotrexate-treated rheumatoid arthritis patients. *Arthritis Rheum* 1995;38:1115.
164. Van Os EC, Zins BJ, Sandborn WJ, et al. Azathioprine pharmacokinetics after intravenous, oral, delayed release oral and rectal foam administration. *Gut* 1996;39:63.
165. Huskisson EC. Azathioprine. *Clin Rheum Dis* 1984;10:325.
166. Elion GB, Hitchings GH. Azathioprine. In: Eichler O, Farah A, Herken H, Welch AD, eds. *Handbuch der experimentellen pharmakologie (handbook of experimental pharmacology)*, vol. XXXVII/2. Berlin: Springer Verlag, 1975:404.
167. Bergan S, Rugstad HE, Bentdal O, et al. Kinetics of mercaptopurine and thioguanine nucleotides in renal transplant recipients during azathioprine treatment. *Ther Drug Monit* 1994;16:13.
168. el-Yazigi A, Wahab FA. Pharmacokinetics of azathioprine after repeated oral and single intravenous administration. *J Clin Pharmacol* 1993;33:522.
169. Chan GL, Erdmann GR, Gruber SA, et al. Azathioprine metabolism: pharmacokinetics of 6-mercaptopurine, 6-thiouric acid and 6-thioguanine nucleotides in renal transplant patients. *J Clin Pharmacol* 1990;30:358.
170. Van Scoik KG, Johnson CA, Porter WR. The pharmacology and metabolism of the thiopurine drugs 6-mercaptopurine and azathioprine. *Drug Metab Rev* 1985;16:157.
171. Bertino JR. Chemical action and pharmacology of methotrexate, azathioprine and cyclophosphamide in man. *Arthritis Rheum* 1973;16:79.
172. Stolk JN, Boerbooms AM, de Abreu RA, et al. Reduced thiopurine methyltransferase activity and development of side effects of azathioprine treatment in patients with rheumatoid arthritis. *Arthritis Rheum* 1998;41:1858.
173. Black AJ, McLeod HL, Capell HA, et al. Thiopurine methyltransferase genotype predicts therapy-limiting severe toxicity from azathioprine. *Ann Intern Med* 1998;129:716.
174. Yates CR, Krynetski EY, Loennechen T, et al. Molecular diagnosis of thiopurine S-methyltransferase deficiency: genetic basis for azathioprine and mercaptopurine intolerance. *Ann Intern Med* 1997;126:608.
175. McLeod HL, Lin JS, Scott EP, et al. Thiopurine methyltransferase activity in American white subjects and black subjects. *Clin Pharmacol Ther* 1994;55:15.
176. Dubinsky MC, Lamothe S, Yang HY, et al. Pharmacogenomics and metabolite measurement for 6-mercaptopurine therapy in inflammatory bowel disease. *Gastroenterology* 2000;118:705.

177. LePage GA. Incorporation of 6-thioguanine into nucleic acids. *Cancer Res* 1960;20:403.
178. Van Scoik KG, Johnson CA, Porter WR. The pharmacology and metabolism of the thiopurine drugs 6- mercaptopurine and azathioprine. *Drug Metab Rev* 1985;16:157.
179. Urowitz MB, Gordon DA, Smythe HA, et al. Azathioprine in rheumatoid arthritis. A double-blind, cross over study. *Arthritis Rheum* 1973;16:411.
180. Urowitz MB, Hunter T, Bookman AAM, et al. Azathioprine in rheumatoid arthritis: a double-blind study comparing full dose to half dose. *J Rheumatol* 1974;1:274.
181. Woodland J, Chaput de Saintonge DM, Evans SJ, et al. Azathioprine in rheumatoid arthritis: double-blind study of full versus half doses versus placebo. *Ann Rheum Dis* 1981;40:355.
182. Paulus HE, Williams HJ, Ward JR, et al. Azathioprine versus D-penicillamine in rheumatoid arthritis patients who have been treated unsuccessfully with gold. *Arthritis Rheum* 1984;27:721.
183. Kruger K, Schattenkirchner M. Comparison of cyclosporin A and azathioprine in the treatment of rheumatoid arthritis—results of a double-blind multicentre study. *Clin Rheumatol* 1994;13:248.
184. Dwosh IL, Stein HB, Urowitz MB, et al. Azathioprine in early rheumatoid arthritis. Comparison with gold and chloroquine. *Arthritis Rheum* 1977;20:685.
185. Berry H, Liyanage SP, Durance RA, et al. Azathioprine and penicillamine in treatment of rheumatoid arthritis: a controlled trial. *BMJ* 1976;1:1052.
186. Currey HL, Harris J, Mason RM, et al. Comparison of azathioprine, cyclophosphamide, and gold in treatment of rheumatoid arthritis. *BMJ* 1974;3:763.
187. Harris J, Jessop JD, Chaput de Saintonge DM. Further experience with azathioprine in rheumatoid arthritis. *BMJ* 1971;4:463.
188. Hunter T, Urowitz MB, Gordon DA, et al. Azathioprine in rheumatoid arthritis: a long-term follow-up study. *Arthritis Rheum* 1975;18:15.
189. Singh G, Fries JF, Spitz P, Williams CA. Toxic effects of azathioprine in rheumatoid arthritis. A national post-marketing perspective [see comments]. *Arthritis Rheum* 1989;32:837.
190. Whisnant JK, Pelkey J. Rheumatoid arthritis: treatment with azathioprine [IMURAN (R)]Clinical side-effects and laboratory abnormalities. *Ann Rheum Dis* 1982;41:44.
191. Jeurissen ME, Boerbooms AM, van de Putte LB, Kruijsen MW. Azathioprine induced fever, chills, rash, and hepatotoxicity in rheumatoid arthritis. *Ann Rheum Dis* 1990;49:25.
192. Lawson DH, Lovatt GE, Gurton CS, Hennings RC. Adverse effects of azathioprine. *Adverse Drug React Acute Poisoning Rev* 1984;3:161.
193. Jeurissen ME, Boerbooms AM, van de Putte LB. Pancytopenia related to azathioprine in rheumatoid arthritis. *Ann Rheum Dis* 1988;47:503.
194. Larvol L, Soule JC, Le Tourneau A. Reversible lymphoma in the setting of azathioprine therapy for Crohn's disease. *N Engl J Med* 1994;331:883.
195. Connell WR, Kamm MA, Dickson M, et al. Long-term neoplasia risk after azathioprine treatment in inflammatory bowel disease. *Lancet* 1994;343:1249.
196. Guidelines for the management of rheumatoid arthritis: update. *Arthritis Rheum* 2002;46:328.
197. Dougados M, Combe B, Cantagrel A, et al. Combination therapy in early rheumatoid arthritis: a randomised, controlled, double blind 52 week clinical trial of sulphasalazine and methotrexate compared with the single components. *Ann Rheum Dis* 1999;58:220.
198. Sharp JT. An overview of radiographic analysis of joint damage in rheumatoid arthritis and its use in metaanalysis. *J Rheumatol* 2000;27:254.

CHAPTER 26

Sulfasalazine

Dinesh Khanna and Daniel E. Furst

Sulfasalazine (SSZ) was designed by Nanna Svartz (1) in 1938 specifically for the treatment of rheumatoid arthritis (RA). The idea behind the creation of the drug was to combine an antibacterial agent (sulfapyridine) and an antiinflammatory agent (salicylic acid). RA was, at that time, believed to have a bacterial etiology, making the combination useful for the treatment of RA. After losing favor as a therapy for RA, SSZ has regained a key role as a disease-modifying antirheumatic drug (DMARD) (Fig. 26.1).

PHARMACOLOGY

Dosage and Administration

The dosage and administration of SSZ are as follows:

- Most common adult dosage is 2 g per day (range, 1.5–3.0 g per day).
- Enteric-coated formulation decreases gastrointestinal (GI) side effects.
- Taken as 1 g, twice a day with meals.
- To minimize the risk of intolerance, start at 500- to 1,000-mg daily dose, increasing by increments of 500 mg per day at intervals of 1 week.

Pharmacokinetics

The pharmacokinetics of SSZ have been investigated extensively in humans (2). Much of the work has been reported in patients with ulcerative colitis rather than RA.

ABSORPTION

SSZ is an azo compound of sulfapyridine and 5-aminosalicylic acid (5-ASA). The percentage of the SSZ dose absorbed as the whole compound from the small intestine is 25% to 33% (3). Detectable blood levels occur within 1 to 2 hours after ingestion of a loading dose (4). Peak plasma levels are reached after 1.5 to 6.0 hours, and the elimination half-life of SSZ is 5 to 8 hours (5).

DISTRIBUTION

Autoradiographic studies have shown a uniform pattern of distribution of SSZ (6). SSZ has a high serum protein (albumin) binding capacity (approximately 99%) (7); it binds to the warfarin site on albumin, which is also the primary binding site of bilirubin. SSZ is found in RA synovial fluid at concentrations similar to those in plasma (8). SSZ and its metabolites equilibrate freely across the human placenta in full-term pregnant women (9) (Table 26.1). Because of the risk of bilirubin displacement by the high-protein binding of SSZ, caution should be taken using SSZ during the latter part of pregnancy. SSZ passes into human milk at approximately 40% of the serum concentration (10). The mean peak serum concentration of SSZ is between 6 and 14 μg per mL, 3 hours after a single 2-g dose in tablet form (approximately 0.025–0.038 mm). Stool concentrations are approximately 1.25 to 2.0 mm (11).

METABOLISM

SSZ is absorbed via the small intestine and is returned to the colon unchanged via the bile (12) (Table 26.1). In the colon, azoreductive cleavage occurs by the intestinal bacteria, resulting in the formation of sulfapyridine and 5-ASA (13). Therefore, coliform bacteria are necessary to reduce the relatively inactive parent drug to its active moieties. Nearly all sulfapyridine is absorbed, whereas 5-ASA (67%) is largely excreted in the feces. The efficacy of SSZ in inflammatory bowel disease may be explained by the fact that 67% of 5-ASA remains in the small and large bowel (14). 5-ASA is inactivated to *N*-acetyl-5-ASA via *N*-acetyl-transferase-1 in the colonic mucosa and excreted in the urine (15). Sulfapyridine is well absorbed from the colon; it does not have beneficial effects in patients with ulcerative colitis (16). Sulfapyridine is inactivated in the liver to *N*-acetyl-sulfapyridine via *N*-acetyl-transferase-2 and, subsequently, hydroxylated and conjugated with glucuronide and excreted in the urine. The metabolism is dependent on the rate of acetylation, which is determined by genetic factors (17).

Possible Drug Interactions

Broad-spectrum antibiotics that alter gut flora may reduce the bioavailability of sulfapyridine and 5-ASA as the azo link between them is cleaved by bacterial metabolism. Concomitant use of cholestyramine is likely to reduce the availability of SSZ as it binds the drug, making it unavailable for bacterial cleavage by the gut flora (18). SSZ binds to the warfarin site on the albumin, causing displacement of warfarin and transiently increasing the prothrombin time and its anticoagulation effect (19). Rarely, SSZ can enhance the action of oral hypoglycemics by displacing them from their protein binding sites, causing life-threatening hypoglycemia in diabetics. Therefore, close monitoring of blood sugar is essential. There is theoretic concern regarding the combination use of methotrexate (MTX) and

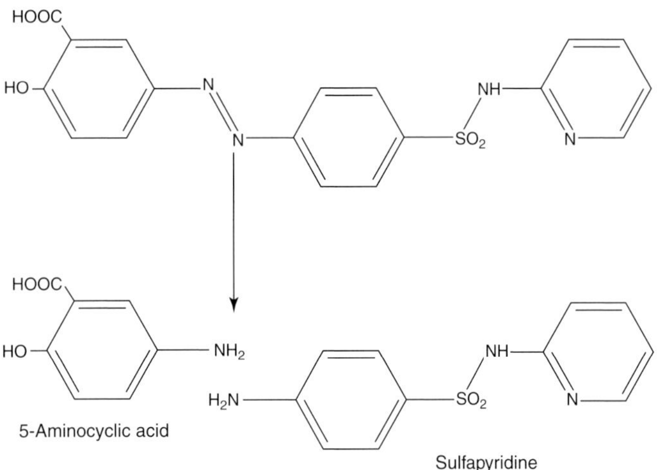

Figure 26.1. Chemical structure of sulfasalazine.

SSZ, as both act by inhibiting folate metabolism. However, combination trials have failed to show an increased risk of folate deficiency (20).

Clinical Consequences

ACTIVE MOIETY OF SULFASALAZINE IN RHEUMATOID ARTHRITIS

Studies in inflammatory bowel disease suggest that 5-ASA is the therapeutically active moiety of SSZ in that disease (21). The nature of the active moiety in RA was investigated in a placebo-controlled trial comparing 2 g per day of sulfapyridine with 1 to 2 g per day of 5-ASA (22). Clinical and laboratory improvement were found in the sulfapyridine group—indicating that it is the active agent—with mild improvement in the 5-ASA group. This observation suggested the use of sulfapyridine in preference to SSZ for treatment of RA. The efficacy of SSZ and sulfapyridine have not been compared directly, but both drugs appear to have broadly similar effects, with sulfapyridine causing more side effects—particularly nausea and vomiting—making SSZ the preferred treatment (23). It has even been suggested that SSZ is a convenient vehicle to deliver sulfapyridine to the large bowel, thus causing fewer GI symptoms. It remains unclear whether the effect of SSZ is mediated entirely through the sulfapyridine component or whether the parent molecule itself also has antirheumatic activity.

ACETYLATOR STATUS OF THE PATIENT

The percent of slow acetylators in RA patients is similar to that in the general white population (24). Fast- and slow-acetylator RA patients do not differ in age, sex, or disease characteristics. A study by Pullar et al. (25) reported a higher incidence of both efficacy and toxicity in patients who were slow acetylators. However, later studies designed to show differences in the slow and fast acetylators in terms of the efficacy and toxicity of SSZ in RA patients have been negative (26,27). Therefore, the routine measurement of the acetylator phenotype has no practical value for determining therapeutic efficacy.

MECHANISMS OF ACTION

Despite decades of research, the etiology of RA is largely unknown. As a result, evaluation of the mode of action of DMARDs can be difficult. SSZ has several biologic activities that might contribute to its beneficial clinical effects in RA (Table 26.2).

Local Gastrointestinal Effects

ANTIBACTERIAL EFFECTS

Several studies have investigated the spectrum of different microorganisms in RA patients compared to that of the healthy population (28,29), and a decrease in several species of gut flora has been observed after treatment with SSZ (30). *In vitro* studies have also shown that SSZ and its metabolites inhibit bacterial growth (31). Although the possibility that RA is an enteropathic arthropathy has been considered (32), no conclusive evidence of an infectious etiology has been presented to date. Although the metabolite sulfapyridine has antibacterial properties, the use of two other sulfonamides, sulfamethoxazole and phthalylsulfathiazole (33,34), have failed to show any clinical efficacy in RA, which argues against an enteropathic etiology of RA. This finding also argues that the mechanism of action of SSZ is not antibacterial, per se.

IMMUNOMODULATORY EFFECTS

Most *in vitro* studies of SSZ have reported immunologic effects at higher concentrations than those attained in the serum of patients

TABLE 26.1. Use of Sulfasalazine (SSZ) in Pregnancy, in Renal/Hepatic Disease, and with Other Comorbid Conditions

Pregnancy
- Category B[a]/D[b] (at term).
- Caution during third trimester due to risk of kernicterus (bilirubin displacement by SSZ).
- Excreted in breast milk (at approximately 40% of serum concentration).
- American Academy of Pediatrics guidelines suggests using SSZ "with caution."

Renal/hepatic disease
- Caution in patients with mild to moderate renal impairment.
- Avoid with a creatinine clearance of <10 mL/min.
- Caution in patients with mild to moderate hepatic disease.

Other comorbid conditions
- Avoid in patients with ileostomy.
- Avoid in patients with glucose-6-phosphate dehydrogenase deficiency (due to increased risk of hemolytic anemia).

[a]No evidence of risk in humans (either animal findings show risk with no findings in humans or, if no adequate human studies have been done, animal findings are negative).
[b]Positive evidence of risk (investigational or post-marketing data show risk to fetus). Nevertheless, potential benefits outweigh the risks.

TABLE 26.2. Mechanisms of Action of Sulfasalazine

Immunomodulation
- Inhibition of T-cell proliferation and natural killer cell activity (not at achievable therapeutic concentrations)
- Suppression of B lymphocyte function—immunoglobulins and immunoglobulin M rheumatoid factor at therapeutic concentrations
- Inhibition of macrophage activation (not at achievable therapeutic concentrations)
- Inhibition of transcription factor nuclear factor–κB
- Inhibition of proinflammatory cytokines—interleukin-1 and tumor necrosis factor α
- Inhibits components of angiogenesis

Antiinflammatory effect
- Inhibition of superoxide production by granulocytes
- Inhibition of granulocyte function, including chemotaxis, degranulation, and random migration
- Impaired folic-acid absorption in the gastrointestinal tract and inhibition of folate metabolizing enzyme—dihydrofolate reductase

Antibacterial effect
- Inhibition of bacterial growth *in vitro* and *in vivo*

receiving therapeutic doses of this agent (Table 26.3). In patients with RA, the concentration of the SSZ within the small intestine is approximately two orders of magnitude higher than serum levels. It has been suggested that these high concentrations of SSZ may suppress the activity of gut-associated lymphoid tissue, affecting lymphocyte traffic and exerting an immunomodulatory effect (35,36). One study evaluated lymphocyte subpopulations and HLA-DR expression in biopsy specimens from the duodenal–jejunal mucosa and in peripheral blood samples obtained from 17 patients with RA, both before and after 16 weeks of SSZ treatment. Samples were also obtained from controls (37). The mucosa of the small intestine in RA patients showed no differences in morphology, HLA-DR expression, or the amounts and distribution of $CD3^+$, $CD4^+$, $CD8^+$, and T-cell receptor γ/δ lymphocytes compared with the control group at second biopsy. However, there was a reduction in mucosal $CD3^+$ and T-cell receptor γ/δ lymphocyte numbers after SSZ therapy. These reductions did not correspond with a change in peripheral blood $CD3^+$ lymphocyte number, suggesting local immunoregulatory effects.

Systemic Effects

EFFECTS ON IMMUNOLOGIC FUNCTIONS

In vitro, SSZ inhibits both T-cell proliferation and natural killer cell activity at higher concentrations (38–40) (Table 26.2). The effects of SSZ and its two metabolites have been studied in cultured peripheral blood lymphocytes from patients with RA and from healthy subjects. At very high concentrations (100 µg) in one study, SSZ, but not its metabolites, inhibited mitogen-induced proliferative responses of peripheral blood lymphocytes and purified B lymphocytes. Immunoglobulin (Ig) and IgM rheumatoid factor (RF) synthesis is also depressed by SSZ in a dose-dependent manner (10–25 µg per mL), indicating an effect on B lymphocyte. Furthermore, no study has assessed the effects of SSZ and its metabolites on the function of human B cells (41). In contrast to the previous study, SSZ (1–10 µg per mL) and both its metabolites, sulfapyridine and 5-ASA, suppressed the production of Igs at pharmacologically attained concentrations. There was no suppression of T-cell function, suggesting that SSZ and its metabolites preferentially suppress B-cell function. A further immunomodulating effect of SSZ is suggested by the observed reduction in serum IgA levels in treated patients (42) and by the reduction in the number of circulating IgA-producing cells that precedes and correlates with clinical improvement (43). *In vitro*, both SSZ and sulfapyridine have been shown to inhibit activation of a mouse macrophage cell line; however, the minimal dose of SSZ needed for inhibition was 50 µg per mL, approximately five times the pharmacologically attainable concentrations (44).

Another potential mode of SSZ action is the inhibition of nuclear factor–κB (NF-κB). This factor, which is also suppressed by corticosteroids, induces the transcription of central mediators of the immune response. An *in vitro* study found that SSZ, but not its metabolites, strongly inhibited NF-κB–dependent transcription in colonic cells, suggesting important antiinflammatory properties (45). Tumor necrosis factor α–induced nuclear translocation of NF-κB was prevented by SSZ through inhibition of NF-κB inhibitor degradation. This response was achieved at approximately ten times the pharmacologically attained concentrations in the serum, although these concentrations were achievable in the intestines. NF-κB activation was blocked in response to three different stimuli, suggesting that SSZ interfered with an early common signal in these different signal transduction cascades. SSZ treatment inhibited translocation of NF-κB into the nucleus. Another study suggested that this beneficial effect may be due to induction of apoptosis and subsequent clearance of activated T lymphocytes (46). These data suggest an immunomodulatory effect on T and B cells—but only in the GI tract. In this case, an effect of SSZ in RA would have to be indirect, as noted earlier.

Part of the action of SSZ may result from the modulation of cytokine production or cytokine activity. Patients treated with SSZ show a progressive decline in serum levels of interleukin-1 and tumor necrosis factor α in association with improvement in clinical measures of disease activity (47). Because the effects on cytokines may be a reflection of disease activity, rather than the cause, this finding may not be relevant to the mechanism of action of SSZ.

Studies in collagen and antigen-induced arthritis in mice have shown significant immunosuppressive effects of SSZ by inhibiting histologic changes and cartilage destruction (48,49).

Because angiogenesis may contribute to proliferation of synovial tissue in RA, the effect of SSZ and its metabolites was assessed on the angiogenic process (50). Volin et al. (50) demonstrated that SSZ and its metabolite, sulfapyridine, may affect the pathogenesis of RA by inhibiting endothelial cell chemotaxis, proliferation, tube formation, and expression of soluble intercellular adhesion molecule-1 and interleukin-8.

ANTIINFLAMMATORY EFFECTS

SSZ inhibits various inflammatory cell functions, such as polymorphonuclear cell chemotaxis and random migration (51,52) (Table 26.2). Superoxide production and enzyme secretion are also inhibited by SSZ (53,54).

SSZ, but not its metabolites, inhibits dihydrofolate reductase (55). This effect is especially interesting, as it is shared with MTX. Its relevance to the therapeutic action of SSZ is uncertain because this enzymatic inhibition only occurs at high drug concentrations.

Despite the wealth of data describing the antibacterial, immunologic, and antiinflammatory activities of SSZ, these effects may be secondary to improvement in disease control, and it remains unclear which is responsible for its antirheumatic effects.

CLINICAL EFFICACY AND SAFETY

Placebo-Controlled Trials

Early results from Svartz's study of SSZ in the treatment of RA were encouraging, with two-thirds of more than 400 patients from a large case series judged to have a good response (56). An open-label North American study also showed positive results (57), but, in the post-war period, a negative British study report (58), along with the discovery of cortisone, eclipsed interest in SSZ for the treatment of RA. Interest in SSZ was renewed within the rheumatology community with the report of an uncontrolled study in 1978 showing marked improvement in RA patients' clinical state and improvement in laboratory indices, which persisted for 22 weeks of therapy in 78% of the patients (59). Another uncontrolled study in 74 patients from the same group 2 years later showed improvement in pain and laboratory indices at a dose of 2 g per day in active RA. The improvement lasted for a period of 52 weeks on continued SSZ therapy (60).

The first placebo-controlled trial of SSZ in modern times was conducted in 1983 (61) (Table 26.3). The trial randomized 30 patients to placebo, intramuscular gold (50 mg per week), or SSZ (3 g per day). The patients in each of the treatment groups had a median disease duration of 6 years. The SSZ group showed significant improvements in erythrocyte sedimentation rate (ESR) (–45 mm per hour), articular index (–19) and grip strength (+ 6 mm Hg), as compared to placebo. However, only

TABLE 26.3. Analysis of Pivotal Trials

Study/yr (Reference)	Type of Study	Dosage	Number of Patients Completing Study	Study Duration (wk)	Change in Tender Joints or Articular Index	Change in Swollen Joints	Change in Pain/Visual Analog Scale	Change in Physician Global Assessment	Change in Patient Global Assessment	Change in Acute Phase Reactants (Erythrocyte Sedimentation Rate)	American College of Rheumatology 20% Response
Placebo trials											
Pullar et al., 1983 (61)	SSZ	3 g/d	18	24	−18	ND	NS	ND	ND	−45	ND
	Placebo	—	19		−5.5	—	—	—	—	−4	—
Pinals et al., 1986 (62)	SSZ	3 g/d	31	15	−13	−12	−23	NS	NS	−16.2	ND
	Placebo	—	31		−8	−6	−4	—	—	−7.1	—
Australian Multicentre Study,	SSZ	2 g/d	29		−6.9	−10.4[a]	−1.2	ND	NS	−16.6	ND
1992 (63)	Placebo	—	36	24	−5	−4.3	−3.6	—	NS	−0.02	—
Hannonen et al., 1993 (64)	SSZ	2 g/d	18	48	−3.6	−2.9	−15	−0.4[b]	−0.5[b]	NI	ND
	Placebo	—	11		−0.4	0.6	−3	0	0	—	—
Smolen et al., 1999 (67)	SSZ	2 g/d	83	24[c]	−8.1	−6.2	−19.8	−1[a]	−1.1[b]	−16.6	56%
Compared to other disease-modifying antirheumatic drugs	Placebo	—	51		−4.3	−3.4	−8.8	−0.3	−0.4	3.4	29%
Haagsma et al., 1997 (81)	SSZ	2–3 g/d	22	52	−9.2	−1.8	−25.2	NI	−15.4	−17	NI
	MTX	7.5–15 mg/wk	33		−12.4	−2	−25.1	NI	−21.3	−21	NI
Dougados, 1999 (82)	SSZ	2–3 g/d	58	52	−7.1	−4.5	NI	−0.7[b]	−0.9[b]	−30	59%
	MTX	7.5–15 mg/wk	62		−4.2	−3.9	NI	−0.7	−0.9	−24	59%
Smolen et al., 1999 (67)	SSZ	2 g/d	83	24[c]	−8.1	−6.2	−19.8	−1	−1.1[b]	−16.6	56%
	Leflunomide	20 mg/d	96		−9.7	−7.2	−27.3	−1.1	−1.1[b]	−7.4	55%
Boers et al., 1997 (89)	SSZ	2 g/d	56	56[c]	−9	−5	−25	−20	−21	−24	49%
	SSZ, prednisone, and MTX	See text	70		−10	−7	−23	−27	−14	−31	72%

MTX, methotrexate; ND, not done; NI, no information; SSZ, sulfasalazine.
[a]Swollen and tender joint.
[b]Likert scale (0–5).
[c]Mean change from baseline.

18 of 30 patients completed the trial in the SSZ group (two stopped due to lack of effect and nine due to side effects), and the benefit fell short of statistical significance. SSZ was, again, compared to placebo in 1987 at the same dosage (62). Eighty-six patients with active RA and mean disease duration of 6.1 years were randomized against placebo for a period of 15 weeks. Thirty-one of 50 patients completed the trial in the SSZ group, with 12 patients having a significant clinical response. There was clinically significant improvement in morning stiffness (–88 minutes), grip strength (–19 mm Hg), tender (–13) and swollen joint counts (–13), ESR (–16 mm per hour), and pain score in patients completing the trial. Laboratory indices showed improvement but fell short of statistical significance. Both trials had relatively high rates of patient withdrawal, 28% in each of the studies, largely due to upper-GI side effects. These studies seemed to show an effect of SSZ on the signs and symptoms of RA in patients able to tolerate the drug, although toxicity appeared to be a significant problem.

Studies in Early Rheumatoid Arthritis

As rheumatologists began using DMARDs early in the disease, two trials were conducted in the early 1990s in patients with less than 12 months of symptomatic RA. The Australian Muticentre Clinical Trial Group (63) randomized 105 patients with early RA to either SSZ or placebo for 24 weeks. Use of nonsteroidal antiinflammatory drugs was permitted. Significant improvement was noted in the number of involved joints, the acute phase reactants, and in morning stiffness. There was also a trend toward less erosion over a 12-month period in the active treatment group. In another study, 80 patients with early RA were assigned to either SSZ or placebo for 48 weeks (64). Use of nonsteroidal antiinflammatory drugs and low-dose prednisone (up to 7.5 mg per day) was permitted. Compared to placebo, the SSZ group had a reduced swollen joint count, Ritchie's articular index, and patient global assessment. The trend in favor of active treatment was already evident at 4 weeks. There was no difference in the physician global assessment and morning stiffness between the two groups at the end of the study. Subgroup analysis suggested a better response in RF-negative patients. This question was assessed in a seronegative RA population in a placebo-controlled trial over a period of 24 weeks (65). There was significant improvement in tender joint count, morning stiffness, grip strength, and ESR, as compared to placebo.

A metaanalysis of eight placebo-controlled, randomized trials, which included 552 patients taking SSZ (2–3 g) and 351 receiving placebo, reported that SSZ therapy was significantly more effective than placebo (66). Compared to placebo, 2 g per day of SSZ reduced the duration of morning stiffness (61% vs. 33%; $p = .008$), number of painful joints (59% vs. 33%; $p = .004$), number of swollen joints (51% vs. 26%; $p < .0001$), amount of joint pain (42% vs. 15%; $p < .0001$), and patient global assessment (26 vs. 14; $p = .02$). Comparison of 2-g doses (eight studies) and 3-g doses (two studies) of SSZ showed no advantage of the higher dose of SSZ in terms of efficacy, as defined by improvement in number of swollen joints (51% vs. 43%) and painful joints (59% vs. 38%) and ESR (37% vs. 25%) (2-g vs. 3-g doses of SSZ). The withdrawals due to lack of efficacy were 11% in the 2-g group, as compared to 4% in the 3-g group; withdrawals due to side effects were 24% and 29%, respectively. Although there were more patients taking 2 g per day (552 patients) than 3 g per day (80 patients), no dose-response effect was seen in the analysis.

The efficacy of leflunomide (LEF) (20 mg per day) was compared to that of SSZ (2 g per day) and placebo in a randomized, double-blind trial (67). The SSZ group (N = 133) had a mean disease duration of 7.4 years, whereas the mean disease duration was 7.6 years in the LEF group (N = 133). There was consistent improvement in tender and swollen joint count, physician and patient global assessment, pain, and acute phase reactants for the LEF and SSZ groups over 24 weeks. LEF, however, had an earlier clinical effect than did SSZ, as assessed by significant differences in tender joint and swollen joint count, patient and physician assessment, and pain intensity. Functional status, as defined by the Health Assessment Questionnaire (HAQ), showed a clinically meaningful improvement in disability index (DI) by –0.29 in the SSZ group and –0.50 in the LEF group versus –0.04 in the placebo-treated group. Seventy-four patients (56%) achieved an American College of Rheumatology (ACR) 20% response—similar to that of LEF (55%) and better than that of placebo (29%) ($p = .0001$ for SSZ and LEF vs. placebo). ACR 50% responder rate for SSZ was 30%, as compared with 33% for LEF 33% and 4% for the placebo. Twenty-five (19%) of 133 patients withdrew due to adverse effects from the SSZ group, as compared to 14% withdrawals in the LEF group (p = not significant). The most common side effects were GI disturbances (36 out of 133) and rashes (9 out of 133). Two patients in the SSZ group developed agranulocytosis with high fevers. Both of them recovered after discontinuation of the therapy. Forty-five percent of patients allocated to placebo and 42% in the SSZ group had less than 2 years of RA, but no analysis was provided for this subset of patients.

Relative Efficacy of Sulfasalazine Compared to Other Disease-Modifying Antirheumatic Drugs

Early randomized controlled trials have been conducted comparing SSZ against hydroxychloroquine (HCQ) (68,69), D-penicillamine (D-Pen) (70–72), and gold sodium thiomalate (73–76). In a metaanalysis of these trials conducted by Weinblatt et al. (66), HCQ was found to be as efficacious as SSZ (37% improvement in swollen joint count for SSZ, as compared to 28% for HCQ; $p = .38$); ESR decreased by 43% in the SSZ group, as compared to 26% in the HCQ group ($p = .10$). The withdrawal rate due to lack of efficacy was 30% in the HCQ group, as compared to 10% in the SSZ group ($p = .06$), and withdrawal due to toxicity was comparable for both groups ($p = .28$) (66). Greater numbers of patients were available for a metaanalysis comparing D-Pen and SSZ. Again, both drugs were equally efficacious (articular index, 36% improvement in the SSZ group, as compared to 31% receiving D-Pen; $p = .70$; ESR, 42% reduction for SSZ group, as compared to 43% taking D-Pen; $p = .93$). There was no difference in the rate of discontinuation, either due to lack of efficacy ($p = .58$) or toxicity ($p = .62$). Comparison to intramuscular gold showed a similar efficacy in terms of swollen and painful joints and ESR. Thirteen percent of the SSZ group withdrew due to lack of efficacy compared to 4% taking gold ($p = .006$), whereas withdrawal due to side effects was higher for patients taking gold (29%) than those taking SSZ (12%; $p < .0001$).

Two large metaanalyses conducted in the early 1990s evaluated 79 trials in RA that included more than 6,500 patients (77,78). The trials showed that SSZ was as effective as D-Pen, intramuscular gold, and MTX with respect to improvements in ESR, tender joint count, and grip strength and significantly better than oral gold, azathioprine, and HCQ.

Controlled clinical trials have shown SSZ to be an effective DMARD. Studies using time-on-drug survival curves in the usual care is another measure of drug effectiveness. However, Aletaha and Smolen (79) examined the effectiveness of traditional DMARDs in two rheumatology practices in Vienna. MTX used at a median dose of 10 mg per week had a higher retention rate (median drug survival time of 40 months), as compared to 2 g per day of SSZ (median drug survival time of 23 months)

(79). The discrepancy was due to inefficacy, more in the SSZ group than the MTX group (p <.001), whereas the withdrawal due to toxicity was similar in both groups. Box and Pullar (80) also found that 25% of patients remained on SSZ after 5 years of initiating treatment.

There has been significant interest in the efficacy of SSZ as compared to MTX, especially in North America. This issue was addressed directly in a controlled, prospective trial in which 105 randomized patients with early RA (<12 months of symptomatic disease) to SSZ alone (2–3 g per day), MTX alone (7.5–15.0 mg per week), or a combination of both drugs (81). All patients were either RF and/or HLA-DR1 or -DR4 positive and were followed for 52 weeks. All three regimens were equally effective, with a trend favoring greater benefits for the combination therapy [mean change in disease activity score (DAS) in combination, –1.9; vs. MTX alone, –1.7; and SSZ alone, –1.6]. Most of the MTX patients received 7.5 mg per week, with 11 patients (31%) increasing their dosage up to 15 mg per week. Another study from Europe compared 205 early RA patients with aggressive disease (RF or HLA-DR1, or both, or HLA-DR4 positivity) in a similar trial, randomized to SSZ (2–3 g per day), MTX (7.5–15.0 mg per day), or a combination (82). The mean baseline HAQ score in the SSZ group was 1.38, and the DAS score was 4.23. The mean improvement in articular index for the SSZ group was 7.1, as compared to 4.2 for the MTX group and 9.4 for the combination group (p = .001 combination vs. SSZ and MTX alone); mean improvement in DAS for the SSZ group was 1.15, as compared to 0.87 for the MTX group and 1.26 for the placebo group (p = .019 combination vs. SSZ and MTX alone). Radiographic progression was similar in all three groups. The combination group experienced more adverse events (91%), as compared to either of the other two groups (75%; p = .025) (Table 26.4). The most common adverse effects were nausea (23–49%), headache (4–12%), and leukopenia (1–10%). Forty-eight percent of patients on MTX had their dosage increased due to lack of efficacy. No analysis was provided in either study to compare the efficacy of this subset of MTX patients with the SSZ group. Because MTX is often used at higher doses when clinically indicated, the relative effectiveness of either medication alone may not have been adequately addressed in these studies.

A well-designed study compared SSZ, LEF, and placebo over 24 weeks (67). Both active drug treatments were similar in efficacy, as described earlier. A 2-year double-blind extension of this study showed continued efficacy in the SSZ group similar to that of patients taking LEF (83). For the SSZ and LEF groups, there was a sustained improvement in ESR (–15.0 vs. 16.1 mm per hour), morning stiffness (–67 vs. –117 minutes), and pain score (–26.6 vs. 141.7 mm visual analog scale). However, physician (50% vs. 32% improvement) and patient (46% vs. 29% improvement) global assessment, ACR 20% (82% vs. 60%), and 50% response (52% vs. 25%) rate were significantly better in the LEF group, as compared to SSZ (p <.05 for all groups).

Radiographic Progression

Prevention or slowing of erosive disease on radiographs is considered by many RA experts as a "true" disease-modifying effect of any antirheumatic agent. Early trials examining SSZ as a DMARD demonstrated its ability to slow the rate of erosions, as compared to placebo. An initial study compared 31 patients with established RA, taking SSZ with ten placebo controls who refused a second DMARD therapy (84). SSZ appeared to slow the progression of radiologic damage over a period of 2 years.

Another study evaluated 60 patients with RA randomly allocated to receive either SSZ (mean disease duration of 15.6 months) or HCQ (mean disease duration of 12.8 months) and looked for new erosions and progression of joint space narrowing on x-rays of the hands and feet (85). The erosion score and total score (erosions and joint space narrowing) increased significantly less in the SSZ group (p <.02) than that of the HCQ group at 48 weeks. This was observed consistently over a 3-year follow-up period (86). Patients randomized to SSZ took a dose of 2 g per day, and patients on HCQ took 200 mg twice a day for 24 weeks, and then the HCQ was decreased to 200 mg once daily to reduce toxic effects, which may have contributed to this difference. At the end of 48 weeks, 68% of patients on SSZ had new erosions, demonstrating its inability to completely halt disease activity. Two well-designed clinical trials in early RA (symptomatic disease, <12 months) have assessed radiographic progression as a secondary measure (62,63). Both studies confirm that SSZ indeed slows the progression of erosive disease compared to placebo; however, a significant number of patients receiving SSZ with no baseline erosions had erosions at the end of the study, again demonstrating that erosions developed despite the SSZ therapy.

The most compelling evidence for a true disease-modifying effect of SSZ is derived from an international study of 358 RA patients who were randomly assigned to LEF, SSZ, or placebo (67). There was significantly less disease progression in the LEF and SSZ groups, as compared to placebo, at the end of 24 weeks. Changes in eroded joint count were similar in the LEF and SSZ groups and fewer in the placebo group. In a 24-month open-label extension of this trial, SSZ treatment showed a continual beneficial effect on erosive disease; however, LEF showed a tendency toward fewer new erosions than SSZ (change in Larsen score of –0.07 in LEF vs. –0.03 in SSZ) (83). A recent analysis compared the radiographic changes in three randomized trials of LEF, SSZ, and MTX (87). All three DMARDs were equally effective in retarding radiographic progression. Possibly, the initial studies may have had a type 2 statistical error due to small sample size, shorter follow-up duration, and high rate of dropouts.

Combination Use

Because the pathophysiology of RA involves multiple inflammatory pathways, two or three drug combinations of DMARDs are increasingly favored over single-DMARD therapy. In principle, combination therapy may allow the use of lower doses of individual DMARD therapy, possibly reducing toxicity.

A series of articles has been published, both in early and established RA, evaluating the benefit of combination therapy over monotherapy. An example of a well-designed trial is a prospective study of 102 RA patients (with mean disease duration of 6–10 years) who had failed to respond to at least one previous DMARD (88). The duration of RA was between 6 and 10 years, and patients had used an average of 1.6 DMARDs before enrolling in the study. The patients were randomized to triple therapy with SSZ (500 mg twice a day), MTX (7.5–17.5 mg titrated to response), and HCQ (200 mg twice a day), to MTX alone or to SSZ and HCQ in combination. The primary end point of the study was the successful completion of 2 years of treatment and a 50% improvement in composite symptoms of arthritis. This triple therapy was able to achieve a 50% response of at least a 2-year duration in 77% of patients, as compared to the same level of durable response in 40% and 33% of patients randomized to double and single agents, respectively (p = .003 comparison with triple therapy). One of the potential limitations of the study was the use of SSZ, at only 1 g per day, which possibly underestimated its efficacy.

Another well-designed prospective study evaluated the response of combination therapy (SSZ, 2 g per day; MTX, 7.5 mg

TABLE 26.4. Data on Radiographic Progression

Study/yr (Reference)	Type of Study, Comparator	Duration of Study	Mean Duration of Disease in SSZ	Dosage of SSZ/d	Number of Patients Treated with SSZ	Baseline Score in SSZ Group	Baseline Score for Placebo/Active Disease-Modifying Antirheumatic Drug Comparator	Δ SSZ	Δ Placebo/ Δ Active Disease-Modifying Antirheumatic Drug Comparator	*p* Value
Pullar et al., 1987[a] (84)	Open-labeled, placebo	104 wk	6 yr	1–4 g	31	NR	NR	5[c]	19[c]	Trend favoring SSZ
Van der Heijce et al., 1989[a] (85)	Blind observer, comparison to hydroxychloroquine	48 wk	15.6 mo	2 g	22	2[c]	3[c]	8	33	<.02
Hannonen et al., 1993[a] (64)	Blind observer, placebo	48 wk	4.7 mo	2 g	38	1.9[d]	2.1[d]	3.5	7.1	.13
Boers et al., 1997[a] (89)	Blind observer, combination (COBRA regimen)	80 wk	4 mo (median)	2 g	79	5[c]	3[c]	12	4	.01
Smolen et al. 1999[b] (67)	Blind observer, placebo	24 wk	7.4 yr	2 g	133	1.39[d]	1.48[d]	0.01	0.05	<.001
Smolen et al.. 1999[b] (67)	Blind observer, leflunomide	24 wk	7.4 yr	2 g	133	1.39[d]	1.48[d]	0.01	0.01	NS
Landewe et al., 2002[a] (90)	Open, combination (extension of Boers et al. trial)	4–5 yr	4 mo (median)	2 g	74	17[d]	6.5[d]	43.4/8.6 per yr	23.4/5.6 per yr	.02

COBRA regimen, sulfasalazine, 2 g per day/methotrexate, 7.5 mg per week/prednisone, initial dosage of 60 mg per day lowered over 6 weeks to 7.5 mg per day; Δ, change in the radiographic progression on total joint score, either by Larsen score or modified Sharp score; NR, not recorded; NS, not significant; SSZ, sulfasalazine.

[a]Modified Sharp score.
[b]Larsen score.
[c]Median score.
[d]Mean score.

per week; and prednisone, initial dosage of 60 mg per day and lowered over 6 weeks to 7.5 mg per day), termed the COBRA regimen, to SSZ alone in early RA (median duration of disease, 4 months) (89). Seventy-eight percent and 72% were RF positive in the combination and SSZ groups, respectively, and 77% had baseline erosions. According to the step-down design, prednisone and MTX were withdrawn at 28 and 40 weeks, respectively. Efficacy was assessed by a pooled index of five measures: tender joint count, physician global assessment, grip strength, ESR, and McMaster-Toronto Arthritis questionnaire (a disease-specific activity of daily living questionnaire). At week 28 (primary end point), the combination therapy was significantly better when clinically compared to SSZ alone (p <.001), although the patients in triple therapy were still taking prednisolone. There was no difference at week 56. Fifty-five (72%) of the combined treatment group compared with 39 (49%) of the SSZ group had a 20% ACR response, and 49% compared to 27% had a 50% ACR improvement at 28 weeks (p = .006). This difference was no longer significant at 56 weeks. The HAQ score and McMaster-Toronto Arthritis questionnaire showed a clinically significant change in the combination group compared to SSZ at 28 weeks (p = .007). The improvement in the HAQ was still significant at week 56, despite that fact that both prednisolone and MTX had been withdrawn by then, favoring the combination group. The radiographic benefits due to this combination therapy were significant at weeks 28, 56, and 80. Because patients had been withdrawn from prednisolone by week 34 and MTX by week 40, the effect on radiographic progression lasted well beyond the withdrawal of prednisolone and MTX. Even at the 5-year follow-up, the patients allocated to combination therapy continued to maintain less progression compared to the SSZ treatment arm (p = .033), independent of subsequent DMARD therapy (90).

In an open-labeled parallel study of early RA (mean duration of disease, 7–9 months), combination therapy with SSZ, MTX, HCQ, and prednisone was significantly better than SSZ therapy, alone or with prednisone, in inducing remission at 1-year (p = .011) and 2-year (p = .003) follow-ups (91). ACR 50% clinical response was achieved after 1 year in 68 patients (75%) with combination therapy and in 56 patients (60%) using single-drug therapy (p = .028); whereas, at the 2-year follow-up, 69 and 57, respectively (71% vs. 58%, p = .058), had improved clinically. These results must be viewed with caution, as the study was not blinded. Together, these data indicate that SSZ is as effective as SSZ and MTX therapy combined but significantly less effective than more intensive combination therapy.

In most trials, there was no statistically increased risk of adverse drug reactions in the combination group compared to SSZ as monotherapy, with a trend toward more events in the combination group. In one trial by Dougados et al. (82), the combination group experienced more adverse events (91%), as compared to either the SSZ or MTX group (75%; p = .025). The most common adverse effects were nausea (23–49%), headache (4–12%), and leukopenia (1–10%). In the trial by Boers et al. (89), the combination group was associated with more weight gain (2.5 kg vs. 0.7 kg; p = .002) and bone loss at the lumbar spine than the SSZ group (0%) (p = .06)—possibly because the combination group was also taking prednisone (–1.2%). Trials by Mottonen et al. (91) and O'Dell et al. (88) did not show any increase in side effects in the combination group when compared to SSZ alone, and more patients continued the study in the combination group because clinical efficacy was maintained in the combination group more so than in the SSZ-treated group (ACR 50% improvement: 71% in the combination group vs. 58% in the SSZ group; p = .058 in the Mottonen et al. trial). The benefit to toxicity ratio favors the combination group, making it an appealing approach.

Impact on Disability and Quality of Life

Important goals of RA therapy are to reduce or prevent functional disability and to improve quality of life. Two validated disease-specific instruments can assess functional status in RA: the HAQ and the modified HAQ—and there are others (92). Functional disability is also a part of ACR response criteria to evaluate efficacy of antirheumatic drugs. In a trial by Smolen et al. (67), 358 RA patients were randomly assigned to LEF, SSZ, or placebo. Approximately 40% of patients had disease duration of less than 2 years, and 55% patients were classified as ACR Functional Class II, with baseline mean HAQ-DI scores of 1.1 (93). At the end of 6 months, the mean and percent change in the SSZ group was –0.29 and 29%, respectively, whereas that for LEF was –0.50 and 45%, and placebo was –0.04 and 4%. The LEF patients improved more than those in the SSZ group at 6 months [p = .0086; confidence interval (CI), –0.28 to 0.04]. The open extension of the trial over 24 months showed continued improvement in the HAQ-DI for both the SSZ (–0.36 and 40% from baseline) and the LEF (–0.65 and 59% from baseline) groups. The improvement was greater in the LEF group than in the SSZ group (p = .01) (83). In a study by Dougados et al. (82), 205 early RA patients with RF positivity and active disease were randomized to SSZ (2–3 g per day), MTX (7.5–15.0 mg per day), or combination therapy. The baseline HAQ-DI was 1.38, 1.25, and 1.32 in the SSZ, MTX, and combination groups, respectively. At the end of 1 year, all three groups had a similar improvement in the HAQ score, –0.74, –0.73, and –0.70, respectively.

Survival Benefit

An important outcome of a chronic disease is mortality. In a cohort study of RA patients over 18 years, MTX was shown to improve survival in patients with active RA when compared to other DMARDs (94). After adjusting for prognostic factors, the mortality hazard ratio for MTX use (mean dose of 13 mg per week, with a maximum dose of 25 mg per week) compared to no use was 0.4 (CI, 0.2–0.8). SSZ (mean dose not mentioned) did not decrease the mortality in this cohort (mortality hazard ratio of 0.9; CI, 0.2–4.2). One possible limitation of this study is that this cohort came from a single clinic practice in the United States, whereas most literature about SSZ-treatment outcomes is from European studies.

Adverse Drug Reactions

The adverse events associated with SSZ can be divided into two categories. The first one is dose dependent, and the second one is composed of hypersensitivity reactions. Knowledge of these classifications is helpful in the management of patients with RA. Dose-related side effects may be resolved with reduction or temporary withholding of the SSZ, whereas hypersensitivity reactions require immediate withdrawal of the drug (Table 26.5).

The following guidelines should be used to monitor SSZ use:

- Full information should be provided to patients regarding common and life-threatening side effects.
- Complete blood cell count, including a differential white blood cell count and liver function tests every 2 to 4 weeks for the first 3 months and once every 3 months thereafter, should be performed.
- Neutropenia, especially agranulocytosis, usually occurs within the first 3 months of treatment. However, it can occur at any time during therapy; monitoring to avoid it is difficult. Patients should know to stop the drug in the event of fevers, sore throat, and/or mouth ulcers.

TABLE 26.5. Toxicity of Sulfasalazine

Side Effects	Range (%)
Dose-related	
Gastrointestinal[a]: nausea, vomiting, dyspepsia, anorexia, abdominal pain	10–25
Central nervous system[a]: dizziness, irritability, headache, malaise, depression	1–10
Hematologic problems	
Leukopenia[b]	1–5
Thrombocytopenia, increase in erythrocyte mean cell volume, hemolysis,[b] methemoglobinemia	Rare
Hypersensitivity reactions	
Skin reactions	
Rash[a] (pruritic, maculopapular)	5–15
Photosensitivity	—
Exfoliative dermatitis, toxic epidermal necrolysis,[b] Stevens-Johnson syndrome[b]	Rare
Hepatitis: rise in hepatic enzymes (3%), fatal hepatic necrosis[b]	0.5–1.0
Pulmonary: eosinophilic pneumonitis, fibrosing alveolitis	Rare
Agranulocytosis[b] and aplastic anemia[b]	0.04–0.6
Other side effects	
Autoimmunity: reversible systemic lupus erythematosus	Rare
Male infertility: reversible oligospermia and abnormal sperm motility	Rare

[a]Common side effects.
[b]Serious, even life-threatening side effects.

In a long-term study of patients taking SSZ for up to 11 years, 26.5% of patients stopped treatment due to an adverse event (95). Seventy-six percent of these events occurred within 3 months, and few occurred beyond the first year. Most events were trivial and self-limiting after withdrawal of the drug; of the potentially more serious adverse effects, 66% occurred within 3 months of treatment. Other observational studies have reported that the majority of the reactions (62%) occurred within 3 to 4 weeks after beginning SSZ therapy (96). UK fatal toxicity reports concerning SSZ therapy from 1963 to 2000 show that most deaths are attributed to hematologic side effects (42 cases), followed by liver failure or hepatitis, or both (eight cases) (97).

GASTROINTESTINAL

Nausea and upper abdominal discomfort are the most common adverse effects of SSZ. Their incidence was between 9% and 23% in one large population study and was the most common cause of withdrawal (61%) in that patient population (95). Their incidence is reduced by increasing the dose of SSZ gradually and by using enteric-coated tablets. Hepatitis, in the form of transient elevations of liver enzymes, is seen in 0.5% to 1.0% of patients (98). The transaminitis usually returns to normal on cessation of the drug. In a study of the toxicity of SSZ therapy in inflammatory bowel disease involving 718 patients using SSZ for 6 months or longer, there were no reported cases of liver dysfunction during treatment (99).

Occasionally, more widespread hypersensitivity occurs, with fevers, rash, lymphadenopathy, and severe hepatitis. Granulomatous hepatitis with noncaseating granulomas is the characteristic pathologic finding, with marked elevations in serum alkaline phosphatase due to SSZ hepatotoxicity (100). The presumed mechanism of liver injury in SSZ hepatotoxicity is an idiosyncratic hypersensitivity response. All of these features are similar to those seen with cases of sulfonamide-induced liver injury, and the sulfapyridine moiety of SSZ is likely to be responsible. Most cases present within 1 month of initiating treatment and resolve quickly on drug withdrawal. Both severe hepatitis and acute liver failure have been attributed to SSZ (101). The syndrome usually reverses after cessation of the drug, although treatment using high-dose systemic pulse steroids may be needed (102). Patients with SSZ hepatotoxicity demonstrate a prompt recurrence of symptoms on rechallenge with SSZ or sulfonamide (103). Rarely, death may occur within 3 weeks of starting SSZ, with evidence of massive hepatocellular necrosis, acute hypersensitivity myocarditis, focal acute tubulointerstitial nephritis, and extensive bone marrow necrosis, thought to be hallmarks of the so-called 3-week SSZ syndrome, a rare, but often fatal, immunoallergic reaction (104).

CENTRAL NERVOUS SYSTEM

Irritability, headaches, depression, and dizziness may affect up to 10% of patients taking SSZ. The symptoms usually occur during the initiation of the drug and respond to dose reduction. Rarely, seizures have been reported in patients taking SSZ, often in the setting of other clinical manifestations of toxicity (102,105).

HEMATOLOGIC

The incidence of leukopenia (white blood cell count $<4 \times 10^9$ per L) and neutropenia varies from 1% to 5% of patients on SSZ (106,107). Observational studies (108) and case reports (109) indicate that the vast majority of cases of SSZ-associated bone marrow suppression occurs within 3 months of starting treatment. Although most often seen during the first 3 months of therapy, leukopenia can occur at any time, necessitating continued surveillance (110). Most studies report spontaneous improvement of leukopenia despite continuation of treatment under close supervision. Other authors have successfully continued the treatment with temporary discontinuation of the drug and reintroduction at a lower dosage.

Agranulocytosis and aplastic anemia are serious and potentially fatal idiosyncratic reactions to SSZ (111). In the Swedish Adverse Drug Advisory Committee report from 1972 to 1989 (111), the incidence of SSZ-induced agranulocytosis was 0.04% during the first 30 days, with a fatality rate of 6.5%. The risk of developing agranulocytosis during SSZ treatment is considerable during the first 3 months of treatment, suggesting that frequent complete blood cell counts, every 2 to 4 weeks for the first 3 to 4 months, is advisable. In a large community-based study of nearly 4,000 patients, there was a 0.6% incidence of agranulocytosis or neutropenia (108). Bone marrow biopsy specimens of patients with SSZ-induced agranulocytosis reveal a paucity of myeloid cells, but full recovery typically occurs within 10 days of drug discontinuation (109). SSZ-induced agranulocytosis is believed to be mediated by immunologic hypersensitivity of myeloid precursors (108). Spontaneous recovery from SSZ agranulocytosis is frequently seen, although fatalities have been reported, and some patients may benefit from granulocyte-macrophage colony-stimulating factor (112).

Another rare side effect of SSZ is hemolytic anemia, especially in patients with glucose-6-phosphate dehydrogenase deficiency (113). It has been suggested (113) that lack of rise in hematocrit levels in RA patients on successful treatment should be considered for subclinical hemolysis. For this reason, some authorities recommend obtaining a blood test for baseline glucose-6-phosphate dehydrogenase before starting therapy. An increase in erythrocyte mean cell volume with rare megaloblastic anemia is occasionally seen with SSZ therapy. SSZ acts as a competitive inhibitor of folate uptake in the small bowel, with the possibility of folate deficiency in RA (95,107). This effect is usually of no clinical significance, although folate deficiency should be considered, particularly in patients with anemia and in those at risk for having a poor diet (114), such as the elderly.

In a prospective study (115), SSZ did not alter the serum or red cell folate level at a dosage of 2 g per day for 24 weeks. Methemoglobinemia and thrombocytopenia have been reported with SSZ, and improvement usually occurs after temporarily stopping the treatment.

SKIN REACTION

Skin rashes occur in approximately 5% to 15% of cases (95,116) and may take the form of a generalized, pruritic, maculopapular rash; urticaria; photosensitivity; or stomatitis. The rash usually disappears after stopping the medication. Patients who have less severe mucocutaneous reactions to SSZ can be desensitized if it is deemed necessary. Initially given as 1-mg doses orally, the SSZ dose is gradually escalated over 25 to 86 days. Successful desensitization has been achieved in as many as 85% of cases (117).

Rarely, severe, life-threatening hypersensitivity reactions can present in the form of toxic epidermal necrolysis (118) or Stevens-Johnson syndrome (119), requiring immediate discontinuation of the drug.

PULMONARY

Rare allergic interstitial pneumonitis with or without eosinophilia has been reported in patients receiving SSZ (120). Parry et al. (97) reviewed the literature of SSZ and pulmonary toxicity. They found 50 cases in the literature from 1972 to 1999. The most common presenting symptoms included cough, dyspnea, and fever. Peripheral eosinophilia was seen in 52% of the cases, with abnormal chest radiographs in all cases, with the majority showing pulmonary infiltrates. The most common histologic diagnosis was interstitial pneumonitis, followed by fibrosing alveolitis. The recovery usually occurs after stopping the medication, with a mean period of 6.5 weeks, and, in 20% of cases, corticosteroids were added. Despite these reports, pulmonary toxicity is very rare and UK fatal toxicity reports for SSZ from 1963 to 2000 have shown only two respiratory deaths attributed to SSZ (97).

AUTOIMMUNE

Several patients taking SSZ have developed evidence of systemic lupus erythematosus (121). The syndrome is usually reversible once SSZ is discontinued but may occur with the rechallenge. A small study suggested that slow acetylators and HLA-DQA1*0501 may be the predisposing factor for development of clinical systemic lupus erythematosus (122); however, this observation has not been confirmed.

MALE FERTILITY

SSZ can cause reversible oligospermia, reduced sperm motility, and cause an increased proportion of abnormal forms (123). These effects are usually seen within 2 months of starting the SSZ treatment and are probably caused by the sulfapyridine moiety (124). The changes are usually reversible within 2 to 3 months of stopping SSZ (123). The mechanism is unclear, but antifolate and antiprostaglandin activities have been suggested (125). Teratogenesis is not associated with SSZ therapy (126).

CONCLUSION

In conclusion, SSZ is an effective DMARD for treatment of RA. It has proven its efficacy in both early and established disease, both as a single agent and in combination use in randomized clinical trials. It has a favorable impact on retardation of the radiographic progression, especially in early RA. Definitive data comparing the therapeutic ratios of SSZ and MTX at equipotent doses are not available in the clinical trials. Efficacy is comparable to intramuscular gold, D-Pen, and MTX. SSZ is associated with relatively more common, non–life-threatening side effects compared to MTX and has a well-defined toxicity profile. SSZ appears to be safe in pregnancy and has significant drug interactions. If introduced properly, it is tolerated well in patients and has a reasonably good safety profile.

ACKNOWLEDGMENTS

We would like to thank Ali Farrokh for his help with producing Figure 26.1 and Tables 26.3 and 26.4 and Jules Kessler for preparation of the manuscript.

REFERENCES

1. Svartz N. Ett nytt sulfonamidpreparat. Förelöpande meddelande. *Nord Med* 1941;9:51.
2. Das KM, Dubin R. Clinical pharmacokinetics of sulfasalazine. *Clin Parmacokinet* 1976;1:406–425.
3. Schröder H. Simplified method for determining acetylator phenotype. *BMJ* 1972;3:506–507.
4. Khan AKA, Truelove SC, Aronson JK. The disposition and metabolism of sulphasalazine (salicylasulphapyridine) in man. *Br J Clin Pharmacol* 1982; 13:523–528.
5. Das KM, Eastwood MA, McManus JP, et al. The metabolism of salicylazosulphapyridine in ulcerative colitis. I. The relationship between metabolites and the response to treatment in inpatients. *Gut* 1973;14:631–641.
6. Peppercorn MA, Goldman P. Distribution studies of salicylazosulfapyridine and its metabolites. *Gastroenterology* 1973;64:240–245.
7. Sjoholm I, Ekman B, Kober A, et al. Binding of drugs to human serum albumin: XI. The specificity of three binding sites as studied with albumin immobilized in microparticles. *Mol Pharmacol* 1979;16:767–777.
8. Farr M, Brodrick A, Bacon PA. Plasma and synovial fluid concentrations of sulphasalazine and two of its metabolites in rheumatoid arthritis. *Rheumatol Int* 1985;5:247–251.
9. Hensleigh PA, Kauffman RE. Maternal absorption and placental transfer of sulfasalazine. *Am J Obstet Gynecol* 1977;15;127:443–444.
10. Jarnerot G, Into-Malmberg MB. Sulphasalazine treatment during breast feeding. *Scand J Gastroenterol* 1979;14:869–871.
11. Peppercorn MA, Goldman P. Distribution studies of salicylazosulfapyridine and its metabolites. *Gastroenterology* 1973;64:240–245.
12. Das KM, Chourdhury JR, Zapp B, et al. Small bowel absorption of sulfasalazine and its hepatic metabolism in human beings, cats, and rats. *Gastroenterology* 1979;77:280–284.
13. Peppercorn MA, Goldman P. The role of intestinal bacteria in the metabolism of salicylazosulfapyridine. *J Pharmacol Exp Ther* 1972;181:555–562.
14. Peppercorn MA, Goldman P. Distribution studies of salicylazosulfapyridine and its metabolites. *Gastroenterology* 1973;64:240–245.
15. Allgayer H, Ahnfelt NO, Kruis W, et al. Colonic *N*-acetylation of 5-aminosalicylic acid in inflammatory bowel disease. *Gastroenterology* 1989;97:38–41.
16. Das KM, Eastwood MA, McManus JP, et al. Adverse reactions during salicylazosulfapyridine therapy and the relation with drug metabolism and acetylator phenotype. *N Engl J Med* 1973;289:491–495.
17. Schröder H, Campbell DE. Absorption, metabolism, and excretion of salicylazosulfapyridine in man. *Clin Pharmacol Ther* 1972;13:539–551A.
18. Haagsma CJ. Clinically important drug interactions with disease-modifying antirheumatic drugs. *Drugs Aging* 1998;13:281–289.
19. Jarnerot G, Into-Malmberg MB. Sulphasalazine treatment during breast feeding. *Scand J Gastroenterol* 1979;14:869–871.
20. Haagsma CJ. Clinically important drug interactions with disease-modifying antirheumatic drugs. *Drugs Aging* 1998;13:281–289.
21. Das KM, Chourdhury JR, Zapp B, et al. Small bowel absorption of sulfasalazine and its hepatic metabolism in human beings, cats, and rats. *Gastroenterology* 1979;77:280–284.
22. Pullar T, Hunter JA, Capell HA Which component of sulphasalazine is active in rheumatoid arthritis? *BMJ* 1985;25;290:1535–1538.
23. Pullar T, Hunter JA, Capell HA. Sulphasalazine in the treatment of rheumatoid arthritis: relationship of dose and serum levels to efficacy. *Br J Rheumatol* 1985;24:269–276.
24. Kitas GD, Farr M, Waterhouse L, et al. Influence of acetylator status on sulphasalazine efficacy and toxicity in patients with rheumatoid arthritis. *Scand J Rheumatol* 1992;21:220–225.
25. Pullar T, Hunter JA, Capell HA. Sulphasalazine in rheumatoid arthritis: a double blind comparison of sulphasalazine with placebo and sodium aurothiomalate. *BMJ (Clin Res Ed)* 1983;287:1102–1104.
26. Pullar T, Hunter JA, Capell HA. Effect of acetylator phenotype on efficacy and toxicity of sulphasalazine in rheumatoid arthritis. *Ann Rheum Dis* 1985; 44:831–837.

27. Bax DE, Greaves MS, Amo RS. Sulphasalazine for rheumatoid arthritis: relationship between dose, acetylator phenotype and response to treatment. *Br J Rheumatol* 1986;25:282–284.
28. Ebringer A, Ptaszynska T, Corbett M, et al. Antibodies to proteus in rheumatoid arthritis. *Lancet* 1985;2:305–307.
29. Shinebaum R, Neumann VC, Cooke EM, et al. Comparison of faecal florae in patients with rheumatoid arthritis and controls. *Br J Rheumatol* 1987;26:329–333.
30. Neumann VC, Shinebaum R, Cooke EM, et al. Effects of sulphasalazine on faecal flora in patients with rheumatoid arthritis: a comparison with penicillamine. *Br J Rheumatol* 1987;26:334–337.
31. Sandberg-Gertzen H, Kjellander J, Sundberg-Gilla B, et al. In vitro effects of sulphasalazine, azodisal sodium, and their metabolites on *Clostridium difficile* and some other faecal bacteria. *Scand J Gastroenterol* 1985;20:607–612.
32. Philips PE. Infectious agents in the pathogenesis of rheumatoid arthritis. *Semin Arthritis Rheum* 1986;16:1–10.
33. Astbury C, Hill J, Bird HA. Co-trimoxazole in rheumatoid arthritis: a comparison with sulphapyridine. *Ann Rheum Dis* 1988;47:323–327.
34. Astbury C, Hill J, Bird HA. Phthalylsulphathiazole in rheumatoid arthritis. *Br J Rheumatol* 1992;31:461–463.
35. Gibson PR, Jewell DP. Sulphasalazine and derivatives, natural killer activity and ulcerative colitis. *Clin Sci (Lond)* 1985;69:177–184.
36. Sheldon P, Webb C, Grindulis KA. Effect of sulphasalazine and its metabolites on mitogen induced transformation of lymphocytes—clues to its clinical action? *Br J Rheumatol* 1988;27:344–349.
37. Kanerud L, Scheynius A, Hafstrom I. Evidence of a local intestinal immunomodulatory effect of sulfasalazine in rheumatoid arthritis. *Arthritis Rheum* 1994;37:1138–1145.
38. Symmons DP, Salmon M, Farr M. Sulfasalazine treatment and lymphocyte function in patients with rheumatoid arthritis. *J Rheumatol* 1988; 15:575–579.
39. Gibson PR, Jewell DP. Sulphasalazine and derivatives, natural killer activity and ulcerative colitis. *Clin Sci (Lond)* 1985;69:177–184.
40. Comer SS, Jaasin HE. In vitro immunomodulatory effects of sulfasalazine and its metabolites. *J Rheumatol* 1988;15:580–586.
41. Hirohata S, Ohshima N, Yanagida T, Aramaki K. Regulation of human B-cell function by sulfasalazine and its metabolites. *Int Immunopharmacol* 2002;2:631–640.
42. Jorgensen C, Bologna C, Anaya JM, et al. Variation in the serum IgA concentration and the production of IgA in vitro in rheumatoid arthritis treated by sulfasalazine. *Rheumatol Int* 1993;13:113–116.
43. Feltelius N, Gudmundsson S, Wennersten L, et al. Enumeration of IgA producing cells by the enzyme linked immunospot (ELISPOT) technique to evaluate sulphasalazine effects in inflammatory arthritides. *Ann Rheum Dis* 1991;50:369–371.
44. Hasko G, Szabo C, Nemeth ZH, Deitch EA. Sulphasalazine inhibits macrophage activation: inhibitory effects on inducible nitric oxide synthase expression, interleukin-12 production and major histocompatibility complex II expression. *Immunology* 2001;103:473–478.
45. Wahl C, Liptay S, Adler G, et al. Sulfasalazine: a potent and specific inhibitor of nuclear factor kappa B. *J Clin Invest* 1998;101:1163–1174.
46. Liptay S, Bachem M, Hacker G, et al. Inhibition of nuclear factor kappa B and induction of apoptosis in T-lymphocytes by sulfasalazine. *Br J Pharmacol* 1999;128:1361–1369.
47. Danis VA, Franic GM, Rathjen DA, et al. Circulating cytokine levels in patients with rheumatoid arthritis: results of a double blind trial with sulphasalazine. *Ann Rheum Dis* 1992;51:946–950.
48. Holmdahl R, Klareskog L, Rubin K, et al. Role of T lymphocytes in murine collagen induced arthritis. *Agents Actions* 1986;19:295–305.
49. Hunneyball IM, Crossley MJ, Spowage M. Pharmacological studies of antigen-induced arthritis in BALB/c mice. II. The effects of second-line antirheumatic drugs and cytotoxic agents on the histopathological changes. *Agents Actions* 1986;18:394–400.
50. Volin MV, Harlow LA, Woods JM, et al. Treatment with sulfasalazine or sulfapyridine, but not 5-aminosalicyclic acid, inhibits basic fibroblast growth factor-induced endothelial cell chemotaxis. *Arthritis Rheum* 1999;42:1927–1935.
51. Rhodes JM, Bartholomew TC, Jewell DP. Inhibition of leucocyte motility by drugs used in ulcerative colitis. *Gut* 1981;22:642–647.
52. Harvath L, Yancey KB, Katz SI. Selective inhibition of human neutrophil chemotaxis to N-formyl-methionyl-leucyl-phenylalanine by sulfones. *J Immunol* 1986;137:1305–1311.
53. McConkey B, Amos RS, Durham S, et al. Sulphasalazine in rheumatoid arthritis. *BMJ* 1980;280:442–444.
54. Neal TM, Winterbourn CC, Vissers MC. Inhibition of neutrophil degranulation and superoxide production by sulfasalazine. Comparison with 5-aminosalicylic acid, sulfapyridine and olsalazine. *Biochem Pharmacol* 1987;36:2765–2768.
55. Franklin JL, Rosenberg HH. Impaired folic acid absorption in inflammatory bowel disease: effects of salicylazosulfapyridine (Azulfidine). *Gastroenterology* 1973;64:517–525.
56. Svartz N. The treatment of rheumatic polyarthritis with acid azo compounds. *Rheumatism* 1948;4:56–60.
57. Kuzzell WC, Gardner GM. Salicyclazosulfapyridine in rheumatoid arthritis. *Calif Med* 1950;73:478–480.
58. Sinclair RJG, Duthie JJR. Salazopyrin in the treatment of rheumatoid arthritis. *Ann Rheum Dis* 1948;8:226–231.
59. McConkey B, Amos RS, Butler EP, et al. Salazopyrin in rheumatoid arthritis. *Agents Actions* 1978;8:438–441.
60. McConkey B, Amos RS, Durham S, et al. Sulphasalazine in rheumatoid arthritis. *BMJ* 1980;280:442–444.
61. Pullar T, Hunter JA, Capell HA. Sulphasalazine in rheumatoid arthritis: a double blind comparison of sulphasalazine with placebo and sodium aurothiomalate. *BMJ (Clin Res Ed)* 1983;287:1102–1104.
62. Pinals RS, Kaplan SB, Lawson JG, et al. Sulfasalazine in rheumatoid arthritis. A double-blind, placebo-controlled trial. *Arthritis Rheum* 1986;29:1427–1434.
63. Sulfasalazine in early rheumatoid arthritis. The Australian Multicentre Clinical Trial Group. *J Rheumatol* 1992;19:1672–1677.
64. Hannonen P, Mottonen T, Hakola M, et al. Sulfasalazine in early rheumatoid arthritis. A 48-week double-blind, prospective, placebo-controlled study. *Arthritis Rheum* 1993;36:1501–1509.
65. Farr M, Waterhouse L, Johnson AE, et al. A double-blind controlled study comparing sulphasalazine with placebo in rheumatoid factor (RF)-negative rheumatoid arthritis. *Clin Rheumatol* 1995;14:531–536.
66. Weinblatt ME, Reda D, Henderson W, et al. Sulfasalazine treatment for rheumatoid arthritis: a metaanalysis of 15 randomized trials. *J Rheumatol* 1999;26:2123–2130.
67. Smolen JS, Kalden JR, Scott DL, et al. Efficacy and safety of leflunomide compared with placebo and sulphasalazine in active rheumatoid arthritis: a double-blind, randomised, multicentre trial. European Leflunomide Study Group. *Lancet* 1999;353:259–266.
68. Faarvang KL, Egsmose C, Kryger P, et al. Hydroxychloroquine and sulphasalazine alone and in combination in rheumatoid arthritis: a randomised double blind trial. *Ann Rheum Dis* 1993;52:711–715.
69. Nuver-Zwart IH, van Riel PL, van de Putte LB, et al. A double blind comparative study of sulphasalazine and hydroxychloroquine in rheumatoid arthritis: evidence of an earlier effect of sulphasalazine. *Ann Rheum Dis* 1989;48:389–395.
70. Capell HA, Marabani M, Madhok R, et al. Degree and extent of response to sulphasalazine or penicillamine therapy for rheumatoid arthritis: results from a routine clinical environment over a two-year period. *QJM* 1990;75: 335–344.
71. Carroll GJ, Will RK, Breidahl PD, et al. Sulphasalazine versus penicillamine in the treatment of rheumatoid arthritis. *Rheumatol Int* 1989;8:251–255.
72. Neumann VC, Grindulis KA, Hubball S, et al. Comparison between penicillamine and sulphasalazine in rheumatoid arthritis: Leeds-Birmingham trial. *BMJ (Clin Res Ed)* 1983;287:1099–1102.
73. Pullar T, Hunter JA, Capell HA. Sulphasalazine in rheumatoid arthritis: a double blind comparison of sulphasalazine with placebo and sodium aurothiomalate. *BMJ (Clin Res Ed)* 1983;287:1102–1104.
74. Raspe HH, Kindel P, Vesterling K, et al. Change in functional capacity and pain intensity of 81 cP patients treated with Azulfidine RA or aurothioglucose. Preliminary statistical assessment of the German multicenter study of the treatment of chronic polyarthritis with Azulfidine RA. *Z Rheumatol* 1987;46:71–75.
75. Schattenkirchner M. Sulfasalazine (Azulfidine RA) versus aurothioglucose in therapy of chronic polyarthritis—status report of an open, comparative, multicenter long-term study. German. *Z Rheumatol* 1987;46:67–70.
76. Williams HJ, Ward JR, Dahl SL, et al. A controlled trial comparing sulfasalazine, gold sodium thiomalate, and placebo in rheumatoid arthritis. *Arthritis Rheum* 1988;31:702–713.
77. Felson DT, Anderson JJ, Meenan RF. The comparative efficacy and toxicity of second-line drugs in rheumatoid arthritis. Results of two metaanalyses. *Arthritis Rheum* 1990;33:1449–1461.
78. Felson DT, Anderson JJ, Meenan RF. Use of short-term efficacy/toxicity tradeoffs to select second-line drugs in rheumatoid arthritis. A metaanalysis of published clinical trials. *Arthritis Rheum* 1992;35:1117–1125.
79. Aletaha D, Smolen JS. Effectiveness profiles and dose dependent retention of traditional disease modifying antirheumatic drugs for rheumatoid arthritis. An observational study. *J Rheumatol* 2002;29:1631–1638.
80. Box SA, Pullar T. Sulphasalazine in the treatment of rheumatoid arthritis. *Br J Rheumatol* 1997;36:382–386.
81. Haagsma CJ, van Riel PL, de Jong AJ, et al. Combination of sulphasalazine and methotrexate versus the single components in early rheumatoid arthritis: a randomized, controlled, double-blind, 52 week clinical trial. *Br J Rheumatol* 1997;36:1082–1088.
82. Dougados M, Combe B, Cantagrel A, et al. Combination therapy in early rheumatoid arthritis: a randomised, controlled, double blind 52 week clinical trial of sulphasalazine and methotrexate compared with the single components. *Ann Rheum Dis* 1999;58:220–225.
83. Scott DL, Smolen JS, Kalden JR, et al. European Leflunomide Study Group. Treatment of active rheumatoid arthritis with leflunomide: two year follow up of a double blind, placebo controlled trial versus sulfasalazine. *Ann Rheum Dis* 2001;60:913–923.
84. Pullar T, Hunter JA, Capell HA. Effect of sulphasalazine on the radiological progression of rheumatoid arthritis. *Ann Rheum Dis* 1987;46:398–402.
85. van der Heijde DM, van Riel PL, Nuver-Zwart IH, et al. Effects of hydroxychloroquine and sulphasalazine on progression of joint damage in rheumatoid arthritis. *Lancet* 1989;1:1036–1038.
86. van der Heijde DM, van Riel PL, Nuver-Zwart IH, et al. Sulphasalazine versus hydroxychloroquine in rheumatoid arthritis: 3-year follow-up. *Lancet* 1990;3;335:539.
87. Sharp JT, Strand V, Leung H, et al. Treatment with leflunomide slows radiographic progression of rheumatoid arthritis: results from three randomized

controlled trials of leflunomide in patients with active rheumatoid arthritis. Leflunomide Rheumatoid Arthritis Investigators Group. *Arthritis Rheum* 2000;43:495–505.
88. O'Dell JR, Haire CE, Erikson N, et al. Treatment of rheumatoid arthritis with methotrexate alone, sulfasalazine and hydroxychloroquine, or a combination of all three medications. *N Engl J Med* 1996;334:1287–1291.
89. Boers M, Verhoeven AC, Markusse HM, et al. Randomized comparison of combined step-down prednisolone, methotrexate and sulphasalazine with sulphasalazine alone in early rheumatoid arthritis. *Lancet* 1997;350:309–318.
90. Landewe RB, Boers M, Verhoeven AC, et al. COBRA combination therapy in patients with early rheumatoid arthritis: long-term structural benefits of a brief intervention. *Arthritis Rheum* 2002;46:347–356.
91. Mottonen T, Hannonen P, Leirisalo-Repo M, et al. Comparison of combination therapy with single-drug therapy in early rheumatoid arthritis: a randomised trial. FIN-RACo trial group. *Lancet* 1999;353:1568–1573.
92. Wolfe F, Pincus T, Fries JF. Usefulness of the HAQ in the clinic. *Ann Rheum Dis* 2001;60:811.
93. Scott DL. Leflunomide improves quality of life in rheumatoid arthritis. *Scand J Rheumatol Suppl* 1999;112:23–29.
94. Choi HK, Hernan MA, Seeger JD, et al. Methotrexate and mortality in patients with rheumatoid arthritis: a prospective study. *Lancet* 2002;359: 1173–1177.
95. Amos RS, Pullar T, Bax DE, et al. Sulphasalazine for rheumatoid arthritis: toxicity in 774 patients monitored for one to 11 years. *BMJ (Clin Res Ed)* 1986;293:420–423.
96. Nakajima H, Munakata A, Yoshida. Adverse effects of sulfasalazine and the treatment of ulcerative colitis with mesalazine. *J Gastroenterol* 1995;30:115–117.
97. Parry SD, Barbatzas C, Peel ET, et al. Sulphasalazine and lung toxicity. *Eur Respir J* 2002;19:756–764.
98. Pullar T, Hunter JA, Capell HA. Sulphasalazine and hepatic transaminases. *Ann Rheum Dis* 1987;46:421.
99. Cunliffe RN, Scott BB. Monitoring for drug side-effects in inflammatory bowel disease. *Aliment Pharmacol Ther* 2002,16:647–662.
100. Fich A, Schwartz J, Braverman D, et al. *Am J Gastroenterol* 1984;79:401–402.
101. Marinos G, Riley J, Painter D, et al. Sulfasalazine-induced fulminant hepatic failure. *J Clin Gastroenterol* 1992;14:132–135.
102. Quallich LG, Greenson J, Haftel HM, et al. Is it Crohn's disease? A severe systemic granulomatous reaction to sulfasalazine in patient with rheumatoid arthritis. *BMC Gastroenterol* 2001;1:8.
103. Gulley RM, Mirza A, Kelley CE. Hepatotoxicity of salicylazosulfapyridine: a case report and review of the literature. *Am J Gastroenterol* 1979;72:561–564.
104. Lau G, Kwan C, Chong SM. The 3-week sulphasalazine syndrome strikes again. *Forensic Sci Int* 2001;122:79–84.
105. Smith MD, Gibson GE, Rowland R. Combined hepatotoxicity and neurotoxicity following sulfasalazine administration. *Aust N Z J Med* 1982;12:76–80.
106. Farr M, Symmons DP, Blake DR, et al. Neutropenia in patients with inflammatory arthritis treated with sulphasalazine. *Ann Rheum Dis* 1986;45:761–764.
107. Pullar T. Adverse effects of sulphasalazine. *Adverse Drug React Toxicol Rev* 1992;11:93–109.
108. Jick H, Myers MW, Dean AD. The risk of sulfasalazine and mesalazine-associated blood disorders. *Pharmacotherapy* 1995;15:176–181.
109. Jacobson IM, Kelsey PB, Blyden GT, et al. Sulfasalazine induced agranulocytosis. *Am J Gastroenterol* 1985,80:118–121.
110. Marabani M, Madhok R, Capell HA, Hunter JA. Leucopenia during sulphasalazine treatment for rheumatoid arthritis. *Ann Rheum Dis* 1989;48:505–507.
111. Keisu M, Ekman E. Sulfasalazine associated agranulocytosis in Sweden 1972–1989. Clinical features, and estimation of its incidence. *Eur J Clin Pharmacol* 1992;43(3):215–218.
112. Roddie P, Dorrance H, Cook M, et al. Treatment of sulphasalazine-induced agranulocytosis with granulocyte macrophage-colony stimulating factor. *Aliment Pharm Ther* 1995;9:711–712.
113. Wijnands MJ, Nuver-Zwart IH, van Riel PL, et al. Hemolysis during low-dose sulfasalazine treatment in rheumatoid arthritis patients. *Scand J Rheumatol* 1991;20:52–57.
114. Swinson CM, Perry J, Lumb M, et al. Role of sulphasalazine in the aetiology of folate deficiency in ulcerative colitis. *Gut* 1981;22:456–461.
115. Grindulis 1985. Does sulphasalazine cause folate deficiency in rheumatoid arthritis? *Scand J Rheumatol* 1985;14:265–270.
116. Zurcher K, Krebs A. *Cutaneous drug reactions: an integral synopsis of today's systemic drugs*, 2nd ed. Basel: Karger, 1992.
117. Bax DE, Amos RS. Sulphasalazine in rheumatoid arthritis: desensitising the patient with a skin rash. *Ann Rheum Dis* 1986;45:139–140.
118. Jullien D, Wolkenstein P, Roupie E, et al. Toxic epidermal necrolysis after sulfasalazine treatment of mild psoriatic arthritis: warning on the use of sulfasalazine for a new indication. *Arthritis Rheum* 1995;38:573.
119. Martin L, Hazouard E, Michalak-Provost S, et al. Fatal toxic respiratory epitheliolysis. Subacute tracheo-bronchial desquamation in Stevens-Johnson syndrome. *Rev Pneumol Clin* 2001;57:297–301.
120. Hamadeh MA, Atkinson J, Smith LJ. Sulfasalazine-induced pulmonary disease. *Chest* 1992;101:1033–1037.
121. Walker E, Carty J. Sulphasalazine-induced systemic lupus erythematosus in a patient with erosive arthritis. *Br J Rheumatol* 1994;33:175–176.
122. Gunnarsson I, Kanerud L, Pettersson E, et al. Predisposing factors in sulphasalazine-induced systemic lupus erythematosus. *Br J Rheumatol* 1997; 36:1089–1094.
123. O'Morain C, Smethurst P, Dore CJ, et al. Reversible male infertility due to sulphasalazine: studies in man and rat. *Gut* 1984;25:1078–1084.
124. Di Paolo MC, Paoluzi OA, Pica R, et al. Sulphasalazine and 5-aminosalicylic acid in long-term treatment of ulcerative colitis: report on tolerance and side-effects. *Dig Liver Dis* 2001;33:563–569.
125. Steeno OP. Side-effects of salazopyrin on male fertility. *Eur J Obstet Gynecol Reprod Biol* 1984;18:361–364.
126. Norgard B, Czeizel AE, Rockenbauer M, et al. Population-based case control study of the safety of sulfasalazine use during pregnancy. *Aliment Pharmacol Ther* 2001;15:483–486.

CHAPTER 27

Gold Compounds and Antimalarials

Alice V. Klinkhoff and Daniel E. Furst

GOLD COMPOUNDS

The first reports of gold use in rheumatoid arthritis (RA) emanated from France in 1929, based on a prevalent theory that tuberculosis and RA were related. In addition, studies indicated that gold cyanide inhibited growth of the tubercle bacilli *in vitro* (1). The beneficial effects of parenteral gold therapy were conclusively documented later in placebo-controlled trials in Europe and in the United States. As the disease-modifying antirheumatic drug (DMARD) with the longest history of use, the spectrum of common and rare side effects of gold is well established, although the mechanism of action has not been definitively elucidated. Since the introduction of methotrexate into common clinical practice in the 1980s, the use of gold has fallen worldwide.

Although intramuscular (IM) gold compounds [gold sodium thiomalate (GST) and gold sodium aurothioglucose (ATG)] and oral gold (auranofin) appear to be similarly beneficial in clinical trials, oral gold has been much less effective than IM gold in standard clinical practice, and it is used very rarely today. For this reason, IM gold will be emphasized in this chapter.

Mechanisms of Action

Numerous immunologic cellular and enzymatic effects are ascribed to gold compounds, but there is uncertainty concerning which mechanisms are responsible for the therapeutic benefits of gold. *In vivo* experiments, including serial synovectomy studies and postmortem studies, have shown selective accumulation of gold in macrophages of many tissues and, in particular, abundance during gold treatment in lysosomes of synovial macrophages of rheumatoid synovium. Although there is progressive reduction of the amount of gold in the macrophages after gold is discontinued, gold has been found in synovial macrophages up to 23 years after treatment is discontinued (2). It is probable that many of the beneficial effects of gold result from its influence on multiple arthritis-perpetuating factors derived from the monocytes and macrophages (3). Monocytes and macrophages are key players in RA pathogenesis. They act as antigen-presenting cells, produce complement, release proteolytic enzymes, and produce and release cytokines. With chronic use, gold reduces cytokine production of synovial macrophages. This effect has been observed in synovial fluid samples and has been demonstrated by reduction in interleukin (IL)-1 staining of the synovium in gold-treated patients (4). In the synovial lining, there is, in addition, a decrease in macrophage numbers and IL-6 and IL-8 production. *In vitro* experiments show a reduction of angiogenic properties of macrophages (8). In monocytes, gold compounds inhibit Fc and C_3 receptor expression and oxygen radical production. Gold compounds inhibit lymphocyte proliferative responses by their action on the monocyte and macrophage (8). GST inhibits incorporation of IL-1 into fibroblasts, reducing basal and IL-1–induced fibroblastic proliferation (5). There is a reduction of immunoglobulin and rheumatoid factor synthesis (6). GST inhibits spontaneous and interferon γ–induced production of the second component of complement by monocytes and macrophages, as well as interferon γ–induced expression of DR antigens (7). Other actions of gold compounds are listed in Table 27.1.

Pharmacokinetics

Two products, each containing 50% gold in solution (GST) or suspension (ATG), are currently available for parenteral administration. GST is water soluble and rapidly absorbed after IM injection. Gold sodium ATG, a suspension in sesame oil, reaches peak levels approximately 24 hours after administration and achieves 30% lower peak serum levels, compared with GST; this difference may account for the observed lower incidence of adverse effects with ATG, as compared to GST. In plasma, approximately 95% of GST is bound to albumin; 70% is eliminated in urine and 30% in feces (8–10). After the standard weekly injection schedule, 40% of the dose is excreted each week, and the remainder is retained or excreted more slowly. The serum elimination half-life of gold, after a single 50-mg IM dose, has been reported to range from 3 to 27 days early in the treatment (8–10). With prolonged administration, gold is stored in bone marrow, liver, spleen, nodes, skin, and kidneys; elimination half-lives of up to 168 days have been documented after 10 weekly injections, with considerable individual variation (8–10). After several months, serum levels stabilize with weekly injections; a steady decline in steady-state serum levels occurs when intervals between injections are increased (9).

Auranofin is a triethylphosphine gold compound, 29% gold by weight that is absorbed orally. First studied in the 1970s, it was found to have substantially different chemical and pharmacologic properties, compared with parenteral gold. After ingestion, 25% to 30% of auranofin is absorbed. Its serum elimination half-life is approximately 1 week, whereas its protein binding is

TABLE 27.1. Mechanisms of Action

Inhibits phagocytic action of macrophages
Inhibits fibroblast proliferation
Decreases immunoglobulin and rheumatoid factor synthesis
Inactivates classic and alternate complement pathways
Inhibits cytokine production, IL-1, IL-6, IFN-γ
Inhibits cellular responses to IL-1, IL-2, IFN-γ
Inhibits acid phosphates, collagenase, protein kinases, and phospholipase C

IFN, interferon; IL, interleukin.
Adapted from Vernon-Roberts B, Doré JL, Jessop JD, et al. Selective concentration & localization of gold in macrophages of synovial and other tissues during and after chrysotherapy in rheumatoid patients. *Ann Rheum Dis* 1976;35:477–486; Kinne RW, Stuhlmuller B, Palombo-Kinne E, et al. The role of macrophages in rheumatoid arthritis. In: Firestein GS, Panay GS, Wollheim FA, eds. *Rheumatoid arthritis: new frontiers in pathogenesis and treatment.* Oxford: Oxford University Press, 2000:80; Kirkham BW, Navarro FJ, Corkill MM, et al. In vivo analysis of disease-modifying drug therapy activity in RA by sequential immunohistological analysis of synovial membrane IL1B. *J Rheumatol* 1994;21:1615–1619; Matsobara T, Saegusa Y, Hirohata K. Low dose gold compounds inhibit fibroblast proliferation and do not affect interleukin secretion by macrophages. *Arthritis Rheum* 1988;31:1272–1280; Gottlieb NL, Kiem IM, Penneys NS, et al. The influence of chrysotherapy on serum protein and immunoglobulin levels, rheumatoid factor, and antiepithelial antibody titers. *J Lab Clin Med* 1975;86:962–970; and Kawakami A, Eguchi K, Migiti K, et al. Inhibitory effects of gold sodium thiomalate on the proliferation and interferon gamma induced HLA DR expression in human endothelial cells. *J Rheumatol* 1990;17:430–435.

only approximately 60%, and, after absorption is complete, auranofin is cleared approximately equally by the gastointestinal tract and kidneys (10a). With the standard dose of 3 mg twice daily, serum gold levels rise gradually over 8 to 12 weeks to a median of 500 ng per mL. This value compares with serum gold levels of 3,000 ng per mL, with weekly IM GST (8).

Efficacy

PLACEBO-CONTROLLED TRIALS

Between 1960 and 1983, there were four prospective, placebo-controlled trials of gold compounds, summarized in Table 27.2. Each trial showed statistically significant improvement in treated patients when gold was compared with placebo in terms of active joint counts and laboratory measures of disease activity. Three of the four trials evaluated radiographic progression; two showed reduction of erosions in gold-treated patients, compared with those assigned to placebo (11–15). The 1960 Empire Rheumatism Council trial entered 200 RA patients (11). The active treatment arm received GST, 50 mg per week, and the placebo was 0.5 mg of GST. After 20 weekly injections, treatment was terminated, and the patients were followed, without additional therapy, for a total of 30 months. Statistically significant clinical benefit was shown at 3, 6, 12, and 18 months. By month 30, 2 years after discontinuation of gold or placebo, there was no longer a difference in clinical measures between the group originally assigned to placebo and the group that had received a 6-month course of gold. X-rays were evaluated at 18 months for the development of new erosions, extension of erosions, and joint space narrowing. Radiographic differences between active and control groups were not statistically significant at 18 months, 12 months after discontinuation of gold or placebo (12).

Sigler evaluated the benefit of 2 years of gold therapy, compared with placebo, in a study that was double blinded for the entire 24-month duration (13). The dose was 50 mg per week for 18 weeks, every 2 weeks for 12 weeks, every 3 weeks for 12 weeks, and, thereafter, every 4 weeks. This is the only adequate controlled trial of monthly maintenance gold therapy. Thirty-two patients were entered, and 27 were analyzed—13 in the gold and 14 in the placebo group. Statistically significantly improvement in clinical outcomes was achieved for gold over placebo at 6, 9, 12, 18, and 24 months. Statistically significantly reduction of joint erosion scores and narrowing scores at 24 months, compared with baseline, was achieved in the gold-treated group. Three of 13 gold-treated, and no placebo-treated, patients achieved a complete remission.

The Cooperating Clinics of the American Rheumatism Association performed two 6-month, placebo-controlled trials, in 1973 and 1983 (14,15). The first Cooperating Clinics trial enrolled 68 patients in seven centers. There were 25 noncompleters who were not evaluated. In patients treated with GST, all clinical measures improved, but statistically significant improvement over placebo was shown only for the erythrocyte sedimentation rate and physician global assessment. Radiographic progression was observed in 3 out of 20 gold-treated patients and nine out of 19 controls ($p = .06$) during a period of 27 weeks. The 1983 Cooperating Clinics trial compared auranofin with GST and placebo in 193 RA patients (15). Important improvement was defined as a 50% improvement in clinical measures. In an intent-to-treat analysis, 4.5% of placebo-, 31% of auranofin-, and 35% of GST-treated patients showed a 50% or greater improvement in pain or tenderness scores. A decrease of 50% or greater in number of swollen joints was seen in 12.5% of placebo, 28% of auranofin, and 37% of GST patients. Overall, statistically significant improvement comparing GST with placebo was seen for four out of ten clinical measures and four out of four laboratory measures (hemoglobin, platelet count, rheumatoid factor, and erythrocyte sedimentation

TABLE 27.2. Summary of Published Trials Comparing Parenteral Gold with Placebo

Trial and References	No. of Patients Enrolled	Month of Treatment/Month of Follow-Up	Improvement versus Placebo	Withdrawals LOE GST/P	Withdrawals SE GST/P
Empire Rheumatism Council (12)	200	20/210	Newly affected and quiescent joints. Grip strength, ESR, Hgb, analgesic use.	3/3	14/4
Sigler et al., 1974 (13)	32	104/104	Active joints, ring size, grip strength, ESR, x-ray progression.	1/8	2/1
American Rheumatism Association 1974 (14)	68	27/27	ESR, physician global assessment, x-ray progression ($p = .06$).	2/12	8/1
Ward et al., 1983 (15)	193 46 placebo 72 auranofin 75 GST	21/21	Both GST and auranofin for tender joints, ESR, and platelets. GST and not auranofin for swelling scores, Hgb, and physician global assessment.	P/A/GST = 5/2/0	P/A/GST = 1/5/22

A, auranofin; ESR, erythrocyte sedimentation rate; GST, gold sodium thiomalate; Hgb, hemoglobin; LOE, lack of effect; P, placebo; SE, side effect.

rate). Comparing auranofin with placebo, improvements were statistically significant for three out of ten clinical measures and one out of four laboratory measures. GST was numerically superior to auranofin in every clinical and laboratory measure and statistically superior for hemoglobin and platelet count.

RADIOGRAPHIC OUTCOME STUDIES

Luukkainen et al. compared radiographic progression, according to the Larsen scale, in patients who had received a total dose of more than 500 mg of IM gold versus those who had received less than 500 mg (16). The mean cumulative dose of gold was 1,858 mg in the high-total-dose gold group, and 254 mg in the low-total-dose gold group. Radiographs were evaluated before start of gold and 5 years later. There were no statistically significant differences between Larsen scores at baseline; the reduction in damage after 5 years in the high-total-dose gold group was statistically better than the low-total-dose group (p <.001).

Buckland-Wright et al. compared joint damage using quantitative microfocal radiography in a group receiving gold early with matched RA patients whose gold therapy was delayed 6 months. There was a decrease in a total erosion area score after 6 months of gold treatment but not in the first 6 months of treatment (17). In a 12-month, prospective, double-blind, parallel study comparing 50 mg GST weekly with 15 mg methotrexate weekly, the slope of x-ray progression was reduced in the second 6 months of therapy for both DMARDs, with no difference between the two regimens (18).

COMPARISON WITH OTHER DISEASE-MODIFYING ANTIRHEUMATIC DRUGS

In a 12-month, double-blind, parallel study of 50 mg GST weekly versus 15 mg IM methotrexate weekly in 174 patients, there was similar improvement, more remissions, and more withdrawals for toxicity in the gold-treated patients (19). A study comparing sulfasalazine with GST showed similar benefits over the short term (20). In a metaanalysis by Felson et al., published in 1990, little difference in efficacy could be found comparing gold, methotrexate, and sulfasalazine therapy (21).

LONG-TERM GOLD THERAPY

Prospective analyses of large numbers of patients on gold have demonstrated acceptable safety in experienced hands but disappointing adherence to therapy in the long term. In a 10-year follow-up of 376 RA patients, the likelihood of discontinuation was 50% by 18 months and 92% by 10 years (22). Mucocutaneous side effects were the main reason for discontinuation within the first 3 years, and loss of effectiveness was the main reason for discontinuation after 3 years. These poor long-term adherence results of life table analysis have been confirmed by others for gold and for other DMARDs.

In patients remaining on gold, improved effectiveness may be seen with long-term therapy. In one study of 111 patients, 47 had an excellent response: Two achieved remission after 20 weeks, eight between 20 and 52 weeks, 31 between 12 and 18 months, and a further six had remitted by 24 months. The authors concluded that, when appropriate, gold should be continued longer than 6 months, even in the face of an equivocal response (23). Wolfe et al. described outcomes in 98 patients followed before 1992, according to usual clinical practice using gold. There investigators concluded that, in patients who had been receiving gold for 12 months, approximately two-thirds achieve substantial improvement, with 41% achieving 50% or greater improvement in global disease severity and 63% achieving more than 50% improvement in joint count (24).

A 1990 Finnish study evaluated mortality in patients with RA who were hospitalized in the years 1961 to 1966. The mortality rate was highest for patients never treated with gold and lowest for patients with the longest duration of IM gold treatment (25). Although effective in clinical trials, auranofin appears to be somewhat less effective compared with parenteral gold (26). Auranofin is rarely used in clinical practice today.

DISEASE-MODIFYING ANTIRHEUMATIC DRUG COMBINATIONS WITH GOLD

Adding cyclosporine (mean dose of 2.5 mg per kg) to baseline gold therapy has shown benefit without unexpected toxicity or drug interaction after 6 months (27). Adding hydroxychloroquine (HCQ) to gold showed no measurable benefit in one study (28). A 48-week double-blind, placebo-controlled trial showed benefit in terms of American College of Rheumatology (ACR) 20% response and no important drug interactions when ATG, 50 mg weekly, was given to partial responders on methotrexate (mean dose of methotrexate, 18.5 mg) (29).

Safety Overview

A number of large series have been published supporting the safety of gold therapy in experienced hands. Lockie and Smith described 47 years of experience in 1,019 patients (30). Skin reactions, including pruritus with or without rash, occurred in 36%, buccal irritation in 22%, proteinuria in 0.9%, immune thrombocytopenia in 1%, transient bone marrow aplasia in 0.8%, low white blood cell count in 0.1%, and postinjection reactions in 6% (Table 27.3) (30). In a 38-year experience with gold use, there was a similar incidence of mucocutaneous reactions, renal toxicity, and immune thrombocytopenia, as well as possible gold-induced interstitial pneumonitis (2 in 1,021) (31). Neither of these large series included a fatality related to gold. Side effects resolved with dose adjustment or gold discontinuation. Rare serious side effects of gold include cholestatic jaundice, enterocolitis, gold lung, and aplastic anemia. Each probably occurs in less than 1 per 1,000 gold courses.

MUCOCUTANEOUS REACTIONS

Mucocutaneous reactions, including dermatitis and stomatitis, are the most common side effects of chrysotherapy and account for premature discontinuation of therapy in 30% of patients. Gold dermatitis can affect any part of the body and is virtually always pruritic (32). Pruritus may be the earliest manifestation of gold toxicity; early in treatment, pruritus involving any part of the body, including the scalp or vagina, may be the first indication of gold toxicity. Klinkhoff and Teufel suggest that continuation of full-dose therapy in the presence of symptoms of drug

TABLE 27.3. Adverse Effects of Intramuscular Gold

Adverse effect	Incidence
Pruritus with or without rash	30–40%
Stomatitis	10%
Proteinuria	2–7%
Thrombocytopenia	1%
Eosinophilia	10–20%
Nitritoid reactions	5% with GST, rare with ATG
Interstitial pneumonitis	<1/1,000
Aplastic anemia	<1/1,000
Granulocytopenia	<1%
Cholestatic hepatitis	<1/1,000
Hypogammaglobulinemia	Rarely reported
Encephalopathy/peripheral neuropathy	Rarely reported
Pancreatitis	Rarely reported
Hemorrhagic colitis	Rarely reported
Chrysiasis	Related to cumulative dosage >8 g
Corneal or lens chrysiasis	Related to cumulative dosage of gold

ATG, gold sodium aurothioglucose; GST, gold sodium thiomalate.

TABLE 27.4. Precautions with Gold Compounds

	Risk
Contraindications	
Blood dyscrasias	Risk if unable to recognize development of gold toxicity.
Baseline proteinuria	Risk if unable to recognize development of gold toxicity.
Renal failure	Drug accumulation and toxicity.
SLE	Increased risk of toxicity.
Drug interaction	
ACE inhibitor	Risk of nitritoid reaction with GST (use of ACE inhibitor not a contraindication).
Precautions	
Anticoagulant	Risk of hematoma with intramuscular injections (not a contraindication).

ACE, angiotensin-converting enzyme; GST, gold sodium thiomalate; SLE, systemic lupus erythematosus.

sensitivity can result in serious gold dermatitis and exfoliation. Management of mucocutaneous reactions should normally include temporary discontinuation of gold, with reinstitution of gold at 50% of the total dose or less. In patients with mucocutaneous reactions or other limiting side effects in spite of appropriate dose reductions, very-low-dose-therapy between 2 mg and 10 mg every 1 to 4 weeks has been used (33). Pathologic features of gold dermatitis are variable, but skin biopsy may help to diagnose confounding dermatologic conditions. Precautions due to comorbidity and concomitant medication use are included in Table 27.4.

Chrysiasis, a gray-blue skin discoloration, may develop with long-term gold therapy and cumulative amounts greater than 10 g (34). Chrysiasis occurs primarily on sun-exposed skin of white subjects and is asymptomatic but may be a cosmetic concern in fair-skinned individuals. Biopsy shows gold particles in the lysosomes of dermal macrophages and an increase in melanin content of sun-exposed skin (34).

Metallic taste is a rare side effect of gold, which typically occurs early and resolves with ongoing therapy (32).

PROTEINURIA

Approximately 2% of patients treated with gold therapy develop proteinuria, due to membranous glomerulonephritis. Ordinarily, proteinuria develops within the first 12 months of therapy, with 50-mg weekly dosing regimens, and resolves without sequelae 3 to 18 months after gold is discontinued (35,36). With appropriate monitoring, nephrotic syndrome occurs rarely. To prevent nephrotic syndrome, clinicians are advised to discontinue gold if proteinuria greater than 500 mg per 24 hours is detected. Once proteinuria has subsided, Klinkhoff and Teufel state that gold may be safely resumed at 50% lower dosage (37). It is said to be rare for proteinuria to recur when gold is resumed at 25 mg weekly (37).

HEMATOLOGIC TOXICITY

The most serious side effect of gold is aplastic anemia, occurring in less than 1 per 1,000 patients. Bone marrow aplasia due to gold is treated similarly to idiopathic and other drug-induced aplastic anemia with immunosuppression, and, when necessary, bone marrow transplantation (38,39). Excellent supportive care has improved the outcome of this condition. Immune thrombocytopenia develops in 1%, typically within the first 6 months of treatment (40). Cases of delayed gold-induced thrombocytopenia have been reported as long as 18 months after drug discontinuation. An association with HLA-DR3 has been reported (40). Appropriate management includes early detection, permanent discontinuation of gold, and the use of prednisone, 30 to 60 mg, until thrombocytopenia resolves. Isolated neutropenia is an uncommon manifestation of myelotoxicity (41). Neutropenia, due to Felty's syndrome, is not a contraindication to gold treatment, because it normally responds well to chrysotherapy, with improvement in neutrophil counts over time (42). A benign and nonprogressive leukopenia may develop in patients on long-term therapy and need not lead to drug discontinuation (41). Pure red cell aplasia has been described (43). Eosinophilia may be an early sign of gold sensitivity and warrants increased vigilance for the common gold side effects, although it is not, in itself, a reason to alter treatment (32). Hypogammaglobulinemia is a rare side effect of gold (32).

POSTINJECTION REACTIONS

The most common postinjection reaction is a nitritoid reaction; vasomotor symptoms occur within minutes after injection and consist of flushing, dizziness with or without nausea, vomiting, sweating, and symptoms of hypotension, including syncope (44). The majority of reactions are benign and transient, and they become milder and disappear with continued therapy. Serious complications have been described, including myocardial infarction and stroke occurring as a result of prolonged hypotension (45,46). Nitritoid reactions occur primarily with GST, probably due to rapid absorption, compared with ATG; the severity of the reaction depends on the severity and duration of hypotension and the susceptibility of the patient to hypotensive episodes. The association of nitritoid reactions when using gold and angiotensin-converting enzyme inhibitors together has been reported (47,48). Management includes lying down; observation for 20 minutes postinjection; dose reduction, which may be temporary; and switching to ATG (44). Postinjection nonvasomotor reactions include arthralgias, myalgias, and flare of RA (49). These typically occur early in the course of therapy with GST, wane with ongoing treatment, and respond with improvement when the dose of gold is temporarily reduced or when the patient is switched to ATG.

PULMONARY, GASTROINTESTINAL, AND NEUROLOGIC TOXICITY

Pulmonary, gastrointestinal (GI), and neurologic toxicity is rare (much less than 0.1%) and serious. Gold must be discontinued at the earliest suggestion of these reactions and appropriate investigations should be initiated urgently. Characteristically, these side effects develop early in the treatment course.

Gold-induced interstitial pneumonitis is an acute fulminant disease. It may be distinguished from rheumatoid lung disease by its acute onset, usually in association with recent initiation of gold therapy (50,51). Management requires intensive care and usually treatment with high-dose steroids, although no controlled trials have documented the efficacy of immunosuppressive interventions. Gold-induced colitis presents with severe bloody diarrhea and ulcerating colitis (52). Cholestatic hepatitis manifests with nausea, weakness, and cholestatic jaundice (52–54). Symptoms resolve with discontinuation of therapy and supportive care. Neurotoxicity is a rare idiosyncratic reaction manifesting with encephalitis or peripheral neuritis early in the gold course (55,56).

Dosage Regimens

When Forrestier first used IM gold in RA, the dose was 250 mg weekly for 12 weeks. Subsequently, he adopted 100 mg weekly for a second series and found it to be less toxic (1). The traditional dosage regimen was developed empirically and adopted from the first Empire Rheumatism Council trial, published in 1960. The test dose of 10 mg occasionally elicits a skin or allergic reaction. As long as the 10-mg dose is tolerated, the second injection is 25 mg, and subsequent doses are normally 50 mg weekly. No dose-finding studies have been done to determine the optimal dose. Nevertheless, both high and low doses of gold have been studied (57–59). It is clear from evaluating the extensive literature on gold that side effects are increased with higher weekly dosage and that all doses studied to date have been shown to have a therapeutic benefit. There is substantial individual variability with regard to tolerability and effectiveness. Comparing 50 mg with 150 mg weekly, effectiveness was similar, but toxicity was greater in the high-dose gold group (57). Comparing 25 mg with 50 mg weekly dosage, there was similarly no difference in effectiveness (58). A single trial reported use of 10-mg doses and found those to be effective (60).

The most effective and least toxic schedule for gold administration has not been established. Thus, a reasonable regimen might allow for flexibility of dosing, depending on effectiveness and side effects, similar to dosing regimens for methotrexate. One regimen suggests using 50-mg weekly injections. Gold injections are held when the patient develops non–life-threatening side effects and reintroduced at a 50% lower dosage once the side effects have subsided (33,44). Following this protocol, it appears that patients who have experienced mucocutaneous reactions and proteinuria can eventually be established on a suitable regimen, and doses as low as 2 to 10 mg every 1 to 4 weeks appear to be effective in selected gold-sensitive patients (44). Although the traditional regimen includes weekly injections to a cumulative dose of 1 g and, thereafter, at increased intervals, this maintenance regimen has not been evaluated well for effectiveness in the long term; loss of effect with increasing dosing interval is such a common scenario that, unless there is limiting toxicity, one author suggests that weekly or every-other-week injections may be administered indefinitely (*author's opinion*).

Pregnancy and Lactation

Gold crosses the placenta and is excreted in mothers' milk (1–37,61–64). There is no evidence for teratogenicity, and women wishing to conceive can safely take gold. Normally, women choose to discontinue gold in pregnancy; however, gold may be safely continued in selected patients whose RA is of such severity as to warrant it (63). The literature is controversial and theoretical regarding risks to a baby exposed to gold while nursing (64).

Summary

Although the mechanisms of action of the gold compounds (aurothiomalate, ATG, or auranofin) are not fully understood, it is probable that they affect macrophage and monocyte functions, such as antigen processing and presentation, cytokine production, angiogenesis, oxygen radical production, and lymphocyte proliferative responses. The IM compounds are well, although slowly, absorbed and can remain in the body for years. The oral compound is more rapidly excreted. A number of trials in the 1960s through the 1980s definitively proved that organic gold compounds are effective for the treatment of symptoms and signs of RA, as well as for decreasing the rate of radiologic damage. IM gold compounds have been shown to be effective for the treatment of RA. In general, auranofin, an oral compound, is less effective than the IM gold medications. Gold compounds cause a significant number of side effects, including rashes, stomatitis, proteinuria, and, rarely, thrombocytopenia, leukopenia, and bone marrow aplasia. Careful follow-up can decrease some of the toxicities of organic gold compounds. Although used infrequently today, IM organic gold compounds may still have a significant role to play in the treatment of patients resistant to other DMARDs.

ANTIMALARIAL COMPOUNDS

The antimalarials consist of two 4-aminoquinolone derivatives, chloroquine and HCQ, and quinacrine. Quinacrine is not an aminoquinolone, but the chloroquine structure is embedded within the structure of the quinacrine molecule.

Aminoquinolone derivatives, such as quinine, were first used in 1894 to treat systemic lupus erythematosus (SLE) (65). An important article by Page in 1951 noted that quinacrine treated both the skin lesions of SLE and RA (66). More recently, a whole range of connective tissue diseases has been treated by aminoquinolones (antimalarials). These include diseases such as dermatomyositis (67), palindromic rheumatism (68), juvenile-onset SLE (69), eosinophilic fasciitis (70), and osteoarthritis (71).

Mechanisms of Action

4-Aminoquinolones are weak bases and, as such, enter the lysosome, where they are protonated and raise the intralysosomal pH. The pH change, in turn, interferes with antigen processing and leads to decreased cytokine production, decreased stimulation of T cells, decreased granulocyte migration, and down-regulation of the autoimmune response (72–74). In SLE, HCQ seems to inhibit apoptosis (75). HCQ may affect platelet activation by inhibiting the expression of platelet surface markers, such as glycoprotein IIb/IIIa, thus potentially explaining the effect of HCQ in SLE-associated antiphospholipid syndrome (76).

Although structures of the antimalarials are very similar, the mechanisms of action may differ. Quinacrine, and, to a lesser extent, chloroquine, have inhibitory effects on lipopolysaccharide-induced expression of IL-1β and tumor necrosis factor α, whereas all three compounds inhibit arachidonate acid release and eicosanoid formation through inhibition of phospholipase A_2 (77). Chloroquine inhibits the proliferative response of human lymphocytes and also inhibits natural killer cell action (72). Antimalarials form complexes with DNA by binding of the quinoline ring to the nucleotide bases, thereby inhibiting nuclear events (78). DNA–anti-DNA complexes may also be inhibited by this drug (79).

Pharmacokinetics

HYDROXYCHLOROQUINE

There is significant interindividual variability of kinetics with HCQ, not surprisingly, because oral bioavailability ranges from 30% to 100% (80). As a weak base, HCQ accumulates in cell lysosomes, and this uptake may account for its large volume of distribution—500 L (81).

The 4-aminoquinolones are concentrated in the pigmented tissues of the eye. In rats, chloroquine concentrations in the pigmented retina are 10 to 20 times greater than that in any other tissue (82).

Although up to 25% of HCQ is cleared renally, most of HCQ is metabolized to desethylhydroxychloroquine, desethylchloroquine, and bisdesethylchloroquine. In a study of 212 patients, there was a positive correlation between a combined measure of response and blood desethylhydroxychloroquine concentrations, whereas the best correlation with adverse events was that between HCQ concentrations and GI adverse effects (83).

HCQ rapidly distributes into the blood, with a half-life of approximately 3 hours. Drug distribution into tissues has a half-life of 40 hours to 5 days, and the final phase of drug elimination has a long half-life of 40 to 50 days (81). HCQ is a racemic mixture; although the racemates are not cleared at an equal rate, there does not appear to be any chiral inversion. HCQ undergoes stereo-selective metabolism and stereo-selectively binds to proteins (81). It is not known whether the stereoisomers differ in activity.

Although few drug interaction studies of HCQ have been published, one study indicated that the bioavailability of metoprolol is increased by 65% after HCQ (84). Another study examined the interaction between methotrexate and HCQ, showing, in ten healthy patients, that HCQ increased the maximum methotrexate concentration and increased the area under the curve for methotrexate by 81%, which is likely to be clinically significant (p <.025) (85).

CHLOROQUINE

The elimination half-life of chloroquine is 3.5 to 12 days; approximately 55% of the total ingested dose is eliminated by urinary excretion (86). One report stated that small amounts of chloroquine may be found in the plasma, red blood cells, and urine for as long as 5 years after the last dose (87). Like HCQ, chloroquine is highly distributed to the tissues and concentrates in the eye.

Efficacy

Several studies starting in the 1960s have documented the effectiveness of HCQ for the treatment of RA (81). In 1993, a 24-week double-blind trial in 126 RA patients with less than 5 years' disease duration documented improvement in the HCQ-treated group in a combined joint swelling and tenderness score, grip strength, and global assessment, compared to the placebo group (93). In 2000, a metaanalysis was performed on all randomized, controlled trials involving HCQ versus placebo or HCQ with other DMARDs (94). Among four trials including 300 patients randomized to HCQ and 292 to placebo, HCQ was statistically better than placebo in most measures (standardized mean differences ranging from –0.33 to –0.52). No differences were observed in withdrawals due to toxicity.

Although the usual dose of HCQ is no more than 6 mg per kg and no higher than 400 mg per day (95), a recent trial indicated that the use of 800 or 1,200 mg daily HCQ for 6 weeks improved the response rate in RA patients (96). Paulus response criteria during the 6-week double-blind portion of that study were 47.9%, 57.7%, and 63.6% in the 400 mg per day, 800 mg per day, and 1,200 mg per day groups, respectively (p = .05). After 6 weeks, the dose of HCQ was reduced to 400 mg. Discontinuations for GI toxicities were increased in a dose-response manner (three, five, and six instances, respectively), but no statistical differences were noted. Ocular abnormalities were not dose related (96).

HCQ is still used frequently for the treatment of patients with recent-onset RA. For example, in a survey in Brittany, HCQ and injectable gold were the most widely used DMARDs in early RA (97). Particularly when taking cost into account, HCQ was the most commonly cited medication for the treatment of patients with mild disease activity severity in a survey of 375 rheumatologists (98). Among 195 patients using 4-aminoquinolones for the treatment of early RA (median duration of 6 months), a delay of therapy by more than 4 months was the only predictor of remission (i.e., delay of treatment predicted fewer remissions) (99). Using a large database collected over 20 years, the cumulative improvement in RA was better for methotrexate and IM gold than for HCQ, but all three drugs were more effective for earlier disease (less than 1 year) (100).

Some patients respond for prolonged periods. In a study of 541 patients in an open, randomized, controlled trial with a flexible dosing regimen, 30% of patients on HCQ were in remission at 5 years (101). Unfortunately, observational studies indicate that discontinuations for inefficacy were also more common among HCQ-treated patients during long-term follow-up, compared to those receiving penicillamine, sulfasalazine, auranofin, IM gold, methotrexate, cyclosporin, or azathioprine (102). Griffiths et al. documented a median duration of initial DMARD therapy for HCQ of 11 months, compared to 5 months for sulfasalazine and 15 months for methotrexate (103).

A trial of chloroquine (250 mg per day) for RA was published in 1960 and included 107 patients given chloroquine, of whom 80% completed 1 year of treatment with "general improvement," compared to 30% improvement for an approximately equal number of patients given placebo (104). In 1994, a somewhat smaller, 6-month trial comprising a total of 44 early RA patients tested chloroquine (300 mg per day decreasing to 100 mg per day) versus cyclosporin A (2.5 mg per kg per day increasing to 3.6 mg per kg per day). Response was equivalent in the two groups, although more paresthesias and increased creatinine levels were noted in the cyclosporin-treated group (not statistically significant) (105).

A retrospective study comparing chloroquine and HCQ was published by Avina-Zubieta et al. in 1998 (106). In a cohort of 940 patients having RA, SLE, palindromic arthritis, or other diagnoses, 57% used chloroquine, and 43% used HCQ. The hazard ratio for discontinuations because of inefficacy was significantly higher for HCQ than for chloroquine [hazard ratio = 1.4 (95% confidence interval: 1.1–1.9)], thus suggesting chloroquine is likely to be more effective than HCQ. Fifteen percent of the HCQ-treated patients had adverse events, compared to 28% of those taking chloroquine. The hazard ratio for discontinuations secondary to toxicity was lower for HCQ (hazard ratio = 0.6), suggesting that HCQ is less toxic than chloroquine.

COMPARISON WITH OTHER DISEASE-MODIFYING ANTIRHEUMATIC DRUGS

Although it is not now ethically appropriate to compare the progression of radiologic damage in patients taking DMARDs versus those receiving a true (i.e., no nonsteroidal antiinflammatory drugs or steroids) placebo, several studies have compared the efficacy of HCQ to other DMARDs. In a 48-week, double-blind, randomized, parallel trial comparing HCQ and sulfasalazine (with an open-label 3-year extension), sulfasalazine reduced radiographic progression significantly more than HCQ (107). This finding supported a metaanalysis of eight trials involving sulfasalazine in 1999, showing a trend for those patients taking sulfasalazine to have fewer inefficacy dropouts (p = .055) and to have a greater improvement in erythrocyte sedimentation rate and morning stiffness than patients treated with HCQ (p = .09 and .10, respectively).

An unexplained difference between HCQ and chloroquine was found in comparisons with D-penicillamine, where x-ray deterioration was less for patients receiving D-penicillamine than for those receiving chloroquine but not less than for HCQ-treated patients (108,109).

In a trial comparing HCQ or auranofin to IM gold or D-penicillamine to methotrexate or sulfasalazine, remission occurred in 16% given HCQ or auranofin, compared to 24% and 31%, respectively, for the other treatments (p <.05 for the group on HCQ or auranofin vs. either of the other two groups) (110). Progression of radiologic damage scores was also less for the IM gold or D-penicillamine group or the methotrexate or sulfasalazine group than for the HCQ or auranofin patients (p <.05).

The clinical impression that HCQ is slightly less effective than some other DMARDs was supported by the metaanalysis of Felson et al. in 1990 (111). Among 66 clinical trials, a composite measure of outcomes revealed that antimalarials were numerically but not statistically better (p =.11) than auranofin but were not statistically less effective than other DMARDs. Thus, antimalarials appeared somewhat less effective than other DMARDs and only slightly more effective than auranofin in the context of a metaanalysis, where dosing and disease severity are not well matched. Chloroquine-treated patients did better than HCQ-treated patients. On the other hand, antimalarials had generally less toxicity than the other DMARDs. Most studies were not large enough to avoid false-negative results (i.e., to avoid the finding of no difference when, in fact, there were differences).

A trial of minocycline versus HCQ was reported by O'Dell et al. in 2001 (112). Sixty early RA patients were randomized to minocycline, 100 mg twice daily, versus HCQ, 200 mg twice daily, a 2-year, double-blind protocol. The primary end point was the ACR 50%, rather than the ACR 20%, responses. Twice as many patients achieved the ACR 50% response at 2 years on the minocycline, compared to the HCQ groups (60% vs. 33%, $p = .04$).

EFFICACY IN JUVENILE RHEUMATOID ARTHRITIS

Although open studies indicated efficacy when using HCQ to treat juvenile RA, a placebo-controlled study found neither HCQ nor D-penicillamine to be more effective than placebo (113,114).

EFFICACY IN SYSTEMIC LUPUS ERYTHEMATOSUS

HCQ or chloroquine, or both, is frequently used to treat the skin lesions of discoid lupus, musculoskeletal symptoms, mucocutaneous signs and symptoms, and fevers associated with SLE (88,88a,89). A well-done, placebo-controlled withdrawal study demonstrated that HCQ decreases the risk of SLE flares (90). It may even prevent some of the osteoporosis associated with steroids in SLE (92). Finally, one small, anecdotal study suggested that using HCQ and quinacrine together may be of benefit in HCQ-resistant SLE (91).

HYDROXYCHLOROQUINE AND CHLOROQUINE IN DISEASE-MODIFYING ANTIRHEUMATIC DRUG COMBINATION STUDIES

Because HCQ and chloroquine have mechanisms of action that appear to differ from other DMARDs and have well-described kinetics and toxicities, it is possible to construct rational matrices for combinations of DMARDs, including the antimalarials. This matrix identifies nonoverlapping mechanisms of action, kinetics, and toxicities of DMARDs, and these aspects of the DMARDs can be used to define DMARD combinations most likely to work well together (115). Based on these matrices, it would be expected that antimalarials plus methotrexate, antimalarials plus azathioprine, and antimalarials plus sulfasalazine would be effective combinations, whereas their combination with cyclosporine and tumor necrosis factor α blockers would probably also be appropriate, although less sure to work. HCQ and gold would not be expected to be a good combination. In fact, a published study shows that HCQ did not add to the efficacy of IM gold (28). In a survey of 160 Canadian rheumatologists, 99% of the rheumatologists used combination DMARDs, the most popular combination being methotrexate with HCQ (116). In 1999, a survey article indicated that 13.4% of RA patients in the United States were taking methotrexate plus HCQ (117). The use of HCQ and methotrexate together increases the area under the curve for methotrexate by 81%. The RA Investigators Network of O'Dell et al. showed that 60% of patients treated with methotrexate and HCQ achieve an ACR 20% response after 2 years, compared to 49% of those treated with methotrexate and sulfasalazine. The ACR 50% responses in this study were 40% and 29%, respectively (118).

A 91-patient, double-blind, 6-month study comparing HCQ, sulfasalazine, and the combination of the two may have been underpowered (only approximately 30 patients per group), and only 62 patients completed the trial (119). Patients in the combination group responded more quickly than those treated with HCQ, but there were no statistical differences between groups.

When 1.25 mg per kg per day or 2.5 mg per kg per day cyclosporin or placebo were added to background chloroquine, ACR 20% responses were achieved by 28% of the patients in the placebo plus chloroquine group, 34% of the patients in the low-dose cyclosporine plus chloroquine group, and 50% of the patients in the 2.5 mg per kg per day cyclosporine plus chloroquine group, demonstrating a clear trend ($p = .07$) (120). The number of patients was too small for adequate statistical power to distinguish clinical efficacy between treatment groups, however. The RA Investigators Network trial included a third arm, methotrexate (7.5 to 17.5 mg per week), sulfasalazine (up to 2 g per day), and HCQ (400 mg per day) (118). The triple therapy arm achieved an ACR 20% response of 78% at 2 years, significantly greater than either of the other two arms (60% and 49%, respectively). The authors of this study concluded that the triple therapy was more effective than methotrexate and sulfasalazine and marginally superior to methotrexate plus HCQ. A cost-effectiveness analysis concluded that this triple therapy combination was more cost-effective than methotrexate continuation, cyclosporine plus methotrexate, or etanercept group monotherapy by a factor of approximately two to three (121).

Consistent with the rationale for combination therapeutics published by Munster and Furst, the combination of HCQ and D-penicillamine was not better than D-penicillamine alone (122).

A postmarketing study of adalimumab versus placebo with standard background DMARD therapy indicated that the addition of adalimumab to antimalarials improved response by approximately 20% in a small number of patients (123).

Safety Overview

In a prospective cohort study of approximately 400 patients, 120 were randomized to HCQ (124). Eight percent of the patients receiving HCQ eventually discontinued this drug, secondary to an adverse event (Table 27.4). In an SLE database of 156 patients receiving antimalarials, 203 courses of antimalarials were documented over an average duration of 6.9 years per patient, of which 97% used HCQ (125). Ten percent had side effects requiring withdrawal. In a study by Fries et al. among 2,747 patients using DMARDs, HCQ was found to have the most favorable side effect profile (126). The same conclusion was reached in a meta-analysis by Felson et al. (111).

In an overview of clinical trials of early RA by van Jaarsveld et al., one group of 120 patients was treated with HCQ plus nonsteroidal antiinflammatory drugs (124). In this subset, 26% had GI side effects, 14% mucocutaneous adverse events, and 12% had renal side effects (increased urinary protein or serum creatinine, usually associated with nonsteroidal antiinflammatory drugs). Other side effects (other than infections) occurred in fewer than 5% of patients. The most common side effects with HCQ are GI, including nausea, vomiting, epigastric pain, cramps, diarrhea, and weight loss (81). Rashes, pruritus, alopecia, and rare side effects, such as third-degree atrioventricular block, blood dyscrasias, and precipitation of porphyria, have occurred. In Wang et al.'s database of SLE patients, 11 of 20 withdrawals among 203 courses of therapy were for GI problems (55%), two patients each withdrew secondary to headache or dizziness (10%), one each withdrew secondary to hearing loss and rash (5%), one developed retinopathy at 6 years at a dose of 6.5 mg per kg per day (0.95 cases per 1,000 patient-years of HCQ), and two patients developed HCQ myopathy (1.9 cases per 1,000 patient-years) (125). Most studies indicate that the side effects of HCQ are infrequent and mild (81,111,126).

Retinopathy remains a concern, although its incidence is quite rare. A prospective cohort study from 1985 to 2000 examined the incidence of retinopathy in 526 Greek patients, 400 of whom had completed at least 6 years of treatment (127). No retinal toxicity was noted in any of the patients during the first 6 years of treatment. Two of the patients developed retinopathy beyond 6 years, one at 6.5 years and one at 8.0 years of treatment. The incidence of

HCQ-related retinopathy was 0.5% for 400 patients who were treated with recommended doses of the drug for a mean of 8.7 years. As of 1993, only four cases of retinopathy have been reported from HCQ at doses less than 6.5 mg per kg per day (128). If retinopathy occurs, the prognosis is excellent if the drug is discontinued when the patient presents with normal central and color vision and only relative scotomata. However, if the vision is less than 20/20 or abnormal color vision or absolute scotomata have occurred, progressive vision loss may occur, even if the drug is discontinued. Most ophthalmologists feel that eye examinations every 6 to 12 months in asymptomatic patients receiving less than 6.5 mg per kg per day HCQ are sufficient for monitoring (128).

The incidence of retinal toxicity after chloroquine may be higher than that for HCQ. Although some studies have found no difference in retinal toxicity, one study of 110 patients who received more than 100 g of HCQ or chloroquine during the previous 15 years reported that seven of 31 chloroquine-treated patients, but none of 66 patients receiving HCQ, exhibited retinopathy (129).

It is appropriate to separate retinal toxicity from defects in accommodation or corneal deposits, which may be associated with the use of HCQ and chloroquine (130,131). These latter effects are easily reversible (accommodation) or appear to have few, if any, consequences (corneal deposits).

Among the very rare side effects of chloroquine is a neuromuscular syndrome that includes proximal lower-extremity weakness, a neurogenic component, abnormal muscle and nerve biopsies, and normal creatine phosphokinase (132). Cardiomyopathy has also been reported (133).

Because HCQ is used for the treatment of SLE, and many SLE patients are women in the childbearing years, the data regarding the use of HCQ during pregnancy have been most extensively studied in this population (134). Based on these observations, as well as others, HCQ can be continued during pregnancy. The rationale is as follows:

- Low doses of antimalarial prophylaxis in pregnant women traveling to malaria-infested areas have long been recommended and appear safe.
- Flares of SLE disease have been documented when antimalarials are discontinued during pregnancy.
- The terminal half-life of HCQ is 40 to 50 days, so discontinuation of HCQ during pregnancy still results in exposure during most of the pregnancy (200–250 days).
- The mechanisms of action of HCQ, including inhibition of platelet aggregation and lowering of serum lipids, promote successful pregnancy and general medical health, respectively.

Summary

HYDROXYCHLOROQUINE, CHLOROQUINE, AND QUINACRINE

HCQ and chloroquine probably work by changing the pH of lysosomes, interfering with antigen processing, decreasing cytokine production, and decreasing T-cell stimulation. Apoptosis as a mechanism of action of antimalarials may also have a role to play, at least for the treatment of SLE. Quinacrine and chloroquine may have additional effects on lymphocyte proliferation and natural killer cell activity. There is significant variability of antimalarial absorption (bioavailability 30% to 100%), and these compounds have a very large tissue distribution, particularly concentrating in the retina. Their serum half-lives are also prolonged, in the range of 42 to 50 days. HCQ, at appropriate doses, is more effective than placebo for the treatment of the signs and symptoms of RA but is generally considered less effective than most other DMARDs, with the exception of auranofin. Chloroquine, on the other hand, appears to be somewhat more effective than HCQ. Most DMARDs are more effective than HCQ in terms of preventing or slowing radiologic damage to joints. HCQ is one of the most commonly used DMARDs in combination with other DMARDs, particularly methotrexate. The antimalarials are generally less toxic than most other DMARDs, with GI toxicity being the most common side effect. When used in appropriate doses and followed with appropriate ocular exams, clinically significant retinal lesions are extremely rare.

REFERENCES

1. Forrestier MJ. L'aurotherapie dans les rhumatismes chroniques. *Bull Mem Soc Med Hop Paris* 1929;53:323–327.
2. Vernon-Roberts B, Doré JL, Jessop JD, et al. Selective concentration & localization of gold in macrophages of synovial and other tissues during and after chrysotherapy in rheumatoid patients. *Ann Rheum Dis* 1976;35:477–486.
3. Kinne RW, Stuhlmuller B, Palombo-Kinne E, et al. The role of macrophages in rheumatoid arthritis. In: Firestein GS, Panay GS, Wollheim FA, eds. *Rheumatoid arthritis: new frontiers in pathogenesis and treatment*. Oxford: Oxford University Press, 2000:80.
4. Kirkham BW, Navarro FJ, Corkill MM, et al. In vivo analysis of disease-modifying drug therapy activity in RA by sequential immunohistological analysis of synovial membrane IL1B. *J Rheumatol* 1994;21:1615–1619.
5. Matsobara T, Saegusa Y, Hirohata K. Low dose gold compounds inhibit fibroblast proliferation and do not affect interleukin secretion by macrophages. *Arthritis Rheum* 1988;31:1272–1280.
6. Gottlieb NL, Kiem IM, Penneys NS, et al. The influence of chrysotherapy on serum protein and immunoglobulin levels, rheumatoid factor, and antiepithelial antibody titers. *J Lab Clin Med* 1975;86:962–970.
7. Kawakami A, Eguchi K, Migiti K, et al. Inhibitory effects of gold sodium thiomalate on the proliferation and interferon gamma induced HLA DR expression in human endothelial cells. *J Rheumatol* 1990;17:430–435.
8. Riestra Noriega JL, Harth M. Pharmacology of gold compounds in rheumatoid arthritis: a review. *Can J Clin Pharmacol* 1997;4:127–136.
9. Repchinsky C, Welbanks L, Bisson R, eds. *Compendium of pharmaceuticals and specialties*. Correction Pharmacists Association. Canadian Pharmacists Association. Ottawa, 2002:1569.
10. Gottlieb NL. Metabolism and distribution of gold compounds. *J Rheumatol* 1979;6:2–6.

10a. Blocka KLN, Paulus HE, Furst DE. Clinical pharmacokinetics of oral and injectable gold compounds. *Clin Pharmacokinet* 1986;11:133–143.

11. The Research Subcommittee of the Empire Rheumatism Council. Gold therapy in rheumatoid arthritis. Report of a multi-centre controlled trial. *Ann Rheum Dis* 1960;19:95–117.
12. Empire Rheumatism Council Research Sub-committee. Gold therapy in rheumatoid arthritis. Final report of a multicentre controlled trial. *Ann Rheum Dis* 1961;20:315–334.
13. Sigler JW, Bluhm GB, Duncan H, et al. Gold salts in the treatment of rheumatoid arthritis. A double blind study. *Ann Intern Med* 1974;80:21–26.
14. The Cooperating Clinics Committee of the American Rheumatism Association. A controlled trial of gold salt therapy in rheumatoid arthritis. *Arthritis Rheum* 1973;16:353–358.
15. Ward J, Williams HJ, Egger MJ, et al. Comparison of auranofin, gold sodium thiomalate and placebo in the treatment of rheumatoid arthritis. A controlled clinical trial. *Arthritis Rheum* 1983;26:1303–1315.
16. Luukkainen R, Kajander A, Isomaki H. Effect of gold on progression of erosions in rheumatoid arthritis. Better results with early treatment. *Scand J Rheumatol* 1977;6:189–192.
17. Buckland-Wright JC, Clarke GS, Chikanza IC, et al. Quantitative microfocal radiography detects changes in erosion area in patients with early rheumatoid arthritis treated with myocrisine. *J Rheumatol* 1993;20:243–247.
18. Rau R, Herborn G, Menninger H, et al. Progression in early erosive rheumatoid arthritis: 12 month results from a randomized controlled trial comparing methotrexate and gold sodium thiomalate. *Br J Rheumatol* 1998;37:1220–1226.
19. Rau R, Herborn G, Menninger H, et al. Comparison of intramuscular methotrexate and gold sodium thiomalate in the treatment of early erosive rheumatoid arthritis: 12 month data of a double-blind parallel study of 174 patients. *Br J Rheumatol* 1997;36:345–352.
20. Williams HJ, Ward JR, Dahl SL, et al. A controlled trial comparing sulfasalazine, gold sodium thiomalate and placebo in rheumatoid arthritis. *Arthritis Rheum* 1988;31:702–713.
21. Felson DT, Anderson JJ, Meenan RF. The comparative efficacy and toxicity of second-line drugs in rheumatoid arthritis. *Arthritis Rheum* 1990;33:1449–1461.
22. Bendix G, Bjelle A. A 10 year follow up of parenteral gold therapy in patients with rheumatoid arthritis. *Ann Rheum Dis* 1996;55:169–176.
23. Srinivasan R, Miller BL, Paulus HE, et al. Long term chrysotherapy in rheumatoid arthritis. *Arthritis Rheum* 1979;22:105–110.
24. Wolfe F, Hawley D, Cathey MA. Measurement of gold treatment effect in clinical practice: evidence for effectiveness of intramuscular gold. *J Rheumatol* 1993;20:797–801.
25. Lehtinen K, Isomaki H. Intramuscular gold therapy is associated with long survival in patients with rheumatoid arthritis. *J Rheumatol* 1991;18:524–529.

26. Rau R, Schlattenkirchner M, Muller-Fassbender H, et al. A three-year study of auranofin and gold sodium thiomalate in rheumatoid arthritis. *Clin Rheumatol* 1990;9:461–474.
27. Bensen W, Tugwell P, Roberts R, et al. Combination therapy of cyclosporine with methotrexate and gold in rheumatoid arthritis (2 pilot studies). *J Rheumatol* 1994;21:2034–2038.
28. Porter DR, Capell HA, Hunter J. Combination therapy in rheumatoid arthritis—no benefit of addition of hydroxychloroquine to patients with suboptimal response to intramuscular gold therapy. *J Rheumatol* 1993;20:645–649.
29. Lehman AF, Esdaile JM, Klinkhoff A, et al. A 48 week double blind double observer placebo controlled multicentre trial of intramuscular gold in combination with methotrexate in rheumatoid arthritis. *Arthritis Rheum* 2002;46:5204.
30. Lockie LM, Smith DM. Forty-seven years experience with gold therapy in 1019 rheumatoid arthritis patients. *Semin Arthritis Rheum* 1985;14:238–246.
31. Klinkhoff A, Teufel A, McCartney C. A review of 38 years of experience with injectable gold. *Clin Invest Med* 1989;12:B95.
32. Gordon DA, Klinkhoff AV. Gold and penicillamine. In: Ruddy S, Harris ED, Sledge CB, eds. *Kelley's textbook of rheumatology*, 6th ed. Philadelphia: WB Saunders, 2000:869–878.
33. Klinkhoff AV, Teufel A. How low can you go? Use of very low dosage of gold in patients with mucocutaneous reactions. *J Rheumatol* 1995;22:1657–1659.
34. Leonard PA, Moatamed FM, Ward JR, et al. Chrysiasis: the role of sun exposure in dermal hyperpigmentation secondary to gold therapy. *J Rheumatol* 1986;13:58–64.
35. Hall CL. The natural course of gold and penicillamine nephropathy: a long term study of 54 patients. *Adv Exp Med Biol* 1989;252:247–256.
36. Katz WA, Blodgett RC, Pietrusko RG. Proteinuria in gold treated rheumatoid arthritis. *Ann Intern Med* 1984;101:176–179.
37. Klinkhoff AV, Teufel A. Reinstitution of gold after gold induced proteinuria. *J Rheumatol* 1997;24:1277–1279.
38. Kay AG. Myelotoxicity of gold. *BMJ* 1976;1:1266–1268.
39. Yan A, Davis P. Gold induced marrow suppression: a review of 10 cases. *J Rheumatol* 1990;17:47–51.
40. Coblyn JS, Weinblatt M, Holdsworth D, et al. Gold induced thrombocytopenia. A clinical and immunogenetic study of twenty-three patients. *Ann Intern Med* 1981;95:178–181.
41. Aaron S, Davis P, Percy J. Neutropenia occurring during the course of chrysotherapy: a review of 25 cases. *J Rheumatol* 1985;12:897–899.
42. Dillon AM, Luthra HS, Conn D, et al. Parenteral gold therapy in the Felty syndrome. *Medicine* 1986;65:107–112.
43. Reid C, Patterson AC. Pure red cell aplasia after gold treatment. *BMJ* 1977;2:1457.
44. Arthur AB, Klinkhoff AV, Teufel A. Nitritoid reactions: case reports, review, and recommendations for management. *J Rheumatol* 2001;28:2209–2212.
45. Gottlieb NL, Brown HE. Acute myocardial infarction following gold sodium thiomalate induced vasomotor (nitritoid) reaction. *Arthritis Rheum* 1977; 20:1026–1028.
46. Tilelli JA, Heinrichs MM. Adverse reactions to parenteral gold salts. *Lancet* 1997;349:853.
47. Healey LA, Backes MB. Nitritoid reactions and angiotensin converting enzyme inhibitors. *N Engl J Med* 1989;321:763.
48. Karrar AA, EC Ramahi KM, Jishi FA. Intramuscular gold, angiotensin converting enzyme inhibitor and anaphylactic reactions. *J Rheumatol* 1996;23:200–201.
49. Halla JT, Hardin JG, Linn JE. Postinjection non vasomotor reactions during chrysotherapy. *Arthritis Rheum* 1977;20:1188–1191.
50. Smith W, Ball GV. Lung injury due to gold treatment. *Arthritis Rheum* 1980;23:351–354.
51. Evans RB, Ettensohn DB, Fawaz-Estrup F, et al. Gold lung: recent development in pathogenesis, diagnosis and therapy. *Semin Arthritis Rheum* 1987; 16:126–205.
52. Rocha MP, Burrichter PJ, Blodgett RC. Effect of chrysotherapy on the lower gastrointestinal tract: a review. *Semin Arthritis Rheum* 1987;16:294–299.
53. Lowthian PJ, Cleland LG, Vernon-Roberts B. Hepatotoxicity with aurothioglucose therapy. *Arthritis Rheum* 1984;27:230–232.
54. Favreau M, Tannenbaum H, Lough J. Hepatic toxicity associated with gold therapy. *Ann Intern Med* 1977;87:717–719.
55. Fam AG, Gordon DA, Sarkozi J, et al. Neurologic complications associated with gold therapy for rheumatoid arthritis. *J Rheumatol* 1984;11:700–706.
56. Schlumpf U, Meyer M, Ulrich J, et al. Neurologic complications induced by gold treatment. *Arthritis Rheum* 1983;26:825–831.
57. Furst DE, Levine S, Srinivasan R, et al. A double blind trial of high versus conventional dosage of gold salts for rheumatoid arthritis. *Arthritis Rheum* 1977;20:1473–1479.
58. Cats A. A multicenter controlled trial of the effects of different dosage of gold therapy followed by a maintenance dosage. *Agents Actions* 1976;6:355–363.
59. Sharp JT, Lidsky MD, Duffy J, et al. Comparison of two dosage schedules in the treatment of rheumatoid arthritis. *Arthritis Rheum* 1977;20:1179–1187.
60. Hart FD. Is gold treatment advisable during pregnancy? *BMJ* 1984;288:1359.
61. Tarp U, Graudal H. A followup study of children exposed to gold compounds in utero. *Arthritis Rheum* 1985;28:235–236.
62. Cohen DL, Orzel J, Taylor A. Infants of mothers receiving gold therapy. *Arthritis Rheum* 1981;24:104–105.
63. Blau SP. Metabolism of gold during lactation. *Arthritis Rheum* 1973;16:777–778.
64. Rooney TW, Lorber A, Veng-Pedersen P, et al. Gold pharmacokinetics in breast milk of a lactating woman. *J Rheumatol* 1987;14:1120–1122.
65. Payne JP. A post-graduate lecture on lupus erythematosus. *Clin J* 1894;4;223.
66. Page F. Treatment of lupus erythematosus with mepacrine. *Lancet* 1951;2:755.
67. Olson NY, Lindlsey CB. Adjunctive use of hydroxychloroquine in childhood dermatomyositis. *J Rheumatol* 1989;16:1545–1547.
68. Youssef W, Yan A, Russell A. Palindromic rheumatism: a response to chloroquine. *J Rheumatol* 1991;18;1.
69. Carreno L, Lopez-Longo FJ, Gonzalez CM, Monteagudo I. Treatment options for juvenile-onset systemic lupus erythematosus. *Paediatr Drugs* 2002;4:241–256.
70. Lakhanpal S, Ginsburg WW, Michet CJ, et al. Eosinophilic fascitis: clinical spectrum and therapeutic response in 52 cases. *Semin Arthritis Rheum* 1988;17:221–231.
71. Thorne C, Weisman M, et al. Hydroxychloroquine versus acetaminophen versus placebo in the treatment of nodal osteoarthritis of the hands. *Arthritis Rheum* 2000;43[Suppl]:932(abst).
72. Ausiello C, Sorrentino V, Ruggiero V, Rossi GB. Action of lysosomotropic amines on spontaneous and interferon-enhanced NK and CTL cytolysis. *Immunol Lett* 1984;8:11–15.
73. Ausiello CM, Barbieri P, Spagnoli GC, et al. In vivo effects of chloroquine treatment on spontatneous and interferon-induced natural killer activities in rheumatoid arthritis patients. *Clin Exp Rheumatol* 1986;1:255.
74. Fox RI. Mechanism of action of hydroxychloroquine as an antirheumatic drug. *Semin Arthritis Rheum* 1993;2[Suppl 1]:82–91.
75. Liu ST, Wang CR, Yin GD, et al. Hydroxychloroquine sulphate inhibits in vitro apoptosis of circulating lymphocytes in patients with systemic lupus erythematosus. *J Allergy Immunol* 2001;19:29–35.
76. Espinola RG, Pierangeli SS, Ghara AE, Harris EN. Hydroxychloroquine reverses platelet activation induced by human IgG antiphospholipid antibodies. *Thromb Haemost* 2002;87:518–522.
77. Bondeson J, Sundler R. Antimalarial drugs inhibit phospholipase A2 activation and induction of interleukin 1 beta and tumor necrosis factor alpha in macrophages: implications for their mode of action in rheumatoid arthritis. *Gen Pharmacol* 1998;30:357–366.
78. Ciak J, Hahn FE. Chloroquine: mode of action. *Science* 1966;151:347–351.
79. Stoller D, Levine L. Antibodies to denatured DNA and lupus erythematosus. *Arch Biochem* 1963;101:355–357.
80. Tett SE. Clinical pharmacology of slow acting antirheumatic drugs. *Clin Pharmacokinet* 1993;25:392–407.
81. Nishihara KK, Furst DE. Hydroxychloroquine and its use in rheumatoid arthritis. *Today's Therapeutic Trends* 1995;13:109–124.
82. Bernstein H, Zvaifler N, Rubin M, Mansour AM. The ocular deposition of chloroquine. *Invest Ophthalmol* 1963;2:384–391.
83. Munster T, Gibbs JP, Shen D, et al. Hydroxychloroquine concentration-response relationships in patients with rheumatoid arthritis. *Arthritis Rheum* 2002;46:1460–1469.
84. Somer M, Kallio J, Pesonen U, et al. Influence of hydroxychloroquine on the bioavailability of oral metoprolol. *Br J Clin Pharmacol* 2000;49:549–554.
85. Carmichael SJ, Beal J, Day RO, Tett SE. Combination therapy with methotrexate and hydroxychloroquine for rheumatoid arthritis increases exposure to methotrexate. *J Rheumatol* 2002;29:2077–2083.
86. McChesney EW, Fasco MJ, Banks WF Jr. The metabolism of chloroquine in man during and after repeated oral dosage. *J Pharmacol Exp Ther* 1967;158:223–332.
87. Rubin M, Bernstein HN, Zvaifler N. The studies on the pharmacology of chloroquine. *Arch Ophthalmol* 1962;70:474–478.
88. DuBois E. Antimalarials in the management of discoid and systemic lupus erythematosus. *Semin Arthritis Rheum* 1978;8:33–38.
88a. Winkleman RF, Mervin CF, Brunsting LA. Anti-malarial use in lupus erythematosus. *Ann Intern Med* 1961;55:772–781.
89. Vitali C, Doria A, Tincani A, et al. International survey on the management of patients with SLE. I. General data on the participating centers and the results of a questionnaire regarding mucocutaneous involvement. *Clin Exp Rheumatol* 1996;14[Suppl 16]:S17–22.
90. The Canadian Hydroxychloroquine Study Group. A randomized study of the effect of withdrawing hydroxychloroquine sulfate in systemic lupus erythematosus. *N Engl J Med* 1991;324:150.
91. Toubi E, Rosner I, Rozenbaum M, et al. The benefit of combining hydroxychloroquine with quinacrine in the treatment of SLE patients. *Lupus* 2000;9:81–82.
92. Lakshminarayanan S, Walsh S, Mohanraj M, Rothfield N. Factors associated with low bone mineral density in female patients with systemic lupus erythematosus. *J Rheumatol* 2001;28:102–108.
93. Clark P, Casas E, Tugwell P, et al. Hydroxychloroquine compared with placebo in rheumatoid arthritis. *Ann Intern Med* 1993;119:1067–1071.
94. Suarez-Almazor ME, Belseck E, Shea B, et al. Antimalarials for treating rheumatoid arthritis. *Cochrane Database Syst Rev* 2000;4:CD000959.
95. Mackenzie AH. Dose refinements in long-term therapy of rheumatoid arthritis with antimalarials. *Am J Med* 1983;75:40–45.
96. Furst DE, Lindsley H, Baethge B, et al. Dose-loading with hydroxychloroquine improves the rate of response in early, active rheumatoid arthritis: a randomized double-blind six-week trial with eighteen-week extension. *Arthritis Rheum* 1999;42:357–365.
97. Saraux A, Berthelot JM, Charles G, et al. Second-line drugs used in recent-onset rheumatoid arthritis in Brittany (France). *Joint Bone Spine* 2002;69:37–42.
98. Erkan D, Yaziei Y, Harrison MJ, Paget SA. Physician treatment preferences in rheumatoid arthritis of differing disease severity and activity: the impact of cost on first line therapy. *Arthritis Rheum* 2002;15:47:285–290.
99. Mottonen T, Hannonen P, Korpela M, et al. Delay to institution of therapy and induction of remission using single-drug or combination-disease-modi-

fying antirheumatic DR therapy in early rheumatoid arthritis. *Arthritis Rheum* 2002;46:894–898.

100. Hurst S, Kallan MJ, Wolfe FJ, et al. Methotrexate, hydroxychloroquine, and intramuscular gold in rheumatoid arthritis: relative area under the curve effectiveness and sequence effects. *J Rheumatol* 2002;29:1639–1645.
101. Jessop JD, O'Sullivan MM, Lewis PA, et al. A long term five-year randomized controlled trial of hydroxychloroquine, sodium aurothiomalate, auranofin and penicillamine in the treatment of patients with rheumatoid arthritis. *Br J Rheumatol* 1998;37:992–1002.
102. Papadopoulos NG, Alamanos Y, Papadopoulos IA, et al. Disease modifying antirheumatic drugs in early rheumatoid arthritis: a long-term observational study. *J Rheumatol* 2002;29:261–266.
103. Griffiths RI, Bar-Din M, MacLean C, et al. Patterns of disease-modifying antirheumatic drug use, medical resource consumption, and cost among rheumatoid arthritis patients. *Ther Apher* 2001;5:92–104.
104. Freedman A, Steinberg VL. Chloroquine in rheumatoid arthritis, a doubleblindfold trial of treatment for one year. *Ann Rheum Dis* 1960;19:243–256.
105. Landewe RB, Goei The HS, van Rijthoven AW, et al. A randomized, doubleblind, 24 week, controlled study of low dose cyclosporine versus chloroquine for early rheumatoid arthritis. *Arthritis Rheum* 1994;37:637–643.
106. Avina-Zubieta JA, Galindo-Rodriquez G, Newman S, et al. Long-term effectiveness of antimalarial drugs in rheumatic diseases. *Ann Rheum Dis* 1998;57:582–587.
107. van der Heijde DM, van Riel PL, Nuver-Zwart IH, van de Putte LB. Alternative methods for analysis of radiographic damage in a randomized, double blind, parallel group clinical trial comparing hydroxychloroquine and sulfasalazine. *J Rheumatol* 2000;27:535–539.
108. Gibson T, Emory P, Armstrong RD, et al. Combined D-penicillamine and chloroquine treatment of rheumatoid arthritis: a comparative study. *Br J Rheumatol* 1987;26:279–284.
109. Bunch TW, O'Duffy JD, Tompkins RB, O'Fallon WM. Controlled trial of hydroxychloroquine and D-penicillamine singly and in combination in the treatment of rheumatoid arthritis group. *Arthritis Rheum* 1984;27:267–279.
110. van Jaarsveld CH, Jahangier ZN, Jacobs JW, et al. Toxicity of anti-rheumatic drugs in a randomized clinical trial of early rheumatoid arthritis. *Rheumatology (Oxford)* 2000;39:374–382.
111. Felson DT, Anderson JJ, Meenan RF. The comparative efficacy and toxicity of second line drugs in rheumatoid arthritis. Results of two meta-analyses. *Arthritis Rheum* 1990;33:1449–1461.
112. O'Dell JR, Blakely KW, Mallek JA, et al. Treatment of early seropositive rheumatoid arthritis: a two-year, double-blind comparison of minocycline and hydroxychloroquine. *Arthritis Rheum* 2001;44:2235–2241.
113. Manners PJ, Ansell BM. Slow acting antirheumatic drugs used in systemic onset juvenile chronic arthritis. *Pediatrics* 1986;77:99–105.
114. Brewer EJ, Giannini EH, Kuzima N, Alekseev L. D-penicillamine and hydroxychloroquine in the treatment of severe rheumatoid arthritis. *N Engl J Med* 1986.
115. Munster T, Furst DE. Pharmacotherapeutic strategies for disease-modifying antirheumatic drug (DMARD) combinations to treat rheumatoid arthritis (RA). *Clin Exp Rheumatol* 1999;17[6 Suppl 18]:S29–36.
116. Pope JE, Hong P, Kochler BE. Prescribing trends in disease modifying antirheumatic drugs for rheumatoid arthritis: a survey of practicing Canadian rheumatologists. *J Rheumatol* 2002;29:255–260.
117. Hawley DJ, Wolfe F, Pincus T. Use of combination therapy in the routine care of patients with rheumatoid arthritis: physician and patient surveys. *Clin Exp Rheumatol* 1999;17[6 Suppl 18]:S78–82.
118. O'Dell JR, Leff R, Paulsen G, et al. Treatment of rheumatoid arthritis with methotrexate and hydroxychloroquine, methotrexate and sulfasalazine or a combination of the three medications: results of a two-year, randomized, double-blind, placebo-controlled trial. *Arthritis Rheum* 2002;46: 1164–1170.
119. Faarvandang KL, Egsmose C, Kryger P, et al. Hydroxychloroquine and sulfasalazine alone and in combination in rheumatoid arthritis: a randomized double-blind trial. *Ann Rheum Dis* 1993;52:711–715.
120. van den Borne BE, Lanadewe RB, Goei The HS, et al. Combination therapy in recent onset rheumatoid arthritis: a randomized double-blind trial of the addition of low dose cyclosporine to patients treated with low-dose chloroquine. *J Rheumatol* 1998;25:1493–1498.
121. Choi HK, Seeger JD, Kuntz KM. A cost-effectiveness analysis of treatment options for patients with methotrexate-resistant rheumatoid arthritis. *Arthritis Rheum* 2000;43:2316–2327.
122. Bunch TW, O'Duffy JD, Tompkins RB, et al. Controlled trial of hydroxychloroquine and D-penicillamine singly and in combination in the treatment of rheumatoid arthritis. *Arthritis Rheum* 1984;27:267–276.
123. Weinblatt M, Keystone E, Furst DE, et al. Adalimumab, a fully human anti-TNF-α monoclonal antibody, and concomitant standard antirheumatic therapy for the treatment of rheumatoid arthritis: results of STAR (Safety Trial of Adalimumab in Rheumatoid Arthritis). *J Rheumatol* 2003;48:855.
124. van Jaarsveld CH, Jahangier ZN, Jacobs JW, et al. Toxicity of anti-rheumatic drugs in a randomized clinical trial of early rheumatoid arthritis. *Rheumatology (Oxford)* 2000;39:1374–1382.
125. Wang C, Fortin PR, Li Y, et al. Discontinuation of antimalarial drugs in systemic lupus erythematosus. *J Rheumatol* 1999;26:808–815.
126. Fries JF, Williams CA, Ramey D. The relative toxicity of disease modifying antirheumatic drugs. *Arthritis Rheum* 1993;36:297–306.
127. Mavrikakis I, Sfikakis PP, Mavrikakis E, et al. The incidence of irreversible retinal toxicity in patients treated with hydroxychloroquine: a reappraisal. *Ophthalmology* 2003;110:1321–1326.
128. Easterbrook M. An ophthalmological view on the efficacy and safety of chloroquine versus hydroxychloroquine. *J Rheumatol* 1999;26:1866–1868.
129. Finbloom DS, Silver K, Newsome DA, et al. Comparison of hydroxychloroquine and chloroquine use and the development of retinal toxicity. *J Rheumatol* 1985;12:692–694.
130. Berliner RW, Earl DP Jr, Taggart JV, et al. Studies on the chemotherapy of human malarious. VI. The physiologic deposition, antimalarial activity and toxicity of several derivatives of 4-aminoquinolones. *J Clin Invest* 1948;27 [Suppl]:98–110.
131. Hobbs HE, Calnan DC. The ocular complications of chloroquine therapy. *Lancet* 1958;1:1207–1209.
132. Estes ML, Ewing-Wilson D, Chou SM, et al. Chloroquine neuromyotoxicity clinical and pathological prospective. *Am J Med* 1987;82:447–459.
133. Ratliff NB, Estes ML, Myles JL, et al. Diagnosis of chloroquine cardiomyopathy by endomyocardial biopsy. *N Engl J Med* 1987;316:191–194.
134. Borden MB, Parke AL. Antimalarial drugs in systemic lupus erythematosus: use in pregnancy. *Drug Saf* 2001;24:1055–1063.

CHAPTER 28

Minocycline

Marcela Juárez and Graciela S. Alarcón

Although the use of minocycline for the treatment of rheumatoid arthritis (RA) dates only to the 1990s (1–3), antibiotics of the tetracycline family have been advocated for the treatment of this disease and other rheumatic disorders as far back as the late 1960s (4); that was done in the belief that mycoplasmas (and perhaps other tetracycline-sensitive microorganisms) were involved in the etiopathogenesis of RA and other chronic arthritides (5,6). The lack of confirmation of the mycoplasma etiology for RA, coupled with a negative (albeit not adequately powered) randomized clinical trial conducted in the early 1970s, contributed to the skepticism about this therapy among mainstream rheumatologists in the United States and abroad (7). Not until the late 1980s to early 1990s did interest in the use of tetracyclines for the treatment of RA resurface (8–10). This interest was due to several reasons: (a) the appreciation of the nonantimicrobial properties of the tetracyclines (antiinflammatory, chondroprotective, and immunomodulatory) (11–13); (b) the demonstration that synthetic tetracyclines devoid of antimicrobial activity retain their antirheumatic properties (14,15); and (c) the continued interest in the possible infectious etiology of RA (13). To date, several well-conducted and adequately powered studies have demonstrated the benefits of minocycline in the treatment of RA (1–3,16). Despite these studies, minocycline and other tetracycline derivatives are used infrequently in the treatment of RA (17,18). The comments that follow apply particularly to minocycline.

PHARMACOLOGY

Minocycline is a semisynthetic tetracycline derivative. The parent compounds, chlortetracycline and oxytetracycline, are produced by the fungi *Streptomyces aureofaciens* and *Streptomyces rimosus*, respectively. The tetracyclines are constituted by a polycyclic core; chemical alterations on the side chains of this core have resulted in different derivatives, minocycline being one of them (a monohydrochloride derivative) (12,13,19). The chemical structure of minocycline is shown in Figure 28.1. Minocycline is readily absorbed (95–100%) by the oral route, and peak serum levels are achieved within 2 hours of its administration; its absorption takes place in the upper small intestine, and, in contrast to other tetracyclines, its absorption is not affected by most nutrients (20), but divalent cations (such as calcium, magnesium, and iron) and aluminum do impair its absorption (19). Thus, food rich in calcium (particularly dairy products or products purportedly enriched with calcium), calcium, magnesium, and aluminum-containing antacids, as well as iron preparations, impair the absorption of minocycline (13,19,21). Once absorbed, minocycline circulates bound to serum proteins; being liposoluble, it is widely distributed to tissues and body fluids, resulting in high concentrations in the bile, tears, saliva, and synovial fluid but not in the cerebrospinal fluid (19). Like other tetracyclines, minocycline crosses the placenta, reaching the fetus; it is also excreted in milk. Chelation with calcium results in the deposit of minocycline (and other tetracycline derivatives) in growing bones and forming teeth, resulting in their permanent damage (19,22).

Minocycline is excreted in the bile and in the urine; some of the compound excreted in the bile (where it achieves very high concentrations) is reabsorbed (enterohepatic circulation), contributing to maintaining adequate serum levels. High lumen levels of minocycline are achieved, resulting in significant changes in the intestinal flora, particularly in subjects taking it for prolonged periods (19). Approximately half of minocycline is excreted in the urine by glomerular filtration and the rest in the feces. The half-life of minocycline varies between 11 and 70 hours, depending on whether renal and hepatic function are normal (11–22 hours) or impaired (11–70 hours) (19). Within the tetracyclines, minocycline is considered a long-acting preparation, and, thus, it is amenable to a once-a-day dosing (12,19), although it has been dosed twice daily in all RA clinical trials.

There is a significant drug interaction with warfarin; thus, patients taking warfarin may require a dose adjustment to maintain the same level of anticoagulation as the one present before minocycline administration (19). For unclear reasons, minocycline (and other tetracycline derivatives) may render oral contraceptives less effective (23). This is particularly important in view of the possible deleterious effect of these compounds on developing bones and teeth (19,22).

MECHANISMS OF ACTION

As already noted, minocycline and other tetracycline derivatives have been found to have antiinflammatory, immunomodulatory, and chondroprotective properties. These data have been directly generated in *in vitro* and *in vivo* studies using canine osteoarthritis and periodontal disease models (8,10,12,24–26); indirect evidence for some of these properties has been obtained during the recently conducted clinical trials (1,2). These data will be now briefly presented.

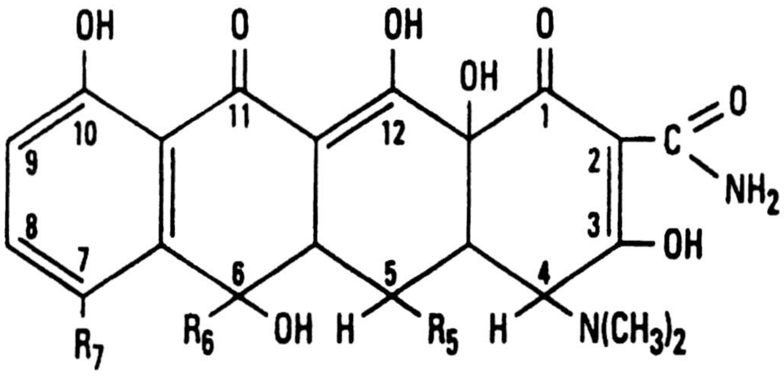

R_7	R_6	R_5
$N(CH_3)_2$	H	H

Figure 28.1. Chemical structure of minocycline. (Modified from Chambers HF. Chloramphenicol, tetracyclines, macrolides, clindamycin and streptogramins. In: Katzung BG, ed. *Basic and clinical pharmacology*. 8th ed. New York: Lange Medical Books/McGraw-Hill, 2001:774–792.)

Antiinflammatory Properties

Both *in vivo* and *in vitro* studies have shown tetracycline derivatives in general, and minocycline in particular, to inhibit phospholipase A_2, resulting in a decreased production of cyclooxygenase and lipoxygenase and their corresponding downstream inflammatory mediators (prostaglandins and leukotrienes) (27). Other proinflammatory mediators, including oxygen radicals and nitric oxide, also have been shown to be released less efficiently in the presence of tetracycline derivatives or to be scavenged in their presence (28–30).

Tetracycline derivatives, minocycline included, have also been shown to up-regulate the production of tissue inhibitors of matrix metalloproteinases; this up-regulation results in a decreased matrix metalloproteinase activity. This effect has been demonstrated both *in vitro* and *in vivo* (10,11,31–33). Initial studies involved the periodontal disease animal model; in such models, a decrease in collagenase activity in the crevicular fluid was observed after the administration of doxycycline (24). Subsequently, Greenwald et al. demonstrated a significant decrease in collagenase activity in synovial tissue (or fluid) samples obtained subsequently to the administration of a short course of minocycline to patients with RA, in comparison to the levels observed in samples obtained before this therapeutic intervention (34). Of interest, these antiinflammatory properties have been described also with chemically synthesized tetracyclines devoid of antibacterial activity (14,15).

Indirect evidence for the antiinflammatory properties of minocycline has been obtained from the human trials to be discussed. For example, a decrease in the levels of C-reactive protein, an increase in hemoglobin levels, and a decrease in erythrocyte sedimentation rate have been observed in the minocycline-treated patients but not in those treated with placebo or with hydroxychloroquine (1,2).

Immunomodulatory Properties

Sera from patients receiving tetracyclines have been shown to impair leukocyte migration and phagocytosis and to arrest lymphocyte proliferation and activation in animal models (35–37). Minocycline has also been shown to impair the proliferation and activation of human lymphocytes and synovial tissue cells, resulting in a decrease in the production of proinflammatory cytokines and the corresponding downstream inflammatory mediators (38).

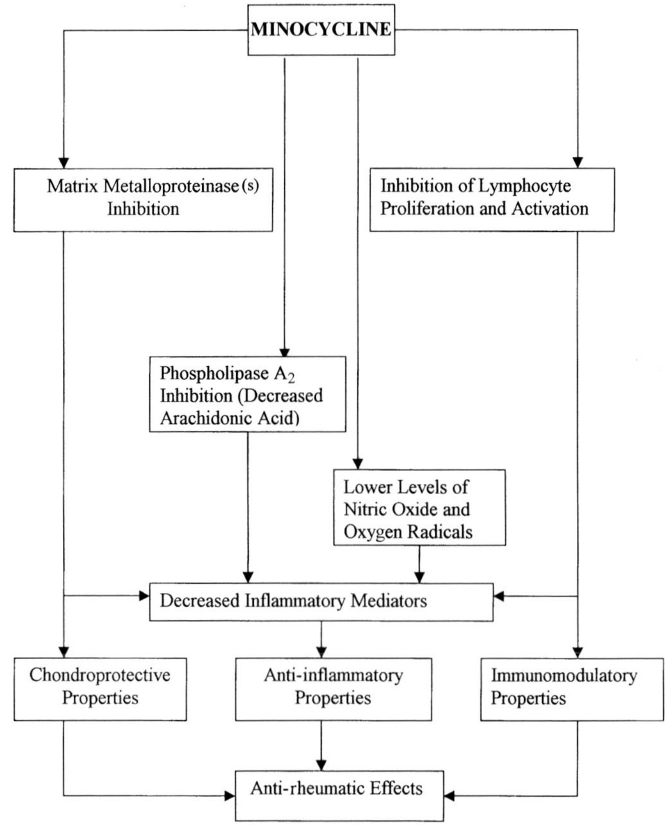

Figure 28.2. Properties of minocycline.

Chondroprotective Properties

As noted above, animal and human studies have shown that minocycline (and other tetracycline derivatives) produces up-regulation of tissue inhibitors of matrix metalloproteinases, which is followed by a decrease in the activity of different mammalian matrix metalloproteinases (10,11,31–33,39). The end result is a decrease in cartilage breakdown. This effect has been used as the basis for animal and human trials of doxycycline in osteoarthritis (25,40).

Although unproven, data from different *in vitro* and *in vivo* studies suggest that the mechanism underlying the antiinflammatory, chondroprotective, and immunomodulatory effects of minocycline and other tetracycline derivatives relates to their ability to chelate heavy metals. In fact, the addition of calcium or zinc may reverse the anticollagenolytic activity of doxycycline, and changes in intracellular calcium levels relate to altered lymphocyte transformation and differentiation, as demonstrated in *in vitro* and *in vivo* models of inflammation (41).

It is still possible that minocycline may exert its antirheumatic effect as an antimicrobial, although such has not been proven. The role of infectious agents in the etiology of RA remains a viable option, periodically reinforced when an infectious agent is shown to induce a rheumatoid-like arthropathy; that has been the case with some viruses, such as parvovirus or rubella, but also with nonviral agents, such as *Borrelia burgdorferi*, the spirochete responsible for Lyme disease (13). Of note, however, none of the microbes rendered bacteriostatic by minocycline (and other tetracycline derivatives), other than mycoplasmas, have been implicated in the etiology of RA, and changes in the intestinal flora that occurred with these antibiotics have not been shown to relate to the antirheumatic effects of these compounds.

Many of the practitioners who endorsed the use of minocycline and other antibiotics for the treatment of RA before the 1990s, and even those who endorse their use at the present time, as well as many of the patients who seek this therapeutic option, do so believing that the antirheumatic properties of minocycline and other tetracycline derivatives are primarily the result of their antimicrobial activity (42). These ideas are now disseminated and advocated via the World Wide Web. Figure 28.2 illustrates the properties of minocycline.

CLINICAL EFFICACY AND SAFETY

The early positive experience with tetracycline derivatives, as reported by Sanchez in Brazil and Brown et al. in the United States, was imperfect and, thus, either open to significant criticism or simply ignored (4,5). Subsequently, Skinner et al. published the results of a small, randomized clinical trial; in this study, 27 of 30 patients completing this 1-year trial received either 250 mg of tetracycline or placebo (7). Although the drug was well tolerated, the dose was probably insufficient to exert any antirheumatic effect; this study, published in *Arthritis and Rheumatism*, was perhaps the main reason why tetracycline derivatives were not used for the treatment of RA for several years afterward. By the 1980s, however, enough data suggesting the antiinflammatory, chondroprotective, and immunomodulatory effects of tetracycline derivatives had been accumulated; experience in the use of minocycline in other chronic inflammatory disorders (such as periodontal disease and acne vulgaris) had also emerged (43,44). These data led to two relatively small open studies, one conducted in the Netherlands and the other in Israel (45,46).

In the first of these two open trials, Breedveld et al. (46) treated ten RA patients with escalating doses of minocycline for a total of 16 weeks; patients were started on 200 mg of minocycline per day. If the clinical response was incomplete and there were no deleterious effects, the dose could be increased to 400 mg per day; however, one patient discontinued minocycline before drug escalation, and six others could not escalate it. Nevertheless, when compared to pretrial parameters, patients experienced significant clinical improvement, while at the same time, laboratory parameters suggestive of ongoing inflammation improved (45). The second open trial was conducted in Israel (46). In this trial, 18 patients were treated with a fixed dose of minocycline (200 mg per day) for approximately 1 year. Of the 18 patients, one was lost to follow-up, two discontinued minocycline because of toxic manifestations, and three more discontinued for lack of efficacy; of the 12 patients completing the trial, three were in near remission, and the remaining nine were significantly improved. As with the first open trial, improvement in laboratory parameters of inflammation was observed, paralleling the clinical response (46).

The first of the two open studies can be truly considered the prelude for the subsequent double-blind randomized clinical trials. The impetus for the first American study was, however, as much science as it was pressure from the community (through Congress) urging the National Institutes of Health to prove the antirheumatic properties of minocycline (and tetracycline derivatives). In fact, this trial was well under way by the time the second open trial was published by Langevitz et al. in 1992 (45).

These trials have clearly demonstrated the benefit of minocycline when used for the treatment of RA. Minocycline, however, has not been compared in an equally careful manner with methotrexate (considered by many rheumatologists to be the gold standard in RA treatment) or with the newer compounds, such as leflunomide, or the biologic compounds (anti–tumor necrosis factor or anti–interleukin-1 receptor antagonist). With most investigators now conducting clinical trials with these and other potentially interesting biologic compounds, it is unlikely that such trials will ever be conducted.

The first randomized clinical trial was conducted in the Netherlands and involved 80 patients with RA of relatively long duration (mean disease duration was ≥10 years) who were treated with either minocycline (200 mg per day) or placebo for a total of 26 weeks (6 months) (1). These patients, who had already failed one disease-modifying antirheumatic drug (DMARD), were continued with their background medication (DMARD included) for the duration of the trial; the large majority of these patients were seropositive for immunoglobulin M rheumatoid factor, had evidence of destructive disease radiographically, and had evidence of active disease, as determined by clinical and laboratory parameters.

The other three large clinical trials were conducted in North America (2,3,16). The first North American study [Minocycline in RA (MIRA)] was published around the same time as the study from the Netherlands and was sponsored by the National Institute of Arthritis and Musculoskeletal and Skin Disorders (2); the MIRA study was conducted in six centers across the United States and involved 219 patients with established RA, yet with much less severe RA than the patients studied by Kloppenburg et al. (1). Patients in the MIRA trial were not continued in a DMARD but had to have failed at least one of them to be included in the study. Patients in the MIRA trial were treated for approximately 1 year (48 weeks), and although they met the inclusion criteria for active disease (a given number of tender and swollen joints), they certainly had less severe disease than the patients treated by Kloppenburg et al. In fact, only approximately two-thirds of the MIRA patients were either seropositive for immunoglobulin M rheumatoid factor or had erosive disease; as a group, they also did not have as severe inflammation as the patients from Holland.

The other two North American studies have been conducted under the leadership of O'Dell from the University of Nebraska (3,16). O'Dell has constituted an investigational network of midwest academic and nonacademic rheumatologists [RA Investigational Network (RAIN)] that has been involved in several large clinical trials (47). The studies from the RAIN group include one placebo-controlled trial and another in which the active comparator was hydroxychloroquine (3,16). Both RAIN studies differ from the studies from the MIRA group and from the Netherlands in that only patients with early and seropositive (for immunoglobulin M rheumatoid factor) disease who had never received a DMARD were included. The first RAIN study involved 46 patients and lasted 6 months, whereas the second study involved 60 patients and lasted 2 years (3). In the second RAIN study, but not in the first, all patients were given a small dose of prednisone, even if they had not been taking any prednisone before the initiation of the study (5.0–7.5 mg per day were given, depending on the patient's weight) (16). Longitudinal data from patients enrolled in the minocycline studies are only available for the studies from O'Dell et al. (48,49).

With the exception of the second RAIN study, the other three studies were planned and conducted before the formulation of the American College of Rheumatology (ACR) and the European League Against Rheumatism response criteria for clinical improvement in RA clinical trials (50–52); these three studies, therefore, do not include the same outcome variables. In the study from Kloppenburg et al., for example, patients improved significantly in terms of duration of morning stiffness, the Ritchie articular index, the number of swollen joints, as well as in their functional capacity. Parameters of inflammation, including hemoglobin, erythrocyte sedimentation rate, and C-reactive protein and platelet counts, also improved (1). In the MIRA study, clinical improvement was defined *a priori* as a reduction of at least 50% in the number of swollen and tender joints. A significantly greater proportion of patients in the minocycline-treated group than in the placebo-treated group met these two primary outcome criteria; in addition, other clinical parameters (considered secondary outcomes by study design) changed in the expected direction in the minocycline-treated but not in the placebo-treated patients. Laboratory parameters of inflammation, including hemoglobin levels, C-reactive protein levels, platelet counts, and erythrocyte sedimentation rate, also improved significantly in the minocycline-treated patients but not in the placebo-treated patients (2).

In the first study from the RAIN group, the primary outcome variable was a 50% clinical improvement by the 6-month evaluation point; this 50% improvement was defined as at least a 50% improvement in three of several clinical variables, including morning stiffness, joint tenderness, joint swelling, and erythrocyte sedimentation rate. Secondary outcome variables included the Ritchie articular index for joint pain and joint swelling, overall pain (as scored by the patient), and the patient and physician global assessments of disease activity. Sixty-five percent of minocycline-treated patients, but only 13% of the placebo-treated patients, achieved the primary outcome. In addition, patients in the minocycline group tended to have improvement in the secondary variables, but that was not the case for patients in the placebo group (3).

In the second study from the RAIN group, there were two primary variables, the ACR 50% response rate and the dose of prednisone reached at the end of the study (2 years). A greater proportion of patients in the minocycline group (60%) achieved an ACR 50% response rate, as compared to those treated with hydroxychloroquine (33%); at the end of 2 years, patients in the minocycline group were taking a much lower daily prednisone dose (0.81 mg) than those in the hydroxychloroquine group (3.21 mg). Moreover, patients in the minocycline group who achieved an ACR 20%/50% response rate were more likely than those in the hydroxychloroquine group, achieving the same ACR responses, to be completely off prednisone (75% vs. 33% for those patients achieving an ACR 20% reponse rate and 71% vs. 25% for those achieving an ACR 50% reponse rate). As in the other studies, parameters of inflammation improved in the minocycline-treated patients, and these changes were of a greater magnitude than in those patients treated with hydroxychloroquine (16).

Despite the differences in these four trials (patient characteristics, trial duration, comparator compound, and different outcome variables), taken together, the data support the efficacy of minocycline for the treatment of RA. The longitudinal data, obtained by the RAIN group in their first study, further indicate that the response to minocycline is sustained and that, over time, patients treated with minocycline were likely to remain on the drug and to not be taking corticosteroids or any other DMARDs (48). In contrast, patients originally randomized to placebo were more likely to be taking a DMARD (minocycline an option), to be taking corticosteroids, and not to be in remission. These longitudinal data are quite relevant; they suggest that patients with early, yet not too aggressive, disease may particularly benefit from the use of minocycline (48). Longitudinal data from the minocycline versus hydroxychloroquine study have not been published in full at the time of this writing; preliminary analyses demonstrate similar sustained long-term benefits from minocycline (49). Despite the data from these four clinical studies, particularly the data from O'Dell, it is the authors' personal experience that most rheumatologists to date will choose hydroxychloroquine (or methotrexate) over minocycline in their daily practice, even in patients with relatively mild to moderate disease; moreover, minocycline is variably mentioned in American and European rheumatology textbooks and even in books dedicated exclusively to RA. Some of these books totally exclude any reference to minocycline, whereas others provide only a very short synopsis of it. Moreover, in a pharmacology textbook published in 2001, compounds introduced into the rheumatologist's armamentarium only relatively recently, such as leflunomide, etanercept, and infliximab, are described, whereas minocycline is described along with the other compounds of the tetracycline family in the antimicrobial section of the book, but not

TABLE 28.1. Demographic and Clinical Features of Rheumatoid Arthritis Patients from Minocycline Double-Blind Studies

	Study Names, Yr (References)			
Feature	Kloppenburg, 1994 (1) (N = 80)	Tilley, 1995, MIRA (2) (N = 219)	O'Dell, 1997 (3) (N = 46)	O'Dell, 2001 (16) (N = 60)
Age (yr), mean	56	54	45	48
Female (%)	68	78	72	73
Ethnicity (%)	—	—	—	—
White	100[a]	55	NA[b]	NA[b]
African-American	0	28	—	—
Hispanic/other	0	6	—	—
Disease duration, yr, mean	13.0	8.6	0.4	0.5
Functional class (%)				
I	18	6	ND	ND
II	63	80	—	—
III	19	14	—	—
Erosive disease (%)	95	68	NA	NA
Previous DMARD use (%)	56[c]	46	0	0
Corticosteroid use (%)	11	31	0	100[d]
Functional capacity, 0–3 scale, mean	1.7	0.9	ND	ND
Patient global assessment, 0–10 VAS, visual analog scale, mean	ND	ND	5.1	5.0
IgM RF positivity (%)	89	56	100	100
ESR mm/h, mean	50	34	32	32

DMARD, disease-modifying antirheumatic drug; ESR, erythrocyte sedimentation rate; IgM, immunoglobulin M; NA, not available or applicable; ND, not done; RF, rheumatoid factor.
[a]Inferred based on country where study was done.
[b]The majority are probably white.
[c]Allowed during study.
[d]Required at study initiation.

TABLE 28.2. Primary Outcomes from Minocycline Double-Blind Studies in Rheumatoid Arthritis

			Number of Patients				Patients Achieving Primary Outcome(s) (%)			
Author, Yr (Reference)	Study Characteristic	Treatment Duration	Placebo	Minocycline	HCQ	Primary Outcome(s)	Placebo	Minocycline	HCQ	*p* Value
Kloppenburg et al., 1994 (1)	Placebo-controlled	26 wk	40	40	NA	≥25% improvement in two of the following three: Ritchie articular index, number of swollen joints, and C-reactive protein levels	18	38	NA	<.005
Tilley et al., 1995 (2)	Placebo-controlled	48 wk	110	109	NA	≥50% improvement in joint swelling	39	54	NA	.023
						≥50% improvement in joint tenderness	41	56	NA	.021
O'Dell et al., 1997 (3)	Placebo-controlled	26 wk (6 mo)	23	23	NA	≥50% improvement in three of the following variables: morning stiffness, joint tenderness, joint swelling, and ESR	13	65	NA	<.001
O'Dell et al., 2001 (16)	Active comparator	96 wk (2 yr)	NA	30	30	ACR 50% improvement	NA	60	33	.04
						Prednisone				
						Not taking it at the end of study	NA	71	23	.03
						Dose achieved mg/d, mean	NA	0.81	3.21	<.01

ACR, American College of Rheumatology; ESR, erythrocyte sedimentation rate; HCQ, hydroxychloroquine; NA, not applicable.

otherwise (53). The levels of improvement observed in the minocycline trials would have been taken more positively by the rheumatology community if they had been obtained with a compound other than minocycline (particularly a biologic compound).

The demographic and clinical features of the patients involved in these four trials and the outcome of these trials are presented in Tables 28.1 and 28.2.

The data relative to drug toxicity are quite divergent in these four trials (1–3,16). The studies from O'Dell et al. report no significant side effects in patients receiving these compounds, particularly during the initial phases of both studies (3,16). In contrast, the data from the MIRA study show an array of relatively minor side effects, although they occurred with comparable frequency in the minocycline-treated and in the placebo-treated patients (2). Finally, in the study from the Netherlands, vestibular reactions leading to falls and fractures were reported with greater frequency in the minocycline-treated than in the placebo-treated patients (1). Discontinuation rates directly attributable to side effects vary between 6% and approximately 13%. In clinical practice, some patients complain of abdominal symptoms (abdominal pain, nausea without vomiting, and diarrhea), and they occur particularly at treatment initiation. These symptoms are, however, rarely severe enough to force discontinuation of the drug; to the contrary, they tend to subside with time. Dizziness, as reported in the trial from the Netherlands, is vestibular in origin and tends to be more frequent in the elderly, particularly in women (54); other central nervous system manifestations include headaches and, occasionally, pseudotumor cerebri, complications that have been described mainly in children (55,56).

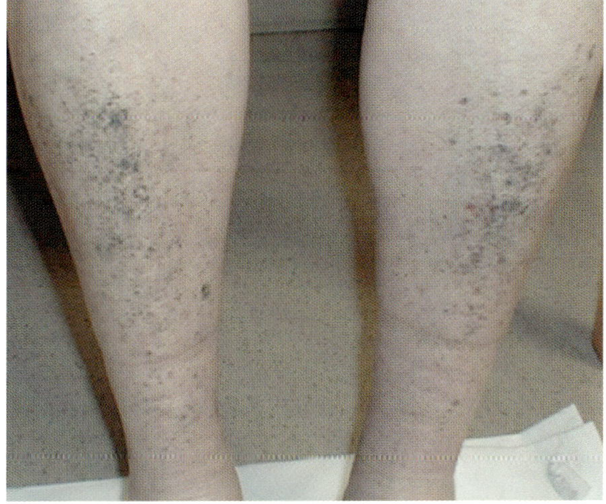

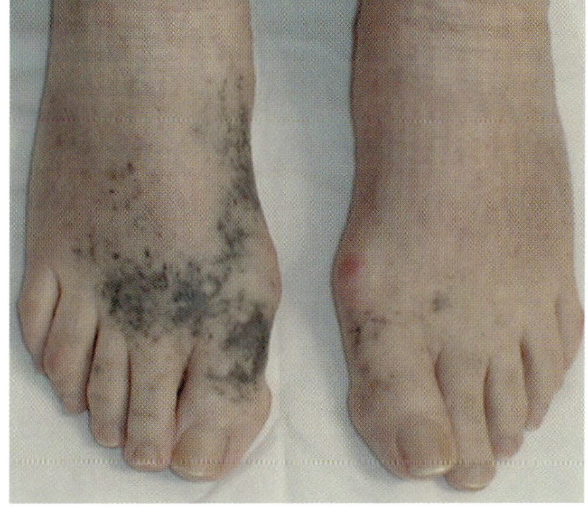

Figure 28.3. Pigmentation occurring around scar from bunionectomy in a patient with rheumatoid arthritis treated with minocycline for more than 5 years.

TABLE 28.3. Adverse Events Reported in Open and Double-Blind Minocycline Studies in Rheumatoid Arthritis

	Open Studies		Double-Blind, Placebo-Controlled Studies			
	Breedveld, 1990 (46)	Langevitz, 1992 (45)[a]	Kloppenburg, 1994 (1)[a]		Tilley, 1995 (MIRA) (2)[a]	
Adverse Event (%)	Minocycline[b] (N = 10)	Minocycline (N = 18)	Minocycline (N = 40)	Placebo (N = 40)	Minocycline (N = 109)	Placebo (N = 110)
Cutaneous						
Rash	0	0	0	3	5	6
Hyperpigmentation	0	22	0	0	0	0
Gastrointestinal	20	6	58	15	24	25
Pulmonary (allergic pneumonitis)	0	0	3	0	0	0
CNS						
Dizziness, vertigo, light-headedness	50	11	40	15	19	20
(Leading to major event)	0	0	5	0	0	0
Headaches	0	0	3	0	20	20
Other (infections)	0	22	0	8	0	0

CNS, central nervous system.
[a]Some patients had more than one adverse event.
[b]Minocycline dose: 200–400 mg/d.

Although not reported in the longitudinal data gathered by O'Dell and his collaborators, there are now a number of small series and clinical cases describing different autoimmune manifestations, which have been related to the use of minocycline (57–69); some of these manifestations have been documented, particularly in younger patients in whom minocycline is prescribed for the treatment of acne (61), but also in patients with RA (70). A clear idea of the frequency of these autoimmune reactions is lacking, given the fact that the denominator (that is, the number of RA patients exposed to minocycline per year) is largely unknown. These autoimmune manifestations are quite diverse and include hepatitis, nephritis, pneumonitis, central nervous system involvement, and a lupus-like systemic disorder characterized by fever, arthritis, photosensitivity, a number of different photosensitive and nonphotosensitive skin rashes (morbilliform, exfoliative, fixed drug eruption), and variable organ system involvement. These patients may exhibit antinuclear antibodies, but, in contrast with what occurs in other drug-induced lupus syndromes, these patients lack antihistone antibodies (62,63,65,71). These manifestations may occur shortly after the initiation of minocycline or on rechallenge; this is particularly the case in adolescents who tend to take minocycline intermittently, as their acne flares and subsides (68).

Cutaneous, mucosal, and organ system pigmentary changes have been reported after prolonged minocycline administration; given the relative short duration of the minocycline RA trials, such changes were not reported in these trials (72–76). During the longitudinal phase of O'Dell's studies, however, such pigmentary changes have been observed (48). The authors also have observed pigmentary changes in three patients in whom minocycline had been administered for longer than 2 years; pigmentation has occurred in the skin (around a scar) in one patient in the palmar aspect of the thenar eminence in another, and in the oral mucosa in the third (Fig. 28.3). The first two patients chose to continue minocycline, whereas the one with pigmentary changes in the oral mucosa chose to discontinue it. Iron in pigmented-laden macrophages has been observed in the subcutaneous tissue from pigmented skin biopsies by light and electron microscopy; whether other pigment may be involved, especially when organ system pigmentation is observed, is unclear to date (73,74). As with any other medication, patients may be willing to continue minocycline

TABLE 28.4. Adverse Events Reported in Other Double-Blind Minocycline Studies in Rheumatoid Arthritis

					Follow-Up, Double-Blind Studies			
	Double-Blind, Placebo-Controlled Studies [O'Dell, 1997 (3)]		Double-Blind, Active Comparator [O'Dell, 2001 (16)]		Placebo-Controlled		Active Comparator	
					O'Dell, 1999 (48)		O'Dell, 2000 (49)	
Adverse Event (%)	Minocycline (N = 23)	Placebo (N = 23)	Minocycline (N = 30)	HCQ (N = 30)	Minocycline (N = 20)	Placebo (N = 18)	Minocycline (N = 30)	HCQ (N = 28)
Cutaneous								
Rash	0	0	0	0	0	0	0	4
Hyperpigmentation	0	0	0	0	20	0	7	0
Gastrointestinal	0	0	0	0	0	0	0	4
Pulmonary (allergic pneumonitis)	0	0	0	0	0	0	0	0
CNS								
Dizziness, vertigo, light-headedness	0	0	0	0	0	0	3	0
(Leading to major event)	0	0	0	0	0	0	0	0
Headaches	0	0	0	0	0	0	0	0
Other (infections)	0	0	0	0	0	0	0	0

CNS, central nervous system; HCQ, hydroxychloroquine.

TABLE 28.5. Adverse Events Secondary to Minocycline and Suggestions for Drug Monitoring

Event Type and Manifestation(s) (References)	Population at Risk	Baseline	Monitoring	Management
Toxic				
Mucocutaneous (2,12,45,48,49,72) Skin hyperpigmentation	All (presence of scars)	History and physical examination	History and physical examination	May continue
Gastrointestinal (1,2,45,46,59) Nausea, vomiting, abdominal pain	All	Increase dose gradually	History	May continue
Hepatotoxicity	Hepatic and renal involvement, impairment	Chemistry profile (liver and kidney)	Chemistry profile (liver and kidney)	Decrease dose or discontinue
Renal (2) Nephrotoxicity	Hepatic and renal involvement, impairment	Chemistry profile (liver and kidney), urinalysis	Chemistry profile (kidney), urinalysis, ABG	Decrease dose or discontinue
CNS (1,2,12,45,46,48) Dizziness, vertigo, headaches	Older women	Increase dose gradually	History (consider fractures)	May continue
Immune or allergic				
Mucocutaneous (61) Sweet's syndrome	NA	—	History and physical examination	Corticosteroids
Gastrointestinal (62,63,71) Autoimmune hepatitis	Younger women	Chemistry profile (liver); hepatitis B, C profile	Chemistry profile (liver), follow up for 1 yr to rule out autoimmune chronic hepatitis	Discontinue corticosteroids, immunosuppressants
Pulmonary (1,57,60) Pneumonitis	Women	Chest x-ray film	History and physical examination, chest x-ray film, ABG, bronchoalveolar lavage	Discontinue corticosteroids
Renal (58) Acute interstitial nephritis	NA	Chemistry profile (liver and kidney), urinalysis	Chemistry (kidney), urinalysis (eosinophils), ABG	Discontinue
Lupus-like syndrome (62,66,70,71)	Younger women	Chemistry profile (liver and kidney), urinalysis, ANA	History, chemistry profile (liver and kidney), urinalysis, chest x-ray film, ANA	Discontinue

ABG, arterial blood gases; ANA, antinuclear antibodies; CNS, central nervous system; NA, not available.

if its beneficial effect appears to be substantial, whereas they will opt for discontinuing it if the benefit is marginal, at best.

If minocycline (and other tetracycline derivatives) are inadvertently administered to young children and pregnant women, a permanent brownish discoloration of all teeth occurs; in addition, skeletal maturation is retarded under these circumstances (12,22).

Tables 28.3 and 28.4 summarize the most common adverse reactions to minocycline, as reported in the context of the initial open studies, the four randomized clinical trials, and the two longitudinal studies. Table 28.5 summarizes the toxic and allergic events described in patients treated with minocycline and how to monitor for their occurrence. Table 28.6 lists the relative and absolute contraindications for the use of minocycline, and Figure 28.4 summarizes minocycline dosage and administration.

CRITICAL ANALYSIS OF THE RESULTS OF CLINICAL TRIALS

As noted in the editorial that accompanied the publication of the MIRA trial (77), the first two large randomized clinical trials (the MIRA trial and the one from Kloppenburg et al.) were well designed and impeccably executed, rendering credibility to the data generated. The data from O'Dell and his RAIN collaborators are equally credible (78,79). Taken together, these four double-blind placebo (or active comparator) studies represent the best effort the rheumatology community could have undertaken to answer the public's request of providing a definitive answer as to whether minocycline (and perhaps other tetracycline derivatives) has antirheumatic properties. Unfortunately, only in the Kloppenburg studies were *in vitro* data obtained in parallel, demonstrating the immunomodulatory effects of minocycline; however, the exact mechanism underlying the antirheumatic effects of minocycline was not pursued further (38).

Radiographic data have now been completed and published only for the MIRA study (80). Like other clinical and laboratory parameters measured in this study, this trial was not powered to detect differences in the rate of progression of joint erosions, joint space narrowing, or the sum of the two in the two treatment groups. Indeed, the rate of progression was not different in the two groups. Newly involved joints (as determined radiographically) were, however, more common in the placebo-treated than in the minocycline-treated patients. When only the data for the white patients were examined, those patients carrying a shared epitope encoding the HLA-DR4 allele (a marker of RA severity) and treated with placebo were more likely to develop new erosions than those treated with minocycline also carrying the epitope (odds ratio, 14; confidence interval: 12.9–215) (81).

TABLE 28.6. Contraindications for the Use of Minocycline

Clinical Situation (Reference)	Absolute	Relative
Patient with known hypersensitivity to tetracycline (1,45,46,82)		✓
Infants and children up to age 8 (22,75,82)	✓	
Women of childbearing age without effective contraception (1,46)	✓	
Pregnancy (19,22,82)	✓	
Renal insufficiency[a] (1,12,45,46,58,59,82)		✓
Hepatic involvement[a] (1,12,45,46,82)		✓

[a]Could be absolute if function or impairment is severe; dose could be adjusted downward, but data are not available (from rheumatoid arthritis studies) on how exactly to do it.

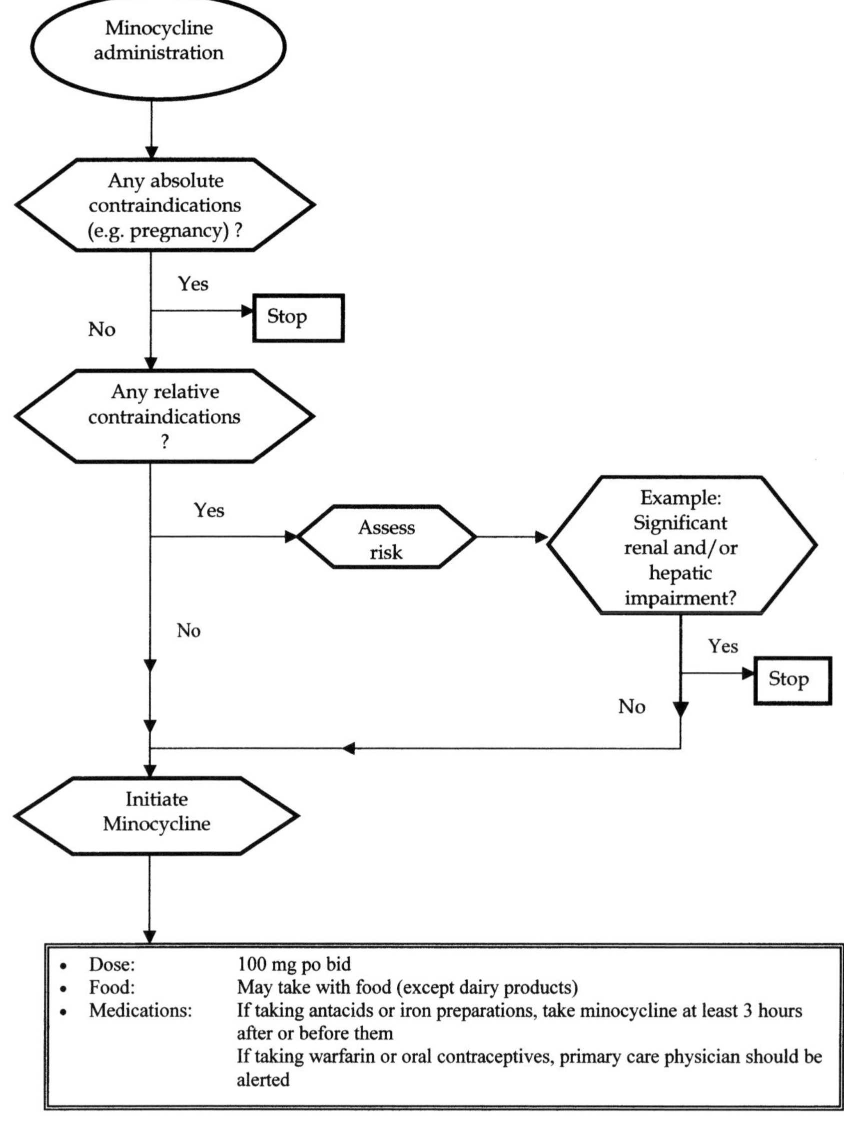

Figure 28.4. Flow diagram for the administration of minocycline.

In short, the quality of the minocycline studies parallels the quality of other recent RA trials; if minocycline had been a new compound with a pharmaceutical company sponsoring it, the data could have been used to gain its approval at the Food and Drug Administration in the United States or its European counterpart.

REFERENCES

1. Kloppenburg M, Breedveld FC, Terwiel JP, et al. Minocycline in active rheumatoid arthritis. A double-blind, placebo-controlled trial. *Arthritis Rheum* 1994;37:629–636.
2. Tilley BC, Alarcón GS, Heyse SP, et al. Minocycline in rheumatoid arthritis: a 48 week, double-blind, placebo-controlled trial. *Ann Intern Med* 1995;122:81–89.
3. O'Dell JR, Haire CE, Palmer W, et al. Treatment of early rheumatoid arthritis with minocycline or placebo: results of a randomized, double-blind, placebo-controlled trial. *Arthritis Rheum* 1997;40:842–848.
4. Sanchez I. As tetraciclinas no tratamento da artrite reumatoid e doencas reumaticas inflamatorias. *Bras Med* 1968;82:22–31.
5. Brown TM, Clark HW, Bailey JS, Gray CW. A mechanistic approach to treatment of rheumatoid type arthritis naturally occurring in a gorilla. *Trans Am Clin Climatol Assoc* 1970;82:227–247.
6. Bartholomew LE. Isolation and characterization of mycoplasmas (PPLO) from patients with rheumatoid arthritis, systemic lupus erythematosus and Reiter's syndrome. *Arthritis Rheum* 1965;8:376–388.
7. Skinner M, Cathcart ES, Mills JA, Pinals RS. Tetracycline in the treatment of rheumatoid arthritis. A double blind controlled study. *Arthritis Rheum* 1971;14:727–732.
8. Golub LM, Lee HM, Lehrer G, et al. Minocycline reduces gingival collagenolytic activity during diabetes. Preliminary observations and a proposed new mechanism of action. *J Periodontal Res* 1983;18:516–526.
9. El Attar TMA, Lin HS, Schulz R. Effect of minocycline on prostaglandin formation in gingival fibroblasts. *J Periodontal Res* 1988;23:285–286.
10. Yu LPJ, Smith GNJ, Hasty KA, Brandt KD. Doxycycline inhibits type XI collagenolytic activity of extracts from human osteoarthritic cartilage and of gelatinase. *J Rheumatol* 1991;18:1450–1452.
11. Golub LM, Wolff M, Lee HM. Further evidence that tetracyclines inhibit collagenase activity in human crevicular fluid and from other mammalian sources. *J Periodontal Res* 1985;20:12–23.
12. Alarcón GS. Tetracyclines for the treatment of rheumatoid arthritis. *Exp Opin Invest Drugs* 2000;9:1491–1498.
13. Alarcón GS, Mikhail IS. Antimicrobials in the treatment of rheumatoid arthritis and other arthritides: a clinical perspective. *Am J Med Sci* 1994;308:201–209.
14. Golub LM, McNamara TF, D'Angelo G, Greenwald RA, Ramamurthy NS. A nonantibacterial chemically modified tetracycline inhibits mammalian collagenase activity. *J Dent Res* 1987;66:1310–1314.
15. Golub LM, Evans RT, McNamara TF, et al. A non-antimicrobial tetracycline inhibits gingival matrix metalloproteinases and bone loss in Porphyromonas gingivalis induced periodontitis in rats. *Ann N Y Acad Sci* 1994;732:96–111.
16. O'Dell JR, Blakely KW, Mallek JA, et al. Treatment of early seropositive rheumatoid arthritis with minocycline or hydroxychloroquine. *Arthritis Rheum* 2001;44:2235–2241.
17. Panush RS, Thoburn R. Should minocycline be used to treat rheumatoid arthritis? *Bull Rheum Dis* 1996;45:2–5.
18. Toussirot E, Despaux J, Wendling D. Do minocycline and other tetracyclines have a place in rheumatology? *Rev Rheum Engl Ed* 1997;64:474–480.
19. Chambers HF. Chloramphenicol, tetracyclines, macrolides, clindamycin and streptogramins. In: Katzung BG, ed. *Basic and clinical pharmacology*. 8th ed. New York: Lange Medical Books/McGraw-Hill, 2001:774–792.

20. Jung H, Peregrina AA, Rodriguez JM, Moreno-Esparza R. The influence of coffee with milk and tea with milk on the bioavailability of tetracycline. *Biopharm Drug Dispos* 1997;18:459–463.
21. Alarcón GS. Minocycline for the treatment of rheumatoid arthritis. *Rheum Dis Clin North Am* 1998;24:489–499.
22. Demers P, Fraser D, Goldbloom RB, et al. Effects of tetracyclines on skeletal growth and dentition. A report by the Nutrition Committee of the Canadian Paediatric Society. *Can Med Assoc J* 1968;99:849–854.
23. Helms SE, Bredle DL, Zajic J, et al. Oral contraceptive failure rates and oral antibiotics. *J Am Acad Dermatol* 1997;36:705–710.
24. Golub LM, Ciancio S, Ramamurthy NS, et al. Low-dose doxycycline therapy: effect on gingival and crevicular fluid collagenase activity in humans. *J Periodontal Res* 1990;25:321–330.
25. Yu LPJ, Smith GNJ, Brandt KD, et al. Reduction of the severity of canine osteoarthritis by prophylactic treatment with oral doxycycline. *Arthritis Rheum* 1992;35:1150–1159.
26. Cole AA, Chubinskaya S, Luchene LJ, et al. Doxycycline disrupts chondrocyte differentiation and inhibits cartilage matrix degradation. *Arthritis Rheum* 1994;37:1727–1734.
27. Pruzanski W, Greenwald RA, Street IP, et al. Inhibition of enzymatic activity of phospholipases A2 by minocycline and doxycycline. *Biochem Pharmacol* 1992;44:1165–1170.
28. Amin AR, Attur MG, Thakker GD, et al. A novel mechanism of action of tetracyclines: effects on nitric oxide synthases. *Proc Natl Acad Sci U S A* 1996;93:14014–14019.
29. Attur MG, Patel RN, Patel PD, et al. Tetracycline up-regulates Cox-2 expression and prostaglandin E2 production independent of its effect on nitric oxide. *J Immunol* 1999;15:3160–3167.
30. Sadowski T, Steinmeyer J. Minocycline inhibits the production of inducible nitric oxide synthase in articular chondrocytes. *J Rheumatol* 2001;28:336–340.
31. Golub LM, Ramamurthy NS, McNamara TF, et al. Tetracyclines inhibit tissue collagenase activity. A new mechanism in the treatment of periodontal disease. *J Periodontal Res* 1984;19:651–655.
32. Greenwald RA, Moak SA, Ramamurthy NS, Golub LM. Tetracyclines suppress matrix metalloproteinase activity in adjuvant arthritis and in combination with flurbiprofen, ameliorate bone damage. *J Rheumatol* 1992;19:927–938.
33. Yu LPJ, Burr DB, Brandt KD, et al. Effects of oral doxycycline and administration on histomorphometric and dynamics of subchondral bone in a canine model of osteoarthritis. *J Rheumatol* 1996;23:137–142.
34. Greenwald RA, Golub LM, Lavietes B, et al. Tetracyclines inhibit human synovial collagenase in vitro and in vitro. *J Rheumatol* 1987;14:28–32.
35. Elewski BE, Lamb BAJ, Sams WMJ, Gammon WR. In vivo suppression of neutrophil chemotaxis by systemically and topically administered tetracycline. *J Am Acad Dermatol* 1983;8:807–812.
36. Naess A, Glette J, Halstensen AI, et al. In vivo and in vitro effects of doxycycline on leucocyte membrane receptors. *Clin Exp Immunol* 1985;62:310–314(abst).
37. Thong YH, Ferrante A. Effect of tetracycline treatment on immunological responses in mice. *Clin Exp Immunol* 1980;39:728–732.
38. Kloppenburg M, Dijkmans BA, Verweij CL, Breedveld FC. Inflammatory and immunological parameters of disease activity in rheumatology patients treated with minocycline. *Immunopharmacology* 1996;31:163–169.
39. Sadowski T, Steinmeyer J. Effects of tetracyclines on the production of matrix metalloproteinases and plasminogen activators as well as of their natural inhibitors, tissue inhibitor of metalloproteinases-1 and plasminogen activator inhibitor-1. *Inflamm Res* 2001;50:175–182.
40. Brandt KD. Modification by oral doxycycline administration of articular cartilage breakdown in osteoarthritis. *J Rheumatol* 1995;43:149–151.
41. Sewell KL, Breedveld F, Furrie E, et al. The effect of minocycline in rat models of inflammatory arthritis: correlation of arthritis suppression with enhanced T cell calcium flux. *Cell Immunol* 1996;167:195–204.
42. Brown TM, Hochberg MC, Hicks JT, Clark HW. Antibiotic therapy of rheumatoid arthritis: a retrospective cohort study of 98 patients with 451 patient-years of follow-up. (Proceedings of Meeting). *Internatl Cong Rheumatol* 1985;S85.
43. Hughes BR, Murphy CE, Barnett J, Cunliffe WJ. Strategy of acne therapy with long-term antibiotics. *Br J Dermatol* 1989;121:623–628.
44. Ciancio SG, Mather ML, McMullen JA. An evaluation of minocycline in patients with periodontal disease. *J Periodontol* 1980;51:530–534.
45. Langevitz P, Bank I, Zemer D, et al. Treatment of resistant rheumatoid arthritis with minocycline: an open study. *J Rheumatol* 1992;19:1502–1504.
46. Breedveld FC, Dijkmans BAC, Mattie H. Minocycline treatment for rheumatoid arthritis: an open dose finding study. *J Rheumatol* 1990;17:43–46.
47. O'Dell JR, Haire CE, Erikson N, et al. Treatment of rheumatoid arthritis with methotrexate alone, sulfasalazine and hydroxychloroquine, or a combination of all three medications. *N Engl J Med* 1996;334:1287–1291.
48. O'Dell JR, Paulsen G, Haire CE, et al. Treatment of early seropositive rheumatoid arthritis with minocycline: four-year followup of a double-blind, placebo-controlled trial. *Arthritis Rheum* 1999;42:1691–1695.
49. O'Dell JR, Blakely KW, Mallek JA, et al. Early sero-positive rheumatoid arthritis treatment: a 2-year, double-blind comparison of minocycline and hydroxychloroquine. *Arthritis Rheum* 2001;44:2235–2241.
50. Felson DT, Anderson JJ, Boers M, et al. American College of Rheumatology preliminary definition of improvement in rheumatoid arthritis. *Arthritis Rheum* 1995;38:727–735.
51. Felson DT. Choosing a core set of disease activity measures for rheumatoid arthritis clinical trials. *J Rheumatol* 1993;20:531–534.
52. van Gestel AM, Prevoo ML, van't Hof MA, et al. Development and validation of the European League Against Rheumatism response criteria for rheumatoid arthritis. Comparison with the preliminary American College of Rheumatology and the World Health Organization/International League Against Rheumatism Criteria. *Arthritis Rheum* 1996;39:34–40.
53. Furst DE. Nonsteroidal antiinflammatory drugs. Disease-modifying antirheumatic drugs, nonopioid analgesics and drug used in gout. In: Katzung BG, ed. *Basic & clinical pharmacology*. 8th ed. New York: Lange Medical Books/McGraw-Hill, 2001:596–623.
54. U.S. Department of Health and Welfare. Vestibular reactions to minocycline after meningococcal prophylaxis. *Morbidity Mortality* 1975;24:10–11.
55. Ang ER, Zimmerman JC, Malkin E. Pseudotumor cerebri secondary to minocycline intake. *J Am Board Fam Pract* 2002;15:229–233.
56. Shiri J, Amichai B. Intracranial hypertension and minocycline. *Ann Intern Med* 1997;127:168.
57. Sitbon O, Bidel N, Dussopt C, et al. Minocycline pneumonitis and eosinophilia. A report on eight patients. *Arch Intern Med* 1994;154:1633–1640.
58. Walker RG, Thomson NM, Dowling JP, Ogg CS. Minocycline-induced acute interstitial nephritis. *Br Med J* 1979;1(6162):524.
59. Burette A, Finet C, Prigogine T, et al. Acute hepatic injury associated with minocycline. *Arch Intern Med* 1984;144:1491–1492.
60. Guillon JM, Joly P, Autran B, et al. Minocycline-induced cell-mediated hypersensitivity pneumonitis. *Ann Intern Med* 1992;117:476–481.
61. Thibault M, Billick RC, Srolovitz H. Minocycline-induced Sweet's syndrome. *J Am Acad Dermatol* 1992;27:801–804.
62. Gough A, Chapman S, Wagstaff K, et al. Minocycline induced autoimmune hepatitis and systemic lupus erythematosus-like syndrome. *BMJ* 1996;312:169–172.
63. Elkayam O, Levartovsky D, Brautbar C, et al. Clinical and immunological study of 7 patients with minocycline-induced autoimmune phenomena. *Am J Med* 1998;105:484–487.
64. Elkayam O, Levartovsky D, Brautbar C, et al. Minocycline (MNC) induced immunologic phenomena: clinical, immunological and genetic characteristics of 6 patients. *Arthritis Rheum* 1997;40:S267(abst).
65. Gough A, Chapman S, Wagstaff K, et al. Minocycline induced autoimmune hepatitis and systemic lupus erythematosus-like syndrome. *BMJ* 1996;312:169–172.
66. Gordon MM, Porter D. Minocycline induced lupus: case series in the West of Scotland. *J Rheumatol* 2001;28:1004–1006.
67. Graham LE, Bell AL. Minocycline-associated lupus-like syndrome with ulnar neuropathy and antiphospholipid antibody. *Clin Rheumatol* 2001;20:67–69.
68. Lawson TM, Amos N, Bulgen D, Williams BD. Minocycline-induced lupus: clinical features and response to rechallenge. *Rheumatol* 2001;40:329–335.
69. Kiessling S, Forrest K, Moscow J, et al. Interstitial nephritis, hepatic failure, and systemic eosinophilia after minocycline treatment. *Am J Kidney Dis* 2001;38:E36.
70. Marzo-Ortega H, Misbah S, Emery P. Minocycline induced autoimmune disease in rheumatoid arthritis: a missed diagnosis? *J Rheumatol* 2001;28:377–378.
71. Angulo JM, Sigal LH, Espinoza LR. Coexistent minocycline-induced systemic lupus erythematosus and autoimmune hepatitis. *Semin Arthritis Rheum* 1998;28:18–92.
72. Angeloni VL, Salasche SJ, Ortiz R. Nail, skin, and scleral pigmentation induced by minocycline. *CUTIS* 1987;40:229–234.
73. Fenske NA, Millns JL, Greer KE. Minocycline-induced pigmentation at sites of cutaneous inflammation. *JAMA* 1980;24:1103–1106.
74. Ridgway HB, Reizner GT. Acquired pseudo-mongolian spot associated with minocycline therapy. *Arch Dermatol* 1992;128:565.
75. Rumbak MJ, Pitcock JA, Palmieri GMA, Robertson JT. Black bones following long-term minocycline treatment. *Arch Pathol Lab Med* 1991;115:939–941.
76. Bell CD, Kovacs K, Horvath E, et al. Histologic, immunohistochemical, and ultrastructural findings in a case of minocycline-associated "black thyroid." *Endocr Pathol* 2001;12:443–451.
77. Paulus HE. Minocycline treatment of rheumatoid arthritis. *Ann Intern Med* 1995;122:147–148.
78. Breedveld FC. Minocycline in rheumatoid arthritis. *Arthritis Rheum* 1997;40:794–796.
79. Cooper SM. A perspective on the use of minocycline for rheumatoid arthritis. *J Clin Rheumatol* 1999;5:233–238.
80. Bluhm GB, Sharp JT, Tilley B, et al. Radiographic results from the minocycline in rheumatoid arthritis trial (MIRA). *J Rheumatol* 1997;24:1295–1302.
81. Reveille JD, Alarcón GS, Fowler SE, et al. HLA-DRB1 genes and disease severity in rheumatoid arthritis. *Arthritis Rheum* 1996;39:1802–1807.
82. Abernethy DRE. *Mosby's drug consult*. Section III ed. Mosby Inc, 2002:1915–1918.

CHAPTER 29

Cyclosporine

David E. Yocum

Cyclosporine (CsA) is an immunomodulatory agent discovered in 1972 and widely used in solid organ transplantation since 1978. It was first used to treat rheumatoid arthritis (RA) in 1979. As monotherapy, it was found effective in treating established RA. More recent studies of the efficacy of CsA for the treatment of early RA alone and in combination with methotrexate (MTX), hydroxychloroquine, and gold have also produced positive results. CsA has also been found to be effective for the treatment of psoriasis, atopic dermatitis, Behçet's disease, and ulcerative colitis.

MECHANISM OF ACTION

CsA is a lipophilic, cyclic polypeptide, purified from fungi (*Tolypoladium inflatum* and *Cylindrocarpon lucidium*) (Fig. 29.1). Although it has variable antifungal properties, it was developed primarily because of its potent immunosuppressive properties (1,2). Most of its effects on immune response are secondary to a selective inhibition of T-cell activation (3,4). CsA inhibits T-cell activation by interfering with calcium-dependent signaling events involved in lymphokine gene transcription (Fig. 29.2).

CsA forms a complex with a 17-kd cytoplasmic-binding protein, called *cyclophilin*, which has peptidyl-prolyl cis-trans isomerase activity (1,2). The binding of CsA to cyclophilin inhibits its enzymatic activity. Binding is not in itself immunosuppressive because the binding of nonimmunosuppressive analogues of CsA inhibits the same enzyme. The common target for the CsA–cyclophilin complex was found to be a serine/threonine phosphatase, calcineurin, which is a heterodimer consisting of a 59-kd catalytic A subunit and a 19-kd regulatory B subunit. Although the specific target for calcineurin has not been identified, the dephosphorylation of the cytosolic form of the transcription factor nuclear factor of activated T cells is required before passage of this transcription factor into the nucleus. Additionally, although more than 100 immunophilins have been described, the reasons for their existence and their physiologic role in immune regulation, if any, are unknown.

The principal mechanism by which CsA exerts its immunosuppressive action is by inhibiting the transcription of a group of T-cell cytokine genes. Although the inhibition of interleukin-2 (IL-2) has been most extensively documented, CsA also inhibits IL-3, IL-4, granulocyte-macrophage stimulating factor, tumor necrosis factor α, and interferon γ expression (1,5,6). The blocking of these key cytokines results in the inhibition of T-cell activation and, ultimately, suppression of T-cell–dependent immune responses, including B-cell activation (7). CsA is not cytotoxic, as other gene products and cellular pathways critical for cell survival remain intact. *In vivo*, only IL-10 levels decrease significantly during CsA therapy (8). Recent data have also demonstrated that CsA inhibits the production of vascular endothelial growth factor by synovial fibroblasts taken from RA patients (9).

OPEN-LABEL STUDIES

The first study of CsA as a treatment for RA was reported by Herrmann and Mueller in 1979 (10). This open-label evaluation involved doses of CsA now considered to be high in seven patients with RA and in one patient with rheumatoid factor (RF)–positive psoriasis. Although the majority of patients achieved a subjective clinical response, unacceptable elevations of serum creatinine (S_{cr}) and the development of herpes zoster in two patients delayed future studies. However, the observations that one patient with vasculitis exhibited a prolonged positive clinical response and that clearing of psoriasis occurred in the patient with psoriatic arthritis led to the use of CsA in several other patients with psoriasis, all of whom experienced significant clearing of skin disease within 2 weeks (11).

Other open-label trials in RA were initiated in the early- to mid-1980s (Table 29.1) (12–17). Although these trials suggested clinical efficacy, elevations of S_{cr} levels were of major concern. The report by Palestine et al. (18), which evaluated nephrotoxicity clinically and histologically in patients with uveitis, helped to establish guidelines for use of CsA by clinicians. These guidelines, in addition to the greater availability of an accurate, reproducible CsA assay, resulted in multiple controlled and double-blind trials in patients with RA that established the clinical efficacy of CsA (Tables 29.2 and 29.3) (19–28).

EARLY DOUBLE-BLIND STUDIES

Van Rijthoven et al. (20) reported the results from a double-blind, placebo-controlled trial in 36 patients with established RA. Patients were started on CsA at 10 mg per kg per day, with planned dosage reductions throughout the trial. There was significant clinical improvement in the patients treated with CsA compared to those treated with placebo, although a 36% increase in S_{cr} over baseline levels was observed. Subsequently, Dougados et al. (21) reported on a double-blind, placebo-controlled trial starting at doses of CsA of 5 mg per kg per day, with the potential

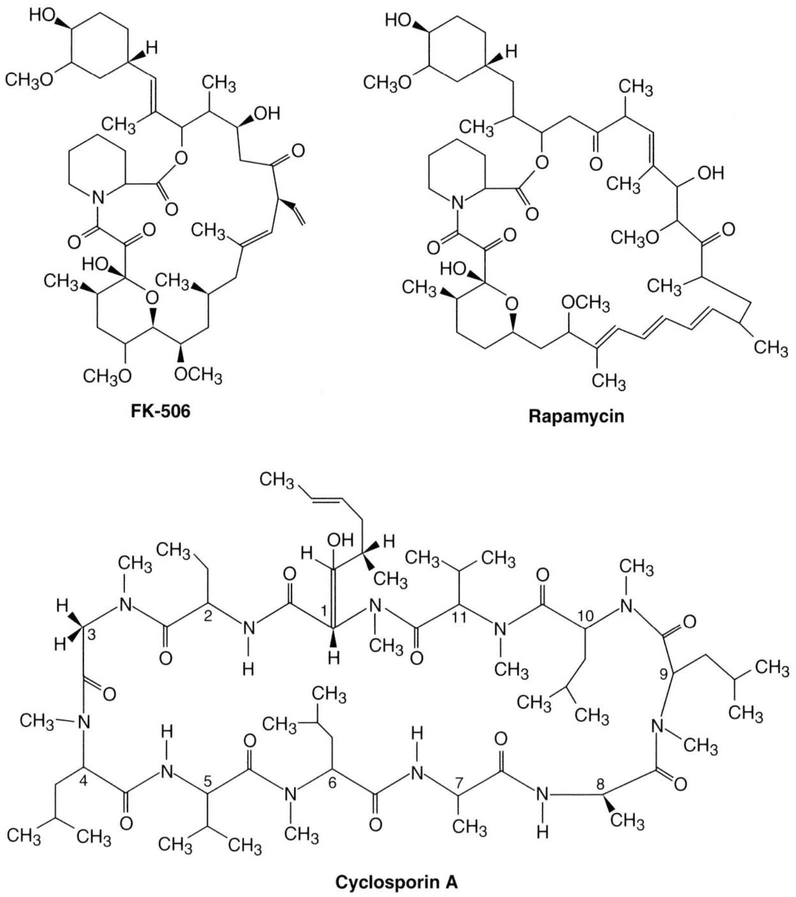

FK-506

Rapamycin

Cyclosporin A

Figure 29.1. Chemical structure of cyclosporine. (Adapted from Sigal NH, Dumont FJ. Cyclosporin A, FK-506, and rapamycin. Pharmacologic probes of lymphocyte signal transduction. *Annu Rev Immunol* 1992;10:519–560.)

of increasing to 7.5 mg per kg per day for efficacy if the S_{cr} allowed. The guideline was to keep increases in S_{cr} to less than 50% of the baseline level. Using this method, clinical efficacy was similar to that reported by Van Rijthoven et al. (20), but S_{cr} rose only 23% above baseline. Long-term renal effects were not reported in either of these studies.

In a study initiated at approximately the same time, Yocum et al. (22) conducted a double-blind, high-dose (10 mg per kg per day) versus low-dose (1 mg per kg per day) trial of CsA using strict guidelines to limit increases in S_{cr} to less than 30% of baseline levels. Although the high-dose group started at 10 mg per kg per day, the titration of dose based on these guidelines resulted in only a 17% mean increase in S_{cr} levels at the end of the trial. Additionally, patients who developed elevated blood pressures while on CsA and who did not respond to dose reduction were removed from the study. Even with these strict guidelines, there was a 60% reduction in active joint scores in the high-dose cohort. This response was maintained during 12 months of therapy without further increases in S_{cr}. In contrast, only 4 of 16 patients had a clinical response to the low-dose cyclosporin. Between 6 and 12 months, all four patients had flares in their arthritis.

Finally, based on a small open-label trial of 40 patients with RA (16), Tugwell et al. (23) conducted a large double-blind, placebo-controlled trial using the "go low, go slow" method. Patients were started on doses of 2.5 mg per kg per day of CsA and escalated to a maximum dose of 5 mg per kg per day using 30% to 50% elevations of baseline S_{cr} levels as a guide. Overall, efficacy was somewhat less than that in other studies but was still significant compared to placebo, and the S_{cr} increased only 17% above entry values. During and after the study, 16 patients who had persistent elevations of S_{cr} underwent renal biopsies, none of which demonstrated histologic changes consistent with CsA-induced effects. Therefore, maximum clinical benefit with minimal renal side effects was achieved by beginning at a dose of 2.5 mg per kg per day and escalating the dose by 0.5 mg per kg per day to a maximum dose of 5 mg per kg per day while maintaining the S_{cr} to within 30% of baseline. The most recent consensus guidelines

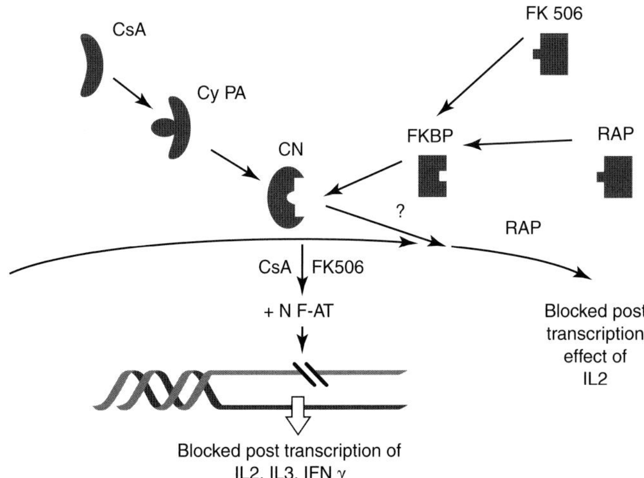

Figure 29.2. Mechanism of action of cyclosporine (CsA), FK-506, and rapamycin. CsA binds to cyclophilin (Cy PA) and binds to calcineurin (CN), ultimately going to the nucleus, blocking translation of interleukin (IL)-2, IL-3, and interferon (IFN)-γ. NF-AT, nuclear factor of activated T cells; RAP, receptor-associated protein.

TABLE 29.1. Uncontrolled Studies of Cyclosporine in Rheumatoid Arthritis

Principal Author	Year	Trial Design	Total Number Treated	Initial Average Dose (mg/kg/d)	Final Average Dose (mg/kg/d)	Number of Months	Reference
Herrmann	1979	Open, uncontrolled	6	10.0	6.0	5–10	10
Amor	1985	Open, uncontrolled	6	8.5	7.8	3	12
Dougados	1987	Open, uncontrolled	12	5.0	5.2	12	13
Weinblatt	1987	Open, uncontrolled	10	6.0	6.1	6	14
Bowles	1989	Open, uncontrolled	10	6.0	3.9	6	15
Tugwell	1987	Open, uncontrolled	20	5.0/2.5	4.3	6	16
Dougados	1989	Open, uncontrolled	49	5.0/2.5	?	12	17

recommend a starting dose of CsA of 2.5 mg per kg per day, with strict adherence to the "30% golden rule" (29).

MONOTHERAPY IN EARLY RHEUMATOID ARTHRITIS

A majority of patients with RA treated with CsA in clinical trials had average disease durations of longer than 10 years and had previously received three or more slow-acting antirheumatic drugs. One would not expect such patients to be especially responsive to CsA, and, in fact, 18 months after starting monotherapy, only 33% remained on CsA (30). It would be desirable to conduct trials in early RA, in which one would expect greater efficacy for longer durations. Few trials using CsA in early RA have been conducted, however.

In an open-label, long-term trial, Madhok et al. (30) studied 20 patients with less than 7 years of disease, and 11 of the 20 patients had less than 3 years of disease. Overall, the average duration of CsA therapy was nearly 2.5 years, whereas patients with less than 3 years of disease received the drug an average of 36 months. Although far from conclusive, such data suggest that CsA might be more efficacious in early disease.

In support of the efficacy of CsA in early disease, Förre et al. (31) reported the results of a double-blind placebo-controlled trial in patients with an average of 8.8 years of disease (31). To reduce the risk of nonsteroidal antiinflammatory drug (NSAID)–related renal side effects, these drugs were generally excluded in favor of low-dose steroids. After 1 year of therapy, 56.8% of patients treated with CsA were significantly better, as measured by the Ritchie index, number of swollen joints, pain score, patient global assessment, and physician global assessment, as compared to the measurements of 39.1% of placebo patients. Furthermore, patients receiving CsA demonstrated lack of progression in the number of erosions and in the Larsen score using hand radiographs, whereas the placebo group exhibited increases in both variables at 48 weeks. These data lend further support to the earlier use of CsA and strongly suggest it may alter the course of joint destruction.

Landewé et al. (32,33) compared CsA and chloroquine in patients with RA with an average of 7 months of disease (all of them with disease for <2 years). More than 70% of the patients tested positive for serum RF and already had erosions on radiographs, pointing to an increased risk for early disability and death. At 6 months, both CsA- and chloroquine-treated patients had significantly improved, with no difference between treatment groups (30). At 12 months, the patients treated with chloroquine demonstrated a worsening in clinical parameters. However, the patients treated with CsA continued to improve (31). The differences between groups at 12 months were statistically significant. Additionally, although there was a disproportionate number of patients with erosive disease randomized to the CsA group, the chloroquine group had greater deterioration, as assessed radiologically, than did the patients treated with CsA.

Pasero et al. (34) reported on an open-label randomized study comparing CsA to other standard disease-modifying antirheumatic drugs (DMARDs). Although there was no significant difference in efficacy between the groups after 1 year, those patients on cyclosporin had significantly fewer erosions and a lower damage score. Patients with no erosions at baseline were less likely to develop erosions on CsA. Similar results were observed at 3 years of follow-up.

In an open-label, randomized study with blinded radiographs as a primary end point, Zeidler et al. (35) compared CsA to parenteral gold in 375 patients with early (average, 1 year) active RA. After 18 months of therapy, there was no difference in the clinical response, except that more patients withdrew from the gold group,

TABLE 29.2. Controlled Studies of Cyclosporine in Established Rheumatoid Arthritis

					Average Dose (mg/kg/d)			
Principal Author	Year	Trial Design	Total Number Treated	Total Number Treated with Cyclosporine	Initial	Final	Number of Months	Reference
Førre	1987	Open, control vs. azathioprine	24	12	10	6.4	6	19
Van Rijthoven	1986	Double-blind placebo controlled	36	17	10	5.0	6	20
Dougados	1988	Double-blind placebo controlled	52	26	5	4.6	4	21
Yocum	1988	Double-blind dose comparison	31	15	10	4.6	6	22
			—	16	1	0.85	—	—
Tugwell	1990	Double-blind placebo controlled	144	72	2.5	3.8	6(+2)	23
Førre	1991	Double-blind placebo controlled	122	61	5	5	12	24
Schattenkirchner	1991	Double-blind vs. azathioprine	117	59	5	4.2	6	25
Van Rijthoven	1991	Double-blind vs. D-penicillamine	93	46	5	4.4	6	26
Cohen	1993	Double-blind vs. methotrexate	264	101	2.5	2.87	8.5	27
Altman	1999	Double-blind placebo controlled	244	138	2.5	2.85	5	28

TABLE 29.3. Studies of Cyclosporine in Early Rheumatoid Arthritis

Principal Author	Year	Trial Design	Total Number Treated	Average Dose (mg/kg/d) Initial	Final	Number of Months	Reference
Madhok	1985	Open, uncontrolled	20	5	6	60	30
Førre	1994	Double-blind placebo controlled	122	5	3.9	12	31
Landewé	1994	Double-blind vs. chloroquine	44	2.5	3.6	0.6	32
Pasero	1996	Open, randomized vs. disease-modifying antirheumatic drugs	361	3.0	2.93	12	34
Zeidler	1998, 2002	Open, randomized vs. gold	375	3.9	3.19	36	35, 36
Drosos	2002	Open, randomized vs. methotrexate	?	?	?	42	37

primarily during the first 6 months, due to adverse events. Using the Larsen-Dale joint damage score, erosion score, and number of erosions, both the CsA and the gold group progressed at the same rate. Only a completers analysis showed statistically less progression in the CsA group using the Larsen-Dale joint damage score. These two groups continued to be followed for 3 years (36). Of the original 187 CsA and 188 gold patients, 84 and 76, respectively, continued therapy in the extension. Only the Health Assessment Questionnaire scores were statistically better in the CsA-treated group. Radiographic progression was similar for both groups.

In an open, randomized trial, Drosos et al. (37) compared CsA to MTX in 103 patients with early, DMARD-naïve RA. After 42 months of therapy, 71% of the CsA group and 76% of the MTX group remained radiographically stable using the Larsen-Dale scoring method.

CsA appears to be more effective as monotherapy in early compared to late RA, as evidenced by better clinical and radiologic outcomes. Although this observation is true of most DMARDs, the postulated mechanism of action of CsA and current views regarding the immunopathogenesis of RA suggest that early disease is the more appropriate time to intervene with an agent that primarily affects T cells (1,3,38,39).

COMBINATION THERAPY WITH CYCLOSPORINE

Although not a new concept in the treatment of RA, the use of combination therapy increased dramatically over the last 5 to 10 years (40). The immunopathology of synovial tissue from patients with RA shows a heterogeneous cell population, which may not be responsive to a single DMARD (38,39). In addition, for most of the older DMARDs used in RA, either the mechanism of action is poorly understood or relatively nonspecific. These are two of the reasons why monotherapy has been a relatively ineffective approach and combinations difficult to rationally develop for the treatment of RA (41). However, this situation has changed over the last few years with the development of targeted biologic agents, a concept that began with studies using the anti–T-cell drug CsA.

CsA has been used successfully in combination with other agents for the treatment of RA (Table 29.4). Not all combinations have produced strikingly positive clinical benefits. Initial studies using MTX plus azathioprine afforded promising results, but double-blind trials did not demonstrate additive effects over MTX alone (42,43). The combinations of MTX with sulfasalazine (SSZ), and hydroxychloroquine, or both, have shown variable efficacy (44,45). In contrast, the combination of CsA and MTX demonstrated positive clinical benefit in several studies. The distinct mechanisms of action of CsA and MTX would suggest combined biologic effects (1,46). Additionally, a study comparing each drug alone to the combination of the two in type II collagen arthritis in mice has demonstrated positive results and suggests true synergism between these agents (47).

Based on this information and a preliminary open-label trial, Tugwell et al. (48) reported on a study in which CsA was given to patients with a partial response to MTX. To enter the study, patients had to be on a stable dose of MTX for at least 3 months. After observation for an additional month to ensure that their arthritis was active but stable, patients were randomized to receive either CsA or placebo in addition to MTX. At the end of 6 months, patients receiving CsA plus MTX had improved significantly in at least three American College of Rheumatology (ACR) criteria plus the number of tender and swollen joints as compared to the placebo plus MTX group. During the second 6 months, patients on placebo were crossed over to CsA and exhibited similar clinical benefit (49).

Whether these observations point to a true biologic synergism remains to be tested. These data were encouraging, and this creative study design established a model to test combinations using fewer patients than required by conventional three-arm study designs.

In support of the preceding findings, Ferraccioli et al. (50) evaluated the use of combined treatment with CsA, MTX, and SSZ in early RA (50). In this unique step-up study design, patients were randomized to either CsA (group 1), MTX (group 2), or SSZ (group 3). After 6 months, patients in groups 1 and 2 who had not achieved an ACR 50% response rate had MTX or CsA added, respectively. At 12 months, SSZ was added to the therapy of those

TABLE 29.4. Combination Studies Using Cyclosporine in Rheumatoid Arthritis

Principal Author	Year	Trial Design	Total Number Treated	Dose of Cyclosporine (mg/kg/d)	Number of Months	Reference
Tugwell	1995	Double-blind, controlled	148	2.5	6	48
Yocum	2000	Double-blind, controlled	505	2.5	12	51, 52
Gerards	2000	Open-label, randomized	120	2.5	12	53
Proudman	2000	Randomized	82	1.5	12	54
Ferraccioli	2002	Randomized, step-up	126	3.0	12	50

patients in groups 1 and 2 who had still not achieved an ACR 50% response rate. At the end of 18 months, 90% in group 1 and 88% in group 2 had achieved an ACR 50% response rate, as compared to 24% in group 3, in which only SSZ was used.

More recently, Yocum et al. (51,52) reported the results of a large, multicenter, multinational, double-blind randomized study comparing CsA and MTX to MTX alone in patients with less than 6 years of disease duration. The odds ratio of achieving ACR 20%, 50%, and 70% response rate with the combination were 1.78, 1.77, and 2.03, respectively. Patients with a high clinical risk indicator (positive RF, high C-reactive protein level, presence of erosions on hand or foot radiographics, high swollen joint count) were more likely to achieve an ACR 20%, 50%, or 70% response rate. The use of low-dose corticosteroids had no effect on clinical response.

Gerards et al. (53) treated 120 RA patients with early disease (mean disease duration, 3 months) with either CsA and MTX or CsA alone in a double-blind, randomized, placebo-controlled trial with radiologic progression as the primary outcome (53). Using the Larsen score to evaluate hand and foot radiographs at 6 and 48 weeks, the combination-treated patients progressed significantly less ($p = .004$) than patients treated with CsA alone (scores, 2–4 vs. 2.5–10.0, respectively).

Finally, in a small, open-label randomized trial, Proudman et al. (54) compared CsA in combination with MTX to SSZ alone. The combination group also received intraarticular steroids. At the end of 48 weeks, the combination group was numerically (58% vs. 45% for SSZ) but not statistically ($p = .28$) better than the monotherapy group. There were many more withdrawals for the monotherapy group, as compared to the combination group (10 out of 42 vs. 1 out of 40, respectively) ($p = .007$). Given the open nature of this study, the potential confounding effect of intraarticular steroids and the small number of patients (only 40 per group), these results are difficult to interpret and, if anything, favor the combination group.

In vitro studies combining CsA and chloroquine suggest biologic interactions between these two drugs (55,56). No combination trials with these agents have been performed, however. Finally, a preliminary trial using CsA in partially responsive parenteral gold–treated patients with RA also appears promising (57).

In summary, the combination of CsA and MTX is better in treating the signs and symptoms of RA than either drug alone. Although each agent alone has been shown to slow radiographic progression, it is not entirely clear whether the combination provides greater effects. Patients with more severe disease appear to do better with the combination.

IMMUNOLOGIC EFFECTS OF CYCLOSPORINE IN RHEUMATOID ARTHRITIS

Despite the large number of studies using CsA in RA and the immunologic effects of CsA, few studies have investigated immune function *in vivo* in patients treated with CsA (58–61). CsA has not been shown to significantly affect RF titers, gammaglobulin levels, or Epstein-Barr virus titers (58,59). Similarly, CsA does not affect proliferation of peripheral lymphocytes to mitogens or deplete T-cell subsets in RA (58–61). It does decrease IL-2 receptor expression by T cells after prolonged therapy, however, and is associated with enhanced proliferation to recall antigen stimulation in patients who respond clinically.

A study demonstrated significant decrease in circulating levels of IL-10 in RA patients receiving CsA (8). One study suggested that patients with peripheral anergy to soluble recall antigens were more likely to respond to CsA (58). Patients who are anergic tend to have greater inflammatory indices in the synovium, with more striking infiltration of lymphocytes, especially the $CD4^+$ subset (62,63). In general, although having significant effects on disease activity, CsA has not been found to produce irreversible, potentially harmful effects on immune function.

ADVERSE EVENTS

Mild Side Effects

The adverse events associated with CsA are well documented and usually reversible with dose reduction or discontinuation of drug (Table 29.5) (22,23,29,36,48,50). Although many consider that the more serious adverse events, such as hypertension and reduced renal function, are the primary reason for discontinuation, gastrointestinal upset is common and often leads to discontinuation (22). Patients complain of bloating, diarrhea, and flatulence symptoms that are uncomfortable or socially unacceptable. It is important to inform patients that these symptoms may occur. Often, taking CsA with meals resolves this issue. The newer formulation of CsA, a microemulsion called *Neoral*, has much more consistent absorption from the gastrointestinal tract. Its bioavailability is not affected by concomitant food, resulting in more consistent blood levels. Neoral should be used whenever possible (64–68).

Another mild, but often unacceptable, side effect is hypertrichosis (10,22). Although it does not cause hirsutism, it does result in rapid hair growth and, often, a darkening of the hair. This side effect can be difficult for women who take this agent. Patients should be informed about its occurrence and possible solutions, such as depilatories.

Severe neurologic side effects are commonly observed with higher doses of CsA (>5 mg per kg per day) and include headaches, paresthesias, and, at very high doses, severe tremors (10). At lower doses, some patients note unusual temperature sensations (hot seems hotter and cold seems colder), and some might note perioral tingling (22).

Early in the course of therapy and at higher doses, some premenopausal women note menstrual irregularities (22). This symptom resolves over time and may be due to the binding of CsA to the prolactin receptor, increasing the free prolactin blood levels. In one study, a female patient noted a brief period of lactation (22).

Finally, a typically mild side effect that can become more of a problem if not recognized is gingival hyperplasia (10,18). The exact mechanism by which this occurs is not known, but is more common at higher doses (>5 mg per kg per day) and, in one study, was reduced by ensuring good dental hygiene (22). Mild gingival hyperplasia at lower doses can be seen and is not a problem.

Renal Toxicity

Probably the most important limitation on the use of CsA is the possibility of renal toxicity (Table 29.6). Although the mechanism of this toxicity is unclear, several potential causes have been suggested (69–71). These include the following: (a) vasoconstriction leading to ischemia; (b) vasoconstriction due to an increased production or activation of renin, or both; and (c) increased responsiveness hypersensitivity to vasoconstrictors, such as angiotensin II, or vasopressin as a result of increased calcium influx.

The renal toxicity of CsA is dose dependent and reversible if strict guidelines are followed (72,73). Overall, up to 35% of patients receiving CsA experience an increase in S_{cr} with a decrease in creatinine clearance. As long as the S_{cr} is maintained at less than 30% above the patient's creatinine on initiation of

TABLE 29.5. Adverse Events Associated with Cyclosporine (CsA)

Adverse Events	Incidence (%)		Withdrawal Rate Due to Adverse Events (%)	
	CsA[a]	CsA + MTX[b]	CsA	CsA + MTX
Gastrointestinal[c]				
Diarrhea	4	3	<1	1
Nausea, bloating	9	9	1	9
Cardiovascular[d]				
Edema	<5	8	—	1
Hypertension	—	—	1	—
Systolic (>140 mm Hg on ≥2 occasions)	11	15	—	—
Diastolic (>90 mm Hg on ≥2 occasions)	11	9	—	—
Central nervous system[c]				
Headache	8	11	<1	—
Paresthesia	7	4	—	—
Tremor	4	4	—	—
Renal[d]				
Serum creatine (≥30% over baseline)	30	36	1	—
Hypertrichosis[c]	16	12	—	—
Gingival hyperplasia[c]	<5	<5	—	—

MTX, methotrexate.
[a]Values in this table are for patients treated with the recommended, low initial CsA dosage of 2.5 mg per kg per day.
[b]Incidence in the CsA (or CsA plus MTX) treatment group minus the incidence in the placebo (or placebo plus MTX) group.
[c]Mild.
[d]Potentially serious.
Adapted from Mueller W, Herrmann B. Cyclosporin A for psoriasis [Letter]. *N Engl J Med* 1979;301:555; Amor B, Dougados M. Cyclosporin in rheumatoid arthritis. Open trials with different dosages. In: Schindler R, ed. *Cyclosporin in autoimmune diseases.* Berlin: Springer, 1985:283–287; Dougados M, Amor B. Cyclosporin A in rheumatoid arthritis. Preliminary clinical results of an open trial. *Arthritis Rheum* 1987;30:83–87; and Bowles CA. Long-term treatment of rheumatoid arthritis with cyclosporin (CsA) [Abstract]. *Arthritis Rheum* 1989;32:S61.

CsA therapy, the effect is nearly always reversible (29). The most common histologic changes are tubular atrophy, arteriolar changes, and interstitial fibrosis (74–78). Risk factors associated with a higher rate of renal toxicity include a higher initial CsA dose, greater maximum S_{cr} over baseline during therapy, and increased age. Age dose not seem to affect the metabolism of CsA. Data from renal biopsy studies have shown lower rates of nephropathy when lower doses of CsA are used.

The recommendation is to start patients at 3 mg per kg per day in split dose after carefully determining the baseline S_{cr} (Fig. 29.3) (29,79). The dose should rarely exceed 4 mg per kg per day. S_{cr} should be monitored initially on a biweekly basis and, once the S_{cr} is stable, on a monthly basis. If the dose is increased, testing should return to a biweekly basis. The dose should be decreased or held for S_{cr} levels greater than 30% above baseline (Fig. 29.4). For S_{cr} levels greater than 50% above baseline, CsA should be held until the S_{cr} level returns to greater than 30% above baseline. Many of the studies previously discussed have followed these guidelines, which have been published (16,22,23,29,48,51).

Hypertension

Several studies have documented the development of new hypertension, as well as exacerbation of existing hypertension, with the use of CsA (80,81). Although the mechanism of this effect is not known, hypertension associated with CsA seems to be salt dependent and associated with low renin as well as prerenal pathophysiology. CsA does induce vasoconstriction in the preglomerular microvasculature, which may be associated with increased thromboxane A_2 and prostacyclin synthesis. Hypertension may also occur as a result of sodium and water retention due to increases in proximal tubule reabsorption of sodium. Some data suggest that the renin-angiotensin system may be involved, as both renal and systemic vasoconstriction occur with CsA use.

Treatment of CsA-associated hypertension should begin with dosage reduction (Fig. 29.5) (29). However, if therapy is just beginning, this may not be possible. In many cases, dose reduction does not work or the patient has a disease flare. Therefore, in some patients, treatment with antihypertensive

TABLE 29.6. Drugs/Food That Affect Cyclosporine (CsA) Concentrations

Will Increase CsA Concentrations	Effect on CsA Concentrations
Antifungals	
Fluconazole	↑
Itraconazole	↑
Ketoconazole	↑
Antibiotics	
Erythromycin	↑
Clarithromycin	↑
Nafcillin	↓
Rifampin	↓
Rifabutin	↓
Calcium channel blockers[a]	
Diltiazem	↑
Nicardipine	↑
Verapamil	↑
Glucocorticoids	
Methylprednisolone[b]	↑
Anticonvulsants	
Carbamazepine	↓
Phenobarbital	↓
Phenytoin	↓
Others	
Allopurinol	↑
Bromocriptine	↑
Danazol	↑
Metoclopramide	↑
Grapefruit	↑
Octreotide	↓
Ticlopidine	↓

↑, increase; ↓, decrease.
[a]Because nifedipine may cause gingival hyperplasia, it is advised that this drug be avoided in patients who develop gingival hyperplasia with CsA therapy.
[b]Interaction observed only with high doses of methylprednisolone.
From references 89–107, with permission.

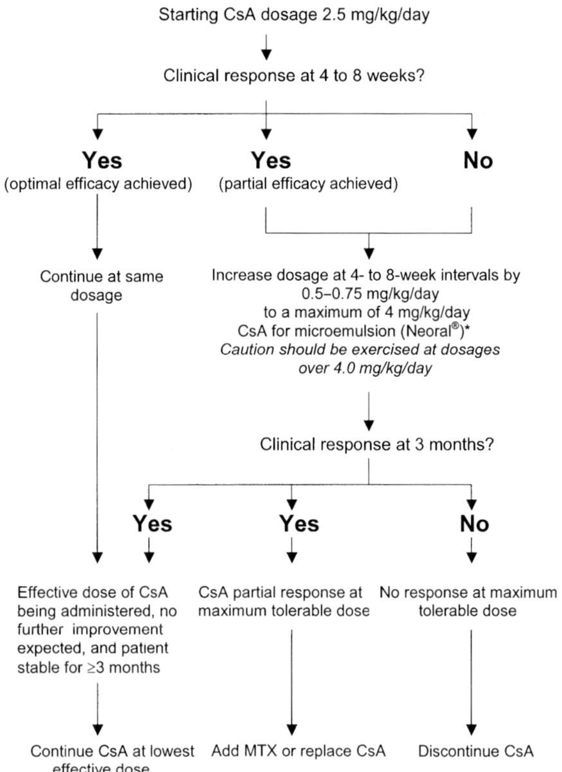

Figure 29.3. Recommended dosing guidelines to optimize treatment with cyclosporine (CsA). *Maximum, 5 mg per kg per day CsA, USP (Sandimmune). MTX, methotrexate. (Adapted from Panayi GS, Tugwell P. *Br J Rheumatol* 1997;36:808–811.)

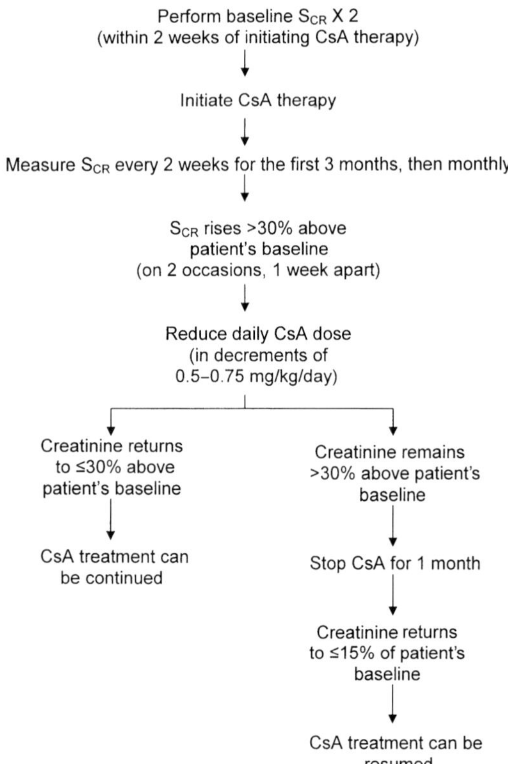

Figure 29.4. Guidelines to minimize or avoid adverse renal effects with cyclosporine (CsA). Also consider reducing or discontinuing nonsteroidal antiinflammatory drugs. S_{CR}, serum creatinine. (Adapted from Panayi GS, Tugwell P. *Br J Rheumatol* 1997;36:808–811.)

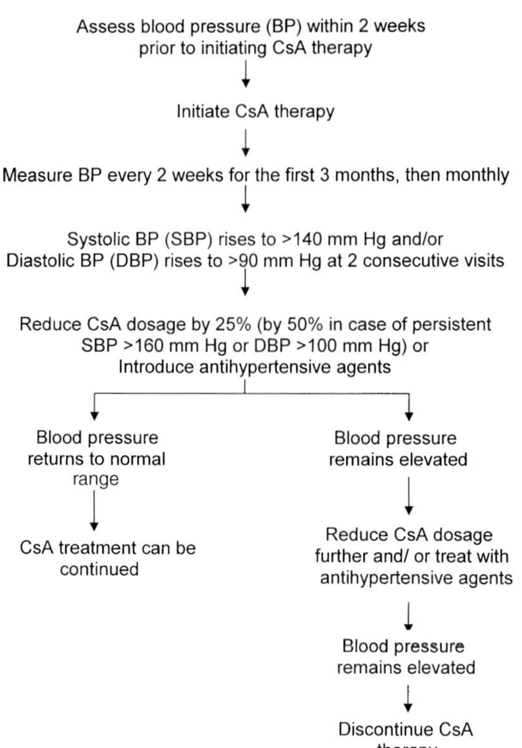

Figure 29.5. Guidelines to manage cyclosporine (CsA)-associated hypertension.

drugs is warranted. Diuretics should be avoided and calcium channel blockers, such as nifedipine or isradipine, are first-line agents, as they do not affect CsA metabolism (82). Blood pressure should be followed in all patients on a regular basis.

Malignancy

CsA is not itself mutagenic but, theoretically, could result in malignancy due to its immunomodulatory activity. Although RA is not associated with an increase in overall malignancies, there is an increase in lymphoproliferative disorders (83,84). So far, studies of CsA in RA have not shown an increase in either overall malignancies or lymphoproliferative cancers (85).

Infections

Similar to lymphoproliferative disorders, the risk of infection is greater in patients with RA (86,87). This risk correlates with duration of disease, age, and immunosuppressive therapy. Steroids, especially in higher doses, are an independent risk. In the early development of CsA, when doses up to 10 mg per kg per day were being used, the incidence of infections appeared greater with CsA than with placebo (10). With the lower doses of CsA presently being used (2.5–4.0 mg per kg per day), the incidence of overall infection and the risk of serious infection does not appear increased over placebo or active comparator (88). However, care should be taken with combination therapy, especially when several agents are being used that target different parts of the immune system.

Drug Interactions

A number of important drug interactions occur with CsA because it is metabolized by the cytochrome P450 enzymes in the liver (Table 29.6) (88–95). As many of these drugs are used

TABLE 29.7. Drugs That May Potentiate Cyclosporine (CsA)-Associated Renal Dysfunction and Those with Special Considerations

Drugs That May Potentiate Renal Dysfunction	Drugs with Special Considerations
Antibiotics	Antiinflammatory agents
Gentamicin	Indomethacin (enhances CsA nephrotoxicity)
Tobramycin	Diclofenac (enhances CsA nephrotoxicity, decreases diclofenac metabolism)
Vancomycin	Cardiovascular agent
Trimethoprim plus sulfamethoxazole	Digoxin (enhances CsA nephrotoxicity)
Antifungals	Hepatic 3-methylglutaryl coenzyme A reductase inhibitor
Amphotericin B	Lovastatin (myopathy)
Ketoconazole	
Antiinflammatory agents	
Nonsteroidal antiinflammatory drugs (including naproxen and sulindac)	
Antineoplastic agent	
Melphalan	
Immunosuppressive agent	
Tacrolimus	

From references 89–105, with permission.

regularly in medical practice, it is important to review a patient's drug list before and during therapy with CsA. One dietary item, grapefruit, can increase blood concentrations of the drug by affecting metabolism via cytochrome P450 (96,97).

Another important area of concern when using CsA is the use of drugs that can potentiate its nephrotoxicity (Table 29.7). One group of agents that is difficult to avoid in the therapy of RA is the NSAIDs (98,99). However, the effect of these agents appears to be marginal, as most patients are already on one of these agents when CsA therapy is initiated. The major time of concern is when a NSAID is switched during therapy. Another group of agents is the antibiotics, of which the aminoglycosides and antifungals are the most important (100–107).

CONCLUSION

CsA is a unique immunomodulatory drug approved in combination with MTX to treat the signs and symptoms of RA. The population that appears most responsive to CsA is patients with earlier, more active disease (persistent swelling, erosions, elevated C-reactive protein, and positive RF). Nearly all studies that have included radiographic analysis have shown a slowing of disease with CsA, although it is not approved by the U.S. Food and Drug Administration as an agent that inhibits disease progression.

The major side effect of CsA is renal, with decreased glomerular filtration rate and, if not properly managed (allowing the S_{cr} level to stay >50% over baseline for more than 3 months), can result in permanent renal toxicity. Monitoring should include measurement of S_{cr} (maintaining the level <30% above baseline), blood pressure, and liver function profile if the patient is on MTX. This monitoring should be done every 2 weeks initially and then every 4 weeks.

REFERENCES

1. Sigal NH, Dumont FJ. Cyclosporin A, FK-506, and rapamycin. Pharmacologic probes of lymphocyte signal transduction. *Annu Rev Immunol* 1992;10:519–560.
2. Braun W, Kallen J, Mikol V, et al. Three-dimensional structure and actions of immunosuppressants and their immunophilins. *FASEB J* 1995;9:63–72.
3. Krönke M, Leonard WJ, Depper JM, et al. Cyclosporin A inhibits T cell growth factor gene expression at the level of mRNA transcription. *Proc Natl Acad Sci U S A* 1984;81:5214–5218.
4. Lin CS, Boltz RC, Siekierka JJ, Sigal NH. FK-506 and cyclosporin A inhibit highly similar signal transduction pathways in human T lymphocytes. *Cell Immunol* 1991;133:269–284.
5. Herold KC, Lancki DW, Moldwin RL, Fitch FW. Immunosuppressive effects of cyclosporin A on cloned T cells. *J Immunol* 1986;136:1315–1321.
6. Granelli-Piperno A. In situ hybridization for interleukin 2 and interleukin 2 receptor mRNA in T cells activated in the presence or absence of cyclosporin A. *J Exp Med* 1988;168:1649–1658.
7. Wicker LS, Boltz RC, Matt V, et al. Suppression of B-cell activation by cyclosporine A, FK506 and rapamycin. *Eur J Immunol* 1990;20:2277–2283.
8. Ferraccioli G, Fallet, E, DeVita S, et al. Circulating levels of interleukin 10 and other cytokines in rheumatoid arthritis treated with cyclosporine A or combination therapy. *J Rheumatol* 1998;25:1874–1879.
9. Cho ML, Cho CS, Min SY, et al. Cyclosporine inhibition of vascular endothelial growth factor production in rheumatoid synovial fibroblasts. *Arthritis Rheum* 2002;46:1202–1209.
10. Herrmann B, Mueller W. Die therapie der chronischen polyarthritis mit Cyclosporin A, einens neuen immun-suppressivum. *Akt Rheumatotol* 1979;4:173–186.
11. Mueller W, Herrmann B. Cyclosporin A for psoriasis [Letter]. *N Engl J Med* 1979;301:555.
12. Amor B, Dougados M. Cyclosporin in rheumatoid arthritis. Open trials with different dosages. In: Schindler R, ed. *Cyclosporin in autoimmune diseases.* Berlin: Springer, 1985:283–287.
13. Dougados M, Amor B. Cyclosporin A in rheumatoid arthritis. Preliminary clinical results of an open trial. *Arthritis Rheum* 1987;30:83–87.
14. Weinblatt ME, Coblyn JS, Fraser PA, et al. Cyclosporin A treatment of refractory rheumatoid arthritis. *Arthritis Rheum* 1987;30:11–17.
15. Bowles CA. Long-term treatment of rheumatoid arthritis with cyclosporin (CsA) [Abstract]. *Arthritis Rheum* 1989;32:S61.
16. Tugwell P, Bombardier C, Gent M, et al. Low dose cyclosporin in rheumatoid arthritis. A pilot study. *J Rheumatol* 1987;14:1108–1114.
17. Dougados M, Duchesne L, Awada J, Amor B. Assessment of efficacy and acceptability of low dose cyclosporin in patients with rheumatoid arthritis. *Ann Rheum Dis* 1989;48:550–556.
18. Palestine AG, Austin HA, Balow JE, et al. Renal histopathologic alterations in patients treated with cyclosporine for uveitis. *N Engl J Med* 1986;314:1293–1298.
19. Förre Ø, Bjerkhoel F, Salvesen CF, et al. An open, controlled, randomized comparison of cyclosporine and azathioprine in the treatment of rheumatoid arthritis. A preliminary report. *Arthritis Rheum* 1987;30:88–92.
20. Van Rijthoven AWAM, Dijkmans BAC, Goei The HS, et al. Cyclosporin treatment for rheumatoid arthritis. A placebo controlled, double-blind, multicentre study. *Ann Rheum Dis* 1986;45:726–731.
21. Dougados M, Awada H, Amor B. Cyclosporin in rheumatoid arthritis. A double blind, placebo controlled study in 52 patients. *Ann Rheum Dis* 1988;47:127–133.
22. Yocum DE, Klippel JH, Wilder RL, et al. Cyclosporin A in severe, treatment-refractory rheumatoid arthritis. A randomized study. *Ann Intern Med* 1988;109:863–869.
23. Tugwell P, Bombardier C, Gent M, et al. Low dose cyclosporin versus placebo in patients with rheumatoid arthritis. *Lancet* 1990;335:1051–1055.
24. Förre Ø, Norwegian Arthritis Disease Study Group. Cyclosporine as a disease modifier in rheumatoid arthritis. 2nd Congress on Immunointervention in Autoimmune Diseases [Abstract 197]. Paris, 1991.
25. Schattenkirchner M, Kruger K. Cyclosporine vs. azathioprine in the treatment of rheumatoid arthritis—a controlled double blind study. 2nd Congress on Immunointervention in Autoimmune Diseases [Abstract 198]. Paris, 1991.
26. Van Rijthoven AWAM, Dijkmans BAC, Goei The HS, et al. Comparison of cyclosporine and D-penicillamine for rheumatoid arthritis: a randomized, double-blind multicenter study. *J Rheumatol* 1991;18:815–820.
27. Cohen S, Rutstein J, Luggen, et al. Comparison of the safety and efficacy of cyclosporine-A and methotrexate in refractory rheumatoid arthritis; a randomized, multi-centered, placebo-controlled trial. *Arthritis Rheum* 1993;36[Suppl]:S56.
28. Altman RD, Schiff M, Kopp EJ. Cyclosporine A in rheumatoid arthritis: randomized, placebo controlled dose finding study. *J Rheumatol* 1999;26:2102–2109.
29. Cush JJ, Tugwell P, Weinblatt M, Yocum D. U S consensus guidelines for the use of cyclosporine A in rheumatoid arthritis. *J Rheumatol* 1999;26:1176–1186.
30. Madhok R, Torley HI, Capell HA. A study of the long-term efficacy and toxicity of cyclosporine A in rheumatoid arthritis. *J Rheumatol* 1991;18:1485–1489.
31. Förre Ø, Norwegian Arthritis Study Group. Radiologic evidence of disease modification in rheumatoid arthritis patients treated with cyclosporine. Results of a 48-week multicenter study comparing low-dose cyclosporine with placebo. *Arthritis Rheum* 1994;37:1506–512.
32. Landewé RBM, Goei The HS, Van Rijthoven AWAM, et al. A randomized, double-blind, 24-week controlled study of low-dose cyclosporine versus chloroquine for early rheumatoid arthritis. *Arthritis Rheum* 1994;37:637–643.
33. Landewé RBM, Goei The HS, Van Rijthoven AWAM, et al. Cyclosporine in early rheumatoid arthritis. Delayed onset of optimal efficacy. In: *Cyclosporine in RA.* Leiden: University of Netherlands, 1994:71–88.

34. Pasero G, Priolo F, Marubini E, et al. Slow progression of joint damage in early rheumatoid arthritis treated with cyclosporine A. *Arthritis Rheum* 1996;39:1006–1115.
35. Zeidler HK, Kvien TK, Harmensen P, et al. Progression of joint damage in early active severe rheumatoid arthritis during 18 months of treatment: comparison of low-dose cyclosporine and parenteral gold. *Br J Rheumatol* 1998;37:874–882.
36. Kvien TK, Zeidler HK, Hannenen P, et al. Long term efficacy and safety of cyclosporine versus parental gold in early rheumatoid arthritis: a three year study of radiographic progression, renal function and arterial hypertension *Ann Rheum Dis* 2002;61:511–516.
37. Drosos AA, Voulgari PV, Katsaraki A, Ziken AK. Influence of cyclosporine A on radiographical progression in early rheumatoid arthritis patients: a 42-month prospective study. *Rheum Int* 2000;19:113–118.
38. Panayi GS. The immunopathogenesis of rheumatoid arthritis. *Br J Rheum* 1993;32[Suppl 1]:4–14.
39. Kurosaka M, Ziff M. Immunoelectron microscopic study of distribution of T cell subsets and HLA-DR expressing cells in rheumatoid synovium. *Arthritis Rheum* 1983;26:S53.
40. Csuka M, Carreara GF, McCarty DJ. Treatment of intractable rheumatoid arthritis with combined cyclophosphamide, azathioprine and hydroxychloroquine. A follow-up study. *JAMA* 1986;255:2315–2319.
41. Amor B, Herson D, Cherot A, et al. Follow-up study of patients with rheumatoid arthritis over a period of more than 10 years (1966–1978). Analysis of disease progression and treatment in 100 cases. *Ann Med Intern* 1981;132:168–173.
42. Biro JA, Segal AM, MacKenzie AH, et al. The combination of methotrexate and azathioprine for resistant rheumatoid arthritis [Abstract]. *Arthritis Rheum* 1987;30:S18.
43. Willkens RF, Urowits MB, Stablei DM, et al. Comparison of azathioprine, methotrexate, and the combination of both in the treatment of rheumatoid arthritis. A controlled clinical trial. *Arthritis Rheum* 1992;35:849–856.
44. Haagsma C, Van Riel P, deRooij DJ, Van de Patte L. Combination therapy in RA. Sulphasalazine and methotrexate [Abstract]. *Arthritis Rheum* 1993;36:S53.
45. O'Dell J, Haire C, Erikson N, et al. Triple DMARD therapy for rheumatoid arthritis. Efficacy [Abstract]. *Arthritis Rheum* 1994;37:S295.
46. Segal R, Mozes E, Yaron M, et al. The effects of methotrexate on the production and activity of interleukin-1. *Arthritis Rheum* 1989;32:370–377.
47. Brahn E, Peacock DJ, Banquerigo ML. Suppression of collagen-induced arthritis by combination cyclosporin A and methotrexate therapy. *Arthritis Rheum* 1991;34:1282–1288.
48. Tugwell P, Pincus T, Yocum D, et al. Combination therapy with cyclosporine and methotrexate in severe rheumatoid arthritis. *N Engl J Med* 1995;333:137–141.
49. Stein CM, Pincus T, Brooks RH, et al. Combination therapy with cyclosporine and methotrexate: results of a 24 week extension study subsequent to a 24 week double-blind study [Abstract]. *Arthritis Rheum* 1994;37:S5252.
50. Ferraccioli GF, Gremese E, Tomietto P. Analysis of improvements, full responses, remission and toxicity in rheumatoid patients treated with step-up combination therapy (methotrexate, cyclosporine A, sulphasalazine) in monotherapy for three years. *Rheumatology* 2002;41:892–898.
51. Yocum D, Allard S, Laasonen L, et al. Pooled 48 week efficacy and safety results of two double blind randomized controlled studies comparing methotrexate plus cyclosporine versus methotrexate plus placebo in patients with early severe RA. *Arthritis Rheum* 2000;43:S344.
52. Yocum D, Allard S, Marubini E, et al. Effect of baseline clinical studies and use of steroids on ACR improvement criteria in early RA patients treated with methotrexate plus cyclosporine. *Arthritis Rheum* 2000;43[Suppl]:S345.
53. Gerards AH, Landeive RBM, Prins APA, et al. Radiological progression in patients with early rheumatoid arthritis is significantly retarded by combination therapy with methotrexate and cyclosporine to cyclosporine alone. *Arthritis Rheum* 2000;43:aS345.
54. Proudman SM, Canagham PG, Richardson C, et al. Treatment of poor-prognosis early rheumatoid arthritis. A randomized study of treatment with methotrexate, cyclosporine A, and intra-articular corticosteroids compared with sulfasalazine alone. *Arthritis Rheum* 2000;43:1809–1819.
55. Landewé RBM, Miltenburg AMM, Breedveld FC, et al. Cyclosporine and chloroquine synergistically inhibit the IFN gamma production by CD4-positive and CD8-positive synovial T cell clones derived from a patient with rheumatoid arthritis. In: *Cyclosporine in RA*. Leiden: University of Netherlands, 1994:111–123.
56. Landewé RBM, Miltenburg AMM, Verdonk MJA, et al. Cyclosporine and chloroquine synergistically inhibit T cell proliferation by interference with IL-2 production and IL-2 responsiveness. In: *Cyclosporine in RA*. Leiden: University of Netherlands, 1994:125–146.
57. Bensen W, Tugwell P, Roberts R, et al. Combination therapy of cyclosporin with methotrexate and gold in rheumatoid arthritis (2 pilot studies) [Abstract]. *Arthritis Rheum* 1994;37:S335.
58. Yocum D. Immunological actions of cyclosporin A in rheumatoid arthritis. *Br J Rheum* 1993;32[Suppl 1]:38–41.
59. Yocum DE, Wilder RL, Dougherty S, et al. Immunological parameters of response in patients with rheumatoid arthritis treated with cyclosporin A. *Arthritis Rheum* 1990;33:1310–1316.
60. Walsh BT, Seaver N, Bennett R, et al. Immunologic profile of rheumatoid arthritis patients treated with cyclosporin A and methotrexate. Results from a double-blind placebo-controlled trial [Abstract]. *Arthritis Rheum* 1992;35:S216.
61. Yocum DE, Cornett M, Olson S, Nordensson K. Effects of methotrexate and methotrexate plus cyclosporine on mononuclear cell proliferation and lymphocyte surface markers in rheumatoid arthritis patients. Results of a double-blind trial. *Arthritis Rheum* 1994;37:S5254.
62. Haraoui B, Wilder RL, Malone DG, et al. Immune function in severe, active rheumatoid arthritis. A relationship between peripheral blood mononuclear cell proliferation to soluble antigens and mononuclear cell subset profiles. *J Immunol* 1984;133:697–701.
63. Malone DG, Wahl SM, Tsokos M, et al. Immune function is severe, active rheumatoid arthritis. A relationship between peripheral blood mononuclear cell proliferation to soluble antigens and synovial tissue immunohistologic characteristics. *J Clin Invest* 1984;74:1173–1185.
64. Kahan BD, Dunn J, Fitts C, et al. Reduced inter- and intrasubject variability in cyclosporine pharmacokinetics in renal transplant recipients treated with a microemulsion formulation in conjunction with fasting, low-fat meals. *Transplantation* 1995;59:505–511.
65. van den Borne BEEM, Landewé RBM, Goei The HS, et al. Relative bioavailability of a new oral form of cyclosporine A in patients with rheumatoid arthritis. *Br J Clin Pharmacol* 1995;39:172–175.
66. Kahan BD, Dunn J, Fitts C, et al. The Neoral formulation: improved correlation between cyclosporine through levels and exposure in stable renal transplant recipients. *Transplant Proc* 1994;26:2940–2943.
67. Mueller EA, Kovarik JM, van Bree JB, et al. Improved dose linearity of cyclosporine pharmacokinetics from a microemulsion formulation. *Pharm Res* 1994;11:301–304.
68. Yocum D. Comparison of the safety, tolerability and efficacy of Sandimmune and Sandimmune Neoral in subjects with severe, active RA: a randomized, double-blind study [Abstract]. *Arthritis Rheum* 1996;39[Suppl]:S105
69. Mason J. The effect of cyclosporine on renal function. *J Autoimmun* 1992;5[Suppl A]:349–354.
70. Schiff M, the 652 Study Group. Dose-dependency of the renal function and blood pressure effects of cyclosporine in severe arthritis patients: a multicenter, placebo-controlled study [Abstract]. *Arthritis Rheum* 1996;39[Suppl]:S105.
71. Mason J, Müller-Schweinitzer E, Dupont M, et al. Cyclosporine and the renin-angiotensin system. *Kidney Int* 1991;39[Suppl 32]:S28–S32.
72. van den Borne BEEM, Landewé RBM, Goei The HS, et al. Low dose cyclosporine in early rheumatoid arthritis: effective and safe after two years of therapy when compared with chloroquine. *Scand J Rheumatol* 1996;25:307–316.
73. Landewé RBM, Dijkmans BAC, van der Woude FJ, et al. Longterm low dose cyclosporine in patients with rheumatoid arthritis: renal function loss without structural nephropathy. *J Rheumatol* 1996;23:61–64.
74. Rodriguez F, Krayenbühl JC, Harrison WB, et al. Renal biopsy findings and followup of renal function in rheumatoid arthritis patients treated with cyclosporine A: an update from the International Kidney Biopsy Registry. *Arthritis Rheum* 1996;39:1491–1498.
75. Feutren G, Mihatsch MJ. Risk factors for cyclosporine induced nephropathy in patients with autoimmune diseases. The International Kidney Biopsy Registry of Cyclosporine in Autoimmune Disease. *N Engl J Med* 1992;326:1654–1660.
76. Mihatsch MJ, Antonovych T, Bohman S-O, et al. Cyclosporin A nephropathy: standardization of the evaluation of kidney biopsies. *Clin Nephrol* 1994;41:23–32.
77. Lundin D, Alexopoulou I, Esdaile JM, Tugwell P. Renal biopsy specimens from patients with rheumatoid arthritis and apparently normal renal function after therapy with cyclosporine. The Canadian Multicentre Rheumatology Group. *Am J Kidney Dis* 1994;23:260–265.
78. Feutren G. Renal morphology after cyclosporine A therapy in rheumatoid arthritis patients. *Br J Rheumatol* 1993;32[Suppl 1]:65–71.
79. Buonpane E. Therapeutic drug monitoring of cyclosporine. *Conn Med* 1990;54:17–19.
80. Lewis RM. Mechanisms of cyclosporine A-associated hypertension and their management. *Transplant Immunol Lett* 1992;8:3,16–18.
81. Cusi D, Barlassina C, Niutta E, et al. Mechanism of cyclosporine-induced hypertension. *Clin Invest Med* 1991;14:607–613.
82. Endresen L, Bergan S, Holdaas H, et al. Lack of effect of the calcium antagonist isradipine on cyclosporine pharmacokinetics in renal transplant patients. *Ther Drug Monit* 1991;13:490–495.
83. Sela O, Shoenfeld Y. Cancer in autoimmune diseases. *Semin Arthritis Rheum* 1988;18:77–87.
84. Katustic S, Beard CM, Kurland LT, et al. Occurrence of malignant neoplasms in the Rochester, Minnesota, rheumatoid arthritis cohort. *Am J Med* 1985;78[Suppl 1A]:50–55.
85. Arellano F, Krupp P. Malignancies in rheumatoid arthritis patients treated with cyclosporine A. *Br J Rheumatol* 1993;32[Suppl 1]:72–75.
86. Yocum DE. Combination therapy: the risks of infection and tumor induction *Springer Semin Immunopathol* 2001;23:63–72.
87. Mitchell DM, Spitzs PW, Young DW, et al. Survival, prognosis, and cause of death in rheumatoid arthritis. *Arthritis Rheum* 1986;29:706.
88. Torley H, Yocum D. Effects of dose and treatment duration on adverse experiences with cyclosporine in RA: analysis of North American Trials [Abstracts]. *Arthritis Rheum* 1994;37[Suppl]:S334.
89. Faulds D, Goa KL, Benfield P. Cyclosporin: a review of its pharmacodynamic and pharmacokinetic properties, and therapeutic use in immunoregulatory disorders [published erratum appears in *Drugs* 1993;46:377]. *Drugs* 1993;45:953–1040.
90. Yee GC, McGuire TR. Pharmacokinetic drug interactions with cyclosporine (part 1). *Clin Pharmacokinet* 1990;19:319–332.

91. Cutler RE, Pettis JL. Cyclosporine drug interactions. *Dial Transplant* 1988;17: 139–141,151.
92. Arnold JC, O'Grady JG, Tredger JM, Williams R. Effects of low-dose prednisolone on cyclosporine pharmacokinetics in liver transplant recipients: radioimmunoassay with specific and non-specific monoclonal antibodies. *Eur J Clin Pharmacol* 1990;39:257–260.
93. Klintmalm G, Säwe J. High dose methylprednisolone increases plasma cyclosporine levels in renal transplant recipients [Letter]. *Lancet* 1984;1:731.
94. Gorrie M, Beaman M, Nicholls A, Backwell P. Allopurinol interaction with cyclosporine. *BMJ* 1994;308:113.
95. Gorrie M. Allopurinol and cyclosporine: elevation of cyclosporine concentration-interaction. *Clin-Alert* 1994;6.
96. Lown KS, Bailey DG, Fontana RJ, et al. Grapefruit juice increases felodipine oral availability in humans by decreasing intestinal CYP3A protein expression. *J Clin Invest* 1997;99:2545–2553.
97. Yee GC, Stanley DL, Pessa LJ, et al. Effect of grapefruit juice on blood cyclosporine concentration. *Lancet* 1995;345:955–956.
98. Kovarik JM, Mueller EA, Gerbeau C, et al. Cyclosporine and nonsteroidal antiinflammatory drugs: exploring potential drug interactions and their implications for the treatment of rheumatoid arthritis. *J Clin Pharmacol* 1997;37:336–343.
99. Altman RD, Perez GO, Sfakianakis GN. Interaction of cyclosporine A and nonsteroidal anti-inflammatory drugs on renal function in patients with rheumatoid arthritis. *Am J Med* 1992;93:396-402.
100. Kramer MR, Marshall SE, Denning DW, et al. Cyclosporine and itraconazole interaction in heart and lung transplant recipients. *Ann Intern Med* 1990;113:327–329.
101. Soto J, Sacristan JA, Alsar MJ. Effect of the simultaneous administration of rifampicin and erythromycin on the metabolism of cyclosporine. *Clin Transplant* 1992;6:312–314.
102. Gersema LM, Porter CB, Russell EH. Suspected drug interaction between cyclosporine and clarithromycin [Letter]. *J Heart Lung Transplant* 1994;13: 343–345.
103. Ferrari SL, Goffin E, Mourad M, et al. The interaction between clarithromycin and cyclosporine in kidney transplant recipients. *Transplantation* 1994;58:725–727.
104. Benedetti MS. Inducing properties of rifabutin, and effects on the pharmacokinetics and metabolism of concomitant drugs. *Pharmacol Res* 1995;32:177–187.
105. Dy GR, Raja RM, Mendez MM. The clinical and biochemical effect of calcium channel blockers in organ transplant recipients on cyclosporine. *Transplant Proc* 1991;23:1258–1259.
106. Kureishi A, Jewwsson PJ, Rubinger M, et al. Double-blind comparison of teicoplanin versus vancomycin in febrile neutropenic patients receiving concomitant tobramycin and piperacillin: effect on cyclosporine A–associated nephrotoxicity. *Antimicrob Agents Chemother* 1991;35:2246–2252.
107. Ringdén O, Andström E, Remberger M, et al. Safety of liposomal amphotericin B (AmBisome) in 187 transplant recipients treated with cyclosporine. *Bone Marrow Transplant* 1994;14[Suppl 5]:S10.

CHAPTER 30

Leflunomide

Josef S. Smolen

Leflunomide (LEF) is a low-molecular-weight compound that has been approved as a disease-modifying antirheumatic drug (DMARD) for rheumatoid arthritis (RA). It has been thoroughly investigated in a series of large clinical trials. Importantly, some of these trials included placebo and active comparators, and in 2000 the LEF database comprised the largest single database of prospectively studied DMARD therapies in RA patients. The compound has also been investigated as a component of combination therapies and in studies of its efficacy in diseases other than RA.

CHEMICAL STRUCTURE AND CLINICAL PHARMACOKINETICS

LEF is the generic name of a compound of 270.2 d molecular weight, N-(4'-trifluoromethylphenyl)-5-methylisoxazole-4-carboxamide (empiric formula: $C_{12}H_9F_3N_{202}$), an isoxazole derivative. Its active metabolite, A77 1726, is formed from the prodrug both in the submucosal wall of the intestinal tract and in the liver during first passage. This conversion is almost complete and results in the opening of the isoxazole ring to form a manolonitrilamide. The structural formulas of LEF and its active metabolite are shown in Figure 30.1. For reasons of consistency and simplicity, the term *LEF* is used in this chapter but essentially denotes qualities of the active metabolite, A77 1726.

LEF is highly bound to plasma proteins (>99%). A dose of 20 mg per day leads to a steady state in approximately 7 weeks, and steady-state plasma concentrations are approximately 35 µg/mL (1,2). The recommended loading dose shortens the time to steady-state. Linear pharmacokinetics are indicated by the linear relationship of trough plasma concentrations to the maintenance dose. The bioavailability is not affected by food intake. LEF undergoes enterohepatic circulation and biliary recycling. The drug is eliminated in the feces (approximately 50%) and in the urine (approximately 40%). In the feces, the primary metabolite is A77 1726 (>80%) with additional hydroxymethyl-A77 1726. In urine, the main metabolites are glucuronide products of LEF and an oxanilic acid derivative of A77 1726 (para-trifluoromethylaniline-oxanilic acid). In patients with renal failure, LEF was eliminated similar to healthy volunteers or more rapidly (3). Because LEF is cleared via hepatic metabolism and biliary secretion, hepatic dysfunction is likely to affect elimination, but such data are not available. Men and women have similar pharmacokinetics, and elderly patients do not appear to require dose adjustments. Smokers may have a faster clearance without consequences for clinical efficacy.

LEF has a long elimination half-life of 14 to 18 days (mean among RA patients, 16 days) (3). Enterohepatic recirculation can be interrupted, and, consequently, drug elimination is enhanced by administration of activated charcoal (50 g every 6 hours) or cholestyramine (8 g every 8 hours). Levels of A77 1726 can be reduced by approximately 50% within 24 hours by such procedures (used in clinical situations of toxicity or when other reasons require rapid elimination).

The high degree of protein binding of LEF leads to a displacement and, consequently, an increase in free drug concentrations of other protein-bound drugs, such as nonsteroidal antiinflammatory drugs or oral antidiabetic agents. Anticoagulants are likely also affected by this protein binding. The antiovulatory action of an oral triphasic contraceptive was not affected, and the pharmacokinetics of methotrexate (MTX) were not altered by LEF, however (4). Concomitant rifampicin therapy increases plasma levels of LEF by approximately 40%. *In vitro*, LEF is an inhibitor of the isoenzyme 2C9 of cytochrome P450 (CYP 2C9), which metabolizes drugs such as phenytoin, tolbutamide, and warfarin. Caution is therefore advised when such drugs are given together with LEF, but, in the *in vivo* situation, the concentration of free LEF is much below the concentration that inhibits 50% for this enzyme. Other cytochrome P450 isoenzymes, such as CYP 1A2, 2D6, or 3A4, are not inhibited by LEF.

LEF is teratogenic and fetotoxic in animals. Women of childbearing potential must practice contraceptive measures. LEF is not mutagenic. Carcinogenicity tests in male mice showed an increased incidence of lymphomas and, in female mice, an increased incidence of bronchoalveolar adenomas (3). The dose of LEF used in these studies was high (15 mg per kg), and the significance of these findings in relation to clinical use are not known. Carcinogenicity tests in rats were negative.

MODE OF ACTION AND EFFECTS IN EXPERIMENTAL MODELS OF ARTHRITIS

The main effect of LEF is the inhibition of dihydroorotate dehydrogenase (DHODH), an enzyme involved in the *de novo* synthesis of uridine monophosphate (5). Uridine monophosphate is a precursor of pyrimidine nucleotides, and a decrease in its levels leads to decreased synthesis of RNA and DNA, cell cycle arrest in the G1 phase, and inhibition of cell proliferation (6–9) (Fig. 30.2). This action affects cell cycling and proliferation in general but may be particularly pronounced among lymphocytes, which require significant increases of the pyrimidine over the purine

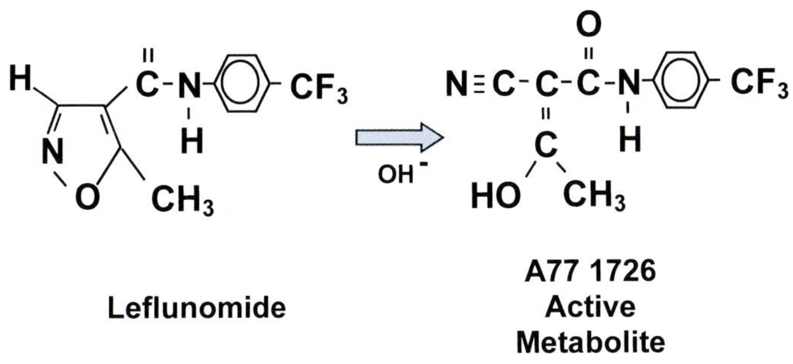

Leflunomide

A77 1726
Active
Metabolite

Figure 30.1. Structure of leflunomide and its active metabolite after conversion.

pool during activation (10,11). The salvage pathway for pyrimidine synthesis, which is effective in resting cells, cannot cope with the demand after activation (11). As expected, exogenous uridine reverses the inhibitory activity of LEF on pyrimidine synthesis and cell proliferation (6,7,10,11). LEF also inhibits the induction of interleukin (IL)-2 and IL-2 receptors (9,12), providing an additional explanation for its effects on T-cell function aside from the antiproliferative effects. The effects of LEF on T cells also lead to modulation of the Th1/Th2 balance, as the compound selectively interferes with Th1 cell activation while fostering Th2 cell differentiation (13).

In addition to its effects on IL-2, LEF affects other cytokines and molecules involved in up- or down-regulation of the inflammatory response: transforming growth factor β, an anti-inflammatory cytokine, IL-1ra, and tissue metalloproteinase-1 are augmented, whereas IL-1β and metalloproteinases are relatively reduced (12,14,15). LEF inhibits tumor necrosis factor α–mediated induction of nuclear factor–κB (NF-κB), a transcription factor importantly involved in cytokine-elicited activation of genes coding for molecules involved in inflammation and tissue destruction (16). This NF-κB inhibition is reversible by uridine, suggesting it is due to inhibition of DHODH. LEF also inhibits JAK and STAT6 tyrosine phosphorylation as well as other protein tyrosine kinase activities (17–19).

LEF may also affect B cells, decreasing immunoglobulin M and immunoglobulin G production (17). It may also inhibit activation of adhesion molecules and thus cell adhesion by restricting the availability of uridine diphosphate sugars, which are required for the glycosylation of these molecules (11). Moreover, LEF inhibits transendothelial monocyte migration, an effect that is reversible by addition of exogenous uridine (20).

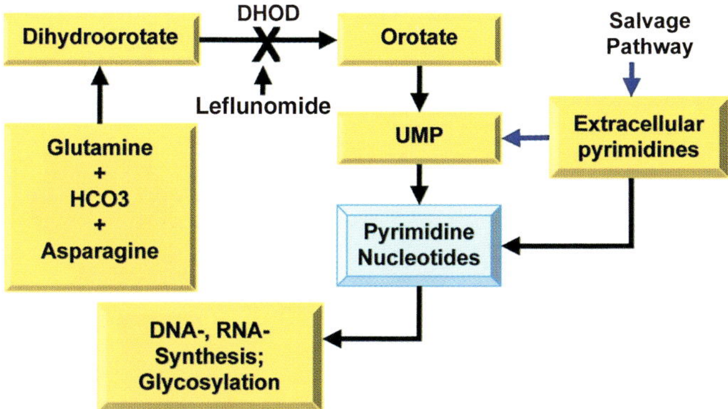

Figure 30.2. Mode of action. Leflunomide inhibits the enzyme dihydroorotate dehydrogenase (DHODH), which is pivotally engaged in the *de novo* pyrimidine pathway. The salvage pathway involving extracellular pyrimidines is not affected. UMP, uridine monophosphate.

These *in vitro* data are mirrored by *in vivo* data indicating that LEF reduces cellular infiltration of the synovial membrane to a larger degree than MTX (15).

Thus, LEF, by virtue of inhibition of DHODH, appears to have multiple effects on the functions of cells of the adaptive and innate immune system, all of which may contribute to the clinical effects described in the following sections.

In accordance with its immunomodulating effects, LEF has been shown to have significant beneficial effects in experimental antigen-induced arthritis as well as adjuvant arthritis (21–24). Moreover, the lupus-like disease of MRL/*lpr* mice, which also have arthritis, is suppressed by LEF treatment (25).

CLINICAL EFFICACY

Rheumatoid Arthritis

MONOTHERAPY

Four large, multicenter, double-blind, randomized controlled trials were performed to evaluate the efficacy of LEF and provide evidence that LEF improves signs and symptoms, radiographic progression, and health-related quality of life in patients with RA. Some of the relevant data are shown in Table 30.1.

In an initial 6-month, dose-ranging, placebo-controlled phase II trial of 402 patients (1), LEF was investigated in doses of 5, 10, and 25 mg per day. Although the 5-mg dose had similar rates of American College of Rheumatology (ACR) 20% responses as placebo (33% and 28%, respectively), the higher doses showed significantly better efficacy than placebo (50% at 10 mg per day, 54% at 25 mg per day). Compared to placebo, the two higher doses led to a significant improvement in swollen joint counts, patient and physician global assessments, Health Assessment Questionnaire score, pain assessment, and acute phase response. The highest dose also produced significant improvement in tender joint count and morning stiffness.

In a subsequent phase III trial of 6 months' duration (MN301), 358 patients were randomized to receive LEF at 20 mg per day (with a loading dose of 100 mg for 3 days), sulfasalazine at 2 g per day (with an initial dose increase from 0.5–2.0 g), or placebo (Fig. 30.3) (26). The ACR 20% response was 55% for LEF and 56% for sulfasalazine, which were significantly higher rates than for placebo (29%) (Fig. 30.3). The improvement of individual clinical and serologic core set variables was similar among the two active drug medications. Perhaps related to the loading dose used, LEF demonstrated a more rapid onset of action as evidenced by significant clinical improvement already after 4 weeks of therapy. Importantly, significant retardation of radiologic progression as determined by the Larsen-Dale joint damage score was already evident after 6 months. These data suggest that (a) the effect of DMARDs on radiographic changes can be evaluated as soon as 6 months after starting treatment, and (b) giving placebo for 6 months constitutes an ethical issue, as within such a short time frame radiographic progression on placebo exceeds that of patients receiving a DMARD by fourfold (27).

A 6-month, double-blind extension study with a switch from placebo to sulfasalazine was allowed for patients completing this 6-month trial. This study showed that the response to LEF was sustained and that patients who switched from placebo to sulfasalazine improved significantly and to a similar degree as seen for DMARD therapy during the first 6-month period (28). This improvement was particularly true also for the progression of radiographic changes, which was low in all groups during the second 6-month term. A further double-blind continuation of the comparison of LEF and sulfasalazine for the subsequent 12 months (i.e., for a total duration of 24 months) was also performed. LEF

TABLE 30.1. Efficacy of Leflunomide (LEF) in Rheumatoid Arthritis

Regimen	Dose	Trial Phase	Duration (mo)	ACR 20% (%)	ACR 50% (%)	Radiographic Progression by Sharp Score	Reference
LEF	10 mg/d	II	6	50	—	ND	1
LEF	25 mg/d	—	—	54	—	ND	1
PL	—	—	—	28	—	ND	1
LEF	20 mg/d[a]	III	6	55	33	1.20	26
SSZ	2 g/d	—	—	56	30	2.30	26
PL	—	—	—	29	14	5.90	26
LEF	20 mg/d[a]	III	12	52	34	0.50	30
MTX	7.5–15.0 mg/wk	—	—	46	23	0.90	30
PL	—	—	—	26	8	2.20	30
LEF	20 mg/d[a]	III	12	51	—	2.50	33
MTX	10–15 mg/wk	—	—	65	—	1.60	33
LEF + MTX	(10–20)mg/d + (15–20) mg/wk	IIIb	6	52	26	ND	42
PL + MTX	15–20 mg/wk	—	—	23	6	ND	42

ACR, American College of Rheumatology; MTX, methotrexate; ND, not determined; PL, placebo; SSZ, sulfasalazine.
[a]With loading dose of 100 mg for 3 consecutive days.

and sulfasalazine demonstrated a sustained response, but the LEF patient cohort had a significantly greater ACR 20% (82% vs. 60%) and ACR 50% (52% vs. 25%) response rate than patients receiving sulfasalazine. Moreover, improvement in Health Assessment Questionnaire scores was significantly greater with LEF than with sulfasalazine. It is important to note that the initial trial and its extension were all performed in a double-blind fashion; however, with each extension, the numbers of patients became smaller, and, in general, extension studies do not allow evaluation of primary end points very well, unless set forth *a priori* (29).

In two large 12-month phase III trials, LEF at 20 mg daily, with a loading dose as above, was also compared to MTX at doses that are regarded as moderate today (Fig. 30.4). In the first of these trials (US301), LEF was evaluated against placebo and MTX (mean dose, 13.5 mg per week) (30). Folate was supplemented in this trial. ACR 20% responses were observed in 52% of the patients on LEF and 46% on MTX, both significantly better than the 26% responders on placebo. Similar changes of clinical and serologic variables were observed with both agents and were significantly greater than those with placebo. Radiographic progression, as determined by Sharp score, was significantly retarded by LEF and MTX when compared to placebo (Fig. 30.5). LEF resulted in significantly more improvement in a number of disability and quality-of-life measures compared to MTX (31). Completers of this study were given the option for a 12-month double-blind extension study, which suggested sustained improvement in signs and symptoms of the disease that were significantly greater with LEF- than MTX-treated patients achieving an ACR 20% response (32).

The second of the trials comparing LEF to MTX was a head-to-head study of 999 patients and did not have a placebo arm (MN302). Moreover, disease duration of these patients was lower (3.7 years) than that of the former trial (7 years). LEF was dosed as in the first of these trials. MTX was dosed at 10 to 15 mg per week; in this trial, only a minority of the patients received folate supplementation. After 52 weeks, more MTX-treated patients (64%) met the ACR 20% criteria than LEF-treated patients (51%) (Fig. 30.4) (33). Retardation of radiographic progression was similar between the two groups at 52 weeks (34). At the end of the extension study,

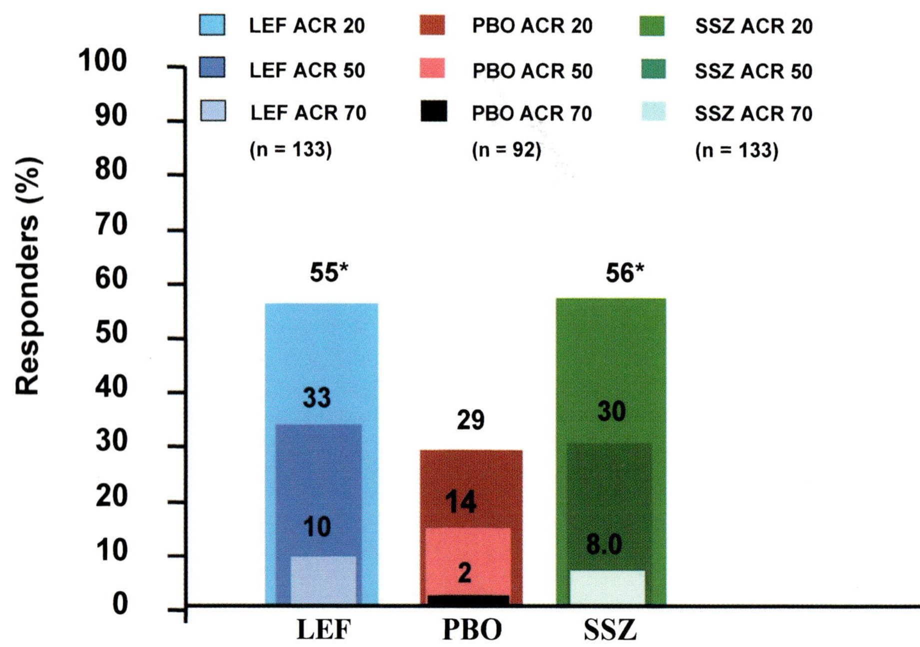

Figure 30.3. Efficacy of leflunomide (LEF) and sulfasalazine (SSZ) over 6-month treatment. American College of Rheumatology (ACR) 20%, 50%, and 70% responses are shown for each of the three groups. *p <.05 compared to placebo (PBO). (Smolen JS, Kalden JR, Scott DL, et al. Efficacy and safety of leflunomide compared with placebo and sulphasalazine in active rheumatoid arthritis: a double-blind, randomised, multicentre trial. *Lancet* 1999;353:259–266.)

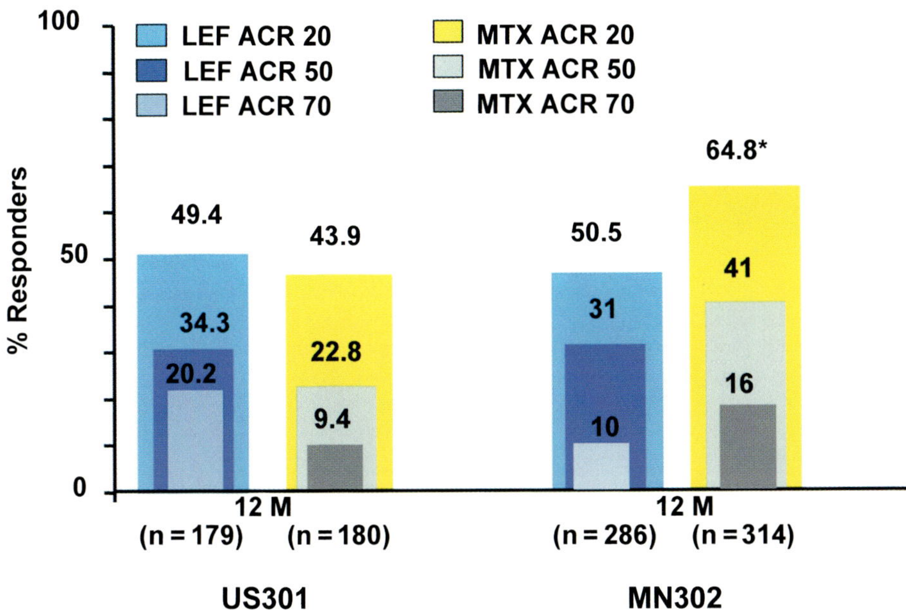

Figure 30.4. Efficacy of leflunomide (LEF) and methotrexate (MTX) over 1-year treatment. Data from two trials comparing LEF with MTX are depicted in terms of American College of Rheumatology (ACR) 20%, 50%, and 70% responses. The US 301 study also involved placebo (not shown). *MTX versus LEF $p < .05$ at 12 months (M). (Adapted from Strand V, Cohen S, Schiff M, et al. Treatment of active rheumatoid arthritis with leflunomide compared with placebo and methotrexate. *Arch Int Med* 1999;159:2542–2550; and Emery P, Breedveld FC, Lemmel EM, et al. A comparison of the efficacy and safety of leflunomide and methotrexate for the treatment of rheumatoid arthritis. *Rheumatology* 2000;39:655–665.)

the ACR 20% response rates were comparable between LEF and MTX, although MTX was more effective in retarding radiographic disease progression than LEF (Fig. 30.5) (34). One reason for the difference in results between the two phase III trials involving MTX as comparator could be the use of folate supplementation in the first but not the second trial: Although folates have been suggested to reduce the toxicity of MTX but not its efficacy (35), higher MTX doses appear to be needed to maintain similar clinical efficacy when folates are supplemented (36).

Thus, taken together, LEF demonstrates a consistent improvement of signs and symptoms of RA, consistent retardation of progression of radiographic damage (Fig. 30.5) (34) and consistent improvement in functional disability and health-related quality of life (37,38). Its onset is rapid, and its efficacy is sustained.

COMBINATION THERAPY

Combination with Methotrexate. Treatment with combinations of DMARDs has become standard for patients with RA who do not respond to monotherapy and commonly involve step-up approaches (i.e., addition of a new DMARD to an existing one). Several combinations have been advocated (39–41), including some with biologic agents (24,25). At present it has not been sufficiently clarified whether adding DMARDs is better than switching from one to another, as several combinations have not proved to be more efficacious than monotherapy and direct comparisons between adding and switching have only rarely been performed (42). MTX is the most commonly used DMARD and, therefore, most combinations include MTX as one of the DMARD partners. The use of MTX and LEF in combination appears rational on the basis of the pharmacologic effects because MTX interferes with purine metabolism whereas LEF interferes with pyrimidine pathways. After an open-label, 52-week trial of LEF in patients who had an insufficient response to continued MTX therapy, which revealed added efficacy with acceptable though added toxicity (4), a 24-week, double-blind, placebo-controlled trial was performed in patients with active disease despite MTX. While continuing MTX, these patients received a loading dose of LEF for only 2 days, and

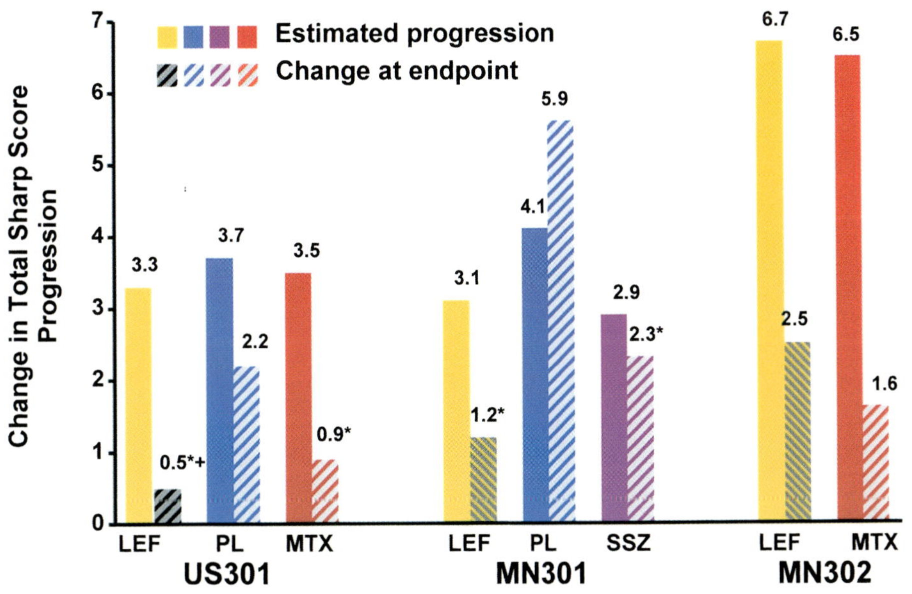

Figure 30.5. Radiographic changes observed in three pivotal trials; the clinical results were shown in Figures 30.3 and 30.4. Radiographic changes were evaluated using the Sharp score. For every arm in each of the three trials, estimated radiographic progression as calculated at baseline is depicted in addition to the progression of radiographic changes during the trials. Note that the estimated radiographic progression was similar among the groups in each trial, and the progression on placebo (PL) approximated the estimated changes, whereas radiographic progression on all active compounds was significantly retarded compared to estimated progression as well as PL (where available). *$p \leq .01$, active versus PL. †$p \leq .05$ versus methotrexate (MTX). LEF, leflunomide; SSZ, sulfasalazine. (From Sharp JT, Strand V, Leung H, et al. Treatment with leflunomide slows radiographic progression of rheumatoid arthritis. Results from three randomized controlled trials of leflunomide in patients with active rheumatoid arthritis. *Arthritis Rheum* 2000;43:495–505, with permission.)

thereafter the drug was continued at 10 mg per day with an option to increase to 20 mg daily after 2 months in patients with persistently active disease (43). LEF provided additional benefit to MTX therapy, as evidenced by the 52% of patients who achieved an ACR 20% response. In an extension for an additional 6 months, the benefit was sustained, and patients who switched from placebo to LEF experienced a similar degree of improvement as seen in the initial part of the trial on combination therapy (44). The issue of liver toxicity with this combination is discussed in the section Safety and Tolerability.

Combination with Sulfasalazine. Patients who did not respond sufficiently to LEF therapy were randomized to receive sulfasalazine in addition to LEF or to switch to sulfasalazine monotherapy. After 24 weeks, 45% of the patients in the combination group achieved a Disease Activity Score 28 response compared to 34% in the sulfasalazine monotherapy group. This difference was not significant due to the low number of patients that could be randomized after the initial open-label LEF part of this study, which showed an unexpectedly low Disease Activity Score 28 nonresponder rate (14%) (45). Nevertheless, this study provided evidence for the potential safety and clinical efficacy of such combination.

Combination with Biologics. Twenty patients with RA received LEF at 20 mg per day (after a loading dose of 10 mg for 3 days) with the addition of infliximab at week 2 after initiation of LEF (46). In this open-label trial, among completers 80% of the patients achieved an ACR 20% response, and more than 45% of the patients achieved an ACR 70% response. Treatment was limited by a high degree of cutaneous adverse events (see the section Cardiovascular, Renal, Skin, Bone Marrow, and Central Nervous System Abnormalities). Combinations with other biologics have not been investigated.

Long-Term Clinical Efficacy in Rheumatoid Arthritis

In addition to extensions of initial clinical trials, longer-term observational studies provide information on drug efficacy and span more than 3 years. These studies suggest that LEF is as effective as MTX (47). Although some studies report somewhat higher termination rates with LEF than with other DMARDs (48–50), this occurrence may be related to the loading dose of 100 mg for the first 3 days. Interpretation of these studies should consider that the initial experience with LEF was derived from patients who had failed to respond to other DMARDs and that its effectiveness in clinical practice is substantial over periods of up to 2 years (51). However, the issue of the loading dose may have to be revisited and, in fact, when rapid effects are not deemed important, it may be sufficient to start with 20 or 40 mg daily for the first few days. Moreover, dosing of LEF may need reconsideration and investigation with respect to occurrence of adverse reactions and failure to achieve responses, particularly as other DMARDs, such as MTX or sulfasalazine, are used in much higher doses today than previously.

LEFLUNOMIDE IN OTHER RHEUMATIC DISORDERS

LEF is currently being investigated in several other rheumatic disorders, including juvenile arthritis, psoriatic arthritis (PsA), ankylosing spondylitis, systemic lupus erythematosus, and Wegener's granulomatosis (52). In all these disorders, this agent has shown some efficacy, but more information is needed from larger clinical trials. In polyarticular juvenile arthritis, 14 of 27 patients with active disease despite MTX therapy were classified as responders to LEF (53). In open trials, LEF also improved both PsA and psoriasis in several patients (54–56) and also had effects on radiographic changes (57). A controlled trial has recently been presented, and similar results were achieved (56). Among patients with lupus arthritis, LEF at 40 mg daily was highly effective in 30% of cases (58). In a two-center pilot study of mildly active systemic lupus erythematosus, the activity score tended to decrease by 25% (59), whereas in another open trial, LEF improved disease activity even more significantly than in the other study (40). Finally, at doses of 30 to 40 mg daily, LEF was effective in maintaining remission of Wegener's granulomatosis in a significant number of patients (39,52). All of these open trials suggest a potential for LEF therapy in inflammatory rheumatic diseases aside from RA; however, controlled trials, such as that performed in PsA, are needed to validate these preliminary observations.

SAFETY AND TOLERABILITY

Organ Systems

GASTROINTESTINAL EVENTS

The most common adverse events from LEF therapy are gastrointestinal symptoms, especially diarrhea, but also nausea, abdominal pain, and dyspepsia. In clinical trials, diarrhea usually occurs within the first 3 months of therapy and tends to resolve within a short time. The overall frequency of diarrhea with LEF is approximately 17%, which is significantly higher than for active comparators or placebo. In approximately one-third of the patients, diarrhea persists for longer than 1 month, but it is a reason for discontinuation in only 2% of the treated patients. LEF can also be associated with significant weight loss (60).

LIVER ABNORMALITIES

Hepatic enzyme elevations (>threefold increase of upper normal levels in serum hepatic enzyme levels) was observed in 2% to 4% of patients treated with LEF, which is generally similar to the frequency observed with MTX. A post-marketing report of the European Medicinal Products Evaluation Agency detailed 129 cases of serious liver disease during more than 100,000 patient-years; most of these abnormalities were observed in patients who took other potential hepatotoxic drugs (including MTX) and/or had additional comorbidities. In fact, almost 30% of patients receiving combination therapy of LEF and MTX had liver enzyme elevations, and in approximately 4% of patients these elevations exceeded threefold the upper limit of the normal level (43). These rates for liver enzyme abnormalities are similar to those reported with MTX (61,62). Mild liver enzyme elevations often improve without change of dose; liver enzyme elevations of more than threefold above the upper limit of normal often decrease with dose reduction. If liver abnormalities persist, LEF should be discontinued and a washout procedure instituted as for serious adverse events (see the section Washout Procedure). LEF is contraindicated in patients with impaired liver function.

CARDIOVASCULAR, RENAL, SKIN, BONE MARROW, AND CENTRAL NERVOUS SYSTEM ABNORMALITIES

Hypertension occurred in approximately 10% of the patients in clinical trials of LEF, most frequently, as an aggravation of preexisting hypertension. LEF has not been associated with renal function abnormalities. However, because it is partly eliminated by the kidney, it is contraindicated in patients with moderately severe impairment of renal function. On the other hand,

LEF reduces serum uric acid levels in approximately one-third of the patients (but does not affect calcium, phosphate, or bicarbonate levels) (3).

Skin reactions were seen in approximately 10% of LEF-treated patients and usually consisted of pruritus or rash. LEF was discontinued in 1.3% of treated patients due to a rash. Alopecia occurred in approximately 10% of the patients but was a reason for discontinuation in less than 1%. Rare cases of Stevens-Johnson syndrome and toxic epidermolysis have been observed, but these patients also received other drugs known to be associated with these skin reactions.

In postmarketing information, patients have been reported with pancytopenia, but they have usually received confounding comedication, including MTX. Transient reductions in leukocytes and thrombocytes are seen with LEF and, therefore, monitoring of blood counts should be performed more frequently in patients with preexisting bone marrow abnormalities or potential myelotoxic combination therapies. CNS effects, such as headache and dizziness, occurred in similar frequencies as with MTX or sulfasalazine and were generally mild; paraesthesias were observed in 3% of the patients. In contrast to MTX therapy, no cases of pneumonitis were observed in the clinical trials, but some cases of pneumonitis have been described in postmarketing observations, especially in Japan.

Immune System and Malignancies

The rate of infections was similar in patients receiving LEF and placebo; no opportunistic infections were reported in any of the clinical trials. However, because LEF is an immunomodulating agent, the potential for increased infections exists, and LEF should not be used in patients with immunodeficiency, preexisting (serious) infections, or significant bone-marrow suppression. If infections occur, particularly if LEF is combined with other immunomodulating agents, prompt treatment of the infection and discontinuation of LEF with washout should be considered. No increases in malignancies, including lymphoproliferative disease, have been observed in patients taking LEF.

LABORATORY MONITORING

Aside from potential changes of liver function tests and blood counts, laboratory abnormalities are usually not observed. However, regular laboratory monitoring, particularly of blood counts and liver function tests, must be performed. The product insert recommends these control examinations frequently (up to every 2 weeks for the first 6 months), but these requirements may change with increasing experience in clinical practice (63).

DRUG INTERACTIONS

No pharmacokinetic interactions were observed when LEF was used in conjunction with MTX, a triphasic oral contraceptive pill, or cimetidine. The free fraction of diclofenac, ibuprofen, and tolbutamide is increased by 13% to 50%. The clearance of LEF is 38% higher in smokers than nonsmokers, but no difference was seen in clinical efficacy between these two groups (3).

TERATOGENICITY

LEF is teratogenic in animals and, therefore, should not be used in women who may become pregnant or who are breast-feeding. Women who wish to become pregnant should either use accelerated removal or wait for 2 years after stopping the drug to ensure that levels of LEF's active metabolite A77 1726 are below 0.02 μg per mL, which is regarded to constitute minimal teratogenic risk. Likewise, although the risk of male-mediated fetal toxicity is unknown, the manufacturer recommends discontinuation and washout procedure in men who wish to father a child.

WASHOUT PROCEDURE

In situations of serious adverse events or when other reasons for accelerating elimination exist, a washout procedure using either activated charcoal or cholestyramine (8 g three times daily for 11 days) should be performed (approximately 40% decrease in blood levels after the first day). After the washout, plasma levels of A77 1726 should be determined and be less than 0.02 μg per mL; this plasma level should be confirmed by a second test at least 2 weeks later. LEF plasma levels are not affected by hemodialysis or chronic ambulatory peritoneal dialysis.

CONCLUSION

LEF is an efficacious DMARD for RA that reduces disease activity, retards radiographic progression, and improves function-related quality of life. Its overall safety profile is comparable to that of other DMARDs. It can be used as mono- and combination therapy and has also been shown to be efficacious in several other disorders, such as PsA.

REFERENCES

1. Mladenovic V, Domljan Z, Rozman B, et al. Safety and effectiveness of leflunomide in the treatment of patients with active rheumatoid arthritis: results of a randomized, placebo-controlled, phase II study. *Arthritis Rheum* 1995;38:1595–1603.
2. Weber W, Harnisch L. Use of a population approach to the development of leflunomide: a new disease-modifying drug in the treatment of rheumatoid arthritis. In: Aarons L, Balant LP, Danhof M, et al. eds. *European cooperation in the field of scientific and technical research*. Brussels: European Commission Directorate-General Science, Research and Developement, 1997:239–244.
3. Investigator's Brochure HWA486 1998:81.
4. Weinblatt ME, Kremer JM, Coblyn JS, et al. Pharmacokinetics, safety and efficacy of the combination of methotrexate and leflunomide in patients with active rheumatoid arthritis. *Arthritis Rheum* 1999;42:1322–1328.
5. Greene S, Watanabe K, Braatz-Trulson J, Lou L. Inhibition of dihydroorotate dehydrogenase by the immunosuppressive agent leflunomide. *Biochem Pharmacol* 1995;50:861–867.
6. Cao WW, Kao PN, Chao AC, et al. Mechanism of the antiproliferative action of leflunomide. *J Heart Lung Transplant* 1995;12:1016–1030.
7. Cherwinski HM, Cohn RG, Cheung P, et al. The immunosuppressant leflunomide inhibits lymphocyte proliferation by inhibiting pyrimidine biosynthesis. *J Pharmacol Exp Ther* 1995;275:1043–1049.
8. Fox RI. Mechanism of action of leflunomide in rheumatoid arthritis. *J Rheumatol* 1998;25[Suppl 53]:20–26.
9. Zielinski T, Herrmann M, Müller HJ, et al. The influence of leflunomide on cell cycle, IL-2-receptor (IL-2R) and its gene expression. *Agents Actions* 1994;41[Spec Iss]:C204–C205.
10. Fairbanks LD, Bofi M, Rückemann K, Simmonds HA. Importance of ribonucleotide availability to proliferating T lymphocytes from healthy humans. *J Biol Chem* 1995:29682–29691.
11. Rückemann K, Fairbanks LD, Carrey EA, et al. Leflunomide inhibits pyrimidine de novo synthesis in mitogen-stimulated T-lymphocytes from healthy humans. *J Biol Chem* 1998:21682–21691.
12. Cao WW, Kao PN, AY, et al. A novel mechanism of the immunomodulatory drug, leflunomide: augmentation of the immunosuppressive cytokine, TGF-beta1, and suppression of the immunostimulatory cytokine, IL-2. *Transplant Proc* 1996:3079–3080.
13. Dimitrova P, Skapenko A, Herrmann ML, et al. Restriction of de novo pyrimidine biosynthesis inhibits Th1 cell activation and promotes Th2 cell differentiation. *J Immunol* 2002;169:3392–3399.
14. Déage V, Burger D, Dayer J-M. Exposure of T lymphocytes to leflunomide but not to dexamethasone favors the production by monocytic cells of interleukin-1 receptor antagonist and tissue inhibitor of metalloproteinases-1 over that of interleukin-1beta and metalloproteinases. *Eur Cytokine Netw* 1998;9:663–668.

15. Kraan MC, Reece RJ, Barg EC, et al. Modulation of inflammation and metalloproteinase expression in synovial tissue by leflunomide and methotrexate in patients with active rheumatoid arthritis. Findings in a prospective, randomized, double-blind, parallel-design clinical trial in thirty-nine patients at two centers. *Arthritis Rheum* 2000;43:1820–1830.
16. Manna SK, Aggarwal BB. Immunosuppressive leflunomide metabolite (A77 1726) blocks TNF-dependent nuclear factor-kappa B activation and gene expression. *J Immunol* 1999;162:2095–2102.
17. Siemasko KF, Chong A-SF, Jäck H-M, et al. Inhibition of JAK3 and STAT6 tyrosine phosphorylation by the immunosuppressive drug leflunomide leads to a block in IgG1 production. *J Immunol* 1998;160:1581–1588.
18. Elder RT, Xu X, Williams JW, et al. The immunosuppressive metabolite of leflunomide, A77 1726, affects murine T cells through two biochemical mechanisms. *J Immunol* 1997;159:22–27.
19. Xu XL, Williams JW, Bremer EG, et al. Inhibition of protein tyrosine phosphorylation in T cells by a novel immunosuppressive agent, leflunomide. *J Biol Chem* 1995;270:12398–12403.
20. Grisar J, Aringer M, Iler K, et al. Leflunomide inhibits transendothelial migration of peripheral blood mononuclear cells. *Ann Rheum Dis* 2004 (*in press*).
21. Glant TT, Mikecz K, Bartlett RR, et al. Immunomodulation of proteoglycan-induced progressive polyarthritis by leflunomide. *Immunopharmacology* 1992;23:105–116.
22. Thoss K, Henzgen S, Petrow PK. Immunomodulation of rat antigen-induced arthritis by leflunomide alone and in combination with cyclosporine. *Inflamm Res* 1996;45:103–107.
23. Pasternak RD, Wadopian NS, Wright RN, et al. Disease-modifying activity of HWA 486 in rat adjuvant-induced arthritis. *Agents Actions* 1987;21:241–243.
24. Arai Y, Ueyama S, Kitagawa H, et al. Leflunomide inhibits bone resorption in vitro and the severity of type II collagen-induced arthritis (CIA) in mice. *Ann Rheum Dis* 2000;59:144(abst).
25. Bartlett RR, Popovic S, Raiss RX. Development of autoimmunity in MRL/lpr mice and the effect of drugs on this murine disease. *Scand J Rheumatol* 75:290–299.
26. Smolen JS, Kalden JR, Scott DL, et al. Efficacy and safety of leflunomide compared with placebo and sulphasalazine in active rheumatoid arthritis: a double-blind, randomised, multicentre trial. *Lancet* 1999;353:259–266.
27. Emery P, Smolen JS. Issues in rheumatoid arthritis. *Lancet* 1999;353:1186.
28. Scott DL, Smolen JS, Kalden JR, et al. Treatment of active rheumatoid arthritis with leflunomide: two year follow up of a double blind, placebo controlled trial versus sulfasalazine. *Ann Rheum Dis* 2001;60:913–923.
29. Landewé R, van der HD. Follow up studies in rheumatoid arthritis. *Ann Rheum Dis* 2002;61:479–481.
30. Strand V, Cohen S, Schiff M, et al. Treatment of active rheumatoid arthritis with leflunomide compared with placebo and methotrexate. *Arch Int Med* 1999;159:2542–2550.
31. Strand V, Tugwell P, Bombardier C, et al. Function and health-related quality of life. Results from a randomized controlled trial of leflunomide versus methotrexate or placebo in patients with active rheumatoid arthritis. *Arthritis Rheum* 1999;42:1870–1878.
32. Cohen S, Cannon GW, Schiff M, et al. Two-year, blinded, randomized, controlled trial of treatment of active rheumatoid arthritis with leflunomide compared with methotrexate. *Arthritis Rheum* 2001;44:1984–1992.
33. Emery P, Breedveld FC, Lemmel EM, et al. A comparison of the efficacy and safety of leflunomide and methotrexate for the treatment of rheumatoid arthritis. *Rheumatology* 2000;39:655–665.
34. Sharp JT, Strand V, Leung H, et al. Treatment with leflunomide slows radiographic progression of rheumatoid arthritis. Results from three randomized controlled trials of leflunomide in patients with active rheumatoid arthritis. *Arthritis Rheum* 2000;43:495–505.
35. Morgan SL BJ, Vaughn WH, et al. Supplementation with folic acid during methotrexate therapy for rheumatoid arthritis. *Ann Intern Med* 1994;121:833–841.
36. van Ede AE, Laan RF, Rood MJ, et al. Effect of folic or folinic acid supplementation on the toxicity and efficacy of methotrexate in rheumatoid arthritis: a forty-eight week, multicenter, randomized, double-blind, placebo-controlled study. *Arthritis Rheum* 2001;44:1515–1524.
37. Kalden JR, Scott DL, Smolen JS, et al. Improved functional ability in patients with rheumatoid arthritis—longterm treatment with leflunomide versus sulfasalazine. *J Rheumatol* 2001;28:1893–1891.
38. Tugwell P, Wells G, Strand V, et al. Clinical improvement as reflected in measures of function and health-related quality of life following treatment with leflunomide compared with methotrexate in patients with rheumatoid arthritis. Sensitivity and relative efficiency to detect a treatment effect in a twelve-month placebo-controlled trial. *Arthritis Rheum* 2000;43:506–514.
39. Metzler C, Fink C, Lamprecht P, et al. Maintenance of remission with leflunomide in Wegener's granulomatosis. *Rheumatology (Oxford)* 2004;43:315–320.
40. Remer CF, Weisman MH, Wallace DJ. Leflunomide in SLE. *Lupus* 2001; 10:483.
41. O'Dell J. Treatment of rheumatoid arthritis with methotrexate alone, sulfasalazine and hydroxychloroquine, or a combination of all three medications. *N Engl J Med* 1996;334:1287–1291.
42. Maini RN, Breedveld FC, Kalden JR, et al. Therapeutic efficacy of multiple intravenous infusions of anti-tumor necrosis factor alpha monoclonal antibody combined with low-dose weekly methotrexate in rheumatoid arthritis. *Arthritis Rheum* 1998;41:1552–1563.
43. Kremer JM, Genovese MC, Cannon GW, et al. Concomitant leflunomide therapy in patients with active rheumatoid arthritis despite stable doses of methotrexate. A randomized, double-blind, placebo-controlled trial. *Ann Intern Med* 2002;137:726–733.
44. Kremer J, Genovase M, Cannon GW, et al. Combination leflunomide and methotrexate therapy for patients with active rheumatoid arthritis failing methotrexate monotherapy: an open-label extension of a randomized, double-blind, placebo-controlled trial. *J Rheumatol* 2004 (*in press*).
45. Dougados M, Emery P, Lemmel EM, et al. Efficacy and safety of leflunomide and predisposing factors for treatment response in patients with active rheumatoid arthritis: RELIEF 6-month data. *J Rheumatol* 2003;30:2572–2579.
46. Kiely PDW, Johnson DM. Infliximab and leflunomide combination therapy in rheumatoid arthritis: an open-label study. *Rheumatology* 2002;41:631–637.
47. Wolfe F, Michaud K, Doyle J, Stephenson B. Toward a definition and method of assessment of treatment failure and treatment effectiveness: the case of leflunomide versus methotrexate. *Arthritis Rheum* 2002;46[Suppl]:S571.
48. Brault I, Gossec L, Pham T, Dougados M. Leflunomide termination rates in comparison with other DMARDs in rheumatoid arthritis. *Arthritis Rheum* 2002;46[Suppl]:S540–S541.
49. Siva C, Shepherd R, Cunningham F, Eisen S. Leflunomide use in the first 33 months after FDA approval: experience in a national cohort of 3325 patients. *Arthritis Rheum* 2002;46[Suppl]:S538.
50. Aletaha D, Stamm T, Kapral T, et al. Survival and effectiveness of leflunomide compared with methotrexate and sulfasalazine in rheumatoid arthritis: matched observational study. *Ann Rheum Dis* 2003;62:944–951.
51. Fries JF, Krishnan E. Estimates of functional disability averted by leflunomide treatment in rheumatoid arthritis. *Arthritis Rheum* 2002;46[Suppl]:S539.
52. Sanders S, Harisdangkul V. Leflunomide for the treatment of rheumatoid arthritis and autoimmunity. *Am J Med Sci* 2002;323:190–193.
53. Fleischmann R. Safety and efficacy of disease-modifying antirheumatic agents in rheumatoid arthritis and juvenile rheumatoid arthritis. *Expert Opin Drug Saf* 2003;2:347–365.
54. Reich K, Hummel KM, Beckmann I, et al. Treatment of severe psoriasis and psoriatic arthritis with leflunomide. *Br J Dermatol* 2002;146:335–336.
55. Scarpa R, Manguso F, Oriente A, et al. Leflunomide in psoriatic polyarthritis: an Italian pilot study. *Arthritis Rheum* 2001;44[Suppl]:S92.
56. Kaltenbach J, et al. Leflunomide in psoriatic arthritis (TOPAS). *Arthritis Rheum* 2002.
57. Cuchacovich M, Soto L. Leflunomide decreases joint erosions and induces reparative changes in a patients with psoriatic arthritis. *Ann Rheum Dis* 2002;61:942–943.
58. Remer CF, Weisman MH, Wallace DJ. Benefits of leflunomide in systemic lupus erythematosus: a pilot observational study. *Lupus* 2001;10:480–483.
59. Petera P, Manger B, Manger K, et al. A pilot study of leflunomide in systemic lupus erythematosus (SLE). *Arthritis Rheum* 2000;43:S241.
60. Coblyn JS, Shadick N, Helfgott S. Leflunomide-associated weight loss in rheumatoid arthritis. *Arthritis Rheum* 2001;44:1048–1051.
61. Wolfe F. Low rates of serious liver toxicity to leflunomide (LEF) and methotrexate (MTX): a longitudinal surveillance study of 14,997 LEF and MTX exposures in RA. *Arthritis Rheum* 2002;46:S375.
62. Cannon G, Schiff M, Strand V, Holden W. Hepatic adverse events and other toxicity during treatment with leflunomide (LEF), methotrexate (MTX), other disease modifying antirheumatic drugs (DMARDs), and combination DMARD therapy: comparison to NSAIDs alone and adjustment for comorbidities. *Arthritis Rheum* 2002;46:S166–S167.
63. Aletaha D, Smolen JS. Laboratory testing in rheumatoid arthritis patients taking disease-modifying antirheumatic drugs: clinical evaluation and cost analysis. *Arthritis Rheum* 2002;47:181–188.

CHAPTER 31

Etanercept

Edward C. Keystone and Boulos Haraoui

Substantial data has accumulated supporting the pivotal role of tumor necrosis factor (TNF) in the pathogenesis of rheumatoid arthritis (RA). As a consequence, TNF has become a prime therapeutic target. One approach has been to mimic nature's own mechanism to maintain TNF homeostasis. After TNF activates its target cells, the TNF-specific cell-surface receptors are released to "mop" up circulating unbound TNF. These so-called circulating soluble TNF receptors (sTNFRs) are thought to lower TNF to homeostatic levels. In RA, the levels of sTNFR appear to be inadequate to reduce the proinflammatory activity of TNF. This provided the rationale for developing, through recombinant DNA technology, a soluble TNF receptor to affect the balance between the proinflammatory cytokine TNF and its natural antagonists. Etanercept was developed to fulfill such a role. It was the first biologic approved by the regulatory agencies for use in RA.

MOLECULAR STRUCTURE AND MODE OF ACTION

Etanercept (ENBREL) is a dimeric human TNFR p75-Fc fusion protein made of two extracellular ligand-binding portions of the human 75-kd (p75) TNFR linked by the constant Fc portion of human immunoglobulin G1 (Fig. 31.1). Etanercept is produced by recombinant DNA technology in the Chinese hamster ovary mammalian cell expression system. It consists of 934 amino acids and has an approximate molecular weight of 150 kd.

TNF is a naturally occurring cytokine produced primarily by activated macrophages and T cells and exists predominantly as a trimer (1–4). TNF is produced in joints predominantly by macrophage-type synoviocytes, resulting in elevated levels in the synovial fluid of RA patients. Two distinct receptors for TNF exist naturally as monomeric molecules on cell surfaces and in soluble forms. One is a 55-kd protein (p55) and the other has a molecular weight of 75 kd (p75). The biologic activity of TNF is dependent on binding to either cell-surface TNFRs. Monomeric fractions of the extracellular portion of the TNFRs that are naturally cleaved from the cell surface are referred to as *sTNFRs*. With high-affinity binding to circulating TNF, sTNFRs act as natural antagonists to TNF, preventing the TNF molecules from binding to cell-bound receptors.

The dimeric structure of etanercept enhances its binding affinity and provides substantially greater competitive inhibition of TNF than monomeric soluble receptors (Fig. 31.2). Use of an immunoglobulin Fc region as a fusion element in this construction imparts a longer serum half-life compared to monomeric soluble receptors.

Etanercept inhibits the activity of human TNF in *in vitro* assays and is efficacious in many *in vivo* models of inflammation, including arthritis. In collagen-induced arthritis in mice, sTNFRs reduced the incidence and severity of arthritis when administered before disease onset and stabilized disease when administered after disease onset (5). sTNFRs was shown to reduce the inflammatory component as well as joint destruction and cartilage depletion.

Etanercept competitively inhibits the binding of both TNF-α and TNF-β (lymphotoxin-α) to cell-surface TNF receptors, rendering TNF biologically inactive (6). Etanercept does not cause lysis of TNF-producing cells *in vitro* in the presence or absence of complement (7).

Etanercept also modulates different biologic responses indirectly by controlling or inhibiting molecules that are induced or regulated by TNF, such as the expression of adhesion molecules E-selectin and, to a lesser extent, intercellular adhesion molecule-1 and serum levels of interleukin-6 (IL-6) and matrix metalloproteinase-3 or stromelysin as well as IL-1 (8,9).

The immune function of patients with RA who were treated with etanercept has been extensively studied (10,11). T-cell responsiveness to microbial antigens as well as to collagen type II is not altered. No significant differences were noted between patients treated with etanercept or placebo in the phenotypes of peripheral blood leukocytes, in T-cell proliferative responses, in neutrophil function, in delayed-type hypersensitivity reactions, or in serum immunoglobulin levels.

HUMAN PHARMACOKINETICS

The pharmacokinetics of etanercept were studied in approximately 300 subjects with doses ranging from 0.125 mg per m^2 to 60 mg per m^2 administered by a single intravenous (i.v.) infusion over 30 minutes or single or multiple subcutaneous injections. After a single administration of 25 mg subcutaneously to 26 healthy volunteers, peak serum concentration is reached after a mean of 51 hours, with a maximal drug concentration of 1.46 μg per mL (range, 0.37–3.47) (12). The elimination half-life is 68 hours. The pharmacokinetic parameters of single and chronic dosing were compared in 25 patients with RA and found to be similar (13). To maintain a steady-state concentration, the twice weekly dosing regimen is indicated. Analyses of serum samples from adult RA patients in long-term treatment trials (6 months of

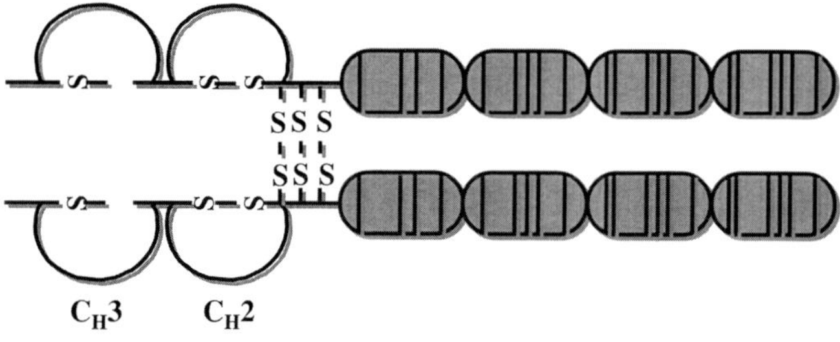

Figure 31.1. Structure of etanercept. Etanercept is made of two extracellular domains of the human p75 tumor necrosis factor (TNF) receptor to increase its affinity. Etanercept is linked to the Fc region of human immunoglobulin G1 (IgG1), which provides a longer half-life.

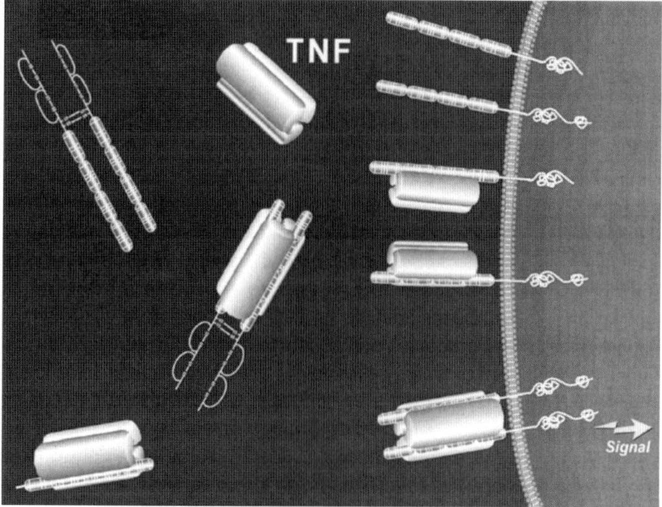

Figure 31.2. Mechanism of action of etanercept. Etanercept binds with high affinity to circulating tumor necrosis factor (TNF) molecules before they attach to cell-bound TNF receptors, thus preventing cell activation.

treatment with etanercept) showed expected steady-state concentrations of etanercept. Recently, studies are being conducted to evaluate the possibility of a once weekly dose of 50 mg.

There is no need for dose adjustment in presence of renal or hepatic impairment, or both. No difference was observed in pharmacokinetics between men and women. Clearance and volume estimates in patients ages 65 to 87 years were similar to those for patients younger than 65 years of age. Concomitant methotrexate (MTX) administration does not alter the pharmacokinetics of etanercept.

ETANERCEPT AND PREGNANCY

Etanercept has not been studied in pregnant women. TNF-α plays a role in pregnancy and parturition (14). Therefore, etanercept has the potential to interfere with these processes. Anecdotal cases of successful pregnancies and deliveries have been reported, but caution should be exercised awaiting definitive confirmation of its safety (15).

ETANERCEPT IN THE TREATMENT OF ADULT-ONSET RHEUMATOID ARTHRITIS

Etanercept was evaluated in several double-blind, randomized, placebo-controlled trials and open-label extensions in patients with RA at different stages of their disease progression.

Etanercept Monotherapy in Established Disease

Two trials were conducted in patients with established disease and who had failed to respond to traditional therapies. To take part, patients had to discontinue all other disease-modifying antirheumatic drugs (DMARDs). Different doses of etanercept were compared to placebo.

In the first placebo-controlled trial, etanercept was administered subcutaneously twice a week for 3 months to 180 patients (44–46 patients per group) using three doses of 0.25, 2.0, and 16.0 mg per m^2 (16). Based on the American College of Rheumatology (ACR) response criteria, a dose-related improvement was observed with the 16 mg per m^2 dose, resulting in 75% of patients achieving an ACR 20% response compared with 14% of the placebo group. Improvement was seen as early as the first month in a majority of patients. No dose-limiting toxic effect was noted, and no antibodies to TNFR:Fc were detected. Patients were followed for 2 more months after cessation of therapy; measures of disease activity gradually returned to base-line levels, and significant loss of efficacy was evident as early as 4 weeks after discontinuing therapy.

In another 6-month trial, 234 patients with RA were randomized to one of three therapeutic groups: placebo, 10 mg or 25 mg of etanercept administered subcutaneously twice a week (17). Patients enrolled in this trial had long-standing severe disease with a mean disease duration of 12 years, having failed to respond to more than three DMARDs; they had an average of 25 swollen and 34 tender joints at baseline. At 3 months, 62% of the patients in the 25-mg group reached the ACR 20% response criteria, compared to 23% in the placebo group. At the 6-month evaluation, the ACR 20% response was maintained in 59% of patients, whereas the placebo group dropped to 11%. Moreover, 40% of patients achieved an ACR 50% response compared to only 5% of the placebo-treated patients. The average reduction in the number of swollen and tender joints was 56% and 46%, respectively, for the 25-mg group compared to 6% and 7% for the placebo group. Other measures of disease activity, such as the C-reactive protein (CRP) and the disability scores measured by the Health Assessment Questionnaire (HAQ), also improved significantly as early as the first month after initiation of therapy. The 25-mg dose was found to be more effective than the 10-mg dose, and both were more effective than placebo. Etanercept was generally well tolerated, with mild injection site reactions (ISRs) being the most frequently reported side effect.

Etanercept/Methotrexate Combination Therapy in Established Disease

Etanercept was evaluated in combination with MTX in a multicenter, double-blind, randomized, placebo-controlled trial in patients with persistently active disease despite treatment with MTX (18). Patients with a mean disease duration of 13 years receiving MTX at an average dose of 18 mg per week (12.5–25.0 mg) were randomized to 25 mg of etanercept (59 patients) or placebo (30 patients) given subcutaneously twice a week. As early as 12 weeks, two-thirds of the patients on etanercept achieved an ACR 20% response compared to one-third of the placebo group. The response was maintained at 6 months with, 71% and 27% of patients achieving an ACR 20% response in the etanercept and placebo groups, repectively. Forty percent and 15% of the etanercept-treated patients reached ACR 50% and

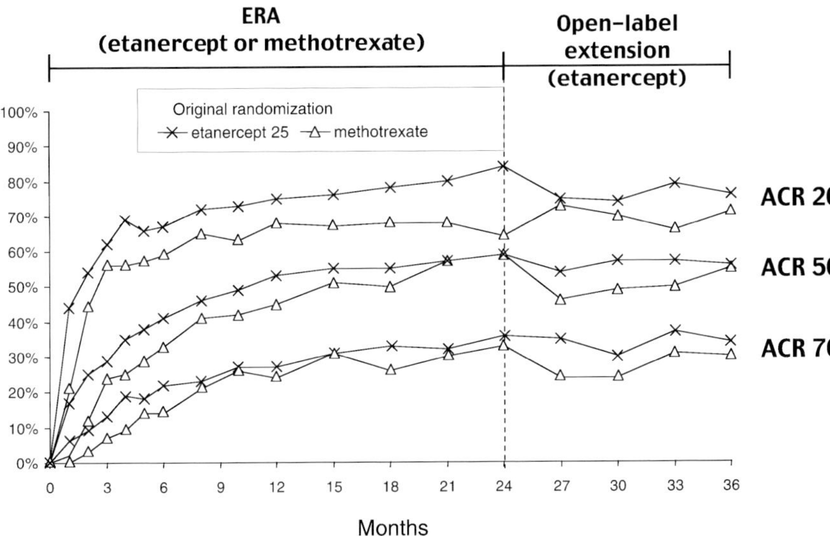

Figure 31.3. American College of Rheumatology (ACR) responses in the early rheumatoid arthritis (ERA) trial. Etanercept has a faster onset of action, but no statistically significant differences are seen with methotrexate beyond the fourth month.

ACR 70% levels, compared to 3% and 0% of patients in the placebo group. All of the components of the ACR response criteria significantly improved. The HAQ disability score was reduced by 47%, dropping from a median of 1.5 to 0.8, and the CRP declined by 62% from a median of 2.2 mg per dL to 0.5.

The addition of etanercept to medium- to high-dose MTX background therapy was well tolerated, with ISR being the only adverse reaction, occurring more frequently in the etanercept group (42% vs. 7%). The infection rate was similar in both groups. The ISRs do not appear to influence the efficacy of the etanercept, with 72% of those patients experiencing ISR achieving an ACR 20% response compared to 71% of those who did not have reactions.

Etanercept Monotherapy in Early Rheumatoid Arthritis

Etanercept was evaluated in patients with early RA (ERA) (i.e., duration of <3 years) in a head-to-head comparison with high-dose MTX (19). In a 52-week, double-blind, randomized, placebo-controlled trial of 632 patients (210 patients per group), subjects were randomized to 10 or 25 mg of etanercept subcutaneously twice a week or MTX (rapidly escalated to 20 mg over an 8-week period) (mean dose, 19 mg per week). The primary efficacy measure was the ACR 20% response at 1 year. Patients also had radiographs of the hands, wrists, and feet taken at baseline and after 1 and 2 years. The x-rays were evaluated according to the modified Sharp scoring technique, with a total score being the sum of the erosion and joint space narrowing scores (20–22).

Etanercept (25 mg) resulted in a rapid clinical improvement compared to MTX, with differences apparent as early as 2 weeks. A greater proportion of patients in the 25-mg etanercept group achieved ACR 20%, ACR 50%, and ACR 70% responses than the MTX group within the first 4 months (Fig. 31.3). By 12 months, the responses between the MTX and etanercept groups were comparable, with 72% of the etanercept (25-mg dose)-treated patients, compared with 65% of the MTX-treated patients, achieving an ACR 20% response. A similar proportion of patients completed the trial: 85% for etanercept, 25 mg, and 79% for MTX.

Overall, the monotherapy and combination therapy studies with etanercept show consistent improvement in ACR responses across all trials (Fig. 31.4).

In terms of radiographic progression, all groups in the ERA trial showed a similar significant reduction in the progression over 12 months in the total Sharp scores compared to the predicted values (19). Etanercept (25-mg dose), however, resulted in significantly less progression of joint erosions compared with MTX (i.e., 0.47-U vs. 1.03-U change in Sharp score erosion, respectively). No differ-

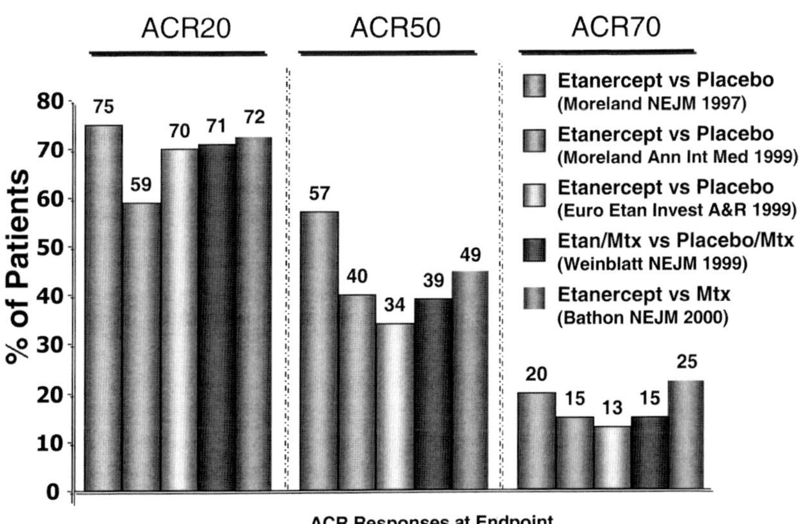

Figure 31.4. Etanercept (Etan) has shown consistent clinical responses across trials and different time points. ACR, American College of Rheumatology; Mtx, methotrexate.

ence in progression of joint space narrowing was observed. Good correlation was noted between the clinical response and the progression of radiographic damage. Patients who had the best clinical improvement had the least x-ray deterioration. When the subsets of patients with radiographic erosions at study entry were retrospectively analyzed, 72% of etanercept (25-mg dose)-treated patients compared with 60% of MTX-treated patients demonstrated no progression in the erosion score at 12 months.

Both treatments were well tolerated and had a similar adverse events profile. ISRs were reported more frequently with etanercept, whereas more patients had the usual side effects of MTX, including nausea, alopecia, mouth ulcers, and rashes.

Patients enrolled in the ERA trial were followed for an additional 12-month period (23). Seventy-five percent of patients taking etanercept, 25 mg, completed the 2-year follow-up compared with 58% of those taking MTX. The ACR 20% response was achieved in, 80% and 63% of patients in the etanercept, 25 mg, and MTX groups, respectively. The rate of progression of radiographic joint damage was slower during the following 2 years. The annual progression fell from 0.9 Sharp units in the first year, 0.57 Sharp units in the second year, and 0.37 Sharp units in the third year (24). Whether the withdrawal rate for lack of efficacy over 3 years accounts for the slower rate of progression with continuous therapy remains unclear.

A retrospective analysis of etanercept controlled trial data was carried out to determine whether etanercept affects disability differentially in early and late RA (25). Disability was evaluated in patients with early RA (N = 207; mean duration, 1 year) as well as long-standing disease (N = 563; mean duration, 12 years). Baseline demographic and disease activity characteristics were comparable. Disability improved more in patients with established RA. Despite comparable baseline characteristics between the groups, the data must be interpreted with caution given that patients were evaluated from two different patient cohorts.

Etanercept Dosing

To determine whether a higher dose of etanercept would yield greater clinical benefit, etanercept, 25 mg twice weekly, was compared with 50 mg twice weekly in a 6-month double-blind, randomized, controlled trial involving 77 patients (26). The results revealed that etanercept, 50 mg, achieved a more rapid response than the 25-mg dose; however, there was no difference in ACR responses by 6 months of therapy. Whether a dose increase is warranted in patients with an inadequate response to 25 mg twice weekly remains unclear.

Etanercept/Anakinra Combination Therapy

Because preclinical data supported an additive effect of a TNF antagonist and IL-1ra (27), an open-label trial of 58 patients was carried out to evaluate the effect of combination anakinra with etanercept in patients who had an inadequate response to the latter alone (28). Addition of anakinra to etanercept resulted in additional clinical benefit, with a 25% and 50% improvement in swollen and tender joints, respectively. However, a higher serious infection rate of 7% was observed. A further controlled trial of a combination of etanercept and anakinra as initial therapy is under way.

Long-Term Open-Label Studies

Patients enrolled in previous etanercept monotherapy or safety trials were followed prospectively (29–31). In the first report, efficacy and safety parameters were assessed in 628 North American patients; 479 received etanercept for at least 12 months, 334 for at least 24 months, and 139 for 30 months (29). Efficacy was sustained during the entire observation period, with median counts of four tender and five swollen joints at 30 months. CRP remained within normal limits throughout. Approximately 73% of patients achieved an ACR 20% response at 30 months. Fifty-five percent of patients were able to reduce their prednisone dose by a mean of 70%, and 25% of patients were able to discontinue it. The incidence of infectious and noninfectious adverse events were in line with those observed during the double-blind controlled phase.

Recently, an update of the long-term follow-up of 2,572 patients receiving etanercept monotherapy in open-label protocols in North American and European trials was reported (30). Follow-up of patients for up to 6 years demonstrated sustained efficacy and a rate of serious infection (requiring hospitalization or i.v. antibiotics) comparable to the rate in the control group from controlled trials (30). In patients receiving a combination of etanercept and MTX (N = 64) who have remained on therapy in the open-label extension for a median duration of 47 months (maximum, 54 months), sustained efficacy was observed. Thirty-one percent of patients have reduced the MTX dose, whereas an additional 24% have discontinued it (31). Of the patients taking corticosteroids, 82% have reduced or discontinued the steroid dose by a mean of 66%, whereas 69% have discontinued steroid use.

The impact of etanercept on health-related quality of life and functional status over time was analyzed in 533 RA patients previously in randomized trials of etanercept (32). Initial improvement in patient-centered outcomes, including HAQ, physical component, and mental component summary scores, was shown to be sustained over time in patients with either long-term or early-stage disease. The impact of etanercept on health care use and employment was also evaluated in 260 patients with ERA (from the ERA trial) (33). Even though the control group of patients who received etanercept only at the termination of the ERA study received it for a mean of 239 days, patients originally randomized to etanercept for a mean of 882 days reported fewer patient visits, outpatient surgeries, and hospital admissions for RA than controls. RA patients who were employed at disease onset and originally randomized to etanercept had more hours of employment compared to controls. These data suggest the possibility of reducing health care utilization and increased employment with the use of etanercept for a relatively short period. Further studies of patients examined in clinical practice are needed to demonstrate cost-effectiveness.

Long-term observational cohorts have also been used to compare the efficacy of etanercept to infliximab. In one study, patients receiving etanercept (N = 88) were compared with those taking infliximab (N = 32) with regards to flares during the first year of therapy relative to the year before their initiation (34). Although biases likely existed regarding selection of the particular agent as well as the infliximab dose and dosing regimen, the results demonstrated no difference in the rate of flare relative to pretreatment between those treated with etanercept compared to infliximab. Confounding factors, such as patient selection and infliximab dosing, have been influential in determining the results of comparative analyses. Efficacy of infliximab compared to etanercept was also recently examined in terms of ACR 20% and Disease Activity Score response in the Stockholm Registry for TNF-α antagonists (35). A comparison of infliximab-treated patients (N = 202) with those treated with etanercept (N = 110) for 3 to 12 months revealed similar responses, with a trend to slightly increased clinical efficacy at 3 months in the infliximab group. A Swedish observational study of etanercept (N = 184), infliximab (N = 223), and leflunomide (N = 114) was also performed using ACR response criteria for evaluation (36). Etanercept appeared somewhat more efficacious than infliximab, with both TNF blockers being superior to leflunomide. Survival on drug as an evaluating tool in the same patient population revealed similar results at 12 months (37).

ETANERCEPT IN THE TREATMENT OF CHRONIC JUVENILE RHEUMATOID ARTHRITIS

The efficacy and safety of etanercept was evaluated in children with polyarticular juvenile RA who did not tolerate or had an inadequate response to MTX (38). Sixty-nine patients were treated for up to 3 months in an open-label fashion with etanercept, 0.4 mg per kg. Fifty-one of the 69 patients (74%) fulfilled the predefined criteria for 30% improvement (39). These patients entered the second double-blind phase and were randomized to either etanercept or placebo and followed for 4 months or until a flare occurred. Twenty-one of the 26 patients (81%) who were in the placebo arm withdrew because of a disease flare, as compared to 7 of 25 (28%) who received etanercept. The median time for a flare was 28 days for the placebo group and more than 116 days for etanercept. Etanercept was generally well tolerated, with no significant differences in the incidence or nature of side effects compared to placebo.

ADULT STILL'S DISEASE

Twelve adult patients with Still's disease and active arthritis at baseline were treated in an open-label clinical trial with etanercept, 25 mg subcutaneously twice a week (40). Two patients withdrew because of a disease flare, and four other patients had to increase the dose to 25 mg 3 times a week. Seven patients met the ACR 20% response criteria, and four were ACR 50% responders.

SAFETY OF ETANERCEPT

Etanercept has been evaluated in approximately 1,100 patients in all clinical trials with long-term follow-up safety studies as noted previously. The most frequent adverse events are summarized in Table 31.1.

TABLE 31.1. Rates of Adverse Events in Controlled and Open-Label Extension Trials

	Controlled Trials		Long-Term Therapy
	Placebo	Etanercept	
	(N = 152)	(N = 349)	(N = 628)
Event	Event/ Patient-Yr	Event/ Patient-Yr	Event/ Patient-Yr
Injection site reactions	0.62	7.73[a]	N/A[b]
Upper respiratory illness	0.68	0.82	0.46
Headache	0.62	0.68	0.27
Sinusitis	0.42	0.31	0.19
Rash	0.12	0.21	0.18
Nausea	0.47	0.30	0.14
Skin infection	0.30	0.16	0.14
Rhinitis	0.35	0.45	0.13
Diarrhea	0.35	0.27	0.13

N/A, not applicable.
[a]$p < .001$ compared to placebo.
[b]Injection site reactions were not required to be reported after 3 months of therapy.
[From Bathon JM, Genovese MC, Martin RW, et al. Etanercept (Enbrel®) in Early Erosive Rheumatoid Arthritis (ERA trial): observations at 3 years. *Ann Rheum Dis* 2002;61[Suppl]:S54, (abstract 0P0072), with permission.]

Injection Site Reactions

The only side effect that was observed more frequently in the etanercept-treated patients (~40%) than in the placebo group (~7%) was ISRs. ISRs usually appeared within the first 3 weeks of therapy. Less than 1% of patients withdrew from therapy because of ISRs, which are usually easily managed with local cold packs; rarely, a topical corticosteroid is warranted. ISRs subsided within 4 weeks in virtually all patients.

Infection

COMMON INFECTION

Blockade of TNF-α poses a theoretic risk of increased infections. However, in all of the etanercept double-blind trials, no increases in the frequency or the nature of infections were noted, including serious infections, between etanercept- and placebo-treated patients. Moreover, in the ERA trial, serious infections were statistically higher in the MTX group compared with the etanercept-treated patients. Because of the potential risk, it is recommended not to administer etanercept to patients with recurrent infectious episodes and to stop in the presence of infections requiring antibiotics until resolved.

Evaluation of 2,572 patients in open-label, long-term North American and European studies of etanercept as monotherapy for up to 5 years revealed a low rate of adverse events, with the frequency of serious infection (requiring hospitalization or i.v. antibiotics) being comparable to the rate in the control group in controlled trials (30). Similar results were observed with a long-term study cohort of 64 patients receiving a combination of etanercept and MTX (31).

Several studies have evaluated the frequency of infections after etanercept administration compared to the frequency before its initiation. In one study, the rate of infection in 90 patients was compared to the rate of infection 1 year before therapy. The results showed a significant (approximately twofold) increase in the incidence of recorded infections after the initiation of therapy (41). Most infections were respiratory, and the majority were nonserious. Similar data were observed in another study of 168 patients followed over 1 year (42). In that study, nonserious infections were seen in 51% of patients during etanercept therapy compared with 19% in the pretreatment period, although the rate of serious infections was comparable (1.8% vs. 2.9%) before and after therapy.

Analysis of post-marketing reports of serious infections in 103,000 etanercept-treated patients (~102,000 patient-years) revealed that 78% were receiving corticosteroids, and patients had multiple comorbidities, including chronic lung disease, ischemic heart disease, and hypertension (43). The types of infection and organisms are consistent with infection in the pre-TNF antagonist era. Etanercept is contraindicated in patients with infections requiring antibiotics and in patients with infected open wounds as well as chronic recurrent infections (e.g., bronchiectasis). It should be used with caution in patients with recurrent infection and conditions increasing the risk of infection such as uncontrolled diabetes. During infections requiring antibiotics, etanercept should be stopped until clinical recovery and restarted after antibiotics are discontinued. It would be prudent to discontinue etanercept 2 weeks preoperatively, especially for gastrointestinal or genitourinary surgery, and restarted 1 to 2 weeks postoperatively. Patients should be advised about the possibility of an increased risk of infection.

It is relevant to note that at least in patients with psoriatic arthritis, pneumococcal vaccine results in normal antibody responses (44).

OPPORTUNISTIC INFECTION

TNF has been shown to be critical to the maintenance of post-infectious granuloma generated in response to microbial agents such as *Mycobacterium tuberculosis* (MTb), histoplasmosis, and other opportunistic infections. Recent post-marketing surveillance data (Wyeth/Immunex: data on file) is available (as of December 2001) for 114,000 etanercept-treated patients (150,000 patient-years) worldwide, of which 108,000 were treated in the United States and approximately 6,000 were treated outside the United States. To date, 20 cases of MTb have been reported worldwide, of which 15 cases were reported in the United States. The pattern of MTb was consistent, with significant immunosuppression and three of the patients exhibiting a miliary pattern. The median time of onset of reactivation was 6 months. Because the expected incidence of MTb in the United States is 6 to 8 per 100,000 patient-years, it is unclear whether MTb is increased in etanercept patients. This is particularly so because underreporting and provision of inaccurate information to the U.S. Food and Drug Administration (FDA) and industry is well documented with post-approval surveillance. It is notable, however, that preliminary data showed that 27 patients with a history of MTb or positive purified protein derivative (PPD) received etanercept for an average of 9 months without reactivation of latent MTb. Further long-term observational studies are critical. Nevertheless, screening for latent MTb with a chest x-ray and PPD skin test is advisable. A positive PPD consistent with local health regulations (5–10 mm) would suggest the need for initiating therapy for latent MTb at least 1 month before etanercept therapy using isoniazid (for 9 months) or rifampin (for 4 months). Combination of rifampin and pyrazinamide has been shown to be hepatotoxic and should be avoided. A chest x-ray consistent with active MTb would necessitate completion of combination antibiotic therapy before initiation of etanercept. Other opportunistic infections have also been reported, including atypical mycobacterium (N = 8), *Pneumocystis carinii* (N = 5), with a few cases of candidiasis (N = 3), cryptococcosis (N = 3), aspergillosis (N = 2), and isolated cases of histoplasmosis (N = 1), and *Listeria monocytogenes* (N = 1). Whether these reflect an increase relative to conventional DMARDs is uncertain.

Demyelinating Disorders

Recent reports on other TNF antagonists have suggested the possibility of induction or aggravation of demyelinating disease (45,46). As of December 2001, 23 cases of multiple sclerosis had been reported, including ten patients with newly diagnosed disease and 13 with relapses. In addition, five patients with optic neuritis had been reported. A causal relationship to etanercept is unclear, nor is it certain whether demyelinating disorders are increased with etanercept therapy.

Hematologic Abnormalities

Pancytopenia (N = 12) and aplastic anemia (N = 5)—some with a fatal outcome—have been described (Wyeth/Immunex: data on file). The majority of patients had concurrent or recent exposure to other myelosuppressive DMARDs. Pancytopenia occurred as early as 2 weeks after initiating therapy. Thrombocytopenia has been observed more frequently than pancytopenia. Rapid reversal is observed with discontinuation of therapy. A causal relationship to hematologic abnormalities is unclear; however, caution should be used in patients who have a previous history of hematologic abnormalities. No monitoring guidelines have been recommended to date; however, periodic complete blood cell counts might be advisable.

Antibodies to Etanercept

Non-neutralizing antibodies to etanercept have been documented at least once in 16% of RA patients. A correlation between the presence of antibodies and efficacy or adverse events has not been observed.

Lupus-Like Syndrome/Autoantibodies

Clinical trial data have shown the development of antinuclear antibodies in 11% of etanercept-treated patients compared with 5% of placebo controls. Fifteen percent of etanercept-treated patients developed new anti–double-stranded DNA antibodies (by radioimmunoassay) compared with 4% of placebo controls. Three percent of etanercept-treated patients developed anti–double-stranded DNA antibodies (by crithidia) versus none in controls. To date, 22 patients have been reported in the literature as new cases of systemic lupus erythematosus (SLE) in RA associated with etanercept therapy (47–49). Initially, two cases of etanercept-induced lupus-like syndrome were described (47). One patient presented with a discoid rash, fatigue, diffuse pain, an elevated creatine phosphokinase, and positive antinuclear antibody (ANA), anti-DNA, and anticardiolipin antibodies. Discontinuation of etanercept resulted in clearing of clinical symptoms and a reduction in creatine phosphokinase and biologic markers. The other patient presented with diffuse erythema and purpuric skin eruption associated with lymphopenia, thrombocytopenia, elevated erythrocyte sedimentation rate, abnormal liver function, and positive ANA. The clinical manifestations resolved after discontinuation of etanercept. Four cases of SLE-like disease were also reported, with at least one sign of disease (rash) associated with ANA positivity and resolution of symptoms after discontinuation of therapy (4). More recently, a report of FDA data described 13 patients, 9 of whom were classified as having definite SLE. SLE developed a median of 4 months after initiating etanercept (49). Various rashes, including discoid (N = 8), photosensitivity (N = 6), and malar (N = 4) were reported. In 12 cases, symptoms completely resolved in 1 to 4 months after withdrawal of etanercept. To date, reports of a total of 43 cases, including some or all of the cases described above, have been received by Wyeth/Immunex. The characteristics of these cases have not been reported.

Lymphoma

Reports from the worldwide etanercept post-marketing safety database of 117,000 patients (~145,000 patient-years) revealed lymphoma rates with etanercept of 0.03 cases per 100 patient-years, comparable to that expected for RA (0.08 cases per 100 patient-years). The time-of-onset distribution of histologic subtypes was comparable to previous observations from RA cohorts in the pre-TNF antagonist literature.

INDICATION

According to FDA recommendations, etanercept is approved for improvement of signs and symptoms in early and established RA as well as delay in radiographic progression of joint damage in patients with ERA. It can be used alone or in combination with MTX in patients with an inadequate response to the latter.

The role of etanercept in the therapeutic paradigm continues to evolve with the acquisition of more information regarding long-term safety and efficacy. Currently, etanercept should be used in patients with moderate to severe RA, especially when there is a partial response to MTX. Although radiographic erosions were fewer with etanercept than MTX in the first 2 years of the ERA trial, the long-term clinical significance of this finding remains unclear. Whether initiation of etanercept in combination with MTX in ERA will provide additional benefit relative to monotherapy is currently being addressed in ongoing clinical studies.

CONCLUSION

The development of etanercept has provided the proof of principle that targeted therapy with biologics have substantial clinical benefit in RA and that TNF is a key cytokine in the pathogenic process. Etanercept has set a new therapeutic standard for the treatment of RA with its substantial reduction in signs and symptoms, disability, and radiographic progression. Etanercept's safety record to date, coupled with its sustained benefit, makes it one of the most important additions to the therapeutic armamentarium of RA.

REFERENCES

1. Beayert R, Fiers W. Tumor necrosis factor and lymphotoxin. In: Mire-sluis AR, Thorpe R, eds. *Cytokines*, 1st ed. London: Academic Press, 1998:235–260.
2. Krakauer T, Vilcek J, Oppenheim JJ. Proinflammatory cytokines: TNF and IL-1 families, chemokines, TGF-β, and others. In: Pauluis WE, ed. *Fundamental immunology*, 4th ed. Philadelphia: Lippincott–Raven, 1999:775–811.
3. McDermott MF. TNF and TNFR biology in health and disease. *Cell Mol Biol* 2001;47:619–635.
4. Locksley RM, Kileen N, Lenardo MJ. The TNF and TNF receptor superfamilies: integrating mammalian biology. *Cell* 2001;104:487–501.
5. Wooley PH, Dutcher J, Widmer MB, et al. Influence of a recombinant human soluble tumor necrosis factor receptor FC fusion protein on type II collagen-induced arthritis in mice. *J Immunol* 1993;151:6602–6607.
6. Mohler KM, Torrance DS, Smith CA, et al. Soluble tumor necrosis factor (TNF) receptors are effective therapeutic agents in lethal endotoxemia and function simultaneously as both TNF carriers and TNF antagonists. *J Immunol* 1993;151:1548–1561.
7. Barone D, Krantz C, Lambert D, et al. Comparative analysis of the ability of etanercept and infliximab to lyse TNF-expressing cells in a complement dependent fashion. *Arthritis Rheum* 1999;42[Suppl]:S90 (abstract 116).
8. Verschueren PC, Markusse H, Smeets TJM, et al. Reduced cellularity and expression of adhesion molecules and cytokines after treatment with soluble human recombinant TNF receptor (p75) in RA patients. *Arthritis Rheum* 1999;42[Suppl]:S197 (abstract 762).
9. Cartina AI, Lampa J, Ernestam S, et al. Anti tumor necrosis factor (TNF)-α therapy (etanercept) down regulates serum matrix metalloproteinase (MMP)-3 and MMP-1 in rheumatoid arthritis. *Rheumatology* 2002;41:484–489.
10. Berg L, Lampa J, van Vollenhoven R, et al. Increased peripheral T cell reactivity to microbial antigens and collagen type II in rheumatoid arthritis after treatment with soluble TNFα receptors. *Ann Rheum Dis* 2001;60:133–139.
11. Moreland LW, Bucy RP, Weinblatt ME, et al. Immune function in patients with rheumatoid arthritis treated with etanercept. *Clin Immunol* 2002;103:13–21.
12. Korth-Bradley JM, Rubin AS, Hanna RK, et al. The pharmacokinetics of etanercept in healthy volunteers. *Ann Pharmacother* 2000;34:161–164.
13. Kremer J, Spencer-Green G, Hanna RK, et al. Enbrel® (etanercept) pharmacokinetics in patients with rheumatoid arthritis. *Arthritis Rheum* 2000;43[Suppl]:S229 (abstract 976).
14. Terranova PF, Hunter VJ, Roby KF, et al. Tumor necrosis factor-α in the female reproductive tract. *Proc Soc Exp Biol Med* 1995;209:325–342.
15. Sills ES. Successful ovulation induction, conception and normal delivery after chronic therapy with etanercept: a recombinant fusion anti-cytokine treatment for rheumatoid arthritis. *Am J Reprod Immunol* 2001;46:366–368.
16. Moreland LW, Baumgartner SW, Schiff MH, et al. Treatment of rheumatoid arthritis with a recombinant human tumor necrosis factor receptor (p75)-Fc fusion protein. *N Engl J Med* 1997;337:141–147.
17. Moreland LW, Schiff MH, Baumgartner SW, et al. Etanercept in rheumatoid arthritis. A randomized, controlled trial. *Ann Intern Med* 1999;130:478–486.
18. Weinblatt ME, Kremer JM, Bankhurst AD, et al. A trial of etanercept, a recombinant tumor necrosis factor receptor:Fc fusion protein, in patients with rheumatoid arthritis receiving methotrexate. *N Engl J Med* 1999;340:253-259.
19. Bathon JM, Martin RW, Fleischmann RM, et al. A comparison of etanercept and methotrexate in patients with early rheumatoid arthritis. *N Engl J Med* 2000;343:1586–1593.
20. Sharp JT, Lidsky MD, Collins LC, et al. Methods of scoring the progression of radiologic changes in rheumatoid arthritis: correlation of radiologic, clinical and laboratory abnormalities. *Arthritis Rheum* 1971;14:706–720.
21. Van der Heijde DMFM, van Leewen MA, van Riel PLCM, et al. Bi-annual radiographic assessments of hands and feet in the three-year prospective follow-up of patients with early rheumatoid arthritis. *Arthritis Rheum* 1991;35:26–34.
22. Plant MJ, Saklatvala J, Borg AA, et al. Measurement and prediction of radiological progression in early rheumatoid arthritis. *J Rheumatol* 1994;21:1808–1813.
23. Genovese M, Martin R, Fleischmann R, et al. Etanercept vs. methotrexate in early rheumatoid arthritis (ERA trial): two-year follow-up. *Arthritis Rheum* 2000;43[Suppl]:S269 (abstract 1217).
24. Bathon, JM, Genovese MC, Martin RW, et al. Etanercept (Enbrel®) in Early Erosive Rheumatoid Arthritis (ERA trial): observations at 3 years. *Ann Rheum Dis* 2002; 61[Suppl]:S54 (abstract 0P0072).
25. Fleischmann RM, Baumgartner SW, Moreland LW, et al. Improvement in disability in rheumatoid arthritis patients with early vs. established disease after treatment with etanercept. *Ann Rheum Dis* 2002;61[Suppl]:168 (abstract FRI 0025).
26. Schiff M, Mease P, Weinblatt M, et al. Randomized controlled trial of 25 mg vs. 50 mg Enbrel® (etanercept) twice weekly in rheumatoid arthritis (RA). *Arthritis Rheum* 2000;43[Suppl]:S391 (abstract 1947).
27. Bendele AM, Chlipola ES, Schever J, et al. Combination benefit of treatment with the cytokine inhibitors interleukin-1 receptor antagonist and PEGylated soluble tumor necrosis factor receptor type I in animal models of rheumatoid arthritis. *Arthritis Rheum* 2000;43:2648–2659.
28. Schiff MH, Bulpitt K, Weaver AA, et al. Safety of combination therapy with anakinra and etanercept in patients with rheumatoid arthritis. *Arthritis Rheum* 2001;44[Suppl]:S79 (abstract 57).
29. Moreland LM, Cohen SB, Baumgartner SW, et al. Long term safety and efficacy of etanercept in patients with rheumatoid arthritis. *J Rheumatol* 2001;28:1238–1244.
30. Klareskog L, Moreland LM, Cohen SB, et al. Global safety and efficacy of up to five years of etanercept therapy in rheumatoid arthritis. *Arthritis Rheum* 2001;44[Suppl]:S77 (abstract 150).
31. Kremer JM, Weinblatt ME, Fleischmann RM, et al. Etanercept in addition to methotrexate in rheumatoid arthritis: long term observations. *Arthritis Rheum* 2001;44[Suppl]:S78 (abstract 152).
32. Yelin E, Katz P, Lubeck D, et al. Impact of Etanercept (Enbrel®) on health care use and employment in early RA. *Arthritis Rheum* 2001;44[Suppl]:S152 (abstract 595).
33. Lubeck DP, Katz P, Yelin E, et al. Long term impact of etanercept (Enbrel®) on health related quality of life and functional status of persons with rheumatoid arthritis. *Arthritis Rheum* 2001:44[Suppl]:S184 (abstract 787).
34. Yazia Y, Eikan D, Kulman I, et al. Etanercept (ETA) vs. infliximab (TNF): a comparison of efficacy in controlling rheumatoid arthritis (RA) flares during the first year of therapy and the year prior to their use. *Arthritis Rheum* 2001;44[Suppl]:S81 (abstract 171).
35. vanVollenhoven RF, Harju A, Bratt J, et al. Etanercept and infliximab treated in the Stockholm TNFα antagonist registry: a comparison of two TNFα antagonists. *Arthritis Rheum* 2001;44[Suppl]:S79 (abstract 162).
36. Geborek P, Crnkic M, Petersson IF, et al. Efficacy of etanercept, infliximab and leflunomide in rheumatoid arthritis (RA). Experience using a clinical protocol on a regional basis. *Arthritis Rheum* 2001;44[Suppl]:S77 (abstract 147).
37. Geborek P, Crukic M, Teleman A, et al. Tolerability using survival on drug as evaluation tool. Experience of etanercept, infliximab and leflunomide in rheumatoid arthritis (RA). *Arthritis Rheum* 2001;44[Suppl]:S77 (abstract 146).
38. Lovell DJ, Gianninni EH, Reiff A, et al. Etanercept in children with polyarticular juvenile rheumatoid arthritis. *N Engl J Med* 2000;342:763–769.
39. Gianninni EH, Ruperto N, Ravelli A, et al. Preliminary definition of improvement in juvenile arthritis. *Arthritis Rheum* 1997;40:1202–1209.
40. Husni ME, Maier AL, Mease PJ, et al. Etanercept in the treatment of adult patients with Still's disease. *Arthritis Rheum* 2002;46:1171–1176.
41. Belostocki KB, Leibowitz E, Tai K, et al. Infections associated with etanercept treatment in rheumatoid arthritis: 2 years of experience in the "real-world." *Arthritis Rheum* 2001;44[Suppl]:S173 (abstract 725).
42. Phillips K, Husni ME, Karlson EW, et al. Experience with etanercept in an academic medical center: are infection rates increased? *Arthritis Care Res* 2002;47:17–21.
43. Wallis WJ, Burge DL, Holman J, et al. Infection reports with etanercept (Enbrel®) therapy. *Arthritis Rheum* 2001;44[Suppl]:S78 (abstract 154).
44. Mease P, Richler C, Martin R, et al. Response to pneumoccocal vaccination in psoriatic arthritis patients treated with etanercept. *Arthritis Rheum* 2002;44 [Suppl]:S91 (abstract 23).
45. Van Ooasten BW, Barkholf F, Truyen L, et al. Increased MRI activity and immune activation in two multiple sclerosis patients treated with monoclonal anti-tumor necrosis factor antibody cA2. *Neurology* 1996;47:1531.
46. Mohan N, Edwards ET, Cupps TR, et al. Demyelination diagnosed during etanercept (TNF receptor fusion protein) therapy. *Arthritis Rheum* 2000;43 [Suppl]:S228.
47. DeBandt M, Descomps V, Meyer O. Two cases of etanercept-induced lupus-like syndrome in RA patients. *Arthritis Rheum* 2001;44[Suppl]:S372 (abstract 1919).
48. Shakoor N, Michalska M, Harris CA, et al. Drug-induced systemic lupus erythematosus associated with etanercept therapy. *Lancet* 2002;359:579–580.
49. Mohan AK, Edwards ET, Cote TR, et al. Drug induced systemic lupus erythematosus and TNF alpha blockers [correspondence]. *Lancet* 2002;360:646.

CHAPTER 32

Antibodies to Tumor Necrosis Factor α: Infliximab and Adalimumab

E. William St. Clair

Antibodies to tumor necrosis factor α (TNF-α) occupy an important place in the treatment of rheumatoid arthritis (RA). In the early 1990s, Marc Feldmann and Ravinder Maini pioneered the initial development of the first successful antibody to TNF-α. This anticytokine antibody joined a new class of highly targeted biologic agents that would revolutionize the treatment of RA. The emergence of biologic therapies paralleled an unprecedented growth in our knowledge of fundamental disease mechanisms beginning in the 1980s with the discovery of cytokines, interleukins (ILs), interferons (IFNs), and colony-stimulating factors (CSFs). The availability of purified cytokines made possible the development of specific monoclonal antibodies (mAbs), which were invaluable probes for unraveling the mechanisms of rheumatoid synovitis. Also, the advances in technology affording the isolation of complementary DNAs encoding cytokines, ILs, IFNs, and growth factors enabled these cellular mediators to be detected in rheumatoid synovium with high sensitivity and specificity. These tools dramatically enhanced our understanding about the role of TNF-α and other mediators in the pathophysiology of RA.

The proinflammatory nature of TNF-α and its abundant expression in the rheumatoid synovium focused early attention on this particular cytokine. Other macrophage-derived proinflammatory cytokines, such as IL-1, were also readily detectable in inflamed synovial tissue, but the T-cell cytokines IFN-γ and IL-2 were notably absent or only minimally expressed (1). Feldmann et al. found that unstimulated short-term cultures of dissociated cells from synovial tissue produced an array of proinflammatory cytokines, including TNF-α, IL-1, IL-6, and granulocyte-macrophage-CSF (GM-CSF). These cultures are considered to be experimental models of synovial inflammation and contain 30% T cells, 30% to 40% macrophages, and lesser proportions of endothelial cells, fibroblasts, dendritic cells, B cells, and plasma cells from synovial tissue. These observations led to the notion that synovial inflammation in RA is a product of a dysregulated cytokine network. The array of proinflammatory cytokines in these cultures emphasized the redundancy of the cytokine response. The cytokine redundancy was initially viewed as a potential barrier to anticytokine therapy. However, further studies suggested that TNF-α was a key regulatory cytokine in the inflammatory cascade. The first clues about the importance of TNF-α in the cytokine cascade came from studies of synovial cell cultures, in which the addition of anti–TNF-α mAb down-regulated the production of other proinflammatory cytokines, such as IL-1, GM-CSF, and IL-6 (2,3). These results, coupled with the observed benefits of anti-TNF-α treatment in animal models of inflammatory arthritis, provided the rationale for testing this approach in the clinic.

The interest in examining the efficacy of anti–TNF-α agents in human disease led to the development of infliximab (initially called *cA2*), a chimeric anti–TNF-α mAb. RA was among the first diseases to be targeted using this approach. In 1999, after a series of controlled clinical trials, infliximab (Remicade, Centocor) was approved for the treatment of RA, verifying the crucial importance of TNF-α in the pathogenesis of this disease. Other anti–TNF-α agents rapidly joined the developmental pipeline. One of these agents, etanercept (Enbrel, Immunex/Amgen), was engineered as a dimer of the p75 TNF receptor (TNFR) linked to the Fc portion of an immunoglobulin (Ig) G molecule. It moved efficiently through development and became in 1998 the first anti–TNF-α drug approved for the treatment, 1 year ahead of infliximab's approval. Etanercept therapy for RA is fully discussed in Chapter 31. Lenercept, a p55 TNFR-Ig-Fc fusion protein, was initially shown to be clinically efficacious for the treatment of RA, but its development was abandoned due to problems with immunogenicity and manufacturing. Amgen has produced a dimeric polyethylene glycolylated truncated p55 TNFR, which has been under investigation for the treatment of RA.

Among the anti–TNF-α mAbs, CDP571 (Celltech), a humanized mAb with engrafted murine hypervariable regions, was initially evaluated as an antirheumatic agent. However, preliminary studies suggested CDP571 was less effective for the treatment of RA than infliximab at equivalent doses, ending its development. Celltech, in collaboration with Pharmacia, produced a polyethylene glycol–linked Fab fragment, CDP870, which has been under investigation for the treatment for RA (4). Another anti–TNF-α mAb, D2E7, was derived by phage display technology with a fully human structure and initially developed by the pharmaceutical company BASF/Knoll. In 2001, Abbott, another pharmaceutical company, purchased BASF/Knoll and successfully completed phase III trials of this anti–TNF-α mAb in RA. D2E7, now known as adalimumab, was approved for the treatment of RA in December of 2002.

This chapter reviews infliximab and adalimumab therapy for RA, focusing on its clinical aspects. The topic of anti–TNF-α therapy is introduced with a discussion of the role of TNF-α and other cytokines in the pathogenesis of chronic inflammatory arthritis. Results from controlled trials are described that provide the evidence attesting to the clinical efficacy and safety of these two anti–TNF-α antibodies. Also included is practical information about the pharmacology of these agents, as well as their mode of administration, use in specific clinical situations, and potential for causing toxicity. Anti–TNF-α therapy has been shown in patients with RA to affect multiple pathways of immune cell function and inflammation, affording insights into treatment mechanisms.

ROLE OF TUMOR NECROSIS FACTOR α IN THE PATHOGENESIS OF RHEUMATOID ARTHRITIS

Abundant expression of TNF-α and other inflammatory procytokines is a hallmark of rheumatoid synovitis (1). TNF-α exhibits many immunostimulatory properties that are consistent with its role in the pathogenesis of RA (5) (Table 32.1). It is a potent activator of macrophages, inducing the production of other proinflammatory mediators such as IL-1, IL-6, GM-CSF, prostaglandins, and nitric oxide. TNF-α further amplifies the inflammatory response by increasing the expression of adhesion molecules, activating endothelial cells and neutrophils, and stimulating the secretion of chemokines. TNF-α also serves as a growth factor for T cells and B cells.

Inflammatory cytokines, such as TNF-α, can also modulate the function of bone marrow hematopoietic progenitor cells. In bone marrow cultures, stromal cells from patients with RA produce high levels of TNF-α and show reduced capacity to support normal hematopoiesis (6). In addition, patients with RA exhibit a low number of $CD34^+$ progenitor cells, with defective clonogenic potential. Moreover, TNF-α–mediated apoptotic deletion of bone marrow progenitor cells is likely an important factor in causing the anemia of chronic disease in RA (7). Infliximab therapy has been shown to reverse these abnormalities of erythropoiesis in patients with RA and boost hemoglobin levels, adding proof that overproduction of TNF-α suppresses bone marrow function (7).

TNF-α bioactivity also has the potential to be immunosuppressive (Table 32.1). T cells chronically exposed to TNF-α *in vitro* show impaired activation by antigen (8). Indeed, chronic TNF-α exposure appears to recapitulate many of the T-cell defects seen in RA. This T-cell hyporesponsiveness may result from down-regulation of $CD_3\zeta$, a critical signaling component of the TCR complex (9), and decreased expression of CD28, a T-cell costimulatory molecule (10). CD28 engagement by CD80 or CD86 on antigen-presenting cells is essential for antigen-induced T-cell proliferation, and its expression is down-regulated after T-cell activation. Notably, $CD4^+CD28^{null}$ T cells occur with increased frequency in the peripheral blood of patients with RA (11), a T-cell phenotype that could result from increased TNF-α production. TNF-α can also promote apoptosis, inhibit dendritic cell costimulation, and induce the production of inhibitory cytokines, such as IL-6, IL-10, and transforming growth factor β (5). Thus, the effect of TNF-α may be inhibitory depending on the timing and duration of exposure.

TABLE 32.1. Biologic Effects of Tumor Necrosis Factor (TNF) α

Stimulatory
- Stimulate release of proinflammatory cytokines (e.g., IL-1, IL-6, GM-CSF), chemokines, and angiogenic factors (e.g., VEGF)
- Activate endothelial cells
- Up-regulate expression of adhesion molecules
- Activate neutrophils
- Promote T- and B-cell growth
- Stimulate bone resorption and release of matrix metalloproteinases

Inhibitory
- Depress T-cell responses
- Induce inhibitory cytokines (e.g., IL-10) and natural cytokine inhibitors (IL-1ra, sTNFRs)
- Induce apoptosis
- Inhibit erythropoiesis

GM-CSF, granulocyte-macrophage colony-stimulating factor; IL, interleukin; IL-1ra, interleukin-1 receptor antagonist; sTNFRs, soluble tumor necrosis factor receptors; VEGF, vascular endothelial growth factor.

Cytokine Network

TNF-α is prominently expressed in the rheumatoid synovium together with other proinflammatory cytokines. It potently induces the production of other cytokines, cytokine receptors, and other mediators. This complex mixture of molecules with multiple biologic activities constitutes a cytokine network, which is a key regulator of inflammatory reactions as well as cellular growth and differentiation, development, and repair (12). TNF-α is an important component of the innate immune system, which functions as the first line of defense against infection. The principal function of TNF is to induce inflammation and activate leukocytes. In a healthy state, the inflammatory response is usually self-limited on elimination of the pathogen and with the subsequent release of antiinflammatory cytokines and other counter-regulatory mediators. However, in RA, the inflammatory response continues unchecked in the joint with persistent up-regulated expression of TNF-α and other proinflammatory cytokines, implying a dysregulated cytokine network.

Regulation of Tumor Necrosis Factor α

TNF-α and most other cytokines function as short-range, intercellular protein mediators. They elicit their multiple effects on different cell types by binding to cytokine receptors. The response to TNF-α is complex and depends on the differential bioactivities of its membrane-bound and secreted forms and differential signaling through its two receptors, TNFR1 and TNFR2 (p55 and p75, respectively). The regulation of TNF-α occurs at multiple points (Table 32.2). Although dysregulation may occur at any of these points and contribute to disease, the timing and site of TNF-α production has also been shown to influence the development of autoimmunity (13).

The transcriptional regulation of the TNF-α gene is complex, and its details are beyond the scope of this chapter. Briefly, many inducers of TNF-α act through converging signaling pathways to generate transcription factors that stimulate expression of the TNF-α gene. The transcription factors bind to sites in the promoter region of the TNF-α gene that coordinately regulate gene expression. The promoter region of the TNF-α gene contains nuclear factor (NF)-κB, κB, κ3 binding sites, and a cyclic adenosine monophosphate responsive element. The cyclic adenosine monophosphate responsive element binds the heterodimer acti-

TABLE 32.2. Regulation of Tumor Necrosis Factor (TNF) α Bioactivity

- Transcriptional regulation
- TNF-α messenger RNA (ARE)
- Cleavage of membrane-bound TNF precursor into soluble form by TACE
- Regulated expression of TNF-α receptors
- Processing of membrane-bound TNF receptors into soluble forms by TACE
- Feedback inhibition on transcription

ARE, AU-rich element; RNA, ribonucleic acid; TACE, TNF-α converting enzyme.

vating transcription factor 2/Jun, and the κ3 site interacts with NF of activating T cells (NF-AT), an important transcription factor regulating T-cell activation. Additionally, the TNF-α promoter is subject to autoregulation, allowing for amplification of the inflammatory response. The TNF-α gene contains single nucleotide polymorphisms of potential functional significance that have been investigated for their association with disease susceptibility and severity (14). Whether these gene variants contribute to the pathophysiology of disease is unknown.

The translational efficiency of TNF-α is regulated by a consensus 3' untranslated AU-rich element (ARE) in messenger RNA. Similar versions of the ARE motif occur in other cytokine and growth factor mRNAs. Transgenic mice bearing a human TNF-α gene without a functioning ARE have been shown to develop inflammatory bowel disease and chronic inflammatory arthritis (15). In contrast, transgenic mice expressing human TNF-α containing an authentic 3' untranslated region show no evidence of arthritis, pointing toward the ARE as an important site of regulation. The ARE is bound by the cytosolic protein tristetraprolin (TTP), which enhances mRNA turnover (16). Notably, mice lacking TTP develop an inflammatory arthritis, cachexia, dermatitis, conjunctivitis, myeloid hyperplasia with extramedullary hematopoiesis, and high titers of anti-DNA antibodies (17). TNF-α induces TTP production, creating a negative feedback loop that destabilizes TNF-α mRNA and decreases TNF-α synthesis. $CD68^+$ macrophages express TTP in rheumatoid synovium, indicating a role for TTP in regulating TNF-α mRNA turnover at this inflammatory site (18). As yet, no studies incriminate ARE dysfunction in the pathogenesis of a human inflammatory disease.

TNF-α is translated as a 26-kd precursor protein with a signal peptide allowing for insertion into the plasma membrane. It associates in the membrane to form a homotrimeric protein. During inflammation, a zinc-dependent metalloproteinase, termed *TNF-α converting enzyme*, cleaves membrane-bound TNF-α into a 17-kd form, which is secreted into the extracellular compartment. Both the membrane-bound and soluble TNF-α molecules are biologically active. The membrane-bound form of TNF-α may act through cell–cell contact with TNFR1 and TNFR2. Indeed, human TNF-α transgenic mice genetically engineered to overexpress only the membrane-bound form of TNF-α develop local TNF-α–mediated pathology (19).

TNF-α mediates its biologic effects through the TNFR1 and -2, which are type 1 transmembrane proteins consisting of an extracellular N terminus and an intracellular C terminus (20). A single TNF-α trimer binds to three receptor molecules. Engagement of TNFR1 is responsible for most of the biologic activity of TNF-α. The binding of TNF-α to the TNFR initiates a series of intracellular signals that activate NF-κB and c-Jun, two major transcription factors. These transcription factors induce genes encoding diverse products involved in inflammation, cellular proliferation and differentiation, and cell death.

The cytoplasmic domains of the TNFRs are docking sites for adapter proteins that mediate the TNF-α response (21). After TNF-α engagement, TNFR1 binds the TNFR-associated death domain (TRADD), which, in turn, recruits additional adapter proteins, including receptor-interacting protein 1 (RIP1), TNFR-associated factor 2 (TRAF2), and the Fas-associated death domain (FADD). FADD recruits caspase 8, which initiates a protease cascade leading to apoptosis. TRAF2 activates the mitogen-activated protein kinase pathway, resulting in the activation of c-Jun. RIP1 is believed to be critical for activating NF-κB. TNFR2 uses TRAF2 and TRAF1 as adapters and transmits signals that are inflammatory and antiapoptotic (22).

The expression of TNFRs may be another point at which TNF-α responsiveness may be controlled at the cellular level. Various cytokines and growth factors can modulate TNFR expression. Another TNF-α regulatory checkpoint is the cleavage of the membrane-bound TNFRs into soluble forms, soluble TNFR1 and soluble TNFR2. This cleavage step is mediated by TNF-α converting enzyme, the same protease that cleaves the precursor membrane-bound TNF-α molecule. Soluble TNFRs are considered to be natural inhibitors of TNF-α activity, although they can also stabilize the trimeric structure of TNF-α and, thereby, potentiate its activity (23). The evidence that cleavage represents an important regulatory checkpoint for TNF-α activity comes from studies of patients with TNFR-associated periodic syndrome (TRAPS). TRAPS, a recurrent inflammatory syndrome, is caused by mutations in the extracellular domain of TNFR1, leading to ineffective receptor shedding (24). The inflammatory manifestations of TRAPS may be inhibited by treatment with subcutaneous injections of etanercept, a genetically engineered form of soluble TNFR2 (25).

Tumor Necrosis Factor α and Arthritis

The pathophysiology of rheumatoid synovitis involves multiple pathways contributing to joint inflammation, proliferation, and destruction. The rheumatoid synovium contains mostly T cells (mainly $CD4^+$ T cells), macrophages/monocytes, and plasma cells, with fewer numbers of B cells, mast cells, and dendritic cells. All of these immune cells participate in the inflammatory response and play at least some role in promoting synovial proliferation and joint destruction. The synovium grows exuberantly in RA and invades into adjacent joint tissue. Such proliferation is supported by marked angiogenesis under the influence of TNF-α as well as other proinflammatory mediators. Fibroblast-like synovial cells, stimulated by TNF-α and other proinflammatory mediators, assume a transformed phenotype and generate increased levels of matrix metalloproteinases (MMPs) and other proteinases that act to degrade the underlying cartilage and bone.

Most, if not all, of the bone damage in RA results from inflammatory osteolysis, a process by which osteoclasts resorb bone. Inflammatory cytokines, especially TNF-α, have been shown to stimulate differentiation of macrophage progenitors into activated osteoclasts. TNF-α stimulates this process through two mechanisms (26). First, it induces the expression of the receptor activator of NF-κB ligand (RANKL) on stromal cells. RANKL can then interact with its receptor RANK on osteoclast precursors to induce the downstream signaling molecule NF-κB, which, in turn, stimulates differentiation of these precursors into osteoclasts. Second, with RANKL expression at permissive levels, TNF-α can also directly induce osteoclastogenesis in a highly synergistic fashion. TNF-α can only induce osteoclast differentiation in the presence of RANKL.

The major sources of TNF-α in the rheumatoid synovium are the cells of the macrophage-monocyte lineage. T cells, neutrophils, mast cells, and endothelial cells produce TNF-α in relatively smaller amounts. The mechanisms responsible for excessive TNF-α production are not known. Studies *in vitro* have shown that stimulated T cells can induce monocytes to release TNF-α through a mechanism dependent on cell–cell contact (27). T cells stimulated with cytokines as well as anti-CD3 mAbs (T-cell receptor–mediated) share this property. Indeed, T cells isolated from rheumatoid synovium have been shown to induce TNF-α by cell contact–dependent mechanisms (28). RA synovial T cells produce only low levels of IFN-γ and IL-2, and in this manner resemble cytokine-activated T cells. IL-15, which is abundantly expressed in the rheumatoid synovium, has the capacity to activate T cells and stimulate cell contact–dependent TNF-α production by macrophages (29).

As noted above, TNF-α appears to be a pivotal regulatory cytokine in short-term cultures of synovial cells from patients with RA (30). The addition of anti–TNF-α mAb to synovial cell cultures decreases the production of IL-1, GM-CSF, IL-6, and IL-8 (2,3,31). In contrast, incubation of synovial cell cultures with the IL-1 receptor antagonist reduces IL-6 and IL-8, but not TNF-α (31). The antiinflammatory cytokines IL-10 and IL-11 are also spontaneously produced in synovial cell cultures. Blockade of TNF-α down-regulates IL-10 (32) and IL-11 (33) production in this culture system. Conversely, IL-10 and IL-11 neutralization leads to increases in TNF-α levels. Although cytokine production in the rheumatoid synovium is complex, TNF-α appears to play a central role in orchestrating the overall inflammatory effect.

Tumor Necrosis Factor α in Animal Models of Arthritis

The results from studies in animal models show the importance of TNF-α in the mechanisms of inflammatory arthritis. Type II collagen-induced arthritis in mice has been widely investigated as an animal model of RA. After the establishment of arthritis, treatment of murine collagen-induced arthritis with a hamster IgG1 mAb to mouse TNF-α (34) or human TNFR1-IgG fusion protein (35) has been shown to decrease paw swelling and the histopathologic severity of disease.

Studies in transgenic mice provide further evidence that TNF-α can provoke an inflammatory arthritis (15). A destructive arthritis develops spontaneously in transgenic mice expressing a 3'-modified human TNF-α transgene. In this model, the 3'-flanking sequences of the human TNF-α gene have been replaced with those of the β-globin gene. As discussed above, the ARE in the 3'-untranslated region of the TNF-α gene confers mRNA instability. Substituting the 3'-untranslated region of the β-globin gene removes the ARE from the human TNF-α transgene, leading to increased mRNA stability and translational efficiency. Treatment of these transgenic mice with a mAb to human TNF-α completely abrogates the arthritis. Also, treatment of these transgenic mice with a mAb to the type 1 IL-1 receptor prevents the development of joint inflammation (36). Thus, in this model, IL-1 appears to act in series with TNF-α, mediating the full pathologic effects of TNF-α. A mutant form of the human TNF-α gene has been engineered to produce a membrane-bound protein that cannot be cleaved by TNF-α converting enzyme. Interestingly, transgenic mice carrying this mutant construct of the human TNF-α gene develop an inflammatory arthritis, suggesting a major role for membrane-bound TNF-α in the triggering of the pathologic process (19). Finally, TNF-α does not appear to be essential for the development of an inflammatory arthritis. Studies have shown that murine collagen-induced arthritis can be induced in TNF-deficient mice, albeit a less severe arthritis than in wild-type mice (37). These immunized TNF-α–deficient mice show evidence of altered humoral and cellular immune responses to type II collagen. Compared with immunized wild-type mice, the immunized TNF-deficient mice exhibit a significantly attenuated IgG response and enlarged spleens and lymph nodes, implying an immunosuppressive role for TNF-α in this model system.

INFLIXIMAB

Isolation and Structure

Infliximab (also referred to as cA2 and Remicade) is a mouse/human IgG1κ chimeric anti–TNF-α mAb (Fig. 32.1). It was derived from a murine anti–human TNF-α mAb isolated from a BALB/c mouse immunized with purified recombinant human TNF-α (38). For therapeutic use, modification of murine antibodies to a more human form is desirable to reduce immunogenicity. Therapeutic antibodies bearing foreign (nonhuman) proteins can elicit antibodies that trigger allergic or hypersensitivity reactions. Murine antibodies have a shorter biologic half-life than chimeric antibodies, limiting therapeutic potency. The human constant region domains of chimeric antibodies also may confer Fc-mediated effector functions, such as complement fixation, antibody-dependent cellular cytotoxicity, and Fc-mediated antibody clearance.

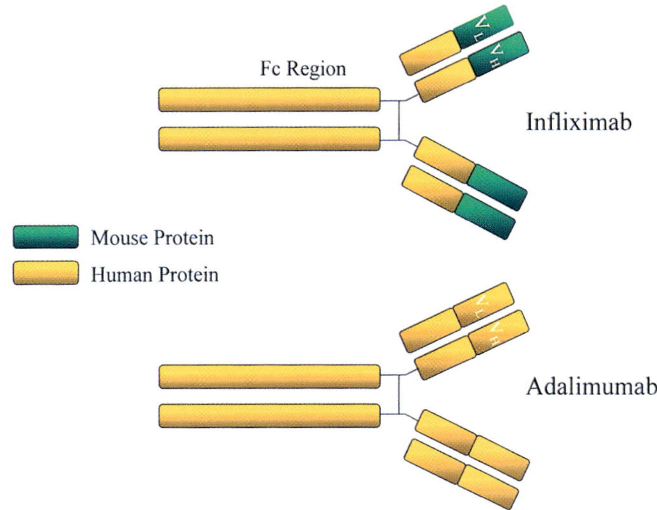

Figure 32.1. Structures of infliximab and adalimumab. Infliximab is a chimeric anti–tumor necrosis factor (TNF) α monoclonal antibody (mAb). It consists of a mouse Fv component, which includes the antigen-binding site, covalently linked to a human Fc region. Adalimumab is a fully humanized anti–TNF-α mAb produced by phage display technology. V_H, variable heavy chain; V_L, variable light chain.

Infliximab binds to both soluble and membrane-bound TNF-α with high specificity and affinity ($K_a = 10^{10}\ M^{-1}$) (39). Infliximab prevents TNF-α from forming a stable complex with TNFR1 and TNFR2. When infliximab is added to preformed TNF-TNFR complexes, TNF-α rapidly dissociates from its receptors. Also, infliximab is cytotoxic against TNF-α, expressing cells *in vitro* (39), but the significance of this effect *in vivo* is unknown.

Infliximab is manufactured by continuous perfusion culture of mammalian cells. It is purified from cell culture supernatants by affinity and ion exchange chromatography. The formulation is supplied as a sterile, white, lypholized powder containing 100 mg of infliximab per vial with no preservatives that is dissolved in 10 mL of sterile water for intravenous use.

Pharmacokinetics

Infliximab has a terminal half-life of approximately 9.5 days (40). For comparison, the terminal half-life of human IgG1 has been estimated to be 21 days (41). The pharmacokinetics of infliximab has been investigated in several clinical trials, including Anti-Tumor Necrosis Factor Trial in Rheumatoid Arthritis with Concomitant Therapy (ATTRACT) (42). In this 54-week trial, infliximab, 3 to 10 mg per kg, was administered intravenously to patients with active RA at weeks 0, 2, and 6, and then every 4 or 8 weeks. All of the patients in this trial were also receiving methotrexate therapy. Clinical response was assessed using the American College of Rheumatology (ACR) criteria for clinical improvement (43) (see Appendix B), a standard composite index for defining responders in clinical trials. Serum levels of infliximab were measured using an enzyme-linked immunosorbent assay. In this study, the median serum concentrations of infliximab 1 hour after a 3 and 10 mg per kg dose were found to be approximately 68 and 217 mg per mL, respectively. Thus, the C_{max} (1-hour postinfusion level) of infliximab is proportional to the intravenous dose over this range. The observed C_{max} for infliximab approximates the predicted serum concentrations, in which the total dose occupies only the plasma volume.

The median trough serum levels of infliximab differed among the four treatment groups. The median trough levels of infliximab were highest for the 10 mg per kg every 4 weeks group, intermediate for the 10 mg per kg every 8 weeks and 3 mg per kg every 4 weeks groups, and lowest for the 3 mg per kg every 8 weeks group (42). In the lowest-dose group, 22% to 30% of patients had trough levels below the detectable limits of the assay (<0.1 mg per mL) from week 22 to 54. The ACR 50% response rates were significantly lower in the 3 mg per kg every 8 weeks group than the other treatment groups, suggesting a dose response across the lower end of the range. Because some patients achieving an ACR 70% response had undetectable trough serum levels, the magnitude of individual responses does not tightly correlate with a trough level above a certain lower limit. Thus, routine measurement of trough serum infliximab levels does not have a useful role in practice.

Pharmacokinetic modeling has been performed to predict trough serum levels of infliximab using doses and dosing intervals not evaluated in ATTRACT (42). These studies were undertaken because of anecdotal reports that some patients were experiencing disease worsening at the end of the treatment interval between infusions, suggesting a waning of TNF-α neutralizing activity. The modeling shows that shortening the dosing interval from 8 to 6 weeks increases the trough serum levels of infliximab more than increasing the dose by 100 mg, or 1 vial. For example, a 70-kg individual receiving 3 mg per kg every 8 weeks would have a predicted trough level of 0.8 mg per mL. Although a 100-mg dose increase would boost the trough level to 1.8 mg per mL, maintaining the same dose and shortening the interval from 8 to 6 weeks would result in a trough level of 2.8 mg per mL. The hypothesis that dose escalation can enhance clinical efficacy of infliximab therapy has not been confirmed in a controlled trial.

Clinical Trials

Elliott et al. from the Kennedy Institute of Rheumatology described in 1993 the results of the first open trial of infliximab therapy for RA (44). In this study, 20 patients with active RA were treated with infliximab infusions and were followed for 8 weeks to assess clinical response, possible toxicity, and immune effects. Fifteen of the patients received infliximab, 10 mg per kg at entry and day 14, whereas five of the patients were given infliximab, 5 mg per kg at entry and at days 4, 8, and 12. Infliximab therapy was associated with improvement in all of the clinical indices of disease activity, including duration of morning stiffness, pain scores, Ritchie Articular Index (45), grip strength, functional disability, and serum levels of erythrocyte sedimentation rate and C-reactive protein. The infliximab treatment was well tolerated, except for two minor infectious episodes. There was a significant decrease in the serum IL-6 levels, and some of the patients showed a drop in their serum rheumatoid factor titer. The results of this trial indicated that the redundancy of the cytokine network would not be a barrier to successful anti–TNF-α therapy.

These initial results were confirmed in a randomized, double-blind, placebo-controlled trial of a single infusion of 1 or 10 mg per kg infliximab in 73 patients with active RA (46). Patients stopped other disease-modifying antirheumatic drugs (DMARDs) at least 4 weeks before study entry. Clinical improvement was determined using the Paulus index (47) (see Appendix C). By week 4, 19 (79%) of 24 patients treated with infliximab 10 mg per kg had achieved a Paulus 20% response, compared with 11 (44%) of 25 responders in the 1 mg per kg group (44%) and 2 (8%) of 24 patients in the placebo group. These results confirmed the clinical benefits of anti–TNF-α therapy for RA.

Initial experience revealed that patients with RA who respond to infliximab therapy almost invariably show a disease flare within approximately 12 to 16 weeks. Subsequently, seven of the patients in the first open trial were retreated with infliximab at a dose of 20 mg per kg for the first infusion and 10 mg per kg for a subsequent infusion (48). After disease flare, each of the patients responded to repeated infusions of infliximab, although the duration of response appeared to shorten after successive cycles of treatment. Four of the seven patients in this retreatment trial developed serum antibodies to infliximab, prompting concerns about the chimeric antibody's immunogenicity.

The efficacy and safety of multiple infusions of infliximab were evaluated in a 26-week, randomized, double-blind, placebo-controlled, multicenter trial in Europe (49). All of the DMARDs, except methotrexate (MTX), were withdrawn before study entry. Patients were eligible if they had active disease and had inadequately responded to 7.5 to 15.0 mg per week of MTX therapy. The 101 study patients recruited into this trial were predominately women (67–86%) and positive for serum rheumatoid factor (67–93%), with a mean disease duration of 7.6 to 14.3 years. The eligible patients were randomly allocated to the following treatment groups: infliximab, 1 mg per kg (with or without MTX), 3 mg per kg (with or without MTX), or 10 mg per kg (with or without MTX), or placebo infusions plus MTX. Patients assigned to the MTX treatment groups were treated with 7.5 mg per week of MTX. Study infusions were administered at weeks 0, 2, 6, and 14, with follow-up through week 26. Seven of the patients withdrew from the trial due to adverse events, including five because of infusion reactions. Seventeen patients withdrew prematurely due to lack of efficacy.

At the 3 and 10 mg per kg dose, infliximab (with or without MTX) produced a significantly higher Paulus 20% response rate than the placebo plus MTX group, with rates approaching 60% for each of the infliximab groups. The duration of response was not significantly different between the 3 mg per kg and 10 mg per kg infliximab plus MTX groups and the corresponding 3 mg per kg and 10 mg per kg infliximab plus placebo groups. However, a trend toward more prolonged responses was observed in the infliximab plus MTX groups than in the infliximab plus placebo groups at comparable doses. In contrast, the 1 mg per kg infliximab group and the infliximab plus MTX group had a statistically shorter duration of response than the placebo plus MTX group. Because the patients were only taking 7.5 mg per week of MTX in this trial, these results may not generalize to MTX doses in the range of 12.5 to 25.0 mg per week, the doses most frequently used in practice.

The most common adverse events in this study were headache (12.6%), diarrhea (9.2%), rash (6.9%), pharyngitis (6.9%), rhinitis (6.9%), and cough (5.7%). There were two serious infections: severe bacterial endophthalmitis and septicemic shock from *Staphylococcus aureus*. Seven (8%) of the patients receiving infliximab developed anti–double-stranded DNA (dsDNA) antibodies, including a patient who experienced a systemic lupus erythematosus–like syndrome characterized by fever, arthralgia, and pleuropericarditis. The illness was treated with an increased dosage of corticosteroids and resolved without sequelae. The overall incidence of antibodies to infliximab in this study was 17.4%, but the rates were less in the groups receiving the combination of infliximab plus MTX, compared to infliximab alone. Higher doses of infliximab were also associated with a lower incidence of antibodies to infliximab. Similar results were found in a smaller, randomized, double-blind, placebo-controlled, dose-finding trial that evaluated the safety and efficacy of a single infusion of infliximab in combination with background MTX therapy (50). These results confirmed the importance of TNF-α as a therapeutic target.

ATTRACT was the pivotal trial for substantiating the clinical and radiologic efficacy of maintenance infliximab therapy for RA (51,52). Patients were eligible for this randomized, double-blind, placebo-controlled, multicenter, international trial if they had active RA despite taking at least 12.5 mg per week of MTX therapy. Treatment with MTX must have been continuous for the 3 months before entry, with stable doses for the 4 weeks before screening. Other DMARDs were withdrawn at least 4 weeks before the screening visit. Patients were allowed to continue taking nonsteroidal antiinflammatory drugs and low doses of oral corticosteroids (prednisone ≤10 mg per day). The study enrolled 428 patients who were randomly allocated to receive placebo, 3 mg per kg, or 10 mg per kg of infliximab every 4 or 8 weeks. All of the patients were administered infliximab or placebo infusions at weeks 0, 2, and 6 and every 4 weeks for 54 weeks. Placebo infusions were given to patients in the infliximab, 3 mg per kg and 10 mg per kg every 8 weeks, groups on alternate 4-week visits to maintain the blinding. The MTX dose was kept the same during the trial, unless it had to be modified because of toxicity.

The results were first reported after the patients had completed 30 weeks of the study (51). The study population was predominately women (73–81%) and more than three-fourths (77–84%) tested positive for serum rheumatoid factor. The mean duration of disease ranged from 9 to 12 years across the five treatment groups. Infliximab therapy was associated with a rapid and significant improvement in the signs and symptoms of RA. At 30 weeks, an ACR 20% response was achieved by 53%, 50%, 58%, and 52% of patients in the 3 mg per kg every 4 or 8 weeks groups and 10 mg per kg every 4 or 8 weeks groups, respectively. Each of the ACR 20% response rates for the infliximab plus MTX treatment groups were significantly better than the ACR 20% response rate of 20% in the placebo group. The infusions were generally well tolerated during the study. These data formed the basis for the U.S. Food and Drug Administration's approval of infliximab therapy for reducing the signs and symptoms of RA.

The ATTRACT trial continued in a blinded fashion through week 54 to evaluate for the first time the impact of infliximab therapy on the progression of radiologic joint damage in RA (52). Withdrawals for lack of efficacy were more frequent in the placebo group (36%) than the infliximab treatment groups (7–20%), attesting to the benefits of maintenance infliximab therapy. However, withdrawal rates for adverse events were the same across the treatment groups (5–10%). Infliximab therapy produced sustained improvement in the signs and symptoms of RA through week 54 (Fig. 32.2). The ACR 20% response rates in the infliximab treatment groups ranged from 42% to 59% and were significantly better than the placebo response rate of 17%. Thus, infliximab therapy produces an absolute treatment benefit (active-control rate) of 25% to 42%. Similarly, ACR 50% and ACR 70% responses were achieved by 21% and 39% and 10% to 25% of patients in the 3-mg and 10-mg infliximab treatment groups, compared with placebo response rates of 8% and 2%, respectively. There was a trend toward a lower response rate in the 3 mg kg every 8 weeks group, compared with the higher-dose groups, although this difference was only statistically significant in comparing the ACR 50% response rates across the infliximab treatment arms.

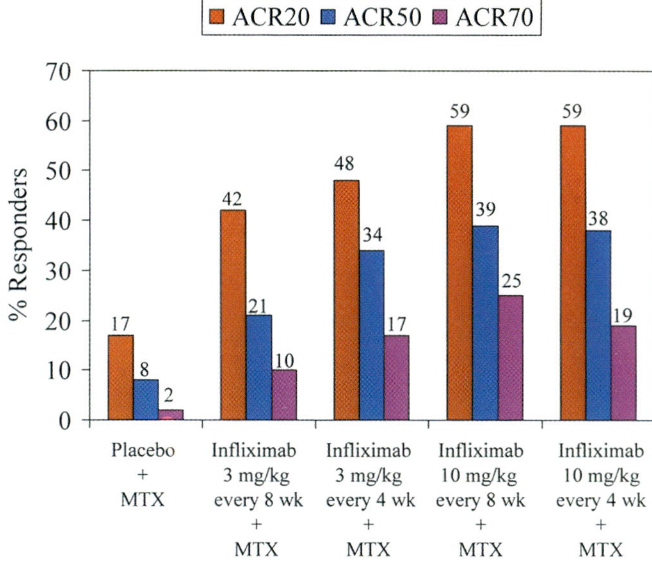

Figure 32.2. Repeated infusions of infliximab produce clinical improvement in patients with rheumatoid arthritis receiving stable doses of methotrexate (MTX) therapy. Results shown are from Anti-Tumor Necrosis Factor Trial in Rheumatoid Arthritis with Concomitant Therapy and compare the rate of American College of Rheumatology (ACR) 20%, ACR 50%, and ACR 70% responses among treatment groups at week 54. For the ACR 20% responder rates, the p values were <.001 for comparisons between each of the infliximab treatment groups and the placebo group. Comparisons were done using a chi-squared test.

Adverse events occurred in 94% of the MTX plus placebo group and 95% of the patients receiving MTX plus infliximab. Serious adverse events were no more frequent in the MTX plus placebo arm (21%), compared with the MTX plus infliximab treatment groups (11–20%). The rates of serious infections were also similar across the treatment groups (2–8%). However, upper respiratory infections tended to occur more frequently in the patients treated with MTX plus infliximab compared with MTX alone (34% vs. 22%). Infusion reactions were mostly mild in severity and occurred in 16% to 20% of patients receiving infliximab compared with 10% of patients receiving MTX alone. Only two patients withdrew from the trial because of an infusion reaction. Cancer was diagnosed in five patients during the trial, all of whom were taking infliximab. Death was reported in eight cases, three (3%) in the MTX plus placebo group, compared with five (1%) in the MTX plus infliximab groups.

To evaluate radiographic progression of joint damage, x-rays of the hands and feet were taken at weeks 0, 30, and 54 and scored according to the van der Heijde modification of the Sharp score (53). In this system, the radiographs are scored for both joint space narrowing and erosion, with scores ranging from 0 to 440. Higher scores denote more severe damage. As a group, the patients in ATTRACT were characterized at entry by advanced disease with total Sharp scores averaging 67 to 82 across the treatment groups. The analysis showed that joint damage progressed significantly more in the patients receiving MTX alone, compared with those in the MTX plus infliximab arms (Table 32.3). However, no significant difference was observed in the rate of radiographic progression among the infliximab treatment groups. Infliximab therapy produced significant benefits in slowing the rate of joint space narrowing and accumulation of erosions. Only a small proportion of patients in the infliximab treatment groups (<10%) showed radiographic progression of joint damage. The results of ATTRACT show that repeated infusions of infliximab, in combination with MTX therapy, not only controls the signs

TABLE 32.3. Infliximab Therapy Slows the Radiographic Progression of Joint Damage

Variable	Placebo + Methotrexate N = 64	3 mg/kg Infliximab Every 8 Wk + Methotrexate N = 71	3 mg/kg Infliximab Every 4 Wk + Methotrexate N = 71	10 mg/kg Infliximab Every 8 Wk + Methotrexate N = 77	10 mg/kg Infliximab Every 4 Wk + Methotrexate N = 66
Total Sharp score					
Mean ± SD change	7.0 ± 10.3	1.3 ± 6.0	1.6 ± 8.5	0.2 ± 3.6	−0.7 ± 3.8
Median (IQR) change	4.0 (0.5, 9.7)	0.5 (−1.5, 3.0)	0.1 (−2.5, 3.0)	0.5 (−1.5, 2.0)	−0.5 (−3.0, 1.5)
p value		<.001	<.001	<.001	<.001
Erosion score					
Mean ± SD change	4.0 ± 7.9	0.2 ± 2.9	0.3 ± 4.7	0.2 ± 2.9	−0.7 ± 3.0
Median (IQR) change	2.0 (0.5, 9.7)	0.0 (−1.4, 1.5)	0.0 (−1.5, 1.5)	0.5 (−1.0, 1.5)	−0.5 (−1.8,0.7)
p value		<.001	<.001	<.001	<.001
Joint space narrowing score					
Mean ± SD change	2.9 ± 4.2	1.1 ± 4.4	0.7 ± 4.3	0.0 ± 3.1	0.0 ± 2.5
Median (IQR) change	1.5 (0.0, 5.8)	0.0 (−1.0, 2.0)	0.0 (−1.0, 2.0)	0.0 (−0.9, 1.0)	0.0 (−1.5, 1.0)
p value		.001	<.001	<.001	<.001

IQR, interquartile range.
Note: Change values are the baseline minus week 54 scores, and *p* values are for the comparison with the placebo + methotrexate group.

and symptoms of RA but also retards the progression of joint damage.

A protocol amendment extended ATTRACT from 54 weeks to 102 weeks to obtain further efficacy data on the radiographic progression of disease (54). This longer-term analysis also focused on the effects of infliximab therapy on functional disability and quality of life. Functional disability was assessed by the Health Assessment Questionnaire (HAQ) (see Appendix E); quality of life was measured using the Short Form-36. Of the 428 study subjects, 259 entered the second year of the trial, including 28 (32%) of the 88 patients in the MTX alone group and 231 (68%) of the 340 patients in the MTX plus infliximab treatment groups. Patients who had increased their corticosteroid dose or changed DMARD therapy were required to resume their baseline dose of corticosteroids and withdraw any new DMARDs before entering this phase of the study. The timing of the amendment and the requisite changes in antirheumatic therapy created a gap in infliximab therapy of more than 8 weeks for slightly more than one-third of patients. The study protocol was unblinded after the results of the 54-week analysis because of ethical considerations and recommendations from a Data and Safety Monitoring Committee. The unblinding afforded patients receiving only MTX therapy the opportunity to begin infliximab treatment; eight patients in the MTX group and 43 patients in the infliximab plus MTX groups were unblinded to treatment assignment before the week 102 visit.

A total of 331 (77%) of the 428 originally randomized patients were available for the week 102 visit. However, only 216 of this group continued study medication through week 102. Similar to the results at week 54, the median change in radiographic scores from week 0 to 102 was significantly lower for the MTX plus infliximab treatment groups, compared with the MTX alone group. Thus, these findings indicate that infliximab therapy has a favorable effect on the progression of radiologic joint damage over 2 years. Infliximab therapy also produces significant improvements in functional disability and quality of life. The median change in HAQ scores from week 0 to 102 was only 0.1 for the infliximab plus MTX treatment groups, compared with 0.4 for the placebo plus MTX arm. Similar beneficial effects favoring the infliximab treatment groups were also observed for the physical component of the SF-36. These changes in physical function and quality of life for patients with RA translate to lower rates of disability, higher employment rates, and lower health care costs (55,56). The ACR 20% response rates trended lower at week 102 for the infliximab treatment groups (40–48%), but they remained significantly higher than the MTX alone group (16%). This decline in response rates from week 54 to 102 could have resulted from the gap in infliximab treatment that occurred for some patients. Overall, the results from ATTRACT provide strong evidence that infliximab therapy produces significant clinical, radiographic, and functional benefits for RA.

Because infliximab contains sequences from a mouse protein, use of this agent has the potential to induce antiinfliximab antibodies. Serum antibodies to infliximab are measured using an enzyme-linked immunosorbent assay. The assay results are inconclusive when infliximab is present in the serum sample and can compete for antiinfliximab antibodies. In ATTRACT, serum antibodies to infliximab were detected in 25 (8.5%) of 295 infliximab-treated patients (57). However, because infliximab was present in 165 of these serum samples, the results were inconclusive in a majority of cases. No evidence has indicated that antiinfliximab antibodies can diminish the extent of clinical improvement in RA, although this potential consequence of immunogenicity remains an open question.

Toxicity

Overall, infliximab therapy has been generally well tolerated in patients with RA. Infliximab therapy has been associated with mild-to-moderate reactions in approximately 10% of patients (58). Usually, these infusion reactions are characterized by headache, pruritus, urticaria, flushing, hypertension, or injection site erythema. Some of these symptoms are suggestive of a type I hypersensitivity-like reaction. More ominous symptoms, such as dyspnea, symptomatic hypotension, low back pain, or throat tightness, have also been reported during infusions. Rarely, infliximab infusions can provoke a severe anaphylaxis-like reaction, with chest pain, bronchospasm, laryngeal edema, and shock (59). Infusion reactions have been successfully managed by slowing or stopping the infusion and, depending on their severity, treating with diphenhydramine, corticosteroids, or epinephrine.

The expanded use of this product in patients has led to a more complete understanding of its potential toxicity. As of October 2001, more than 170,000 patients with RA or Crohn's disease worldwide had been treated with infliximab. In the United States, these adverse events have been primarily generated through the Adverse Events Reporting System of the U.S. Food and Drug Administration, a passive surveillance system for detecting unexpected adverse events. This system of detection has many limitations, including the likelihood of underreporting of adverse events, the little information that often accompanies these reports, the lack of a denominator (e.g., number of patients exposed to the therapy), and a suitable comparison group of nonexposed patients. These limitations frequently prevent making definite conclusions regarding causality, but certain findings and patterns may signal a possible cause-and-effect relationship.

Between August 1998 and June 2001, 84 cases of tuberculosis were reported worldwide in association with infliximab therapy, according to the U.S. Food and Drug Administration. Keane et al. (60) analyzed 70 of these cases (47 patients with RA, 18 patients with Crohn's disease, five with other forms of arthritis) and found that 48 (69%) of the patients developed tuberculosis after three or fewer infliximab infusions. The median interval was 12 weeks (range, 1–52 weeks) from the start of infliximab therapy to the diagnosis of tuberculosis. Among this group, 40 (57%) of the patients had extrapulmonary disease, including 17 (24%) with disseminated disease. Notably, 55 (79%) of the 70 patients were reported to be taking other immunosuppressive medications that would have increased the risk of tuberculosis. The relatively high number of reports and the temporal association between infliximab therapy and the diagnosis of tuberculosis prompted the U.S. Food and Drug Administration to issue a Black Box Warning, notifying prescribers about this finding. The issuance recommended that patients should be evaluated for the possibility of latent or active tuberculosis before initiating infliximab therapy. In the United States and most European countries, tuberculin skin testing is done to screen for latent tuberculosis. If the tuberculin skin test is positive, then the patient should receive appropriate antituberculosis prophylaxis before initiating anti–TNF-α therapy.

Other opportunistic infections have been reported in association with infliximab therapy, including histoplasmosis (61), listeriosis (60), pulmonary aspergillosis (62), and *Pneumocystis carinii* pneumonia (60). The nine cases of histoplasmosis have been analyzed and found to occur within 6 months of starting infliximab therapy. Each of the cases of histoplasmosis was diagnosed in residents of a geographic region endemic for this infection (e.g., Ohio and Mississippi River valleys in the United States). All of the patients had been taking at least one other immunosuppressive medication. Whether these cases represent reactivation of latent infection, primary infection, or recurrent infection is not known. After this initial report, the U.S. Food and Drug Administration was notified of ten additional cases of histoplasmosis in the United States, one case in Canada, and one case in Switzerland in association with infliximab therapy. Because *Histoplasma capsulatum* is transmitted by inhalation of mycelial fragments and microconidia of the organism from contaminated soil, patients receiving TNF-α antagonists in endemic areas should avoid activities that increase the risk for *H. capsulatum* exposure, such as cleaning chicken coops and exploring caves.

The occurrence of opportunistic infections during treatment with potent TNF-α antagonists is not unexpected given the role played by TNF-α in host defense. Studies in animal models show that TNF-α is critical in the mechanisms of granuloma formation and protecting against infection with tuberculosis (63). In mice, TNF-α is also a key mediator of immunity against *H. capsulatum* (64), *Listeria monocytogenes* (65), and *P. carinii* (66). Thus, the development of tuberculosis, histoplasmosis, and listeriosis in patients receiving infliximab therapy is consistent with the data from animal models and confirms the importance of TNF-α in combating these intracellular pathogens.

Treatment with TNF-α antagonists, including infliximab, has been associated with neurologic events exhibiting clinical and radiographic features of demyelination. Among 20 patients reported with neurologic events, the most common clinical manifestations were paresthesias, gait disturbance, apraxia, facial palsy, and Guillain-Barré syndrome (67). Magnetic resonance imaging scans have shown evidence of demyelination in the brain and spinal cord. The neurologic events resolved in most cases after stopping the anti–TNF-α therapy. The occurrence of these neurologic events raises the possibility of a true association between anti–TNF-α therapy and demyelinating syndromes, but proof of a cause-and-effect relationship is lacking.

Antinuclear antibodies develop in approximately one-half to two-thirds of patients receiving anti–TNF-α therapy. A subset of these patients developed serum antibodies to dsDNA, but only rarely do such patients develop a systemic lupus erythematosus–like syndrome. In a retrospective study, Charles et al. (68) tested multiple sera from 156 patients for the presence of anti-dsDNA antibodies before and after treatment with infliximab. Three different assays were used in this study. Twenty-two (14.1%) of the 156 patients developed a positive test for anti-dsDNA antibodies, including eight (5%) that were positive at a level of more than 25 units per mL. The anti-dsDNA antibodies were all of the IgM isotype except for one case. The patient with serum anti-dsDNA antibodies of the IgG isotype also developed a lupus-like syndrome. Among the four infliximab-treated groups in ATTRACT, the incidence was 7% to 11% for developing a positive test for anti-dsDNA antibodies at a level of more than 25 units per mL (52). One of the patients in ATTRACT developed a rash, accompanied by an increase in antinuclear antibody (ANA) titer from 1:40 to 1:80 and low complement levels, but no anti-dsDNA antibodies (51). A patient with Crohn's disease developed an inflammatory polyarthritis, leukopenia, and antibodies to dsDNA after receiving two infusions of 5 mg per kg infliximab (69). The polyarthritis and leukopenia resolved after stopping the infliximab therapy.

In ATTRACT, elevations in serum transaminases were observed more frequently in patients receiving infliximab plus methotrexate than in patients taking methotrexate alone. These elevations were mostly mild and transient. Infliximab has been associated with reversible cholestatic liver disease in two cases. In one case, a 36-year-old woman with RA developed an exacerbation of arthritis, jaundice, elevated serum transaminases, hyperbilirubinemia, and a positive test for anti-dsDNA antibodies after three infusions of infliximab (70). Serologic testing was negative for antibodies to hepatitis B and C and smooth muscle and mitochondria. A liver biopsy revealed moderate-to-severe portal inflammation and ductal damage. Despite persistence of anti-dsDNA antibodies, the serum transaminase and bilirubin levels returned to normal after the patient discontinued infliximab and was treated with high doses of methylprednisolone. Another case of reversible cholestatic liver disease has been described after a single infusion of infliximab in a patient with Crohn's disease (71). In contrast, serum testing for anti-dsDNA antibodies was negative, and the liver biopsy showed cholestasis without an appreciable inflammatory infiltrate. Because these patients were also receiving other potentially hepatotoxic medications, a causative relationship between infliximab therapy and liver disease is not certain.

A variety of skin lesions have been associated with infliximab therapy. Although rashes may appear during infusions, some have occurred with latencies of 24 hours or more. An erythema multiforme–like rash was observed 2 to 4 weeks after two to four infusions in three cases; a lichenoid eruption was noted in another case 3 weeks after a second infusion (72). Bullous skin lesions developed 24 hours after a fourth dose of infliximab in a 72-year-old man with RA (73). Immunofluorescence findings were not typical for pemphigus vulgaris or bullous pemphigoid in this case.

Studies in animals suggest that elevated TNF-α levels can cause left ventricular dysfunction (74), prompting studies to examine the possible efficacy of anti–TNF-α for heart failure. Analysis of the results from the ATTACH (Anti–TNF-α Therapy Against Chronic Heart Failure) trial has revealed an excess number of deaths and hospitalization for worsening of heart failure among patients receiving 5 mg per kg and 10 mg per kg doses of infliximab (75). As a result of this information, the U.S. Food and Drug Administration issued an alert in October 2001 to physicians about the possible association between infliximab therapy and heart failure. However, these data are insufficient to demonstrate a cause-and-effect relationship between infliximab therapy and adverse cardiac outcomes.

Brown et al. identified 39 cases of lymphoma associated with infliximab therapy (76). For RA specifically, four cases have been reported in trials involving 2,458 patient-years. This rate of lymphoma can be compared with that of the general population using the Surveillance, Epidemiology, and End Results database. In infliximab-treated patients from RA trials, the standardized incidence ratio for lymphoma is 6.4 [95% confidence interval (CI): 1.7–16]. This finding should be interpreted with caution because lymphomas occur two to three times more commonly in patients with RA than the general population and the rate of lymphoma may be even higher in RA patients with high inflammatory activity. Current evidence is insufficient to conclude that infliximab therapy leads to the development of lymphoma.

Recommendations for Clinical Use of Infliximab

DOSAGE AND ADMINISTRATION

Infliximab is administered by the intravenous route according to the following schedule: first dose (time 0), second dose (week 2), third dose (week 6), fourth dose (week 14), and subsequent doses every 8 weeks. For the treatment of RA, the usual starting dose is 3 mg per kg. Depending on the extent of improvement, physicians may elect to increase the dose of infliximab or shorten the interval between infusions. Dosage adjustment is not usually considered until after the interval between infusion has been extended to every 8 weeks (e.g., after week 14). Dosage adjustment is usually deferred until this point because the serum levels of infliximab are relatively high during the initial induction phase, even at the 3 mg per kg dose. Initial responders to infliximab therapy may show an exacerbation of disease activity before the next infusion. In such cases, increasing the dose or shortening the interval between infusions may improve disease control.

The product labeling calls for concomitant administration of MTX, which aligns with the study design for ATTRACT. Clinical experience suggests infliximab may be also given safely without MTX and in combination with sulfasalazine, leflunomide, azathioprine, and cyclosporine. Concerns have been raised about using a TNF-α antagonist, such as infliximab, with anakinra (IL-1 receptor antagonist) because of the possible increased risk of serious infection using this combination. A small open study of 58 patients with RA found a 7% incidence of serious infection over 6 months after the addition of anakinra to maintenance etanercept therapy (77). This rate contrasts with a 1.5% and 2.1% incidence of serious infections for patients taking anakinra (with or without MTX) alone and a 0.7% incidence of serious infections in placebo controls.

Infliximab infusions are typically administered over 2 hours in an outpatient clinical or hospital setting. Because infliximab therapy has been associated with infusion reactions, the site should be equipped to monitor the patient's vital signs and treat any infusion reactions. Diphenhydramine, epinephrine, and corticosteroids should be available for managing any reactions. Figure 32.3 diagrams a procedure for managing infusion reactions. Infliximab therapy should be discontinued for any patient experiencing a severe reaction, such as anaphylaxis, profound hypotension, or severe respiratory distress. There has been a single report of successful desensitization (78).

INDICATIONS, CONTRAINDICATIONS, WARNINGS, AND PRECAUTIONS

According to the product labeling, infliximab is indicated for the treatment of patients with moderate to severe RA who have had an inadequate response to MTX therapy. Infliximab is contraindi-

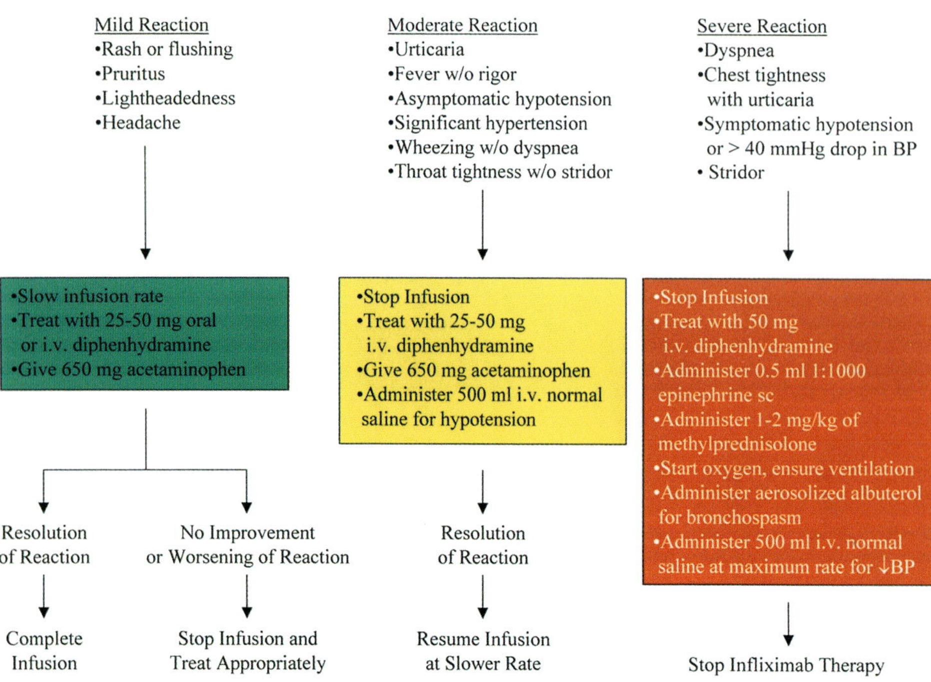

Figure 32.3. Protocol for management of infliximab infusion reactions. Facilities that administer infliximab should be equipped with the appropriate emergency drugs and have trained personnel available to monitor and treat any infusion reactions. Infliximab infusions are generally administered intravenously over 2 hours in 250 mL of fluid. After resolution of an infusion reaction, infusion can be restarted at 10 mL per hour and the rate gradually increased to 250 mL per hour in 10-mL-per-hour increments every 10 to 15 minutes, as tolerated. In the setting of a relatively mild infusion reaction, a physician may choose to continue the infusion with close monitoring. Patients with a history of a mild to moderate infusion reaction are usually treated 30 to 60 minutes before infusions with 650 mg acetaminophen and an oral antihistamine for prophylaxis against subsequent reactions. BP, blood pressure; w/o, without.

cated for patients with moderate or severe congestive heart failure and should be administered cautiously to patients with signs of left ventricular dysfunction. Infliximab should be stopped in patients with new or worsening congestive heart failure. Patients considered for infliximab therapy should be appropriately evaluated for the possibility of opportunistic infection, including latent tuberculosis. Therefore, patients should have a tuberculin skin test before infliximab therapy. A positive test (>5 mm of induration) calls for further evaluation and the initiation of antituberculosis prophylaxis. With appropriate antituberculosis prophylaxis, the risk for subsequent reactivation of latent tuberculosis from infliximab therapy is not known.

Patients with an active infection should not start infliximab therapy. If a patient develops a clinically significant infection during infliximab therapy, then he or she should be monitored closely by a physician. The physician must decide about the clinical significance of any acute or chronic infection, but any infection requiring antimicrobial therapy would probably be of concern. Because infliximab has a relatively long half-life (e.g., approximately 9.5 days), it often persists at detectable serum levels until the next infusion, during which time host defense may be impaired.

Many patients with RA and other rheumatic disorders are infected with hepatitis C due to its increasing incidence in the population. The decision to use infliximab therapy for patients with hepatitis C infection must be made carefully. It depends on the importance of this therapy to the patient, and the suitability of therapeutic alternatives. A small study found that patients with RA and hepatitis C who are treated with TNF-α antagonists do not worsen their liver function tests over the short term (79). Thus, limited data suggest anti–TNF-α therapy may not exacerbate hepatitis C infection, but further studies are needed to evaluate its long-term effects on the outcomes of this chronic viral infection.

Live vaccines are not recommended for patients receiving infliximab therapy. There are no data about the risk for secondary transmission of infection by live vaccines in patients taking this agent.

USE IN PREGNANCY

Infliximab is labeled pregnancy category B, which means that no maternal toxicity, embryotoxicity, or teratogenicity has been observed in animal studies. The evidence that infliximab does not cause fetal harm in humans is limited. Antoni et al. (80) have described pregnancy outcomes for a series of 59 women with RA and Crohn's disease who had received infliximab therapy before pregnancy and during the first trimester. The rates of live births and miscarriages were similar to those of healthy women. Therefore, the decision to continue infliximab therapy in a pregnant woman should be carefully weighed according to its relative benefits and risks.

There are no published data regarding the concentrations of infliximab in the breast milk of nursing mothers receiving this agent. However, some Igs are excreted in breast milk. The decision to discontinue infliximab in this setting must be individualized and based on the importance of nursing and the treatment benefit of this agent to the mother.

USE IN PATIENTS WITH HEPATIC AND RENAL INSUFFICIENCY

The pharmacokinetic profile of infliximab in hepatic or renal failure is not known. However, a patient with RA receiving hemodialysis has been safely treated with infliximab, with dramatic improvement in her arthritis activity (81).

DRUG INTERACTIONS

There have been no investigations of possible drug interactions between infliximab and other medications.

ADALIMUMAB

Isolation and Structure

In January 2003, adalimumab became available for commercial use in the United States. Adalimumab (D2E7, Humira) is a fully human IgG1κ anti–TNF-α mAb (Fig. 32.4). It was produced by phage display technology, using a murine antihuman TNF-α mAb as a template. During this process, the murine sequences are completely replaced with their human counterparts. Because this method mimics natural human Ig rearrangement, adalimumab should be virtually indistinguishable from naturally occurring IgG1 and, in theory, should exhibit minimal, if any, immunogenicity in humans.

Like infliximab, adalimumab binds *in vitro* with high affinity ($K_a = 6 \times 10^{10}\ M^{-1}$) and high specificity to TNF-α, and inhibits TNF-α binding with TNFR1 and TNFR2 (82). Adalimumab is produced in a mammalian culture system and undergoes a purification process with the necessary steps for virus inactivation. It is supplied in both single-use 1-mL prefilled sterile syringes and 2-mL glass vials (0.9 mL of drug product) for subcutaneous administration. Each syringe and glass vial is designed to deliver 0.8 mL (40 mg) of drug.

Pharmacokinetics

The pharmacokinetics of subcutaneous injections of adalimumab allow for weekly or every other week administration. After a single 40-mg subcutaneous injection of adalimumab, the maximum serum concentration is 4.7 ± 1.6 μg per mL, and the time to reach the maximum concentration is 131 ± 56 hours. The average bioavailability of adalimumab is 64% for a single 40-mg subcutaneous injection.

The pharmacokinetics of adalimumab has also been evaluated after a single intravenous infusion at doses of 0.25, 0.5, 1.3, and 5 mg per kg (83). The observed serum levels were most consistent with a two-compartment model and increased proportionately with dose. The mean terminal half-life ranged from 14.7 to 19.3 days. Based on data from five patients with RA, the concentrations of adalimumab in the synovial fluid are 31% to 96% of that found in serum.

Clinical Trials

Initial clinical trials of adalimumab therapy for RA were performed in Europe testing both the intravenous and subcutaneous route of administration (84). Single and multiple infusions of adalimumab ranging from 0.5 to 10 mg per kg were evaluated in a randomized, double-blind, placebo-controlled, dose-escalation trial involving 120 patients with active RA. All DMARDs were withdrawn before receiving adalimumab. In the three highest dosage groups, ACR 20% responses were achieved by 56% to 80% of patients, with a plateau of the dose response at 1 mg per kg. Weekly subcutaneous administration of 0.5 to 1.0 mg per kg adalimumab was evaluated in a 3-month, randomized, double-blind, placebo-controlled trial in 24 patients with active RA. Approximately 70% of patients met criteria for an ACR 20% response at the end of this study. A single 1 mg per kg intravenous or subcutaneous injection of adalimumab was evaluated in 54 patients who had inadequate responses to MTX therapy. The combination produced ACR 20% response rates of 72% and 67%, respectively. Subcutaneous dosing was associated with mild injection site reactions. In an extension study, 66 of the 120 patients with RA in the original controlled trial were treated with adalimumab in an open-label fashion for 12 months and evaluated for radiographic progression of joint damage. The median

Sharp score did not change significantly from baseline to month 12 in this subset, suggesting that adalimumab therapy slows radiographic progression of disease.

The Anti-TNF Research Study Program of the Monoclonal Antibody Adalimumab in Rheumatoid Arthritis trial investigated the clinical efficacy and safety of subcutaneous injections of adalimumab in combination with MTX therapy (85). To be eligible, patients must have had active RA and had been treated with MTX for at least 6 months, with a stable dose of 12.5 to 25 mg per week for at least 4 weeks before entry. Other DMARDs were withdrawn before the study, although patients were permitted to continue treatment with nonsteroidal antiinflammatory drugs and low doses of oral corticosteroids (prednisone, ≤10 mg per day). Patients were randomly allocated to receive placebo or 20-mg, 40-mg, 60-mg, or 80-mg adalimumab injections every 2 weeks for 24 weeks. In the absence of an ACR 20% response at week 16, patients were eligible to roll over into an open-label continuation study.

Among the 271 patients randomly allocated to the four treatment groups (62, placebo; 69, 20 mg adalimumab; 67, 40 mg adalimumab; 73, 80 mg adalimumab), 161 (59%) patients completed the 24 weeks of treatment. The withdrawals included 92 patients who rolled over into the open-label study (35, placebo; 23, 20 mg adalimumab; 27, 40 mg adalimumab; 27, 80 mg adalimumab), seven patients with adverse events, five patients who withdrew consent, three patients with lack of efficacy, one patient with a protocol violation, and two patients who were lost to follow-up. The study population was predominately female, with a disease duration of 11 to 13 years. The mean MTX dose ranged from 16 to 17 mg per week across the four treatment groups. At week 24, ACR 20% response rates in the 20 mg, 40 mg, and 80 mg adalimumab treatment groups were 48%, 67%, and 66%, respectively, significantly greater than the ACR 20% response rate of 14.5% in the placebo group. ACR 50% response rates were also significantly higher in the 20 mg, 40 mg, and 80 mg adalimumab groups (32% to 55%) than in the placebo group (8%). Most of the responders had achieved a response to adalimumab therapy by 4 weeks, indicative of a rapid response. Adalimumab therapy also produced significant improvements in the disability index of the HAQ, SF-36 scores, and the fatigue scale of the Functional Assessment of Chronic Illness Therapy instrument. Treatment with adalimumab increased hemoglobin levels over the treatment period, consistent with the known effects of TNF-α on hematopoiesis. Serum levels of pro-MMP-1 and pro-MMP-3, potential markers of cartilage destruction, also decreased in association with adalimumab therapy.

Adalimumab therapy was generally well tolerated in this study. Pain or reaction at the injection site occurred in 12% to 22% of the adalimumab-treated patients, compared with 3.2% of patients in the placebo group. The rate of infections was similar across treatment groups. Two patients receiving adalimumab developed a serious infection (pneumonia), and one patient was diagnosed with adenocarcinoma of the colon. Three of the patients in the study (1, placebo; 1, 20 mg adalimumab; 1, 80 mg adalimumab) tested positive for serum antiadalimumab antibodies, but the assay methodology and details of this analysis were not described.

Three other randomized, double-blind trials have assessed the clinical efficacy and safety of subcutaneous adalimumab therapy for RA. A 26-week, placebo-controlled study investigated the clinical benefits of adalimumab monotherapy in 544 patients with active RA who failed treatment with at least one DMARD (86). Eligible patients were randomized into five treatment groups: placebo, 20 mg adalimumab every week or every other week, and 40 mg adalimumab every week or every other week. ACR 20% and ACR 50% response rates were significantly higher in the adalimumab treatment groups compared with the placebo group (Fig. 32.4). The ACR 20% response rates for the patients receiving adalimumab, 40 mg every week and every other week, were numerically superior to those in the 20 mg adalimumab-treatment groups. Injection site reactions occurred in 19.4% of adalimumab-treated patients. Thus, adalimumab monotherapy can produce significant improvement in the signs and symptoms of RA.

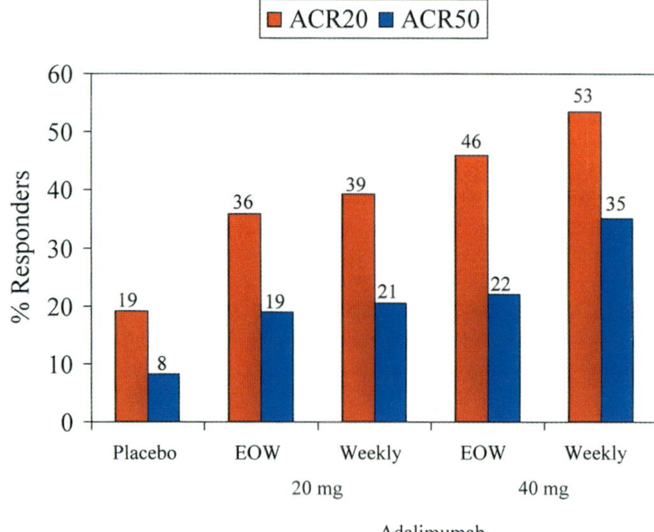

Figure 32.4. Adalimumab monotherapy is effective for the treatment of rheumatoid arthritis. Results shown are from a 26-week, randomized, double-blind, placebo-controlled trial comparing the clinical efficacy of four different adalimumab treatment regimens with placebo. The p values were <.01 for comparisons of the American College of Rheumatology (ACR) 20% response rates between each of the adalimumab treatment groups and placebo group. For ACR 50% response rates, the p values were <.01 for comparisons between the 20 mg weekly, 40 mg every other week (EOW), and 40 mg weekly adalimumab treatment groups and placebo group. The p value was <.05 for the comparison of the ACR 50% response rates between the 20-mg EOW adalimumab and placebo groups.

A 52-week placebo-controlled trial evaluated the effect of adalimumab therapy on radiographic progression of joint damage in RA (87). In this study, 619 patients taking stable doses of MTX were randomly assigned to receive placebo, 20 mg adalimumab weekly, or 40 mg adalimumab every other week. At week 52, significantly more patients had no erosions in the 20 mg of adalimumab weekly group (57.9%) and 40 mg of adalimumab every other week group (61.8%) than patients in the placebo group (46%). Also, the median change from baseline to week 52 in the total Sharp scores was significantly lower for the adalimumab treatment groups (0.0 for both) than the placebo group (1.0). ACR 20% and ACR 50% response rates were 54.7% and 37.7% for the 20 mg adalimumab every week group and 58.9% and 41.5% for the 40 mg adalimumab every other week group, which were significantly greater than the corresponding rates in the placebo group (24.0% and 9.5%). Adalimumab therapy also produced significant improvements in the disability index of the HAQ, SF-36 scores, and the Functional Assessment of Chronic Illness Therapy fatigue scale scores (88). Injection site reactions were reported for 22.9% of the patients in the adalimumab-treatment groups. Infection rates were similar among the treatment groups. Like infliximab therapy, subcutaneous injections of adalimumab in combination with MTX therapy can slow the radiographic progression of joint disease in RA.

The safety of adalimumab was evaluated in a 24-week, placebo-controlled trial involving 636 patients with active RA (89). In this trial, patients continued to receive their prestudy antirheumatic medications, including nonsteroidal antiinflammatory drugs, low doses of oral corticosteroids, and DMARDs. Eligible subjects were randomly allocated to receive placebo (N = 318) or 40 mg of adalimumab every other week (N = 318). Injection site reactions occurred more frequently in the 40 mg adalimumab every other week group than the placebo group (19.5% vs. 11.6%). The rate of serious adverse events was similar between the placebo and adalimumab groups (6.9% vs. 5.3%). Also, no difference was found in the frequency of serious infections for the two groups (1.9% vs. 1.3%). These results show that adalimumab 40 mg every other week added to standard of care does not produce a significant increase in the frequency of adverse events over a 24-week treatment period.

Adverse Events

The most frequent adalimumab-related toxicity in clinical trials was injection site reaction. Most of these reactions were mild and only rarely led to study withdrawal. Rates of infection were similar for adalimumab-treated and placebo-treated patients (approximately one per patient per year). Like other TNF-α antagonists, adalimumab therapy has been associated in clinical trials with tuberculosis, mostly within the first 8 months of treatment. Other opportunistic infections, such as histoplasmosis, aspergillosis, and nocardiosis, have also been reported in trials of adalimumab therapy.

As described above, treatment with infliximab and etanercept has been associated with the production of autoantibodies and, rarely, the onset of autoimmune disease. In the Anti-TNF Research Study Program of the Monoclonal Antibody Adalimumab in Rheumatoid Arthritis trial, 18 (11.1%) of the adalimumab-treated patients and 3 (6.1%) of the 49 placebo-treated patients converted from ANA negative at entry to ANA positive at some point during the study (85). Also, in the Anti-TNF Research Study Program of the Monoclonal Antibody Adalimumab in Rheumatoid Arthritis trial, 8 (3.9%) of the 204 adalimumab-treated patients and none of the placebo-treated patients developed antibodies to dsDNA. One of 2,334 patients in clinical trials of adalimumab therapy developed systemic lupus erythematosus–like manifestations. The exposure of larger numbers of patients to adalimumab therapy will likely uncover rare instances of serious toxicity similar to that observed with other TNF-α antagonists.

According to the product information, 2,468 patients in clinical trials of adalimumab therapy have developed 48 malignancies, including 10 cases of lymphoma. In this sample, the Standardized Incidence Ratio for all malignancies was 1.0 (95% CI: 0.7–1.3) and for lymphoma was 5.4 (95% CI: 2.6–10.0). Importantly, patients with RA have a several-fold increased incidence of lymphoma, which may account for the increased rate of lymphoma in this study population.

Recommended Clinical Use of Adalimumab

DOSAGE AND ADMINISTRATION

Adalimumab is given by the subcutaneous route. The recommended dose of adalimumab is 40 mg every other week. Patients not receiving MTX may receive additional benefit by increasing the dose to 40 mg every week.

INDICATIONS, CONTRAINDICATIONS, WARNINGS, AND PRECAUTIONS

Adalimumab is indicated for reducing the signs and symptoms of RA, as well as retarding the radiographic progression of joint damage. Patients may receive adalimumab injections with or without MTX therapy.

Because serious infections have occurred in patients receiving TNF-α antagonists, the same warnings and precautions described for infliximab therapy apply to the use of adalimumab.

USE IN PREGNANCY

Like infliximab, adalimumab is classified as pregnancy category B, indicating no evidence of harm to the fetus in animal studies. No human studies have been reported assessing the impact of adalimumab on pregnancy. It is not known if adalimumab is excreted in human milk.

USE IN PATIENTS WITH HEPATIC OR RENAL INSUFFICIENCY

There are no studies of adalimumab therapy in patients with hepatic or renal insufficiency.

DRUG INTERACTIONS

MTX reduces the clearance of single and multiple doses of adalimumab by 29% and 44%, respectively, according to the product information.

MECHANISMS OF ANTI–TUMOR NECROSIS FACTOR α THERAPY

Treatment with TNF-α antagonists broadly ameliorates the disturbances in the cytokine network that contribute to the pathogenesis of RA. Most of the published studies have evaluated the mechanisms by which infliximab therapy down-regulates the inflammatory response. Infliximab therapy has been shown to reduce serum levels of C-reactive protein, IL-6, and IL-18, as well as serum levels of natural cytokine inhibitors, such as soluble TNFR1, soluble TNFR2, and IL-1 receptor antagonist (90,91). However, serum levels of IL-12 and IL-13 are not affected by infliximab therapy. Treatment with adalimumab appears to have a similar effect on serum levels of acute phase reactants and cytokines (92), but such studies have been much more limited using this anti–TNF-α agent. Apart from cytokines, other proinflammatory mediators are influenced by the anti–TNF-α effect. For example, a single infusion of 5 to 20 mg per kg of infliximab treatment can reduce the overexpression of nitric oxide synthase type 2 by peripheral blood monocytes and, thereby, inhibit inducible nitric oxide production (93).

Treatment with TNF-α antagonists decreases the expression of proinflammatory cytokines in rheumatoid synovium. Using immunohistochemical techniques, Ulfgren et al. (94) have shown that a single infusion of infliximab, 10 mg per kg, reduces the synovial expression of TNF-α and, in a subgroup of patients, IL-1 expression as well. The decrease in TNF-α expression occurs within 2 weeks, simultaneous with the rapid onset of clinical improvement.

In synovial tissue, anti–TNF-α therapy inhibits the expression of adhesion molecules and deactivates endothelium. Tak et al. (95) have shown that treatment with 10 mg per kg or 20 mg per kg of infliximab diminishes the synovial tissue expression of vascular cell adhesion molecule-1 (VCAM-1) and E-selectin. The reduced expression of adhesion molecules was accompanied in this study by a decrease in the number of infiltrating $CD3^+$ T cells. Because VCAM-1 and E-selectin are TNF-α inducible and mediate leukocyte adherence to endothelial cells, the antiinflammatory effect of infliximab therapy may result from decreased leukocyte recruitment to the joint.

In RA, the synovial inflammatory response may depend on the increased expression of chemokines, which regulate the trafficking of leukocytes to sites of inflammation. In one study, synovial biopsy specimens were obtained before and after infliximab therapy and analyzed for the expression of IL-8, monocyte chemotactic protein 1 (MCP-1), macrophage inflammatory protein 1α, macrophage inflammatory protein 1β, Gro-α, and regulated on activation, normal T cell–expressed and –secreted (RANTES) (96). A single infusion of infliximab produced a significant reduction in the expression of IL-8 and MCP-1 and numbers of infiltrating $CD3^+$ T cells, $CD22^+$ B cells, and $CD68^+$ macrophages. MCP-1, a potent monocyte and T-cell chemoattractant, was diminished in expression in both the synovial lining and sublining layers. Additionally, the drop in MCP-1 expression in the synovial lining layer significantly correlated with a decrease in the numbers of $CD68^+$ macrophages. Although the expression of Gro-α, RANTES, and macrophage inflammatory protein 1β trended lower after infliximab therapy, these changes were not statistically significant. Thus, TNF-α may differentially regulate the expression of the various members of the chemokine family. Taken together, the evidence suggests that the clinical benefits of anti–TNF-α therapy result, at least in part, from decreased recruitment of leukocytes to the inflamed joint. This notion is supported by a study showing that infliximab treatment is associated with a significant reduction in the migration of indium-111–labeled granulocytes to inflamed joints (96).

A single infusion of infliximab, 1 or 10 mg per kg, decreases serum levels of E-selectin and intracellular adhesion molecule-1 (ICAM-1), but not serum levels of VCAM-1 (97). Insofar as soluble adhesion molecules are shed from the vasculature, elevated circulating levels of adhesion molecules are believed to reflect endothelial activation, although only levels of ICAM-1 and VCAM-1 appear to correlate with disease activity. In parallel with the decreased serum levels of E-selectin and ICAM-1, infliximab treatment led to an increase in circulating lymphocytes. This effect on leukocyte trafficking could be the result of an anti–TNF-α effect on endothelial activation or chemokine production, or both.

Formation of new blood vessels contributes to rheumatoid synovitis by regulating the supply of nutrients as well as providing a conduit for the ingress of inflammatory cells into the joint. Several lines of evidence suggest VEGF plays a role in this process. VEGF has been detected in synovial tissue from patients with RA. In addition, serum levels of VEGF are markedly elevated in patients with RA, compared with those of healthy individuals. Infliximab treatment has been shown to reduce the serum levels of VEGF in patients with RA, implying that TNF-α mediates production of this angiogenic mediator *in vivo* (98).

TNF-α up-regulates the expression of MMPs and stimulates osteolysis, leading to cartilage and bone destruction. In placebo-controlled studies, infliximab therapy has been shown to lower serum levels of MMP-1 and MMP-3 in patients with RA (99). Therefore, anti–TNF-α therapy may partly confer protection against joint damage by this mechanism, although MMP-1 and MMP-3 are not validated serum markers of cartilage and bone damage. TNF-α influences the regulation of osteoprotegerin (OPG) and soluble RANKL (sRANKL), which are critically involved in osteoclastogenesis. Serum levels of OPG and sRANKL levels are higher in patients with RA than in healthy controls (100). Because OPG and sRANKL are much higher in synovial fluid than serum, the elevated levels in serum probably represent a spillover from local joint production. Infliximab infusions have been shown to normalize serum OPG and sRANKL levels, providing evidence that TNF-α, either directly or indirectly, mediates these effects.

CONCLUSION

The beneficial effects of infliximab and adalimumab therapy on the clinical, laboratory, and radiographic manifestations of RA verify the key role played by TNF-α in the pathogenesis of this disease. These anti–TNF-α therapies represent a major breakthrough in the treatment of RA. Despite this advance, anti–TNF-α therapy only partially controls disease activity in most patients, and withdrawal of these agents can lead to a disease flare. Moreover, in clinical trials, nonresponder rates using anti–TNF-α therapies are as high as 40%. These findings strongly suggest TNF-α is not solely responsible for driving the inflammatory response in RA despite its prominence in the cytokine cascade and the impressive clinical benefits of anti–TNF-α therapies.

Prospects exist for improving the effectiveness of anti–TNF-α therapy for RA. Genetic polymorphisms within the TNF-α and TNFR genes may have functional significance and correlate with individual responses to anti–TNF-α therapy. The identification of such polymorphisms could allow for selection of patients with a high likelihood of responding to anti–TNF-α therapy. Additionally, the use of anti–TNF-α agents in novel combination therapies may lead in the future to improved clinical efficacy. Hypothetically, there may be a window of opportunity during the early stages of RA, during which time the use of anti–TNF-α agents may produce superior outcomes. Regardless, infliximab and adalimumab are likely to be valuable agents in our therapeutic armamentarium for years to come.

REFERENCES

1. Chu CQ, Field M, Feldmann M, Maini RN. Localization of tumor necrosis factor α in synovial tissues and at the cartilage-pannus junction in patients with rheumatoid arthritis. *Arthritis Rheum* 1991;34:1125–1132.
2. Brennan FM, Chantry D, Jackson A, et al. Inhibitory effect of TNF α antibodies on synovial cell interleukin-1 production in rheumatoid arthritis. *Lancet* 1989;2:244–247.
3. Haworth C, Brennan FM, Chantry D, et al. Expression of granulocyte macrophage colony-stimulating factor in rheumatoid arthritis: regulation by tumor necrosis factor α. *Eur J Immunol* 1991;21:2575–2579.
4. Choy EH, Hazleman B, Smith M, et al. Efficacy of a novel PEGylated humanized anti-TNF fragment (CDP870) in patients with rheumatoid arthritis: a phase II double-blinded, randomized, dose-escalating trial. *Rheumatology* 2002;41:1133–1137.
5. O'Shea JJ, Ma A, Lipsky P. Cytokines and autoimmunity. *Nat Rev Immunol* 2002;2:37–45.
6. Papadaki HA, Kritikos HD, Gemetzi C, et al. Bone marrow progenitor cell reserve and function and stromal cell function are defective in rheumatoid arthritis: evidence for a tumor necrosis factor α–mediated effect. *Blood* 2002;99:1610–1619.
7. Papadaki HA, Kritikos HD, Valatas V, et al. Anemia of chronic disease in rheumatoid arthritis is associated with increased apoptosis of bone marrow erythroid cells: improvement following anti-tumor necrosis factor-α antibody therapy. *Blood* 2002;100:474–482.
8. Cope AP, Londei M, Chu NR, et al. Chronic exposure to tumor necrosis factor (TNF) in vitro impairs the activation of T cells through the T cell receptor/CD3 complex: reversal in vivo by anti-TNF antibodies in patients with rheumatoid arthritis. *J Clin Invest* 1994;94:749–760.
9. Isomäki P, Panesar M, Annenkov A, et al. Prolonged exposure of T cells to TNF down-regulates TCRζ and expression of the TCR/CD_3 complex at the cell surface. *J Immunol* 2001;166:5495–5507.
10. Bryl E, Vallejo AN, Weyand CM, Goronzy JJ. Down-regulation of CD28 expression by TNF-α. *J Immunol* 2001;167:3231–3238.
11. Martens PB, Goronzy JJ, Schaid D, Weyand CM. Expansion of unusual CD4+ T cells in severe rheumatoid arthritis. *Arthritis Rheum* 1997;40:1106–1114.
12. Feldmann M, Brennan FM, Maini RN. Role of cytokines in rheumatoid arthritis. *Annu Rev Immunol* 1996;14:397–440.
13. Grewal IS, Grewal KD, Wong FS, et al. Local expression of transgene encoded TNF-α in islets prevents autoimmune diabetes in nonobese diabetic (NOD) mice by preventing the development of auto-reactive islet-specific T cells. *J Exp Med* 1996;184:1963–1974.
14. Verweij CL. Tumour necrosis factor gene polymorphisms as severity markers in rheumatoid arthritis. *Ann Rheum Dis* 1999;58[Suppl]:I20–I26.
15. Keffer J, Probert L, Cazlaris H, et al. Transgenic mice expressing human tumour necrosis factor: a predictive genetic model of arthritis. *EMBO J* 1991;19:4025–4031.

16. Carballo E, Lai WS, Blackshear PJ. Feedback inhibition of macrophage tumor necrosis factor-α production by tristetraprolin. *Science* 1998;281:1001–1005.
17. Taylor GA, Carbello E, Lee DM, et al. A pathogenic role for TNF α in the syndrome of cachexia, arthritis, and autoimmunity regulating from tristetraprolin (TTP) deficiency. *Immunity* 1996;4:445–454.
18. Brooks SA, Connolly JE, Diegel RJ, et al. Analysis of the function, expression, and subcellular distribution of human tristetraprolin. *Arthritis Rheum* 2002;46:1362–1370.
19. Georgopoulos S, Plows D, Kollias G. Transmembrane TNF is sufficient to induce localized tissue toxicity and chronic inflammatory arthritis in transgenic mice. *J Inflamm* 1996;46:86–97.
20. Locksley RM, Killeen N, Lenardo MJ. The TNF and TNF receptor superfamilies: integrating mammalian biology. *Cell* 2001;104:487–501.
21. Chen G, Goeddel DV. TNF-R1 signaling: a beautiful pathway. *Science* 2002;296:1634–1635.
22. Baud V, Karin M. Signal transduction by tumor necrosis factor and its relatives. *Trends Cell Biol* 2001;11:372–377.
23. Aderka D, Engelmann H, Maor Y, et al. Stabilization of the bioactivity of tumor necrosis factor by its soluble receptors. *J Exp Med* 1992;175:323–329.
24. Aksentijevich I, Galon J, Soares M, et al. The tumor-necrosis-factor receptor–Associated periodic syndrome: new mutations in TNFRSFiA, ancestral origins, genotype-phenotype studies, and evidence for further genetic heterogeneity of periodic fevers. *Am J Hum Gen* 2001;69:301–314.
25. Drewe E, McDermott EM, Powell RJ. Treatment of the nephrotic syndrome with etanercept in patients with the tumor necrosis factor receptor–associated periodic syndrome (correspondence). *N Engl J Med* 2000;343:1044–1045.
26. Lam J, Abu-Amer Y, Nelson CA, et al. Tumour necrosis factor superfamily cytokines and the pathogenesis of inflammatory osteolysis. *Ann Rheum Dis* 2002:61[Suppl II]:ii82–ii83.
27. Burger D. Cell contact-mediated signaling of monocytes by stimulated T cells: a major pathway for cytokine induction. *Eur Cytokine Netw* 2000;11:346–353.
28. Brennan FM, Haynes AL, Ciesielski CJ, et al. Evidence that rheumatoid arthritis synovial T cells are similar to cytokine-activated T cells. *Arthritis Rheum* 2002:46:31–41.
29. McInnes IB, Leung BP, Sturrock RD, et al. Interleukin-15 mediates T cell-dependent regulation of tumor necrosis factor-α production in rheumatoid arthritis. *Nat Med* 1997;3:189–195.
30. Feldmann M, Maini RN. Anti-TNFα therapy of rheumatoid arthritis: what have we learned? *Annu Rev Immunol* 2001;19:163–196.
31. Butler DM, Maini RN, Feldmann M, Brennan FM. Modulation of proinflammatory cytokine release in rheumatoid synovial membrane cell cultures. Comparison of monoclonal anti-TNF-α antibody with the interleukin-1 receptor antagonist. *Eur Cytokine Netw* 1995;6:225–230.
32. Katsikis PD, Chu CQ, Brennan FM, et al. Immunoregulatory role of interleukin 10 in rheumatoid arthritis. *J Exp Med* 1994;179:1517–1527.
33. Hermann JA, Hall MA, Maini RN, et al. Important immunoregulatory role of interleukin-11 in the inflammatory process in rheumatoid arthritis. *Arthritis Rheum* 1998;41:1388–1397.
34. Williams RO, Feldmann M, Maini RN. Anti-tumor necrosis factor ameliorates joint disease in murine collagen-induced arthritis. *Proc Natl Acad Sci U S A* 1992;89:9784–9788.
35. Williams RO, Ghrayeb J, Feldmann M, Maini RN. Successful therapy of collagen-induced arthritis with TNF receptor-IgG fusion protein and combination with anti-CD4. *Immunology* 1995;84:433–439.
36. Probert L, Plows D, Kontogeorgos G, Kollias G. The type I interleukin-1 receptor acts in series with tumor necrosis factor (TNF) to induce arthritis in TNF-transgenic mice. *Eur J Immunol* 1995;25:1794–1797.
37. Campbell IK, O'Donnell K, Lawlor KE, Wicks IP. Severe inflammatory arthritis and lymphadenopathy in the absence of TNF. *J Clin Invest* 2001;107:1519–1527.
38. Knight DM, Trinh H, Le J, et al. Construction and initial characterization of a mouse-human chimeric anti-TNF antibody. *Mol Immunol* 1993;30:1443–1453.
39. Scallon BJ, Moore MA, Trinh H, et al. Chimeric anti-TNF-α monoclonal antibody cA2 binds recombinant transmembrane TNF-α and activates immune effector functions. *Cytokine* 1995;7:251–259.
40. Cornille F, Shealy D, D'Haens D, et al. Infliximab induces potent anti-inflammatory and local immunomodulatory activity but no systemic immune suppression in patients with Crohn's disease. *Aliment Pharmacol Ther* 2001;15:463–473.
41. Morell A, Terry WD, Waldmann TA. Metabolic properties of IgG subclasses in man. *J Clin Invest* 1970;49:673–680.
42. St. Clair EW, Wagner CL, Fasanmade AA, et al. The relationship of serum infliximab concentrations to clinical improvement in rheumatoid arthritis. Results from ATTRACT, a multicenter, randomized, double-blind, placebo-controlled trial. *Arthritis Rheum* 2002;46:1451–1459.
43. Felson DT, Anderson JJ, Boers M, et al. American College of Rheumatology preliminary definition of improvement in rheumatoid arthritis. *Arthritis Rheum* 1995;38:727–735.
44. Elliott MJ, Maini RN, Feldmann M, et al. Treatment of rheumatoid arthritis with chimeric monoclonal antibodies to tumor necrosis factor α. *Arthritis Rheum* 1993;36:1681–1690.
45. Ritchie DM, Boyle JA, McInnes JM, et al. Clinical studies with an articular index for the assessment of joint tenderness in patients with rheumatoid arthritis. *QJM* 1968;147:393–406.
46. Elliott MJ, Maini RN, Feldmann M, et al. Randomized double-blind comparison of chimeric monoclonal antibody to tumor necrosis factor α (cA2) versus placebo in rheumatoid arthritis. *Lancet* 1994;344:1105–1110.
47. Paulus HE, Egger MJ, Ward JR, et al. Analysis of improvement in individual rheumatoid arthritis patients treated with disease-modifying antirheumatic drugs, based on the findings in patients treated with placebo. *Arthritis Rheum* 1990;33:1443–1453.
48. Elliott MJ, Maini RN, Feldmann M, et al. Repeated therapy with monoclonal antibody to tumor necrosis factor α (cA2) in patients with rheumatoid arthritis. *Lancet* 1994;344:1125–1127.
49. Maini RN, Breedveld FC, Kalden JR, et al. Therapeutic efficacy of multiple intravenous infusions of anti-tumor necrosis factor α monoclonal antibody combined with low-dose weekly methotrexate in rheumatoid arthritis. *Arthritis Rheum* 1998;41:1552–1563.
50. Kavanaugh A, St. Clair EW, McCune WJ, et al. Chimeric anti-tumor necrosis factor-α monoclonal antibody treatment of patients with rheumatoid arthritis receiving methotrexate therapy. *J Rheumatol* 2000;27:841–850.
51. Maini RN, St. Clair EW, Breedveld F, et al. Infliximab (chimeric anti-tumor necrosis factor α monoclonal antibody) versus placebo in rheumatoid arthritis patients receiving concomitant methotrexate: a randomized phase III trial. *Lancet* 1999;354:1932–1939.
52. Lipsky PE, van der Heijde DMFM, St. Clair EW, et al. Infliximab and methotrexate in the treatment of rheumatoid arthritis. *N Engl J Med* 2000;343:1594–1602.
53. Lipsky P, van der Heijde D, St. Clair EW, et al. 102-wk clinical and radiologic results from the ATTRACT trial: a 2 year, randomized, controlled, phase 3 trial of infliximab (Remicade™) in patients with active rheumatoid arthritis despite methotrexate. *Arthritis Rheum* 2000;43[Suppl]:S269(abst).
54. Van der Heijde D. Plain x-rays in rheumatoid arthritis: overview of scoring methods, their reliability and applicability. *Baillieres Clin Rheumatol* 1996;10:435–453.
55. Wolfe F. A reappraisal of HAQ disability in rheumatoid arthritis. *Arthritis Rheum* 2000;43:2751–2761.
56. Kosinski M, Zhao SZ, Dedhiya S, et al. Determining minimally important changes in generic and disease-specific health-related quality of life questionnaires in clinical trials of rheumatoid arthritis. *Arthritis Rheum* 2000;43:1478–1487.
57. Wagner CL, St. Clair EW, Han C, et al. Effects of antibodies to infliximab on ACR response in patients with rheumatoid arthritis in the ATTRACT study. *Arthritis Rheum* 2002;46(suppl):S132 (abst).
58. Shergy WJ, Isern RA, Cooley DA, et al. Open label study to assess infliximab safety and timing of onset of clinical benefit among patients with rheumatoid arthritis. *J Rheumatol* 2002;29:667–677.
59. O'Connor M, Buchman A, Marshall G. Anaphylaxis-like reaction to infliximab in a patient with Crohn's disease. *Dig Dis Sci* 2002;47:1323–1325.
60. Keane J, Gershon S, Wise RP, et al. Tuberculosis associated with infliximab, a tumor necrosis factor (alpha)-neutralizing agent. *N Engl J Med* 2001;345:1098–1104.
61. Lee JH, Slifman NR, Gershon SK, et al. Life-threatening histoplasmosis complicating immunotherapy with tumor necrosis factor α antagonists infliximab and etanercept. *Arthritis Rheum* 2002;46:2565–2570.
62. Warris A, Bjorneklett A, Gaustad P. Invasive pulmonary aspergillosis associated with infliximab therapy (correspondence). *N Engl J Med* 2001;344:1099–1100.
63. Flynn JL, Chan J. Immunology of tuberculosis. *Annu Rev Immunol* 2001;19:93–129.
64. Zhou P, Miller G, Seder RA. Factors involved in regulating primary and secondary immunity to infection with *Histoplasma capsulatum*: TNF-α plays a critical role in maintaining secondary immunity in the absence of IFN-γ. *J Immunol* 1998;160:1359–1368.
65. White DW, Harty JT. Perforin-deficient CD8+ T cells provide immunity to *Listeria monocytogenes* by a mechanism that is independent of CD95 and IFN-γ but requires TNF-α. *J Immunol* 1998;160:898–905.
66. Chen W, Havell EA, Harmsen AG. Importance of endogenous tumor necrosis factor α and γ interferon in host resistance against Pneumocystis carinii infection. *Infect Immun* 1992;60:1279–1284.
67. Mohan N, Edwards ET, Cupps TR, et al. Demyelination occurring during anti-tumor necrosis factor α therapy for inflammatory arthritides. *Arthritis Rheum* 2001;44:2862–2869.
68. Charles PJ, Smeenk RJT, De Jong J, et al. Assessment of antibodies to double-stranded DNA induced in rheumatoid arthritis patients following treatment with infliximab, a monoclonal antibody to tumor necrosis factor α. Findings in open-label and randomized placebo-controlled trials. *Arthritis Rheum* 2000;43:2383–2390.
69. Ali Y, Shah S. Infliximab-induced systemic lupus erythematosus (letter). *Ann Intern Med* 2002;137:625–626.
70. Saleem G, Li S, MacPherson BR, Cooper SM. Hepatitis with interface inflammation and IgG, IgM, and IgA anti-double-stranded DNA antibodies following infliximab therapy: comment on the article by Charles et al (letter). *Arthritis Rheum* 2001;44:1966–1968.
71. Menghini VV, Arora AS. Infliximab-associated reversible cholestatic liver disease. *Mayo Clin Proc* 2001;76:84–86.
72. Vergara G, Silvestre JF, Betloch I, et al. Cutaneous drug eruption to infliximab: report of 4 cases with an interface dermatitis pattern. *Arch Dermatol* 2002;138:1258–1259.
73. Kent PD, Davis JM III, Davis MDP, Matteson EL. Bullous skin lesions following infliximab infusion in a patient with rheumatoid arthritis (letter). *Arthritis Rheum* 2002;46:2257–2258.
74. Bradham WS, Bozkurt B, Gunasinghe H, et al. Tumor necrosis factor-α and myocardial remodeling in progression of heart failure: a current prospective. *Cardiovasc Res* 2002;53:822–830.

75. Coletta AP, Clark AL, Banarjee P, Cleland JGF. Clinical trials update: RENEWAL (RENAISSANCE and RECOVER) and ATTACH. *Eur J Heart Fail* 2002;4:559–561.
76. Brown SL, Greene MH, Gershon SK, et al. Tumor necrosis factor antagonist therapy and lymphoma development. Twenty-six cases reported to the Food and Drug Administration. *Arthritis Rheum* 2002;46:3151–3158.
77. Schiff MH, Bulpitt K, Weaver AA, et al. Safety of combination therapy with anakinra and etanercept in patients with rheumatoid arthritis. *Arthritis Rheum* 2001;44[Suppl]:S79(abst).
78. Puchner TC, Kugathasan S, Kelly KJ, Binion DG. Successful desensitization and therapeutic use of infliximab in adult and pediatric Crohn's disease patients with prior anaphylactic reaction. *Inflamm Bowel Dis* 2001;7:34–37.
79. Peterson JR, Wener MH, Hsu FC, Simkin PA. Safety of TNF-α antagonists in patients with rheumatoid arthritis and chronic hepatitis C. *Arthritis Rheum* 2001;44[Suppl]:S78(abst).
80. Antoni CE, Furst D, Lichtenstein GR, et al. Outcome of pregnancy in women receiving Remicade® (infliximab) for the treatment of Crohn's disease. *Arthritis Rheum* 2001;44[Suppl]:S152(abst).
81. Singh R, Cuchacovich R, Huang W, Espinoza LR. Infliximab treatment in a patient with rheumatoid arthritis on hemodialysis. *J Rheumatol* 2002;29:636–637.
82. Salfeld J, Kaymakcalan Z, Tracy D, et al. Generation of fully human anti-TNF antibody D2E7. *Arthritis Rheum* 1998;41[Suppl]:S57(abst).
83. Velagaudi RB, Noerteshauser P, Bankmann Y, et al. Pharmacokinetics of adalimumab (D2E7), a fully human anti-TNF-α monoclonal antibody, following a single intravenous injection in rheumatoid arthritis patients treated with methotrexate. *Arthritis Rheum* 2002;46[Suppl]:S133(abst).
84. Kempeni J. Update on D2E7: a fully human anti-tumour necrosis factor α monoclonal antibody. *Ann Rheum Dis* 2000;59[Suppl I]:i44–i45.
85. Weinblatt ME, Keystone EC, Furst DE, et al. Adalimumab, a fully human anti-tumor necrosis factor α monoclonal antibody, for the treatment of rheumatoid arthritis in patients taking concomitant methotrexate. *Arthritis Rheum* 2003;48:35–45.
86. Van de Putte LBA, Atkins C, Malaise M, et al. Adalimumab (D2E7) monotherapy in the treatment of patients with severely active rheumatoid arthritis. *Arthritis Rheum* 2002;46[Suppl]:S205(abst).
87. Keystone E, Kavanaugh AF, Sharp J, et al. Adalimumab (D2E7), a fully human anti-TNF-α monoclonal antibody, inhibits the progression of structural joint damage in patients with active RA despite concomitant methotrexate therapy. *Arthritis Rheum* 2002;46[Suppl]:S205(abst).
88. Welborne F, Keystone EC, Kivitz A, et al. Adalimumab (D2E7), a fully human anti-TNF-α monoclonal antibody, improved health-related quality of life in patients with active rheumatoid arthritis despite concomitant methotrexate therapy. *Arthritis Rheum* 2002;46[Suppl]:S518(abst).
89. Furst DE, Schiff M, Fleischmann R, et al. Safety and efficacy of adalimumab (D2E7), a fully human anti-TNF-α monoclonal antibody, given in combination with standard antirheumatic therapy: safety trial of adalimumab in rheumatoid arthritis. *Arthritis Rheum* 2002;46[Suppl]:S572(abst).
90. Charles P, Elliott MJ, Davis D, et al. Regulation of cytokines, cytokine inhibitors, and acute-phase proteins following anti-TNF-α therapy in rheumatoid arthritis. *J Immunol* 1999;163:1521–1528.
91. Pittoni V, Bombardieri M, Spinelli FR, et al. Anti-tumour necrosis factor (TNF) α treatment of rheumatoid arthritis (infliximab) selectively down regulates the production of interleukin (IL) 18 but not of IL12 and IL13. *Ann Rheum Dis* 2002;61:723–725.
92. Barrera P, Joosten LAB, den Broeder AA, et al. Effects of treatment with a fully human anti-tumour necrosis factor α monoclonal antibody on the local and systemic homeostasis of interleukin 1 and TNFα in patients with rheumatoid arthritis. *Ann Rheum Dis* 2001;60:660–669.
93. Perkins DJ, St. Clair EW, Misukonis MA, Weinberg JB. Reduction of NOS2 overexpression in rheumatoid arthritis patients treated with anti-tumor necrosis factor α monoclonal antibody (cA2). *Arthritis Rheum* 1998;41:2205–2210.
94. Ulfgren AK, Andersson U, Engström M, et al. Systemic anti-tumor necrosis factor α therapy in rheumatoid arthritis down-regulates synovial tumor necrosis factor α synthesis. *Arthritis Rheum* 2000;43:2391–2396.
95. Tak PP, Taylor PC, Breedveld FC, et al. Decrease in cellularity and expression of adhesion molecules by anti-tumor necrosis factor α monoclonal antibody treatment in patients with rheumatoid arthritis. *Arthritis Rheum* 1996;39:1077–1081.
96. Taylor PC, Peters AM, Paleolog E, et al. Reduction of chemokine levels and leukocyte traffic to joints by tumor necrosis factor α blockade in patients with rheumatoid arthritis. *Arthritis Rheum* 2000;43:38–47.
97. Paleolog EM, Hunt M, Elliott MJ, et al. Deactivation of vascular endothelium by monoclonal anti-tumor necrosis factor α antibody in rheumatoid arthritis. *Arthritis Rheum* 1996;39:1082–1091.
98. Paleolog EM, Young S, Starck AC, et al. Modulation of angiogenic vascular endothelial growth factor by tumor necrosis factor α and interleukin-1 in rheumatoid arthritis. *Arthritis Rheum* 1998;41:1258–1265.
99. Brennan FM, Browne KA, Green PA, et al. Reduction of serum matrix metalloproteinase 1 and matrix metalloproteinase 3 in rheumatoid arthritis patients following anti-tumour necrosis factor-α (cA2) therapy. *Br J Rheumatol* 1997;36:643–650.
100. Ziolkowska M, Kurowska M, Radzikowska A, et al. High levels of osteoprotegerin and soluble receptor activator of nuclear factor κB ligand in serum of rheumatoid arthritis patients and their normalization after anti-tumor necrosis factor α treatment. *Arthritis Rheum* 2002;46:1744–1753.

CHAPTER 33

Anakinra (Interleukin-1 Receptor Antagonist)

William P. Arend and Cem Gabay

Interleukin (IL)-1 mediates inflammation and tissue destruction in rheumatoid arthritis (RA), as well as in other autoimmune and chronic inflammatory diseases. IL-1 receptor antagonist (IL-1Ra) is a naturally occurring structural variant of IL-1 that binds to receptors but does not activate target cells. Thus, IL-1Ra is a competitive inhibitor of receptor binding of IL-1 and functions as an important endogenous antiinflammatory molecule. The therapeutic agent anakinra is identical to human IL-1Ra, with the addition of an extra amino acid (methionine) at the NH_2-terminal end. The daily subcutaneous administration of anakinra has proven efficacious in the treatment of RA, leading both to clinical improvement and to a decrease in cartilage and bone destruction.

PHYSIOLOGY OF INTERLEUKIN-1 AND RECEPTORS

The IL-1 system plays important roles in host defense and in the pathophysiology of RA and of other autoimmune and inflammatory diseases. This family consists of two agonists, IL-1α and IL-1β; a specific antagonist, IL-1Ra; two receptors, IL-1 receptor type I (IL-1RI) and IL-1 receptor type II (IL-1RII); and an IL-1R accessory protein (IL-1RAcP) (Table 33.1) (1). Homeostatic or regulatory mechanisms exist within this family to maintain a balance between proinflammatory and antiinflammatory molecules. When this balance is disturbed, chronic inflammatory diseases, such as RA, may develop. Anakinra represents a unique therapy for this disease, based on the administration of the recombinant human IL-1Ra molecule.

IL-1α and IL-1β are synthesized as 31-kd precursor molecules in the cytoplasm of many human cells (pro–IL-1α and pro–IL-1β), but predominantly in cells of the mononuclear phagocyte system. Most pro–IL-1α in the human is either transported to the nucleus, where it exhibits oncogenic properties, or moves to the plasma membrane, where it may be biologically active. Some IL-1α may be cleaved by a specific enzyme into a 17-kd mature form, found in the microenvironment of cells. In contrast, pro–IL-1β is biologically inactive and is cleaved by a specific enzyme, IL-1β converting enzyme (caspase 1), at the plasma membrane and released extracellularly as a biologically active 17-kd mature form. The precursor forms of both IL-1 agonists lack signal peptides, and the mechanisms of secretion from the cytoplasm of cells remain unclear; however, secretion of mature IL-1β is not necessarily linked to processing.

The two IL-1 receptors are present on many cells and play different roles in biology. IL-1RI possesses a long cytoplasmic domain and is biologically active in inducing intracellular signals after receptor binding by IL-1α or IL-1β. In contrast, the IL-1RII possesses a short cytoplasmic domain and is biologically inactive. The major role of IL-1RII appears to be as an inhibitor of IL-1 either at the plasma membrane or in the fluid phase. IL-1RII on the cell surface may bind IL-1 and prevent binding to IL-1RI. In addition, IL-1RII is enzymatically cleaved from the cell, existing in tissues and in the circulation as a soluble receptor. Soluble IL-1RII in the microenvironment of cells or in body fluids may also bind IL-1, preventing interaction with IL-1RI on cells and, thus, functioning as an IL-1 inhibitor.

After binding of IL-1α or IL-1β to IL-1RI, a second molecule, the IL-1RAcP, is incorporated into the complex on the cell surface. Although IL-1 interacts with IL-1RAcP secondarily, IL-1 does not bind to IL-1RAcP primarily without initial interaction with IL-1RI. However, many investigators would consider IL-1RAcP to be the second chain of the IL-1R. The intracellular domains of both IL-1RI and the IL-1RAcP then initiate a signal transduction pathway involving a series of molecules, including MyD88, IL-1 receptor-associated kinase, tumor necrosis factor (TNF) receptor–associated factor 6, the mitogen-activated protein kinase kinase kinase TAK1, and the inhibitor of κB kinases. The end result is activation of both nuclear factor–κB and AP-1 transcription factors that move to the nucleus and bind to DNA. This cell response leads to transcriptional up-regulation of a variety of proteins, including IL-1α and IL-1β themselves, other cytokines, such as IL-6 and IL-8, matrix metalloproteinases (MMPs), and other inflammatory molecules.

IL-1 plays an important role in mechanisms of host defense and in normal physiology. IL-1 enhances host resistance to pathogens that reside within cells, such as *Mycobacteria*, *Listeria*, and various fungi. IL-1 is also a potent endogenous pyrogen, traveling through the circulation to the brain and inducing a fever response, and, along with IL-6, stimulating synthesis of acute phase proteins in the liver. Physiologic functions of IL-1 include increased neutrophil production and migration into tissues, as well as regulation of both the sleep–wake cycle in the central nervous system and the endometrial cycle in the uterus. Individuals deficient in IL-1 have not been described. However, the cytokine network is sufficiently redundant so that in the possible hereditary absence of IL-1 other cytokines may substitute for critical functions.

INTERLEUKIN-1 RECEPTOR ANTAGONIST AND MECHANISM OF ACTION

The IL-1 family of molecules also includes a specific receptor antagonist, IL-1Ra (Table 33.2) (2,3). This structural variant of

TABLE 33.1. Members of the Interleukin-1 (IL-1) Family

Ligands
  Agonists: IL-1α and IL-1β
  Antagonist: IL-1 receptor antagonist
    Three isoforms (1 secreted and 2 intracellular)
Receptors
  IL-1 receptor type I (biologically active)
  IL-1 receptor type II (biologically inactive)
  IL-1 receptor accessory protein

IL-1 binds to both types of IL-1R but fails to induce intracellular responses. Anakinra is a therapeutic agent created by recombinant DNA technology that is identical to native human IL-1Ra, except for the addition of an NH_2-terminal methionine. The genes for IL-1α, IL-1β, and IL-1Ra are located within a small region on human chromosome 2q14, with the gene structures suggesting an origin by duplication from a primordial IL-1 gene. The proteins of the IL-1 family are also closely related, with 18% amino acid identity between human IL-1α and IL-1Ra, 26% between IL-1β and IL-1Ra, and 22% between the two forms of IL-1. The IL-1 family of molecules also is well conserved across species as, for example, the human molecules exhibit a high degree of activity in the mouse.

IL-1Ra is produced by most of the same cells that make IL-1 in response to a variety of stimuli including adherent immune complexes, bacterial lipopolysaccharide (LPS), leptin, and other cytokines, such as IL-1 itself, IL-4, IL-6, IL-10, IL-13, transforming growth factor β, and granulocyte-macrophage colony-stimulating factors. IL-1Ra is produced in a delayed fashion by most cells, after IL-1, suggesting that an important role for IL-1Ra may be in the immediate regulation of IL-1 effects. Early studies on IL-1 inhibitors; the discovery, purification, and cloning of IL-1Ra; and characterization of receptor binding have all been reviewed (2–4).

IL-1Ra is now known to comprise a family of molecules. The original isoform was a secreted molecule (sIL-1Ra), described as exhibiting IL-1 inhibitory bioactivities, in the urine of a patient with monocytic leukemia (5) and in the supernatant of human monocytes cultured on adherent human immunoglobulin G (6). The purified 17-kd molecule from both sources was subsequently demonstrated to function as a specific receptor antagonist of IL-1 (7,8). Three intracellular isoforms of IL-1Ra have subsequently been described. Intracellular IL-1Ra type 1 (icIL-1Ra1) is created by an alternative transcriptional splice and is synthesized as an 18-kd molecule in the cytoplasm of epithelial cells, endothelial cells, fibroblasts, and monocytes/macrophages (9). icIL-1Ra1 is a major protein in the skin, in the upper and lower respiratory tract, and throughout the gastrointestinal tract from the mouth to the large intestine. The second intracellular isoform, icIL-1Ra2, has been described at the messenger RNA (mRNA) level but may not be translated into a protein *in vivo* (10). icIL-1Ra3 can be created by both alternative transcriptional splicing and by alternative translational initiation and is found as a 16-kd molecule primarily inside hepatocytes and neutrophils (11,12). icIL-1Ra3 is created primarily from the sIL-1Ra complementary DNA (cDNA), and its presence has been described *in vivo* in the liver and in other organs where sIL-1Ra is synthesized.

TABLE 33.2. Anakinra: Recombinant *N*-Methionyl Human Interleukin-1 Receptor Antagonist (IL-1Ra)

Protein originally isolated from human monocyte supernatant
Complementary DNA cloned from a library prepared from immunoglobulin G–induced monocytes
Secreted isoform of IL-1Ra
Addition of an N-terminal methionine to native IL-1Ra
153–amino acid protein, 17.3 kd
Nonglycosylated
Manufactured by recombinant DNA technology

The major role in biology of sIL-1Ra is to inhibit the inflammatory effects of IL-1 in the microenvironment of cells. sIL-1Ra is also synthesized as an acute phase protein by hepatocytes and may be present in the serum in high concentrations in patients with acute and chronic inflammatory diseases, infections, tumors, or postsurgery (13). icIL-1Ra1 binds to IL-1R with equal avidity as IL-1 and sIL-1Ra and may be released from keratinocytes under certain conditions, possibly functioning as an extracellular receptor antagonist. icIL-1Ra3 binds to IL-1R more weakly and has not been described to be released from cells. However, the intracellular isoforms of IL-1Ra may carry out additional roles within cells that do not involve binding to IL-1R; these possible unique functions of icIL-1Ra remain largely uncharacterized.

High concentrations of IL-1Ra are necessary to inhibit the biologic effects of IL-1 *in vitro* and *in vivo* because of the spare receptor effect (14). Most cells are very sensitive to IL-1 and exhibit full biologic responses to occupancy of only a few IL-1RI per cell. Because the numbers of IL-1RI on each cell are in great excess, IL-1Ra must be present in 100-fold or higher concentrations over IL-1 to block the binding of only a few molecules of IL-1. Thus, the use of IL-1Ra for *in vivo* treatment has required administration by intravenous infusion or intraperitoneal injection in experimental animal models of disease, frequent subcutaneous injections in humans, or continuous production after gene therapy studies in animals or humans.

The mechanism of action of IL-1Ra has been determined through studies on receptor binding of the IL-1 ligands. The binding of both IL-1 and IL-1Ra to IL-1RI is mediated by the same structural elements in both molecules (2,3). However, the structural variations in IL-1Ra prevent interaction of the IL-1RAcP molecule with the ligand-receptor complex, leading to a failure of initiation of intracellular responses (Fig. 33.1). Thus,

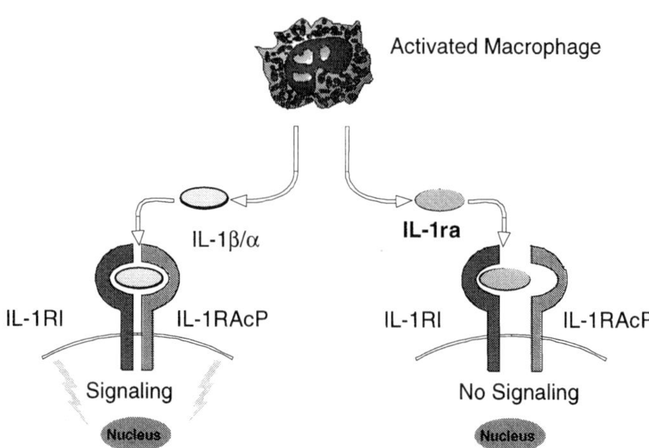

Figure 33.1. Mechanism of action of interleukin-1 receptor antagonist (IL-1Ra). IL-1β and IL-1Ra are produced by macrophages, and both bind with high avidity to IL-1 receptor type I (IL-1RI). IL-1β binding to IL-1RI leads to engagement of the IL-1 receptor accessory protein (IL-1RAcP), resulting in intracellular signaling and cell activation. In contrast, IL-1Ra binding blocks the binding site for IL-1β and prevents engagement of IL-1RAcP. As a result, intracellular signaling and cell activation do not occur. (From Bresnihan B. The prospect of treating rheumatoid arthritis with recombinant human interleukin-1 receptor antagonist. *BioDrugs* 2000;15:87–97, with permission.)

as opposed to the existing TNF-blocking agents that bind TNF in the fluid phase, IL-1Ra exhibits a unique function as a competitive inhibitor of IL-1 receptor binding. IL-1Ra represents the first described naturally occurring receptor antagonist of any cytokine or hormone-like molecule.

Detailed studies have been carried out on the binding of the three members of the IL-1 family to soluble forms of the two IL-1R, and on the relevance of this binding to measurement of these molecules in body fluids (15,16). IL-1β binds more avidly than does IL-1α or IL-1Ra to the soluble IL-1RII, and IL-1Ra binds more avidly to soluble IL-1RI than do the two agonists. Low levels of soluble IL-1RI (1.0–2.5 ng per mL) are present in inflammatory synovial fluids and appear to interfere with quantification of IL-1Ra by enzyme-linked immunosorbent assay. In contrast, high concentrations of soluble IL-1RII (10–20 ng per mL) are present in these synovial fluids and are correlated with IL-1Ra levels. IL-1β protein cannot be detected in these fluids, suggesting that the presence of soluble IL-1RII interferes with this enzyme-linked immunosorbent assay. The combination of soluble IL-1RII and IL-1Ra exhibits additive IL-1 inhibitory effects *in vitro*, whereas the presence of soluble IL-1RI actually reduces the antiinflammatory effects of IL-1Ra. Thus, soluble IL-1RI released *in vivo* may reduce the IL-1 inhibitory effects of endogenously produced IL-1Ra, whereas soluble IL-1RII and IL-1Ra may be additive in blocking the *in vivo* effects of IL-1.

INTERLEUKIN-1 AND INTERLEUKIN-1 RECEPTOR ANTAGONIST IN ANIMAL MODELS OF ARTHRITIS

Abundant evidence indicates an important role for IL-1 in the pathophysiology of RA (2,3,17,18). Studies in animal models of inflammatory arthritis have emphasized the importance of IL-1 in inducing inflammation and tissue destruction. Injections of IL-1 into animal joints have led to reduced proteoglycan synthesis, enhanced proteoglycan degradation, increased release of MMP into the synovial fluid, and enhanced expression of MMP mRNA in both the synovium and cartilage. A single injection of IL-1 into rat joints leads to transient inflammation, but multiple injections of IL-1 lead to a chronic destructive arthritis. Constitutive production of high levels of IL-1β in rabbit knee joints through gene therapy lead to a chronic destructive arthritis exhibiting the multiple pathologic features of RA (19). IL-1 is present in the synovial tissue in many different induced animal models of experimental arthritis, such as collagen-induced arthritis in rats and mice, wherein the presence of IL-1 is correlated with damage to cartilage and bone. Antibodies to IL-1 are effective in preventing both inflammation and tissue destruction in multiple experimental animal models of arthritis. Thus, IL-1 appears to be involved both in the acute inflammatory phase of arthritis in animals as well as in the chronic destructive phase.

Animal studies have also indicated the potency of endogenous and exogenous IL-1Ra in inhibiting arthritis. IL-1Ra blocks the effects of IL-1 on production of prostaglandins and collagenase by explants of bovine cartilage, as well as prostaglandin E_2 production and bone resorption in cultured mouse and rat bones. Administration of antibodies to IL-1Ra exacerbates inflammation and tissue destruction in LPS-induced arthritis in rabbits, indicating the importance of endogenous IL-1Ra production in reducing the severity of arthritis (20). The exogenous administration of IL-1Ra also ameliorates inflammation and tissue destruction in various animal models, including streptococcal cell-wall–induced arthritis in rats and mice (21,22), antigen-induced and collagen-induced arthritis in mice (23,24), and antigen-induced arthritis in rabbits (25). Further studies in collagen-induced arthritis in mice indicate that inhibition of TNF-α with monoclonal antibodies is less effective in ameliorating established arthritis than is IL-1 inhibition with specific monoclonal antibodies or a continuous infusion of IL-1Ra (26). Other work has suggested that complete inhibition of animal models of arthritis requires sustained blood levels of IL-1Ra (27).

The importance of a balance between IL-1 and IL-1Ra is indicated by studies in mice overexpressing IL-1Ra (transgenic mice) and in mice deficient in production of IL-1Ra (knockout mice). Mice transgenic for IL-1Ra exhibit a significant reduction in the incidence and severity of collagen-induced arthritis, whereas knockout mice for IL-1Ra show the opposite pattern (28). Furthermore, IL-1Ra–deficient mice, when bred on a BALB/cA background, spontaneously develop an inflammatory arthritis closely resembling RA (29). During the healing phase of collagen-induced arthritis in mice, icIL-1Ra1 production by synovial cells is greatly enhanced, whereas IL-1β production progressively decreases (30). The production of IL-1Ra by cultured synovial cells from rheumatoid patients with continuously active disease is inadequate in relationship to the levels of IL-1 production (31). These observations all suggest that maintenance of physiologic levels of IL-1Ra may be important in preventing the development or progression of inflammatory arthritis, particularly in the presence of other, as-yet-unknown genes that may predispose to this disease.

Studies in animal models of arthritis also suggest that the combined administration of IL-1Ra with other therapeutic agents may be particularly efficacious. Combination therapy with methotrexate and IL-1Ra give additive or synergistic benefits in adjuvant arthritis in rats (32). Furthermore, the combined blockade of IL-1 and TNF-α using both IL-1Ra and a preparation of soluble TNF receptors leads to greater efficacy in collagen-induced arthritis or adjuvant-induced arthritis in rats than treatment with either agent alone (33,34). The beneficial effects of combined inhibition of both IL-1 and TNF-α are particularly evident when the dose of each agent alone is subtherapeutic. These results suggest that it may be possible to treat patients with RA using combination anticytokine therapy at lower doses that may exhibit less toxicity.

Treatment of inflammatory arthritis through delivery of agents by gene therapy has been thoroughly developed using experimental animal models (35). Local delivery of IL-1Ra using a retroviral vector in an *ex vivo* approach has been successfully adapted in multiple animal models, including collagen-induced arthritis, zymosan-induced arthritis, adjuvant arthritis, and streptococcal cell-wall–induced arthritis. A surprising result is that amelioration of arthritis occurs not only in the treated joint but also in other nearby joints, probably secondary to transfer of the IL-1Ra cDNA via trafficking cells. This observation suggests that treatment of inflammatory arthritis through gene therapy administration to a single joint may benefit multiple joints.

INTERLEUKIN-1 AND INTERLEUKIN-1 RECEPTOR ANTAGONIST IN RHEUMATOID ARTHRITIS

IL-1 is an important proinflammatory cytokine in the pathophysiology of various inflammatory conditions. IL-1 induces several systemic manifestations that can be present in RA patients, such as fever, anemia, anorexia, bone loss, and the increased production of acute phase proteins by the liver (1). However, the local effects of IL-1 may be more important in the pathophysiology of RA (18). The results of many studies strongly suggest that IL-1 is involved in the pathophysiology of arthritis both in early events and in subsequent tissue damage. IL-1 induces the chemotaxis of neutrophils, lymphocytes, and monocytes by increasing the expression of both chemokines and adhesion molecules, enhances the proliferation of fibroblasts leading to the pannus formation, and stimulates the production of prostaglandin E_2. IL-1 also contributes to the destruction of cartilage, bone, and periarticular tissues through effects on both synovial fibroblasts and chondrocytes. The effects of IL-1 on cartilage include an increase in proteoglycan degradation, through inducing the production of neutral MMPs such as collagenase and stromelysin, and a decrease in proteoglycan synthesis by chondrocytes. IL-1 also alters the production of collagen by chondrocytes, decreasing the production of collagen type II, the main constituent of cartilage, and increasing the production of collagen type I. IL-1 stimulates the formation of new blood vessels and, hence, contributes to the development of pannus mass through the release of vascular endothelial growth factor by synovial cells (36).

Periarticular bone loss and bony erosions are typical features of RA. IL-1 has a catabolic effect on bone, primarily through the maturation and activation of osteoclasts. This effect may be mediated in part by up-regulating the expression of receptor activator of nuclear factor–κB ligand, an essential cytokine for osteoclast maturation and activation (37). In addition, IL-1 enhances the stimulatory effect of activated T lymphocytes on osteoclasts (38). IL-1 also stimulates the production of osteoprotegerin, a soluble receptor that binds receptor activator of nuclear factor–κB ligand and inhibits its biologic effect on osteoclasts (39,40). Thus, IL-1 stimulates both an agonist and an antagonist of osteoclast activation. In addition, IL-1 induces osteoclast activation through a receptor activator of nuclear factor–κB ligand–independent pathway.

The results of many studies indicate that endogenous IL-1Ra is produced in human forms of arthritis and may represent an important natural antiinflammatory mechanism. Elevated synovial fluid levels of IL-1Ra are found primarily in RA, although soluble IL-1RI may have obscured accurate measurement of IL-1Ra by enzyme-linked immunosorbent assay (15). Neutrophils may be the major source of IL-1Ra in synovial fluids, although these cells produce relatively less IL-1Ra and more IL-1β than do peripheral blood neutrophils (41,42). Synovial fluid mononuclear cells, as well as synovial tissue macrophages, are also potential sources of IL-1Ra (31). An important antiinflammatory role for endogenous IL-1Ra is suggested by a study that compared the clinical course of knee arthritis in patients with Lyme disease. Patients with high concentrations of synovial fluid IL-1Ra and low concentrations of IL-1β exhibit rapid resolution of acute attacks of arthritis, whereas patients with the reverse pattern of cytokine concentrations have a more protracted course (43). These results suggest either that synovial fluid IL-1Ra is able to penetrate the synovial tissue and counterbalance the proinflammatory effects of IL-1 or that IL-1Ra in the synovial fluid is derived primarily from the tissue.

In the rheumatoid synovium, IL-1Ra mRNA and protein are found primarily in the sublining and perivascular areas and are present at lower levels in the intimal lining layer (44,45). Macrophages cultured from synovial tissue produce primarily sIL-1Ra, whereas synovial fibroblasts are the main source of icIL-1Ra1 (31). However, the production of IL-1Ra *in vitro* by cultured rheumatoid synovial cells is relatively low, in comparison to IL-1. Furthermore, isolated CD14+ synovial macrophages produce much lower amounts of IL-1Ra than do alveolar or *in vitro*–derived macrophages (31). Up to 90% of the cells at the cartilage–pannus interface in the rheumatoid synovium stain for IL-1α, but fewer than 10% of these cells express IL-1Ra protein (44). These observations all indicate that macrophages in the rheumatoid synovium may be relatively poor producers of IL-1Ra.

The production of IL-1Ra has also been investigated in articular chondrocytes and fibroblasts in culture. Chondrocytes produce low amounts of sIL-1Ra in response to IL-1 or to the combination of IL-1 and IL-6 (40). Although relatively weak, the synthesis of IL-1Ra by chondrocytes may be sufficient to exert a protective effect against IL-1–mediated cartilage lesions that occur in RA. Synovial fibroblasts produce both sIL-1Ra and intracellular species of IL-1Ra in response to various cytokines present in rheumatoid joints, including IL-1, TNF-α, and interferon-γ (46–48).

Elevated serum levels of IL-1Ra are found both in adults with RA and in children with juvenile RA. Circulating levels of IL-1Ra are higher in patients with active RA than in those with inactive disease (49). Results from *in vitro* and *in vivo* studies suggest that serum IL-1Ra may be derived primarily from hepatocytes as an acute phase protein in response to stimulation with IL-1β and IL-6 (13,50). Interestingly, RA patients exhibit a lower ratio of IL-1Ra to IL-1β in plasma at both baseline and after surgery, in comparison to patients with osteoarthritis or osteomyelitis (51). Peripheral blood mononuclear cells (PBMCs) from RA patients produce significantly higher amounts of IL-1Ra than do cells from healthy controls. However, the ratios of IL-1 to IL-1Ra produced are higher from rheumatoid cells than from control PBMCs. In addition, this ratio is significantly higher in RA patients with active disease than in patients in remission (52). The results of these studies suggest that a relatively deficient local and systemic production of IL-1Ra, in comparison to that of IL-1, may predispose to the perpetuation of inflammatory mechanisms in the rheumatoid joint, leading to progressive tissue destruction.

Disease-modifying antirheumatic drugs (DMARDs) used in the treatment of RA can influence the ratio of IL-1 to IL-1Ra. PBMCs from RA patients treated with methotrexate produce less IL-1 *in vitro*; this decrease is correlated with clinical improvement (49). Methotrexate has been shown to act as a differentiation factor for monocytic U937 cells, associated with a decrease in IL-1β production and an up-regulation of IL-1Ra release and, thus, modifying favorably the balance between pro- and antiinflammatory mediators (53). Gold sodium thiomalate or auranofin inhibit the production of IL-1 by LPS-stimulated PBMCs and increase the production of IL-1Ra (52).

PHARMACOLOGY OF INTERLEUKIN-1 RECEPTOR ANTAGONIST IN HUMANS

A phase I clinical trial examined the pharmacokinetics and possible consequences of intravenous infusion of IL-1Ra into 25 healthy volunteers (54). Total doses ranging between 1 and 10 mg per kg were administered over 3 hours of continuous infusion. The circulating levels of IL-1Ra were between 3.1 and 28.0 mg per mL at 3 hours. The plasma levels declined rapidly over 9 hours after the infusion, with an initial half-life of 21 minutes and a terminal half-life of 108 minutes. The plasma clearance of IL-1Ra was 2.0 ± 0.3 mg per minute per kg, and less than 3.2% of the administered dose was detected in the urine. These pharmacokinetic characteristics suggest that IL-1Ra is widely distributed in the body after intravenous infusion. In addition, IL-1Ra administration in humans appeared to be safe, as no changes were observed regarding symptoms, complete blood cell count, plasma chemistry, and cortisol levels. PBMC collected after completion of the IL-1Ra infusion produced significantly less IL-6 *ex vivo* than PBMC from saline-injected subjects. This *in vivo* study further documented that IL-1Ra has no agonist effects (54).

The effect of intravenous infusion of IL-1Ra on low-dose endotoxemia was also examined in 14 healthy volunteers. Concurrent to the LPS injections, nine subjects received a 3-hour IL-1Ra infusion, and five were given an infusion of saline.

Endotoxin induced a neutrophilia that was significantly reduced (48%) by the administration of IL-1Ra. The inhibitory effect of LPS on the *ex vivo* mitogen-induced PBMC proliferation was reversed in patients treated with IL-1Ra. In contrast, endotoxin-induced symptoms, such as fever and tachycardia, were unaffected by IL-1Ra, suggesting that cytokines other than IL-1 are involved in the clinical manifestations of gram-negative–induced sepsis (55).

The circulating levels of IL-1Ra were also examined in RA patients receiving a single subcutaneous injection of 0.5, 1.0, 2.0, 4.0, and 6.0 mg per kg. Peak plasma levels of IL-1Ra were detected at 5.9 ± 3.2 hours after injection and averaged between 440 ± 30 and 3,250 ± 370 ng per mL for the 0.5 and 6.0 mg per kg doses, respectively. At 24 hours postinjection, mean plasma concentrations of IL-1Ra were 39 ± 36 and 660 ± 240 ng per mL for the 0.5 and 6.0 mg per kg doses, respectively. There was no accumulation at the low dose but some accumulation at the higher dose. The results of this study indicated that once-daily subcutaneous administration of IL-1Ra provides adequate circulating levels of IL-1Ra for 24 hours (56). Experimental data obtained in the rat after intravenous injection of IL-1Ra showed that the kidney is responsible for 80% of the plasma clearance of IL-1Ra. Because very little IL-1Ra appeared in the urine of subjects after intravenous infusion (10% of the dose administered), it was postulated that IL-1Ra is filtered at the glomeruli, then reabsorbed in the proximal tubules, where it is metabolized (57).

Subjects with end-stage renal failure treated with hemodialysis or continuous ambulatory peritoneal dialysis demonstrated a substantially lower plasma clearance of IL-1Ra (reduction of 86%) and a longer half-life (9.7 ± 3.44 hours) than healthy subjects (5.2 ± 0.4 hours) after intravenous administration. The removal of IL-1Ra by dialysis (both methods) was less than 2.5% of the dose administered, indicating that dialysis has a minimal effect on the pharmacokinetics of IL-1Ra (58). Plasma clearance of IL-1Ra was also decreased in subjects with hepatic dysfunction. However, the decreased plasma clearance correlated with a decrease in estimates of creatinine clearance in this population. Results obtained from 341 RA patients treated with subcutaneous injections of IL-1Ra in a monotherapy clinical trial showed that the plasma clearance was reduced in subjects with lower estimates of creatinine clearance and lower body weight. Mean estimates of circulating half-life of IL-1Ra were 12% lower in women than in men and 9% lower in subjects 65 years of age or older than in younger individuals; again, these differences could be explained by differences in the estimated creatinine clearance.

Interactions between IL-1Ra and a polyethylene glycolylated TNF-α soluble receptor type I (pegsunercept) were examined in a randomized, double-blind, placebo-controlled dose-escalation trial in 16 RA patients. These patients received daily subcutaneous injections of IL-1Ra in combination with different doses of pegsunercept or placebo. The results showed that coadministration of IL-1Ra and pegsunercept did not appear to alter the pharmacodynamics of either agent when compared to each agent administered separately (59).

RESULTS OF CLINICAL TRIALS WITH INTERLEUKIN-1 RECEPTOR ANTAGONIST

Administration of Interleukin-1 Receptor Antagonist in Patients with Sepsis

On the basis of extensive data on the role of IL-1 in the inflammatory response and on the beneficial effect of IL-1Ra in experimental models of septic shock, studies were carried out on the therapeutic use of IL-1Ra in patients with sepsis. These clinical trials were preceded by studies on the levels of IL-1 and IL-1Ra in the circulation of LPS-injected healthy volunteers. Plasma IL-1β levels were first detected at 1 hour after LPS injection, reached a maximum after 2 hours, and decreased during the next 22 hours. In contrast, IL-1Ra concentrations were first detected at 2 hours, peaked at 3 to 6 hours, and slowly declined thereafter. The circulating levels of IL-1Ra after LPS injection were almost 100-fold higher than those of IL-1β and were certainly sufficient to block IL-1 biologic activities.

An initial phase II open-label, placebo-controlled multicenter trial in patients with sepsis syndrome showed that a dose-dependent 28-day survival benefit was associated with IL-1Ra treatment (60). However, subsequent trials with IL-1Ra in patients with sepsis syndrome did not change the overall survival, leading to the discontinuation of these studies (61). Sepsis syndrome in humans is a more complex disease than in experimental animals, and interference in the inflammatory response with cytokine inhibitors may be too late for certain patients with advanced organ dysfunction.

Interleukin-1 Receptor Antagonist As Monotherapy in Patients with Rheumatoid Arthritis

Recombinant human sIL-1Ra (anakinra) has recently been approved for the treatment of RA in the United States and in Europe and is now commercially available as Kineret. IL-1Ra was examined in phase I and II clinical trials in patients with RA. An initial randomized, double-blind study was performed in 172 patients with RA divided into nine different treatment groups. The patients received subcutaneous injections of recombinant IL-1Ra, 20, 70, or 200 mg once, three times, or seven times each week for 3 weeks, followed by a 4-week maintenance phase of once-weekly injections (62). The treatment was well tolerated, the most frequent adverse effect being injection site reactions, reported in 62% of patients and causing 5% to withdraw from the study. Because of the multiple, small treatment groups and the lack of placebo control, it was impossible to draw any firm conclusion concerning efficacy from this first trial. However, the patients receiving the daily injections appeared to exhibit some clinical improvement that was associated with decreased serum levels of C-reactive protein.

A subsequent randomized, double-blind, placebo-controlled multicenter trial was performed in which 472 patients with RA were randomized into four different groups to receive daily subcutaneous injections of placebo or three different doses of IL-1Ra (30, 75, 150 mg) for 24 weeks (63). Any DMARDs previously administered were discontinued for a period of at least 6 weeks before entering patients into the trial. Nonsteroidal antiinflammatory drugs and prednisone (≤10 mg per day) were continued at their previous doses. After 24 weeks, the American College of Rheumatology (ACR) 20% response was achieved by 43% of the patients receiving the largest dose (150 mg per injection) of IL-1Ra, in comparison to 27% of those in the placebo group (Fig. 33.2A). The clinical responses in the 150 mg per day group were superior to the other treatment groups and were significantly better than patients receiving placebo, with respect to a reduction in the number of swollen joints, tender joints, functional disability as assessed by the Health Assessment Questionnaire, erythrocyte sedimentation rate, and C-reactive protein.

A comparison of hand radiographs between baseline and week 24 demonstrated less progression of joint damage among patients receiving the highest dose of IL-1Ra, as compared with the placebo group (63) (Fig. 33.2B). A subsequent evaluation was performed using a scoring system (Genant method) that distinguishes joint space narrowing and the presence of bony erosions. The results of this study showed greater reduction in joint space

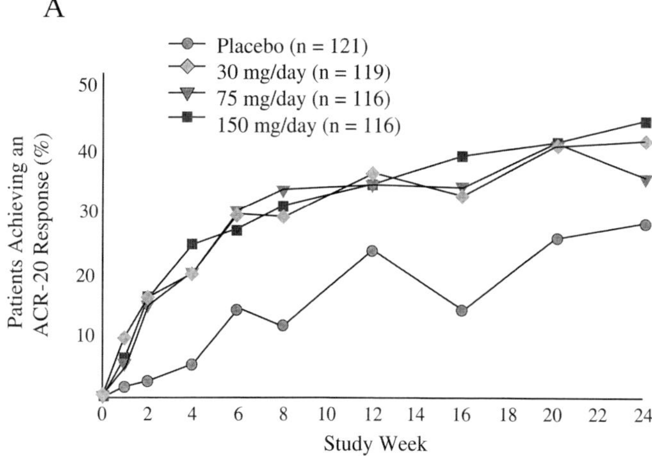

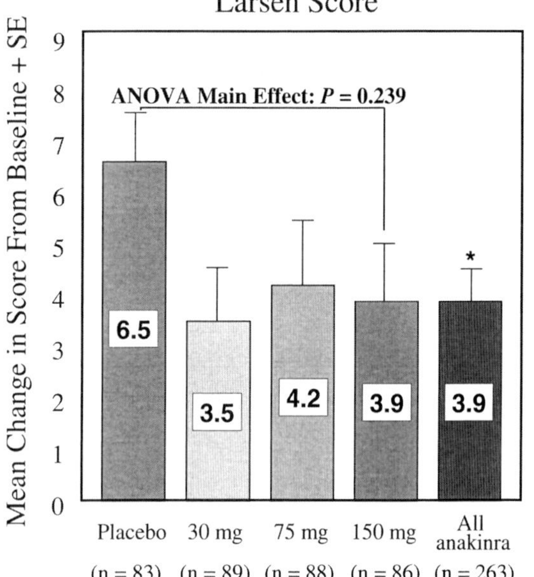

Figure 33.2. Results of a 24-week, double-blind, randomized, placebo-controlled anakinra monotherapy study in patients with rheumatoid arthritis. **A:** The results represent the percentage of patients in each treatment group who achieved the American College of Rheumatology (ACR) 20% response criteria (63). **B:** Evolution of the radiologic signs of structural damage according to Larsen and Genant scores (64). ANOVA, analysis of variance; SE, standard error (*$p < .05$; **$p < .01$, all vs. placebo).

narrowing (58% compared with placebo) than in erosion (38% vs. placebo), raising the possibility that IL-1 inhibition provides greater protection for cartilage than for subchondral bone (64). Although further studies need to be performed to confirm these interesting findings, these results are encouraging for minimizing the tissue destruction that occurs in RA.

Recombinant human IL-1Ra was well tolerated, except for the occurrence of injection site reactions causing a 5% rate of discontinuation in the 150 mg per day group, as compared to 2% in the patients receiving placebo. These reactions were usually mild, appeared within the first 4 weeks of treatment, and tended to regress with time. In conclusion, this study demonstrated that IL-1Ra is effective in reducing the clinical parameters of disease activity in RA patients and is the first biologic agent that demonstrates a beneficial effect on joint damage. A total of 454 patients were screened at baseline and at follow-up for the presence of anti–IL-1Ra antibodies; only one patient in each treatment group developed a positive reaction, whereas none were observed in the placebo group.

A 24-week extension of this study was carried out in which IL-1Ra was given to both active treatment and placebo groups. The results of this extension study showed that administration of IL-1Ra to the placebo patients resulted in clinical improvement and that the patients who previously received IL-1Ra maintained the improvement seen in the first 24-week trial (65). Days of work and domestic activity were quantified in the patients included in this clinical trial. As compared with placebo controls, the results showed that a greater percentage of patients treated with IL-1Ra did not report any missed days of work after 6 and 12 months (66).

Serial synovial biopsies were performed in the 24-week randomized trial of IL-1Ra and in the extension study. The 12 patients included were divided into three groups: placebo (N = 3), IL-1Ra, 30 mg per day (N = 6), and 150 mg per kg (N = 3). Cellular infiltration and expression of adhesion molecules on synovial cells were assessed before and after 24 weeks of IL-1Ra treatment. The results showed a reduction in intimal macrophages, a decrease in subintimal macrophages and lymphocytes, and a down-regulation in expression of E-selectin and vascular cell adhesion molecule-1 on synovial cells in patients receiving 150 mg per day IL-1Ra. The absence of progression in radiologic signs of joint damage seen in some patients correlated with the decrease in intimal macrophages (67). Although this study included only a limited number of patients, the results further demonstrated the beneficial therapeutic effects of IL-1Ra in the rheumatoid synovium, with a possible decrease in joint damage.

Studies on Combination Therapy

There has been a growing interest since the early 1990s in the combined use of several antirheumatic drugs in the treatment of RA, based on the results of studies in experimental animal models of arthritis. The effect of IL-1Ra in combination with methotrexate has been studied recently in a randomized, double-blind, placebo-controlled, multicenter trial (68) in which 419 patients with active RA, despite treatment with methotrexate for 6 consecutive months with stable doses for 3 months or more, were randomized into six groups: placebo or 0.04, 0.1, 0.4, 1.0, or 2.0 mg per kg IL-1Ra administered in a single, daily subcutaneous injection. The primary end point was the proportion of subjects who met the ACR 20% improvement criteria after 24 weeks. Methotrexate was continued, and the mean dose ranged from 16.3 to 17.6 mg per week among the six groups. The results demonstrated that the ACR 20% scores were significantly better in patients who received the combination of methotrexate and 1 mg per kg IL-1Ra than in those who received methotrexate and placebo only (42% vs. 23%) (Fig. 33.3). Subjects treated with IL-1Ra, 0.4 and 2.0 mg per kg, also had higher rates of ACR 20% responses (36% and 35%, respectively) than the placebo group, although these values were not significantly different from the placebo group. The effect of IL-1Ra, according to the time of onset of the ACR 20% response, was already significant at week 4. The percentages of patients who achieved more stringent response criteria, such as ACR 50% and ACR 70% scores, were also significantly higher after treatment with 1 mg per kg and 2 mg per kg IL-1Ra than after treatment with placebo.

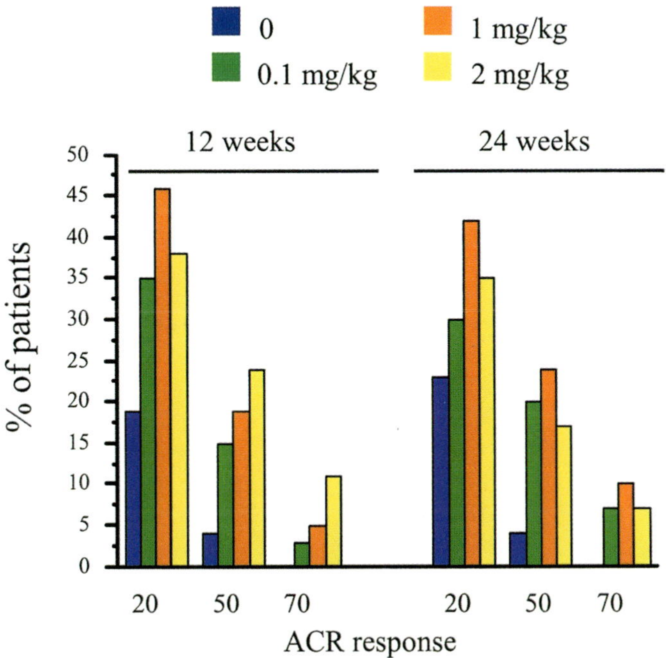

Figure 33.3. Results of a 24-week, multicenter, randomized, double-blind, placebo-controlled trial of anakinra in combination with methotrexate in patients with rheumatoid arthritis (RA). Patients with active RA, despite treatment with methotrexate, were randomized into different groups, including placebo or 0.04, 0.1, 0.4, 1.0, or 2.0 mg/kg anakinra administered in a single, daily subcutaneous injection (68). The results represent the percentage of American College of Rheumatology (ACR) responders in the different treatment groups (results of 0.04 and 0.4 mg/kg groups not shown).

The most common causes of withdrawal from this study were lack of efficacy and adverse events. Most of the withdrawals in the IL-1Ra 1 mg per kg and 2 mg per kg groups were due to injection site reactions (6.8% and 9.7%, respectively). Five patients withdrew from the study because of leukopenia; white blood cell counts returned to normal values after discontinuation of IL-1Ra treatment. Leukopenia was not associated with episodes of infection. No serious infections or deaths were noted during this study. Eight of the 297 tested IL-1Ra–treated patients exhibited anti–IL-1Ra antibodies at some point during the study, but none were positive at more than one time point. One of the 57 tested placebo-treated patients demonstrated anti–IL-1Ra antibodies, and this patient was positive at baseline only. These anti–IL-1Ra antibodies did not neutralize IL-1Ra effects *in vitro* and were not associated with a higher frequency of side effects. The results of this clinical trial indicated that IL-1Ra added to methotrexate was safe and provided a beneficial effect in RA patients exhibiting incomplete responses to methotrexate alone (68) (Table 33.3).

Safety of IL-1Ra was also assessed in a large placebo-controlled population of RA patients seen in clinical practice (69) in which 1,414 patients were randomized to receive either a combination of DMARDs and 100 mg per day IL-1Ra (N = 1,116) or DMARDs and placebo (N = 283). Patients had received stable doses of DMARDs (alone or combination) before inclusion in the study. The rates of serious adverse events were comparable in the two groups. The rate of serious infections was slightly higher in the IL-1Ra than in the placebo group (2.1% vs. 0.4%). However, none of these serious infections resulted in deaths, and none were attributed to opportunistic microorganisms or tuberculosis. These results from a large population indicated that IL-1Ra in association with one DMARD or a combination of DMARDs was safe (69).

The results of studies on combination therapy directed toward both IL-1 and TNF-α in experimental animal models of arthritis indicated additive or synergistic suppression of both inflamma-

TABLE 33.3. Adverse Events and Contraindications to Treatment of Rheumatoid Arthritis with Interleukin-1 Receptor Antagonist (IL-1Ra) and Procedure for Drug Monitoring

Increased occurrence of adverse events
- Injection site reaction (64% vs. 28% in controls).
- Neutropenia (1.8% vs. 0.6% in controls).
- Serious infection (2% vs. <1% in controls). (Patients with asthma may be at higher risk of developing serious infections.)

Contraindications
- Contraindicated in patients with hypersensitivity reaction to anakinra, to any of the materials in the vehicle, or to *Escherichia coli*–derived proteins.
- Should not be initiated in patients with active infections.
- Should not be initiated in patients with neutropenia $<1.5 \times 10^9$/L.
- Live vaccines should not be given in patients treated with anakinra.
- Should not be administered concurrently with a tumor necrosis factor–blocking agent.

Drug monitoring
- History and clinical examination (allergy, injection site reaction, infection).
- Neutrophil counts before the initiation of anakinra, monthly for 3 mo and then quarterly for a period up to 1 yr.
- Serum creatinine in patients with impaired renal function.

Adapted from Cohen S, Hurd E, Cush JJ, et al. Treatment of rheumatoid arthritis with anakinra, a recombinant human interleukin-1 receptor antagonist, in combination with methotrexate. Results of a twenty-four-week, multicenter, randomized, double-blind, placebo-controlled trial. *Arthritis Rheum* 2002;46:614–624.

tion and cartilage damage (33,34). A phase II open trial was recently conducted in 58 RA patients with active disease, despite treatment with etanercept (a fusion protein containing the extracellular domain of TNF receptor p75 and the Fc region of human immunoglobulin G1). These patients received IL-1Ra at a dosage of 1 mg per kg per day, in addition to continuation of etanercept, 25 mg twice weekly, both administered by subcutaneous injection. After 24 weeks, some clinical and biologic parameters of disease activity were ameliorated by the combination of IL-1Ra and etanercept. However, approximately one-third of the patients discontinued this treatment, and 11 out of 58 patients developed serious side effects, including four cases of severe infection (70). Of note, no cases of tuberculosis or opportunistic infections were reported. This increased frequency of infectious adverse events is a concern regarding the possible use of combinations of cytokine inhibitors in human diseases. An objective of future clinical trials will be to define appropriate doses of combinations of cytokine inhibitors that will be effective in the treatment of RA but with minimal toxicity.

A further evaluation of the safety of combined anticytokine therapy was recently carried out in an 8-week, phase I, double-blind, placebo-controlled, dose-escalation clinical trial with IL-1Ra and different dose of pegsunercept (soluble p55 TNF receptors). A total of 16 patients with RA received a combination of 100 mg per kg per day IL-1Ra and placebo or different doses of pegsunercept. Five out of 16 patients with the combination regimen experienced mild infectious episodes, and one patient in the control group reported a mild infection. No serious infectious adverse events were reported (71). These encouraging results should be further confirmed in a larger study with a longer follow-up.

To summarize, IL-1Ra is indicated for the treatment of RA in combination with methotrexate for patients with an incomplete response to methotrexate. Recent data indicate that IL-1Ra is safe when used in combination with other DMARDs. IL-1Ra should be given as a 100-mg, once-daily subcutaneous injection. The current guidelines for use of IL-1Ra in pregnancy, in renal or liver diseases and in other comorbid conditions, are summarized in Table 33.4.

Gene Therapy

The administration of recombinant IL-1Ra to treat human diseases may be limited by the requirement for high amounts of protein to effectively block the effects of IL-1. Thus, investigators have evaluated delivery of IL-1Ra by local gene therapy into arthritic joints, as successfully used in several experimental animal models of arthritis. The results of an initial clinical trial of gene therapy with IL-1Ra in patients with RA demonstrated the successful transfer of *ex vivo* transduced synoviocytes, resulting in abundant intraarticular expression of IL-1Ra mRNA and protein (72). Clinical efficacy could not be assessed in this first clinical trial of gene therapy with IL-1Ra in RA because of its preliminary nature. However, the two important problems of the safety and transient nature of cDNA expression in transduced cells need to be resolved before gene therapy can be further considered in the treatment of RA.

TABLE 33.4. Use of Interleukin-1 Receptor Antagonist (IL-1Ra) in Pregnancy, in Renal or Liver Diseases, and in Other Comorbid Conditions

Not recommended during pregnancy.[a]
Women with childbearing potential should use effective contraception.
Not recommended during lactation.
Plasma clearance of IL-1Ra decreased 70–75% in normal subjects with severe renal failure (estimated creatinine clearance <30 mL/min). No formal studies have been conducted in rheumatoid arthritis patients with impaired renal function.
No formal studies have been conducted in rheumatoid arthritis patients with impaired liver function.
No adjustment of dose is necessary in elderly patients.
Caution should be exercised in patients with preexisting malignancy.
Caution in patients with history of recurrent infection or in chronic illnesses that may predispose to infections.

[a]Animal studies have not demonstrated any harmful effect of IL-1Ra with respect to pregnancy, fetal development, or postnatal outcome.

CONCLUSION

The IL-1 family consists of two agonists (IL-1α and IL-1β), a receptor antagonist (IL-1Ra) with three or more structural variants, two receptors (IL-1RI and IL-1RII), and a receptor accessory protein (IL-1RAcP). Extensive evidence obtained in experimental animal models of arthritis and in clinical trials in patients with RA indicates that IL-1 plays a major role in articular inflammation and in the subsequent events leading to joint damage. The delivery of IL-1Ra in RA by daily subcutaneous injection of recombinant protein was effective in decreasing joint inflammation, as well as in preventing cartilage and bone destruction. The administration of IL-1Ra either alone or in combination with methotrexate has recently been approved for the treatment of patients with RA both in the United States and in Europe. IL-1Ra provides an important addition to other currently used biologic therapies. In addition, additional strategies for targeting IL-1, either at the level of production, in the extracellular space, or in the cell after IL-1 induction of signal transduction pathways, might hold future promise for the treatment of RA.

REFERENCES

1. Dinarello CA. Biologic basis for interleukin-1 in disease. *Blood* 1996;87:2095–2147.
2. Arend WP. Interleukin-1 receptor antagonist. *Adv Immunol* 1993;54:167–227.
3. Arend WP, Malyak M, Guthridge CJ, et al. Interleukin-1 receptor antagonist: role in biology. *Annu Rev Immunol* 1998;16:27–55.
4. Arend WP. Interleukin 1 receptor antagonist. A new member of the interleukin 1 family. *J Clin Invest* 1991;88:1445–1451.
5. Balavoine J-F, de Rochemonteix B, Cruchaud A, et al. Collagenase- and PGE_2-stimulating activity (interleukin-1-like) and inhibitor in urine from a patient with monocytic leukemia. In: Kluger MJ, Oppenheim JJ, Powanda MC, eds. *The physiologic, metabolic, and immunologic actions of interleukin-1.* New York: Alan R. Liss, 1985:429–436.
6. Arend WP, Joslin FG, Massoni RJ. Effects of immune complexes on production by human monocytes of interleukin 1 or an interleukin 1 inhibitor. *J Immunol* 1985;134:3868–3875.
7. Seckinger P, Lowenthal JW, Williamson K, et al. A urine inhibitor of interleukin 1 activity that blocks ligand binding. *J Immunol* 1987;139:1546–1549.
8. Arend WP, Joslin FG, Thompson RC, et al. An IL-1 inhibitor from human monocytes. Production and characterization of biologic properties. *J Immunol* 1989;143:1851–1858.
9. Haskill S, Martin G, Van Le L, et al. cDNA cloning of an intracellular form of the human interleukin 1 receptor antagonist associated with epithelium. *Proc Natl Acad Sci U S A* 1991;88:3681–3685.
10. Muzio M, Polentarutti N, Sironi M, et al. Cloning and characterization of a new isoform of the interleukin 1 receptor antagonist. *J Exp Med* 1995;182:623–628.
11. Malyak M, Guthridge JM, Hance KR, et al. Characterization of a low molecular weight isoform of IL-1 receptor antagonist. *J Immunol* 1998;161:1997–2003.
12. Malyak M, Smith MF Jr., Abel AA, et al. The differential production of three forms of IL-1 receptor antagonist by human neutrophils and monocytes. *J Immunol* 1998;161:2004–2010.
13. Gabay C, Smith MF Jr., Eidlen D, et al. Interleukin 1 receptor antagonist (IL-1ra) is an acute phase protein. *J Clin Invest* 1997;99:2930–2940.
14. Arend WP, Welgus HG, Thompson RC, et al. Biological properties of recombinant human monocyte-derived interleukin 1 receptor antagonist. *J Clin Invest* 1990;85:1694–1697.
15. Arend WP, Malyak M, Smith MF Jr., et al. Binding of IL-1α, IL-1β, and IL-1 receptor antagonist by soluble IL-1 receptors and levels of soluble IL-1 receptors in synovial fluids. *J Immunol* 1994;153:4766–4774.
16. Burger D, Chicheportiche R, Giri JG, et al. The inhibitory activity of human interleukin-1 receptor antagonist is enhanced by type II interleukin-1 soluble receptor and hindered by type I interleukin-1 soluble receptor. *J Clin Invest* 1995;96:38–41.

17. Arend WP, Dayer J-M. Cytokines and cytokine inhibitors or antagonists in rheumatoid arthritis. *Arthritis Rheum* 1990;33:305–315.
18. Arend WP, Dayer J-M. Inhibition of the production and effects of interleukin-1 and tumor necrosis factor α in rheumatoid arthritis. *Arthritis Rheum* 1995;38:151–160.
19. Ghivizzani SC, Kang R, Georgescu HL, et al. Constitutive intra-articular expression of human IL-1β following gene transfer to rabbit synovium produces all major pathologies of human rheumatoid arthritis. *J Immunol* 1997;159:3604–3612.
20. Fukumoto T, Matsukawa A, Ohkawara S, et al. Administration of neutralizing antibody against rabbit IL-1 receptor antagonist exacerbates lipopolysaccharide-induced arthritis in rabbits. *Inflamm Res* 1996;45:479–485.
21. Schwab JH, Anderle SK, Brown RR, et al. Pro- and antiinflammatory roles of interleukin-1 in recurrence of bacterial wall-induced arthritis in rats. *Infect Immun* 1991;59:4436–4442.
22. Kuiper S, Joosten LAB, Bendele AM, et al. Different roles of tumour necrosis factor α and interleukin 1 in murine streptococcal cell wall arthritis. *Cytokine* 1998;10:690–702.
23. Wooley PH, Whalen JD, Chapman DL, et al. The effect of an interleukin-1 receptor antagonist protein on type II collagen-induced arthritis in mice. *Arthritis Rheum* 1993;36:1305–1314.
24. van Lent FLEM, van de Loo FAJ, Holthuysen AEM, et al. Major role for interleukin 1 but not tumor necrosis factor in early cartilage damage in immune complex arthritis in mice. *J Rheumatol* 1995;22:2250–2258.
25. Arner EC, Harris RR, diMeo TM, et al. Interleukin-1 receptor antagonist inhibits proteoglycan breakdown in antigen induced but not polycation induced arthritis in the rabbit. *J Rheumatol* 1995;22:1338–1346.
26. Joosten LAB, Helsen MMA, van de Loo FAJ, et al. Anticytokine treatment of established type II collagen-induced arthritis in DBA/1 mice. *Arthritis Rheum* 1996;39:797–809.
27. Bendele A, McAbee T, Sennello G, et al. Efficacy of sustained blood levels of interleukin-1 receptor antagonist in animal models of arthritis. *Arthritis Rheum* 1999;42:498–506.
28. Ma Y, Thornton S, Boivin GP, et al. Altered susceptibility to collagen-induced arthritis in transgenic mice with aberrant expression of interleukin-1 receptor antagonist. *Arthritis Rheum* 1998;41:1798–1805.
29. Horai R, Daijo S, Tanioka H, et al. Development of chronic inflammatory arthropathy resembling rheumatoid arthritis in interleukin 1 receptor antagonist-deficient mice. *J Exp Med* 2000;191:313–320.
30. Gabay C, Marinova-Mutachieva L, Williams RO, et al. Increased production of intracellular interleukin-1 receptor antagonist type I in the synovium of mice with collagen-induced arthritis. A possible role in resolution of arthritis. *Arthritis Rheum* 2001;44:451–462.
31. Firestein GS, Boyle DL, Yu C, et al. Synovial interelukin-1 receptor antagonist and interelukin-1 balance in rheumatoid arthritis. *Arthritis Rheum* 1994;37:644–652.
32. Bendele A, Sennello G, McAbee T, et al. Effects of interleukin 1 receptor antagonist alone and in combination with methotrexate in adjuvant arthritic rats. *J Rheumatol* 1999;26:1225–1229.
33. Bendele A, Chlipala ES, Scherrer J, et al. Combination benefit of treatment with the cytokine inhibitors interleukin-1 receptor antagonist and PEGylated soluble tumor necrosis factor receptor type I in animal models of rheumatoid arthritis. *Arthritis Rheum* 2000;43:2648–2659.
34. Feige U, Hu Y-L, Campagnuolo G, et al. Anti-interleukin-1 and anti-tumor necrosis factor-α synergistically inhibit arthritis in Lewis rats. *Cell Mol Life Sci* 2000;57:1457–1470.
35. Evans CH, Ghivizzani SC, Kang R, et al. Gene therapy for rheumatic diseases. *Arthritis Rheum* 1999;42:1–16.
36. Paleolog EM, Young S, Stark AC, et al. Modulation of angiogenic vascular endothelial growth factor by tumor necrosis factor alpha and interleukin-1 in rheumatoid arthritis. *Arthritis Rheum* 1998;41:1258–1265.
37. Hofbauer LC, Heufelder AE. The role of osteoprotegerin and receptor activator of nuclear factor κB ligand in the pathogenesis and treatment of rheumatoid arthritis. *Arthritis Rheum* 2001;4:253–259.
38. Horwood NJ, Kartsogiannis V, Quinn JMW, et al. Activated T cells support osteoclast formation in vitro. *Biochem Biophys Res Commun* 1999;265:144–150.
39. Hofbauer LC, Lacey DL, Dunstan CR, et al. Interleukin-1β and tumor necrosis factor-α, but not interleukin-6, stimulate osteoprotegerin ligand gene expression in human osteoblastic cells. *Bone* 1999;25:255–259.
40. Palmer G, Guerne P-A, Mezin F, et al. Production of interleukin-1 receptor antagonist by human articular chondrocytes. *Arthritis Res* 2002;4:226–231.
41. Malyak M, Swaney RE, Arend WP. Levels of synovial fluid interleukin-1 receptor antagonist in rheumatoid arthritis and other arthropathies. Potential contribution from synovial fluid neutrophils. *Arthritis Rheum* 1993;36:781–789.
42. Malyak M, Smith Jr MF, Abel AA, et al. Peripheral blood neutrophil production of interleukin-1 receptor antagonist and interleukin-1β. *J Clin Immunol* 1994;14:20–30.
43. Miller LC, Lynch EA, Isa S, et al. Balance of synovial fluid IL-1β and IL-1 receptor antagonist and recovery from Lyme arthritis. *Lancet* 1993;341:146–148.
44. Deleuran BW, Chu CQ, Field M, et al. Localization of interleukin-1 alpha, type 1 interleukin-1 receptor and interleukin-1 receptor antagonist in the synovial membrane and cartilage/pannus junction in rheumatoid arthritis. *Br J Rheumatol* 1992;31:801–809.
45. Firestein GS, Berger AE, Tracey DE, et al. IL-1 receptor antagonist protein production and gene expression in rheumatoid arthritis and osteoarthritis synovium. *J Immunol* 1992;149:1054–1062.
46. Martel-Pelletier J, McCollum R, Pelletier J-P. The synthesis of IL-1 receptor antagonist (IL-1ra) by synovial fibroblasts is markedly increased by cytokines TNF-alpha and IL-1. *Biochim Biophys Acta* 1993;1175:302–305.
47. Krzesicki RF, Hatfield CA, Bienkowski MJ, et al. Regulation of expression of IL-1 receptor antagonist protein in human synovial and dermal fibroblasts. *J Immunol* 1993;150:4008–4018.
48. Seitz M, Loetscher P, Dewald B, et al. Production of interleukin-1 receptor antagonist, inflammatory chemotactic proteins, and prostaglandin E by rheumatoid and osteoarthritic synoviocytes. Regulation by IFN-γ and IL-4. *J Immunol* 1994;152:2060–2065.
49. Seitz M, Loetcher P, Dewald B, et al. Interleukin 1 (IL-1) receptor antagonist, soluble tumor necrosis factor receptors, IL-1β, and IL-8—markers of remission in rheumatoid arthritis during treatment with methotrexate. *J Rheumatol* 1996;23:1512–1516.
50. Gabay C, Gigley JP, Sipe J, et al. Production of interleukin-1 receptor antagonist by hepatocytes is regulated as an acute-phase protein in vivo. *Eur J Immunol* 2001;31:490–499.
51. Chikanza IC, Roux-Lombard P, Dayer J-M, et al. Dysregulation of the in vivo production of interleukin-1 receptor antagonist in patients with rheumatoid arthritis. *Arthritis Rheum* 1995;38:642–648.
52. Shingu M, Fujikawa Y, Wada T, et al. Increased IL-1 receptor antagonist (IL-1ra) production and decreased IL-1β/IL-1ra ratio in mononuclear cells from rheumatoid arthritis patients. *Br J Rheumatol* 1995;4:24–30.
53. Seitz M, Zwicker M, Loetscher P. Effects of methotrexate on differentiation of monocytes and production of cytokine inhibitors by monocytes. *Arthritis Rheum* 1998;41:2032–2038.
54. Granowitz EV, Porat R, Mier JW, et al. Pharmacokinetics, safety and immunomodulatory effects of human recombinant interleukin-1 receptor antagonist in healthy humans. *Cytokine* 1992;4:353–360.
55. Granowitz EV, Porat R, Mier JW, et al. Hematologic and immunomodulatory effects of an interleukin-1 receptor antagonist coinfusion during low-dose endotoxinemia in healthy humans. *Blood* 1993;82:2985–2990.
56. Lebsack ME, Bloedow DC, Paul CC, et al. Plasma levels of interleukin-1 receptor antagonist following subcutaneous injection in patients with rheumatoid arthritis. *Clin Pharmacol Ther* 1992;192(abst).
57. Kim D-C, Reitz B, Carmichael DF, et al. Kidney as a major clearance organ for recombinant human interleukin-1 receptor antagonist. *J Pharma Sci* 2002;84:575–580.
58. Yang B, Baughman S, Sullivan JT. The kidney is the major organ of elimination of Kineret (anakinra). *Ann Rheum Dis* 2002;61[Suppl I]:203(abst).
59. Martin SW, Nguyen L, Stouch BJ, et al. Pharmacokinetics (PK) of anakinra and PEGylated soluble tumor necrosis factor receptor type I (pegsunercept) were not altered after combination treatment in subjects with rheumatoid arthritis (RA). *Ann Rheum Dis* 2002;61[Suppl I]:205(abst).
60. Fisher CJ Jr., Slotman GJ, Opal SM, et al. Initial evaluation of human recombinant interleukin-1 receptor antagonist in the treatment of sepsis syndrome: a randomized, open-label, placebo-controlled multicenter trial. *Crit Care Med* 1994;22:12–21.
61. Fisher CJ, Dhainaut J-F, Opal SM, et al. Recombinant human interleukin-1 receptor antagonist in the treatment of patients with sepsis syndrome. Results from a randomized, double-blind, placebo-controlled trial. *JAMA* 1994;271:1836–1843.
62. Campion GV, Lebsack ME, Lookabaugh J, et al. Dose-range and dose-frequency study of recombinant human interleukin-1 receptor antagonist in patients with rheumatoid arthritis. *Arthritis Rheum* 1996;39:1092–1101.
63. Bresnihan B, Alvaro-Gracia JM, Cobby M, et al. Treatment of rheumatoid arthritis with recombinant human interleukin-1 receptor antagonist. *Arthritis Rheum* 1998;41:2196–2204.
64. Jiang Y, Genant HK, Watt I, et al. A multicenter, double-blind, dose-ranging, randomized, placebo-controlled study of recombinant human interleukin-1 receptor antagonist in patients with rheumatoid arthritis. *Arthritis Rheum* 2000;43:1001–1009.
65. Bresnihan B, Newmark RD, Robbins S, et al. Anakinra reduces the rate of joint destruction after 1 year of treatment in a randomized controlled cohort of patients with rheumatoid arthritis. *Ann Rheum Dis* 2001;60[Suppl I]:168.
66. Bresnihan B, Chan WW, Woolley JM. Productivity improvement in patients with rheumatoid arthritis receiving anakinra treatment. *Ann Rheum Dis* 2002;61[Suppl I]:182(abst).
67. Cunnane G, Madigan A, Murphy E, et al. The effects of treatment with interleukin-1 receptor antagonist on the inflamed synovial membrane in rheumatoid arthritis. *Rheumatology* 2001;40:62–69.
68. Cohen S, Hurd E, Cush JJ, et al. Treatment of rheumatoid arthritis with anakinra, a recombinant human interleukin-1 receptor antagonist, in combination with methotrexate. Results of a twenty-four-week, multicenter, randomized, double-blind, placebo-controlled trial. *Arthritis Rheum* 2002;46:614–624.
69. Fleishman R, Tesser J, Schechtman J, et al. A safety trial of anakinra: recombinant interleukin-1 receptor antagonist (IL-1ra), in a large, placebo-controlled heterogeneous population of patients with rheumatoid arthritis. *Arthritis Rheum* 2001;44:S84(abst).
70. Schiff MH, Bulpitt K, Weaver AA, et al. Safety of combination therapy with anakinra and etanercept in patients with rheumatoid arthritis. *Arthritis Rheum* 2001;44:S83(abst).
71. Caldwell JR, Offenberg H, Furst D, et al. A phase I safety study of combination treatment with pegylated soluble tumor necrosis factor receptor type I (PEG sTNF-RI) and anakinra (interleukin-1 receptor antagonist, IL-1ra) in patients with rheumatoid arthritis. *Ann Rheum Dis* 2002;61[Suppl I]:186(abst).
72. Ghivizzani SC, Kang R, Muzzonigro T, et al. Gene therapy for arthritis treatment of the first three patients. *Arthritis Rheum* 1997;40:S223(abst).

CHAPTER 34

Staphylococcal Protein A Columns

Grant W. Cannon and Allen D. Sawitzke

Rheumatoid arthritis (RA) is characterized by multiple abnormalities of the immune system (1). Considerable focus has recently been directed at the abnormalities in cytokine production and their regulation through macrophage activities and T-cell functions. In addition to these important facets of the disease, B-cell abnormalities and autoantibodies, such as rheumatoid factor (RF), have long been recognized in RA (1). Although the removal of immunoglobulins (Igs) or the selective removal of RF, or both, has been hypothesized as a potential treatment for RA, results with plasmapheresis were discouraging (2–4).

The gram-positive bacteria *Staphylococcus aureus* (*S. aureus*) produces a surface protein designated *Staphylococcal Protein A* (SpA). SpA binds to Igs (5,6). Columns containing fixed SpA were developed on the hypothesis that the removal of Igs from patients affected by autoimmune diseases via extracorporeal pheresis of plasma over the SpA column could provide clinical benefit. This methodology was initially approved for the treatment of refractory immune thrombocytopenia purpura (ITP) (7–11) and was subsequently approved for the treatment of RA (11–14).

Although the clinical efficacy of SpA column therapy has been documented in a double-blind sham-controlled clinical trial, the mechanism of action of this therapy has not been clearly established. This chapter reports the clinical experience of extracorporeal treatment of RA patients with SpA columns and the possible mechanisms by which this therapy may act in RA patients.

STAPHYLOCOCCAL PROTEIN A

A description of the physical and immunologic characteristics of SpA is important in understanding the rationale for the development of the SpA column treatment and exploring potential mechanisms of actions for this therapy. The most important factors are the binding of SpA to Ig, the function of SpA as a B-cell superantigen, and the potential for SpA to induce alterations in lymphocyte populations, in their regulation, or in both (Table 34.1).

Physical Characteristics

SpA is a 42-kd membrane protein produced by *S. aureus* (6). The SpA gene has been cloned and sequenced (15,16). The protein is encoded by a single gene to produce a single polypeptide chain composed of six domains (17). Five Ig-binding domains are external to the cell wall and are named *C*, *B*, *A*, *D*, and *E*, starting from the cell wall (16,18,19). Each of these domains is 7 kd (5), with 56 to 61 amino acids and more than 80% homology to each other at a protein level (6). Structural studies have determined tertiary configurations for certain components of the SpA molecule (20–22). The transmembrane domain is the X domain at the carboxyl terminus of the molecule (16,18).

The processing and purification of SpA is affected by the means used to isolate the protein. If surface cleavage procedures are used, only the extra membrane portions of the protein may be collected (5,23). Another complication in evaluating SpA properties has been the potential for contamination of some SpA preparations with other *S. aureus* products, which can include enterotoxins capable of acting as T-cell superantigens (24–27). Although SpA used in commercially available SpA columns for treatment of RA and autoimmune diseases are free from such contaminants, some studies may attribute effects to SpA, which are, in fact, the result of other *S. aureus* products (28).

Although SpA may not play any apparent role in metabolic functions of *S. aureus*, SpA is produced by virtually every clinical isolate of *S. aureus* (6). Although not involved in fundamental biologic pathways, SpA appears to enhance the virulence of *S. aureus* (29). SpA production by *S. aureus* may actually be increased in response to infection, as suggested by the induction of SpA production in hypoxic conditions similar to those within an infectious environment (6). Mechanisms through which SpA may act to influence host immune responses are discussed later.

Binding to Immunoglobulin

SpA has two specific and different sites for binding to Ig, one for the Fab and the other for Fcγ. The two SpA binding sites are structurally and functionally unique. The distinct nature of these binding sites is confirmed by the noncompetitive nature for Fab and Fcγ binding, even within a single domain (30,31), and by recent data demonstrating different structural features favoring either Fab or Fcγ binding. Furthermore, SpA can be chemically altered to produce a modified SpA that will only bind to the Fab component of Ig without any Fcγ binding (32), thus demonstrating site specificity.

The Fab binding of SpA occurs to the V_H region of 10% to 50% of human antibodies and involves multiple antibody classes, including IgM, IgA, IgG, and IgE (33–37). In humans, the binding is restricted to the V_HIII gene family (20,21). Similar restriction in antibody binding is found in mice with a limita-

TABLE 34.1. Possible Mechanisms of Action for Extracorporeal Pheresis Therapy with Staphylococcal Protein A (SpA) Columns

Properties of SpA
- Binding to immunoglobulin
- Binding to circulating immune complexes
- Activation of complement
- B-cell superantigen
- Selective depletion of V_HIII-bearing lymphocytes (via superantigen function)

Possible actions of SpA column extracorporeal pheresis therapy
- Current evidence suggests minimal removal of immunoglobulins, circulating immune complexes, or rheumatoid factor.
- Small amounts of SpA may enter the circulation during the pheresis procedure.
- Exact mechanism of action remains unknown.

tion of binding to the V_HIII gene family (38). The binding of SpA to the Fab portion of the V_H regions is not associated with any alteration of the binding of the antibody to its specific ligand (39), confirming that the Fab binding site for SpA does not involve the traditional peptide antigen binding sites (40). Studies to identify the specific sites on the Fab fragment that bind SpA suggest that tertiary structure or multiple V_HIII binding sites, or both, are involved in interactions with SpA (6,41).

The Fcγ binding involves the CH2-CH3 regions of IgG subtypes 1, 2, and 4 and the IgG subtype 3 that bears the Gm3(s+) allotype (19,23,42,43). This binding site has been used extensively for Ig detection and purification (6). In addition, it has been shown that this site binds to circulating immune complexes and can then result in activation of complement (44). Although the binding of SpA to the Fcγ site of Igs has been a useful tool for the purification of Igs, its functional importance is less clear (5). However, the presence of two unique binding sites provides for multiple, potential SpA host interactions.

Immunologic Actions of Staphyloccocal Protein A Columns

SpA is a B-cell superantigen (6,45,46). Superantigens are characterized by their ability to activate large numbers of lymphocytes (generally >5% of the host's entire population) (45) through binding to immunologically conserved sites other than the specific antigen binding site. Conventional peptide antigens function through the binding of an antigen to an antigen-specific binding site, resulting in activation of less than 0.01% of the lymphocyte pool. As described earlier, SpA binds to Igs at two binding sites. The Fab binding results in the activation of large numbers of B cells and, in clonal deletion, through apoptosis, as is described later. The B-cell binding is not without specificity, as only cells with V_HIII families of Ig are recognized. Most typical T-cell superantigens activate B cells through T-cell–dependent bridge formation (47). Some, such as the *Mycoplasma arthritidis* mitogen, are potent stimulators of Ig production, especially of polyvalent antigens, suggesting a non–T-cell–dependent mechanism (48).

In murine models, *in vivo* SpA infusion is associated with specific B-cell depletion of lymphocytes analogous to the human V_HIII family. The infusion of SpA into neonatal or adult mice results in a decrease in SpA binding of mature B cells within 16 hours (6), with a continued decrease over the next 3 days, resulting in an ultimate loss of more than 80% of mature splenic, peritoneal, and bone marrow SpA-reactive B-cell subsets. No impact of SpA infusion was seen in T cells or macrophages in these murine models. The relevance of these findings to human rheumatic disease or the mechanisms of action of SpA, or both, is currently unknown.

Because the SpA molecule contains two bindings sites, the potential exists for SpA to cross-link surface B-cell receptors. This cross-linking can activate complement (49). Increases in C3a, C4a, and C5a are observed in patients after pheresis with SpA columns (44). These increases in complement fragments are likely based on the binding properties of SpA and not on the column, as it is not seen in sham-pheresis–treated patients (50). In addition, complement modification of SpA may allow interactions between the complement receptor CD21 and the B-cell receptor complex. The overall effect of these interactions is the potential for enhanced cellular activation (6). The activation could produce regulatory cytokines, pathogenic antibodies, idiotypic regulatory antibodies, or clonal deletion of pathogenic cell lines. This possibility may occur because not all B cells are activated by SpA. For example, B cells bearing V_HIII are preferentially activated by SpA, and evidence for a role of this population of B cells in RF production and RA has been shown (47). Similarly, a role for Fc receptors in RA has long been postulated and has garnered some support from genetic studies showing association between this disease and specific polymorphisms of the Fc receptor (48). Normally, binding of FcγRII and B-cell antigen receptor results in down-regulation of the B-cell activities. Thus, SpA may have a regulatory role expressed through its Fc binding interaction as well, but this possibility has not been examined.

These data suggest that, in addition to the simple binding property of SpA to Ig, SpA is able to impact immune function through B-cell superantigenic functions, resulting in alterations of lymphocyte function, complement activation, and, ultimately, depletion of SpA reactive cells.

Staphylococcal Protein A Columns

Two types of SpA columns have been used in the treatment of autoimmune diseases. The column approved for the treatment of RA binds SpA to an inert silica matrix (Prosorba) (11). This device is the only SpA column approved by the U.S. Food and Drug Administration (FDA) for the treatment of RA (11). A second column uses SpA coupled to agarose beads (Sepharose; Immunosorba) (5). This SpA column system has not been systematically evaluated for the treatment of RA and is not approved for treatment of RA patients in the United States.

Possible Mechanisms of Action

As stated earlier, the initial hypothesis for the use of SpA columns was their potential to remove Ig from RA patients. Several lines of evidence suggest that this action does not explain the observed clinical efficacy with this therapy. The observations discussed below are from experience with the use of the inert silica matrix (Prosorba) column. It is recognized that the agarose beads (Sepharose; Immunosorba) system may be more effective at removing Ig than the silica matrix (Prosorba) system (5). The clinical trials of RA demonstrate efficacy with use of the silica matrix (Prosorba) system (12–14). Arguments against the removal of Ig or RF, or both, as the mechanism of action for this therapy are discussed below (Table 34.1).

The first observation suggesting that the removal of Ig is not the mechanism through which SpA columns provide their clinical efficacy is that the volume of plasma exposed to the SpA column during a single pheresis episode is generally less than 1,250 cc, only a fraction of total plasma volume (11). The second finding is that the amount of Ig removed by a single pheresis procedure averages only 462 g (50), again, a small fraction representing only approximately 1.5% of a patient's total serum Ig during each treatment. The third observation is that the measured serum Ig levels and RF levels in patients treated with SpA columns are not changed from baseline and, in some cases, actually increase during therapy (5,12). The preceding observations must also be considered in light of the other methods for Ig removal, such as plasmapheresis, which have been proven to reduce Ig levels and yet have not had a significant impact on RA disease activity (2–4). These findings suggest that the removal of Ig is not the means through which the SpA column provides its clinical benefit.

SpA has other potential effects in addition to Ig binding. As discussed above, the superantigen activity and modulation of lymphocyte population can be exerted by small quantities of SpA. *In vitro* studies have demonstrated that SpA can be released from silica matrix (Prosorba) columns on exposure to plasma and serum (51). The exact mechanism for this process is unknown but may involve proteolytic activity of the human serum or plasma used in these experiments, as the release of SpA can be decreased after treatment of the system with protease inhibitors. The amount of SpA released in these experiments was used to predict a potential release of 1.3 μg SpA per kg or approximately 100 μg (51). Mouse studies of *in vivo* SpA activity have generally used injections of 100 μg SpA per mouse (46). An evaluation of ITP patients treated with SpA columns showed that 1 hour after the column treatment SpA was detectable in the patients' serum, with a mean concentration of 4 μg per mL and levels as high as 9 μg per mL noted (51). Of interest, the SpA level in serum did not correlate with clinical response outcomes (51). The amount of SpA released into RA patients is unknown. However, the potential exists that SpA columns may exert their effects by the introduction of SpA into RA patients. However, this observation will require significant work to determine if SpA release into the circulation accounts for its therapeutic effects.

CLINICAL TRIALS WITH STAPHYLOCOCCAL PROTEIN A

Uncontrolled experience and controlled trials have both reported clinical improvement in the subjective and objective measures of RA with the use of SpA columns (12–14). SpA columns have been approved for the treatment of RA patients with specific treatment guidelines (Table 34.2) and with contraindications, which are as follows:

TABLE 34.2. Dosage and Administration of Staphylococcal Protein A (SpA)

Dosage
- The SpA column (Prosorba) approved for the treatment of rheumatoid arthritis (RA) contains approximately 200 mg of SpA bound covalently to 123 ± 2 g of an inert silica matrix contained within a 300-mL polycarbonate housing.

Procedure
- The use of the SpA column in RA patients involves the following steps:
  - The column must be primed with saline and heparin.
  - Two venous access sites are established.
  - Blood from the patient is separated using the apheresis apparatus and plasma passed over the SpA column.
  - 1,250 ± 250 mL of plasma is passed over the SpA column over the course of the procedure.
  - Effluent plasma is reconstituted with red cells and returned to the patient.
  - During the procedure, the patient should have vital signs monitored every 15 min.
  - The patient should be observed for 30–60 min after completion of the procedure.

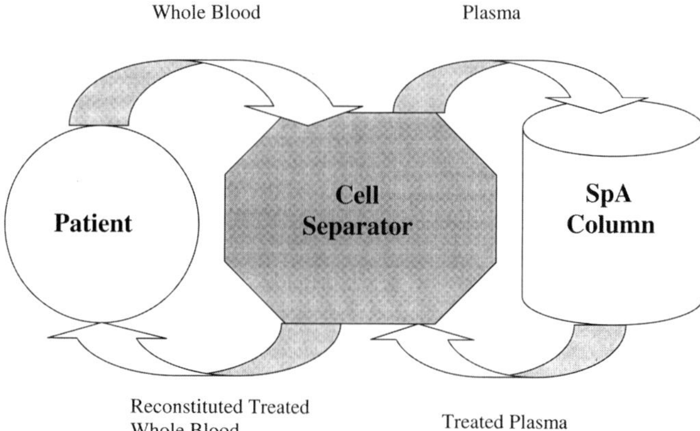

Figure 34.1. Extracorporeal pheresis therapy with a staphylococcal protein A (SpA) column.

- Treatment with angiotensin converting enzyme inhibitors (72-hour withdrawal period required before therapy).
- Inability to tolerate apheresis procedures, including prior hypersensitivity associated with therapeutic apheresis.
- Conditions that could be harmed by acute fluid shifts, such as congestive heart failure, impaired renal function, hypotension, or vascular disease.
- Systemic infection.
- Hypercoagulable state.
- Anticoagulation therapy.
- Inability to tolerate anticoagulation associated with apheresis procedure.
- Severe anemia.
- Inadequate vascular access.
- Safety has not been established in subjects younger than 18 years of age or in pregnancy.

The use of SpA columns involves the extracorporeal pheresis with SpA columns (Fig. 34.1). The approval was based on uncontrolled and controlled clinical trials in RA patients. These studies have reported consistent efficacy outcomes (Fig. 34.2) and similar adverse event experience (Table 34.3). In addition to

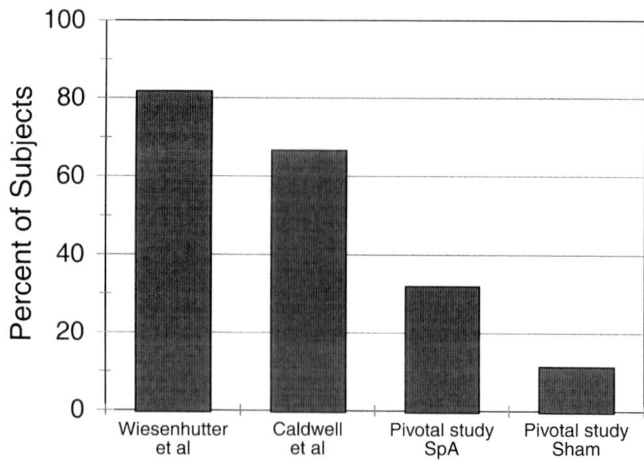

Figure 34.2. Results of clinical trials of extracorporeal pheresis therapy with staphylococcal protein A (SpA) columns. Percent of subjects in three clinical trials experiencing >20% improvement in rheumatoid arthritis composite index 8 weeks after completion of 12 weekly SpA or sham-column treatments. The trials by Wiesenhutter et al. (12) and Caldwell et al. (13) reported 20% response using the Paulus criteria. The double-blind sham-controlled trial (14) evaluated the 20% American College of Rheumatology response criteria.

TABLE 34.3. Adverse Events in Staphylococcal Protein A Therapy[a,b]

Event	Staphylococcal Protein A Column (%)[c] (N = 56)	Sham Therapy (%)[c] (N = 53)	Combined Experienced (%)[d] (N = 82)
Arthritis flare	82	70	74
Fatigue	55	43	63
Hypotension	38	28	34
Blood pressure changes	38	28	30
Nausea	36	28	43
Abdominal pain	30	23	21
Flushing	29	15	22
Hematoma	25	19	17
Headache	25	19	32
Paresthesia	25	23	27
Dizziness	23	34	22
Diarrhea	21	15	21
Rash	21	8	20
Sore throat	21	13	15
Edema	20	25	13
Dry mouth	18	0	12
Chills/rigor	18	13	24
Pain	18	17	37
Hypertension	18	11	12
Anxiety/nervousness	16	21	13
Chest pain	14	4	12
Anemia	14	15	26
Shortness of breath/respiratory difficulties	13	9	16
Fever	13	23	22
Infection	11	9	7
Muscle tightness	11	11	7
Hives/itching	11	6	9
Twitching	4	11	2

[a]Other reported adverse events are as follows: anorexia, bloating, bruising, catheter access and catheter-related infection, constipation, depression, diaphoretic, dyspepsia, facial edema, flatus, insomnia, leg cramp, menses changes, respiratory infection, stiffness, urinary tract infection, and vomiting.
[b]Adverse events with greater than 10% frequency in double-blind sham-controlled trial in either treatment or control group.
[c]Percentage rate is percent of enrolled subjects experiencing the adverse event.
[d]Combined adverse events experience reported in double-blind sham-controlled trial (14) and observational studies (12,13).

RA, the use of SpA column treatments has been reported in other diseases. Currently, treatment with the Prosorba column is approved by the FDA for the treatment of ITP and RA (11). Clinical experience with SpA columns has been reported for thrombotic thrombocytopenia purpura (7,9,10,52), thrombocytopenia associated with human immunodeficiency virus (53), hemolytic uremic syndrome (53), hemophilia (54), and malignancies (52,55–59). This chapter is limited to the evaluation of SpA column treatment in RA patients.

CLINICAL EFFICACY

Uncontrolled Clinical Experience

Two uncontrolled clinical trials have reported experience with extracorporeal pheresis therapy using an SpA column in RA patients (12,13). Both investigations were prospective protocols in patients with severe RA refractory to conventional therapies. Both studies treated patients weekly for 12 weeks. Clinical outcome measures were similar in the two studies with evaluation of traditional outcome measure of joint tenderness, joint swelling, morning stiffness, physician global assessment, patient global assessment, and measurement of erythrocyte sedimentation rate (ESR). The composite outcome measure used was the Paulus criteria (60) for 20% improvement and 50% improvement. Both reports provided detailed individual patient data on the clinical experience.

The report by Wiesenhutter et al. (12) enrolled 11 patients with severe RA characterized by mean baseline parameters of 12.4 years' disease duration, previous treatment with 4.8 different disease-modifying antirheumatic drugs (DMARDs), 44 tender joints, 22 swollen joints, and an ESR equal to 44 mm per hour. After 12 weekly treatments, nine patients (82%) achieved a 50% improvement by Paulus criteria (see Appendix C). Improvement in all component features of the Paulus criteria was also observed and achieved statistical significance, except that there was not a statistically significant change in the ESR. The response observed immediately after the 12 weekly treatments was persistent over the subsequent 12 weeks after the completion of therapy in four patients (36%) who maintained a 50% improvement and in two patients (18%) who maintained a 20% improvement by Paulus criteria. Five patients (45%) regressed to a clinical disease activity level below the 20% Paulus improvement criteria. Two subjects met the American College of Rheumatology (ACR) criteria for remission immediately after the completion of the 12 therapy treatments and continued to meet ACR criteria for remission for an additional 5 and 6 months, respectively, after the completion of treatment.

The study conducted by Caldwell et al. (13) enrolled 15 patients with severe RA characterized by mean baseline parameters of 10.8 years' disease duration, previous treatment with 3.7 DMARDs, 28 tender joints, 18 swollen joints, and an ESR equal to 47 mm per hour. After 12 weekly treatments, five patients (33%) achieved a 50% improvement by Paulus criteria and an additional eight (53%) achieved a 20% improvement by Paulus criteria. Improvement in all component features of the Paulus criteria was also observed and achieved statistical significance, including a statistically significant decrease in the ESR. The response observed immediately after the 12 weekly treatments was persistent over the subsequent

3 months of follow-up for five patients (33%) who maintained a 50% improvement and seven patients (47%) who maintained a 20% improvement by Paulus criteria. Five other patients (45%) regressed to a clinical disease activity level below the 20% Paulus improvement criteria. No specific report is made in this study of patients achieving the ACR criteria for remission.

Controlled Clinical Experience

The double-blind sham-controlled trial of the extracorporeal pheresis with SpA columns (Prosorba) in RA was a multiple center trial comparing pheresis with the SpA column to sham pheresis (14). Patients with severe RA and refractory disease defined as a joint tenderness count of greater than or equal to 20 and a joint swelling count of greater than or equal to10 who had failed at least two previous DMARD courses were eligible candidates. All study subjects underwent similar evaluation and pheresis procedures, with the components of the SpA column apparatus concealed behind a curtain. In patients randomized to SpA column treatment, plasma was passed through the SpA column before being returned to the patient. In patients randomized to sham treatment, plasma was diverted around the SpA column. Only one pheresis technician was aware of the treatment assignment and directed plasma through the column or diverted the plasma around the column. Other personnel involved in the study, including patients and investigators, were blinded to the treatment randomization of study subjects. Patients received once-weekly pheresis treatments for 12 weeks. After completion of the 12-week treatment period, patients were followed for an additional 8 weeks. The primary outcome measure was the ACR 20% response at 20 weeks (8 weeks after completion of pheresis therapy).

This double-blind sham-controlled trial was monitored by a data safety monitoring board. The data safety monitoring board terminated the study early, after an interim analysis demonstrated that the efficacy end point had been successfully achieved. There were 109 (56 SpA-treated subjects and 53 sham-treated subjects) subjects who were entered into the trial and were available for safety evaluation. With the early termination procedures, there were 47 SpA-treated subjects and 44 sham-treated subjects available for efficacy analysis. In the SpA-treated group, 15 (31.9%) of 47 subjects achieved an ACR 20% response in comparison to 5 (11.4%) of 44 sham-treated subjects ($p = .019$) at the 20-week end point. Greater improvement in all elements of the ACR core set measures was seen in the SpA-treated group in comparison to the sham-treated group. No patients fulfilled ACR remission criteria during the double-blind sham-controlled trial. The data generated by the double-blind sham-controlled trial led to FDA approval of the Prosorba device for use in the treatment of RA.

Retreatment Experience

Patients enrolled in the double-blind sham-controlled trial were offered the opportunity for open-label SpA pheresis if they completed the 20-week study follow-up (61). Patients and investigators were not unblinded as to the treatment received by the patient during the initial double-blind phase of the study. To qualify for open-label treatment with SpA, in addition to having completed the double-blind study, the patient had to lack a clinical response or have a relapse after a clinical response during initial therapy. This lack of response was defined as failure to achieve an ACR 20% response (compared to baseline measurement at entry into the clinical trial) at the time of initiation of SpA column treatment. During the open treatment, patients received 12 weekly SpA column treatments in a manner similar to that in the double-blind phase of the study. Thirteen subjects initially treated with SpA columns during the double-blind phase entered the open study either because of an initial failure to respond (N = 4) or a relapse (N = 9). During retreatment, seven of the nine subjects (77%) with an initial ACR response of at least 20% had a second ACR response of at least 20%. The four subjects who failed initial therapy on SpA columns without an ACR 20% response during the initial phase of the study did not have clinical improvement during the open phase of treatment. Eleven patients entered the open-label phase after having received sham therapy during the double-blind phase. Five (45%) of these sham-treated subjects experienced at least a 20% ACR response during open therapy. This rate was similar to the rate of response seen during the double-blind phase. These data suggest that patients without an initial response to therapy will not respond to a subsequent treatment course. In contrast, patients with clinical improvement during SpA column therapy may experience a significant clinical response to retreatment.

Adverse Events

The studies of Wiesenhutter et al. (12) and Caldwell et al. (13), and the double-blind sham-controlled trial (14) showed similar adverse event experiences. Adverse events were common (Table 34.3). All patients in both the observational studies and the double-blind sham-controlled studies reported at least one adverse event. In the double-blind sham-controlled trial, patients receiving SpA treatment reported an average of 27 adverse events, whereas patients receiving sham therapy reported an average of 26 adverse events (not statistically significantly different). During the double-blind sham-controlled trial, 22% of adverse events occurred during treatment and 78% after or in the interval between treatments. For SpA-treated patients, 29 of 47 subjects reported adverse events as severe, whereas 24 of 43 patients on sham therapy reported a severe adverse event. It should be noted that this was a patient/investigator designation of severity and not the clinical trial definition of a serious adverse event. There was an average of 2.8 events reported during each treatment cycle in both the SpA- and sham-treated groups. Caldwell et al. (13) reported an average of 2.5 adverse events per treatment cycle. The number of adverse events per treatment cycle was not reported by Wiesenhutter et al. (12).

In most cases, adverse events did not interrupt the treatment protocol. Wiesenhutter et al. (12) had two patients who had modifications of their treatment schedules. One patient needed to delay treatment because of hypotensive episodes during the pheresis treatments. Caldwell et al. (13) reported that one patient terminated early because of lingular pneumonia. During the double-blind sham-controlled trial (14), three subjects on SpA treatment withdrew because of adverse events—one subject each with abdominal pain and anxiety, petechiae, and septic arthritis after hip surgery. In the sham-treated group, four subjects withdrew for adverse events—one subject each with line-related emboli, necrotizing fasciitis, central-line infection, and change in mental status.

A broad variety of adverse events has been reported (Table 34.3). The adverse events that require specific discussion are problems associated with disease flares during therapy and venous access. Flares in arthritis activity were often seen in patients both immediately and during the 72 hours after pheresis treatments. These episodes were common in both SpA- and sham-treated subjects. Disease flares were managed with analgesia and rest in most cases, with subsequent resolution and without sequelae. Another common problem associated with pheresis therapy was related to vascular access. In the double-blind sham-controlled trial, two subjects in the SpA group and two subjects in the sham group were not able to complete the study because of loss of venous access. Five of nine subjects with central venous catheters placed for access during treatment experienced complications secondary to these catheters. All five of these subjects were withdrawn from the protocol (including three in the sham group). There were three subjects with thrombosis of the catheter and three central-line infections (one of the subjects had combined thrombosis and infection).

Overall, adverse events are common and often severe during SpA column treatments. The similar rates of adverse events in the SpA and sham groups during the double-blind sham-controlled trial suggest that the majority of adverse events are related to the pheresis procedure and not the SpA column. Irrespective of the cause for the adverse event, these episodes are a significant management challenge for the physician and patient receiving extracorporeal pheresis therapy with the SpA column.

Cost

The current cost of SpA column therapy is approximately $25,000 for a 12-course cycle (62). The cost-effectiveness of the procedure for the treatment of RA has not been formally studied. A recent manuscript reviewed the factors that would be required for such an analysis, but did not reach any conclusions or provide an estimate of the cost-effectiveness of this procedure (62).

CONCLUSION

Clinical trials have demonstrated that extracorporeal pheresis with SpA columns is effective in some patients with severe RA refractory to DMARD therapy. The significant expense, logistical issues associated with the administration of the therapy, and associated adverse events are significant barriers to this therapy. Currently, it would appear most prudent to reserve this modality for patients with severe, persistent, aggressive RA who have failed available therapies, including aggressive combination DMARD programs. However, in subjects who have not responded to these other means for the control of RA, pheresis with SpA columns is an alternative worth consideration.

ACKNOWLEDGMENTS

This chapter was supported in part by a research grant from the Western Institute for Biomedical Research, the Veterans Affairs Medical Research Program, and the National Institutes of Health RO1-AR47423, and also by a biomedical research grant from the Arthritis Foundation, the Nora Eccles Treadwell Foundation, and the Valois Egbert Endowment.

REFERENCES

1. Smith JB, Haynes MK. Rheumatoid arthritis—a molecular understanding. *Ann Intern Med* 2002;136:908–922.
2. Wallace DJ, Barnett EV, Nichols S. Immunologic dynamics in cryapheresis for rheumatoid arthritis. *J Rheumatol* 1983;10:894–900.
3. Wallace D, Goldfinger D, Lowe C, et al. A double-blind, controlled study of lymphoplasmapheresis versus sham apheresis in rheumatoid arthritis. *N Engl J Med* 1982;306:1406–1410.
4. Wallace DJ, Goldfinger D, Gatti R, et al. Plasmapheresis and lymphoplasmapheresis in the management of rheumatoid arthritis. *Arthritis Rheum* 1979;22: 703–710.
5. Matic G, Bosch T, Ramlow W. Background and indications for protein A-based extracorporeal immunoadsorption. *Ther Apher* 2001;5:394–403.
6. Silverman GJ. B cell superantigens: possible roles in immunodeficiency and autoimmunity. *Semin Immunol* 1998;10:43–55.
7. Howe RB, Christie DJ. Protein A immunoadsorption treatment in hematology: an overview. *J Clin Apheresis* 1994;9:31–32.
8. Christie DJ, Howe RB, Lennon SS, et al. Treatment of refractoriness to platelet transfusion by protein A column therapy. *Transfusion* 1993;33:234–242.
9. Snyder HW Jr, Cochran SK, Balint JP Jr, et al. Experience with protein A-immunoadsorption in treatment-resistant adult immune thrombocytopenic purpura. *Blood* 1992;79:2237–2245.
10. Snyder HW Jr, Bertram JH, Channel M, et al. Reduction in platelet binding immunoglobulins and improvement in platelet counts in patients with HIV associated idiopathic thrombocytopenic purpura (ITP) following extracorporeal immunoadsorption of plasma over staphylococcal protein A-silica. *Artif Organs* 1989;13:71–77.
11. Prosorba column [package insert]. Redmond, WA: Fresenius HemoCare, Inc.
12. Wiesenhutter CW, Irish BL, Bertram JH. Treatment of patients with refractory rheumatoid arthritis with extracorporeal protein A immunoadsorption columns: a pilot trial. *J Rheumatol* 1994;21:804–812.
13. Caldwell J, Gendreau RM, Furst D, et al. A pilot study using a staph protein A column (Prosorba) to treat refractory rheumatoid arthritis. *J Rheumatol* 1999;26:1657–1662.
14. Felson DT, LaValley MP, Baldassare AR, et al. The Prosorba column for treatment of refractory rheumatoid arthritis. *Arthritis Rheum* 1999;42:2153–2159.
15. Patel Ah, Nowlan P, Weavers ED, et al. Virulence of protein A-deficient and alpha-toxin-deficient mutants of staphylococcus aureus isolated by allele replacement. *Infect Immunol* 1987;55:3103–3110.
16. Uhlen M, Guss B, Nillson B, et al. Complete sequence of the staphylococcal gene encoding protein A. A gene evolved through multiple duplications. *J Biol Chem* 1984;259:1695–1702.
17. Moks T, Abrahmsen L, Nilsson B, et al. Staphylococcal protein A consists of five IgG-binding domains. *Eur J Biochem* 1986;156:637–643.
18. Lofdahl S, Guss B, Uhlen M, et al. Gene for staphylococcal protein A. *Proc Natl Acad Sci U S A* 1983;80:697–701.
19. Alonso DO, Daggett V. Staphylococcal protein A: unfolding pathways, unfolded states, and differences between the B and E domains. *Proc Natl Acad Sci U S A* 2000;97:133–138.
20. Deisenhofer J, Jones TA, Huber R, et al. Crystallographic refinement and atomic models of a human Fc fragment and its complex with fragment B of protein A from staphylococcus aureus at 2.9- and 2.8-resolution. *Hoppe-Seylers Z Physiol Chem* 1978;359:975–985.
21. Gouda H, Torigoe H, Saito A, et al. Three-dimensional solution structure of the B domain of staphylococcal protein A: comparisons of the solution and crystal structures. *Biochemistry* 1992;31:9665–9672.
22. Kato K, Gouda H, Takaha W, et al. C NMR study of the mode of interaction in solution of the B fragment of staphylococcal protein A and the Fc fragments of mouse immunoglobulin G. *FEBS Lett* 1993;328:49–54.
23. Potter KN, Li Y, Mageed RA, et al. Anti-idiotypic antibody D12 and superantigen SPA both interact with human VH3-encoded antibodies on the external face of the heavy chain involving FR1, CDR2, and FR3. *Mol Immunol* 1998;35:1179–1187.
24. Terman DS. Protein A and staphylococcal products in neo-plastic disease. *Crit Rev Oncol Hematol* 1985;4:103–124.
25. Balint J Jr, Totorica C, Stewart J, et al. Detection, isolation and characterization of staphylococcal enterotoxin B in protein A preparations purified by immunoglobulin G affinity chromatography. *J Immunol Methods* 1989;116:37–43.
26. Schrezenmeier H, Fleischer B. Mitogenic activity of staphylococcal protein A is due to contaminating staphylococcal enterotoxins. *J Immunol Methods* 1987;105:133–137.
27. Das C, Langone JJ. Dissociation between murine spleen cell mitogenic activity of enterotoxin contaminants and anti-tumor activity of staphylococcal protein A. *J Immunol* 1989;142:2943–2948.
28. Persson U, Inganas M, Smith CI, et al. Recombinant protein A of non-staphylococcal origin is not mitogenic for human peripheral lymphocytes. Mitogenicity of natural protein A is caused by a contaminant. *Scand J Immunol* 1989;29:151–158.
29. Foster TJ, McDevitt D. Surface-associated proteins of staphylococcus aureus; their possible roles in virulence. *FEMS Microbiol Lett* 1994;118:199–205.
30. Inganas M, Johansson SG, Sjoquist J. Further characterization of the alternative protein-A interaction of immunoglobulins: demonstration of an Fc-binding fragment of protein A expressing the alternative reactivity. *Scan J Immunol* 1981;14:379–388.
31. Erntell M, Myhre EB, Kronvall G. Non-immune F(ab')2- and Fc-mediated interactions of mammalian immunoglobulins with S. aureus and group C and G streptococci. *Acta Pathol Microbiol Immunol Scand [B]* 1986;94:377–385.
32. Silverman GJ, Sasano M, Wormsley SB. Age-associated changes in binding of human B lymphocytes to a Vh3-restricted unconventional bacterial antigen. *J Immunol* 1993;151:5840–5855.
33. Silverman GJ. Human antibody responses to bacterial antigens: studies of a model conventional antigen and a proposed model B cell superantigen. *Int Rev Immunol* 1992;9:57–78.
34. Johansson SG, Inganas M. Interaction of polyclonal hum IgE with protein-A from staphylococcus aureus. *Immunol Rev* 1978;41:248–260.
35. Sasso EH, Silverman GJ, Mannik M. Human IgA and IgG G(ab')2 that bind to staphylococcal protein A belong to the VHIII subgroup. *J Immunol* 1991; 147:1877–1883.

36. Sasso EH, Silverman GJ, Mannik M. Human IgM molecules that bind staphylococcal protein A contain V_HIII H chains. *J Immunol* 1989;142:2778–2783.
37. Harboe M, Folling I. Recognition of two distinct groups of human IgM and IgA based on different binding to staphylococci. *J Immunol* 1974;3:471.
38. Seppala I, Kaartinen M, Ibrahim S, et al. Mouse Ig coded by V_H families S107 or J606 bind to protein A. *J Immunol* 1990;145:2989–2993.
39. Young WW, Tamura Y, Wolock DM, et al. Staphylococcal protein A binding to the Fab of mouse monoclonal antibodies. *J Immunol* 1984;133:3163–3166.
40. Pullen AM, Wade T, Marrack P, et al. Identification of the region of T cell receptor beta chain that interacts with self-superantigen MIs-1a. *Cell* 1990;61:1365–1374.
41. Potter KN, Li Y-C, Capra JD. Staphylococcal protein A simultaneously interacts with framework 1, complementarity region 2, and framework 3 on human V_H3 encoded immunoglobulins. *J Immunol* 1996;157:2982–2988.
42. Graille M, Stura EA, Corper AL, et al. Crystal structure of a staphylococcus aureus protein. A domain complexed with the Fab fragment of a human 1gM antibody: structural basis for recognition of B-cell receptors and superantigen activity. *Proc Natl Acad Sci U S A* 2000;97:5399–5404.
43. Ljungberg UK, Jansson B, Niss U, et al. The interaction between different domains of staphylococcal protein A and human polyclonal 1gG, 1gA, 1gM and F(ab')2: separation of affinity from specificity. *Mol Immunol* 1993;30:1279–1285.
44. Snyder HW Jr, Balint JP, Jones FR. Modulation of immunity in patients with autoimmune disease and cancer treated by extracorporeal immunoadsorption with PROSORBA columns. *Semin Hematol* 1989;[Suppl 1]:21–41.
45. Silverman GJ, Nayak JV, La Cava A. B-cell superantigens: molecular and cellular implications. *Intern Rev Immunol* 1997;14:259–290.
46. Silverman GJ, Cary S, Graille M, et al. A B-cell superantigen that targets B-1 lymphocytes. *Curr Top Microbiol Immunol* 2000;252:251–263.
47. Sawitzke A, Joyner D, Knudtson K, et al. Anti-MAM antibodies in rheumatic disease: evidence for a MAM-like superantigen in rheumatoid arthritis? *J Rheumatol* 2000 Feb;27:358–364.
48. Cole BC, Mu HH, Sawitzke AD. The mycoplasma superantigen MAM: role in arthritis and immune-mediated disease. *Int J Med Microbiol* 2000;290:489–490.
49. Kozlowski LM, Soulika AM, Silverman GJ, et al. Complement activation by a B cell superantigen. *J Immunol* 1996;157:1200–1206.
50. Sasso EH, Merrill C, Furst DE. Immunoglobulin binding properties of the Prosorba immunoadsorption column in treatment of rheumatoid arthritis. *Ther Apher* 2001;5:84–91.
51. Balint JP Jr, Jones FR. Evidence for proteolytic cleavage of covalently bound protein A from a silica based extracorporeal immunoadsorbent and lack of relationship to treatment effects. *Transfus Sci* 1995;16:85–94.
52. Snyder HW Jr, Mittelman A, Oral A, et al. Treatment of cancer chemotherapy-associated thrombotic thrombocytopenic purpura/hemolytic uremic syndrome (C-TTP/HUS) by protein A immunoadsorption of plasma. *Cancer* 1993;71:1882–1892.
53. Mittelman A, Bertram J, Henry DH, et al. Treatment of patients with HIV thrombocytopenia and hemolytic uremic syndrome with protein A (Prosorba column) immunoadsorption. *Semin Hematol* 1989;26[Suppl 1]:15–18.
54. Nilsson IM, Jonsson S, Sundgist S-B, et al. A procedure for removing high titer antibodies by extracorporeal protein A–sepharose absorption in hemophilia: substitution therapy and surgery in a patient with hemophilia B and antibodies. *Blood* 1981:58:38–44.
55. Messerschmidt GL, Henry DH, Snyder HW Jr, et al. Protein A immunotherapy in the treatment of cancer: update. *Semin Hematol* 1989;26[Suppl 1]:31–41.
56. Messerschmidt GL, Henry DH, Snyder HW Jr, et al. Protein A immunoadsorption in the treatment of malignant disease. *J Clin Oncol* 1988;6:203–212.
57. Ainsworth SK, Pilia PA, Pepkowitz SH, et al. Toxicity following protein A treatment of metastatic breast adenocarcinoma. *Cancer* 1988;61:1495–1500.
58. Hakansson L, Jonsson S, Soderberg M, et al. Tumor regression after extracorporeal affinity chromatography of blood plasma across agarose beads containing staphylococcal protein A. *Eur J Cancer* 1984;20:1377–1388.
59. Kiprov DD, Lippert R, Jones FR, et al. Extracorporeal perfusion of plasma over immobilized protein A in a patient with Kaposi's sarcoma, and acquired immunodeficiency. *J Biol Response Modifiers* 1984;3:341–346.
60. Paulus HE, Egger MJ, Ward JR, et al. Analysis of improvement in individual rheumatoid arthritis patients treated with disease-modifying antirheumatic drugs, based on the findings in patients treated with placebo. The Cooperative Systematic Studies of Rheumatic Diseases Group. *Arthritis Rheum* 1990;33:477–484.
61. Furst DE, Felson D, Gendreau M. Patients with severe rheumatoid arthritis responding to treatment respond again on retreatment. *Arthritis Rheum* 1998;41:S316.
62. Griffiths RI, Slurzberg JF. Cost-effectiveness of Prosorba column therapy for rheumatoid arthritis: a framework for analysis. *Ther Apher* 2001;5:105–110.

CHAPTER 35

Combination Disease-Modifying Antirheumatic Drug Therapy

James R. O'Dell

Since the early 1990s, dramatic changes have occurred in how combinations of disease-modifying antirheumatic drugs (DMARDs) are used to treat patients with rheumatoid arthritis (RA). Then, the use of more than one DMARD was rare, but the practice is now commonplace. Other significant paradigm shifts in how we think about and treat patients with RA have also occurred. These have included the general acceptance that early therapy is critical in preventing irreversible damage, the recognition that steroids are indeed disease modifying and their subsequent rebirth as a bridge to effective DMARD therapy, the common use of combinations of DMARDs, and the introduction of biologic therapies that target specific cytokines. The role of comorbidities has also been recognized as critical. Although the role of combinations of DMARDs may not be as compelling as the biologic treatments of RA, they have arguably made a bigger impact because of the frequency of their use. This is particularly true when one considers difficult-to-manage RA, in which the vast majority of patients, at least in the United States, are taking combinations of DMARDs. Currently, the timing and make-up of combinations selected to treat RA are some of the most important decisions that clinicians confront as they care for patients with RA.

Methotrexate remains the current gold standard DMARD and is considered by most as the initial drug of choice for the treatment of early RA. Methotrexate continues to demonstrate superior long-term efficacy, compared with other conventional DMARDs (1,2) and, in the treatment of early RA, with etanercept (3) at a fraction of the cost (4); it has also recently been shown to significantly reduce mortality in patients with RA (5). However, therapy combining methotrexate with other DMARDs is now used to treat a growing number of patients with RA who have not achieved optimal disease control with methotrexate alone. A 1999 survey of U.S. rheumatologists revealed that 99% used combinations of DMARDs to treat an estimated 24% of all patients (6). This number has gone up dramatically from less than 15% of rheumatologists using combinations in 1995. Recently, four major studies (7–10) have demonstrated the superiority of combinations of DMARDs over monotherapy in head-to-head comparisons; three of these studies were done in early RA. Methotrexate, in combination with biologic agents (etanercept, infliximab, adalimumab, or anakinra), is also a common strategy. Clinical studies of multiple agents in patients who had less than optimal responses to methotrexate have shown each of them to be more effective than placebo when added to the baseline methotrexate (11–19). With very few exceptions, all of the clinical trials that have demonstrated the success of combination therapy for RA have included methotrexate as part of the combination. Thus, methotrexate remains the cornerstone of combination therapy (20).

HISTORY OF COMBINATION DISEASE-MODIFYING ANTIRHEUMATIC DRUG THERAPY

Many credit the pioneering studies of McCarty et al., initiated in the late 1970s, for showing both the promise and perils of combination DMARD therapy in patients with RA. Of course, if steroids are considered as DMARDs, thousands of patients with RA have been treated with combination DMARD therapy since the early 1950s. In McCarty's original publication, the combination of cyclophosphamide, azathioprine, and hydroxychloroquine produced dramatic responses in an open-label trial of 17 patients with severe refractory RA (21). Remission was reported in five patients, and an additional two patients achieved near remissions, with excellent responses reported in all but three patients. The investigators cautioned against general adoption of this protocol until further data were available on toxicities. Indeed, 4 years later, this group expanded their report to 31 patients with spectacular clinical responses (22). Remissions were reported in 52%, near remission in 23%, and only one patient failed to have at least a good response. Unfortunately, Csuka et al. reported the development of five malignancies in four patients, with three related deaths. This study simultaneously demonstrated both the promise and pitfalls of combination therapy.

The combinations studied from 1986 to 1995 were shown, for the most part, to have limited efficacy. These results occurred for several reasons, including inadequate dosing, the use of DMARDs with marginal efficacy, and problematic trial design. Suboptimal dosing of methotrexate and azathioprine in the combination arms of studies reported by Willkens et al. was the likely explanation for the inability of these trials to show a significant benefit of combination therapy (23). In this trial, the dose of methotrexate and azathioprine in the combination group was one-half of what it was in the monotherapy groups. Trials that combined oral gold with other DMARDs were examples of the use of DMARDs with marginal efficacy (24). Finally, in the European combination trials of methotrexate and sulfasalazine, only a marginal benefit of this combination over monotherapy was seen (25,26). This lack of significant benefit was largely because of trial design issues, wherein doses of the medications were escalated without clear guidelines or end points. The result was lower doses of the medications in the combination arms, but efficacy was only marginally better. A summary of the results of this phase of trials was published as a metaanalysis, with the conclusion that combination therapy was no better, and perhaps more toxic, than monotherapy (27). Nonetheless, these trials laid the foundation for the success of the next group of trials.

In 1994, the first trial to convincingly show the superiority of combination DMARD therapy in a head-to-head comparison with state-of-the-art DMARD monotherapy was published in abstract form (28); the manuscript was subsequently published in the *New England Journal of Medicine* (7). In this 2-year randomized double-blind parallel study of 102 patients (mean disease duration, 8.6 years), triple-drug therapy with methotrexate-sulfasalazine-hydroxychloroquine (Fig. 35.1) was superior to the combination therapy of hydroxychloroquine-sulfasalazine and monotherapy with methotrexate (7). Seventy-seven percent of patients receiving the triple-drug therapy achieved a Paulus 50% composite response (29) (see Appendix C), compared to 40% of the sulfasalazine-hydroxychloroquine patients and 33% of the methotrexate alone patients ($p = .003$). This combination was well tolerated, with numerically fewer withdrawals in the combination group, compared to the other two groups.

Triple-drug therapy was shown to be durable; follow-up of the patients who continued receiving this combination over a 5-year period revealed that 62% (36 of 58) maintained a 50% efficacy response and tolerated therapy well (30). A similar long-term response rate (67%) occurred in 15 patients who switched to triple-drug therapy after suboptimal response to monotherapy with methotrexate (17.5 mg per week) (31). Remission, as defined by American College of Rheumatology (ACR) criteria (32), was uncommon in this study (12%), and patients tended to deteriorate when any of the components of the triple-drug therapy were discontinued. Importantly, radiographic progression, measured by a modified Sharp method of hand films, demonstrated a significant advantage of triple-drug therapy, compared

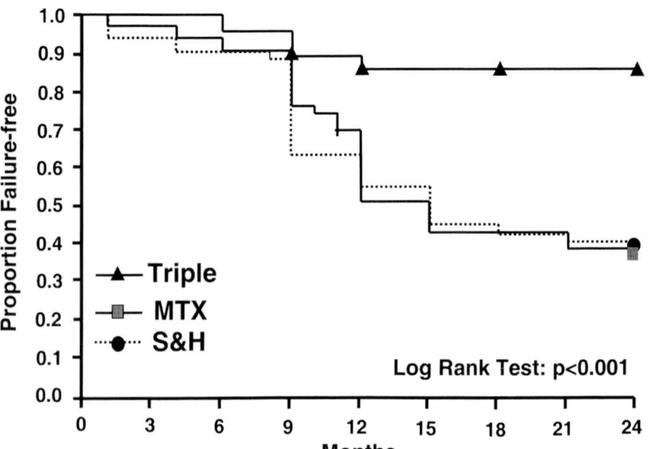

Figure 35.1. Proportion of patients who met Paulus 50% improvement criteria at 9 months and maintained at least this level of response to 24 months. MTX, methotrexate; S&H, sulfasalazine and hydroxychloroquine. (Adapted from O'Dell JR, Haire CE, Erikson N, et al. Treatment of rheumatoid arthritis with methotrexate alone, sulfasalazine, and hydroxychloroquine, or a combination of all three medications. *N Engl J Med* 1996;334:1287–1291.)

to methotrexate alone or the combination of sulfasalazine-hydroxychloroquine; mean progression per year was 1.8 ± 1.95, 5.66 ± 6.09, and 8.3 ± 6.81, respectively. This trial, which began enrollment in 1989, helped set the stage and standards for trials that followed.

COMBINATION DISEASE-MODIFYING ANTIRHEUMATIC DRUG TRIALS: DESIGN AND INTERPRETATION ISSUES

Design and interpretation of studies of combination therapy in the treatment of RA have been problematic; some examples of trials in which design issues have led to difficult interpretation of results have been discussed (inadequate dosing, dose escalation problems, and the use of marginally effective DMARDs). RA is a lifelong disease, and a sufficiently long duration of therapy (≥1 year) during the blinded portion of the trials is essential, especially when dose escalation of medications is required. This minimum duration allows sufficient time for dose escalation and for assessment of longer-term efficacy and safety, thereby allowing differences to manifest themselves between treatments. Drug dosage is critical to study design; in particular, automatic dose escalation on failure to achieve a predetermined level of clinical success that assures comparability of dose escalation between treatment arms is critical for meaningful trial interpretation. The recognition that the population of patients studied may significantly influence results is also important. Responsiveness to therapy may be affected by previous treatment failures with specific DMARDs and by the duration of disease, with late disease being less responsive than early disease.

Combinations can be evaluated by one of three methods: the step-down approach, the step-up approach, or the parallel approach. The step-down approach is one in which two or more DMARDs are administered initially; individual agents are then removed according to protocol or after symptoms are controlled (8). The step-up approach has one DMARD administered initially and another added if the first agent is insufficient (11–19). The parallel approach evaluates two treatment approaches head to head (7,9,10,12). Because placebo trials raise ethical concerns, most new therapies should be compared against active therapies, if such therapies exist, for the patient group being studied. As discussed later, there are at least seven different that treatments have been shown to be effective when added to methotrexate in suboptimal responders (11–19), but there is no information on how these therapies compare to each other.

Finally, the critical issue of generalizability of trial results to patients seen in routine clinical practice needs to be considered. Pincus recently reported that the vast majority of patients seen in rheumatologists' offices do not meet entry criteria of major published clinical trials. The percentage of patients who were seen in various Vanderbilt sites who would qualify for trials in early RA was approximately 30%, whereas the percentage of those who would qualify for trials in later disease (trials usually done in methotrexate suboptimal responders) was as low as 5% (33). The most common reason for patients failing to qualify was disease that was less active than that required for inclusion. These data raise significant questions about the knowledge obtained from classic randomized double-blind trials and its relevance and application to clinical practice.

COMBINATION THERAPY: TIMING

The critically important decision of when in the course of RA to use combination therapy continues to be controversial. This is true in large part because studies that compare regimens using combinations of DMARDs, versus rapid step-up approaches, as initial therapy remain to be done. Recent studies (8–10) suggest that combination therapy may be the best initial therapy for RA. Further, studies clearly demonstrate the benefit of combination DMARD therapy in patients who have not had an optimal response to methotrexate (11–19). Studies in both of these two distinct categories of patients will be reviewed.

EARLY DISEASE TREATMENT: STEP-UP OR STEP-DOWN APPROACHES?

Studies have clearly shown that delays in disease-modifying therapy for as little as 8 to 9 months may result in less optimal outcomes for patients (34–36). Therefore, it makes sense to consider the most potent therapy as an initial treatment (37). In the late 1980s, Wilske and Healey proposed a step-down bridge approach for the treatment of early RA (38). The central tenet of this approach was to completely control disease as early as possible. To achieve this goal, the authors proposed that multiple therapies be started simultaneously as initial therapy for RA, to ensure the quickest possible control of disease, and the patient would be tapered off a number of these drugs, leaving him or her on the simplest possible long-term maintenance regimen. This is clearly an attractive hypothesis, but until 1997, there were little or no data to support it.

COMBINATIETHERAPIE BIJ REUMATOIDE ARTRITIS TRIAL

Researchers in the Netherlands reported on the step-down bridge approach: the Combinatietherapie Bij Reumatoide Artritis (COBRA) trial (8). In this trial, 155 patients with early disease (<2 years) were randomly assigned to two groups (Fig. 35.2). The first group was treated with a combination of prednisolone, methotrexate, and sulfasalazine; the second group was treated with sulfasalazine alone. Prednisolone was started at 60 mg a day and was rapidly tapered to 7.5 mg a day over the course of several weeks; it was discontinued completely by week 28. The dose of methotrexate was 7.5 mg and remained at that level until week 40, when patients were tapered off this medication. The dose of sulfasalazine was the same in both groups and was rapidly accelerated to 2 g per day. At 28 weeks, the combination group was significantly better than the sulfasalazine alone group, with an ACR 20% response rate (39) of 72% versus 49% ($p = .006$) and an ACR 50% response rate of 49% versus 27% ($p = .007$). As the prednisolone and methotrexate were tapered, the response rates became similar in the two groups. However, it is important to note that, in terms of a number of important parameters, significant benefits were observed for patients in the combination-treated group at 54 weeks, at 80 weeks, and at 4 to 5 years (40). The initial trial reported that the progression of total Sharp scores and erosion scores was less in the combination group ($p < .01$) than in the sulfasalazine alone group, and that patients in the combination group were more likely to be employed and were working more hours. Importantly, the withdrawal rate was much higher in the sulfasalazine alone group (39% vs. 8%), demonstrating that combination therapy was not more toxic (as defined by the number of patients who were withdrawn from the protocol by their treating physician for possible toxicity). The authors of the COBRA study have reported that the radiographic benefits conferred by COBRA in the initial trial extend at least 5 years (40) (Fig. 35.2). Radiographs from this follow-up trial continued to be read in a blinded fashion. It is important to note that this radiographic benefit is presumably conferred by the initial 40 weeks of combination therapy, as therapy for these patients did not differ after that point.

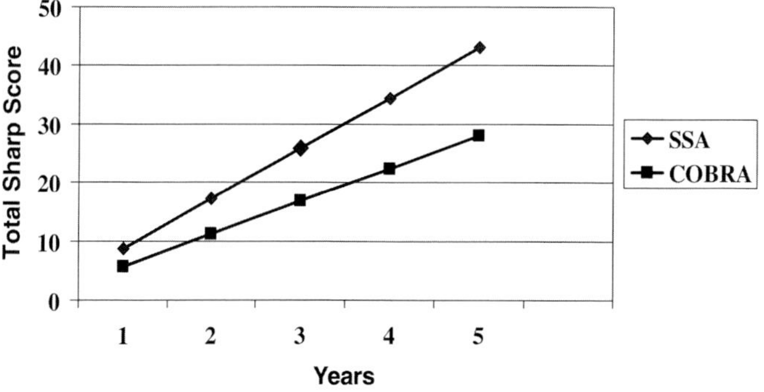

Figure 35.2. Comparison of total Sharp score progression rates in those patients who originally received monotherapy with sulfasalazine (SSA), compared with those who received the Combinatietherapie Bij Reumatoide Artritis (COBRA) therapy. COBRA consisted of high-dose prednisolone tapered off by 28 weeks, low-dose methotrexate tapered off by 40 weeks, and continuous SSA therapy. (Adapted from Landewe RBM, Boers M, ver Hoeven AC, et al. COBRA combination therapy in patients with early rheumatoid arthritis. *Arthritis Rheum* 2002;46:347–356.)

The rapid onset of action of the relatively high doses of prednisolone that was used in the COBRA trial may be the first successful report of induction therapy in RA (37). This study demonstrates that, if an effective induction regimen is used, patients with RA can gain long-term (at least 5 years) benefits. COBRA therapy was clearly effective in rapidly suppressing acute phase reactants. In this trial, the mean erythrocyte sedimentation rate was suppressed by 75% after 2 weeks of treatment, compared to the more than 24 weeks necessary for the monotherapy group to achieve this degree of suppression (Boers M, *personal communication, 2002*).

FINNISH RHEUMATOID ARTHRITIS COMBINATION THERAPY TRIAL

The Finnish Rheumatoid Arthritis Combination (Fin-RA) therapy trial group has reported another important study in patients with early RA (9). In this study, 199 patients were randomized to receive combination DMARD therapy versus monotherapy with sulfasalazine (Table 35.1). The patients had less than 2 years of disease and had not received previous DMARD therapy. The combination used in this study was methotrexate, sulfasalazine, hydroxychloroquine, and low-dose prednisolone. Patients in the sulfasalazine alone group had the option of receiving prednisolone as well, and also of switching to methotrexate if they had suboptimal responses to sulfasalazine alone. Importantly, the major end point of this study was remission. Unlike the COBRA trial, this prospective ran-

TABLE 35.1. Early Rheumatoid Arthritis: The Finnish Rheumatoid Arthritis Combination Trial

199 patients, early rheumatoid arthritis (<2 yr)
Open, 2-yr, randomized
Sulfasalazine (SSA) ± prednisolone vs. methotrexate-SSA-hydroxychloroquine + prednisolone
Major end point: remission
Results
Triple therapy, 37% remissions $p = .003$
Monotherapy, 18% remissions

domized study was an open trial. At 2 years, it was determined that the only factor that predicted remission in this group of patients was whether they had received combination therapy in the beginning (odds ratio, 2.7; $p = .003$). At 2 years, 37% of the combination-treated patients, compared to 18% of the monotherapy group, were in remission. Rheumatoid factor status, number of swollen joints, number of tender joints, disease duration, and gender were not predictive of remission at 2 years. Significantly, the authors of this trial have also reported that, at 5 years, patients treated initially with combination therapy were less likely to have evidence of C1-C2 subluxation on cervical spine x-rays (41).

In the Fin-RA trial, as in the COBRA study, patients tolerated combination therapy well. It is also important to note that secondary end points in this trial, including ACR 20% and 50% response rates, were better than, but not statistically different from, those patients who received monotherapy with sulfasalazine.

TABLE 35.2. Clinical Trials Needed

Initial Therapy	Methotrexate Suboptimal Responders
Combinations vs. step-up Induction: high-dose vs. low-dose steroids Induction: steroids vs. anti-TNF Delineation of factors that predict response Long-term outcomes, including toxicities and costs	Head-to-head comparisons: Anti-TNF vs. triple Leflunomide vs. triple Anti-TNF vs. leflunomide Anti-TNF vs. another Delineation of factors that predict response Long-term outcomes, including toxicities and costs

TNF, tumor necrosis factor.

EFFICACY OF MULTIDRUG COMBINATIONS

A trial from Turkey compared two and three drug combinations. This trial had 180 patients with early RA (mean duration, 2.3 years) who were randomized equally to single DMARD therapy (20 patients each to methotrexate, sulfasalazine, and hydroxychloroquine), two-drug therapy (30 patients each to methotrexate-sulfasalazine and methotrexate-hydroxychloroquine), or three-drug therapy [60 patients to all three drugs (10)]. This trial was an open 2-year trial with end points of Paulus 50% composite response, ACR remission, and no radiographic progression. Because it was an open trial, it may have been subject to some bias that double-blind trials are not, but, of critical importance, the x-rays were read blinded. For all end points measured, two drugs were shown to be statistically superior to monotherapy ($p = .007$ or better). The three-drug regimen was statistically superior to the two-drug regimens for Paulus 50% response rate and ACR remission end points ($p = .007$ or better) and showed a trend for no x-ray progression (Fig. 35.3). The results of this trial show that 88% of patients with early RA who are treated with triple therapy (methotrexate-sulfasalazine-hydroxychloroquine) fulfill Paulus 50% improvement criteria, and 69% have no radiographic progression.

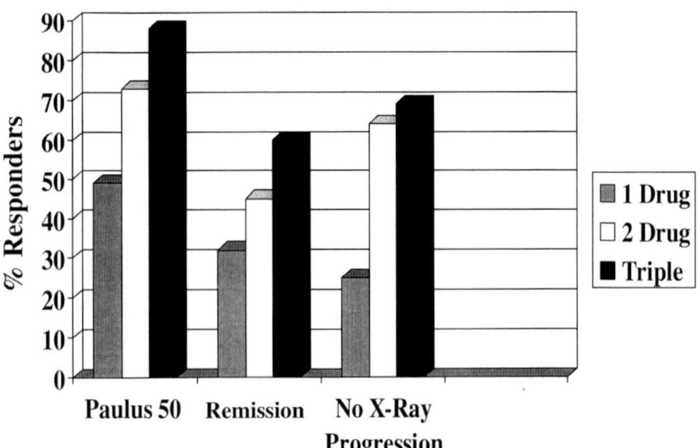

Figure 35.3. Comparison of percentage of responders for Paulus 50% composite response, complete American College of Rheumatology (ACR) remission, or no radiographic progression of patients treated with monotherapy [methotrexate (MTX), 20 patients; sulfasalazine (SSA), 20 patients; hydroxychloroquine, 20 patients)], double therapy (MTX-SSA, 30 patients; MTX-hydroxychloroquine, 30 patients), versus those treated with all three drugs (MTX-SSA-hydroxychloroquine, 60 patients). RA, rheumatoid arthritis. (From Calguneri M, Pay S, Caliskaner Z, et al. Combination therapy versus monotherapy for the treatment of patients with rheumatoid arthritis. *Clin Exp Rheumatol* 1999;17:699–704, with permission.)

With the data provided from the COBRA trial, the Fin-RA trial, and the Turkish trial, a convincing case can be made to treat most patients initially with combination therapy. However, trials to define whether an approach that uses combinations initially is superior to rapid step-up programs have not been done. Additionally, every clinician knows many patients who have done very well with DMARD monotherapy. The question remains, however, whether all patients need combinations at the beginning or whether patients who benefit the most can be selected. Until the studies outlined in Table 35.2 are done or factors are identified that predict differential responses to therapy, recommendations for treating this group of patients will continue to be empiric. Rapid escalation of methotrexate monotherapy as needed to doses of 25 mg per week, with a switch to parenteral administration (42) if oral treatment is not optimal, would appear to be the most effective approach. If patients continue to have active disease, they should be started on combination DMARD therapy, and the studies described below for methotrexate suboptimal responders should dictate future therapeutic choices.

APPROACH TO PATIENTS WITH SUBOPTIMAL RESPONSE TO METHOTREXATE

Methotrexate has gained wide acceptance in the United States as the initial DMARD of choice to treat patients with RA (6). Unfortunately, many patients do not have a complete response and are characterized as incomplete or suboptimal responders. Usually, these patients are described by the weekly dose of methotrexate they have received, and, currently, patients who have received somewhere between 15 mg and 25 mg per week of methotrexate have been described as suboptimal responders. The response to parenteral methotrexate is superior to oral methotrexate in some patients, because oral absorption is highly variable (42); therefore, it would seem prudent to give most patients a trial of subcutaneous or intramuscular methotrexate before abandoning this form of therapy. Further, it is widely recognized that methotrexate can be safely used, particularly in combination with folic acid, in doses up to 25 mg per week. Therefore, a currently acceptable definition of methotrexate suboptimal responders might include increasing the dose to 25 mg per week, switching to parenteral administration (intramuscular or subcutaneous) if oral therapy is not maximally effective, and the use of folic acid (up to 4 mg per day) supplementation to help patients tolerate higher doses of methotrexate. However, it is important to point out that the studies reviewed, in all

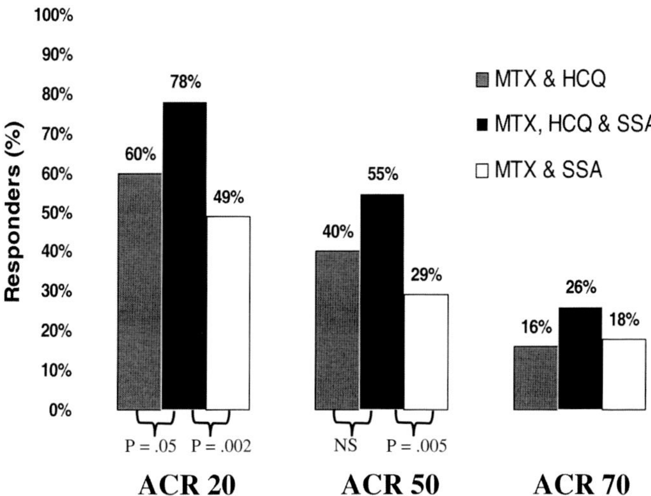

Figure 35.4. Percentage of patients meeting American College of Rheumatology (ACR) 20%, 50%, or 70% response rate by drug treatment. HCQ, hydroxychloroquine; MTX, methotrexate; SSA, sulfasalazine. (Adapted from O'Dell J, Leff R, Paulsen G, et al. Treatment of rheumatoid arthritis with methotrexate and hydroxychloroquine, methotrexate and sulfasalazine, or a combination of the three medications. *Arthritis Rheum* 2002;46:1164–1170.)

cases, used different and less rigorous definitions of suboptimal responders.

Because partial responses to methotrexate are a common clinical problem, a host of trials have been directed at this clinical situation (11–19). Other studies have been designed to compare combination therapy head to head with methotrexate therapy (7). These studies have validated the usefulness of all three combination DMARD trial designs: step-up, step-down, and parallel. However, patient characteristics that predict response remain to be fully clarified and will be the key to future optimal treatment. All the trials that compare an active drug to placebo in methotrexate suboptimal responders (Fig. 35.4) have a significant limitation, because clinicians need head-to-head comparisons with active products to make critical clinical judgments for their patients.

METHOTREXATE AND CYCLOSPORINE COMBINATION

The first study to show that combination therapy with methotrexate and another DMARD, compared with continued therapy with methotrexate alone in this group of patients, was advantageous was the cyclosporine-methotrexate trial (11) (Table 35.3). In this trial, 148 patients with active disease (despite methotrexate in doses up to 15 mg per week; mean dose of methotrexate 10.2 mg per week) were randomized to receive either cyclosporine in low to moderate doses or placebo, in addition to their baseline methotrexate. Forty-eight percent of the patients in the cyclosporine treatment group had achieved an ACR 20% response rate by 6 months, compared with 16% of the patients in the placebo group ($p = .001$). Creatinine elevations did occur in some patients in the cyclosporine group, and dosage adjustments were necessary, with creatinines at the end of the trial being higher in the cyclosporine-treated group than in those treated with placebo ($p = .02$). More importantly, long-term use of cyclosporine was associated with a high rate of withdrawal, most commonly because of elevated creatinine levels, hypertension, and lack of efficacy, or all three. Of the 335 patients enrolled in an open-label extension study, only 22% continued cyclosporine for 3 years (43). The main reasons for discontinuation were hypertension, increasing creatinine values, and inefficacy.

METHOTREXATE AND LEFLUNOMIDE COMBINATION

Among DMARDs, leflunomide is comparable in efficacy to other conventional therapies, such as methotrexate (44) and sulfasalazine (45). The low level of major hematologic and renal and pulmonary toxicity with leflunomide monotherapy suggests its use after or together with methotrexate. A double-blind placebo-controlled trial (14) has compared the addition of leflunomide or placebo to baseline methotrexate in 266 patients selected for suboptimal responses to methotrexate (mean, 16.4 mg per week) (Table 35.3). Leflunomide (10 mg per day) or placebo was added to methotrexate, and the dose of leflunomide could be increased to 20 mg per day. The ACR 20% criteria for clinical response were met by 46% of the group randomized to receive leflunomide at 24 weeks, compared to 20% of the placebo-treated patients ($p < .0001$). The combination was well tolerated clinically, but side effects were increased in the combination arm, with 22% of patients reporting diarrhea, 12% reporting nausea, and 5% reporting dizziness. Elevated levels of alanine aminotransferase occurred frequently (numbers not published) with increases of more than three times normal occurring in 2.3% of patients who received the combination. In a previous small open-label trial of 30 patients who received this combination, 60% of patients had liver enzyme elevations at some time during the trial, but only two patients were withdrawn (13). Reports of liver toxicity with leflunomide have come from Europe (European Agency for the Evaluation of Medicinal Products) and Australia (46). Whether these liver blood test abnormalities will limit the clinical use of this combination remains to be seen.

TABLE 35.3. Combination Trials

Author, Reference	Disease Duration [Mean (Yr)]	N	Double-Blind	Efficacy	Toxicity
McCarty (21,22)	9.9	31	No	++++	>>>
O'Dell (7,28,30)	8.6	102	Yes	++++	<
Kirwan (49,50)	1.3	128	Yes	++	NR
Tugwell (11)	10.3	148	Yes	++	>
Boers (8,40)	0.3	155	Yes	+++	<
Mottonen (9,41)	0.7	199	No	++	=
Calguneri (10)	2.3	180	No	++++	=
Kremer (14)	11.6	266	Yes	++	>
O'Dell (12)	6.9	171	Yes	+++	=

NR, not reported; ++++, very high efficacy; +++, high efficacy; ++, moderate efficacy; <, less toxicity than background or monotherapy; =, toxicity equal to background or monotherapy; >, greater toxicity than background or monotherapy; >>>, much greater toxicity than background or monotherapy.

METHOTREXATE-SULFASALAZINE-HYDROXYCHLOROQUINE

Therapy with the combination of methotrexate, sulfasalazine, and hydroxychloroquine, called *triple therapy*, has been shown by three different groups (four different trials) to not only be well tolerated (7,9,10,12), but also to be more effective than methotrexate monotherapy (7,10), sulfasalazine monotherapy (9), and, in an open trial of patients with early disease, more effective than the double combinations of methotrexate-sulfasalazine or methotrexate-hydroxychloroquine (10).

In a 2-year double-blind trial of patients with moderately advanced disease, the triple combination was compared with the two double combinations (methotrexate-sulfasalazine and methotrexate-hydroxychloroquine) in a head-to-head fashion (12). Patients were eligible for this trial if they had active RA of at least 6 months' duration. Patients were stratified for previous methotrexate use, and the previous user had to have active disease despite 17.5 mg per week.

Triple therapy and both double therapy groups tolerated their treatments well, with only 8% withdrawing for toxicities, which were mostly minor. Triple therapy was shown to be superior to either of the double combinations (Fig. 35.4). The primary outcome variable for this trial was ACR 20% response rate at 2 years, and it was achieved by 78% of the triple therapy patients, 60% of those on methotrexate-hydroxychloroquine ($p = .05$ for triple comparison), and 49% of those on methotrexate-sulfasalazine ($p = .002$, compared to triple) (Fig. 35.4). In a subanalysis of the methotrexate naïve and the methotrexate suboptimal responders, the investigators were able to show that in the methotrexate naïve group of patients, methotrexate-sulfasalazine–treated patients did better than methotrexate-hydroxychloroquine–treated patients (ACR 20% response rate of 71% vs. 56%). However, in the patients who entered the study as methotrexate suboptimal responders, the methotrexate-hydroxychloroquine combination was superior to the methotrexate-sulfasalazine combination (ACR 20% response rate of 55% vs. 36%). This latter observation is notable because the methotrexate-hydroxychloroquine combination has been a very popular combination, used by clinicians for years. These data lend support to this long-standing clinical preference.

NONCONVENTIONAL DISEASE-MODIFYING ANTIRHEUMATIC DRUGS

Although corticosteroids have not traditionally been considered DMARDs, they fulfill all the criteria for DMARDs, including retarding radiographic progression (47–50). Few clinicians who care for patients with RA dispute their efficacy. Indeed, corticosteroids have been used as baseline therapy for well over one-half of the patients included in most of the combination trials discussed earlier. This fact, more than any study, attests to their current usefulness, or at least perceived usefulness, in the treatment of RA.

Prednisolone appears to have been critical to the success of the COBRA protocol (8) and may have contributed to the success of the combination group in the Fin-RA trial (9). Kirwan et al.'s report on the ability of prednisolone to significantly retard radiographic progression of RA, compared to placebo (49,50), is evidence of the efficacy of steroids when used in combination with other DMARDs; all patients in the Kirwan trial were receiving routine background DMARD therapy. In this 2-year double-blind trial, 128 patients with early RA were randomized to receive prednisolone, 7.5 mg per day, or placebo in addition to background DMARD therapy (49). At the end of the 2 years, Larsen scores had increased by 0.72 units for the prednisolone group and by 5.37 units in the placebo group ($p = .004$). In a follow-up study, prednisolone was tapered, and the rate of radiographic progression increased and matched that of the placebo-treated group (50), further supporting the efficacy of prednisolone in this cohort.

The role of corticosteroids as a component of combination therapy remains to be defined. The COBRA trial, particularly the follow-up report of this group of patients (40), as well as the data from Kirwan et al., have raised the issue of whether short courses of high-dose corticosteroids should be used as a form of induction therapy (37).

OTHER COMBINATIONS WITH METHOTREXATE

After their combination therapy protocols of the early 1980s, which showed efficacy, but also toxicity, McCarty et al. reported on a cohort of patients treated with combinations that did not include cyclophosphamide (51). In an observation study of 169 patients followed in their clinic, McCarty et al. reported a complete remission rate of 43% when methotrexate, hydroxychloroquine, and azathioprine were added in a sequential as-needed fashion. In general, patients were started on either hydroxychloroquine or methotrexate alone or a combination of these two medications; azathioprine was added for patients who were not optimally controlled. Overall, they reported satisfactory control of inflammatory disease in 167 of 169 patients. The triple combination of methotrexate, hydroxychloroquine, and azathioprine was well tolerated and was needed in 69 patients (41% of the cohort). The remission rate in this group that needed three-drug therapy was 45%, similar to the overall rate of 43%.

As with all observational studies, the strength of this report is the inclusion of all patients from a particular clinical setting; thus, selection bias of those who do and do not qualify for the study were avoided. However, the weakness of this observation study is the introduction of evaluation bias that could only be controlled for by blinding.

Doxycycline has demonstrated efficacy in animal models of inflammatory arthritis and osteoarthritis (52,53). This efficacy appears to result because of its ability to inhibit metalloproteinases and, presumably, in this way, prevent or inhibit joint destruction. Studies in patients with RA with the closely related compound minocycline have also demonstrated efficacy (54–57). In two studies in patients with advanced disease (duration, 9 and 13 years), a similar degree of modest, but statistically significant, benefit was seen (54,55). A much more significant effect has been seen in the two double-blind studies that were done in patients with early disease (56,57). In the first of these studies, patients with seropositive early RA (<1 year) who had not previously received DMARDs or steroids were randomized into a double-blind trial; 65% of patients randomized to minocycline treatment achieved 50% improvement, compared to only 13% of those in the placebo group ($p < .005$). This response to minocycline when used in early disease was shown to be durable in a 4-year follow-up study (58). Recently, data have been published that compare minocycline to hydroxychloroquine as initial DMARD therapy for patients with early (<1 year) seropositive RA. In a 2-year double-blind protocol, minocycline was superior for both primary outcomes, ACR 50% response rate (60% vs. 33%, $p = .04$), and prednisone dose (mean, 0.81 mg per day vs. 3.21 mg per day, $p < .01$). Recent evidence strongly suggests that minocycline is working in RA because of its ability to upregulate interleukin-10 production (59). Trials are currently in progress to address the use of minocycline in combination with methotrexate in early RA.

BIOLOGICS IN COMBINATION

One of the major developments in the treatment of RA has been the introduction into clinical practice of biologic agents that target specific cytokines. These agents include etanercept and infliximab, which block the action of tumor necrosis factor α (TNF-α) and anakinra, which blocks interleukin-1. Both of the agents that block TNF-α have shown substantial efficacy in advanced RA as monotherapy, when compared to placebo (60,61). Additionally, both etanercept and infliximab have been shown to work well when used with methotrexate (15–17) in patients who have suboptimal responses to methotrexate (again, in comparison to methotrexate-plus-placebo–treated patients). In the case of infliximab, the combination with methotrexate may be particularly important as a possible way to decrease antibodies to the mouse component that may develop to this compound. In this regard, this agent is currently recommended by the Food and Drug Administration as combination therapy (with methotrexate) only. Figure 35.5 shows the percent of ACR 20% responders in the published trials that have been done on patients defined as methotrexate suboptimal responders. This figure is not an attempt to directly compare these therapies to each other; all of these trials defined suboptimal responses differently, were of different length, were done on patients with different disease duration, and had different designs. Figure 35.5 shows the effective therapies for this group of patients, and comparison trials are still needed (Table 35.3). Studies that have included etanercept, infliximab, and anakinra in combination with methotrexate are discussed in more detail in Chapters 31, 32, and 33.

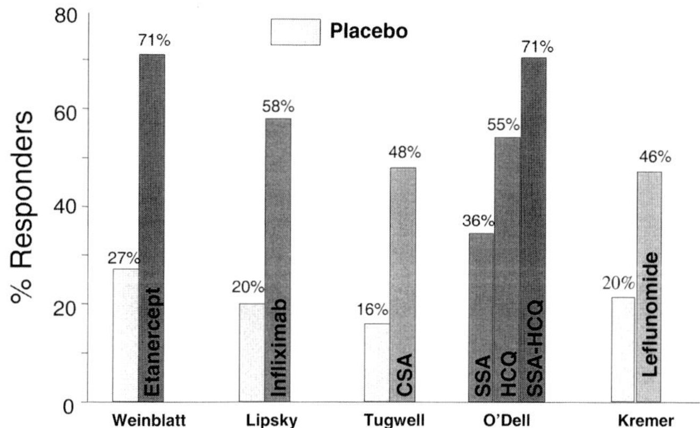

Figure 35.5. American College of Rheumatology (ACR) 20% response rates in five different trials that shared the common characteristic of enrolling patients who were defined as methotrexate (MTX) suboptimal responders or active disease despite MTX therapy. CSA, cyclosporin A; HCQ, hydroxychloroquine; SSA, sulfasalazine. [Adapted from Tugwell P, Pincus T, Yocum D, et al. Combination therapy with cyclosporine and methotrexate in severe rheumatoid arthritis. *N Engl J Med* 1995;333:137–141; O'Dell J, Leff R, Paulsen G, et al. Treatment of rheumatoid arthritis with methotrexate and hydroxychloroquine, methotrexate and sulfasalazine, or a combination of the three medications. *Arthritis Rheum* 2002;46(5):1164–1170; Kremer JM, Genovese MC, Cannon GW, et al. Concomitant leflunomide therapy in patients with active rheumatoid arthritis despite stable doses of methotrexate. A randomized, double-blind, placebo-controlled trial. *Ann Intern Med* 2002;137:726–733; Weinblatt ME, Kremer JM, Bankhurst AD, et al. A trial of etanercept, a recombinant tumor necrosis factor receptor: Fc fusion protein, in patients with rheumatoid arthritis receiving methotrexate. *N Engl J Med* 1999;340:253–259; and Lipsky P, et al. Infliximab and methotrexate in the treatment of rheumatoid arthritis. *N Engl J Med* 2000;343:1594–1602.]

SELECTING THE RIGHT PATIENTS FOR DIFFERENT THERAPIES

The key to improving care of patients with RA lies in selecting the optimal therapies for different patients. Factors that predict a poor prognosis for patients with RA are well accepted and include rheumatoid factor, elevated erythrocyte sedimentation rate and C-reactive protein, the number of joints involved, erosions, the presence of certain genetic markers, and so forth. Therefore, some clinicians have advocated that patients with certain combinations of these factors should be treated more aggressively. However, unless these factors can be shown to predict response to certain therapies in a differential fashion, their use should not be advocated. For example, it is conceivable that patients in an intermediate or even low-risk group may benefit the most from the early use of certain aggressive therapies, whereas patients with the worst prognostic marks will do poorly, regardless of therapy.

Although patient characteristics recommending one therapeutic regimen over another remain to be fully elucidated, genetic differences among individuals may influence outcomes. In an attempt to predict response to specific RA treatment regimens, patients with late disease (7) were tested for the presence of shared HLA-DRB1 epitope alleles (62). Patients who were shared-epitope positive were much more likely to achieve a 50% response if treated with triple therapy (methotrexate-sulfasalazine-hydroxychloroquine), compared with methotrexate alone (94% vs. 32% responders, $p < .0001$). In contrast, shared-epitope–negative patients did equally well, regardless of the treatment provided (88% responders for triple-drug therapy vs. 83% for methotrexate monotherapy). This observation has been supported by data from the Fin-RA trial that suggests that those patients who were DR-4 positive benefitted the most from combination therapy.

FUTURE RESEARCH

Treatment of RA using methotrexate combinations should be the gold standard against which future therapies are compared; overwhelming evidence has been discussed that clearly demonstrates that a variety of DMARD combinations are more effective than methotrexate alone. Many questions remain to be answered (Table 35.2) regarding the appropriate timing of combination therapy and the optimal combinations for specific patients (e.g., differentiated according to clinical or genetic features) and for specific clinical situations (e.g., induction, maintenance therapy, suboptimal response to methotrexate, etc.). Other unanswered questions regarding combination therapy, especially as biologic response modifiers are added, involve appropriate monitoring and long-term safety, particularly as they relate to risk for infection, lymphoma, and hepatotoxicity. Furthermore, the cost–benefit implications of long-term combination therapy and any additional monitoring have yet to be addressed. Future research is needed to clarify the role of steroids and, particularly, biologic response modifiers, specifically anti-TNF therapies, both as components of and alternatives to methotrexate combination regimens.

REFERENCES

1. Pincus T, Marcum SB, Callahan LF. Long-term drug therapy for rheumatoid arthritis in seven rheumatology private practices: II. Second line drugs and prednisone. *J Rheumatol* 1992;19:1885–1894.
2. Wolfe F. The epidemiology of drug treatment failure in rheumatoid arthritis. *Baillieres Clin Rheumatol* 1995;9:619–632.
3. Bathon J, Martin RW, Fleischmann RM, et al. A comparison of etanercept and methotrexate in patients with early rheumatoid arthritis. *N Engl J Med* 2000;343:1586–1593.

4. Choi HK, Seeger JD, Kuntz KM. A cost effectiveness analysis of treatment options for methotrexate-naive rheumatoid arthritis. *J Rheumatol* 2002;29:1156–1165.
5. Choi HK. Methotrexate and mortality in patients with rheumatoid arthritis: a prospective study. *Lancet* 2002;359:1173–1177.
6. Mikuls T, O'Dell J. The treatment of rheumatoid arthritis: current trends in therapy. *Arthritis Rheum* 1999;42:S79.
7. O'Dell JR, Haire CE, Erikson N, et al. Treatment of rheumatoid arthritis with methotrexate alone, sulfasalazine, and hydroxychloroquine, or a combination of all three medications. *N Engl J Med* 1996;334:1287–1291.
8. Boers M, Verhoeven AC, Markusse HM, et al. Randomized comparison of combined step-down prednisolone, methotrexate and sulphasalazine with sulphasalazine alone in early rheumatoid arthritis. *Lancet* 1997;350:309–318.
9. Mottonen T, Hannonsen P, Leirasalo-Repo M, et al. Comparison of combination therapy with single-drug therapy in early rheumatoid arthritis: a randomised trial. *Lancet* 1999;353:1568–1573.
10. Calguneri M, Pay S, Caliskaner Z, et al. Combination therapy versus monotherapy for the treatment of patients with rheumatoid arthritis. *Clin Exp Rheumatol* 1999;17:699–704.
11. Tugwell P, Pincus T, Yocum D, et al. Combination therapy with cyclosporine and methotrexate in severe rheumatoid arthritis. *N Engl J Med* 1995;333:137–141.
12. O'Dell J, Leff R, Paulsen G, et al. Treatment of rheumatoid arthritis with methotrexate and hydroxychloroquine, methotrexate and sulfasalazine, or a combination of the three medications. *Arthritis Rheum* 2002;46:1164–1170.
13. Weinblatt ME, Kremer JM, Coblyn JS, et al. Pharmacokinetics, safety, and efficacy of combination treatment with methotrexate and leflunomide in patients with active rheumatoid arthritis. *Arthritis Rheum* 1999;48:1322–1328.
14. Kremer JM, Genovese MC, Cannon GW, et al. Concomitant leflunomide therapy in patients with active rheumatoid arthritis despite stable doses of methotrexate. A randomized, double-blind, placebo-controlled trial. *Ann Intern Med* 2002;137:726–733.
15. Maini RN, Breedveld FC, Kalden JR, et al. Therapeutic efficacy of multiple intravenous infusions of anti-tumor necrosis factor alpha monoclonal antibody combined with low-dose weekly methotrexate in rheumatoid arthritis. *Arthritis Rheum* 1998;41:1552–1563.
16. Weinblatt ME, Kremer JM, Bankhurst AD, et al. A trial of etanercept, a recombinant tumor necrosis factor receptor: Fc fusion protein, in patients with rheumatoid arthritis receiving methotrexate. *N Engl J Med* 1999;340:253–259.
17. Lipsky P, et al. Infliximab and methotrexate in the treatment of rheumatoid arthritis. *N Engl J Med* 2000;343:1594–1602.
18. Cohen S, Hurd E, Cush J, et al. Treatment of rheumatoid arthritis with anakinra, a recombinant human interleukin-1 receptor antagonist, in combination with methotrexate. *Arthritis Rheum* 2002;46:614–624.
19. Keystone E, Weinblatt M, Furst D, et al. The ARMADA trial: a double-blind placebo controlled trial of the fully human anti-TNF monoclonal antibody, adalimumab (D2E7), in patients with active RA on methotrexate (MTX). *Arthritis Rheum* 2001;44:S213.
20. Kremer JM. Combination therapy with biologic agents in rheumatoid arthritis: perils and promise. *Arthritis Rheum* 1998;41:1548–1551.
21. McCarty DJ, Carrera GF. Treatment of intractable rheumatoid arthritis with combined cyclophosphamide, azathioprine, and hydroxychloroquine. *JAMA* 1982;248:1718–1723.
22. Csuka ME, Carrero GF, McCarty DJ. Treatment of intractable rheumatoid arthritis with combined cyclophosphamide, azathioprine, and hydroxychloroquine. A follow-up study. *JAMA* 1986;255:2315–2319.
23. Willkens RF, Sharp JT, Stablein D, et al. Comparison of azathioprine, methotrexate, and the combination of the two in the treatment of rheumatoid arthritis. *Arthritis Rheum* 1995;38:1799–1806.
24. Williams HJ, Ward JR, Reding JC, et al. Comparison of auranofin, methotrexate, and the combination of both in the treatment of rheumatoid arthritis: a controlled clinical trial. *Arthritis Rheum* 1992;35:259–269.
25. Haagsma CJ, van Riel PL, de Rooj DJ, et al. Combination of methotrexate and sulphasalazine vs methotrexate alone. A randomized open clinical trial in rheumatoid arthritis patients resistant to sulphasalazine therapy. *Br J Rheumatol* 1994;33:1049–1055.
26. Dougados M, Combe B, Cantagrel A, et al. Combination therapy in early rheumatoid arthritis: a randomized, controlled, double blind 52 week clinical trial of sulphasalazine and methotrexate compared with the single components. *Ann Rheum Dis* 1999;58:220–225.
27. Felson DT, Anderson JJ, Meenan RF. The efficacy and toxicity of combination therapy in rheumatoid arthritis. A meta-analysis. *Arthritis Rheum* 1994;37:1487–1491.
28. O'Dell J, Haire C, Erickson N, et al. Triple DMARD therapy for rheumatoid arthritis: efficacy. *Arthritis Rheum* 1994;37:S295.
29. Paulus HE, Egger MJ, Ward JR, William JH. Analysis of improvement in individual rheumatoid arthritis patients treated with disease-modifying antirheumatic drugs, based on the findings in patients treated with placebo. *Arthritis Rheum* 1990;33:477–484.
30. O'Dell J, Paulsen G, Haire C, et al. Combination DMARD therapy with methotrexate (M) - Sulfasalazine (S) - Hydroxychloroquine (H) in rheumatoid arthritis (RA): continued efficacy with minimal toxicity at 5 years. *Arthritis Rheum* 1998;41[Suppl 9]:S132.
31. O'Dell JR, Haire C, Erikson N, et al. Efficacy of triple DMARD therapy in patients with RA with suboptimal response to methotrexate. *J Rheumatol* 1996;23[Suppl 44]:72–74.
32. Pinals RS, Masi AT, Larsen RA. Subcommittee for Criteria of Remission in Rheumatoid Arthritis of the American Rheumatism Association Diagnostic and Therapeutic Criteria Committee. Preliminary criteria for clinical remission in rheumatoid arthritis. *Arthritis Rheum* 1981;24:1308–1315.
33. Sokka T, Pincus T. Eligibility of patients in routine care for major clinical trials of anti-tumor necrosis factor-alpha (TNF-α) agents in rheumatoid arthritis. *Arthritis Rheum* 2003;48:313–318.
34. Egsmose C, Lung B, Borg G, et al. Patients with rheumatoid arthritis benefit from early second-line therapy: 5-year follow-up of a prospective double-blind placebo-controlled study. *J Rheumatol* 1995;22:2208–2213.
35. Tsakonas E, Fitzgerald AA, Fitzcharles MA, et al. Consequences of delayed therapy with second-line agents in rheumatoid arthritis: a 3 year followup on the hydroxychloroquine in early rheumatoid arthritis (HERA) study. *J Rheumatol* 2000;27:623–629.
36. Lard LR. Early versus delayed treatment in patients with recent-onset rheumatoid arthritis: comparison of two cohorts who received different treatment strategies. *Am J Med* 2001;111:446–451.
37. O'Dell JR. Treating rheumatoid arthritis early: a window of opportunity. *Arthritis Rheum* 2002;46:283–285.
38. Wilske KR, Healey LA. Remodeling the pyramid—a concept whose time has come. *J Rheumatol* 1989;16:565–567.
39. Felson DT, Anderson JJ, Boers M, et al. American College of Rheumatology preliminary definition of improvement in rheumatoid arthritis. *Arthritis Rheum* 1995;38:727–735.
40. Landewe RBM, Boers M, Verhoeven AC, et al. COBRA combination therapy in patients with early rheumatoid arthritis. *Arthritis Rheum* 2002;46:347–356.
41. Neva MH. FIN-RACo Trial Group. Combination drug therapy retards the development of rheumatoid atlantoaxial subluxations. *Arthritis Rheum* 2000; 43:2397–2401.
42. Herman RA, Veng-Pedersen P, Hoffman J, et al. Pharmacokinetics of low-dose methotrexate in rheumatoid arthritis patients. *J Pharm Sci* 1989;78:165.
43. Yocum DE, Stein M, Pincus T. Long-term safety of cyclosporin/Sandimmune™ (CsA/SIM) alone and in combination with methotrexate (MTX) in the treatment of active rheumatoid arthritis (RA): analysis of open-label extension studies. *Arthritis Rheum* 1998;41[Suppl]:S364(abst).
44. Strand V, Cohen S, Schiff M, et al., for the Leflunomide Rheumatoid Arthritis Investigators Group. Treatment of active rheumatoid arthritis with leflunomide compared with placebo and methotrexate. *Arch Intern Med* 1999;159:2542–2550.
45. Smolen JS, Kalden JR, Scott DL, et al. Efficacy and safety of leflunomide compared with placebo and sulphasalazine in active rheumatoid arthritis: a double-blind, randomized, multicentre trial. *Lancet* 1999;353:259–266.
46. Leflunomide—serious hepatic, blood, skin and respiratory reactions. *Aust Adverse Drug React Bull* 2001;20.
47. The Joint Committee of the Medical Research Council and Nuffield Foundation on Clinical Trials of Cortisone, ACTH, and Other Therapeutic Measures in Chronic Rheumatic Diseases. A comparison of prednisolone with aspirin or other analgesics in the treatment of rheumatoid arthritis. *Ann Rheum Dis* 1959;18:173–187.
48. A comparison of prednisolone with aspirin or other analgesics in the treatment of rheumatoid arthritis. *Ann Rheum Dis* 1960;19:331–337.
49. Kirwan JR and the Arthritis and Rheumatism Council Low-Dose Glucocorticoid Study Group. The effect of glucocorticoids on joint destruction in rheumatoid arthritis. *N Engl J Med* 1995;333:142–146.
50. Hickling P, Jacoby RK, Kirwan JR. Joint destruction after glucocorticoids are withdrawn in early rheumatoid arthritis. *Br J Rheumatol* 1998;37:930–936.
51. McCarty DJ, Harman JG, Grassanovich JL, et al. Combination drug therapy of seropositive rheumatoid arthritis. *J Rheumatol* 1995;22:1636–1645.
52. Greenwald RA, Moak SA, Ramamurthy NS, Golub LM. Tetracyclines suppress matrix metalloproteinase activity in adjuvant arthritis and in combination with flurbiprofen ameliorate bone damage. *J Rheumatol* 1992;19:927–938.
53. Yu LP, Smith GN, Brandt K, et al. Reduction of the severity of canine osteoarthritis by prophylactic treatment with oral doxycycline. *Arthritis Rheum* 1993;35: 1150–1159.
54. Kloppenburg M, Breedveld FC, Terwiel J, et al. Minocycline in active rheumatoid arthritis. *Arthritis Rheum* 1994;37:629–636.
55. Tilley BC, Alarcon GS, Heyse SP, et al. Minocycline in rheumatoid arthritis. *Ann Int Med* 1995;122:81–89.
56. O'Dell JR, Haire CE, Palmer W, et al. Treatment of early rheumatoid arthritis with minocycline or placebo. *Arthritis Rheum* 1997;40:842–848.
57. O'Dell JR, Blakely KW, Mallek JA, et al. Treatment of early seropositive rheumatoid arthritis. A two-year, double-blind comparison of minocycline and hydroxychloroquine. *Arthritis Rheum* 2001;44:2235–2241.
58. O'Dell JR, Paulsen G, Haire CE, et al. Treatment of early seropositive rheumatoid arthritis with minocycline: four-year followup of a double-blind, placebo-controlled trial. *Arthritis Rheum* 1999;42:1691–1695.
59. Ritchlin CT, Haas-Smith SA, Schwartz EM, Greenwald RA. Minocycline but not doxycycline upregulates IL-10 production in human synoviocytes, mononuclear cells and synovial explants. *Arthritis Rheum* 2000;43:S345.
60. Elliott MJ, Maini RN, Reldmann M, et al. Randomised double-blind comparison of chimeric monoclonal antibody to tumor necrosis factor alpha (cA2) versus placebo in rheumatoid arthritis. *Lancet* 1994;344:1105–1110.
61. Moreland LW, Baumgartner SW, Schiff MH, et al. Treatment of rheumatoid arthritis with a recombinant human tumor necrosis factor receptor (p75)-Fc fusion protein. *N Engl J Med* 1997;337:141–147.
62. O'Dell JR, Nepom BS, Haire C, et al. HLA-DRB1 typing in rheumatoid arthritis: predicting response to specific treatments. *Ann Rheum Dis* 1998;57:209–213.

CHAPTER 36

Treatment of Early Disease

Ferdinand C. Breedveld

Research on the clinical course of large cohorts of patients with rheumatoid arthritis (RA) support the view that the consequences of RA (joint damage and loss of function) are due to persistent, inadequately controlled inflammation. Therefore, a goal of treatment with the currently available interventions is not to decrease signs and symptoms of disease but to return the patient to normal physical and vocational function. Given the role of inflammation in disease pathogenesis, early interventions, shown to prevent irreversible joint damage, disability, a decrease in quality of life, hospitalizations, and premature mortality, are directed against cellular and soluble mediators of this process. Recent findings increasingly support an early, agressive approach. In addition, data obtained from early arthritis clinics challenge previous notions on pathogenesis and disease classification. Progression toward persistent destructive synovitis may involve several steps. Therefore, it can be hypothesized that early intervention affects a pathophysiology that differs from late-stage disease and that this difference creates a window of opportunity not only to prevent destructiveness but also to achieve long-lasting remission. Recognition of RA as early as possible is important. Data from cohorts of patients referred to an early arthritis clinic have revealed that a significant proportion of patients do not fulfill classification criteria for RA initially, but nevertheless develop a chronic erosive disease. These findings highlighted the need for diagnostic and prognostic criteria that would be useful early in the course of RA. Such criteria may also form the scientific basis for referral criteria that have already been shown to be helpful in enabling the rapid diagnosis of active RA and the subsequent initiation of disease-modifying antirheumatic drug (DMARD) treatment.

CHANGING CONCEPTS IN RHEUMATOID ARTHRITIS TREATMENT

An impetus to changing the strategy for treating RA came with reports in the late 1980s of the increased mortality associated with RA (1–3). In many diseases, premature death has served as a benchmark for severity, a rationale for aggressive therapy, and a baseline for improved outcomes. In those studies, premature mortality risks were primarily associated with more severe manifestations of joint destruction and function loss rather than with drugs to treat RA. Therefore, an important question to analyze is whether an improvement in the scores for destruction or functional disability is associated with an improvement in long-term survival. Documentation of such an association needs large-scale longitudinal follow-up studies. The most frequently used methods of assessing structural damage and function loss associated with RA is radiographic quantification of joint damage and questionnaires, such as the Health Assessment Questionnaire (HAQ), specifically designed to monitor functional status in RA patients. Many clinical studies, including cross-sectional studies, prospective studies of patients with varying disease duration, and prospective follow-up studies of patients with early RA, have illustrated the gradually progressive nature of the disease. Although epidemiologic studies indicated that many people who met criteria for RA had a self-limiting process, later studies showed that most patients with RA seen in clinical settings have a persistent inflammatory symmetric arthritis—a progressive disease that does not respond completely to traditional therapies (4,5).

A comprehensive evaluation of published papers has concluded that a large majority found a relation between the rate of progression of structural damage as determined by joint radiography and progression of disability (6). In a 12-year prospective follow-up study of early RA patients, the statistical association between radiographic damage and disability was weak in the early years but became stronger over time (7) (Table 36.1). The disease activity was strongly associated with disability throughout the disease course. These results indicate that the variable course of the HAQ score in individual patients is due to its continuous strong correlation with the variable course of disease activity. Destruction contributes increasingly to the loss of functional capacity, but the disease activity is a strong determinant at all stages of the disease.

Summarizing prospective studies of radiographic progression of patients with early RA, Van der Heijde (8) concluded that 75% of patients with early RA develop the initial erosions in the first 2 years of the disease. However, other investigators have reported that RA patients who are free of erosions at 3 years may nevertheless develop erosions later in their disease course (9). The inherent variability in disease progression among RA patients underscores the need to identify predictors of radiographic damage. Evaluations of predictive factors in early arthritis clinics report common elements in the baseline risk factors for both radiographic progression and disability, which include involvement of large joints, disease duration of 3 months or longer, involvement of hand joints, high disease activity at baseline, increased levels of rheumatoid factor and C-reactive protein levels, as well as radiologic damage (9–12). Although combinations of risk factors for progressive disease may predict various categories of outcome with 35%

TABLE 36.1. Correlation between Functional Capacity and Disability in Rheumatoid Arthritis[a]

Health Assessment Questionnaire	Disease Activity Score	Sharp Score	Erythrocyte Sedimentation Rate	Ritchie	Swollen Joints
0 yr	0.68[b]	0.22[c]	0.24[c]	0.70[b]	0.33[b]
3 yr	0.51[b]	0.29[b]	0.18	0.55[b]	0.36[b]
6 yr	0.52[b]	0.41[b]	0.45[b]	0.51[b]	0.40[b]
12 yr	0.61[b]	0.57[b]	0.38[b]	0.55[b]	0.44[b]

[a]Destruction in hands and feet (Sharp score), erythrocyte sedimentation rate, Ritchie score, and swollen joint count at four points in time in a 12-year follow-up cohort of 112 rheumatoid arthritis patients.
[b]$p < .001$.
[c]$p < .05$.

to 83% accuracy, assessment of risk factors is not sufficient for decision making at the individual patient level to avoid overtreatment or missing an opportunity to prevent irreversible destruction.

In this respect, new techniques, particularly magnetic resonance imaging, ultrasonography, and biochemical or immunologic markers, have shown potential to improve outcome prediction. New hardware, new software, and falling costs will enhance the usefulness and availability of these techniques. By providing more accurate information on prognosis, such predictors offer the prospect of tailoring DMARD therapy to the individual patient. However, selecting the appropriate patients for early and aggressive therapy is far from clear. Möttönen et al. (13) have argued that a good prognosis of RA does not exist, only slow versus rapid progression. Given the relative safety of the current aggressive therapies, their use in patients with mild disease may be successful, perhaps reducing the need for selection of patients for particular treatments based on disease outcome parameters.

EARLY DISEASE-MODIFYING ANTIRHEUMATIC DRUG TREATMENT IMPROVES RHEUMATOID ARTHRITIS OUTCOME

The options for treating a patient with early-onset RA include traditional DMARDs, such as hydroxychloroquine, sulfasalazine, gold salts, and methotrexate, and newer agents such as leflunomide and the inhibitors of the proinflammatory cytokines interleukin-1 and tumor necrosis factor (TNF) (14). These agents have been shown to reduce the signs and symptoms of RA in all stages of the disease and have a considerably greater efficacy to toxicity ratio than traditional agents such as gold salts, penicillamine, and azathioprine. Nonetheless, sustained remission is unusual. Reported remission rates for patients 6 months to 2 years after diagnosis of RA treated by either a single DMARD or placebo have varied between 12% and 27% (15–17). In patients who responded to DMARDs and reached a partial remission, discontinuation of treatment led to a flare within 2 years in more than 50% of the studied patients (18).

Methotrexate has been the most frequently used DMARD in early RA patients with high disease activity. Numerous studies have shown that methotrexate is effective and is generally well tolerated over long periods. Because of the abundant information on the use of methotrexate, evidence-based approaches can be used to avoid many problems. The recommended dosages were increased during the 1990s, and parenteral administration is frequently used (19,20). Several clinical trials have been able to show that DMARDs can reduce radiologic progression. Reduction of radiologic progression has been demonstrated for intramuscular gold (21,22). More recently, sulfasalazine was shown to decrease the rate of radiologic progression more than hydroxychloroquine at 48 weeks in patients with early RA (23). In a metaanalysis, patients treated with methotrexate and patients treated with DMARDs other than methotrexate had similar rates of progression (24).

Low dosages (<10 mg per day) of oral glucocorticoids are considered by many physicians to be an effective symptomatic drug regimen, but their usage has given rise to continuous debate. A metaanalysis of effectiveness suggested that glucocorticoids appear to be more effective than placebo and are nearly equivalent to traditional DMARDs in improving most of the conventional outcome measures (25,26). In patients with early RA, Kirwan (27) demonstrated a significant reduction in radiographic damage if low-dose glucocorticoids were added to antirheumatic treatment in a placebo-controlled study among patients with early RA. Patients received prednisone (7.5 mg per day) or placebo for 2 years in addition to nonsteroidal antiinflammatory drugs (NSAIDs) (95% of patients) and DMARDs (71% of patients). After 2 years, both the mean number of erosions and the number of patients with erosions were significantly lower in the group treated with glucocorticosteroids.

In a placebo-controlled trial, van Everdingen et al. (28) reported that 10 mg of oral prednisone per day without DMARDs produced more clinical improvement than placebo and delayed radiographic progression in early RA. In the first 3 months, patients taking prednisone showed significant clinical improvement compared to those taking placebo. The significance of most differences disappeared at 6 months. However, the usage of additional therapies was significantly lower in the prednisone group. From 12 months on, radiologic scores showed significantly less progression of joint damage compared to placebo. No clinically relevant differences in side effects were observed except for a higher incidence of new osteoporotic fractures in the prednisone group. These investigators concluded that given the limited disease-modifying effects of 10 mg prednisone per day this treatment should be combined with other DMARDs.

Analysis of delayed treatment trials (extensions of placebo-controlled investigations in which the placebo group is switched to active treatment at some point in time) has clearly shown the efficacy of early DMARD treatment for early RA (29,30). In each trial, the group treated at presentation with DMARDs showed significantly more improvement in efficacy parameters than the groups for whom treatment was delayed. In a placebo-controlled study, Borg et al. (29) found significantly higher improvement in joint swelling, HAQ, and mental state as well as less progression of radiographic joint damage after 2 years when RA patients were treated promptly with auranofin. Van der Heijde et al. (30) compared the outcome of NSAID treatment alone with that of DMARDs in early RA and reported more disease activity in the NSAID group. Statistically significant advantages at 12 months for patients receiving DMARDs

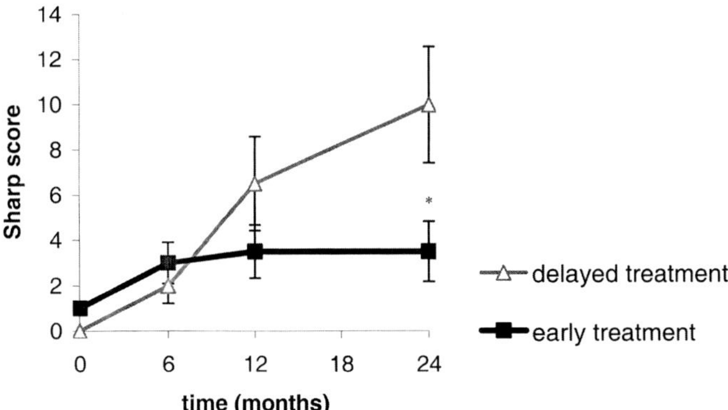

Figure 36.1. Median Sharp score (standard error) during follow-up. * $p < .05$ compared with the delayed treatment group.

immediately with regard to all primary end points were indicated by differences in improvement from baseline. These differences were 0.3 for disability (range, 0–3), 10 mm for pain (range, 0–100), 39 for joint score (0–534), and 11 mm per hour for erythrocyte sedimentation rate (range, 0–140). Radiologic abnormalities progressed at a statistically equal rate in this study but were numerically worse in the non-DMARD group. Another study has independently demonstrated that even a brief delay of 3 to 6 months in starting DMARD therapy has a significant impact on radiographic outcome 2 years later (Fig. 36.1) (31). Importantly, most of these data came well before the impact of biologic treatments. At present, there is little question that biologic treatment can not only halt radiographic progression of established disease but can also alter the 2-year trajectory of radiographic damage in patients with early disease (32).

Early treatment with effective DMARDs may also have effect on long-term outcome and mortality in RA. The studies of Egsmose et al. (33) and Munro et al. (34) indicate that early initiation of DMARDs results in a statistically significant better long-term functional capacity than with a delayed start. Symmons et al. (35) examined the long-term mortality outcome of RA patients divided into late and early presenter groups. Mortality among RA patients who presented early was found to be lower than that for those who presented late in the course of the disease. The study concluded that early treatment results in a milder disease and thereby in improved survival. Dutch patients identified after 1985 and enrolled in a prospective cohort for 10 years did not die any sooner than controls matched for age and sex (36). In addition to considering efficacy of therapy and its effects on mortality, the investigators presented evidence that DMARD toxicity is not worse than that found with long-term NSAID use. These findings provide rheumatologists with additional confidence in their approach to patients with early-onset disease.

COMBINATION THERAPY

When the initial aim of therapeutic approach of RA is the control of disease activity to prevent irreversible damage, combining DMARDs may provide additive effects. High-quality trials have provided evidence of additive therapeutic effects of DMARD combinations, and toxicity remains at an acceptable level. In combining DMARDs, three main strategies can be distinguished: parallel, step-up, and step-down regimens (37–39). In patients with established (or advanced) disease, TNF-α antagonists (40), cyclosporin (41), and leflunomide (42) improve suboptimal clinical responses to methotrexate; the triple combination of methotrexate, sulfasalazine, and hydroxychloroquine also appears clinically better than the components alone (43).

Boers et al. (44) compared the combination of sulfasalazine (2 g per day), methotrexate (7.5 mg per day), and prednisolone (initially 60 mg per day, tapered in six weekly steps to 7.5 mg per day) with sulfasalazine alone in 155 patients with early, active RA. At week 28, significantly better outcomes in the combined treatment group were seen in all composite measures than in the sulfasalazine-alone arm. The clinical difference between the two groups was no longer present after prednisolone was stopped. In addition to the clinical results, progression of radiographically quantified joint damage in the combined group was one-third of that in the sulfasalazine group. Furthermore, radiologic progression in the following 4 years was less progressive in the combination therapy group. Significantly fewer patients were withdrawn from the combined treated than from sulfasalazine treatment due to either inefficacy or toxicity. This study, with its step-down combination treatment strategy, indicated that a combination of relatively high-dose corticosteroid therapy with two DMARDs improves clinical outcome. The problem with this treatment schedule is the rapid loss of the initially achieved advantage due to the cessation of prednisolone.

Efficacy of combination DMARD therapy in early RA was also shown by Möttönen et al. (45) who reported that the combination of methotrexate (7.5–15.0 mg per week), sulfasalazine (1–2 g per day), hydroxychloroquine (300 mg per day), and prednisolone (5–10 mg per day) was superior to sulfasalazine with or without prednisone. After 2 years, remission was achieved in 36% of the patients taking combination therapy and 18% of the patients taking single-drug therapy. At 2 years, the percentages of American College of Rheumatology (ACR) 50% responders was 71% versus 58%, respectively. Significantly more new erosions developed in the single-treatment group compared to the combination group. The frequency of adverse events was similar in both groups. Calguneri et al. (46) studied prospectively the efficacy of single DMARD (methotrexate, sulfasalazine, or hydroxychloroquine) or two DMARDs (methotrexate and sulfasalazine or methotrexate and hydroxychloroquine) and a combination of all three drugs in a prospective randomized trial of 2 years' duration. At the end of the trial, there were significant improvements in the clinical and laboratory parameters in all three groups. However, improvements were greater in the patients taking combination therapies. The triple therapy was more effective than the two-drug combinations (46). Furthermore, the study by Kirwan (27), in which the addition of prednisolone to conventional DMARD therapy showed less radiographic progression compared to conventional DMARD therapy alone, also supports the use of combination therapy.

Not all studies on combination DMARD therapy in early RA show superior efficacy compared to monotherapy. Haagsma et al. (47) and Dougados et al. (48) found that methotrexate and sulfasalazine therapy in combination produced no additional clinical benefits compared to single-drug treatment in randomized, controlled, double-blind clinical studies of 1 year in early RA. The development of joint damage was also assessed, and progression was found to be similar in each treatment arm. Van den Borne et al. (49) enrolled early RA patients with a suboptimal response to chloroquine into a randomized, placebo-controlled, double-blind study comparing the addition of cyclosporin A (1.25–2.50 mg per day) with placebo. No significant benefits were found. Information regarding the reviewed studies is summarized in Table 36.2.

The data available at present suggest that, in early RA, step-down DMARD therapy that includes corticosteroids leads to enhanced efficacy with acceptable toxicity. According to surveys, however, the majority of rheumatologists use combina-

TABLE 36.2. Randomized Controlled Trials of Combination Treatment Strategy with Early Rheumatoid Arthritis Patients

Trial (Reference)	No. of Patients, Selection Criteria	Symptom Duration at Baseline	Drugs Compared	Corticosteroid Use during Trial	Combination Treatment Strategy	Evaluation at (Time)	Clinical Efficacy and (X-Ray Significance)
COBRA trial [Boers et al. (44)]	155, previous treatment with HCQ in 23% of patients	Median 4 mo (≤2 yr)	SSZ + MTX + Prd vs. SSZ	Combi: Prd 60 mg/day tapered to 7.5 mg and stopped after 28 wk	Step-down	28 wk	ACR 50%: 49% vs. 27% (p = .007) Rem[a]: 28% vs. 16% (p = .14) [x-ray (p ≤.0001)]
				Single: not allowed		56 wk	ACR, Rem NS; efficacy withdrawal 5% vs. 15% [x-ray (p = .004)]
FINRACo trial [Möttönen et al. (13)]	199, DMARD naïve	Mean 8 mo (<2 yr)	Combi: mainly SSZ + MTX + HCQ + Prd vs. single DMARD ± Prd	Combi: up to 10 mg/day Single: 0–10 mg/day	Tailored steps with flexible dose adjustment	2 yr	ACR 50%: 71% vs. 58% (p = .058) Rem[b]: 37% vs. 18% (p = .003) [x-ray (p = .002)]
Haagsma et al. (47)	105, DMARD naïve	Mean 3 mo (≤1 yr)	MTX + SSZ vs. MTX vs. SSZ	Not allowed	Parallel with dose adjustment	52 wk	ACR 20%: 78% vs. 74% vs. 71% (NS)
Dougados et al. (48)	209, DMARD naïve	Mean 13 mo (RA diagnosis <1 yr)	MTX + SSZ vs. MTX vs. SSZ	Not reported	Parallel with dose adjustment	52 wk	ACR 20%: 65% vs. 59% vs. 59% [x-ray (NS)]
Van den Borne et al. (49)	88, suboptimal responders to CQ	Mean 4 mo (<3 yr)	CQ + Pl vs. CQ + CSA 1.25 mg/kg/day vs. CQ + CSA 2.5 mg/kg/day	Not reported	Parallel	24 wk	ACR 20%: 28% vs. 34% vs. 50% (p = .07)

ACR 20/50%, fulfilling American College of Rheumatology response criteria; Combi, combination therapy group; CQ, chloroquine; Cs, corticosteroids; CSA, cyclosporine A; DMARD, disease-modifying antirheumatic drug; HCQ, hydroxychloroquine; MTX, methotrexate; NS, not significant; Pl, placebo; Prd, prednisone/prednisolone; Rem, remission rate; Single, single therapy group; SSZ, sulfasalazine; x-ray, radiographic analysis.
[a]ACR criteria for probable or definite remissions.
[b]ACR criteria for definite remission (fatigue and duration excluded, but all others had to be fulfilled).

tion therapy, and they favor the approach of rapidly stepping up DMARD therapy in those patients who have suboptimal responses to DMARD monotherapy. The critically important trial comparing these combination approaches has not been undertaken. Most of these data came from trials designed well before the introduction of biologic treatments. At present, there is little question that biologic treatment can not only halt radiographic progression of established disease (39), but after 2 years can reduce radiographic damage in patients with early-onset disease (32). Studies that compare the efficacy of TNF antagonists with combination DMARD therapy in early RA are in progress.

Importantly, DMARD combination therapy in early RA has been well tolerated in all studies. This finding implies that the fear of overtreatment is unjustified as is the policy to introduce DMARD therapy only when NSAIDs no longer offer adequate disease control. In contrast, evidence demonstrates considerable toxicity of chronic treatment with NSAIDs. Comparison of the quantitative toxicity estimates of NSAIDs and DMARDs indicates that there are no substantial differences between these drug categories (50,51). In parallel with these findings, the simultaneous use of more than one DMARD for the treatment of RA has increased dramatically. Surveys of physicians indicate that approximately 25% of patients are prescribed one or more DMARDs (52). The most commonly used two-drug combinations are methotrexate plus hydroxychloroquine in the United States and methotrexate and sulfasalazine in Europe, according to this survey. These combinations are frequently given with low dosages of prednisone. Further clinical trials and long-term observational studies of various drug combinations (including biologics) and prescription strategies should help to clarify the optimal approaches toward improved outcomes for patients with RA.

EARLY TREATMENT: A WINDOW OF OPPORTUNITY?

An understanding of the type of patient most likely to respond to treatment would have large implications for the treatment choices for individual patients. Anderson et al. (53) have analyzed the results of 14 randomized, controlled clinical trials to identify factors that affect the response. They found that patients with longer disease duration do not respond as well to treatment as do those with earlier disease and that prior DMARD use and worse functional class also, and independently, reduce the likelihood of patient response. In these trials, they found a 10% probability of response among patients who had not previously been treated with DMARDs. This suggests that RA patients who have previously been treated with DMARDs may have a more recalcitrant disease. These findings are indications that the biologic process of RA varies with the stage of the disease.

Experiences of early arthritis clinics have shown that RA may be difficult to diagnose in its very early stages. When all patients who recently developed oligoarthritis (one joint) are taken into account, the arthritis disappears in 60% of patients within 2 years of follow-up. Of patients with persistent arthritis, 60% develop the full RA picture with erosions within the first 2 years (54). Other observations have shown that the majority of RA patients develop specific autoantibodies in the months to years preceding the occurrence of symptoms (55).

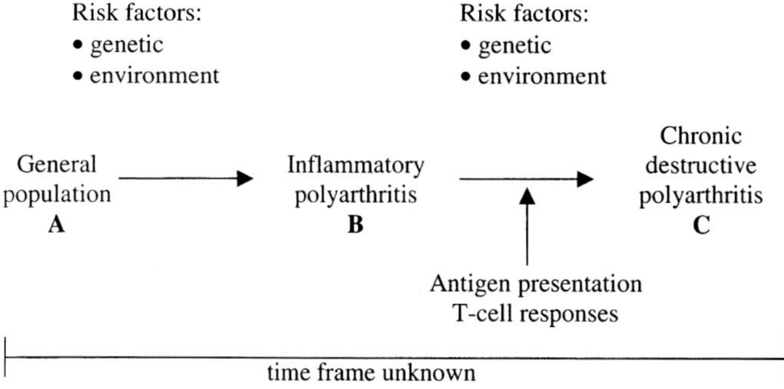

Figure 36.2. Prognostic model of progression to chronic, destructive polyarthritis in a hypothetical patient who begins in the general population (*A*), and then develops, with the influence of genetic and environmental factors, inflammatory polyarthritis (*B*), which subsequently leads to chronic, destructive disease, given the right mode of antigen presentation and T-cell responses (*C*).

Based on these observations, Huizinga et al. (56) has hypothesized that various forms of arthritis may progress in RA (Fig. 36.2). Environmental triggers (micro-organisms, toxins) may, given the right genetic framework, induce an inflammatory polyarthritis. In some of these patients, different factors may become involved. Based on the various forms of antigen presentation, particular B- and T-cell responses may be able to support the synovial inflammation process. The elucidation of $CD4^+$ T-cell responses in this phase of the disease may lead to an understanding of the bias toward a T-helper 1 type of T-cell response, which is supposed to underlie the chronicity of the synovial inflammation. Subsequently, the patients' condition can be characterized by a true autoimmune response that progresses toward a destructive form of arthritis, which rarely can be brought into remission.

A suggestion that disease modification occurs in early RA has been explored in two studies (57). In the patients treated early, HLA alleles had no effect on joint destruction; whereas, in the patients treated conservatively, the $DR4^+$ patients progressed much faster than the $DR4^-$ patients. This interaction was independent of other prognostic factors such as rheumatoid factor and baseline disease activity. This finding suggests that early and aggressive DMARD treatment can affect the dysregulated immune process, for example, by modulating the presentation of autoantigens by antigen-presenting cells or by inhibiting the response of autoantigen-reactive T cells, or both.

Diagnostic tools that identify steps in the development of arthritis that varies in outcomes are not yet available but may emerge from longitudinal studies of patients who present with arthritis of very recent (days) onset. At present, autoantibodies, such as rheumatoid factors, anticitrullinated peptides, and anti-Sa, are known to confer less favorable outcomes over the first year (58). Studies of synovial tissue in early RA have not yet identified a unique pathologic feature that differentiates RA from other forms of synovitis. Further study may open the way for interventions that not only delay or prevent destruction but also increase the chance of long-lasting remission.

EARLY ACCESS TO SYNOVITIS

RA may be difficult to diagnose on presentation, as is the prediction of outcome. Outcome-related diagnoses are of more relevance to the patient. These include self-limiting disease; persistent, nonerosive disease; and persistent, erosive disease. The ACR criteria for RA classification do not perform well for identifying which patients with early inflammatory polyarthritis will later develop RA (60). Visser et al. (61) have tried to identify determinants of the disease course in patients with early RA using the 2-year outcome as the gold standard. In a cohort of 524 patients with arthritis of recent onset, data from patient history, physical examination, blood testing, and imaging were entered in a continuation ratio model to predict outcome after 2 years. In this model, seven variables were found to be optimal for predicting persistent or erosive disease. These seven variables were symptom duration, morning stiffness, polyarthritis, compression pain of metatarsophalangeal joints, positive test for serum rheumatoid factor or anticitrullinated peptide, and the presence of erosions in the hands and feet. Depending on the outcome, different weight factors were assigned to these items, and the sum of these weight factors yielded a probability for persistent or erosive disease. The model developed is being validated in other early arthritis populations.

The probability of disease as estimated by a test result is dependent on the prevalence of a positive test result as well as the prevalence of the disease. The prevalence of disease as well as test results, such as morning stiffness, will differ between rheumatologic practices, and, therefore, the model may vary in reliability elsewhere. As such, diagnostic criteria developed in a research setting is more difficult to translate to clinical practice than classification criteria. However, the availability of a widely accepted set of criteria indicative of probabilities for chronic destructive arthritis would be of great advantage. It would allow the design of algorithms of individualized therapies in early RA. In addition, these criteria would allow the design of methods or early referral for an initiation of treatment. Many rheumatologists accept the assumption that inadequately controlled inflammation leads to permanent destruction and consider that the referral process requires medical urgency. Therefore, Emery et al. (54) have advocated referral criteria based on clinical signs and symptoms that early in the course of arthritis differentiate best between self-limiting and chronic destructive disease. The criteria include the presence of three or more swollen joints, a positive metatarsophalangeal/metacarpophalangeal squeeze test, and morning stiffness of 30 minutes or longer.

The goal of initiating treatment in early disease requires an effective health care system. Despite sincere cooperation in primary and specialist patient care, experience indicates that a patient with recent-onset arthritis may not see a specialist for as long as 6 months from the start of symptoms. In the United States, the diagnostic delay frequently is longer than 6 months (62). Introduction of early arthritis clinics to provide direct service for such patients has already been shown to decrease diagnostic delay and to improve access to rheumatology care (63).

CONCLUSION

Studies of the benefits of early treatment of RA support early referral. Referral to a relevant specialist for appropriate choices in the diagnostic/therapeutic algorithm is important given the information that this type of care is of higher quality than the care provided by primary care physicians (64). The weak performance of the ACR classification criteria in the diagnosis of early RA favors the development of a new set of criteria. These criteria as well as new techniques that will possibly emerge should also allow the identification of a subset of patients at high risk of severe disease. Prediction of arthritis outcome is not an aim in itself, however, and is only relevant if it leads to treatment decisions.

Because the DMARD armamentarium of the rheumatologist is steadily increasing, treatment choices should be individualized to the patient. Many patients with persistent disease develop function losses and radiographic damage. Furthermore, present therapies, including available DMARDs as single agents, are usually insufficient to completely prevent these untoward outcomes. The use of DMARDs in various combinations may result in the more effective slowing of disease progression. In addition, data indicate that treatment of RA of recent onset provides an opportunity for better response when compared to treatment of established RA. In this arena, considerable work has to be done to optimize disease outcome. Future trials should include early RA patients even before they meet the ACR criteria, and the effect of interventions should be studied in subgroups formed on the basis of prognostic markers.

REFERENCES

1. Pincus T, Brooks RH, Callahan LF. Prediction of long-term mortality in patients with rheumatoid arthritis according to simple questionnaire and joint count measures. *Ann Intern Med* 1994;120:26–34.
2. Ward MM. Recent improvements in survival in patients with rheumatoid arthritis: better outcomes or different study designs? *Arthritis Rheum* 2001;44:1467–1469.
3. Gabriel SE, Crowson CS, O'Fallon WM. Mortality in rheumatoid arthritis: have we made an impact in 4 decades? *J Rheumatol* 1996;26:2529–2533.
4. Pincus T, Callahan LF. How many types of patients meet classification criteria for rheumatoid arthritis? *J Rheumatol* 1995;21:1385–1389.
5. Van der Horst-Bruinsma IE, Speyer I, Visser H, et al. Diagnosis and course of early-onset arthritis: results of a special early arthritis clinic compared to routine patient care. *Br J Rheumatol* 1998;37:1084–1088.
6. Scott DL, Pugner K, Kaarela K, et al. The links between joint damage and disability in rheumatoid arthritis. *Rheumatology (Oxford)* 2002;39:122–132.
7. Drossaers-Bakker KW, de Buck M, van Zeben D, et al. Long-term course and outcome of functional capacity in rheumatoid arthritis: the effect of disease activity and radiologic damage over time. *Arthritis Rheum* 1999;42:1865–1860.
8. Van der Heijde DM. Joint erosions and patients with early rheumatoid arthritis. *Br J Rheumatol* 1995;34[Suppl 2]:74–78.
9. Brennan P, Harrison B, Barrett E, et al. A simple algorithm to predict the development of radiological erosions in patients with early rheumatoid arthritis: prospective cohort study. *BMJ* 1996;313:471–476.
10. Van Leeuwen MA, van Rijswijk MH, Sluiter WJ, et al. Individual relationship between progression of radiological damage and the acute phase response in early rheumatoid arthritis: towards development of a decision support system. *J Rheumatol* 1997;24:20–27.
11. van Zeben D, Hazes JMW, Zwindermans AH, et al. The severity of rheumatoid arthritis: a 6-year followup study of younger women with symptoms of recent onset. *J Rheumatol* 1994;21:1620–1625.
12. Green M, Marzo-Ortega H, McGonagle D, et al. Persistence of mild, early inflammatory arthritis: the importance of disease duration, rheumatoid factor, and the shared epitope. *Arthritis Rheum* 1999;42:2184–2188.
13. Möttönen TT, Hannonen PJ, Boers M. Combination DMARD therapy including corticosteroids in early rheumatoid arthritis. *Clin Exp Rheumatol* 1999;17[Suppl 18]:S59–S68.
14. Moreland LW, Bridges SL Jr. Early rheumatoid arthritis: a medical emergency? *Am J Med* 2001;111:498–500.
15. Prevoo MLL, van Gestel AM, van't Hof MA, et al. Remission in a prospective study of patients with rheumatoid arthritis. ARA preliminary remission criteria in relation to the disease activity score. *Br J Rheumatol* 1996;35:1101–1105.
16. Eberhardt K, Rydgren L, Fex B, et al. D-Penicillamine in early rheumatoid arthritis: experience from a 2-year double blind placebo controlled study. *Clin Exp Rheumatol* 1996;14:625–631.
17. Möttönen T, Paimela L, Ahonen J, et al. Outcome in patients with early rheumatoid arthritis treated according to the "sawtooth" strategy. *Arthritis Rheum* 1996;39:996–1005.
18. Ten Wolde S, Breedveld FC, Hermans J, et al. Randomised placebo-controlled study of stopping second-line drugs in rheumatoid arthritis. *Lancet* 1996;347:347–352.
19. Furst DE, Erikson N, Clute L, et al. Adverse experience with methotrexate during 176 weeks of a long-term prospective trial in patients with rheumatoid arthritis. *J Rheumatol* 1990;17:1628–1635.
20. Weinblatt ME, Weissman BN, Holdsworth DE, et al. Long-term prospective study of methotrexate in the treatment of rheumatoid arthritis: 84-month update. *Arthritis Rheum* 1992;35:129–137.
21. Sigler JW, Bluhm GB, Duncan H, et al. Gold salts in the treatment of rheumatoid arthritis. A double-blind study. *Ann Intern Med* 1974;80:21–26.
22. Luukkaainen R. Chrysotherapy in rheumatoid arthritis with particular emphasis on the effect of chrysotherapy on radiographical changes and on the optimal time of initiation of therapy. *Scand J Rheumatol* 1980;34[Suppl]:1–56.
23. Van der Heijde DM, van Riel PL, Nuver-Zwart IH, et al. Effects of hydroxychloroquine and sulphasalazine on progression of joint damage in rheumatoid arthritis. *Lancet* 1989;1:1036–1038.
24. Alarcon GS, Lopez-Mendez A, Walter J, et al. Radiographic evidence of disease progression in methotrexate treated and nonmethotrexate disease modifying antirheumatic drug treated rheumatoid arthritis patients: a meta-analysis. *J Rheumatol* 1992;19:1868–1873.
25. Joint Committee of the Medical Research Council and Nuffield Foundation on Clinical Trials of Cortisone, ACTH, and Other Therapeutic Measures in Chronic Rheumatic Diseases. A comparison of prednisone with aspirin and other analgesics in the treatment of rheumatoid arthritis. *Ann Rheum Dis* 1959;18:173–187.
26. Saag KG, Criswell LA, Sems KM, et al. Low-dose corticosteroids in rheumatoid arthritis: a meta-analysis of their moderate-term effectiveness. *Arthritis Rheum* 1996;39:1818.
27. Kirwan JR. Arthritis and Rheumatism Council Low-dose Glucocorticoid Study Group. The effect of glucocorticoid on joint destruction in RA. *N Engl J Med* 1995;333:142–146.
28. van Everdingen AA, Jacobs JWG, Siewertsz van Reesema DR, et al. Low-dose prednisone therapy for patients with early active rheumatoid arthritis: clinical efficacy, disease-modifying properties, and side effects: a randomized, double-blind, placebo-controlled clinical trial. *Ann Intern Med* 2002;136:1–12.
29. Borg G, Allander E, Lund B, et al. Auranofin improves outcome in early rheumatoid arthritis: results from a 2-year, double-blind placebo controlled study. *J Rheumatol* 1988;15:1747–1754.
30. Van der Heijde DM, Jacobs JW, Bijlsma JW, et al. The effectiveness of early treatment with "second-line" antirheumatic drugs: a randomized, controlled trial. *Ann Intern Med* 1996;124:699–707.
31. Lard LR, Visser H, Speyer I, et al. Early versus delayed treatment in patients with recent-onset rheumatoid arthritis: comparison of two cohorts who received different treatment strategies. *Am J Med* 2001;111:446–451.
32. Bathon JM, Martin RW, Fleischmann RM, et al. A comparison of etanercept and methotrexate in patients with early rheumatoid arthritis. *N Engl J Med* 2000;343:1586–1593.
33. Egsmose C, Lund B, Borg G, et al. Patients with rheumatoid arthritis benefit from early 2nd line therapy: 5 year follow up of a prospective double blind placebo controlled study. *J Rheumatol* 1995;22:2208–2213.
34. Munro B, Hampson R, McEntegart A, et al. Improved functional outcome in patients with early rheumatoid arthritis treated with intramuscular gold: results of a 5-year prospective study. *Ann Rheum Dis* 1998;57:88–93.
35. Symmons DPM, Jones MA, Scott DL, et al. Long-term mortality outcome in patients with rheumatoid arthritis: early presenters continue to do well. *J Rheumatol* 1998;25:1072–1077.
36. Kroot EJ, van Leeuwen MA, van Rijswijk MH, et al. No increased mortality in patients with rheumatoid arthritis: up to 10 years of follow up from disease onset. *Ann Rheum Dis* 2000;59:954–958.
37. Goekoop YP, Allaart CF, Breedveld FC, et al. Combination therapy in rheumatoid arthritis. *Curr Opin Rheumatol* 2001;13:177–183.
38. Verhoeven A, Boers M, Tugwell P. Combination therapy in rheumatoid arthritis: updated systematic review. *Br J Rheumatol* 1998;37:612–619.
39. Pincus T, Breedveld FC, Emery P. Does partial control of inflammation prevent long-term joint damage? Clinical rationale for combination therapy with multiple disease-modifying antirheumatic drugs. *Clin Exp Rheumatol* 1999;17[Suppl 18]:S2–S7.
40. Lipsky PE, Van der Heijde DM, St. Clair EW, et al. Infliximab and methotrexate in the treatment of rheumatoid arthritis. Anti-tumor necrosis factor trial in rheumatoid arthritis with concomitant therapy study group (see comments). *N Engl J Med* 2000;343:1594–1602.
41. Tugwell P, Pincus T, Yocum D, et al. Combination with cyclosporin and methotrexate in severe rheumatoid arthritis. *N Engl J Med* 1995;333:137–141.
42. Kremer JM, Genovese MC, Cannon GW, et al. Concomitant leflunomide therapy in patients with active rheumatoid arthritis despite stable doses of methotrexate. A randomized, double-blind, placebo-controlled trial. *Ann Intern Med* 2002;137:726–733.
43. O'Dell JR. Anticytokine therapy: a new era in the treatment of rheumatoid arthritis. *N Engl J Med* 1999;340:310–312.
44. Boers M, Verhoeven AC, Markusse HM, et al. Randomised comparison of combined step-down prednisolone, methotrexate and sulphasalazine with sulphasalazine alone in early rheumatoid arthritis. *Lancet* 1997;350:309–318.
45. Möttönen R, Hannone P, Leirisalo-Repo M, et al. Comparison of combination therapy with single-drug therapy in early rheumatoid arthritis: a randomised trial. *Lancet* 1999;353:1568–1573.
46. Calguneri M, Pay S, Caliskaner Z, et al. Combination therapy versus monotherapy for the treatment of patients with rheumatoid arthritis. *Clin Exp Rheumatol* 1999;17:699–704.
47. Haagsma CJ, van Riel PL, de Jong AJ, et al. Combination of sulphasalazine and methotrexate versus the single components in early rheumatoid arthritis: a randomized controlled, double-blind, 52 week clinical trial. *Br J Rheumatol* 1997;36:1082–1088.
48. Dougados M, Combe B, Cantragrel A, et al. Combination therapy in early rheumatoid arthritis: a randomised, controlled, double blind 52 week clinical trial of sulphasalazine and methotrexate compared with the single components. *Ann Rheum Dis* 1999;58:220–225.

49. Van den Borne BEEM, Landewé RBM, Goei Thè HS, et al. Combination therapy in recent onset rheumatoid arthritis: a randomized double blind trial of the addition of low dose cyclosporine to patients treated with low dose chloroquine. *J Rheumatol* 1998;25:1493–1498.
50. Fries JF, Williams CA, Bloch DA. The relative toxicity of nonsteroidal antiinflammatory drugs. *Arthritis Rheum* 1991;34:1353–1360.
51. Fries JF, Williams CA, Ramey D, et al. The relative toxicity of disease-modifying antirheumatic drugs. *Arthritis Rheum* 1993;36:297–306.
52. Hawley DJ, Wolfe F, Pincus T. Use of combination therapy in the routine care of patients with rheumatoid arthritis: physician and patient surveys. *Clin Exp Rheumatol* 1999;17[Suppl 18]:S78–S82.
53. Anderson J, Wells G, Verhoeven A, et al. Factors predicting response to treatment in rheumatoid arthritis: the importance of disease duration. *Arthritis Rheum* 2000;43:22–29.
54. Emery P, Breedveld FC, Dougados M, et al. Early referral recommendation for newly diagnosed rheumatoid arthritis: evidence based development of a clinical guide. *Ann Rheum Dis* 2002;61:290–297.
55. Nielen MMJ, van Schaardenburg D, van de Stadt RJ, et al. Autoantibodies in serum of blood donors precede symptoms of rheumatoid arthritis (RA) by 1 to 6 years. *Arthritis Rheum* 2002;46[Suppl]:S370.
56. Huizinga TWJ, Machold KP, Breedveld FC, et al. Criteria for early rheumatoid arthritis. From Bayes law revisited to new thoughts on pathogenesis. *Arthritis Rheum* 2002;46:1155–1159.
57. Lard LR, Boers M, Verhoeven A, et al. Early and aggressive treatment of rheumatoid arthritis patients affects the association of HLA class II antigens with progression of joint damage. *Arthritis Rheum* 2002;46:899–905.
58. El-Gabalawy HS, Goldbach-Mansky R, Smith D, et al. Association of HLA alleles and clinical features in patients with synovitis of recent onset. *Arthritis Rheum* 1999;42:1696–1705.
59. Reference deleted.
60. Harrison BJ, Symmons DPM, Barrett EM, et al. The performance on the 1987 ARA classification criteria for rheumatoid arthritis in a population based cohort of patients with early inflammatory polyarthritis. *J Rheumatol* 1998; 25:2324–2330.
61. Visser H, le Cessie S, Vos K, et al. How to diagnose rheumatoid arthritis early. A prediction model for persistent (erosive arthritis). *Arthritis Rheum* 2002;46:357–365.
62. Chan KW, Felson DT, Yood RA, et al. The lag time between onset of symptoms and diagnosis of rheumatoid arthritis. *Arthritis Rheum* 1994;37:814–820.
63. Speyer I, Hazes JMW, Breedveld FC. Recruitment of patients with early rheumatoid arthritis—The Netherlands experience. *J Rheumatol* 1996;23[Suppl 44]:84–85.
64. Maclean CH, Louie R, Leake B, et al. European Leflunomide Study Group. Quality of care for patients with rheumatoid arthritis. *JAMA* 2000;284:984–992.

CHAPTER 37

Cognitive-Behavioral Therapy

Sandra J. Waters, Lisa C. Campbell, and Francis J. Keefe

Rheumatoid arthritis (RA) is a serious and complex disease that taxes patients' coping resources (1–6). Patients with RA are faced not only with the task of coping with pain, but also with major life stresses, including disruptions in their health, work, family, and marital functioning (7–10). Medical interventions for RA primarily focus on disease management and do not directly address the challenges of coping with this disease.

Patients vary in their abilities to cope with the challenges posed by RA (11,12). Those who cope well are able to maintain a sense of well-being and are often able to maintain a productive and rewarding lifestyle (13). Those who cope poorly become depressed, decrease their physical activity level, and may develop a sedentary lifestyle (14).

Since the early 1980s, psychosocial researchers have developed and refined cognitive-behavioral therapy (CBT) protocols designed to systematically train RA patients in cognitive and behavioral strategies for coping with their disease. The purpose of this chapter is to provide an overview and critical analysis of these CBT protocols. The chapter is divided into four sections. The first section discusses the basic concepts and elements of CBT. The second section reviews studies examining the efficacy of CBT for RA patients. The third section highlights novel applications of CBT. In the final section, the authors identify and discuss a number of emerging issues in this area of clinical research and practice.

COGNITIVE-BEHAVIORAL THERAPY: BASIC CONCEPTS AND ELEMENTS

CBT approaches to RA are based on a biopsychosocial model (15). As shown in Figure 37.1, this model emphasizes that, to understand pain and disability in RA patients, one needs to attend to psychological factors and social factors, as well as to underlying biologic factors (e.g., changes in immune system activity, joint damage). The model also posits reciprocal relationships between biopsychosocial factors and arthritis pain and disability. Arthritis pain and disability can influence, as well as be influenced by, psychological and social factors.

A large body of research has emerged documenting the importance of psychological and social influences in arthritis (16). Empiric studies support the role of a number of psychological factors in understanding pain and disability in arthritis (Fig. 37.1). First, it is now evident that many patients with RA are prone to experience a sense of helplessness with regard to their ability to manage their disease. Studies have shown that RA patients who score high on standard measures of helplessness [e.g., the Arthritis Helplessness Index (17,18)] are more likely to feel depressed (19), experience impairment in daily activities (20), respond poorly to a disease-modifying drug regimen (21), and be at risk for early mortality (22). Second, empirical studies provide strong support for the role of depression in RA pain and disability. RA patients who are depressed report higher levels of pain, fatigue, and disability (23). Third, there is growing evidence that stress is important in understanding disease activity in RA. Studies by Zautra et al. (24) have demonstrated that RA patients are particularly likely to experience increases in disease activity after a period of high interpersonal stress. Finally, the use and perceived efficacy of patients' coping strategies appear to be very important in understanding pain and disability. RA patients who use more active coping strategies and who have a high sense of self-efficacy with regard to their coping abilities report much lower levels of pain, psychological disability, and physical disability (25,26).

Studies have also underscored the importance of social factors in RA (Fig. 37.1). First, RA patients who report higher satisfaction with their social support show better psychological functioning and overall health (27). Second, RA patients with little formal education and low socioeconomic status are much more prone to depression and poorer health status (28). Third, spousal responses, such as criticism, appear to be related to the psychological functioning (e.g., anxiety and depression) in RA patients (29).

As depicted in Figure 37.2, CBT protocols are based on the notion that one can alter arthritis pain and disability by systematically modifying the psychological and social factors that contribute to arthritis pain and disability. CBT protocols have three major aims (30). First, they are designed to help RA patients understand how psychological responses (e.g., changes in thoughts and feelings) and social responses (e.g., interactions with spouse and family) can influence pain and disability. Second, they help patients learn specific cognitive skills (e.g., imagery) and behavioral skills (e.g., activity pacing) for managing pain and disability. Finally, CBT protocols are designed to enhance patients' sense of self-efficacy in managing their own disease (31).

The CBT protocols developed for RA patients share several basic elements. First, patients are provided with a rationale for training in coping skills. The rationale typically takes the form of a simplified biopsychosocial model that emphasizes how the mind and body interact to influence pain. This rationale is particularly important because it underscores the key role that patients can play in managing their arthritis pain and disability. Second, a series of individual or group therapy sessions is used to systematically train patients in cognitive and behavioral coping skills. Each session typically lasts 60 to 90 minutes and consists of introduction of the skill,

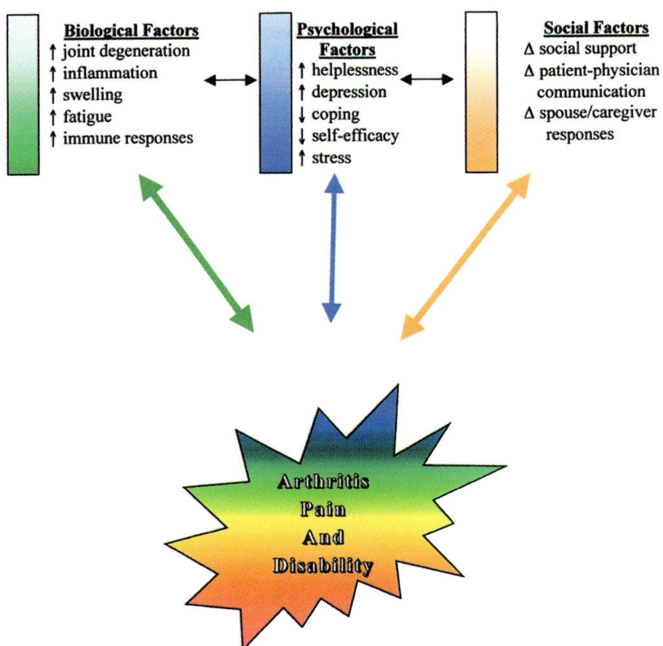

Figure 37.1. The biopsychosocial model of arthritis pain and disability. (Adapted from Keefe FJ, Bonk V. Psychosocial assessment of pain in patients having rheumatic diseases. In: *Rheumatic disease clinics of North America*, 25th ed. Philadelphia: W.B. Saunders, 1999:82.)

guided practice with the skill, and development of a home practice plan. The training typically focuses on training in a variety of coping skills, including progressive relaxation training, activity-pacing methods, pleasant-activity scheduling, imagery, problem solving, and cognitive therapy methods for dealing with overly negative thought patterns. Table 37.1 contains a brief description of skills typically used in CBT protocols and their potential benefits for RA patients. Finally, CBT helps patients plan for maintaining coping skills practice once formal training is completed.

EFFICACY OF COGNITIVE-BEHAVIORAL THERAPY

The first studies to test the efficacy of CBT in RA were conducted in the latter part of the 1980s [e.g., Bradley et al. (32), Applebaum et al. (33), and Parker et al. (34)]. Bradley et al. (32), for example, conducted a study in which they randomly assigned 53 RA patients to one of three conditions: CBT for pain management, social support, or a standard care condition. In the CBT for pain management condition, patients received training in pain coping skills that were presented in a structured group format and participated in a series of biofeedback sessions that focused on reducing pain by enhancing control over muscle tension and vascular responses. Patients in the social support condition attended group sessions that provided educational information about RA and encouraged group discussions and interactions. Patients in the control group continued their regular care. Outcome analyses revealed that CBT produced significant reductions in pain, pain behavior, depression, disease activity, and joint tenderness. No improvements were noted for patients in the social support or standard care conditions. These findings are consistent with other early studies testing the efficacy of CBT for RA (33,34).

Subsequently, Leibing et al. (35) conducted a study testing the effects of an extensive CBT intervention with routine medical care for RA. Patients in the CBT condition received information about the gate-control theory of pain and were given training in relaxation, imagery, pleasant-activity scheduling, and pain management

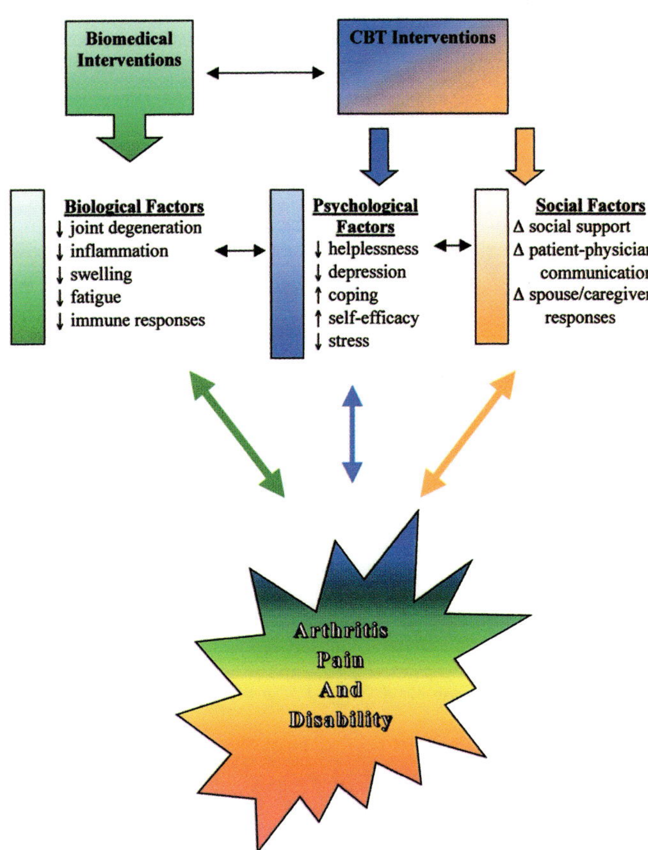

Figure 37.2. The relationship between biomedical and cognitive-behavioral therapy (CBT) interventions and arthritis pain and disability. (Adapted from Keefe FJ, Bonk V. Psychosocial assessment of pain in patients having rheumatic diseases. In: *Rheumatic disease clinics of North America*, 25th ed. Philadelphia: W.B. Saunders, 1999:82.)

strategies for changing maladaptive thinking (e.g., catastrophizing and helplessness). Particularly noteworthy was the finding that, although all participants demonstrated an increase in disease activity over the course of the study, patients in the CBT condition showed less disease progression (i.e., less worsening of inflamed joints and fewer requirements for new or stronger medication) than patients in the routine medical care control condition. Compared to patients in the routine medical care condition, patients in the CBT condition also showed significant decreases in depression, anxiety, helplessness, and resignation coping, and increases in positive acceptance coping. The results of this study suggest that, in addition to improving emotional functioning and coping, CBT interventions may have an impact on RA disease activity.

Other controlled studies have directly compared CBT to other treatments for RA. Kraaimaat et al. (36), for example, directly tested the relative efficacy of CBT and occupational therapy in a sample of RA patients who were experiencing significant progression of disease during the course of the study. Data analyses revealed that both interventions increased patients' knowledge about their disease. However, patients in the CBT condition showed significant improvements in active pain coping (i.e., use of distraction by pleasant activities), whereas those in the occupational therapy condition did not.

In summary, a number of studies have demonstrated the efficacy of CBT in patients with RA. These findings are noteworthy for several reasons. First, the benefits of CBT are consistent across several studies (35,36), despite the fact that the patient populations studied showed significant worsening of their disease status during the course of the study. Second, the results obtained

TABLE 37.1. Cognitive-Behavioral Techniques Used in Cognitive-Behavioral Therapy Protocols for Rheumatoid Arthritis Patients: Brief Description and Potential Benefits

Technique	Description	Potential Benefits
Progressive relaxation training	A technique designed to teach patients to relax deeply, involving a series of exercises in which the individual tenses and then slowly relaxes major muscle groups.	Decreased muscle tension Increased awareness of tension Distraction from pain and other symptoms Reduction in emotional distress Improved ability to rest and sleep
Brief muscle scan	A 30-sec exercise that teaches patients to quickly identify and release muscle tension throughout the body. This exercise can be done up to 20 times a day.	Generalizing learned relaxation skills to daily situations Increased awareness of tension during daily activities Reduced build-up of muscle tension
Activity pacing	A technique that teaches patients to carry out daily activities with less stress and strain. This involves alternating periods of limited activity with limited rest. Over time, patients gradually increase their activity periods and decrease their rest periods.	Increased level and range of activity over time Decreased tendency to rely on prolonged rest breaks to cope with pain Less avoidance of effortful tasks Less physical impairment and deconditioning from disuse of joints
Pleasant-activity scheduling	A method that encourages patients to engage regularly in pleasant activities by identifying pleasant-activity goals and then setting meaningful daily and weekly pleasant-activity goals.	Increased frequency and variety of enjoyable activities Distraction from pain and other symptoms Increased social involvement Decreased depression
Imagery	A technique that teaches patients to generate detailed mental images of pleasant scenes.	Increased relaxation Distraction from pain and other symptoms Increased self-efficacy for symptom control
Cognitive restructuring	A skill used to help patients identify and alter overly negative and distorted thoughts that increase pain and emotional distress and lead to maladaptive behaviors that exacerbate pain.	Reduced anxiety Reduced depression Promotes problem solving Increased adherence to self-care and coping skill regimens
Problem solving	A technique that teaches patients to identify actual or potential problems that may exacerbate pain and other symptoms, generate solutions to address problems, and implement solutions with increasing mastery until problem resolution is achieved.	Increased self-efficacy for symptom control Improved ability to anticipate and prevent problems
Communication and assertiveness skills	Systematic training in social skills that help patients to better communicate their needs to health care providers, family caregivers, and members of their social support network. Typically uses a role-play format with extensive rehearsal of skills and therapist feedback and guidance.	More active role in health care decision making Reduced interpersonal stress and conflict
Relapse prevention training	A strategy that teaches awareness and modification of situations that interrupt continued practice of cognitive-behavioral therapy skills.	Ongoing practice and improved mastery of cognitive-behavioral therapy skills Long-term symptom management

with CBT cannot be attributed to changes in patients' medication intake because, in most studies, medication intake stayed the same or decreased slightly. Finally, these findings appear to generalize other rheumatic disease populations, considering that several randomized controlled studies have shown the efficacy of CBT for patients with osteoarthritis (OA) (37,38).

NOVEL APPLICATIONS OF COGNITIVE-BEHAVIORAL THERAPY IN RHEUMATOID ARTHRITIS PATIENTS

Given the potential benefits of CBT, there is growing interest in developing novel ways to apply it to the management of RA. Novel applications include tailored CBT, CBT as an early intervention, and the use of CBT as a stress management protocol.

Tailored Cognitive-Behavioral Therapy

Two of the most challenging aspects of CBT for RA are the variability of individual patient problems (39) and the readiness of patients to engage in self-management efforts (40). Typically, CBT protocols are delivered in a standardized fashion that limits the flexibility of the therapist in addressing individual variations. It is important to determine whether CBT can be individualized to extend the utility of this approach.

Evers et al. (41) conducted a randomized controlled trial testing the efficacy of a CBT intervention that used treatment modules tailored to address specific problems that patients had prioritized as being most important to them. In this study, 64 adults having RA for less than 8 years were randomized into either a tailored CBT condition or standard care control condition. Patients in both conditions received standardized medical care and scheduled consultations with a rheumatology nurse consultant. Patients in the tailored CBT condition received ten biweekly individualized CBT treatment sessions using treatment modules chosen by the patients. Each patient chose two modules corresponding to their most frequently experienced problems. Selections were made from modules addressing the following conditions: fatigue, negative mood, social relationships, and pain and functional disability. Data analyses revealed that, at the completion of treatment, patients in the tailored CBT condition showed significant decreases in fatigue and depression and increases in active coping. At 6-months' follow-up, patients in the tailored CBT condition maintained their reductions in fatigue and depression and also showed significant improvements in perceived social support and medication compliance. Taken together, these findings suggest that tailored CBT may have promise as an intervention for RA patients.

Cognitive-Behavioral Therapy for Early Rheumatoid Arthritis

With a few exceptions [e.g., the Evers et al. (41) study, previously cited, in which the average disease duration was 3.19 years], most studies of CBT have been conducted with patients with RA of long duration. For example, the average disease duration in the Kraaimaat et al. (36) study was 15.6 years [standard deviation (SD) ± 12.4] and the Leibing et al. (35) study was 9.4 years (SD ± 9.3). The success of CBT in patients with long disease duration raises the question of whether CBT interventions would be even more beneficial if they were introduced early in the disease course when RA patients are still developing their coping styles and may be more open to learning new techniques (25).

Sharpe et al. (42) conducted a controlled study testing the efficacy of CBT in patients with early RA. A sample of 53 patients with RA for less than 2 years (mean, 12.63 months; SD ± 8.22) were randomly assigned to either standard care or standard care plus a CBT intervention. All patients received the routine care provided to early RA patients. Patients in the CBT condition, however, also received systematic training in relaxation techniques, attention diversion, goal setting, pacing, problem solving, cognitive restructuring, assertiveness and communication, and strategies for managing pain flares and high-risk situations likely to lead to setbacks in coping. Data analyses revealed that, after treatment, patients in the CBT condition showed significant improvements in depression and pain coping. CBT also produced significant improvements in joint symptoms (i.e., based on level of pain and inflammation at each joint) at 6-months' follow-up. Finally, CBT was associated with a significant immediate reduction in serum levels of C-reactive protein, although this improvement was not maintained at follow-up. These findings suggest that offering CBT as an adjunct to medical intervention may be beneficial for early RA patients in reducing both psychological distress and physical disability.

Cognitive-Behavioral Therapy for Stress Management

As noted earlier, RA patients report high levels of interpersonal stress (43,44) and show increases in disease activity during periods of high interpersonal stress (45). Based on these findings, one might expect that RA patients may particularly benefit from techniques designed to enhance stress management skills (46).

Parker et al. (9) have conducted one of the few studies designed to directly test the use of a CBT stress management protocol for RA patients. In this study, 141 RA patients were randomly assigned to a CBT stress management protocol, an attention control (patient education) condition, or a standard care control condition. The CBT stress management protocol provided educational information about stress and stress coping and provided systematic training in stress management skills. CBT training included a computer-based, multimedia presentation. Stress management skills included self-monitoring techniques to track stressful events and responses, relaxation techniques, pain coping skills, and cognitive and behavioral strategies for coping with mood and interpersonal problems. Adherence was high and dropout rates were low for patients in the CBT condition, suggesting that participants found the computer-based format used in this condition engaging. Data analyses showed that patients receiving the CBT stress management protocol showed significant long-term (1 year) improvements in pain and lower extremity impairment (based on joint counts). In addition, the CBT stress management protocol led to significant long-term reductions in feelings of helplessness and increases in self-efficacy and coping attempts.

EMERGING ISSUES

The increasing use of CBT in arthritis patients has raised a number of issues. In this section we address the following: Can CBT be conducted by lay persons? How can the long-term benefits of CBT be enhanced? Can CBT be adapted for delivery by telephone-based or Internet-based formats? Can partners assist patients in CBT? What is the effect of emotional disclosure in patients with RA?

Lay-Led Cognitive-Behavioral Therapy Intervention

CBT is typically delivered by a Ph.D.-level psychologist with training in cognitive and behavioral therapy. The CBT protocols tested in RA patients, however, are highly standardized, raising the possibility that CBT could be conducted by individuals having considerably less training.

Since the late 1980s, Lorig et al. have conducted a series of studies in which lay leaders have been used to teach self-help methods to arthritis patients (47,48). Lorig et al. have increasingly incorporated CBT methods into their arthritis self-management course. In one test of this intervention by Lorig et al. (14), a sample of adults having arthritis, heart disease, lung disease, or stroke were randomly assigned to a lay-led self-management intervention or a wait-list control group. The self-management intervention was led by peer leaders (i.e., people who were, themselves, patients), who had received 20 hours of training and followed a detailed session-by-session training manual. These lay leaders delivered the training in seven 2.5-hour weekly sessions. Educational information was provided, along with training in a variety of CBT techniques, such as relaxation, distraction, communication skills, and problem solving. In this study, the self-management training was conducted at various community sites (e.g., churches, senior centers) and was open to family members who wanted to attend. Data analyses revealed that, compared to the wait-list controls, patients in the self-management condition had significant improvements in their health behaviors (increased exercise, increased practice of cognitive symptom management, and improved patient–physician communication), health status (energy vs. fatigue, self-rated health, health distress, disability, and social role and activities limitations) and had fewer hospitalizations. A 2-year follow-up study revealed that patients receiving the self-management training showed long-term reductions in emergency department and outpatient visits and health distress, and improvements in self-efficacy (49). Although the use of a mixed sample of patients precludes analysis of the specific effects of the lay-led intervention for RA patients, these findings are consistent with those obtained in Lorig's prior studies of lay-led self management training for patients with RA and osteoarthritis (47,48).

Lorig et al. (50) have extended their research on the efficacy of lay-led and community-based interventions to address the needs of monolingual Spanish-speaking arthritis patients. In one study, a modified version of the Arthritis Self-Management Program was delivered over 6 weeks to Hispanic patients with RA, OA, and other musculoskeletal or rheumatic diseases. To enhance the cultural sensitivity of the program (i.e., provide a specialized format based on the needs of specific participant groups), all interactions with participants were conducted in Spanish, including recruitment, data collection, training of lay leaders, and delivery of the intervention. Educational materials and audiotapes for home practice of relaxation and exercise were also in Spanish. Results revealed that, compared to wait-listed controls, participants who underwent the Arthritis Self-Management Program reported improvements in exercise,

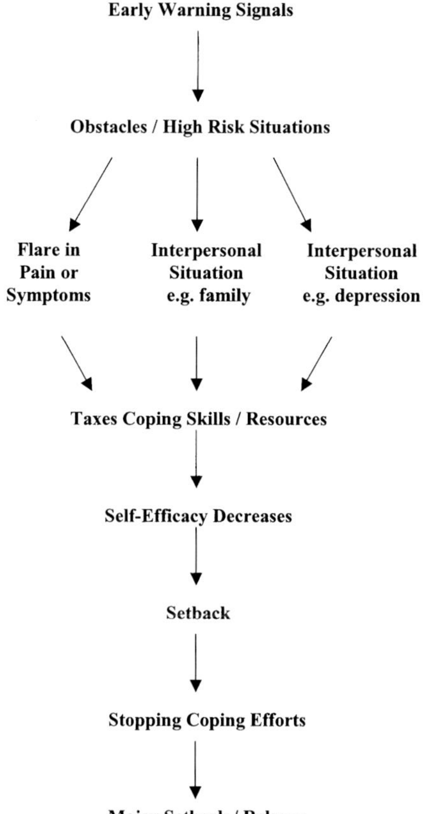

Figure 37.3. A model of the relapse process in coping with pain. (Adapted from Keefe FJ, Van Horn Y. Cognitive-behavioral treatment of rheumatoid arthritis pain. In: *Arthritis care & research*, 6th ed. Atlanta: Arthritis Foundation, 1993:217.)

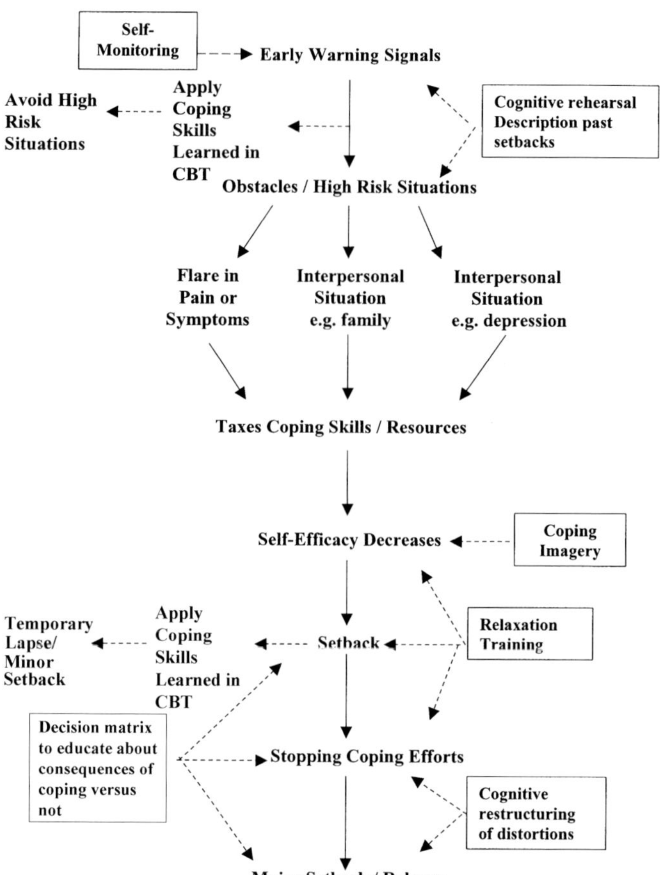

Figure 37.4. Techniques for preventing relapse in pain coping. CBT, cognitive-behavioral therapy. (Adapted from Keefe FJ, Van Horn Y. Cognitive-behavioral treatment of rheumatoid arthritis pain. In: *Arthritis care & research*, 6th ed. Atlanta: Arthritis Foundation, 1993:218.)

self-efficacy, disability, and pain. It appears that lay-led programs delivered in the community can be successfully modified to address language differences and other cultural needs of ethnic minority arthritis patients.

Considered overall, it is likely that, with training, lay leaders may be able to train RA patients in many coping skills, such as relaxation training, problem solving, imagery, activity pacing, and goal setting. Trained clinicians, however, are likely to be required to train RA patients in coping skills derived from cognitive therapy, such as cognitive restructuring (identifying and altering distorted thoughts that contribute to emotional distress, including depression and anxiety). Having a trained professional deliver CBT is particularly important when working with RA patients who are experiencing high levels of emotional distress.

Enhancing Long-Term Outcome

Long-term follow-up studies have shown that, although some RA patients are able to maintain reductions in pain, psychological disability, and physical disability after CBT, others are not (51). Several factors appear to be important in predicting long-term outcomes of CBT. First, there is evidence that patients who continue to practice and apply coping skills learned in CBT are more likely to show long-term gains than those who do not (34). Second, changes in perceived control over pain and negative pain-related thinking appear to be related to long-term outcome. Several studies have found that arthritis patients who show increases in their ability to control pain and reduce their tendency to engage in catastrophizing over the course of CBT are more likely to report improvements in pain and disability (9,37,38). Finally, studies by Lorig et al. have revealed that increases in self-efficacy that occur during the course of training in self-management methods are related to long-term improvements in pain and disability (50).

The findings regarding predictors of long-term CBT outcomes have led to the development of a model of the relapse process in coping with arthritis pain that has important implications for the design of CBT interventions (51). This model, depicted in Figure 37.3, is based on the relapse prevention model developed by Marlatt and Gordon (52). This model maintains that relapses are specific events from which patients can anticipate, prevent, and recover. To prepare patients to cope with relapses, it is important to understand the sequence of events leading up to a relapse. An RA patient, for example, might have early warning signs (e.g., increased joint swelling, disrupted sleep), indicating that they are risk for a setback in coping efforts. These warning signs are often evident in specific high-risk situations that in the past have led to a lapse in coping efforts. These situations might include a pain flare or an interpersonally stressful event, such as an argument with a family member, or an intrapersonal event, such as an episode of depression. Exposure to such events often taxes patients' coping skills and decreases a sense of ability to control pain, reduces self-efficacy with regard to coping with arthritis, and increases overly negative thinking (i.e., catastrophizing). The end result is a cessation of coping efforts that, in turn, can lead to a major setback or relapse.

The relapse prevention model, suggests targets for CBT intervention (Fig. 37.4). Self-monitoring strategies, such as daily diary records, can be incorporated into CBT to help patients become more aware of early warning signs of lapses and setbacks. Early identification of warning signs can enable patients to avoid high-risk situations or alter the way they deal with them. Patients can also be encouraged to describe past setbacks and use cognitive rehearsal to review how they coped with these setbacks. Such a review can further increase patients' awareness of early warning signs and high-risk situations. Patients can also be taught to use positive coping imagery to help them deal with decreases in self-efficacy. Such imagery focuses on prior successes in coping with difficult and challenging events. Relaxation training can also be very helpful in reducing the emotional distress and depression that occurs during a setback. Prompt application of skills learned in CBT can prevent a setback from progressing to a full-blown relapse and ensure that the lapse in coping efforts is only temporary. When patients are tempted to stop coping efforts, they can be encouraged to use a decision matrix, in which they write down the positive and negative consequences of continuing versus failing to continue their coping skills. Finally, cognitive restructuring techniques that modify overly negative and distorted thoughts are particularly useful in coping with the mood changes that come with a major setback or relapse. Although cognitive restructuring techniques may be integrated into clinical practice, the systematic training needed to effectively alter patients' thought patterns may be more easily administered by trained specialists in formal sessions.

The relapse prevention model maintains that one must anticipate and prepare for the long-term maintenance of CBT, rather than simply expect that it will occur. In the future, interventions for RA need to systematically address issues of maintenance early in treatment and need to make greater use of CBT techniques that can foster maintenance.

Telephone-Based and Internet-Based Cognitive-Behavioral Therapy

One factor that has limited the widespread dissemination of CBT is the requirement that patients participate in a series of face-to-face sessions typically conducted by a psychologist in a specialized tertiary care setting. Many RA patients have mobility problems or financial limitations that interfere with their ability to travel. Others are uncomfortable with what they perceive as the psychotherapy-like setting of CBT.

The telephone may offer a useful alternative to traditional face-to-face CBT training. The telephone is relatively low cost and widely available, even in rural areas.

No studies have specifically tested the efficacy of a telephone-based CBT protocol for RA patients. Studies by Weinberger (53), however, have suggested that telephone-based medical advice and support is helpful for RA patients. Maisiak et al. (54) have conducted a controlled trial testing a telephone-based psychosocial intervention based on reality therapy (55). Reality therapy specifically encourages behavior change, rather than change in cognition or emotion. In this study (54), a sample of 204 RA and 175 OA patients was randomly assigned to a telephone counseling condition, a symptom monitoring control condition, or a usual care control condition. Patients in the telephone counseling condition received a series of 11 phone calls over 9 months. In these calls, a trained counselor asked a series of questions about the patient's interaction with the medical care system (e.g., patient–physician communication and medication compliance) and encouraged the patient to engage in self-care activities (e.g., activity pacing, diet, and exercise) and methods for controlling stress (e.g., relaxation strategies and stress coping techniques). Assessments of health status were performed at baseline and at 3-, 6-, and 9-months' follow-up. Results indicated that the RA patients who received telephone-based counseling showed significant improvements in overall health status during the 9-month period, when compared to the symptom monitoring and usual care control conditions. The greatest improvements with the telephone counseling intervention were found for measures of affect and physical functioning, rather than for pain. CBT protocols, in contrast, have had fairly consistent effects on pain outcomes. Nevertheless, the findings in the study suggest that telephone-based intervention may benefit RA patients.

The rapid development of Internet technology offers new opportunities for delivering health services to patients (56). For example, Lorig et al. (57) conducted a randomized study testing the effects of a novel e-mail discussion group for patients with chronic low back pain. A sample of 580 persons with chronic back pain were randomized to a self-care intervention or to a usual care group. Patients in the self-care intervention were provided with access to an e-mail discussion group, a book about pain, and a videotape of appropriate care behaviors for back pain. The e-mail intervention consisted of a closed discussion group in which all participants received all e-mails sent by group members. A moderator prompted and monitored the discussion group, and content experts were available to answer questions several hours each week. Participants who received the self-care intervention showed significant improvements in pain, disability, role function, and health distress. In addition, physician visits declined significantly by 1.5 visits over a 6-month period for patients in the treatment group, compared to that of participants in the control group. Although the focus of this study was on low back pain, Internet-based interventions may be potentially helpful in providing coping skills training to RA patients.

Partner-Assisted Cognitive-Behavioral Therapy

There is growing recognition that RA occurs in a social context and that individuals in the patient's social network (e.g., spouse, family members) are influenced by the life changes associated with RA, and, in turn, these individuals can have an impact on how the patient copes with RA (27). As noted earlier, studies have shown that social support (29) and spousal responses (e.g., critical vs. supportive responses) are related to psychological functioning in RA patients.

Despite evidence for the role of social factors in RA, there have been few studies on interventions that involve members of the patient's social network in CBT. Involving a spouse or partner, for example, could have many benefits. First, the spouse or partner could become more familiar with the goals of CBT and, thus, better support the patient as he or she pursues these goals. Second, the spouse or partner could practice CBT techniques with the patient, thereby increasing their own knowledge of important coping skills and providing a buddy system that supports practice efforts. Third, the spouse or partner might directly benefit from learning CBT techniques that reduce their own emotional distress. Finally, involving a spouse or partner in CBT training may enhance their confidence that they can effectively assist the patient in coping with pain and other challenges of RA.

One study has tested a family-assisted CBT intervention for RA patients (58). This study compared the effects of CBT alone to a CBT plus family support and a control condition without treatment. The CBT and CBT plus family support interventions were both found to be superior to the control condition in reducing pain and improving joint swelling. Although no differences were obtained between CBT alone versus CBT plus family support, this study did demonstrate the feasibility of involving family members of RA patients in treatment.

Keefe et al. conducted a randomized clinical trial testing the effects of a spouse-assisted CBT intervention for patients with OA of the knees (59). A sample of 88 patients having persistent OA knee pain were randomly assigned to spouse-assisted CBT, a conventional CBT condition (patient seen alone), or an arthritis education and social support condition. Like the study of Radojevic et al. (58), there were no significant differences between spouse-assisted CBT and conventional CBT. However, data analyses revealed a consistent pattern in which patients in the spouse-assisted CBT condition showed the best outcomes, conventional CBT the next best outcomes, and the arthritis education and social support condition the worst outcomes. A follow-up study (60) revealed that patients in the spouse-assisted CBT condition who showed the largest initial increases in self-efficacy had the best long-term outcomes.

Emotional Self-Disclosure

Patients with RA frequently experience emotional distress related to disruptions in their health, work, and family life (9,61). However, RA patients often find it difficult to discuss their thoughts and feelings associated with the stress they are experiencing (62,63). A growing body of research has shown that the inability or reluctance to process emotionally stressful events may lead to increases in symptom complaints and poor immune functioning (64,65), outcomes that could adversely impact RA.

Studies conducted primarily in normal healthy populations have shown that emotional self-disclosure about stressful life events may be beneficial. In the emotional disclosure paradigm developed by Pennebaker and Beall (66), participants are asked to attend a series of four daily laboratory sessions, in which they write or talk about the thoughts and feelings associated with a stressful life experience. Research has shown that, during the course of disclosure sessions, fragmented and poorly articulated recollections of stressful events are restructured into more coherent and less emotionally laden recollections (67). It has been suggested that emotional expression facilitates psychological adjustment to stressors by reducing the frequency (68) or impact (69) of intrusive thoughts that create further distress and may usurp cognitive resources necessary for coping.

A systematic review of the literature on emotional disclosure found that this intervention improves a variety of outcomes, including physical health, psychological well-being, and general functioning (70). Furthermore, there is evidence that emotional self-disclosure has physiologic benefits, including increases in immunocompetence [e.g., heightened blastogenic responses to mitogens (64), responses to Epstein-Barr antibodies (71), and higher antibody responses to hepatitis B vaccinations (72)].

Two controlled studies have tested the efficacy of emotional self-disclosure in patients with RA. In the first study, Kelley, Lumley, and Leisen (73) randomly assigned 72 RA patients [average disease duration of 13.39 years (SD ± 10.48)] to either an emotional disclosure intervention or attention control condition. For 4 consecutive days, patients in the emotional disclosure condition spoke privately into a tape recorder for 15 minutes about a stressful event they were currently experiencing or had experienced at some other time in their lives. Participants in the attention control condition were given four color landscape pictures and were instructed to provide an audiotape of a 15-minute detailed description of one picture each day for 4 days. Data analyses revealed that, at the completion of treatment, participants in the emotional disclosure condition experienced a significant increase in negative mood. When assessed 3 months later, however, patients in the emotional disclosure condition showed significantly lower levels of physical dysfunction (i.e., fewer problems with activities of daily living) and affective disturbance (i.e., negative mood and tension) than patients in the control condition. The transient increase in negative mood immediately after emotional disclosure (found in previous research with healthy adults [e.g., Pennebaker (68)]) suggests that the process of restructuring negative emotional memories is difficult for RA patients. Those patients who showed the largest initial increases in negative affect showed the best outcomes at 3-months' follow-up.

The second study testing the potential benefits of emotional disclosure paradigm in patients having RA was conducted by Smyth et al. (70). In this study, a sample of RA patients (N = 51) and asthma patients (N = 61) was randomly assigned to emotional disclosure intervention or a neutral control intervention. All patients spent 20 minutes daily for 3 days involved in a writing task. Those in the emotional disclosure intervention wrote about the most stressful experience in their life. Those in the neutral writing control group wrote about their plans for each day. Data analyses revealed that the RA patients who disclosed information about a stressful event showed a 28% improvement in overall disease activity, an index based on a physician's evaluation of pain, joint swelling, and other factors that assess current clinical status. Patients in the control group showed no significant improvements.

Emotional disclosure and CBT represent different psychosocial approaches for helping patients cope with RA. Emotional disclosure encourages patients to focus on negative and stressful events and to confront their thoughts and feelings about these events. It is based on the notion that exposure to stressful memories can lead to improvements in RA symptoms and function. CBT, on the other hand, is designed to teach patients specific cognitive and behavioral skills for coping with pain and stress. CBT proponents maintain that the development and mastery of these coping skills are important to therapeutic outcome. Although no studies have directly compared and contrasted the effects of emotional disclosure and CBT, it is possible that patients who do not respond to CBT may benefit from emotional disclosure. It is also possible that a treatment protocol that combines emotional disclosure with CBT is more effective than either intervention alone.

CONCLUSION

The studies described in this chapter suggest that CBT interventions are effective. Controlled studies have demonstrated that CBT interventions are superior to standard care and occupational therapy interventions. Patients undergoing CBT have shown improvements in a wide variety of outcomes, including pain, pain coping, emotional stability, depression, helplessness, health distress, self-efficacy, functional impairment, and social relationships (9,14,25,29,35,41,42,49). With regard to disease activity, there is evidence that CBT interventions are associated with slower disease progression (35), a reduction in the number of inflamed and painful joints (42), and reduced fatigue (14,41). CBT interventions have also been found to be associated with reduced health care use among RA patients, including fewer hospitalizations (14) and fewer emergency department and outpatient visits (49). Finally, CBT interventions appear to improve health behaviors among RA patients, including medication compliance (41) and increased use of stretching or strengthening exercises and aerobic exercise (14).

Although many RA patients can benefit from CBT interventions, CBT techniques, like most pain management approaches, are not equally effective for all patients. For example, in patients involved in ongoing litigation or disability or compensation claims, the potential financial gain may influence treatment progress. Also inappropriate for CBT interventions are patients with certain types of severe psychopathology (e.g., psychosis) or addiction problems (e.g., drug or alcohol addiction). In general, CBT interventions are appropriate for the vast majority of arthritis patients. Those patients who are experiencing behavioral or emotional problems in coping with their disease are particularly appropriate referrals. Many tertiary pain management programs have psychologists who have training in delivering CBT for pain management. To obtain names and contact information for therapists having training in CBT, patients or health professionals can contact the Association for the Advancement of Behavior Therapy, located at 305 Seventh Avenue, 16th Floor, New York, NY, 10001-6008. Its telephone number is (212) 647-1890, FAX number is (212) 647-1865, and Web site is www.aabt.org.

ACKNOWLEDGMENTS

This chapter was supported, in part, by grants from the National Institute of Arthritis and Musculoskeletal Diseases (NIAMS AR46305 and NIAMS AR47218) and the Arthritis Foundation and support from the Fetzer Institute.

REFERENCES

1. Egmose C, Lund B, Borg G, et al. Patients with rheumatoid arthritis benefit from early 2nd line therapy: 5 year follow-up of prospective double blind placebo controlled study. *J Rheumatol* 1995;22:2208–2213.
2. Masi AT, Medsger TA. Epidemiology of the rheumatic diseases. In McCarty DJ, ed. *Arthritis and allied conditions*, 9th ed. Philadelphia: Lea & Febiger, 1979:11–30.
3. Meenan RF, Yelin EH, Nevitt M, Epstein WV. The impact of chronic disease: a sociomedical profile of rheumatoid arthritis. *Arthritis Rheum* 1988;25:544–548.
4. Parker JC, Buckelew SP, Smarr KL, et al. Psychological screening in rheumatoid arthritis. *J Rheumatol* 1990;17:1016–1024.
5. Pincus T, Callahan LF, Sale WG, et al. Severe functional declines, work disability, and increased mortality in seventy-five rheumatoid arthritis patients studied over nine years. *Arthritis Rheum* 1984;27:864–872.
6. Wright V. Pain, forward. *Bailliere's Clin Rheumatol Int Pract Res* 1987;1:ix.
7. Kazis L, Meenan RF, Anderson J. Pain in the rheumatic diseases: investigations of a key health status component. *Arthritis Rheum* 1983;26:1017–1022.
8. O'Dell JR. Treating rheumatoid arthritis early: a window of opportunity. *Arthritis Rheum* 2002;46:283–285.
9. Parker JC, Smarr KL, Buckelew SP, et al. Effects of stress management on clinical outcomes in rheumatoid arthritis. *Arthritis Rheum* 1995;38:1807–1818.
10. Van der Heide A, Jacobs JW, Bijlsma JW, et al. The effectiveness of early treatment with "second-line" antirheumatic drugs. A randomized, controlled trial. *Ann Intern Med* 1996;124:699–707.
11. Bathon JM, Martin RW, Fleishchmann RM, et al. Randomised comparison of combined step-down prednisolone, methotrexate and sulphasalazine with sulphasalazine alone in early rheumatoid arthritis. *Lancet* 1997;350:309–318.
12. Landewe RBM, Boers M, Verhoeven AC, et al. COBRA combination therapy in patients with early rheumatoid arthritis: long-term structural benefits of a brief intervention. *Arthritis Rheum* 2002;46:347–356.
13. Zautra AJ, Burleson MH, Matt KS, et al. Interpersonal stress, depression, and disease activity in rheumatoid arthritis and osteoarthritis patients. *Health Psychol* 1995;13:139–148.
14. Lorig K, Sobel D, Stewart AL, et al. Evidence suggesting that a chronic disease self-management program can improve health status while reducing hospitalization: a randomized trial. *Med Care* 1999;37:5–14.
15. Engel GL. The need for a new medical model: a challenge for biomedicine. *Science* 1997;196:129–136.
16. Keefe FJ, Smith SJ, Buffington ALH, et al. Recent advances and future directions in the biopsychosocial assessment and treatment of arthritis. *J Consult Clin Psychol* 2002;70:640–655.
17. Nicassio PM, Wallston KA, Callahan LF, et al. The measurement of helplessness in rheumatoid arthritis: the development of the Arthritis Helplessness Index. *J Rheumatol* 1985;12:462–467.
18. Stein MJ, Wallston KA, Nicassio PM. Factor structure of the Arthritis Helplessness Index. *J Rheumatol* 1988;15:427–432.
19. Smith TW, Christensen AJ, Peck JR, Ward JR. Cognitive distortion, helplessness, and depressed mood in rheumatoid arthritis: a four-year longitudinal analysis. *Health Psychol* 1994;13:213–217.
20. Schoenfeld-Smith K, Petroski GF, Hewett JE, Johnson JC, et al. A biopsychosocial model of disability in rheumatoid arthritis. *Arthritis Care Res* 1996;9:368–375.
21. Nicassio PM, Radojevic V, Weisman MH, et al. The role of helplessness in the response to disease modifying drugs in rheumatoid arthritis. *J Rheumatol* 1993;20:1114–1120.
22. Callahan LF, Cordray DS, Wells G, Pincus T. Formal education and five-year mortality in rheumatoid arthritis: mediation by helplessness scale scores. *Arthritis Care Res* 1996;9:463–472.
23. Thacher I, Haynes SN. A multivariate time series regression study of pain, depression symptoms, and social interaction in rheumatoid arthritis. *Int J Clin Health Psychol* 2001;1:159–180.
24. Zautra AJ, Hoffman J, Potter P, et al. Examination of changes in interpersonal stress as a factor in disease exacerbations among women with rheumatoid arthritis. *Ann Behav Med* 1997;19:279–286.
25. Sinclair VG, Wallston KA. Predictors of improvement in a cognitive-behavioral intervention for women with rheumatoid arthritis. *Ann Behav Med* 2001;23:291–297.
26. Smarr KL, Parker JC, Wright GE, et al. The importance of enhancing self-efficacy in rheumatoid arthritis. *Arthritis Care Res* 1997;10:18–26.
27. Doeglas D, Suurmeijer T, Krol B, et al. Social support, social disability, and psychological well-being in rheumatoid arthritis. *Arthritis Care Res* 1994;7:10–15.
28. Brekke M, Hjortdahl P, Thelle DS, Kvien TK. Disease activity and severity in patients with rheumatoid arthritis: relations to socioeconomic inequality. *Soc Sci Med* 1999;48:1743–1750.
29. Kraaimaat FW, Van Dam-Baggen RM, Bijlsma JW. Association of social support and the spouse's reaction with psychological distress in male and female patients with rheumatoid arthritis. *J Rheumatol* 1995;22:644–648.
30. Keefe FJ, Caldwell DS. Cognitive behavioral interventions. In Wegener S, Belza B, Gall E, eds. *Primer on clinical care in rheumatoid disease*. Atlanta: Arthritis Foundation, 1996:59–63.
31. Schiaffino KM, Revenson TA. Relative contributions of spousal support and illness appraisals to depressed mood in arthritis patients. *Arthritis Care Res* 1995;8:80–87.
32. Bradley VA, Young LD, Anderson JO, et al. Effects of psychological therapy on pain behavior of rheumatoid arthritis patients: treatment outcome and six-month follow-up. *Arthritis Rheum* 1987;30:1105–1114.
33. Applebaum KA, Blanchard EB, Hickling EJ, et al. Cognitive-behavioral treatment of a veteran population with moderate to severe rheumatoid arthritis. *Behav Ther* 1988;19:489–502.
34. Parker J, Frank R, Beck N, et al. Pain management in rheumatoid arthritis: a cognitive-behavioral approach. *Arthritis Rheum* 1988;31:593–601.
35. Leibing E, Pfingsten M, Bartmann U, et al. Cognitive-behavioral treatment in unselected rheumatoid arthritis outpatients. *Clin J Pain* 1999;15:58–66.
36. Kraaimaat FW, Brons MR, Geenen R, et al. The effect of cognitive behavior therapy in patients with rheumatoid arthritis. *Behav Res Ther* 1995;33:487–495.
37. Keefe FJ, Caldwell DS, Williams DA, et al. Pain coping skills training in the management of osteoarthritic knee pain: I. A comparative study. *Behav Ther* 1990;21:49–62.
38. Keefe FJ, Caldwell DS, Williams DA, et al. Pain coping skills training in the management of osteoarthritic knee pain: II. Follow-up results. *Behav Ther* 1990;21:435–447.
39. Affleck G, Tennen H, Urrows S, Higgins P. Individual differences in the day-to-day experience of chronic pain: a prospective daily study of rheumatoid arthritis patients. *Health Psychol* 1991;10:419–426.
40. Keefe FJ, Lefebvre JC, Kerns RD, et al. Understanding the adoption of arthritis self-management: stages of change profiles among arthritis patients. *Pain* 2000;87:303–314.
41. Evers AWM, Kraaimaat FW, van Riel PLCM, et al. Tailored cognitive-behavioral therapy in early rheumatoid arthritis for patients at risk: a randomized controlled trial. *Pain* 2002;100:141–153.
42. Sharpe L, Sensky T, Timberlake N, et al. A blind, randomized, controlled trial of cognitive-behavioral intervention for patients with recent onset rheumatoid arthritis: preventing psychological and physical morbidity. *Pain* 2001;89:275–283.
43. Zautra AJ, Hoffman JM, Matt KS, et al. An examination of individual differences in the relationship between interpersonal stress and disease activity among women with rheumatoid arthritis. *Arthritis Care Res* 1998;11:271–279.
44. Zautra AJ, Smith BW. Depression and reactivity to stress in older women with rheumatoid arthritis and osteoarthritis. *Psychosom Med* 2001;63:687–696.
45. Zautra AJ, Hamilton NSA, Potter P, Smith B. Field research on the relationship between stress and disease activity in rheumatoid arthritis. *Ann N Y Acad Sci* 1999;876:397–412.
46. Stewart MW, Knight RG, Palmer DG, et al. Differential relationships between stress and disease activity for immunologically distinct subgroups of people with rheumatoid arthritis. *J Abnorm Psychol* 1994;103:251–258.
47. Lorig KR, Lubeck D, Kraines R, et al. Outcomes of self-help education for patients with arthritis. *Arthritis Rheum* 1985;28:680–685.
48. Lorig KR, Mazonson P, Holman H. Evidence suggesting that health care education for self-management in patients with chronic arthritis has sustained health benefits while reducing health care costs. *Arthritis Rheum* 1993;36:439–446.
49. Lorig KR, Ritter P, Stewart AL, et al. Chronic disease self-management program. 2-Year health status and health care utilization outcomes. *Med Care* 2001;39:1217–1223.

50. Lorig K, Gonzalez VM, Ritter P. Community-based Spanish language arthritis education program: a randomized trial. *Med Care* 1999;37:957–963.
51. Keefe FJ, Van Horn Y. Cognitive-behavioral treatment of rheumatoid arthritis pain: understanding and enhancing maintenance of treatment gains. *Arthritis Care Res* 1993;6:213–222.
52. Marlatt GA, Gordon JR. Distraction and coping with pain. *Psychol Bull* 1984;95:516–533.
53. Weinberger M. Telephone-based interventions in ambulatory care. *Ann Rheum Dis* 1998;57:196–197.
54. Maisiak R, Austin J, Heck L. Health outcomes of two telephone interventions for patients with rheumatoid arthritis or osteoarthritis. *Arthritis Rheum* 1996;39:1391–1399.
55. Glasser W. *Reality therapy*. New York: Harper & Row, 1975.
56. Maheu M, Gordon B. Counseling and therapy on the internet. *Prof Psychol Res Pr* 2000;31:484–489.
57. Lorig KR, Laurent DD, Deyo RA, et al. Can a back pain e-mail discussion group improve health status and lower health care costs? *Arch Intern Med* 2002;162:792–796.
58. Radojevic V, Nicassio PM, Weisman MH. Behavioral intervention with and without family support for rheumatoid arthritis. *Behav Ther* 1992;23:13–30.
59. Keefe FJ, Caldwell DS, Baucom D, et al. Spouse-assisted coping skills training in the management of osteoarthritis knee pain. *Arthritis Care Res* 1996; 9:279–291.
60. Keefe FJ, Caldwell DS, Baucom D, et al. Spouse-assisted coping skills training in the management of osteoarthritis knee pain: long-term follow-up results. *Arthritis Care Res* 1999;12:101–111.
61. Bellamy N, Bradley LA. Workshop on chronic pain, pain control, and patient outcomes in rheumatoid arthritis and osteoarthritis. *Arthritis Rheum* 1996; 39:357–362.
62. Fernandez A, Sriram TG, Rajkumar S, et al. Alexithymic characteristics in rheumatoid arthritis: a controlled study. *Psychother Psychosom* 1989;51:45–50.
63. Moos RH, Solomon GF. Psychological comparisons between women with rheumatoid arthritis and their nonarthritic sisters. I. *Psychosom Med* 1965;27: 135–149.
64. Pennebaker JW, Kiecolt-Glaser JK, Glaser R. Disclosure of traumas and immune function: health implications for psychotherapy. *J Consult Clin Psychol* 1988;56:239–245.
65. Schwartz GE. Psychobiology of repression and health: a systems approach. In: Singer JL, ed. *Repression and dissociation: implications for personality theory, psychopathology, and health*. Chicago: University of Chicago Press, 1990:405–434.
66. Pennebaker JW, Beall SK. Confronting a traumatic event: toward an understanding of inhibition and disease. *J Abnorm Psychol* 1986;95:274–281.
67. Krystal JH, Southwick SM, Charney DS. Post-traumatic stress disorder: psychobiological mechanisms of traumatic remembrance. In: Schacter DL, ed. *Memory distortion: how minds, brains, and societies reconstruct the past*. Cambridge, MA: Harvard University Press, 1995:150–172.
68. Pennebaker JW. Putting stress into words: health, linguistic, and therapeutic implications. *Behav Ther Res* 1993;31:539–548.
69. Lepore SJ. Expressive writing moderates the relation between intrusive thoughts and depressive symptoms. *J Pers Soc Psychol* 1997;73:1030–1037.
70. Smyth JM, Stone AA, Hurewitz A, et al. Effects of writing about stressful experiences on symptom reduction in patients with asthma or rheumatoid arthritis: a randomized trial. *JAMA* 1999;281:1304–1309.
71. Esterling BA, Antoni MH, Fletcher MA, et al. Emotional disclosure through writing or speaking modulates latent Epstein-Barr virus antibody titers. *J Consult Clin Psychol* 1994;62:130–140.
72. Petrie KJ, Booth RJ, Pennebaker JW, et al. Disclosure of trauma and immune response to a hepatitis B vaccination program. *J Consult Clin Psychol* 1995;63:787–792.
73. Kelley JE, Lumley MA, Leisen JCC. Health effects of emotional disclosure in rheumatoid arthritis patients. *Health Psychol* 1997;16:331–340.

CHAPTER 38

Physical Therapy

Christina H. Stenström

DEFINITION OF PHYSICAL THERAPY

Physical therapy aims to promote health through movement and includes a variety of treating and rehabilitating interventions to reduce or compensate for problems with health or functioning after diseases or injuries, including physical and psychological overload and stress. Physical therapy includes knowledge and study of humans in movement with regard to individuals' ability to experience, take advantage of, and control their bodies in ways that correspond with their goals and the demands from the surrounding world.

Physical therapists perform independent assessment of movement and functioning, and they plan, implement, and evaluate health promotion, prevention, treatment, and rehabilitation interventions for individuals and groups of individuals. Consultation, supervision, and teaching patients, relatives, and other professionals are also important tasks for physical therapists (1).

INTERNATIONAL CLASSIFICATION OF FUNCTIONING, DISABILITY, AND HEALTH: A COMMON LANGUAGE

The International Classification of Functioning, Disability, and Health (ICF) is a framework to describe components of health, rather than consequences of disease (2). It is, thus, well suited for rehabilitation (including physical therapy), which is dedicated to optimizing patient functioning and health. The ICF includes a number of terms that might also be used or understood differently in other contexts. Appropriate use of these terms in rehabilitation is important, as the ICF is likely to become the generally accepted framework for use in needs assessment, matching interventions to specific health states, rehabilitation, and outcome evaluation (3). Some definitions will be given in the following sections. Two umbrella terms, *functioning* and *disability*, are used in the framework (Fig. 38.1).

Functioning refers to unproblematic, neutral aspects of health and includes *body functions* and *body structures* and the life areas *activity* and *participation*. Body functions include physiologic and psychological functions, whereas body structures include anatomic parts. *Activity* and *participation* refer to aspects of functional state from individual and societal perspectives, respectively. Distinctions are made between capacity, the highest level reached at a given moment and in a standard environment, and performance, what is actually done in the current environment.

Disability refers to problems related to health. Thus, *impairments* indicate problems of deviation or loss of body function or body structure. *Activity limitation* indicates difficulties a person might have on a personal level, and *participation restriction* refers to those in life situations.

Environmental factors are physical, social, or attitudinal factors in a person's environment that facilitate disability or represent barriers to functioning. *Personal factors*, such as age, gender, social status, or life experiences, are not classified, but still need to be taken into account when assessing an individual's functioning and health.

DISABILITY IN RHEUMATOID ARTHRITIS

Pain and fatigue are major complaints in rheumatoid arthritis (RA) and may seriously impact functioning and health. The symptoms may often be related to the disease process, but also to various social and psychological factors or to physical inactivity.

The most commonly found physical impairments in individuals with RA are limited joint range of motion (ROM), reduced muscle function, and decreased aerobic fitness. Possible reasons for limited joint mobility are pain, joint effusion, soft tissue contractures, and the destruction of cartilage and bone. Decreased muscle function may be multifactorial and related to pain, reflex inhibition, changes in muscle metabolism, disuse and type II muscle atrophy, reduced number of functioning muscle fibers, peripheral nerve impairment, and medication (4). Physical inactivity possibly plays a role in the process of deconditioning in individuals with RA.

Impairments in RA have been investigated in a number of studies (5). One-half of patients with RA show limited mobility in the hands at the first clinical presentation, whereas loss of joint motion is present in approximately 25% to 35% of larger joints 2 years later (6). The muscle strength of knee and hip has been found in various studies to be reduced by 25% to 50% in patients with mild disability, compared to healthy age-matched controls (7–10). In patients with severe RA, the muscle strength has been reported to be reduced to 30% to 45% of that of healthy volunteers (11). The reduction is more pronounced in patients using corticosteroids (12,13). Muscle endurance may be even more affected than muscle strength and has been reported to be reduced to a level of 45% in patients with RA, compared to that of age-matched healthy individuals (9). The reported reduction of aerobic capacity in patients with RA varies between 20% and 30% in different studies (7,9,14,15). The decrease is probably

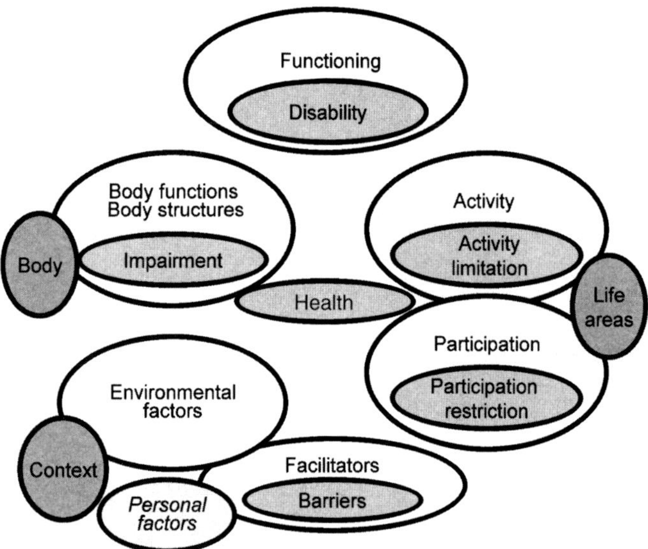

Figure 38.1. The World Health Organization's International Classification of Functioning, Disability, and Health.

more pronounced among patients who are unable to perform ergometer tests.

PHYSICAL THERAPY ASSESSMENT AND EVALUATION

Physical therapy assessment includes patient history, clinical evaluation, and analysis. It is focused on body functions and structures, as well as on activities and participation. The history includes present and past health problems, resources, individual goals, and motivation for physical therapy. The clinical evaluation includes observation, palpation, and standardized clinical tests. The analysis of the patient history and the clinical evaluation form the basis for setting goals, planning, implementing, assessing, and evaluating the physical therapy intervention (1).

The physical therapy assessment of the patient with RA is necessary for decision making and evaluation of interventions, but the physical therapist will also be able to provide the physician and other members of the health care team with useful information on various aspects of the patient's functioning and health. Similarly, the physical therapist will receive information from other team members on the patient's disease activity, difficulty in daily activities, psychological state, and social circumstances.

The American Rheumatism Association (ARA) classification of functional loss among individuals with RA (16) is a helpful tool in the communication between health professionals. Functional class (FC) I includes individuals without difficulties in daily life; FC II, those with symptoms but only minor limitations; FC III, those who are partly dependent; and FC IV, those who are totally dependent on other persons in daily life. The vast majority of individuals with RA belong to FC II (17). The classification system was revised later by the American College of Rheumatology to include vocational activities (18).

The body functions and structures and activities most commonly assessed by physical therapists in rheumatology are listed in Table 38.1. Pain intensity is evaluated, but evaluation of movement-induced pain, affective aspects of pain, and the influence of pain on daily activities are also often included. Aerobic fitness is most often evaluated with submaximal tests on bicycle ergometers or treadmills to estimate the maximum oxygen uptake. Active and passive

TABLE 38.1. Body Functions and Structures and Activities Commonly Assessed by Physical Therapists

Body Functions and Structures	Activity
Pain	Changing body position
Exercise tolerance	Maintaining body position
Mobility of joint	Lifting and carrying objects
Stability of joint	Walking
Muscle power	Moving around
Muscle endurance	Using transport
Gait pattern	Work and employment
	Recreation and leisure

joint ROM are measured in all planes of each joint with a goniometer. Active ROM can also be screened and estimated during functional movements, such as reaching for the neck, back, or feet. Joint stability is tested manually. Static and dynamic muscle strength and endurance are assessed with technical equipment to determine one repetition maximum or one maximal voluntary contraction. Muscle function can also be screened with standardized functional tests, such as timed standing. Gait and posture may be assessed with force plates, optoelectronics systems, or electromyography, but, in a clinical context, they are usually only observed to detect deviations from normal. Physical therapists generally assess capacity, rather than performance, which means that they do not observe the patient performing in daily life, but, rather, the capacity he or she reaches in a standardized environment.

Most aspects of activity and participation can be evaluated by simply asking the patient, but use of standardized questionnaires is generally preferred. Inquiry about exercise habits and motivation for physical activity is of utmost importance in the physical therapy assessment of patients with RA.

PHYSICAL THERAPY INTERVENTIONS

The aim of physical therapy to promote health through movement places physical activity and exercise at the center. Activity and exercise may serve as either prevention or treatment, most often as both. In fact, exercise is the only physical therapy intervention for which there is fairly good scientific evidence of benefits. This does not necessarily mean that manual techniques, physical modalities, or assistive devices are without value, but, rather, that too little research has yet been carried out to establish their efficacy. At present, physical activity and exercise should be viewed as the core physical therapy intervention. Other types of treatments should be prescribed with the objective to reduce symptoms and impairments that may be barriers to adequate levels of physical activity and exercise (Fig. 38.2).

Patient Education

Physical therapists often take part in formalized educational programs and also constantly educate their patients with RA about the structure and function of the human body as a regular part of assessment and treatment. Cognitive-behavioral strategies that may help overcome barriers to physical activity are frequently applied. Various types of self-management, such as muscle relaxation techniques, work and rest positions, home exercise, or application of cold or heat, are also taught.

Physical Activity

Physical activity is defined as "any bodily movement produced by skeletal muscles that results in energy expenditure." It is

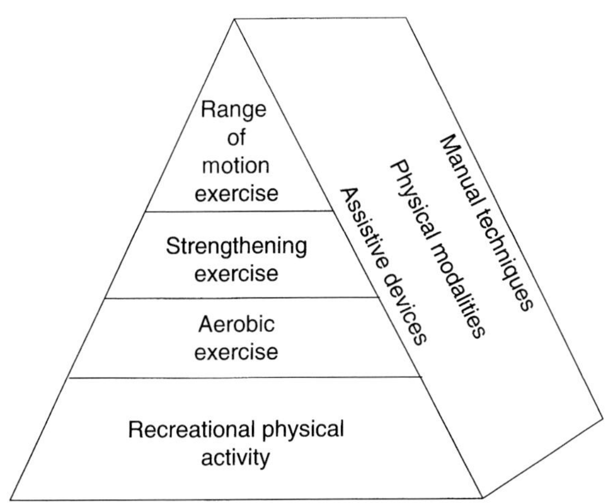

Figure 38.2. Movement is central in physical therapy. Physical activity in daily life should always be encouraged. Various types of exercise may be prescribed and adjusted according to the patient's health status. Interventions with manual techniques, physical modalities, and assistive devices are viewed as temporary and aimed at enhancing physical activity and exercise.

closely related to, but distinct from, exercise (see Exercise). *Physical inactivity* indicates a level lower than that necessary to maintain good health (19).

Physical inactivity has been identified in epidemiologic studies as one of the most, if not the most, important predictor of poor public health and premature death (20,21). Experimental studies also indicate that exercise decreases the risk for coronary heart disease and poor health due to other physical and mental conditions (22). Despite this evidence and recommendations about increased physical activity (23,24), an estimated one-half of the world's population remains essentially sedentary. It has also been found that, independent of the presence of disability, persons with arthritis have substantially lower rates of leisure time physical activity, compared with persons without arthritis (25).

To improve public health, it is recommended that adults be encouraged to increase regular activity gradually, aiming to perform every day at least 30 minutes of physical activity of moderate intensity, such as brisk walking and stair climbing. Further, people with disabilities or chronic diseases should be provided with advice on exercise and facilities appropriate to their needs. The fact that there are benefits to be gained at any age also deserves attention (24). There is also some evidence to suggest that daily physical activity may be carried out in 10-minute periods accumulated during the day (23). This strategy is particularly important to individuals who have difficulties with being active for longer periods.

There is yet no research to indicate that physical activity decreases the risk of comorbidity or premature death among individuals with RA. However, the above recommendations are directed toward the general population, which also includes people with arthritis, and indicate that patients with arthritis, despite old age or disability, need to be physically active to maintain good physical and mental health. Thus, leisure time physical activity should be encouraged from initiation of treatment and considered a preventive measure. Any daily physical activity, such as walking, biking, gardening, or vacuuming, might be beneficial if performed at a moderate level, at least 10 minutes at a time accumulated to 30 minutes a day most days of the week.

Physicians' recommendations on a healthy lifestyle, including appropriate levels of physical activity, may be sufficient to make an individual adopt or maintain an adequate behavior. However, continuous reinforcement of these recommendations and problem solving is often necessary. People with arthritis face the difficulties of overcoming pain, fatigue, impaired body functions, and maybe a fear of aggravating their disease. Physical therapists have the necessary skills to support the individual with RA in the process of identifying possibilities, overcoming barriers, and setting goals for their physical activity. They will also be able to provide continuous feedback and be available to the patients for problem solving and goal revision on a regular basis.

EXERCISE

Exercise is a subset of physical activity defined as "planned, structured, and repetitive bodily movement done to improve or maintain one or more components of physical fitness." Physical fitness is "a set of attributes that people have or achieve that relates to the ability to perform physical activity" (19).

Whereas physical activity is encouraged to improve or maintain general health, the rationale for exercise in RA relates to the impaired body functions described earlier in this chapter. These reasons for exercise have long been recognized, but there have been fears in the past that exercise would aggravate symptoms, increase disease activity, and accelerate joint destruction (26,27). However, a growing body of well-designed studies appears to support the benefit and safety of aerobic and strengthening exercise (4,28–30), which has now become an integrated and self-evident part of the rehabilitation of people with RA.

The documented benefits of exercise in RA are increased aerobic fitness and improved muscle function without any concomitant increase of pain or disease activity. Although exercise produces specific and predictable effects in healthy individuals, more general adaptations to training take place in a deconditioned state. An exercise program designed to improve aerobic fitness in patients with RA may thus also result in increased muscle function and vice versa. It still remains unclear whether exercise influences bone mineral density (31–33), activities of daily living, or health-related quality of life. Generally, no signs of increased joint destruction after exercise programs have been found (30,34–36). However, individuals with initially high joint destruction might be at greater risk for further damage when exercising intensively (30).

The effects of exercise on metabolic, physiologic, or mechanical factors are crucial to our understanding of the mechanisms through which exercise produces benefit. It is tempting to speculate about how aerobic exercise may reduce joint swelling in RA or why strengthening exercise reduces pain reports. Rheumatology-specific research suggests the possibility of exercise-related changes in synovial circulation (37), immune response and inflammatory factors (38–40), and neuropeptide levels (41). General exercise research also may pertain to this population in terms of the benefits of neuromuscular learning and improved elasticity and strength of periarticular structures.

As for exercise prescription, each individual with RA should be instructed to check regularly his or her ROM in each extremity joint and all planes at appropriate intervals that may vary between individuals. Generally, these checks should be performed daily in periods of disease exacerbation with inflamed joints but be reduced during remission phases. For individuals with a persistently active disease or with severe disability (ARA FC III–IV), ROM exercise is the first-line type of exercise therapy, preferably in combination with contractions of large trunk and thigh muscle groups.

Evidence-based guidelines for exercise prescription of aerobic and muscle function exercise are given in Table 38.2. They have been derived from studies mainly of patients with stable RA of ARA FC II (29) but may also be applicable to those in FCs I or III. There is also some support in the literature for the safety and benefit of similar exercise regimens for patients with a

TABLE 38.2. Guidelines for Prescription of Physical Activity and Exercise for Individuals with Rheumatoid Arthritis

Aim	Frequency (Times/Wk)	Duration (Min/Time)	Intensity (% of APM)	Load (% of 1 RM)
Improve or maintain general health	4–7	30	50–70	—
Increase aerobic fitness	3	30–60	60–85	—
Increase muscle strength	2–3	—	—	50–80
Increase muscular endurance	2–3	—	—	30–40

APM, age-predicted maximum heart rate (220 – age); RM, repetition maximum.

recent diagnosis of RA (31,32), active disease (42), or fragile bones (33). Moreover, it has been suggested that even individuals with very severe rheumatic diseases may be motivated to exercise and, with professional guidance, may benefit emotionally as well as physically (43).

The guidelines derived from exercise studies including patients with RA (Table 38.2) are very similar to exercise guidelines given for healthy adults, although some extra attention is needed for people with RA. First, initial increases in pain may be expected. They are, however, generally temporary, resulting from unfamiliar strain on previously unexercised joints, tendons, and muscles; they do not normally prevent continued exercise. Nevertheless, to decrease the risk of aggravated symptoms when introducing exercise programs, they should be started on levels much below those recommended in Table 38.2 but be continuously upgraded over a few weeks' time. Secondly, health professionals should be aware that their attitude toward exercise-induced pain might influence their patients' further exercise behavior. It has been suggested, for example, that an attitude focusing on the goal of the exercise, rather than on increased symptoms, would be a more successful strategy than the reverse (44). However, the use of the 24-hour rule, wherein increased pain exceeding this amount of time should lead to a decrease in exercise dose, is still common. Lastly, because of unpredictable exacerbations and remissions of the disease, upgrading cannot be expected to occur, as in healthy individuals, but needs to be constantly adjusted with the disease course in mind.

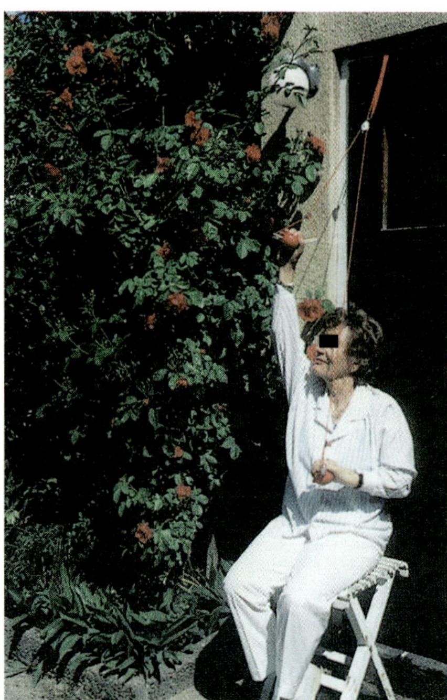

Figure 38.3. Supported range-of-motion exercise of shoulders in a simple pulley apparatus.

Aerobic exercise can be performed in water or on land and can be performed in a clinical environment with continuous supervision or in a community-based environment with professional support. There is not enough research to indicate that any setting or equipment is more efficient than the other. Typical activities might include aquatics, walking, cycling, or aerobic class participation. Strengthening exercises may be static or dynamic and performed against body weight or with various types of equipment, including resistance training equipment, a pulley apparatus, dumbbells, or elastic bands (Figs. 38.3 and 38.4). Progressive adjustment of the load is recommended, and exercises may be performed in a supervised clinical environment or at home with professional support.

Physical Modalities and Manual Techniques

Heat, cold, and electrical stimulation have long been used to reduce pain, stiffness, and swelling in individuals with RA. More recently, acupuncture has been recognized in the Western world as potentially beneficial in reducing RA symptoms. Also, low-level laser therapy has been introduced. Superficial heat is applied by using hot packs, wax baths, heat lamps, or hydrotherapy, deep heat through short-wave diathermy and ultrasound. Cold is usually applied through ice packs, cold packs, or vapo-coolant sprays. The most common modes of transcutaneous electrical nerve stimulation (TENS) are high-frequency TENS, low-frequency or acupuncture-like TENS, and burst mode TENS. Acupuncture is administered through thin needles inserted in specific documented points. Low-level laser therapy

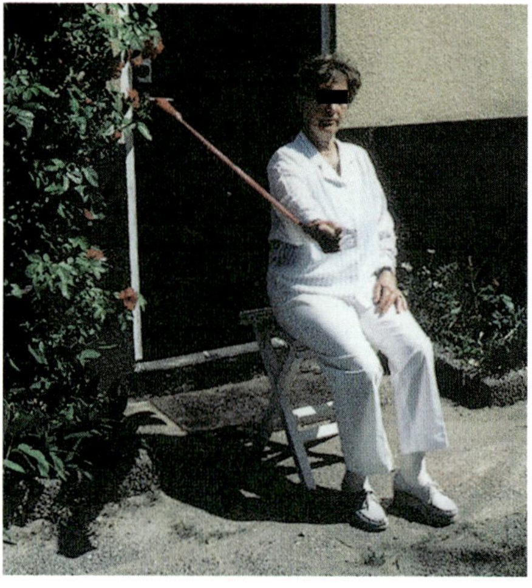

Figure 38.4. Strength training with resistive rubber bands.

is a light source generating extremely pure light of a single wavelength.

Generally, the effectiveness of physical modalities in RA is difficult to evaluate because of a lack of well-designed studies (45–49). Nevertheless, many of these treatments are attractive to the patients, and some useful guidelines for prescription can be derived from a literature review by Hayes (50). Superficial heat may be helpful in reducing symptoms, and there is no reason to avoid its use if the patient benefits from it. However, with adequate use of exercise, superficial heat is usually not necessary. There is little reason to use deep heat, as it is costly, potentially hazardous, and requires clinical visits, and because other, safer means, such as exercise, can result in similar effects. Patients should be encouraged to try cold treatments, especially when joints are acutely inflamed, as cooling may decrease the destructive inflammatory process, as well as symptoms. Use of high-frequency or burst mode TENS seems most effective in decreasing pain and stiffness without negative side effects. It is also important that appropriate professional supervision and instruction accompany the use of any type of physical modality, as they may be harmful if improperly applied (50).

The most commonly used manual techniques to reduce symptoms and increase flexibility in patients with RA are massage, traction, and muscle stretching. The empiric efficacy of these treatments is poorly evaluated in well-conducted studies.

Pre- and Postoperative Assessment and Exercise

Assessment and exercise before and after surgical procedures are important parts of physical therapy. Total joint arthroplasty, in particular that of the lower extremity, is highly successful, and the importance of pre- and postsurgical physical therapy management is widely recognized, despite lack of scientific evidence on its efficacy for patients with RA (51).

Preoperative physical therapy evaluation is performed to identify and address potentially problematic areas. Assessment of movement patterns, including gait, ROM, muscle function, respiration, and activity and participation is performed to enhance rehabilitation and the planning of home care postoperatively. Patients should also be taught and encouraged to exercise preoperatively, as better preoperative function is associated with improved postoperative outcomes (52).

The primary goals of postoperative physical therapy, regardless of surgical procedure, are to decrease pain, gain muscle control, and restore previous levels of functioning (51). In the early postoperative period, the routine after lower extremity total joint arthroplasty includes therapeutic exercise, transfer training, gait training, and activities of daily living instruction. After discharge from the hospital, the long-term goal is to improve ambulation to a normal gait. A general impression among physical therapists and patients is that a prolonged period of physical therapy after discharge from the hospital would improve the results of the surgical procedures by increasing ROM, muscle function, and activity and participation. The scientific evidence for this is, unfortunately, still lacking.

CONCLUSION

Referrals to physical therapy are indicated whenever a patient with RA has difficulties in achieving the levels of physical activity that are required to maintain good health. The physical therapist will not only be able to analyze the patient's level of functioning, but also to prescribe exercise of adequate intensity and frequency to obtain maximum benefit and safety for each individual. Physical modalities, manual techniques, and the prescription of walking aids, including appropriate footwear, are used by the physical therapists to enhance physical activity. The physical therapist will also be able to assist the patient in identifying and overcoming cognitive-behavioral barriers to exercise. There is a special case for physical therapy in connection with surgical procedures as, pre- and postoperative information and exercise might optimize the outcome.

ACKNOWLEDGMENTS

The author thanks Ingmarie Apel Eriksson and Ulla Levin for kind assistance with figures.

REFERENCES

1. Broberg C. *Physical therapy and classification*. Stockholm: Swedish Physical Therapy Association, 1997.
2. ICF resources page. World Health Organization Web site. Available at: www.who.int/classification/icf. Accessed March 24, 2004.
3. Stucki G, Cieza A, Ewert T. Application of the international classification of functioning, disability and health (ICF) in clinical practice. *Disabil Rehabil* 2002;24:281–282.
4. Stenström CH. Therapeutic exercise in rheumatoid arthritis. *Arthritis Care Res* 1994;7:190–197.
5. van den Ende CHM. *Exercise therapy in rheumatoid arthritis*. [doctoral thesis]. Leiden: Rijksuniversiteit te Leiden; 1997.
6. Eberhardt KB, Fex E. Functional impairment and disability in early rheumatoid arthritis: development over 5 years. *J Rheumatol* 1995;22:1037–1042.
7. Ekblom B, Lövgren O, Alderin M, et al. Physical performance in patients with rheumatoid arthritis. *Scand J Rheumatol* 1974;3:121–125.
8. Hsieh LF, Didenko B, Schumacher HR. Isokinetic and isometric testing of knee musculature in patients with rheumatoid arthritis with mild knee involvement. *Arch Phys Med Rehabil* 1987;68:294–297.
9. Ekdahl C, Broman G. Muscle strength, endurance, and aerobic capacity in rheumatoid arthritis: a comparative study with healthy subjects. *Ann Rheum Dis* 1992;51:35–40.
10. Häkkinen A, Hannonen P, Häkkinen K. Muscle strength in healthy people and in patients suffering from recent-onset inflammatory arthritis. *Br J Rheumatol* 1995;34:355–360.
11. Nordesjö LO, Nordgren B, Wigren A, Kolstad K. Isometric strength and endurance in patients with severe rheumatoid arthritis or osteoarthritis in the knee joints. *Scand J Rheumatol* 1983;12:152–156.
12. Danneskiold-Samsoe B, Grimby G. Isokinetic and isometric muscle strength in patients with rheumatoid arthritis: the relationship to clinical parameters and the influence of corticosteroid. *Clin Rheumatol* 1986;5:459–467.
13. Danneskiold-Samsoe B, Grimby G. The relationship between the leg muscle strength and physical capacity in patients with rheumatoid arthritis, with reference to the influence of corticosteroids. *Clin Rheumatol* 1986;5:468–474.
14. Beals CA, Lampman RM, Banwell BF, et al. Measurement of exercise tolerance in patients with rheumatoid arthritis and osteoarthritis. *J Rheumatol* 1985;12:458–461.
15. Minor MA, Hewett JE, Webel RR, et al. Exercise tolerance and disease related measures in patients with rheumatoid arthritis and osteoarthritis. *J Rheumatol* 1988;15:905–911.
16. Steinbrocker O, Traeger CH, Batterman RC. Therapeutic criteria in rheumatoid arthritis. *JAMA* 1949;140:659–662.
17. Allander E. A population survey of rheumatoid arthritis: epidemiological aspects of the syndrome, its pattern, and effect on gainful employment. *Acta Rheumatol Scand* 1970;[Suppl 15]:1.
18. Hochberg MC, Chang RW, Dwosh I, et al. The American College of Rheumatology 1991 revised criteria for the classification of global functional status in rheumatoid arthritis. *Arthritis Rheum* 1992;35:498–502.
19. Caspersen CJ, Powell KE, Christenson GM. Physical activity, exercise, and physical fitness. *Public Health Rep* 1985;100:125–131.
20. Pfaffenberger RS, Hyde RT, Wing AL, Hsieh C-G. Physical activity, all-cause mortality, and longevity of college alumni. *N Engl J Med* 1986;314:606–613.
21. Blair SN, Kohl HW, Pfaffenberger RS, et al. Physical fitness and all-cause mortality. *JAMA* 1989;262:2395–2401.
22. Pate RR, Pratt M, Blair SN, et al. Physical activity and public health: a recommendation from the Centers for Disease Control and Prevention and the American College of Sports Medicine. *JAMA* 1995;273:402–407.
23. National Institute of Health. Physical activity and cardiovascular health. *NIH Consens Statement* 1995;13:1–33.
24. WHO/FIMS Committee on physical activity for health. Exercise for health. *Bull World Health Organ* 1995;73:135–136.
25. Centers for Disease Control and Prevention. Prevalence of leisure-time physical activity among persons with arthritis and other rheumatic conditions—United States 1990-1991. *MMWR Morb Mortal Wkly Rep* 1997;46:389–393.

26. Smith RD, Polley HF. Rest therapy for rheumatoid arthritis. *Mayo Clin Proc* 1978;53:141–145.
27. Alexander GJM, Hortas C, Bacon PA. Bed rest, activity and the inflammation of rheumatoid arthritis. *Br J Rheumatol* 1983;22:134–140.
28. van den Ende CHM, Vilet Vlieland TPM, Munneke M, Hazes JMW. Dynamic exercise therapy in rheumatoid arthritis: a systematic review. *Br J Rheumatol* 1998;37:677–687.
29. Stenström CH, Minor MA. Evidence for the benefit of aerobic and strengthening exercise in rheumatoid arthritis. *Arthritis Rheum* 2003;49:428–434.
30. DeJong Z, Munneke M, Zwinderman AH, et al. Is a long-term high-intensity exercise program effective and safe in patients with rheumatoid arthritis? Results of a randomized controlled trial. *Arthritis Rheum* 2003;48;2415–2424.
31. Häkkinen A, Sokka T, Kotaniemi A, et al. Dynamic strength training in patients with early rheumatoid arthritis increases muscle strength but not bone mineral density. *J Rheumatol* 1999;26:1257–1263.
32. Häkkinen A, Sokka T, Kotaniemi A, Hannonen P. A randomized two-year study of the effects of dynamic strength training on muscle strength, disease activity, functional capacity, and bone mineral density in early rheumatoid arthritis. *Arthritis Rheum* 2001;44:515–522.
33. Westby MD, Wade JP, Rangno KK, Berkowitz J. A randomized controlled trial to evaluate the effectiveness of an exercise program in women with rheumatoid arthritis taking low dose prednisone. *J Rheumatol* 2000;27:1674–1680.
34. Nordemar R, Ekblom B, Zachrisson L, Lundgvist K. Physical training in rheumatoid arthritis. A long-term controlled study, I. *Scand J Rheumatol* 1981; 10:17–23.
35. Hansen TM, Hansen G, Langgard AM, Rasmussen JO. Long-term physical training in rheumatoid arthritis: a randomized trial with different training programs and blinded observers. *Scand J Rheumatol* 1993;22:107–112.
36. Stenström CH. Radiologically observed progression of joint destruction and its relationship with demographic factors, disease severity, and exercise frequency in patients with rheumatoid arthritis. *Phys Ther* 1994;74:32–39.
37. James MJ, Cleland LG, Gaffney RD, et al. Effect of exercise on 99Tc-DTPA clearance from knees with effusions. *J Rheumatol* 1994;21:501–504.
38. Rall LC, Roubenoff R, Cannon JG, et al. Effects of progressive resistance training on immune response in aging and chronic inflammation. *Med Sci Sports Exerc* 1996;28;1356–1365.
39. Shephard RJ, Shek PN. Autoimmune disorders, physical activity, and training, with particular reference to rheumatoid arthritis. *Exerc Immunol Rev* 1997;3:53–67.
40. Lemmey A, Maddison P, Breslin A, et al. Association between insulin-like growth factor status and physical activity levels in rheumatoid arthritis. *J Rheumatol* 2001;28:29–34.
41. Stenström CH, Alexanderson H, Lundberg I, et al. Exercise and variations in neuropeptide concentrations in rheumatoid arthritis. *Neuropeptides* 1999;33:260–264.
42. van den Ende CHM, Breedveld FC, le Cessie S, et al. Effect of intensive exercise on patients with active rheumatoid arthritis: a randomized clinical trial. *Ann Rheum Dis* 2000;59:615–621.
43. Marley WP, Santilli TF. A 15-year exercise program for rheumatoid vasculitis. *Scand J Rheumatol* 1998;27:149–151.
44. Stenström CH. Home exercise in rheumatoid arthritis functional class II: goal-setting versus pain attention. *J Rheumatol* 1994;21:627–634.
45. Brosseau L, Welch V, Wells G, et al. Low level laser therapy (classes I, II and III) for treating rheumatoid arthritis (Cochrane review). In: The Cochrane Library, Issue 4. Oxford: Update Software, 2002.
46. Casimiro L, Brosseau L, Milne S, et al. Acupuncture and electroacupuncture for the treatment of RA. In: the Cochrane Library, Issue 4. Oxford: Update Software, 2002.
47. Casimiro L, Brosseau L, Robinson V, et al. Therapeutic ultrasound for the treatment of rheumatoid arthritis. In: The Cochrane Library, Issue 4. Oxford: Update Software, 2002.
48. Pelland L, Brosseau L, Casimiro L, et al. Electrical stimulation for the treatment of rheumatoid arthritis. In: The Cochrane Library, Issue 4. Oxford: Update Software, 2002.
49. Robinson V, Brosseau L, Casimiro L, et al. Thermotherapy for treating rheumatoid arthritis. In: The Cochrane Library, Issue 4. Oxford: Update Software, 2002.
50. Hayes KW. Physical modalities. In: Robbins L, ed. *Clinical care in the rheumatic diseases*. Atlanta: American College of Rheumatology, 2001.
51. Ganz SB, Viellion G. Pre- and post-surgical management of the hip and knee. In: Robbins L, ed. *Clinical care in the rheumatic diseases*. Atlanta: American College of Rheumatology, 2001.
52. Fortin PR, Clarke AE, Joseph L, et al. Outcomes of total hip and knee replacement: preoperative functional status predicts outcomes at six months after surgery. *Arthritis Rheum* 1999;42:1722–1728.

CHAPTER 39

Occupational Therapy

Catherine L. Backman, Angela Fairleigh, and Gay Kuchta

WHAT IS OCCUPATIONAL THERAPY?

Occupational therapy involves assessment and intervention strategies to help people maintain, restore, or improve their ability to engage in the occupations of daily life. Daily occupations are typically grouped into three main occupational performance areas: self-care (e.g., eating, dressing, bathing, mobility), productivity (e.g., employment, household work, parenting, going to school, volunteering), and leisure (social and recreational activities) (1). Typically, patients with rheumatoid arthritis (RA) are referred to an occupational therapist by their rheumatologist or another health care provider because they have cited specific functional problems at home, work, or school. The cited problems are often just the tip of the iceberg, because some patients are reluctant to mention problems that seem insignificant (e.g., putting on cosmetics) or too shy about others (e.g., managing personal hygiene or perineal care). An occupational therapy assessment will identify and prioritize problems in all aspects of self-care, productivity, and leisure and lead to an action plan to resolve those of greatest impact for the patient.

Referrals to occupational therapy are appropriate throughout the disease process in RA and are part of a comprehensive team approach to management (2). Early referral helps patients learn about the disease process and apply strategies to minimize pain and fatigue while preserving function. Occupational therapists provide a thorough evaluation of functional status to monitor disease progression and make recommendations for adapting activities or the home and work environment to enable participation in activities that are at risk or may have been curtailed by RA symptoms. Later in the disease process, occupational therapists offer assistive devices and strategies to compensate for functional impairment and provide pre- and postoperative rehabilitation for patients undergoing reconstructive surgery.

FUNCTIONAL LIMITATIONS IN RHEUMATOID ARTHRITIS

Despite advances in medical therapy to control arthritis symptoms, some people with RA will experience significant impairment and disability. Recent estimates of the prevalence of work disability in RA range from 22% to 38% (3–5). Adults with RA report working fewer hours of both paid and unpaid (household) work than healthy controls (6). In a survey of 142 women with RA, more than half reported limitations in household tasks (cleaning, doing laundry, and shopping), and, among those with young children, 29% reported limitations in caring for them (7). Lower functional status and pain are associated with both household work limitations (8,9) and limitations in paid work (3,5,9). RA has an adverse affect on participation in a range of productivity and leisure activities (10), and decreased functional abilities have been associated with depression (11). Because the domain of concern for occupational therapy is to maintain, restore, or improve performance in everyday activity, the prevalence of functional limitations in RA provides a strong rationale for inclusion of occupational therapy in the comprehensive management of the disease.

ASSESSMENT AND EVALUATION

The occupational therapist works collaboratively with the patient to identify problems in self-care, productivity, and leisure; identify the underlying causes of these problems; and propose solutions to restore or improve occupational performance. A patient-centered approach (termed *client-centered* in occupational therapy literature) (12,13) is helpful to gain insight into individual beliefs, fears, knowledge of RA, and what techniques have been successful or ineffective in the past. Understanding the patient's perspective provides the basis for a collaborative relationship that often spans many years. The patient-centered approach respects the individual views of people seeking health care and recognizes that their choices and decisions are the ones that direct the care plan (14). An individualized approach helps the therapist to understand the influence of culture, family, community networks, and other environmental factors, as illustrated by a qualitative case study (15). Although not specific to managing RA, increasing evidence indicates that patient-centered approaches improve communication between health care providers and patients and result in greater patient satisfaction with care (13,16). Additionally, approaches based on individualized, collaborative goal-setting with patients result in improved functional outcomes (16).

Once occupational performance problems have been identified, the occupational therapist assesses the *performance components* and *environmental conditions* that may be contributing to the problems (12). Performance components include *physical, affective,* and *cognitive* abilities. The physical assessment is comprised of functional range of motion and strength, observation and palpation of joint swelling, and deformity or instability, especially in the hand and wrist. For example, can patients reach to shampoo their hair or to their feet to pull on socks? Pull files from the back of the filing cabinet at work? Grip tools needed for the job? Evaluation of the affective component considers perceived pain and fatigue, self-efficacy, and general motivation and mood. For example, what activities cause pain or discomfort? How long can one work before requiring a rest? What activities are most important and rewarding? Cognitive performance components are not usually an issue for people with RA, unless comorbidities are present that affect memory, attention, perception, and learning.

During the formal evaluation, particular attention is given to assessing hand function, as RA typically involves the hands, and the hands are involved in almost all daily activities. Questionnaires measuring overall function may not be sensitive enough to capture specific problems with using the hands in everyday activity, based on one correlational study (17). Detailed observations of joint effusions, synovial proliferation, ligamentous integrity, and deformity also contribute to a comprehensive hand assessment (18).

When the patient identifies significant difficulties performing household tasks or paid work, a home or work site visit is indicated. Depending on funding circumstances, such a visit may be provided by a home health occupational therapist, by occupational therapists affiliated with outpatient rehabilitation programs, or a therapist in private practice. Home visits focus on ensuring safe access within the home and recommending adaptations to overcome impairments. Work site visits permit a comprehensive job analysis and observation of the fit between job demands and individual functional capacity. The occupational therapist incorporates recommendations during the visit and demonstrates alternative methods of doing work-related tasks, proposes necessary changes to the physical environment to accommodate pain or functional limitations, and advocates on behalf of the patient for employer support to implement accommodations. One example of the key components in a workplace assessment, compatible with recommendations for reasonable accommodation under the Americans with Disabilities Act, is provided by Jacobs (19) as an appendix within a textbook on ergonomics.

Ideally, the functional assessment is conducted using objective, reliable, and valid instruments, supplemented with skilled observation and informal, qualitative information that acknowledges how RA affects the individual patient. Suggested instruments for measuring occupational performance areas and performance components are listed in Table 39.1.

TABLE 39.1. Selected Instruments Used for Assessing Occupational Performance and Physical Components in Patients with Rheumatoid Arthritis

Test Title and Reference	Description
Canadian Occupational Performance Measure (20)	Individualized outcome measure Semistructured interview rating (on a 1–10 scale) Performance and satisfaction with performance in self-care, productivity, leisure
McMaster-Toronto Arthritis Patient Function Preference Questionnaire (21)	Individualized outcome measure Structured interview to identify and rank physical activities limited by arthritis Improvement rated on a 3-point scale (worse, no change, improved)
Assessment of Motor and Process Skills (22)	Structured observation permitting simultaneous evaluation of performance in instrumental activities of daily living (IADL) tasks selected by the patient and the underlying motor and process skills required to perform the tasks (requires completion of 5-day training program to administer)
Functional Status Index (23)	Self-report questionnaire addressing basic activities of daily living
Work Limitations Questionnaire (24)	Self-report questionnaire rating difficulty performing 25 specific job demands
Safety Assessment of Function and Environment for Rehabilitation Tool (25)	Observational assessment of the home environment and the patient's ability to safely navigate within it, from entering the home to accessing kitchen, bath, and bedroom
Arthritis Hand Function Test (26,27)	Observational assessment of hand strength, dexterity, and ability to perform functional tasks (e.g., fastening buttons, using a knife and fork, pouring water)
Disabilities of the Arm, Shoulder and Hand (28)	Self-report questionnaire identifying limitations in IADL, work, and leisure activities as a result of hand, arm, or shoulder impairment
Michigan Hand Questionnaire (29)	Self-report questionnaire for assessing hand function and esthetics pre- and postoperatively
Sequential Occupational Dexterity Assessment (30)	An observational assessment of bilateral hand dexterity

INTERVENTIONS

Occupational therapy interventions are directed at resolving functional limitations identified by the patient while managing symptoms such as pain and fatigue. Suggested solutions for specific problems related to self-care, productivity, and leisure occupations are summarized in Tables 39.2, 39.3, and 39.4. Key interventions are clustered into five categories: joint protection and energy conservation, splinting, assistive devices, environmental modifications, and modification of daily routines. For each category, we offer a description followed by existing evidence of efficacy.

Joint Protection and Energy Conservation Principles and Techniques

Joint protection principles are recommendations for alternative methods of doing activities based on biomechanical and ergonomic guidelines. Joint protection techniques aim to reduce pain and local inflammation during the performance of tasks, preserve the integrity of vulnerable joint structures, and improve function (31). Energy conservation principles involve planning and pacing activities within the limits of one's capacity to perform. Energy conservation techniques focus on recognizing and managing fatigue to pursue priority activities. Joint protection and energy conservation principles are generic and, to be effective, require demonstration and application to specific roles and activities of the patient (Table 39.5). A simple example of a joint protection technique for a gardener is to reduce effort and avoid stress on the small joints of the hand by supporting a watering can with an upturned flower pot, instead of holding it up to the water faucet.

Joint protection and energy conservation are mainstays of occupational therapy's contribution to patient-education programs, although evidence is just beginning to accumulate. A pretest and posttest study demonstrated that knowledge of joint protection and energy conservation principles applied to 12 activities of daily living was significantly improved in 55 adults with RA after a 1-hour instructional session with an occupational therapist. Improvements were sustained at 6 months (32). The study did not examine changes in behavior.

TABLE 39.2. Resolving Self-Care Performance Limitations: Examples of Impairments, Problems, and Potential Solutions

Signs and Symptoms	Functional Problems	Solutions
Patient complains of shoulder pain with limited range of motion and weakness.	Unable to sustain shoulder elevation to complete hair washing and styling Patient wishes to function independently	Assess extent of disability and establish specific needs Review equipment available at home Try assistive devices, such as long-handled scalp massager or handheld shower on adjustable bracket Suggest use of easy shampoo dispenser Review alternative positioning methods, such as supporting arms on a table or vanity to blow dry hair
Patient complains of knee pain and swelling. There is limited flexion and quadriceps weakness.	Unable to get in and out of the bathtub Patient afraid of falling	Assess upper and lower limb strength and flexibility (to ensure recommendations are within limits of physical ability) Discuss bathroom safety procedures Suggest use of bath stool or bench, grab bars, handheld shower, and nonskid mat Assess home situation to establish available family or outside help Review joint protection techniques
Patient complains of painful fingers and thumb. There is instability of the proximal interphalangeal joints of all fingers and the thumb.	Unable to manipulate buttons	Assess hand range of motion and strength (to ensure recommendations are within limits of physical ability) Discuss the use of alternative fastenings, such as Velcro, and clothing styles without buttons Assess desire and ability to use a buttonhook Splint to control pain and instability of affected joints

Behavior change did occur, however, in a crossover trial comparing group education in joint protection versus no treatment in 35 patients with RA (33). In this study, the intervention was provided in weekly sessions of 2 hours for 4 weeks, with an optional home visit by the occupational therapist. Sessions included written and audiovisual materials describing joint protection methods, group discussion, contracting, and practice with alternative methods and assistive devices. Joint protection behaviors, measured objectively, increased significantly after the program, and changes were maintained at 6 months. In a subsequent trial comparing the joint protection program to a standard arthritis education program of the same duration, the joint protection group (N = 65) demonstrated significant improvement in joint protection behaviors and reported less hand pain and overall pain, less morning stiffness, and improved performance of activities of daily living, compared to the standard care group (N = 62, matched for age and disease duration) (34). The joint protection group also reported fewer doctor visits. These effects were sustained for 1 year and indicate that joint protection education helps to mediate the effects of RA over and above the effects of drug therapy.

A small (N = 16) randomized trial investigated the effect of completing a workbook on energy conservation principles and techniques, compared to standard occupational therapy (35). Twice as many patients completing the workbook program achieved a better balance of rest and activity than those undergoing standard care (50% of the experimental group, compared to 22% of the usual care group). Although this was a small pilot study, it suggested that patients using energy conservation techniques, specifically interspersing rest with activity, increased their overall physical activity.

In a systematic review of 24 studies of patient education for adults with RA, Reimsma et al. found that education was effective in reducing active joint counts and disability and improved psychological status and patient global assessment of disease status, at least in the short term (36). Patient education was defined as any

TABLE 39.3. Resolving Limitations in Productivity: Examples of Impairments, Problems, and Potential Solutions

Signs and Symptoms	Functional Problems	Solutions
Patient complains of bilateral wrist pain, especially at the end of the workday.	Difficulty managing at work. Prolonged use of keyboard and mouse exacerbates wrist symptoms. Patient anxious about ability to continue to function in present job situation.	Assess wrists for pain, range, and strength Conduct ergonomic assessment of work station Select modifications to reduce wrist joint stress Discuss disease management principles, including joint protection, energy conservation, pain management, pacing, positioning, and problem-solving techniques Discuss need of vocational rehabilitation consultation
Patient presents with swelling of MCP joints. There is slight ulnar drift and weak grip strength.	Meal preparation difficult. Difficulty lifting pots and pans, turning taps, and handling utensils for peeling and chopping. Patient concerned about maintaining traditional role in family group.	Conduct hand assessment Instruct in joint protection techniques, including alternative hand positions when lifting or using kitchen tools Offer equipment suggestions, such as the use of power tools, lever taps, and enlarged handles In-home functional assessment Establish the availability of family support and help MCP protection splints
Patient complains of thumb pain. There is involvement of the MCP and interphalangeal joints with instability and weak pinch strength.	Driving problems. Difficulty opening the car door, turning the ignition key, and handling the seat belt.	Splint to support unstable joints Assess car for adaptations—supply key turner and car door opener Refer to registered mechanic to assess for major alterations or car selection advice

MCP, metacarpophalangeal.

TABLE 39.4. Pursuing Leisure Activities: Examples of Impairments, Problems, and Potential Solutions

Signs and Symptoms	Functional Problems	Solutions
Patient complains of generalized fatigue.	Unable to maintain backyard garden	Assess work habits. Discuss disease-management principles. Review the principles of energy conservation, pacing individual tasks, alternating heavy and light jobs. Offer tool selection advice. Consider tools with longer handles for better leverage, lighter weight, and mechanical advantages, such as ratchet mechanisms. Discuss alternatives to standard garden designs, such as raised flowerbeds and low-maintenance plant selection.
Patient presents with neck and upper limb pain and muscle weakness.	Unable to enjoy reading for pleasure	Assess body mechanics. Assess reading habits, preferred location, positions, and type of materials. Check lighting. Review the principles of good posture. Discuss the principles of joint protection. Assess book rest alternatives; see Fig. 39.4D for positioning with lap desk. Consider the use of neck and upper limb support from pillows, selected chairs, or collars. Consider prism glasses to accommodate positioning advice.
Patient complains of rear-foot joint pain. There is evidence of subtalar joint instability.	Unable to play golf	Foot assessment to establish the need for strengthening exercises, footbed orthoses, or foot/ankle support. Assess shoes for suitability. Review the principles of joint protection. Consider the use of a golf cart.

intervention with formal, structured instruction on RA and ways to manage symptoms. Joint protection and energy conservation were explicit components of 14 of the studies reviewed. Although the effect of joint protection and energy conservation cannot be separated from other components of the programs, there is at least some suggestion that they contribute to desirable outcomes.

Splinting

There are at least four purposes of splinting applications in RA:

- To provide localized rest to reduce pain and inflammation—for example, a night resting splint to position and support wrist and hand joints.
- To stabilize joints and enhance function—for example, a splint that immobilizes the wrist and improves grip.
- To realign or position joints in a stable anatomical plane to minimize deformity and stretching of periarticular structures—for example, an anti–swan-neck splint that repositions the proximal interphalangeal joint of the finger in slight flexion.

TABLE 39.5. Joint Protection and Energy Conservation Principles and Sample Techniques

Principle	Sample Techniques or Application
Respect your pain	Reduce time or effort spent on an activity if pain occurs and lasts for more than 2 h after the activity has been discontinued. Avoid nonessential activities that aggravate your pain.
Balance rest and work	Take short breaks during your work. For example, take a 5-min rest at the end of 1 h of work. Intersperse more active tasks with more passive or quiet work.
Reduce the amount of effort needed to do the job	Use assistive devices, such as a jar opener or lever taps. Slide pots across the counter instead of lifting. Use a trolley to transport heavy items. Use a raised toilet seat and seat cushion to reduce stress on hips, knees, and hands. Use frozen vegetables instead of peeling or chopping.
Avoid staying in one position for prolonged periods of time	Change position frequently to avoid joint stiffness and muscle fatigue. For example, take a 30-sec range of motion break after 10–20 min of typing or holding a tool; after standing for 20 min, perch on a stool for the next 20 min; walk to the mailroom after 20–30 min sitting at your desk.
Avoid activities that cannot be stopped immediately if you experience pain or discomfort	Plan ahead. Be realistic about your abilities so you do not walk or drive too far or leave all your shopping and errands to a single trip.
Reduce unnecessary stress on your joints while sleeping	Use a firm mattress for support. Sleep on your back with a pillow to support the curve in your neck. If you prefer to lay on your side, place a pillow between your knees and lay on the least painful side.
Maintain muscle strength and joint range of motion	Do your prescribed exercises regularly. Strong muscles will help support your joints. Regular exercise will reduce fatigue.
Use a well-planned work space	Organize your work space so that work surfaces and materials are at a convenient height for you, to ensure good posture. Place frequently used items within close reach. Reduce clutter by getting rid of unnecessary items or storing less frequently used items away from the immediate work space.

From Mary Pack Arthritis Program, Vancouver Hospital and Health Sciences Centre, Occupational Therapy Department: "Joint Protection Principles and How to Apply Them," with permission.

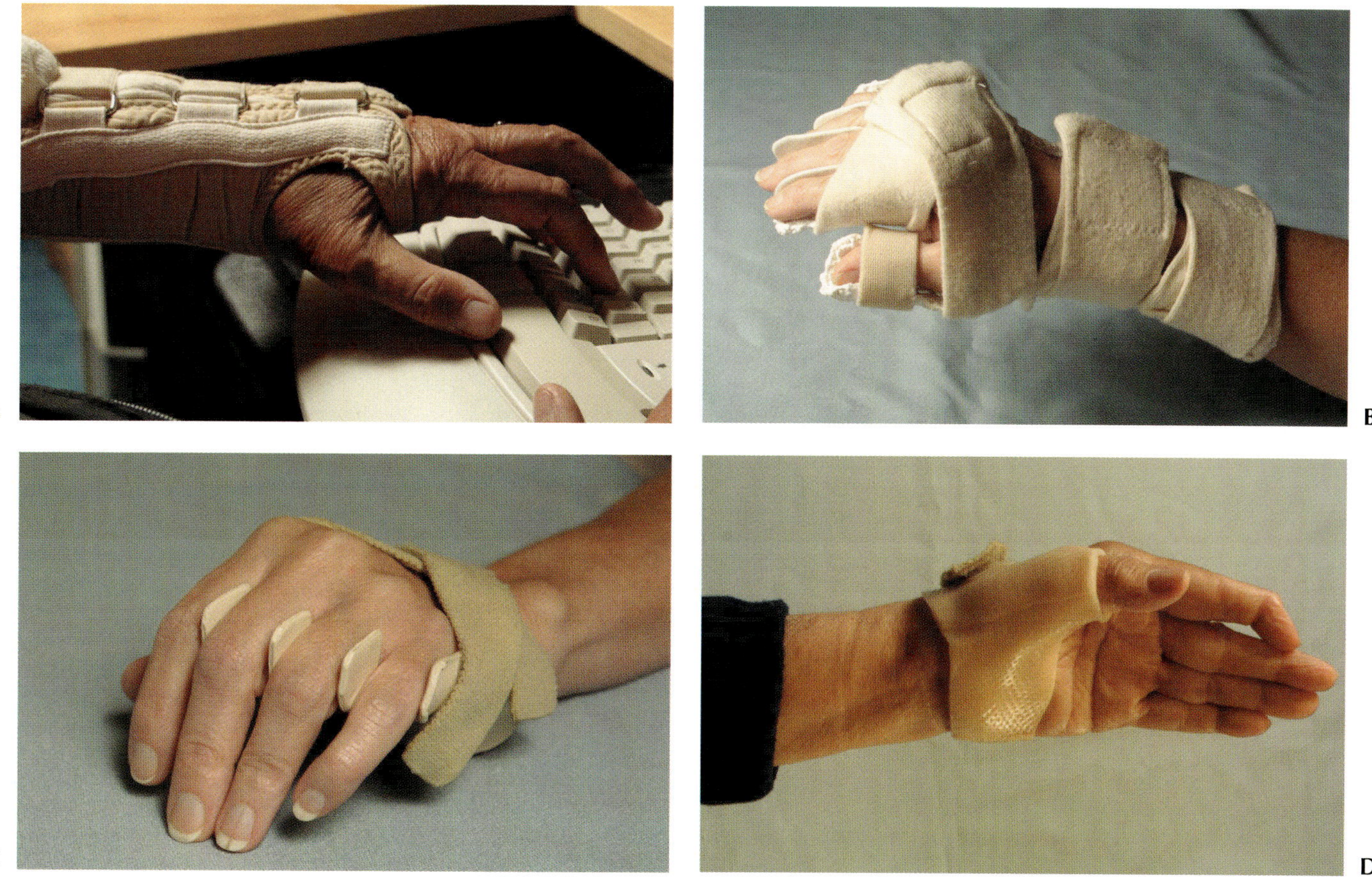

Figure 39.1. Selected splints used in rheumatoid arthritis. **A:** Prefabricated wrist splint immobilizes the wrist while still permitting hand function in daily activities. **B:** Night resting splint with large, soft straps to position the hand and wrist during periods of synovitis. **C:** Metacarpophalangeal protection splint. **D:** Thumb splint.

- To facilitate postoperative recovery—for example, a dynamic extension splint applied after metacarpophalangeal (MCP) arthroplasty, encouraging early finger motion in a controlled range.

Many body parts can be splinted. Commonly used splints include wrist splints, hand resting splints, MCP protection splints, silver ring splints, and thumb splints.

Wrist splints (Fig. 39.1A) are used to reduce pain, support the joint, and facilitate functional performance, such as lifting and carrying. They may also be used to reduce repetitive flexion and extension of the wrist associated with carpal tunnel syndrome. The efficacy of wrist splints in patients with RA has been well documented, including comparisons among different styles of splints. Wrist splints have consistently demonstrated improved hand strength in single subject, repeated measures designs (37) and small clinical trials (38–40), as well as improved ability to lift and carry (37) and reduce pain (38,41). Although wrist splints may compromise hand dexterity when first applied (38), it appears to be a time-limited effect while patients become accustomed to wearing the splints (41). In a crossover trial comparing custom-made splints with commercially available (prefabricated) splints, significantly greater pain relief was achieved with the custom-made splints, although both types of splints improved pain, compared to baseline (41). The difference may be due to improved fit, because commercially available splints have a limited range of sizes that may not achieve optimal wrist stabilization in all patients.

Night resting splints (Fig. 39.1B) are recommended when there is acute pain and swelling of the joints in the hands and wrists. They are designed to support the limb in a loose-packed resting position and prevent deformity that may otherwise occur if the limb rests in a flexed position to accommodate joint effusions. They are worn all or part of the night while sleeping or for short rest periods during the day when synovitis or tenosynovitis is present (18). The use of resting splints is common practice, based on investigations conducted from the late 1960s to the early 1980s, suggesting that splinting achieves the goal of reducing inflammation and pain (42,43). A more recent small trial (N = 39) comparing soft versus hard resting splints found that both effectively reduced pain and that individual preference influenced compliance with instructions for splint use (44). It is recommended that gentle range of motion exercises be done after removing splints to maintain mobility and flexibility (18).

The effect of other splints has not been as well studied. MCP protection splints are provided to limit the amount of flexion and ulnar deviation at the MCP joints (Fig. 39.1C). They are intended to reduce pain and minimize deformity, and x-rays of 27 RA hands wearing such a splint demonstrated correction of the subluxed position in all but the index finger (45). That is, the splint maintained a neutral position at the MCP joints as long as it was worn. Thumb splints (Fig. 39.1D) are provided to stabilize one or more joints in the thumb to reduce pain and improve opposition. They improved symptoms in a retrospective review of 130 thumbs with osteoarthritis (46). A splinting option for realigning finger joints with flexible boutonnière or swan-neck deformities is the silver ring splint. This is an esthetically pleasing splint that reduces the disabled appearance of the hand with a splint that looks like jewelry (Fig. 39.2). Positioning splints like the silver ring splint help

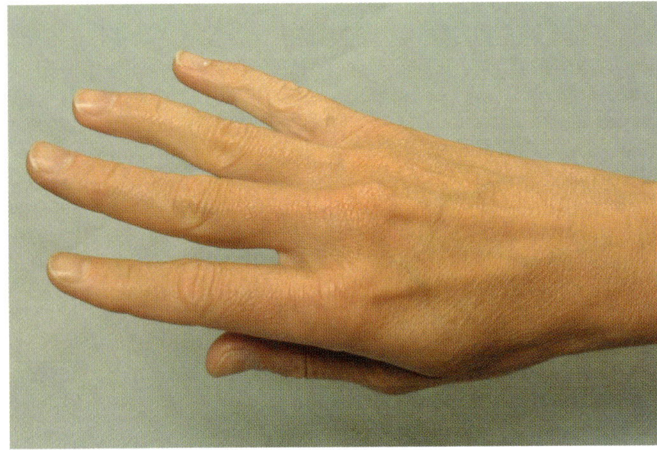

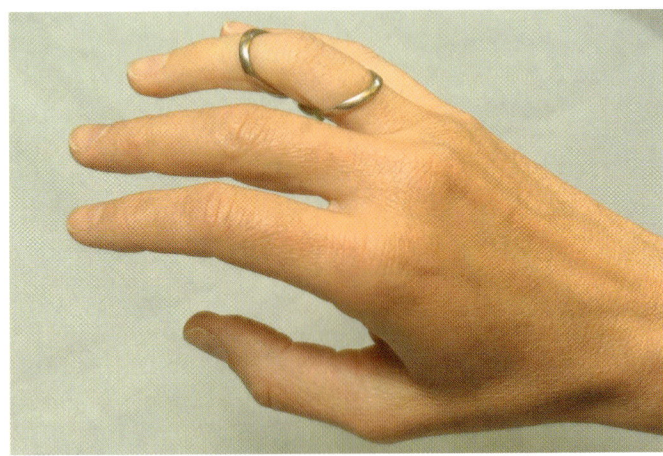

Figure 39.2. Swan-neck deformity uncorrected **(A)** and corrected **(B)** with a silver ring splint.

control the muscle imbalance around a joint and are believed to prevent permanent or fixed deformity if worn continuously. A regime of resting splints alternating with dynamic extension splints enhanced functional recovery after MCP joint arthroplasties (47). No evidence was found to indicate that splints prevent the progression of deformity, most likely because this would require a controlled longitudinal study, and this level of rigorous research has not yet been conducted in the field.

Supportive shoes and foot orthoses are also a type of splint that enhances people's ability to walk comfortably by appropriately positioning the foot and subtalar joint during weightbearing (48). More information on foot orthoses is in Chapter 38, Physical Therapy.

Assistive Devices

An assistive device is any product used to maintain or improve function (49). Assistive devices may compensate for a physical limitation or encourage adherence to joint protection principles for reducing pain. For example, elastic shoelaces and a long-handled shoe horn enable a patient with restricted hip and knee range of motion to put on his or her shoes independently, and a raised toilet seat means less joint stress and pain in hips, knees, and hands. A wide range of devices is available in medical supply catalogs and stores, and many devices are becoming available in regular shops as universal accessibility becomes more prevalent; for example, culinary shops stocking kitchen gadgets now carry utensils with large grips, which are easier for all people to grasp, not just those with RA. Additionally, the *Arthritis Storefront* at The Arthritis Society's Web site (www.arthritis.ca) enables patients worldwide to view more than 250 assistive devices and products available for online purchase.

When suitable devices or equipment are not readily available, the occupational therapist may modify existing equipment or arrange for a carpenter or handyperson to make adjustments. An example is changing the height of work surfaces to ensure safe body mechanics and proper posture, as well as to enhance function by accommodating limitations in range of motion or strength. Assistive devices vary in effectiveness and utility. An occupational therapist will help the patient with RA select the device that is most appropriate for his or her abilities and task requirements. The jar opener that is suitable for one person may be inappropriate for another. Likewise, hands and locks come in different sizes, and the extended key grip prescribed for one person may be ineffective for another person with smaller hands or different locks to open (Fig. 39.3). Additional assistive devices examples are illustrated in Figure 39.4.

Assistive devices are sometimes solutions for short-term limitations. For example, after hip arthroplasty, a long-handled reacher, extended shoe horn, and raised toilet seat are recommended to enable the patient to perform activities of daily living while adhering to postoperative instructions limiting hip

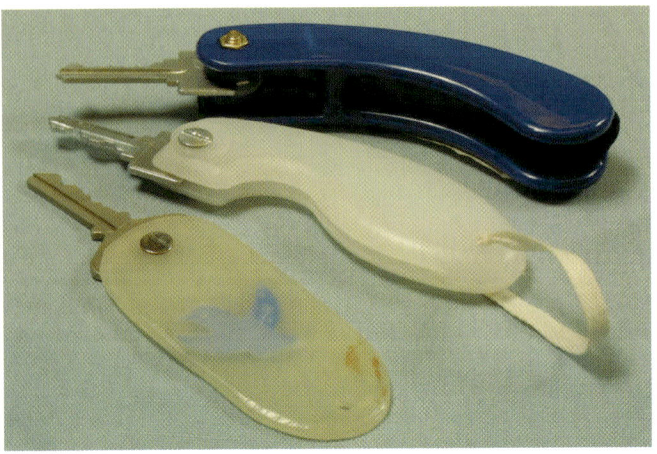

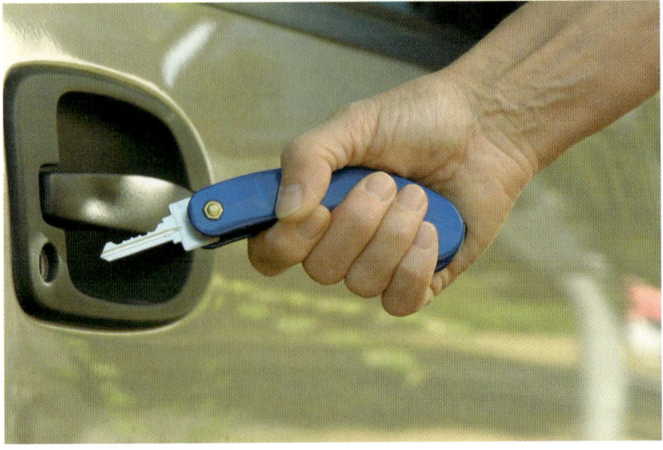

Figure 39.3. Assistive devices come in many models. A selection of key extenders **(A)** and the one the patient found most effective for unlocking a car door **(B)**.

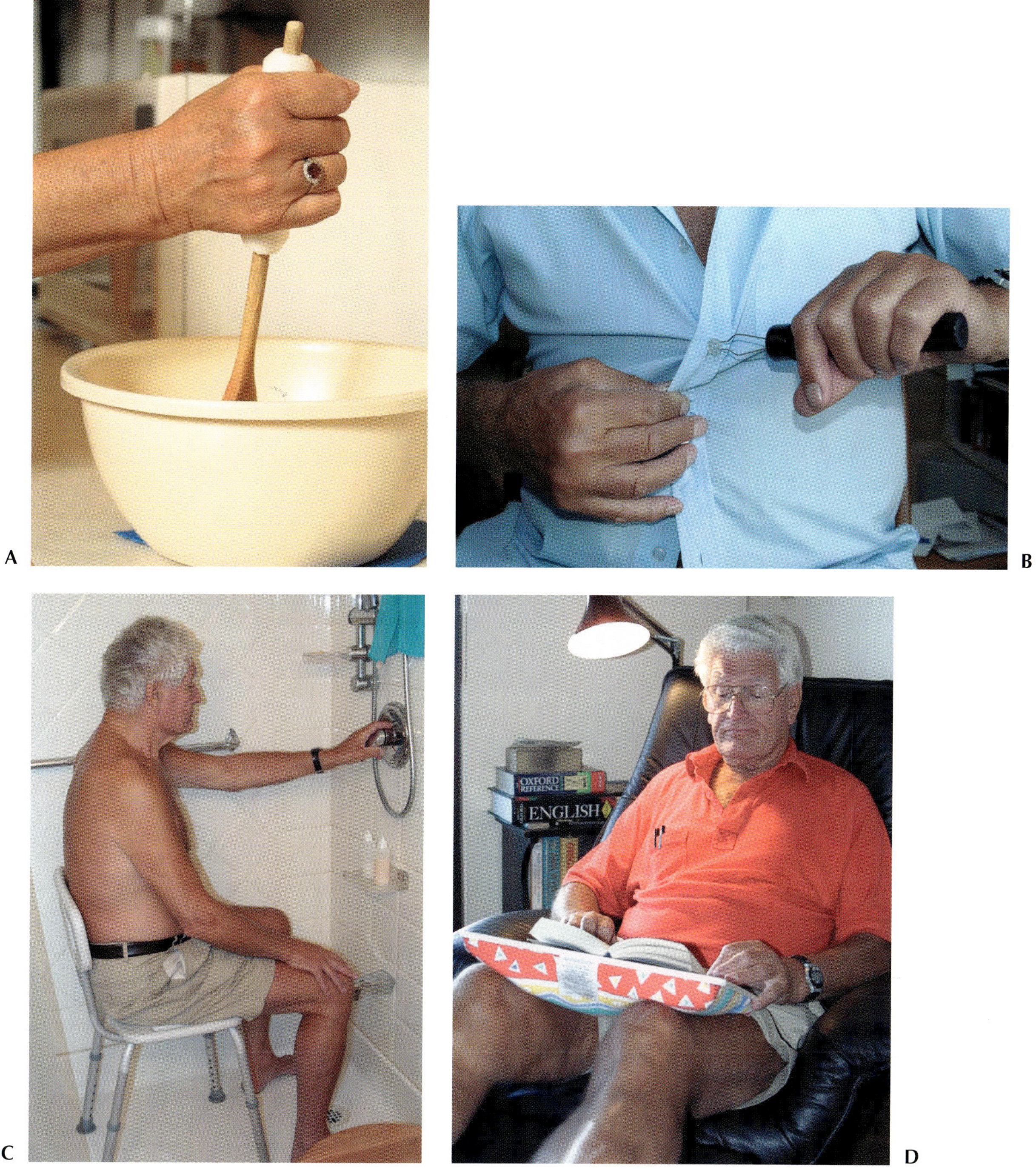

Figure 39.4. Assistive devices enable patients to perform activities and protect vulnerable joints. **A:** An enlarged handle, alternative grip, and nonskid mat placed under the mixing bowl reduce strain on painful hand joints during cooking. **B:** Button hook in use with small shirt buttons. **C:** A walk-in shower with bath seat and adjustable-height shower fixture enables independence in bathing in the presence of hip and knee pain, reduced range of motion, and reduced strength. **D:** A lap desk is one alternative to maintaining a static grip on a book while reading.

flexion and rotation. For other patients, devices are useful over the long term as a compensatory strategy to overcome permanent physical impairments.

The efficacy of an assistive device can be measured by the immediate resolution of a specific problem for the individual patient, for example, a patient who is unable to turn the car ignition key is enabled to do so with the appropriate device. Devices that fail to resolve the functional problem are not used. A follow-up study of 53 women with RA reported that 91% of the recommended devices were still being used 6 to 12 months later (50). Devices such as a special knife, cheese slicer, potato peeler, and scissors, compared to ordinary tools, significantly reduced pain as measured by a visual analog scale (50). A literature review of assistive devices used by people with RA and osteoarthritis reported that the majority of recommended devices are used, but a substantial proportion is not (51). A model was presented to assist in identifying factors related to the patient, his or her living environment, the therapist, and the device itself, to identify nondevice users, and to improve assistive device recommendations. The model lists numerous conditioning and predictor variables to be assessed and methods for calculating an assistive device usage outcome variable; however, the model has not been empirically tested.

Environmental Modifications at Home and Work

Modifications to the living environment may increase independence and functional capacity. Physical environment modifications can be divided into three groups (52):

- Rearranging the living environment, such as moving dishes to lower shelves.
- Adding to the environment, such as the placement of hooks and storage bins to keep frequently used supplies within easy reach.
- Structurally modifying the environment, such as installing a walk-in shower or ramps in place of stairs. See Figure 39.4C for an example of shower modifications.

The need for home modifications was the focus of a 3-year longitudinal study of 61 older adults with arthritis living in the community (53). Functional status declined over 3 years, and participants relied on assistive devices and home modifications to compensate for declining function. The number of assistive devices used in the home increased significantly, from a mean of 15 at baseline to 20 devices at 3 years. Participants made an average of 11 home modifications to resolve problems, such as difficulty accessing areas within the home, difficulty using home appliances, and reducing the risk of falls.

In a qualitative study exploring home environments of women with RA, Moss described in-depth maps of how three women negotiated the spaces in their homes (54). Each of the women studied incorporated additions to the physical environment, such as stair glides and grab bars. They also made modifications in the social environment to compensate for limitations attributed to RA, such as establishing a network of friends and family to assist with chores such as yardwork, or arranging for groceries to be delivered. Their environmental adaptations explain, in part, how they cope with their RA.

Modifying Daily Routines and Problem Solving

RA symptoms can have a significant impact on daily routines. It is not uncommon for morning stiffness, for example, to present a challenge to getting to work on time. Mothers report being unable to enjoy leisure activities with their families after a day's housework, or employees describe spending the weekend recovering from the workweek and are unable to do household chores or enjoy recreation. The occupational therapist works with the patient to find solutions and identify a reasonable approach to plan ahead and adjust routines where possible. Sometimes, finding a solution involves several members of the health care team, as in the example of morning stiffness. Adjusting morning routines may be insufficient to resolve the problem, and referral back to the rheumatologist to re-assess disease activity and medications, or to the physical therapist regarding range of motion exercises to "get going" in the morning, may be useful.

Although RA presents challenges to the patient, most valued activities may still be enjoyed. A consultation with an occupational therapist will generate suggestions for maintaining participation in family outings, recreational sailing, yoga, crafts, or whatever leisure activities the patient wishes to pursue. New activities may be proposed to substitute for former ones, and it is also possible to incorporate self-care principles necessary to managing RA into these activities. For example, range of motion exercises may be incorporated into a gentle dance routine, or hand exercises may be done while washing dishes in warm water.

Only some of the preceding interventions have been the subject of efficacy studies, and, clearly, further studies meeting criteria for higher levels of evidence are required. However, the provision of a comprehensive occupational therapy program has been evaluated. In a well-designed, randomized controlled trial of home-based occupational therapy involving 105 patients with RA, statistically significant and clinically important gains in functional status were obtained after 6 weeks of treatment (55). The experimental group (N = 53) received occupational therapy for 6 weeks, including a comprehensive physical and functional assessment and any of the following treatments indicated by the assessment results: education in joint protection and energy conservation; provision of resting splints and wrist splints; training in alternative methods for gripping, pushing, and holding objects; provision of assistive devices; home adaptations; workplace assessment and adaptations; and counseling on leisure activities and socializing. The control group (N = 52) remained on a waiting list for 6 weeks before being provided with the same 6-week occupational therapy intervention. Function was measured using a validated functional capacity scale (measuring dressing, hygiene, household work, and mobility) designed before the study. The mean improvement measured by this scale was one-half standard deviation. Statistically significant improvements were also noted in a pooled index of number of active joints, grip strength, erythrocyte sedimentation rate, and morning stiffness. Similar results were achieved by control subjects when they received occupational therapy after the 6-week delay. Experimental subjects maintained their functional gains at 12 weeks. Subjects were maintained on a steady regimen of medications, and no competing interventions were provided. Although this is a single study, its rigor offers compelling evidence that a comprehensive occupational therapy intervention will improve function in everyday activities.

Steultjens et al. (56) published a systematic review of occupational therapy for RA, using strict criteria for selection, inclusion, and evaluation of the quality of studies. They reviewed the effect of comprehensive occupational therapy, joint protection techniques, and use of assistive devices, splints, and training in motor function. For each of these five intervention categories, the outcome was classified as strong evidence, limited evidence, indicative findings, or no evidence. Their conclusions concur with the evidence presented in this chapter. Steultjens et al. state there is limited evidence that comprehensive occupational therapy programs and joint protection techniques improve functional status, there is indicative evidence that splints reduce pain, and there is no evidence regarding the effect of assistive devices and training in motor function (56).

CONCLUSION

Occupational therapists collaborate with patients to identify issues impeding performance in self-care, productivity, and leisure occupations. Comprehensive assessment of functional performance leads to practical suggestions for overcoming impairment and maintaining or improving occupational performance while managing the symptoms of RA. Interventions, such as joint protection, energy conservation, splinting, assistive devices, and modifications of the physical environment, all assist people with RA to actively participate in the activities they need and want to do.

ACKNOWLEDGMENT

The authors thank Wendy D. Photography for photographs.

REFERENCES

1. Canadian Association of Occupational Therapists. *Enabling occupation: an occupational therapy perspective*. Ottawa, ON: CAOT Publications, 1997.
2. American College of Rheumatology Subcommittee on Rheumatoid Arthritis Guidelines. Guidelines for the management of rheumatoid arthritis: 2002 update. *Arthritis Rheum* 2002;46:328–346.
3. Allaire SH, Anderson JJ, Meenan RF. Reducing work disability associated with rheumatoid arthritis: identification of additional risk factors and persons likely to benefit from intervention. *Arthritis Care Res* 1996;9:349–357.
4. Lacaille D, Sheps S, Spinelli J, Esdaile JM. Work-related factors that determine risk of work disability (WD) in rheumatoid arthritis (RA). *Arthritis Rheum* 1999;42[Suppl]:S238(abst).
5. Wolfe F, Hawley DJ. The longterm outcomes of rheumatoid arthritis: work disability: a prospective 18 year study of 823 patients. *J Rheumatol* 1998;25: 2108–2117.
6. MacKinnon JR. Occupational profiles: individuals with rheumatoid arthritis and a matched comparison sample. *Work* 1992;2:39–49.
7. Reisine ST, Goodenow C, Grady KE. The impact of rheumatoid arthritis on the homemaker. *Soc Sci Med* 1987;25:89–95.
8. Allaire SH, Meenan RF, Anderson JJ. The impact of rheumatoid arthritis on the household work performance of women. *Arthritis Rheum* 1991;34:669–678.
9. Backman CL. *Participation in paid and unpaid work by adults with rheumatoid arthritis* [doctoral thesis]. Vancouver: University of British Columbia; 2001.
10. Katz PP, Yelin EH. Life activities of persons with rheumatoid arthritis with and without depressive symptoms. *Arthritis Care Res* 1994;7:69–77.
11. Katz PP, Yelin EH. Prevalence and correlates of depressive symptoms among persons with rheumatoid arthritis. *J Rheumatol* 1993;20:790–796.
12. Fearing VG, Clark J, eds. *Individuals in context: a practical guide to client-centered practice*. Thorofare, NJ: Slack, 2000.
13. Lewin SA, Skea ZC, Entwistle V, et al. Interventions for providers to promote a patient-centred approach in clinical consultations. In: The Cochrane Library, Issue 2. Oxford: Update Software, 2002.
14. Law M, Mills J. Client-centered occupational therapy. In: Law M, ed. *Client-centered occupational therapy*. Thorofare, NJ: Slack, 1998:1–18.
15. Dyck I. Managing chronic illness: an immigrant woman's acquisition and use of health care knowledge. *Am J Occup Ther* 1992;46:696–705.
16. Law M. Does client-centred practice make a difference? In: Law M, ed. *Client-centered occupational therapy*. Thorofare, NJ: Slack,1998:19–27.
17. O'Connor D, Kortman B, Smith A, et al. Correlation between objective and subjective measures of hand function in patients with rheumatoid arthritis. *J Hand Ther* 1999;12:323–329.
18. Harrell PB. Splinting of the hand. In: Robbins L, Burckhardt CS, Hannan MT, DeHoratius RJ, eds. *Clinical care in the rheumatic diseases*, 2nd ed. Atlanta: Association of Rheumatology Health Professionals, 2001:191–196.
19. Jacobs K, ed. *Ergonomics for therapists*, 2nd ed. Boston: Butterworth-Heinemann, 1999.
20. Law M, Polatajko H, Carswell A, et al. *The Canadian occupational performance measure*, 3rd ed. Ottawa: CAOT Publications, 1998.
21. Tugwell P, Bombardier C, Buchanan WW, et al. The MACTAR patient preference disability questionnaire: an individualized functional priority approach for assessing improvement in physical disability in clinical trials in rheumatoid arthritis. *J Rheumatol* 1987;14:446–451.
22. Fisher A. *The assessment of motor and process skills*. Fort Collins, CO: Three Star Press, 1995.
23. Jette AM. The functional status index: reliability and validity of a self-report functional disability measure. *J Rheumatol* 1987;[Suppl15]14:15–19.
24. Lerner D, Amick BC, Rogers WH, et al. The work limitations questionnaire. *Med Care* 2001;39:72–85.
25. Letts L, Scott S, Burtney J, et al. The reliability and validity of the safety assessment of function and the environment for rehabilitation (SAFER) tool. *Br J Occup Ther* 1998;61:127–132.
26. Backman C, Mackie H, Harris J. Arthritis hand function test: development of a standardized assessment tool. *Occup Ther J Res* 1991;11:245–256.
27. Backman C, Mackie H. Arthritis hand function test: inter-rater reliability among self-trained raters. *Arthritis Care Res* 1995;8:10–15.
28. Beaton DE, Katz JN, Fossel AH, et al. Measuring the whole or the parts? Validity, reliability, and responsiveness of the disabilities of the arm, shoulder and hand outcome measure in different regions of the upper extremity. *J Hand Ther* 2001;14:128–146.
29. Chung KC, Pillsbury MS, Walters MR, et al. Reliability and validity testing of the Michigan Hand Outcomes Questionnaire. *J Hand Surg [Am]* 1998;23:575–587.
30. van Lankveld W, van't Pad Bosch P, Bakker J, et al. Sequential occupational dexterity assessment (SODA): a new test to measure hand disability. *J Hand Ther* 1996;9:27–32.
31. Luck JN. Enhancing functional ability. In: Robbins L, Burckhardt CS, Hannan MT, DeHoratius RJ, eds. *Clinical care in the rheumatic diseases* 2nd ed. Atlanta: Association of Rheumatology Health Professionals, 2001:196–202.
32. Barry MA, Purser J, Hazleman R, et al. Effect of energy conservation and joint protection education in rheumatoid arthritis. *Br J Rheumatol* 1994;33:1171–1174.
33. Hammond A, Lincoln N, Sutcliffe L. A crossover trial evaluating an educational-behavioural joint protection programme for people with rheumatoid arthritis. *Patient Educ Couns* 1999;37:19–32.
34. Hammond A, Freeman K. One-year outcomes of a randomized controlled trial of an educational-behavioural joint protection programme for people with rheumatoid arthritis. *Rheumatology* 2001;40:1044–1051.
35. Gerber L, Furst G, Shulman B, et al. Patient education program to teach energy conservation behaviors to patients with rheumatoid arthritis: a pilot study. *Arch Phys Med Rehabil* 1987;68:442–445.
36. Riemsma RP, Kirwan JR, Taal E, et al. Patient education for adults with rheumatoid arthritis. In: The Cochrane Library, Issue 2. Oxford: Update Software, 2002.
37. Backman CL, Deitz JC. Static wrist splint: its effect on hand function in three women with rheumatoid arthritis. *Arthritis Care Res* 1988;1:151–160.
38. Stern EB, Ytterberg SR, Krug HE, et al. Finger dexterity and hand function: effect of three commercial wrist extensor orthoses on patients with rheumatoid arthritis. *Arthritis Care Res* 1996;9:197–205.
39. Kjeken I, Moller G, Kvien TK. Use of commercially produced elastic wrist orthoses in chronic arthritis: a controlled study. *Arthritis Care Res* 1995;8:108–113.
40. Pagnotta A, Baron M, Korner-Bitensky N. The effect of a static wrist orthosis on hand function in individuals with rheumatoid arthritis. *J Rheumatol* 1998;25:879–885.
41. Haskett S, Backman C, Porter B, et al. A crossover trial of commercial versus custom-made wrist splints in the management of inflammatory polyarthritis [abstract]. *Arthritis Rheum* 46[suppl]:S556–S557.
42. Gault SS, Spyker JM. Beneficial effects of immobilization of joints in rheumatoid arthritis and related arthritides: a splint study using sequential analysis. *Arthritis Rheum* 1969;12:34–44.
43. Feinberg J, Brandt KD. Use of resting splints by patients with rheumatoid arthritis. *Am J Occup Ther* 1981;35:173–178.
44. Callinan NJ, Mathiowetz V. Soft versus hard resting hand splints in rheumatoid arthritis: pain relief, preference and compliance. *Am J Occup Ther* 1996;50:347–353.
45. Rennie RJ. Evaluation of the effectiveness of a metacarpophalangeal ulnar deviation orthosis. *J Hand Ther* 1996;9:371–377.
46. Swigart CR, Eaton RG, Glickel SZ, et al. Splinting in the treatment of arthritis of the first carpometacarpal joint. *J Hand Surg [Am]* 1999;24:86–91.
47. Burr N, Pratt AL, Smith PJ. An alternative splinting and rehabilitation protocol for metacarpophalangeal joint arthroplasty in patients with rheumatoid arthritis. *J Hand Ther* 2002;15:41–47.
48. Chalmers AC, Busby C, Goyert J, et al. Metatarsalgia and rheumatoid arthritis: a randomized, single blind, sequential trial comparing 2 types of foot orthoses and supportive shoes. *J Rheumatol* 2000;27:1643–1647.
49. Mann W. Assistive technology for persons with arthritis. In: Melvin J, Jensen G, eds. *Rheumatologic rehabilitation series volume 1 assessment and management*. Bethesda, MD: American Occupational Therapy Association, 1998:369–392.
50. Nordenskiold U. Evaluation of assistive devices after a course in joint protection. *Int J Technol Assess Health Care* 1994;10:293–304.
51. Rogers JC, Holm MB. Assistive technology device use in patients with rheumatic disease: a literature review. *Am J Occup Ther* 1992;46:120–127.
52. Barnes K. Modification of the physical environment. In: Christiansen C, Baum C, eds. *Occupational therapy: overcoming human performance deficits*. Thorofare, NJ: Slack Inc, 1991:700–745.
53. Mann WC, Tomita M, Hurren D, et al. Changes in health, functional and psychosocial status and coping strategies of home-based older persons with arthritis over three years. *Occup Ther J Res* 1999;19:126–146.
54. Moss P. Negotiating spaces in home environments: older women living with arthritis. *Soc Sci Med* 1997;45:23–33.
55. Helewa A, Goldsmith CH, Lee P, et al. Effects of occupational therapy home service on patients with rheumatoid arthritis. *Lancet* 1991;337:1453–1456.
56. Steultjens EMJ, Dekker J, Bouter LM, et al. Occupational therapy for rheumatoid arthritis: a systematic review. *Arthritis Rheum* 2002;47:672–685.

CHAPTER 40

Medical Aspects of Surgery

Paola de Pablo, Ronald J. Anderson, and Jeffrey N. Katz

Rheumatoid arthritis (RA) is a common inflammatory joint disease that affects approximately 1% of the general population and up to 3% of the population over age 65 (1,2). It is associated with marked disability and decreased life expectancy. The articular symptoms associated with synovitis and the structural damage that results from the inflammatory process often require surgical management. Although the level of inflammation may vary over time, structural damage is an irreversible and additive process that reflects accumulated preexisting synovitis. Thus, surgical interventions tend to occur later in the disease in severely damaged joints. In fact, orthopedic surgery may be considered as a marker of disease severity (3).

Progress in orthopedics has helped to improve the overall function and quality of life of patients with RA. The most successful surgical procedures are performed for disease in the hips and knees. Hand surgery may lead to cosmetic improvement and some functional benefit. Part of the complexity in assessing the potential benefit of a surgical procedure for the rheumatoid patient is the lack of uniform methods of pre- and postoperative assessment. Critical evaluation of the outcome in patients with RA who undergo joint replacement is lacking.

FREQUENCY OF ORTHOPEDIC SURGERY IN RHEUMATOID ARTHRITIS

A recent study reported the use of orthopedic surgery in a well-defined population-based cohort of 424 patients with RA (4). Surgical procedures involving joints for RA-related disease were performed in 35% of these patients during their disease course. Orthopedic surgeries for non-RA–related causes (including trauma, sepsis, and revision surgeries) were performed in 11%. The most frequently performed procedure was total joint replacement (TJR), with an estimated cumulative incidence at 30 years of 32%. The most frequently involved joint was the knee. The likelihood of surgery was higher in patients who were younger at the time of diagnosis. Among patients with RA, women were twice as likely to have an orthopedic procedure as men, and the risk of having joint surgery was higher in patients with positive rheumatoid factor and subcutaneous nodules (4), confirming previous findings (5). The types of surgery performed in RA are shown in Table 40.1.

INDICATIONS FOR SURGERY

Orthopedic surgery is generally performed electively in patients with RA, with several notable exceptions. The orthopedic emergencies are joint infection, rupture of finger extensors, and cervical spine instability. Patients with RA are at risk for septic arthritis, involving both native joints and prosthetic joints. Drainage of infected joints is critical and must be done quickly. Percutaneous approaches often suffice in some situations in which access for drainage is easy (e.g., septic native knee arthritis) but surgery is needed for treatment of other infections (prosthetic joint septic arthritis, native hip joint septic arthritis) in which observation or access for drainage is difficult. Rupture of the ulnar finger extensor tendons at the wrist, generally due to attrition from dorsal wrist synovitis, also merits urgent surgery to repair the ruptured tendon. Finally, cervical spine instability may lead to myelopathy and radicular neurologic symptoms, including weakness. The findings of myelopathy (not radiculopathy) also merit urgent surgical evaluation, particularly if they arise acutely.

In the absence of emergent or urgent indications, the primary reasons that patients with RA elect surgery are to relieve pain, improve functional status, or both. Patients differ widely in the amount of pain and functional limitation they are willing to tolerate before electing surgery. Therefore, it is difficult to define the level of pain or functional loss that should prompt referral for surgery. Traditionally, physicians have been taught to save major surgeries, such as TJR, until the patient has exhausted conservative measures and believes he or she can no longer tolerate pain. This prescription may be outmoded. There is growing evidence in the joint replacement literature (6) that poor preoperative functional status is a major risk factor for worse postoperative functional status, suggesting that surgery might have better outcomes if patients are operated on at an earlier stage in the trajectory of functional decline.

Furthermore, the patient may have multiple joints with advanced structural damage, requiring thoughtful staging of two or more surgeries. In these circumstances, it may be preferable to operate earlier on a particular joint than would otherwise be indicated, to stage several procedures over a reasonable period of time and preserve function. Finally, the patient should ultimately decide on the right time for a surgical intervention. The physician's role is to guide and present data on risks and benefits of surgery, both short-term and long-term. Ideally, the patient will integrate this information with his or her own preferences for functional improvement and pain relief and his or her degree of risk aversion to make an informed decision of when surgery is appropriate.

The physician's major role, aside from educating the patient about options, is to establish that the symptoms and disability arise from a surgically amenable lesion. Pain may arise from a variety of mechanisms, not all of which can be addressed by

TABLE 40.1. Orthopedic Procedures in the Treatment of Rheumatoid Arthritis (RA)

Purpose	Type of Procedure	Examples	Goals
Diagnostic and therapeutic	Arthroscopy	Sites: knee, shoulder, hip, ankle, wrist Examples: knee synovectomy (débridement, biopsy), meniscus resection and repair, rotator cuff repair, and carpal tunnel release	Identify source of joint disorder, improve or restore function, decrease disability, and eliminate severe pain
Prophylactic and therapeutic	Soft tissue procedures	Synovectomy and tenosynovectomy Tendon repair, tendon transfer, tendon release, and ligament release	Removal of inflamed synovium to prevent subsequent destruction of the articular cartilage Correct malalignment, restore function, arrest deterioration of tendons, and relieve mechanical symptoms
	Arthrodesis	Joint fusion: wire arthrodesis (e.g., wrist, ankle, talonavicular, subtalar, base of the thumb) Atlanto-axial fusion: fusion of the first and second cervical vertebrae, performed for RA cervical spine disease Multiple-level cervical fusions: performed for RA cervical spine disease	Stabilize joint, improve joint or limb alignment to redistribute forces, prevent further malalignment or compression of neural elements
Therapeutic	Fracture repair	Open reduction and internal fixation; fracture repair with implant total joint arthroplasty	Heal fracture, restore or maintain alignment, restore joint function
	Resection arthroplasty	Radial head resection, Girdlestone procedure	Partial removal of a damaged joint
	Implant arthroplasty	Total joint arthroplasty, hemiarthroplasty with an implant component	Improve or restore function, decrease disability, eliminate severe pain
	Revision arthroplasty	Revision surgery for the other arthroplasty procedures	Restore function, reduce pain, repair failed primary arthroplasty, avert major bone loss from osteolysis

surgery. For example, hip girdle pain in a patient with RA can arise from RA involvement of the hip as well as from the spine and the trochanteric bursa. Commonly, it arises from a combination of the three. Thus, it is critically important, and often challenging, for the physician to demonstrate that the symptoms arise from a problem that can be corrected with surgery.

PREOPERATIVE MANAGEMENT

In general, preoperative evaluation and perioperative medical management should focus on optimizing the patient's medical condition to reduce the risk of perioperative complications. The specific needs will depend on a variety of factors, such as age, comorbidities, disease severity, functional status, the type of anesthesia, and the surgery to be performed (7). In addition to a comprehensive history and physical examination to assess the overall general surgical risks, patients should also be examined for skin ulcerations, carious teeth, periodontal disease, and symptoms of urinary tract infection or prostatism, as these problems could increase the risk of postoperative infection (8). Discussion of the generic issues in preoperative medical evaluation can be found in standard medical texts (Table 40.2).

Cervical Spine Involvement

A specific issue that merits special attention in patients with RA is evaluation of the rheumatoid cervical spine (9,10). The cervical spine is significantly affected in 30% to 40% of patients with RA (9,11). Involvement of the rheumatoid cervical spine is often asymptomatic, and, thus, the patient may not be aware of it. An unstable cervical spine arising from atlanto-axial or subaxial subluxation places the patient at risk for potentially severe neurologic complications, particularly if endotracheal intubation is required (12). Atlanto-axial instability may predispose to damage to the medullary respiratory center and long spinal tracts with excessive manipulation of the neck during intubation (13). Therefore, cervical spine instability should be ruled out with lateral flexion and extension films of the cervical spine before surgery, and epidural or spinal anesthesia should be used whenever possible. It has been suggested that patients with cervical spine involvement should wear a soft cervical collar for neck immobilization and also avoid flexion of the cervical spine when asked to curl up for insertion of the spinal needle during spinal anesthesia (14–16,92).

The temporomandibular joint and the cricoarytenoid joints are frequently affected in patients with RA (17,18). Temporoman-

TABLE 40.2. Preoperative Recommendations

Tests
- ECG
- PT, PTT (anticoagulation therapy)
- CBC (rule out anemia, thrombocytopenia)
- Consider electrolytes, renal and liver function tests

Rule out infection
- Skin infection, urinary tract infection, oral cavity infection

Dental evaluation
- Carious teeth should be filled out or extracted before surgery

Lung
- Evaluate lung disease (symptoms, signs)
- Obtain chest films

Cervical spine
- Evaluate rheumatoid cervical spine
- Obtain lateral cervical spine flexion and extension films
- Rule out cervical spine instability: atlanto-axial or subaxial subluxation

Skin
- Rule out skin infection related to nodules, vasculitic ulcerations, and skin breakdown

Corticosteroids
- Aim for lowest possible maintenance dose before surgery

NSAIDs
- Discontinue ≥5 d before surgery

Second-line therapies
- Discontinue 2 wk before surgery

CBC, complete blood cell count; ECG, electrocardiograph; NSAIDs, nonsteroidal antiinflammatory drugs; PT, prothrombin time; PTT, partial thromboplastin time.

dibular joint arthritis and cricoarytenoid arthritis should also be addressed preoperatively, because they may prevent endotracheal intubation by limiting the mandibular opening (19). Careful preoperative evaluation by the anesthesiologist may prevent complications at the time of intubation (14). Fiber-optic intubation minimizes trauma and postoperative laryngeal edema and is also useful in preventing postoperative airway obstruction in patients undergoing cervical spine fusion for RA (20).

Lung Involvement

Respiratory insufficiency is common in RA and may not be apparent to the patient or physician if the patient's arthritis limits functional status more than the patient's pulmonary disease. Thus, lung involvement in RA should also be addressed before surgery. There are at least six forms of rheumatoid lung disease that may complicate perioperative recovery. These include pleural disease, interstitial fibrosis, nodular lung disease, bronchiolitis, pulmonary arteritis with pulmonary hypertension, and small airways disease. Pulmonary nodules may appear singly or in coalescent clusters. Nodules may cavitate, creating a bronchopleural fistula. Pleural effusion most commonly appears in older patients and may be transient, chronic, relapsing, or complicated by the development of empyema or hydropneumothorax. The effusions are characteristically small, may be unilateral or bilateral, and are frequently asymptomatic. However, pleuritic pain may occur, and large effusions may cause dyspnea (21). In cases of interstitial fibrosis, radiographs show a diffuse reticular or reticulonodular pattern in lung fields that can progress to a honeycomb appearance on plain radiographs. The rheumatoid patient is at increased risk of developing pulmonary problems if interstitial fibrosis is present. The principal functional defect is impairment of alveolocapillary gas exchange with decreased diffusion capacity (22). The clinician should be aware that RA patients may have asymptomatic disease because their arthritis limits their respiratory demands.

Blood Loss

Blood loss is an inevitable consequence of surgery. A preoperative hemoglobin level of less than 13 g per dL predicts a twofold increase in the need for transfusion in patients undergoing orthopedic surgery (23). Because anemia predicts morbidity (24) and the need for transfusion, a baseline hematocrit or hemoglobin level should be obtained. The patient can be given the option to donate autologous blood before surgery, reducing the risk of transfusion reactions and blood-borne viral illnesses. However, patients with RA may have anemia of chronic disease, sometimes to the extent that preoperative deposit of autologous blood for intraoperative and postoperative use is not possible. Because it is advantageous to have autologous blood available, the use of erythropoietin to increase hemoglobin levels to a point that allows for patients to donate blood before surgery should be considered (25–27). In addition, red blood cells may be salvaged by suction intraoperatively or retrieved by surgical drains postoperatively using a cell saver. Sufficient blood loss must be present for postoperative reinfusion of filtered or washed red cells to be considered (28,29).

Medication Use

An important task in the care of RA patients undergoing surgery is to recommend the safest and most effective use of medication in the perioperative period (30). Because nonsteroidal antiinflammatory drugs (NSAIDs) inhibit thromboxane A_2 synthesis, a prolongation in the bleeding time may occur, presenting a risk of bleeding for surgical procedures. Ideally, antiinflammatory drugs should be discontinued preoperatively in time to allow total elimination of the drug and its effects before the joint replacement. In particular, aspirin should be discontinued at least 5 days before the surgical procedure because its antiplatelet effects may increase the risk of bleeding. Patients taking glucocorticoids should receive the lowest possible maintenance dose before surgery. Treatment with second-line agents, such as methotrexate, leflunomide, and biologics, may be interrupted 1 to 2 weeks before surgery.

Ocular Involvement

Patients with RA frequently have concomitant Sjögren's syndrome, requiring artificial tears before, throughout, and after surgery to prevent perioperative conjunctival injury. Also, patients taking chronic optic medication should have their eye drops administered before the surgical procedure, especially if a prolonged surgical time is anticipated.

The anesthesiologist must take particular care to position the patient, carefully avoiding excessive pressure on the eye and providing appropriate eye protection, as patients in the prone position are at risk for ocular injury secondary to external pressure (31).

Skin Involvement

Skin integrity may be compromised before and after orthopedic surgical procedures in patients with RA, as a result of chronic therapy with corticosteroids and immunosuppressive agents or as a manifestation of the disease process itself. Localized areas of infection related to nodules, vasculitic ulcerations, and skin breakdown over areas of deformity could be sources of infection and should be treated before surgery (32). The early use of measures to prevent the development of decubitus ulceration is essential to preclude postoperative complications.

Infection

In general, infection rates are significantly higher in RA patients, partly because of the disease process and partly because of the immunosuppressive drugs used to control it (33–40). RA patients may be relatively malnourished, which also predisposes them to infection. Poor nutrition is particularly worrisome in patients undergoing TJR, as deep infections in TJR usually result in failure of the initial operation and the need for extensive débridement and revision.

Three main portals of entry for infection after TJR have been suggested: contamination at the time of surgery, postoperative inoculation of the joint by a puncture wound or wound dehiscence, and hematogenous seeding from a nonorthopedic source. Bacteremias can cause hematogenous seeding of joint implants, both in the early postoperative period and several years after TJR (41). It is likely that bacteremias associated with acute infection in the oral cavity, skin, respiratory system, gastrointestinal and urogenital systems, or other sites can cause late implant infection (37,42,43). Risk of hematogenous total joint infection is increased in immunocompromised patients. Patients with diabetes mellitus, hemophilia, sickle cell disease, and malnutrition are also at increased risk, as are patients with a prior history of prosthetic joint infections or revision surgery (44–46). The risk of prosthetic infection is highest in the first 2 years after joint replacement. Maderazo et al., in a review of 67 cases of joint infections developing more than 1 year after total joint arthroplasty, found that the most common site of origin was the skin and soft tissue (46%), followed by the mouth (15%) and the urinary tract (13%). The most common pathogen responsible for late prosthetic joint infections was *Staphylococcus* (54%) (47).

Patients undergoing TJR should be in good dental health before surgery and should be encouraged to seek professional dental care if necessary, as the risk of bacteremia is increased in patients with ongoing oral inflammation (48). Carious teeth should be filled or extracted before joint surgery. Urinary tract infections should be identified and treated preoperatively. Many female patients have asymptomatic bacteriuria. Urine culture before surgery is required to identify such patients. In male patients, prostatic hypertrophy, if severe, should be treated before surgery to avoid postoperative catheterization, with its attendant risk of infection and bacterial seeding. In general, catheters should be removed at the earliest possible time after surgery, and a surveillance urine culture should be performed to rule out the development of a urinary tract infection.

Prophylactic antibiotics are given to decrease the likelihood of infection. The objective is to eradicate bacteria originating from the air of the operating room, the surgical team, or the patient's own flora. Antibacterial agents are administered just before and during the surgical procedure to ensure high levels in serum and tissues during surgery. Prophylactic antibiotic therapy should commence shortly (less than 2 hours) before surgery and be continued for at least a 24-hour period. Prophylaxis is primarily directed against staphylococci, with the goal of preventing wound infection or infection of implanted devices. Cefazolin, 1 g every 8 hours for 24 hours, or vancomycin, 1 g every 12 hours for 24 hours (in penicillin-allergic patients), is recommended (7). Other means to lower the risk of infection include the use of unidirectional airflow operating rooms, body exhaust systems, ultraviolet light, and double gloves.

Risk Factors Affecting Outcome

Risk factors for postoperative complications include those inherent to the procedure itself and those related to the patient. General health status is a predictor of postoperative complications. Potential patient-related risk factors for postoperative pulmonary complications, in addition to the disease itself and its therapy, include advanced age, poor functional status, smoking, chronic obstructive pulmonary disease, rheumatoid lung disease, and asthma. However, most of the risk attributed to age is due to the effects of associated comorbidities. Smoking increases the risk of postoperative pulmonary complications threefold and is a risk factor, even in patients without established chronic lung disease (49). Pulmonary embolism and deep venous thrombosis (DVT) are common complications after TJR. Their treatment and management are discussed in standard medical texts.

Complications after Total Joint Replacement

Numerous potential complications may result from TJR. These can be divided into medical complications, implant-related complications, and infection. Medical complications are those that may occur after any major reconstructive surgery, including such major complications as cardiac arrhythmias, myocardial infarction, thrombophlebitis, and pulmonary emboli, as well as atelectasis, anemia, and urinary tract infection. Good preoperative medical evaluation and management, plus aggressive prophylactic measures, will minimize the occurrence of these medical problems. Implant-related complications consist primarily of implant wear, breakage, and loosening. Modern materials and designs have diminished remarkably the incidence of implant wear and breakage. Better cementing techniques and the use of alternative fixation methods have decreased greatly the problems of early loosening. The predominant long-term cause of failure of hip or knee replacement appears to be particulate wear debris, which stimulates macrophages to produce substances eliciting osteoclastic bone resorption, producing osteolysis. Wear debris also may contribute to the loosening of total knee and other joint arthroplasty components in a similar fashion. Another implant-related complication is infection. Implant surfaces and metallic wear debris and corrosion products may lower the local resistance to infection (50).

Other complications that may occur after TJR include fat embolism syndrome—distal embolization of fatty tissue arising from bone marrow (51)—particularly in patients undergoing simultaneous bilateral procedures. Fat embolism syndrome presentation may vary from a subclinical state to fulminant respiratory failure. The amount of manipulation of tissue and degree of hypovolemia or hypoperfusion are thought to predispose to fat embolism syndrome. Theories about the origin of fat deposits in the pulmonary vasculature include venous fat embolization originating from traumatized bone marrow or excessive mobilization of free fatty acids from peripheral tissue secondary to stress hor-

TABLE 40.3. Perioperative and Postoperative Recommendations

- Antibiotics
  - Prevent infection:
    - Use of prophylactic antibiotics 2 h before surgery: cefazolin, 1 g every 8 h for 24 h
    - In penicillin-allergic patients: vancomycin, 1 g every 12 h for 24 h
- Eyes
  - Eye drops, artificial tears
  - Avoid increased pressure
- Skin
  - Prevent development of decubitus ulcerations
- TMJ arthritis
  - Use of fiber-optic intubation
- Cervical spine
  - Avoid excessive manipulation of the neck
  - Avoid intubation whenever possible
  - Use a soft cervical collar for neck immobilization
  - Use epidural or spinal anesthesia
  - Avoid flexion of cervical spine when applying spinal anesthesia
- Corticosteroids
  - Stress dose:
    - Hydrocortisone, 100 mg IV before surgery
    - Hydrocortisone, 100 mg IV intraoperatively
    - Hydrocortisone, 100 mg IV every 8 h for 24 h
    - Hydrocortisone, 50 mg IV every 8 h for 24 h
    - Hydrocortisone, 100 mg IV single dose
    - Continue with patient's usual dose
- Disease flares
  - Control with corticosteroids
- Prevent thromboembolism
  - Pneumatic compression devices
  - Early postoperative mobilization
  - Antithrombotic prophylaxis: anticoagulation therapy during hospitalization
    - Warfarin
    - Low-molecular-weight heparin
  - Therapy recommended for ≥7–10 d after surgery and longer for high-risk patients
  - Many clinicians routinely anticoagulate for 4–6 wk postop
- Second-line therapies
  - Resume 2 wk after surgery
- Rehabilitation
  - Rehabilitation program after surgery
- Follow-up after TJR
  - Follow-up with orthopedic surgeon for clinical evaluation
    - Routine appointments at 6 wk, 3 and 6 mo, 1 yr and every 2 yr afterward
  - Radiographic follow-up
    - Screening follow-up radiographs
    - Immediate postoperative and at 2 yr follow-up
  - If osteolysis becomes apparent, the intervals between examinations should be shortened

TJR, total joint replacement; TMJ, temporomandibular joint.

mones (52). These acids coalesce in the blood and form fat aggregates. Regardless of the site of origin of fat emboli, the pulmonary capillaries act as filters and the emboli are carried to the lungs, where they lodge in the pulmonary capillaries and increase the resistance to flow. The lung parenchyma produces lipase to remove emboli. However, hydrolysis of the fat emboli may induce chemical pneumonitis (53). Hemodynamic instability may develop almost immediately or more insidiously during the first 2 to 3 postoperative days. Hematologic abnormalities, such as transient thrombocytopenia, may occur. Frank adult respiratory distress syndrome may develop and become life-threatening. Treatment is supportive and includes the administration of increased concentrations of inspired oxygen, the prevention of pulmonary hypertension by fluid restriction, and the use of diuretics and venodilators. Pulmonary artery catheterization may be helpful to guide therapy; if the pulmonary artery diastolic pressure is maintained at less than 20 mm Hg, respiratory insufficiency is usually prevented. In severe cases, systemic manifestations of fat embolization may occur and become associated with myocardial infarction or severe neurologic damage (Table 40.3).

Rheumatoid Arthritis Flares

Acute disease flares resulting from the abrupt discontinuation of disease-modifying antirheumatic drugs and other immunosuppressive therapies for brief perioperative periods are unusual and can usually be managed with corticosteroids (31). On the other hand, acute cessation of NSAIDs or an error in the administration of corticosteroids may be associated with a disease flare.

PERIOPERATIVE MANAGEMENT

Complications Related to Nonsteroidal Antiinflammatory Drugs

The most common type of toxicity seen in the patient receiving NSAIDs in the postoperative period is renal dysfunction, as the inhibition of prostaglandin synthesis may lead to a decline in renal perfusion and glomerular filtration rate. Other potential effects that may occur include inhibition of tubular sodium and water reabsorption, leading to fluid retention, impaired responsiveness to diuretic therapy, and hyperkalemia. Because NSAIDs inhibit thromboxane A_2 synthesis, a prolongation in the bleeding time may occur, presenting a risk of bleeding for surgical procedures. In patients receiving anticoagulation therapy with warfarin, antiinflammatory drugs are generally discontinued because of the increased potential for bleeding when these drugs are combined (54). NSAIDs may also be associated with gastrointestinal and hepatic toxicity. For all these reasons, NSAIDs should be used cautiously, if at all, in the perioperative period. Acetaminophen and other non-NSAID analgesics are safer choices.

Selective Cyclooxygenase-2 Inhibitors

The identification of cyclooxygenase-2 (COX-2) inhibitors (celecoxib, rofecoxib) in the mid-1990s has been followed by an unprecedented period of discovery and drug development. Celecoxib has been shown to have comparable analgesic and antiinflammatory effects in patients with RA but with lower incidence of endoscopically proven gastroduodenal ulcers, compared with traditional NSAIDs (55,56). Among patients with a recent history of ulcer bleeding, treatment with celecoxib has been shown to be as effective as treatment with diclofenac plus omeprazole, with respect to the prevention of recurrent ulcer bleeding (57). Rofecoxib is also used for the management of acute pain at a dose of 50 mg daily (double the dose recommended for arthritis), with a recommended maximum duration of treatment of 5 days. The COX-2 inhibitors do not interfere with the coagulation system as much as traditional NSAIDs do and may represent a safer option for patients undergoing joint replacement. Although initial clinical trials of COX-2 inhibitors have been consistent and encouraging, recent case reports have described severe NSAID-induced gastropathy with celecoxib and highlighted the possibility of a role for COX-2 in mucosal protection and repair mechanisms (58,59). In addition, COX-2 inhibitors are associated with fluid retention, heart failure, hypertension, renal dysfunction, and hyperkalemia and, thus, must be used carefully (57,60). COX-2 inhibitors are frequently discontinued before elective total joint arthroplasty because of the increased incidence of perioperative bleeding. For the reasons previously given, COX-2 inhibitors should be used cautiously, if at all, in the perioperative setting in patients with RA.

CORTICOSTEROIDS

A common problem in RA patients on chronic corticosteroid therapy undergoing surgery is prophylaxis against adrenal insufficiency. The degree of adrenal suppression in a patient with RA who has received corticosteroid therapy is difficult to predict. Generally, for patients who have stopped corticosteroid treatment within 1 year before joint surgery, replacement therapy with corticosteroids is recommended. Patients taking a dose of more than 10 mg per day of prednisone, those who have taken such dosages for more than 2 weeks in the preceding year, and those who are receiving replacement corticosteroid therapy for known adrenal insufficiency usually receive a stress dose therapy in the perioperative period. A widely used regimen is the parenteral administration of 100 mg of hydrocortisone, where the first dose is administered before surgery, with a second 100-mg dose administered intraoperatively. This is followed by 100 mg intravenously every 8 hours for 24 hours and 50 mg every 8 hours the next day. On the third day, a single intravenous dose of 100 mg is given, after which the patient's usual dose of corticosteroid is restarted. In this fashion, the hydrocortisone dose is tapered rapidly over 48 to 72 hours after the surgical procedure. The usual maintenance dose may be prescribed afterward. In patients undergoing minor surgical procedures, a single preoperative dose of 100 mg is sufficient, as the normal metabolic response to minor surgery is minimal (7).

DISEASE-MODIFYING THERAPIES

In RA patients, little data exist to guide management of disease-modifying and immunosuppressive therapy in the perioperative setting. This issue is increasingly important as patients are treated more aggressively, particularly with methotrexate, combination therapies, and biologic agents. Generally, clinicians stop the medication 2 weeks before and 2 weeks after surgery (31).

This convention was tested in a prospective randomized trial of 388 patients with RA who had elective orthopedic surgery. The study compared the risk of infections and early postoperative complications within 1 year of surgery in patients on continued methotrexate therapy, patients who discontinued methotrexate from 2 weeks before surgery until 2 weeks after surgery, and in patients who were not receiving methotrexate and were receiving other treatments. This study showed that continuation of methotrexate therapy does not increase the risk of either infections or surgical complications. In addition, patients who continued methotrexate in the perioperative period did not have rheumatoid disease flares, in contrast to patients who discontinued methotrexate or patients with other treatments; however, this difference did not reach statistical significance (61). Discontinuation for 2 weeks preoperatively and postoperatively would be reasonable, but this study also suggests that methotrexate can be continued carefully throughout the perioperative period.

ANTICOAGULATION THERAPY

DVT is the most common complication in patients having elective TJR. Without prophylaxis, the incidence of DVT is reported to be as high as 88% after total knee replacement (TKR) (62), and 54% after total hip replacement (THR) (63). Pulmonary embolism (PE) is a major cause of mortality after major orthopedic surgery (64). Approximately 1% of patients experience PE within 90 days of THR (65).

The prevention of thromboembolic events after orthopedic surgery has been studied extensively. Venous thromboembolic disease after THR is largely associated with postoperative immobilization and venous stasis. Therefore, a prevention strategy should include mechanical as well as pharmacologic measures. The concomitant use of epidural anesthesia, pneumatic compression devices (66), and early postoperative mobilization may be effective in reducing the incidence of DVT after surgery.

The risks of DVT and PE can be further reduced by effective antithrombotic prophylaxis. A logical approach is to maximize the prophylaxis intraoperatively, followed by continued prophylaxis using agents that are easily administered and carry minimal bleeding risk. The number of agents that prevent thromboembolism has increased dramatically in the past few years. Unfractionated heparin was for many years the mainstay of acute anticoagulation therapy, with warfarin as the choice for long-term anticoagulation. Currently, the indications for unfractionated heparin are declining as the use of low-molecular-weight heparin (LMWH) increases.

Low-Molecular-Weight Heparin

The first advance over unfractionated heparin was the development of low-molecular-weight forms of heparin that, because of their predictable pharmacology, can be safely administered once a day without laboratory monitoring. LMWH is safe and effective prophylaxis after total knee and hip arthroplasties. These compounds have a predictable dose response, offer high bioavailability at low doses, and have a half-life of approximately 4.5 hours, providing effective dosing every 12 to 24 hours with rapid antithrombotic action. Routine prophylaxis with LMWH seems to be effective in decreasing the occurrence of venous thromboembolism. However, venographic prevalence of DVT among patients undergoing TKR and receiving prophylaxis remains substantial at 30.6% (67).

Only a few studies have compared the efficacy of LMWH with that of warfarin in preventing DVT after total joint arthroplasty. A study found that LMWH resulted in a significantly lower rate of DVT than that noted for warfarin (31.4% vs. 37.4%) but also had a significantly higher bleeding complication rate (2.8% vs. 1.2%) (68). Further studies comparing warfarin and LMWH are needed to investigate their relative efficacy and complication rates.

THROMBOSIS AFTER TOTAL JOINT REPLACEMENT: RISKS AND RECOMMENDATIONS

Because hospital length of stay has decreased considerably after joint replacement, inpatient prophylaxis now covers a shorter fraction of the at-risk period. Thus, patients are discharged while still at risk of venous thromboembolism. Johnson et al. found that, of 83 of fatal PEs after THR, 9.7% occurred during the first postoperative week, 54.2% during the second, 22.9% during the third, 8.4% during the fourth, and 4.8% during the fifth week (69). Another study showed that only 26% of all pulmonary emboli occurring within 6 months of primary THR occurred in the acute inpatient stay (70). Other studies have also reported that the period of risk for thrombosis persists beyond the first postoperative week (71–73).

Risk factors for symptomatic venous thromboembolism after THR include female sex, age older than 85 years, history of venous thromboembolism, body mass index (25 kg/m^2), and delay in ambulation after surgery (74). Factors associated with lower risk include Asian or Pacific Islander ethnicity, use of pneumatic compression among nonobese patients after surgery, and extended thromboprophylaxis after hospital discharge (73). Despite the existence of established risk factors, all patients are eligible candidates for extended prophylaxis, because this surgical procedure is a dominant high-risk factor for postoperative venous thromboembolism (73).

A systematic review of extended out-of-hospital LMWH against DVT in patients after elective hip arthroplasty showed consistent effectiveness and safety in trials. In most studies, LMWH was initiated before surgery. The duration of out-of-hospital prophylaxis evaluated in randomized clinical trials ranged from 19 to 29 days (68). This interval is consistent with studies that found that patients with venographically confirmed symptomatic DVT after hip surgery, in whom prophylaxis was stopped at hospital discharge, were readmitted, on average, between 17 and 27 days after surgery (75,76). In summary, this topic has been reviewed extensively, and the evidence suggests that all patients undergoing elective hip arthroplasty should receive extended thromboprophylaxis after hospital discharge (64,73–83).

TKR is associated with a very high incidence of asymptomatic calf vein thrombosis, with almost all symptomatic DVT events diagnosed in the first 21 days postoperatively (73). The recommendations for prophylaxis after TKR are less well established, but many physicians also treat for at least 4 weeks' post-discharge with anticoagulation.

The U.S. Hip and Knee Registry data indicate that the percentage of patients who receive prophylaxis for longer than 21 days is gradually increasing. In 2000, 53% of THR patients and 47% of TKR patients received prophylaxis for longer than 21 days (84).

Antibiotic Prophylaxis for Dental Patients

Because of evidence that patients with TJR are at increased risk of hematogenous infectious seeding of the prosthetic joint, careful attention must be devoted to the prevention of infection anywhere in the body and its prompt recognition and treatment. Transient bacteremia after a dental procedure may be a source of infection in TJR both in the early postoperative period and for many years after implantation (85). It appears that the most critical period is up to 2 years after joint placement (86,87). Guidelines recommend antibiotic prophylaxis for immunocompromised patients, patients with RA, and patients using corticosteroids (38,88). More extensive dental procedures may increase the potential for infection, as well as procedures lasting more than 45 minutes (88,89). Additionally, bacteremias may occur concurrently with dental and medical procedures, and it is likely that many more oral bacteremias are spontaneously induced by daily events, such as tooth brushing and flossing, than are dental treatment induced (88,90–92). Furthermore, infection of a TJR after a dental procedure is more common than has previously been suspected (93). Therefore, antibiotic prophylaxis should be considered for RA patients with TJR before dental treatment or procedures (89).

The suggested antibiotic prophylaxis regimens in patients with TJR not allergic to penicillin are amoxicillin, cephalexin, or cephradine, 2 g, orally 1 hour before the dental procedure. In patients unable to take oral medications, cefazolin, 1 g, or ampicillin, 2 g, can be given intravenously or intramuscularly 1 hour before the procedure. Patients allergic to penicillin can take clindamycin, 600 mg orally or intravenously, 1 hour before the dental procedure (89). However, other authors consider that there is limited evidence to suggest that patients with RA may be more susceptible to dental-induced bacteremia. Thus, there is some controversy regarding the need for antibiotic coverage (88).

Rehabilitation

Rehabilitation is an important part of the acute and subsequent care program. The overall objective of rehabilitation after orthopedic surgery is to return the patients to their optimal level of function in the shortest possible time, without compromising the surgical outcomes. Physical therapy is an essential treatment strategy for patients with RA. Generally, the objectives of physical therapy in rheumatoid patients are to control pain, increase and maintain joint mobility and muscle strength, maintain cardiopulmonary fitness, protect joints, conserve energy, and preserve function (94). Ideally, the rehabilitation program starts before surgery with a complete assessment of the patient's status. After surgery, an early rehabilitation program during the hospital stay is aimed at restoration of function and range of motion. This must be continued after discharge, whether to a nursing skilled facility, an inpatient rehabilitation facility, or home. Approximately 50% of patients are discharged to an inpatient rehabilitation facility after THR. Factors associated with discharge to a rehabilitation facility after elective THR are female sex, older age, living alone, a low level of education, and obesity. However, the most important factor defining discharge destination after elective THR is the ability to walk without assistance before discharge from the acute care setting (95).

A dynamic rehabilitation program after discharge from the hospital is necessary for patients with TKR to maintain and improve range of motion and function. Continuous passive motion (CPM) is widely used after TKR, especially during the hospitalization period. The effectiveness of CPM in the rehabilitation period is debated. A randomized controlled evaluation of CPM plus conventional rehabilitation, compared with conventional rehabilitation alone, showed that CPM is more effective in improving range of motion, decreasing swelling, and reducing the need for manipulation than is conventional rehabilitation therapy. CPM also lowers cost at 6 weeks after surgery in patients with osteoarthritis and RA undergoing TKR (96). Another controlled trial of CPM after TKR showed that CPM is efficacious in increasing short-term flexion and decreasing the need for knee manipulation without increasing costs (97). A study of an outpatient rehabilitation program comparing home CPM versus professional physical therapy after TKR in osteoarthritis patients showed that CPM is an adequate rehabilitation alternative, with no difference in results but with lower costs, compared with professional therapy continued at home (98).

Radiographic Evaluation

Early radiographs after TJR are done to assess alignment of components and check for postoperative heterotopic ossification (99). Longitudinal radiographic evaluation, critical in the preoperative assessment of the need for surgery and proper technical approach, is essential to short- and long-term postoperative evaluation. Several parameters have to be assessed, such as alignment of the prosthetic components, adequacy of cement fixation, restoration of joint alignment, and detection of osteolysis and postoperative loosening. Prolonged follow-up is necessary, as infection may occur late, and loosening and osteolysis are time-related complications (100,101). If early signs of loosening develop, a decrease in joint loading by avoiding strenuous activities and appropriate use of crutches may prevent or slow the process of loosening (99).

CONCLUSION

In general, preoperative evaluation and perioperative medical management should focus on optimizing the patient's medical condition to reduce the risk of perioperative complications. The specific needs will depend on several factors, such as age, disease severity, medications, functional status, comorbidities, the type of anesthesia, and the specific surgery to be performed. In addition to a comprehensive history and physical examination to assess the overall general surgical risks, specific preoperative recommendations should include blood tests to rule out cytopenias, as well as coagulation disorders and electrolytic imbalances. Infections should be identified and treated before surgery. Carious teeth should be filled out or extracted before surgery. Radiographs should be obtained to evaluate lung disease, as well as rheumatoid cervical spine disease. Among the medications used in the treatment of RA, corticosteroid dose should be reduced to maintain the lowest possible maintenance dose before surgery. For those patients who have stopped corticosteroid treatment within 1 year before joint surgery, the use of a stress dose is recommended. The usual maintenance dose may be prescribed afterward. Second-line agents should be discontinued 2 weeks before surgery and may be resumed 2 weeks postoperatively. NSAIDs should be discontinued at least 5 days before surgery and should be used cautiously in the perioperative period. Prophylactic antibiotics use is recommended, starting 2 hours before surgery and continuing for the first 24 hours postoperatively. Measures to prevent thromboembolism include pneumatic compression devices, early postoperative mobilization, and antithrombotic prophylaxis. Anticoagulation therapy is recommended for at least 7 to 10 days after joint replacement and longer for high-risk patients. Disease flares in the perioperative period may be controlled with corticosteroids. A rehabilitation program after surgery is encouraged, as is long-term follow-up with the orthopedic surgeon for clinical and radiographic evaluation.

REFERENCES

1. Mitchell DM, Spitz PW, Young DY, et al. Survival, prognosis, and causes of death in rheumatoid arthritis. *Arthritis Rheum* 1986;29:706–714.
2. Gabriel SE, Crowson CS, O'Fallon WM. Mortality in rheumatoid arthritis: have we made an impact in 4 decades? *J Rheumatol* 1999;26:2529–2533.
3. Anderson RJ. The orthopedic management of rheumatoid arthritis. *Arthritis Care Res* 1996;9:223–228.
4. Massardo L, Gabriel SE, Crowson CS, et al. A population based assessment of the use of orthopedic surgery in patients with rheumatoid arthritis. *J Rheumatol* 2002;29:52–56.
5. Wolfe F, Zwillich SH. The long-term outcomes of rheumatoid arthritis: a 23-year prospective, longitudinal study of total joint replacement and its predictors in 1,600 patients with rheumatoid arthritis. *Arthritis Rheum* 1998;41:1072–1082.
6. Fortin PR, Clarke AE, Joseph L, et al. Outcomes of total hip and knee replacement: preoperative functional status predicts outcomes at six months after surgery. *Arthritis Rheum* 1999;42:1722–1728.
7. MacKenzie CR, Sharrock NE. Perioperative medical considerations in patients with rheumatoid arthritis. *Rheum Dis Clin North Am* 1998;24:1–17.
8. Glynn MK, Sheehan JM. The significance of asymptomatic bacteriuria in patients undergoing hip/knee arthroplasty. *Clin Orthop* 1984:151–154.
9. Clark CR. Rheumatoid involvement of the cervical spine. An overview. *Spine* 1994;19:2257–2258.
10. Keersmaekers A, Truyen L, Ramon F, et al. Cervical myelopathy due to rheumatoid arthritis. Case report and review of the literature. *Acta Neurol Belg* 1998;98:284–288.

11. Boden SD, Dodge LD, Bohlman HH, Rechtine GR. Rheumatoid arthritis of the cervical spine. A long-term analysis with predictors of paralysis and recovery. *J Bone Joint Surg Am* 1993;75:1282–1297.
12. Cooper RM. Rheumatoid arthritis is a common disease with clinically important implications for the airway. *J Bone Joint Surg Am* 1995;77:1463–1465.
13. Kwek TK, Lew TW, Thoo FL. The role of preoperative cervical spine X-rays in rheumatoid arthritis. *Anaesth Intensive Care* 1998;26:636–641.
14. Sharrock NE. Anesthetic considerations. In: Kelley WN, Ruddy S, Harris ED Jr, Sledge CB, eds. *Textbook of rheumatology*, 5th ed. Philadelphia: WB Saunders, 1997.
15. Skues MA, Welchew EA. Anaesthesia and rheumatoid arthritis. *Anaesthesia* 1993;48:989–997.
16. Campbell RS, Wou P, Watt I. A continuing role for pre-operative cervical spine radiography in rheumatoid arthritis? *Clin Radiol* 1995;50:157–159.
17. Tegelberg A, Kopp S. Clinical findings in the stomatognathic system for individuals with rheumatoid arthritis and osteoarthrosis. *Acta Odontol Scand* 1987;45:65–75.
18. Goupille P, Fouquet B, Cotty P, et al. The temporomandibular joint in rheumatoid arthritis. Correlations between clinical and computed tomography features. *J Rheumatol* 1990;17:1285–1291.
19. Lawry GV, Finerman ML, Hanafee WN, et al. Laryngeal involvement in rheumatoid arthritis. A clinical, laryngoscopic, and computerized tomographic study. *Arthritis Rheum* 1984;27:873–882.
20. Wattenmaker I, Concepcion M, Hibberd P, Lipson S. Upper-airway obstruction and perioperative management of the airway in patients managed with posterior operations on the cervical spine for rheumatoid arthritis. *J Bone Joint Surg Am* 1994;76:360–365.
21. Payne CR. Pulmonary manifestations of rheumatoid arthritis. *Br J Hosp Med* 1984;32:192–197.
22. Frank ST, Weg JG, Harkleroad LE, Fitch RF. Pulmonary dysfunction in rheumatoid disease. *Chest* 1973;63:27–34.
23. Faris PM, Spence RK, Larholt KM, et al. The predictive power of baseline hemoglobin for transfusion risk in surgery patients. *Orthopedics* 1999;22:S135–S140.
24. Carson JL, Poses RM, Spence RK, Bonavita G. Severity of anaemia and operative mortality and morbidity. *Lancet* 1988;1:727–729.
25. Goodnough LT, Rudnick S, Price TH, et al. Increased preoperative collection of autologous blood with recombinant human erythropoietin therapy. *N Engl J Med* 1989;321:1163–1168.
26. Mercuriali F, Gualtieri G, Sinigaglia L, et al. Use of recombinant human erythropoietin to assist autologous blood donation by anemic rheumatoid arthritis patients undergoing major orthopedic surgery. *Transfusion* 1994;34:501–506.
27. Saikawa I, Hotokebuchi T, Arita C, et al. Autologous blood transfusion with recombinant erythropoietin treatment. 22 Arthroplasties for rheumatoid arthritis. *Acta Orthop Scand* 1994;65:15–19.
28. Keating EM. Current options and approaches for blood management in orthopaedic surgery. *Instr Course Lect* 1999;48:655–665.
29. Martin JW, Whiteside LA, Milliano MT, Reedy ME. Postoperative blood retrieval and transfusion in cementless total knee arthroplasty. *J Arthroplasty* 1992;7:205–210.
30. Weinblatt M. Antirheumatic drug therapy and the surgical patient. In: Sledge CB, Ruddy S, Harris ED Jr, Kelley WN, eds. *Arthritis surgery*. Philadelphia: WB Saunders, 1994:771–786.
31. MacKenzie CR. Perioperative medical care of rheumatic disease patients having orthopaedic surgery. Available at: www.rheumatology.hss.edu/phys/diseaseReviews/perio/perio.asp. Accessed August 9, 2002.
32. Sculco T. Introduction to the rheumatoid patient undergoing surgical treatment. In: Sculco TP, ed. *Surgical treatment of rheumatoid arthritis*. St. Louis: Mosby Year Book Inc, 1992.
33. Baum J. Infection in rheumatoid arthritis. *Arthritis Rheum* 1971;14:135–137.
34. Goldenberg DL. Infectious arthritis complicating rheumatoid arthritis and other chronic rheumatic disorders. *Arthritis Rheum* 1989;32:496–502.
35. Harris ED, Jr. Rheumatoid arthritis. Pathophysiology and implications for therapy. *N Engl J Med* 1990;322:1277–1289.
36. Perhala RS, Wilke WS, Clough JD, Segal AM. Local infectious complications following large joint replacement in rheumatoid arthritis patients treated with methotrexate versus those not treated with methotrexate. *Arthritis Rheum* 1991;34:146–152.
37. van Albada-Kuipers GA, Linthorst J, Peeters EA, et al. Frequency of infection among patients with rheumatoid arthritis versus patients with osteoarthritis or soft tissue rheumatism. *Arthritis Rheum* 1988;31:667–671.
38. Deacon JM, Pagliaro AJ, Zelicof SB, Horowitz HW. Prophylactic use of antibiotics for procedures after total joint replacement. *J Bone Joint Surg Am* 1996;78: 1755–1770.
39. Charnley J, Eftekhar N. Postoperative infection in total prosthetic replacement arthroplasty of the hip-joint. With special reference to the bacterial content of the air of the operating room. *Br J Surg* 1969;56:641–649.
40. Doran MF, Crowson CS, Pond GR, et al. Frequency of infection in patients with rheumatoid arthritis compared with controls. *Arthritis Rheum* 2002;46:2287–2293.
41. Wilson MG, Kelley K, Thornhill TS. Infection as a complication of total knee-replacement arthroplasty. Risk factors and treatment in sixty-seven cases. *J Bone Joint Surg Am* 1990;72:878–883.
42. Blomgren G. Hematogenous infection of total joint replacement. An experimental study in the rabbit. *Acta Orthop Scand* 1981;[Suppl]187:1–64.
43. Southwood RT, Rice JL, McDonald PJ, et al. Infection in experimental hip arthroplasties. *J Bone Joint Surg Br* 1985;67:229–231.
44. Carpiniello VL, Cendron M, Altman HG, et al. Treatment of urinary complications after total joint replacement in elderly females. *Urology* 1988;32:186–188.
45. Vannini P, Ciavarella A, Olmi R, et al. Diabetes as pro-infective risk factor in total hip replacement. *Acta Diabetol Lat* 1984;21:275–280.
46. Acurio MT, Friedman RJ. Hip arthroplasty in patients with sickle-cell haemoglobinopathy. *J Bone Joint Surg Br* 1992;74:367–371.
47. Maderazo EG, Judson S, Pasternak H. Late infections of total joint prostheses. *Clin Orthop* 1988;229:131–142.
48. Pallasch TJ, Slots J. Antibiotic prophylaxis and the medically compromised patient. *Periodontology* 2000;10:107–138.
49. Smetana GW. Concise review: risk factors for postoperative pulmonary complications. Available at www.harrisonsonline.com/server-java/Arknoid/amed/harrisons/ex_editorials/edl2318_p01.html. Accessed August 15, 2002.
50. Daniels AUD, Tooms RE, Harkess JW. Arthroplasty. In: Canale TS, ed. *Campbel's operative orthopaedics*, 9th ed. St. Louis: Mosby, 1998.
51. Arroyo JS, Garvin KL, McGuire MH. Fatal marrow embolization following a porous-coated bipolar hip endoprosthesis. *J Arthroplasty* 1994;9:449–452.
52. Fabian TC. Unraveling the fat embolism syndrome. *N Engl J Med* 1993;329:961–963.
53. Acosta J. Fat embolism syndrome. In: Schwartz GR, ed. *Principles and practice of emergency medicine*, 4th ed. Philadelphia: Lippincott Williams & Wilkins, 1999.
54. Shorr RI, Ray WA, Daugherty JR, Griffin MR. Concurrent use of nonsteroidal anti-inflammatory drugs and oral anticoagulants places elderly persons at high risk for hemorrhagic peptic ulcer disease. *Arch Intern Med* 1993; 153:1665–1670.
55. Emery P, Zeidler H, Kvien TK, et al. Celecoxib versus diclofenac in long-term management of rheumatoid arthritis: randomized double-blind comparison. *Lancet* 1999;354:2106–2111.
56. Simon LS, Weaver AL, Graham DY, et al. Anti-inflammatory and upper gastrointestinal effects of celecoxib in rheumatoid arthritis: a randomized controlled trial. *JAMA* 1999;282:1921–1928.
57. Chan FKL, Hung LCT, Suen BY, et al. Celecoxib versus Diclofenac and Omeprazole in reducing the risk of recurrent ulcer bleeding in patients with arthritis. *N Engl J Med* 2002;347:2104–2110.
58. Mohammed S, Croom DW. Gastropathy due to celecoxib, a cyclooxygenase-2 inhibitor. *N Engl J Med* 1999;340:2005.
59. Linder JD, Monkemuller KE, Davis JV, Wilcox CM. Cyclooxygenase-2 inhibitor celecoxib: a possible cause of gastropathy and hypoprothrombinemia. *South Med J* 2000;93:930–932.
60. Hawkey CJ. Gastrointestinal safety of COX-2 specific inhibitors. *Gastroenterol Clin North Am* 2001;30:921–936.
61. Greenan DM, Gray J, Loudon J, Fear S. Methotrexate and early postoperative complications in patients with rheumatoid arthritis undergoing elective orthopaedic surgery. *Ann Rheum Dis* 2001;60:214–217.
62. McKenna R, Bachmann F, Kaushal SP, Galante JO. Thromboembolic disease in patients undergoing total knee replacement. *J Bone Joint Surg Am* 1976;58:928–932.
63. Johnson R, Carmichael JH, Almon HG, Loynes RP. Deep venous thrombosis following Charnley arthroplasty. *Clin Orthop* 1978;132:24–30.
64. Campling EA, Devlin HB, Lunn JN. Reporting to NCEPOD. *BMJ* 1992;305 (6847):252.
65. Katz JN, Losina E, Barrett J, et al. Association between hospital and surgeon procedure volume and outcomes of total hip replacement in the United States medicare population. *J Bone Joint Surg Am* 2001;83A:1622–1629.
66. Bottner F, Sculco TP. Nonpharmacologic thromboembolic prophylaxis in total knee arthroplasty. *Clin Orthop* 2001;392:249–256.
67. Colwell CW Jr. Low molecular weight heparin prophylaxis in total knee arthroplasty: the answer. *Clin Orthop* 2001;392:245–248.
68. Hull RD, Pineo GF, Stein PD, et al. Extended out-of-hospital low-molecular-weight heparin prophylaxis against deep venous thrombosis in patients after elective hip arthroplasty: a systematic review. *Ann Intern Med* 2001;135:858–869.
69. Johnson CF, Convery FR. Preventing emboli after total hip replacement. *Am J Nurs* 1975;75:804–806.
70. Phillips CB, Barrett JA, Losina E, et al. Trends in incidence rates of dislocation, pulmonary embolism and deep hip infection during the first six months after elective total hip replacement. *J Bone Joint Surg Am* 2003;85-A:20–26.
71. Sikorski JM, Bradfield JW. Fat and thromboembolism after total hip replacement. *Acta Orthop Scand* 1983;54:403–407.
72. Kakkar VV, Stringer MD. Prophylaxis of venous thromboembolism. *World J Surg* 1990;14:670–678.
73. White RH, Herderson MC. Risk factors for venous thromboembolism after total hip and knee replacement surgery. *Curr Opin Pulm Med* 2002;8:365–371.
74. White RH, Gettner S, Newman JM, et al. Predictors of rehospitalization for symptomatic venous thromboembolism after total hip arthroplasty. *N Engl J Med* 2000;343:1758–1764.
75. White RH, Romano PS, Zhou H, et al. Incidence and time course of thromboembolic outcomes following total hip or knee arthroplasty. *Arch Intern Med* 1998;27;158:1525–1531.
76. Dahl OE. Continuing out-of-hospital prophylaxis following major orthopaedic surgery: what now? *Haemostasis* 2000;30[Suppl 2]:101–105; discussion 82–83.
77. Geerts WH, Heit JA, Clagett GP, et al. Prevention of venous thromboembolism. *Chest* 2001;119:132S–175S.
78. Lie SA, Engesaeter LB, Havelin LI, et al. Mortality after total hip replacement: 0-10-year follow-up of 39,543 patients in the Norwegian Arthroplasty Register. *Acta Orthop Scand* 2000;71:19–27.

79. Seagrott V, Tan HS, Goldacre M, et al. Elective total hip replacement: incidence, emergency readmission rate, and postoperative mortality. *BMJ* 1991;303:1431–1435.
80. Fender D, Harper WM, Thompson JR, Gregg PJ. Mortality and fatal pulmonary embolism after primary total hip replacement. Result from a national hip register. *J Bone Joint Surg Br* 1997;79:896–899.
81. Warwick DJ. Prophylaxis of deep-vein thrombosis. *J Bone Joint Surg Br* 1995;77:334.
82. McGrath D, Dennyson WG, Rolland M. Death rate from pulmonary embolism following joint replacement surgery. *J R Coll Surg Edinb* 1996;41:265–266.
83. Planes A, Vochelle N, Darmon JY, et al. Risk of deep-venous thrombosis after hospital discharge in patients having undergone total hip replacement: double-blind randomised comparison of enoxaparin versus placebo. *Lancet* 1996;348:224–228.
84. Anderson FA, White K; Hip and Knee Registry Investigators. Prolonged prophylaxis in orthopedic surgery: insights from the US. *Seminars Thromb Hemost* 2002;28:43–46.
85. Rubin R, Salvati EA, Lewis R. Infected total hip replacement after dental procedures. *Oral Surg Oral Med Oral Pathol* 1976;41:18–23.
86. Hanssen AD, Osmon DR. Prevention of deep wound infection after total hip arthroplasty: the role of prophylactic antibiotics and clean air technology. *Semin Arthroplasty* 1994;5:114–121.
87. Hanssen AD, Osmon DR, Nelson CL. Prevention of deep periprosthetic joint infection. *Instr Course Lect* 1997;46:555–567.
88. Seymour RA, Whitworth JM. Antibiotic prophylaxis for endocarditis, prosthetic joints and surgery. *Dent Clin North Am* 2002:635–651.
89. Advisory statement. Antibiotic prophylaxis for dental patients with total joint replacements. American Dental Association and American Academy of Orthopaedic Surgeons. *J Am Dent Assoc* 1997;128:1004–1008.
90. Bender IB, Naidorf IJ, Garvey GJ. Bacterial endocarditis: a consideration for physician and dentist. *J Am Dent Assoc* 1984;109:415–420.
91. Everett ED, Hirschmann JV. Transient bacteremia and endocarditis prophylaxis. A review. *Medicine (Baltimore)* 1977;56:61–77.
92. Guntheroth WG. How important are dental procedures as a cause of infective endocarditis? *Am J Cardiol* 1984;54:797–801.
93. LaPorte DM, Waldman BJ, Mont MA, Hungerford DS. Infections associated with dental procedures in total hip arthroplasty. *J Bone Joint Surg Br* 1999;81:56–59.
94. Helewa A, Smythe HA, Goldsmith CH. Can specially trained physiotherapists improve the care of patients with rheumatoid arthritis? A randomized health care trial. *J Rheumatol* 1994;21:70–79.
95. De Pablo P, Losina E, Phillips CB, et al. Determinants of discharge destination following elective total hip replacement. (*manuscript submitted*).
96. McInness J, Larson MG, Daltroy LH, et al. A controlled evaluation of continuous passive motion in patients undergoing total knee arthroplasty. *JAMA* 1992;268:1423–1428.
97. Ververeli PA, Sutton DC, Hearn SL, et al. Continuous passive motion after total knee arthroplasty. *Clin Orthop* 1995;321:208–215.
98. Worland RL, Arredondo J, Angles F, et al. Home continuous passive motion machine versus professional physical therapy following total knee replacement. *J Arthroplasty* 1998;13:784–787.
99. Sledge CB. Reconstructive surgery for rheumatic disease. Introduction to surgical management of patients with arthritis. In: Ruddy S, Harris ED, Sledge CB, eds. *Kelley's textbook of rheumatology*, 6th ed. Philadelphia: WB Saunders, 2001.
100. Howe JG, Lambert B. Critical pathways in total hip arthroplasty. In: Callaghan JJ, Rosenberg AG, Rubash HE, eds. *The adult hip*. Philadelphia: Lippincott-Raven Publishers, 1998.
101. Iwase T, Wingstrand I, Person BM, et al. The ScanHip total arthroplasty. *Acta Orthop Scand* 2002;73:54–59.

CHAPTER 41

Total Joint Arthroplasty

Christopher Glen Richardson and Thomas Parker Vail

Total joint arthroplasty (TJA) is one of the great surgical advances of the past century. TJA is a highly successful treatment for end-stage degenerative joint disease caused by progressive nonresponsive cartilage degradation in patients with posttraumatic arthritis, osteoarthritis (OA), and rheumatoid arthritis (RA). The goal of any joint replacement is the restoration of function and the elimination of pain. The elimination of pain remains the primary indication for joint replacement, followed by progressive bone loss, malalignment of an extremity, or loss of motion due to joint space deterioration. For patients with monoarticular disease, a joint replacement can result in return to near normal age-adjusted functional status. When an arthritic condition affects multiple joints, the impact of TJA on pain relief can be equally dramatic, but normal function may still be limited. The goals of performing TJA in patients who experience pain with loss of function in multiple joints are preservation of independence, ability to perform self-care, and quality of life. The most commonly performed joint replacement procedures in RA in order of occurrence are total knee arthroplasty (TKA), total hip arthroplasty (THA), total shoulder arthroplasty (TSA), and total elbow arthroplasty (TEA) (1). Metacarpophalangeal arthroplasty and total ankle arthroplasty (TAA) are less common. According to information from the American Academy of Orthopaedic Surgeons, more than 168,000 total hip replacements are performed each year in the United States (1a). There are a number of unique considerations for RA patients that are key to achieving a successful total joint replacement. This chapter will outline those important considerations and detail outcomes for the most commonly performed joint arthroplasty procedures.

GENERAL CONSIDERATIONS

It is estimated that 25% of RA patients can expect to have TJA performed within 21.8 years of disease onset (1). Candidates for TJA can be predicted based on disease severity questionnaires, high white blood counts, anemia, high erythrocyte sedimentation rate, high C-reactive protein, and the need for more aggressive medical therapy to control disease (1). However, most physicians would agree that institution of one or several of many available nonoperative therapies is indicated before recommending joint replacement. These therapies include, but are not limited to, anti-inflammatories or other disease-modifying drugs, analgesic medication, support groups, rest, walking aids, splints, orthotics, weight loss, and physical therapy.

Failure of medical management is one indication for surgery, but there are other factors that must be considered (2). First, a thorough evaluation of the pain pattern, including duration, location, severity, and the inciting and relieving factors, is warranted. Patients who complain of constant and severe pain, especially at rest, are often candidates for TJA. Secondly, determining the functional status of patients defined by walking distance, stair climbing, and ability to perform activities of daily living is important in deciding whether a patient would achieve a functional benefit from TJA. In some cases of severe deforming RA, the functional considerations pale in comparison to the need for pain relief. The physical examination provides information about the objective deficits, such as the amount of angular and rotational deformity, stiffness, instability, and weakness.

The general medical status of patients, including obesity and other comorbidities, may impact the outcome of a major surgical procedure. For example, although infection after primary joint arthroplasty is an uncommon event (<0.5%), the risk may be substantially increased when there is a history of previous joint infection, prior major surgical procedure on the affected joint, a diagnosis of rheumatoid or psoriatic arthritis, or other systemic condition that affects the patient's immune system (3). Finally, correlating the history and physical with radiographic changes is important for determining the need for TJA. Radiographs allow confirmation of the clinical diagnosis of degenerative joint disease and delineation of the pathoanatomy. With the exception of bone loss or severe deformity, it is the desire for functional improvement, relief from pain, or better quality of life that drives the decision to replace a joint (Table 41.1).

UNIQUE PROBLEMS WITH RHEUMATOID ARTHRITIS

Multijoint Involvement

Commonly, more than one joint will be affected in RA patients, and, therefore, the surgeon cannot treat a particular joint in isolation. Determining which joint to replace in an RA patient with severely involved joints can be difficult. Generally, the hip joint is addressed first, as the hip often impacts independent ambulation the most (2). Moreover, stiffness or hip flexion contracture must often be addressed to consider other joints for surgical reconstruction. For example, it is difficult to rehabilitate a TKA in a patient with a diseased hip when a hip flexion contracture prevents the patient from standing upright. Additionally, pain from a diseased hip can refer to the ipsilateral knee. Thus, treating the knee first may not relieve all knee symptoms when the

TABLE 41.1. Specific Criteria for Joint Replacement

Pain resistant to medical management
Progressive angular deformity of an extremity
Loss of joint motion
Radiographic evidence of advanced degenerative joint disease

hip is affected. A possible exception to treating the hip first is the presence of bone loss or malalignment of the knee. A severe valgus, internally rotated rheumatoid knee may affect the stability of an ipsilateral THA (2).

Frequently, the use of walking aids is required after a lower-extremity TJA. However, shoulder and elbow disease may make rehabilitation with walking aids extremely difficult or impossible. Consequently, a rheumatoid patient with severe upper-extremity involvement is faced with the prospect of more prolonged immobilization to adequately protect the joint, or the acceptance of earlier weightbearing after surgery when possible. Often, platform walkers and other assistive devices can be used to protect the shoulders and elbows during rehabilitation. Likewise, the condition of severely affected upper-extremity joints may need to be optimized through therapy or other management before the lower-extremity joint replacement.

Finally, RA can involve the cervical spine, which should be assessed for instability and range of motion before TJA. A review of patients undergoing THA and TKA demonstrated radiographic evidence of cervical spine instability in 50% of cases, despite a lack of symptoms (3). Severe instability may require surgical stabilization before TJA is performed to diminish the risk of spinal cord trauma during intubation at the time of surgery. Simple dynamic flexion-extension lateral radiographs of the cervical spine can be used as a screening test for atlanto-axial and midcervical instability. Stiffness in the cervical spine may make intubation particularly difficult because extension of the cervical spine is required to view the vocal cords, allowing safe passage of the endotracheal tube. In the absence of cervical spine mobility allowing direct visualization of the airway, fiber-optic endoscopic assistance is required to direct the endotracheal tube safely into the appropriate position within the airway.

Chronic Anemia

Many rheumatoid patients, especially those with more active disease, experience anemia. Etiology of the anemia can be attributed to chronic nonsteroidal antiinflammatory drug (NSAID) use or suppressed erythropoietin response to low hemoglobin (4). Anemia in RA patients is problematic, as blood loss from TJA may require blood transfusions. The traditional use of homologous blood transfusions risks disease transmission and sensitization in these patients. Preoperative autologous blood donation is used to avoid homologous blood transfusion for patients with preoperative hemoglobin between 10 and 14, but its use in anemic RA patients may be very limited or even not possible. Recombinant human erythropoietin therapy has been successfully used to increase hemoglobin levels before autologous donation in anemic RA patients (5). Other ways to decrease homologous blood use include preoperative iron therapy, meticulous surgical technique, and decreased operative time.

Medications

Medical therapy is the primary treatment modality for RA. NSAIDs, cyclooxygenase-2 inhibitors, methotrexate (MTX), and, increasingly, anti–tumor necrosis factor (TNF) α drugs are widely used in RA. The side effects of gastric mucosal damage, immune system suppression, and platelet inhibition related to some of these drugs can have important surgical consequences. The platelet or anticoagulation effect is important, especially with anemic RA patients. Minimizing intraoperative blood loss ideally involves the preoperative cessation of medications affecting platelet function. The adverse consequence of stopping medications is that the absence of NSAIDs can make patients uncomfortable until the medication is started postoperatively. The newer cyclooxygenase-2 inhibitors are effective in decreasing inflammation associated with RA and have fewer gastrointestinal complications without the antiplatelet effect (6,7). Thus, it may be possible to continue these medications up until the time of surgery.

Glucocorticoids are potent antiinflammatory drugs that have several deleterious effects related to surgery, including adrenal suppression, osteopenia, soft tissue atrophy, gastric stress ulcers, immunosuppression, and avascular necrosis. Patients taking higher oral doses may require perioperative bolus infusion of corticosteroid to avoid addisonian crises, but lower chronic dosing does not require bolus infusion. Likewise, short-term use to suppress rheumatoid flare-ups is also associated with fewer adverse effects than long-term consumption of glucocorticoids. Currently, recommendations for perioperative coverage with stress doses of steroids should be correlated with the preoperative glucocorticoid dose, the preoperative duration of glucocorticoid administration, and the magnitude of the proposed operation (7a). Intraarticular corticosteroid injections are not associated with adverse systemic effects perioperatively. However, anecdotal evidence suggests that intraarticular injections should be avoided within the weeks before surgery because of the potential for surgical site infection.

MTX is a commonly used disease-modifying antirheumatic drug for treatment of RA that has demonstrated the ability to alter the natural history of RA. The historical concern with the perioperative administration of MTX is the development of wound complications postoperatively related to fibroblast inhibition. Increased postoperative complications have been reported with continued use of MTX in the perioperative period versus discontinuing MTX the week before and the week of surgery (8). More recent larger studies have demonstrated no increase in postoperative complications with use of perioperative MTX (9,10). The effects of newer therapies, such as TNF-α inhibitors, on the outcome of TJA are not known. Early studies suggest that overall immune function may not be affected (11), but there exist no large studies comparing the incidence of postoperative infections in patients receiving TNF-α inhibitors to those treated with other disease-modifying antirheumatic drugs.

Osseous Changes

RA affects not only the articular cartilage but also the underlying bone structure, which is a critical issue for orthopedic surgeons who are implanting a TJA. The initial stability of a joint replacement depends on the mechanical interface between the implant and the cortical cancellous bone, as well as the structural support of the bone. Anything that interferes with this interface, including structurally weakened bone, can potentially lead to early TJA failure. The bone in RA is osteopenic, characterized by the thinning of cortical bone, a larger-diameter medullary canal, decreased cancellous bone density, and, consequently, decreased overall strength. Several studies have shown decreased trabecular bone strength in RA, compared to normal and osteoarthritic bone (12–14). Clinically, the abnormal rheumatoid bone can present as uncomplicated osteoporosis, or with deformity related to marginal bone erosion, localized osteonecrosis, and subchondral plate collapse. Examples of skeletal deformity patterns seen in RA include progressive acetabular protrusio, medial protrusion of the humeral head, and valgus deformity of the knee with lateral femoral condyle deficiency (12). The cause of abnormal bone may be related to steroid use, chronic disease, inactivity, or increased osteoblastic and osteoclastic activity due to inflammation and repair. Bone deficiencies in patients with RA can create technical challenges in TJA and may necessitate the use of specialized implants, polymethylmethacrylate (PMMA) cement, or bone grafts.

Soft Tissues

The RA inflammatory process has profound effects on soft tissues, including synovium, joint capsules, tendons, and ligaments. Soft tissue changes contribute to the deformities that are classically associated with RA. The hand, with its swan-neck and boutonnière deformities, is a well-known example, but soft tissue abnormalities are also found in the lower extremities. The valgus knee deformity presents with an atrophied and weak medial collateral ligament combined with tight contracted lateral structures, such as the lateral collateral ligament, lateral capsule, iliotibial band, and popliteus. This imbalance from angular deformity can make stable balancing of a TKA more difficult. The pes planus deformity in the foot and ankle often has atrophy or failure of the posterior tibial tendon. If the pes planus deformity is chronic, a stiff contracture develops.

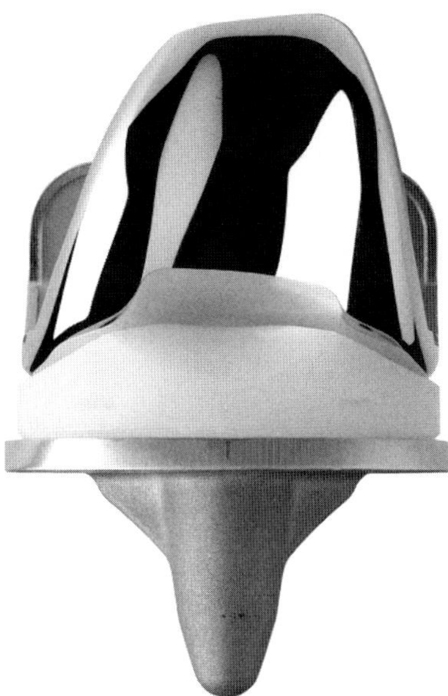

Figure 41.1. Total knee arthroplasty. (Courtesy of DePuy Inc., a Johnson & Johnson company.)

TOTAL KNEE ARTHROPLASTY

The classic presentation in RA is a valgus knee with medial laxity, tight lateral soft tissues, and a flexion contracture. The extent of this deformity will vary. This valgus, or *knock-knee*, presentation of inflammatory arthropathy is in contrast to the more common varus, or *bow-legged*, deformity, caused by medial compartment disease in OA. As RA is often tricompartmental and progressive, other more conservative operations, such as osteotomies and unicondylar knee replacements, will not provide lasting benefits for the large majority of patients. As a result, TKA is the preferred surgical choice in RA and other inflammatory arthropathies, in which the entire joint surface is frequently pathologic.

TKA can be conceptualized as a resurfacing operation of the distal femur, proximal tibia, and articular surface of the patella (Fig. 41.1). The bone cuts are planned to correct any deformity and create an osseous surface that allows for stable fixation of the implants. Fixation can be aided with the use of PMMA cement, or the implants can be cementless. Cementless TKA, less commonly performed than cemented TKA, relies on bony ingrowth into the prosthesis to give lasting stability. Currently, most surgeons prefer cemented total knee prosthesis because of the excellent clinical record of cemented implants, the inferior bone found in rheumatoid patients, and the immediate fixation cementing provides (15).

Occasionally, RA involves both knees severely, to the extent that patients are unable to distinguish which knee is worse. In this situation, the surgeon can consider performing simultaneous bilateral TKA. The benefits of bilateral TKA, including decreased rehabilitation time and decreased cost, must be tempered with increased morbidity and mortality from bilateral procedures. The 30-day mortality is significantly higher in patients of all diagnoses (0.49% vs. 0.17%) who undergo bilateral versus unilateral TKA (16). Even in the face of chronic disease, however, the 30-day mortality of TKA in RA is not significantly different than that of TKA in OA.

TKA relies on the capsule, medial collateral ligament, lateral collateral ligament complex, and the extensor mechanism for stability and function. Depending on the implant, the posterior cruciate ligament (PCL) can be retained or sacrificed. The fate of the PCL in TKA is controversial. When the PCL is sacrificed, a PCL-substituting total knee design is used. The PCL-substituting design includes more articular conformity between the femoral and tibial components, with a central cam mechanism that provides femoral rollback on the tibial surface as the knee is flexed. Rollback of the femur on the tibia is a feature of normal knee kinematics. When intact, the PCL can provide the rollback function. Proponents of sacrificing the PCL claim that proper soft tissue balancing is achieved by removal of a diseased PCL and that a cam mechanism compensates for the absence of the PCL. Advocates of preserving the PCL claim that more normal biomechanics of the knee are retained when a contracted or diseased PCL is surgically balanced. In rheumatoid patients, the PCL is shown to have altered collagen structure and weakened mechanical properties (17,18). Due to these changes, some surgeons recommend sacrificing the PCL, because of the potential for development of posterior instability and recurvatum deformity if it is retained (19). A criticism of the PCL-substituting TKA is the increase in stress transfer to the implant bone interface (20,21). Theoretically, increased stress transfer to the bone–cement interface could increase loosening of the implant (20,21) in a PCL-substituting design. Nevertheless, other studies of RA patients with PCL-retaining TKA report implant survival rates of 81% to 97% at 10- to 13-year follow-up (20,21). Most revisions in these studies were because of failure of the metal-backed patellar components (now largely obsolete), not instability.

The long-term results of TKA in RA are generally favorable. Several studies report 10-year survival rates of the prosthesis ranging from 83% to 97% (20–24). Furthermore, good to excellent clinical results are reported in 83% to 95% of these cases (20,24). Rheumatoid TKA survival rates compare favorably with survival rates of TKA in patients who have OA, and several studies show no significant difference (19,22,25,26). Aside from aseptic loosening, the most concerning complication is infection. Several studies present infection rates as high as 4.1% (24,27,28). The treatment of this complication is difficult, often requiring a two-stage reimplantation, with inferior functional results.

TOTAL HIP ARTHROPLASTY

THA is a successful treatment for many types of end-stage hip disease. Rheumatoid patients frequently develop hip joint involvement. Approximately 28% of RA patients will be symptomatic, and 13% will require hip arthroplasty within 5 years of diagnosis of disease (29). A long-term study of RA patients reported that approximately 44 years after disease onset, 25% of RA patients would have had a THA (1).

The THA implant consists of four component parts. First, the acetabulum is resurfaced with either a cemented or cementless hemispheric shell. A cemented component involves the use of PMMA bone cement as a grout to hold an ultra-high-molecular-weight hemispheric polyethylene shell in the acetabulum. An uncemented acetabular component involves the use of a metallic hemispheric cup, usually constructed of titanium or cobalt chromium alloy with a porous external surface that allows osseous attachment to the cup at its interface with the pelvis (Fig. 41.2). Initial stability of these cups is obtained by press-fitting the component into the shaped acetabular socket. Further fixation can be achieved by using screws placed through the dome of the cup into the pelvis. Secondly, a liner, constructed of ultra-high-molecular-weight polyethylene, is fitted into the metal shell. Historically, wear of the polyethylene liner of the total hip has led to osteolysis, aseptic loosening, and failure of the implants over the long term. Concerns over polyethylene wear debris have led to improvements in polyethylene wear resistance by manufacturing processes such as radiation cross-linking of the polyethylene material. In addition, other bearing materials, including hard bearing surfaces, such as metal-on-metal and ceramic bearings, are being developed as options to metal-on-polyethylene bearings.

Modern THA uses modularity of the components to provide off-the-shelf customization for each patient. Modularity allows the surgeon to match the stem size with the appropriate neck length, head size, and socket diameter to meet the patient's individual anatomy and activity requirements. Additionally, modularity allows the surgeon to revise the bearing surface without removing the entire total hip at the time of revision or alter the neck length on the femoral component to best obtain intraoperative soft tissue tension and stability. The femoral head is typically made of a highly polished cobalt chromium ferrous metal alloy. Ceramic femoral heads are available as an alternative bearing surface for use against polyethylene acetabular liners. Ceramic-on-ceramic bearings have recently been approved by the U.S. Food and Drug Administration for general use in hip replacement.

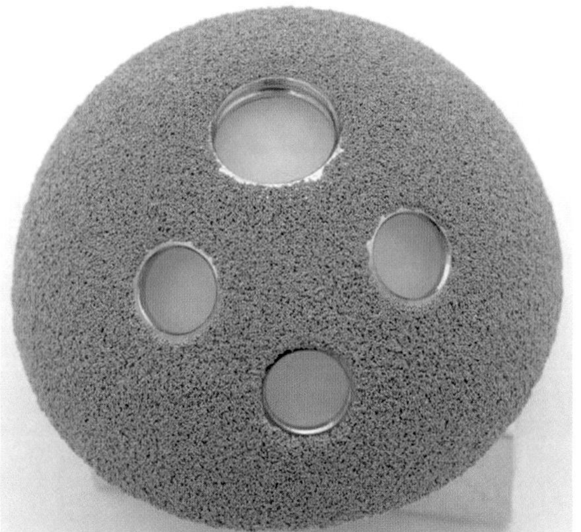

Figure 41.2. A porous-coated cementless hip socket. (Courtesy of DePuy Inc., a Johnson & Johnson company.)

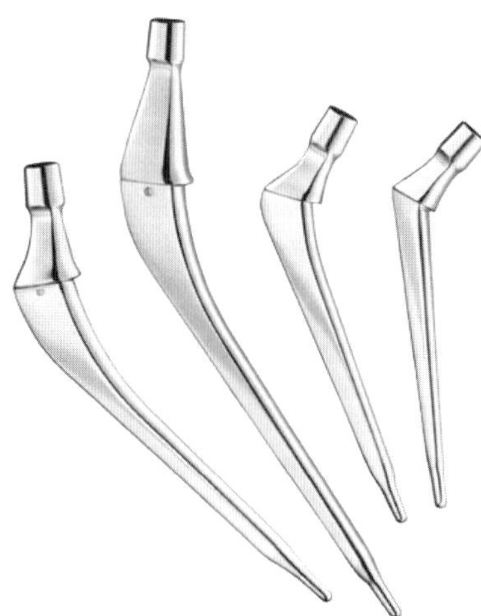

Figure 41.3. Total hip stems designed for insertion with cement. (Courtesy of Zimmer, Inc.)

The femoral stem can be cemented or cementless. The cemented component uses PMMA (bone cement) injected into the prepared femoral canal under pressure. The femoral stem is placed into the cement-filled canal, further pressurizing the cement into the cancellous bone. Cemented stems are generally made of cobalt chrome (Fig. 41.3). The cementless femoral stems are press-fitted into an undersized prepared femoral canal. The roughened surface of the cementless femoral component allows for the bone to attach to the stem directly. The cementless components are made of cobalt chromium alloy or titanium alloy. A hybrid THA is one in which one component is cemented and the other is cementless. The most common combination is a cemented femoral component and cementless acetabular shell.

It is a matter of debate about which implant to use as well as in which patient it should be used. As THA has evolved, a number of trends have emerged. Initially, THA was cemented with a metal-on-polyethylene bearing surface and a small femoral head diameter (22.25 mm). It became evident that results in younger patients were inferior to those in older patients. This fact, as well as the concern of cement disease (later recognized as polyethylene-induced osteolysis) led to the development of cementless implants. Traditionally, cementless THA has been reserved for younger patients but is seeing broader use in all patients as its performance in less dense bone is proven. Furthermore, the bearing surface has also evolved. Metal-on-metal, ceramic-on-ceramic, and ceramic-on–ultra-high-molecular-weight polyethylene are examples of new material combinations designed to decrease wear debris production and decrease the incidence of aseptic loosening of total hip implants. Usually, these alternative bearing surfaces are used in more active patients.

Due to the frequent incidence of osteopenic bone in rheumatoid patients, the standard hip replacement has been the cemented THA. Long-term results of cemented THA have demonstrated survival rates for rheumatoid patients, comparable to those of patients with OA using similar techniques (30,31) (Fig. 41.4). Ten-year implant survival rates of 93% are reported, but it is clear that the acetabular component is the main cause of failure. Cemented acetabular components have failure rates of 8% to 20% when the failure includes revised and radiographically loose cups. These acetabular failure rates are in contrast to femoral stem failure rates of 2% (30–32). Acetabular failure rates are lower if the functioning but radiographically loose implants are excluded (30–32). Loosening of the femoral implant is also observed (Fig. 41.5).

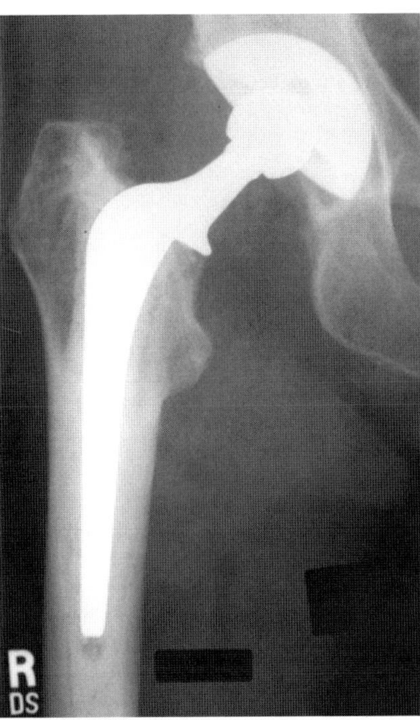

Figure 41.4. Radiograph of a patient with a well-functioning total hip replacement at 7 years after implantation. There are no radiographic signs of implant loosening, bone loss, or wear.

The high failure rates documented with the cemented acetabular components in RA and the promising results of cementless acetabular components led to the use of uncemented THA. Cementless implants require the ability to achieve bone ingrowth for long-term stability. An early study with short-term follow-up of 4.5 years demonstrated that only one in 35 acetabular components had evidence of radiographic loosening (33). A 10-year follow-up study demonstrated a 98.1% survivorship of porous-coated femoral stems, 93.8% for porous-coated cups, and 84.3% for cemented cups (34). Early results suggest that cementless acetabular components are an improvement over cemented cups.

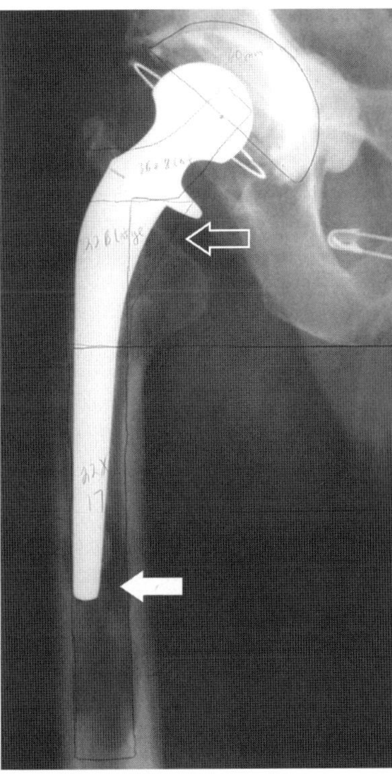

Figure 41.5. Radiograph of a patient with a loose cemented total hip implant. The radiograph has been measured for a revision hip stem that will extend below the bone lysis. The white arrow indicates a radiolucent line between the implant and bone. There is loss of bone beneath the collar of the femoral implant (*open arrow*).

Occasionally, juvenile RA (JRA) can lead to joint destruction severe enough to warrant joint replacement. JRA patients are more complicated from the joint reconstruction perspective because of their small stature and general fragility. It is not uncommon for a JRA patient to require customized or unusually small implants. Nevertheless, long-term studies have demonstrated successful treatment of JRA with cemented THA. Acetabular survival rates are reported from 70% to 87.8% at 15 years, which are less than femoral component survival rates of 85% to 91.9% at 15 years (35,36). Improvements in components and technique should improve implant survival in these patients. The use of cementless implants awaits long-term reports.

There are a number of complications that can occur after THA in any group of patients. The development of postoperative infections is a particular concern in patients with RA because of the increasing use of medications that suppress the immune system. Nevertheless, recent studies have failed to demonstrate an increased infection rate attributable to RA (37,38). Another important complication of THA is instability or dislocation of the femoral head from the acetabular socket postoperatively. However, RA does not seem to decrease stability because revision rates for instability are only 1% to 2%, with a linear rate of increase as length of follow-up increases (30,34). Other perioperative complications include deep venous thrombosis, pulmonary embolus, nerve injuries, and periprosthetic fractures. Periprosthetic fracture, dislocation, loosening of the implant, wear of the implant bearing surface, and infection can also present as late complications of THA. Despite the frailty of RA patients, the 30-day mortality after THA is not significantly different than that for OA patients (39).

TOTAL SHOULDER ARTHROPLASTY

RA affecting the shoulder leads to severe pain and limitation of motion. The shoulder is important for everyday activities and is often a weightbearing joint for RA patients who have lower-extremity involvement requiring assistive devices to walk. Once the disease has progressed to the point where conservative measures no longer provide adequate pain relief or function, the next step is TSA (40).

There are two approaches to surgical replacement of the shoulder. The first involves removing the diseased humeral head and press-fitting or cementing a humeral stem with an articulating surface against the natural glenoid, without resurfacing the glenoid. This is referred to as *hemiarthroplasty*. *TSA* refers to replacing the articular surface of the humerus as well as the glenoid (Fig. 41.6). Due to the inflammatory nature of RA, it is preferable to perform a TSA, versus a hemiarthroplasty, in most cases, as there is more predictable pain relief and function (40–43). Hemiarthroplasty is indicated if erosion of the glenoid prevents adequate fixation of the implant or there is deficiency of the rotator cuff (42,43). The decision to use a cemented or cementless implant is usually based on patient age and bone quality. Generally, a cemented implant is used for older patients with poor bone quality, often the case with RA.

TSA is indicated in an RA patient when the pain is not manageable with medications and function is curtailed. The contraindications for a TSA include ongoing infection elsewhere in

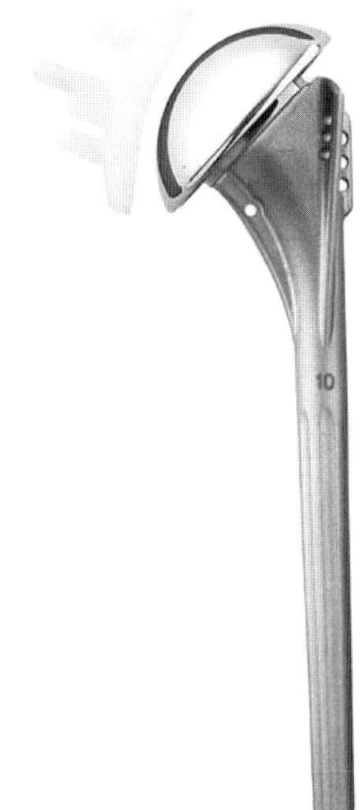

Figure 41.6. Total shoulder arthroplasty. (Courtesy of DePuy Inc., a Johnson & Johnson company.)

the body, ongoing shoulder sepsis, complete loss of deltoid muscle function, and joint paralysis (40). Relative contraindications would be a painless arthrodesis or a well-functioning resection arthroplasty (40).

Long-term results of TSA in RA have demonstrated good pain relief. Pain relief has lasting results, with 89% of patients showing good results at a mean of 7.7 years in one study (41). Another study reported 78% of patients with no or slight pain at a mean of 9.5 years (44). In both studies, there was significant improvement in range of motion compared to the preoperative state, but range of motion was not normal (41,44). The revision rate varies depending on implants and time of follow-up. A revision rate of 4% with predominately cemented prosthesis at 7.7 years was shown, versus 8% with a cementless humeral component and cemented glenoid at 9.5 years (41,44). The predominant cause of failure for TSA is glenoid loosening, with rates of 25% at 9.5 years to 40% at 7.7 years (41,44). Clearly, not all the shoulders required revision, which shows the ability of the patient to compensate with the other arm, ipsilateral wrist, and elbow.

Another important finding of long-term follow-up is the development of progressive proximal migration of the implant in 40% to 50% of patients (41,44). Proximal migration of the implant is directly related to the quality of the rotator cuff at the time of TSA. The consequence of proximal migration is a rocking effect on the eccentrically loaded glenoid component as the prosthetic humeral head moves upward away from the intended point of contact with the glenoid (41). The eccentric loading of the glenoid by the proximally migrated humeral head leads to loosening of the glenoid and possibly the humeral component as well (41,44).

There are several complications that can occur after TSA that require special surveillance (40,45). As with all TJA, infection is a serious complication, occurring in approximately 1% of cases (40,45). The treatment of this complication in TSA is not as thoroughly studied as in TKA or THA but usually requires a resection arthroplasty followed by a course of antibiotic therapy. Once removal of the implant is completed, the patient can be reimplanted or left without a shoulder prosthesis. Other complications of TSA include instability (1–2%), nerve injury (axillary nerve is most common), and recurrent rotator cuff tears leading to TSA proximal migration (40,45).

TOTAL ELBOW ARTHROPLASTY

As many as 50% of patients with RA will have elbow involvement (46). Nevertheless, TEA is not a common procedure, compared to other arthroplasties, such as THA and TKA (1,46). The lower incidence of TEA reflects the ability of the RA patient to accommodate for impaired elbow function. The main indication for surgery is incapacitating pain, which is not controlled effectively with medications. A relative indication would be a stiff elbow with a nonfunctional range of motion.

Unlike THA and TKA, there are two designs of TEA that can be broadly grouped under partially constrained unlinked and semiconstrained linked. The capitellocondylar TEA is an example of a partially constrained, unlinked TEA. The stability of the elbow relies on the integrity of the soft tissues, including the capsule, medial, and lateral collateral ligaments, for stability (46). The Coonrad-Morrey TEA is an example of the linked semiconstrained type of TEA. The link is a loose hinge that allows medial-lateral movement, which decreases the stress transferred to the implant bone interface and provides necessary stability (46).

Success with both types of TEA has been demonstrated. A study of capitellocondylar prostheses at 5.8 years reported 87% good results, with an aseptic revision rate of 1.5% and 5% radiographic loosening rate (47). Despite the overall satisfactory results, the patients in this series had a complication rate of 34%, which included minor wound problems, heterotopic bone formation, nerve injury, and stiffness. The Coonrad-Morrey TEA had 98% pain relief at 10 years, with 7.6% aseptic revision rate (48). The authors also had a high complication rate of 14%. Complication rates are high after TEA, compared to other TJAs. There are several reasons for a higher complication rate, including the relatively poor soft tissues in RA coupled with the already thin subcutaneous tissue over the elbow, the proximity of nerves and vessels, and usually poor bone stock (46). Infection rates run from 1% to 3% (46–48). Nerve palsies can occur after TEA, with the ulnar nerve being most vulnerable. It is not uncommon for the ulnar nerve to show signs of compression preoperatively and, thus, should be decompressed at the time of surgery (46). Triceps muscle avulsion is a serious complication, with surgical reattachment as soon as possible (46). Instability after surgery is a complication associated with the partially constrained unlinked TEA. Mechanical failure can occur with the linked semiconstrained TEA.

TOTAL ANKLE ARTHROPLASTY

Replacement of the ankle joint has proven more difficult to accomplish than the other joints discussed. Earlier designs had good results, initially; however, longer follow-up revealed unacceptable failure rates (49–51). Complications included infection, poor wound healing, and loosening (51). Failure of a TAA is a problem because salvage operations are extremely difficult. The alternative operation or salvage procedure in end-stage ankle disease is an ankle arthrodesis. This procedure is not without complications, including nonunion, malunion, and infection. Furthermore, fusion of the ankle can lead to arthrosis in the subtalar and midtarsal joints (49).

Improvements in the design of TAA have led to second-generation implants (Fig. 41.7). Uncemented implants are more

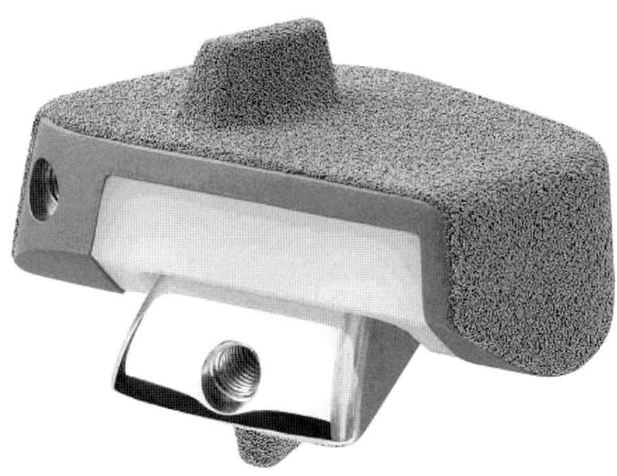

Figure 41.7. Total ankle arthroplasty. (Courtesy of DePuy Inc., a Johnson & Johnson company.)

commonly used because better results have been reported with cementless implants (49,52). The results of the newer implants are short-term but are improved (52), and longer follow-up is needed to evaluate their clinical utility.

CONCLUSION

For the rheumatoid patient with a painful stiff joint, TJA has been shown in many cases to be the best treatment option. There are many very exciting areas of ongoing development in TJA, including new bearing surfaces, new metals with improved bone fixation potential, bone conservation techniques, minimally invasive techniques, and revision techniques. Improved medical therapy of RA and the development of successful cartilage repair strategies may eventually have the largest impact by obviating the need for a TJA.

REFERENCES

1a. American Academy of Orthopaedic Surgeons website. http://www.AAOS.org. 2002. Accessed April 19, 2004.
1. Wolfe F, Zwillich S. The long-term outcomes of rheumatoid arthritis: a 23-year prospective, longitudinal study of total joint replacement and its predictors in 1,600 patients with rheumatoid arthritis. *Arthritis Rheum* 1998;416:1072–1082.
2. Stuchin SA, Johanson NA, Lachiewcz PF. Surgical management of inflammatory arthritis of the adult hip and knee. *Instr Course Lect* 1999;48:93–109.
3. Collins DN, Barnes Lowry C, FitzRandolph RL. Cervical spine instability in rheumatoid patients having total hip or knee arthroplasty. *Clin Orthop* 1991;272:127–135.
4. Takashima N, Kondo H, Kashtwazaki S. Suppressed serum erythropoietin response to anemia and the efficacy of recombinant erythropoietin in anemia of rheumatoid arthritis. *J Rheumatol* 1990;17:885–887.
5. Matsuda S, Kondo M, Mashima T, et al. Recombinant human erythropoietin therapy for autologous blood donation in rheumatoid arthritis patients undergoing total hip or knee arthroplasty. *Orthopedics* 2001;241:41–44.
6. Langenegger T, Michel BA. Drug treatment for rheumatoid arthritis. *Clin Orthop* 1999;366:22–30.
7a. Salem M, Tainsh RE Jr, Bromberg J, et al. Perioperative glucocorticoid coverage: a reassessment 42 years after emergence of a problem. *Ann Surg* 1994; 219:416–425.
7. Lane JM. Anti-inflammatory medications: selective COX-2 inhibitors. *J Am Acad Orthop Surg* 2002;10:75–78.
8. Carpenter MT, West SG, Vogelgesang SA, et al. Postoperative joint infections in rheumatoid arthritis patients on methotrexate therapy. *Orthopedics* 1996;193:207–210.
9. Perhala RS, Wilke WS, Clough JD, et al. Local infectious complications following large joint replacement in rheumatoid arthritis patients treated with methotrexate vs those not treated with methotrexate. *Arthritis Rheum* 1991; 34:146–152.
10. Grennan DM, Gray J, Loudon J, et al. Methotrexate and early postoperative complications in patients with rheumatoid arthritis undergoing elective orthopaedic surgery. *Ann Rheum Dis* 2001;603:214–217.
11. Moreland LW, Bucy RP, Weinblatt ME, et al. Immune function in patients with rheumatoid arthritis treated with etanercept. *Clin Immunol* 2002;103 (1):13–21.
12. Bogoch ER, Moran EL. Bone abnormalities in the surgical treatment of patients with rheumatoid arthritis. *Clin Orthop* 1999;366:8–21.
13. Hvid I. Trabecular bone strength at the knee. *Clin Orthop* 1998;227:210–221.
14. Yang JP, Bogoch ER, Woodside TD, et al. Stiffness of trabecular bone of the tibial plateau in patients with rheumatoid arthritis of the knee. *J Arthroplasty* 1997;12:798–803.
15. Chmell MJ, Scott RD. Total knee arthroplasty in patients with rheumatoid arthritis: an overview. *Clin Orthop* 1999;366:54–60.
16. Parvizi J, Sullivan T, Trousdale RT, et al. Thirty-day mortality after total knee arthroplasty. *J Bone Joint Surg Am* 2001;83-A8:1157–1161.
17. Neurath MF. Detection of loose bodies, spiraled collagen, dysplastic collagen, and intracellular collagen in rheumatoid connective tissues: an electron microscopic study. *Ann Rheum Dis* 1993;52:285–291.
18. Hagena FW, Hoffman GO, Mittlemeier T, et al. The cruciate ligaments in knee replacement. *Int Orthop* 1989;13:13–16.
19. Laskin R, O'Flynn H. Total knee replacement with posterior cruciate ligament retention in rheumatoid arthritis: problems and complications. *Clin Orthop* 1997;345:24–28.
20. Archibeck MJ, Berger RA, Barden R, et al. Posterior cruciate ligament-retaining total knee arthroplasty in patients with rheumatoid arthritis. *J Bone Joint Surg Am* 2001;83-A8:1231–1236.
21. Schai PA, Scott RD, Thornhill TS. Total knee arthroplasty with posterior cruciate retention in patients with rheumatoid arthritis. *Clin Orthop* 1999;367:96–106.
22. Weir DJ, Moran CG, Pinder IM. Kinematic condylar total knee arthroplasty: 14-year survivorship analysis of 208 consecutive cases. *J Bone Joint Surg Br* 1996;78-B6:907–911.
23. Rand JA, Ilstrup DM. Survivorship analysis of total knee arthroplasty. *J Bone Joint Surg Am* 1991;73-A(3):397–409.
24. Rodriguez JA, Saddler S, Edelman S, et al. Long-term results of total knee arthroplasty in class 3 and 4 rheumatoid arthritis. *J Arthroplasty* 1996;112: 141–145.
25. Elke R, Meier G, Warnke K, et al. Outcome analysis of total knee replacements in patients with rheumatoid arthritis versus osteoarthritis. *Arch Orthop Trauma Surg* 1995;114:330–334.
26. Scuderi GR, Insall JN, Windsor RE, et al. Survivorship of cemented knee replacement. *J Bone Joint Surg* 1989;71-B:798–803.
27. Kristensen O, Kjaergaard-Anderson P, Hvid I, et al. Long-term results of total condylar knee arthroplasty in rheumatoid arthritis. *J Bone Joint Surg* 1992;74B:803.
28. Laskin RS. Total condylar knee replacement in patients who have rheumatoid arthritis. *J Bone Joint Surg* 1990;72A:529.
29. Eberhardt K, Fex E, Johnsson K, et al. Hip involvement in early rheumatoid arthritis. *Ann Rheum Dis* 1995;54:45–48.
30. Creighton MG, Callaghan JJ, Olejniczak JP, et al. Total hip arthroplasty with cement in patients who have rheumatoid arthritis: a minimum ten-year follow-up study. *J Bone Joint Surg Am* 1998;80-A10:1439–1446.
31. Severt R, Wood R, Cracchiolo A, et al. Long-term follow-up of cemented total hip arthroplasty in rheumatoid arthritis. *Clin Orthop* 1991;265:137.
32. Unger AS, Inglis AE, Ranawat CS, et al. Total hip arthroplasty in rheumatoid arthritis: a long-term follow-up study. *J Arthroplasty* 1987;23:191–197.
33. Lachiewicz PF. Porous-coated total hip arthroplasty in rheumatoid arthritis. *J Arthroplasty* 1994;91:9–15.
34. Jana AK, Engh CA Jr, Lewandowski PJ, et al. Total hip arthroplasty using porous-coated femoral components in patients with rheumatoid arthritis. *J Bone Joint Surg Br* 2001;83-B5:686–690.
35. Chmell MJ, Scott RD, Thomas WH, et al. Total hip arthroplasty with cement for juvenile rheumatoid arthritis. *J Bone Joint Surg Am* 1997;79-A1:44–52.
36. Lehtimaki MY, Lehto MUK, Kautiainen H, et al. Survivorship of the Charnley total hip arthroplasty in juvenile chronic arthritis. *J Bone Joint Surg Br* 1997;79-B5:792–795.
37. Sochart DH, Porter ML. The long-term results of Charnley low friction arthroplasty in young patients who have congenital dislocation, degenerative osteoarthrosis, or rheumatoid arthritis. *J Bone Joint Surg Am* 1997;79-A:1599–1617.
38. Furnes O, Lie SA, Espehaug B, et al. Hip disease and the prognosis of total hip replacements: a review of 53,698 primary total hip replacements reported to the Norwegian Arthroplasty Register 1987–99. *J Bone Joint Surg Br* 2001;83-B4:579–586.
39. Parvizi J, Johnson BG, Rowland C, et al. Thirty-day mortality after elective total hip arthroplasty. *J Bone Joint Surg Am* 2001;83-A10:1524–1528.
40. Waldman BJ, Figgie MP. Indications, technique and results of total shoulder arthroplasty in rheumatoid arthritis. *Orthop Clin North Am* 1998;293: 435–444.
41. Sojbjerg JO, Frich LH, Johannsen HV, et al. Late results of total shoulder replacement in patients with rheumatoid arthritis. *Clin Orthop* 1999;366:39–45.
42. Bell SN, Gschwend N. Clinical experience with total shoulder and hemiarthroplasty of the shoulder using the Neer prosthesis. *Int Orthop* 1986;6104: 217–222.
43. Boyd AJ, Thomas WH, Scott RD. Total shoulder arthroplasty versus hemiarthroplasty. *J Arthroplasty* 1990;5:329–336.

44. Stewart MP, Kelly IG. Total shoulder replacement in rheumatoid disease: 7 to 13-year follow-up of 37 joints. *J Bone Joint Surg Br* 1997;79-B1:68–72.
45. Cofield RH. Degenerative and arthritic problems of the glenohumeral joint. In: Rockwood CA, Matsen FA III, eds. *The shoulder*. Philadelphia: WB Saunders, 1990:740–745.
46. Hargreaves D, Emery R. Total elbow replacement in the treatment of rheumatoid arthritis. *Clin Orthop* 1999;366:61–71.
47. Ewald FC, Simmons ED, Sullivan JA, et al. Capitellocondylar total elbow replacement in rheumatoid arthritis: long term results. *J Bone Joint Surg* 1993;75-A:498–507.
48. Gill DRJ, Morrey BF. The Coonrad-Morrey total elbow arthroplasty in patients who have rheumatoid arthritis: a 10-15 year follow-up study. *J Bone Joint Surg* 1998;80-A:1327–1335.
49. Saltzman CL. Total ankle arthroplasty: state of the art. *Instr Course Lect* 1999;48:263–268.
50. Kitaoka HB, Patzer GL. Clinical results of the Mayo total ankle arthroplasty. *J Bone Joint Surg Am* 1996;78-A:1658–1664.
51. Conti SF, Wong YS. Complications of total ankle replacement. *Clin Orthop* 2001;391:105–114.
52. Pyevich MT, Saltzman CL, Callaghan JJ, et al. Total ankle arthroplasty: a unique design: two to twelve-year follow-up. *J Bone Joint Surg Am* 1998;80A:1410–1420.

CHAPTER 42

Hand and Wrist Surgery

Philip E. Blazar, Peter D. Pardubsky, and Barry P. Simmons

The hand is the primary mode of physical interaction with our environment. Therefore, even minor alterations of the function of the hand and wrist resulting from rheumatoid arthritis (RA) can affect activities of daily life and the ability to function occupationally and recreationally. A multidisciplinary approach involving rheumatologist, hand surgeon, and hand therapist is advisable for the optimal care of patients with these disorders. Because delays in surgical and nonsurgical treatment may lead to further disease progression, joint destruction, and loss of function, early intervention is imperative. Both the initial evaluation of a patient's problem and its treatment are challenging because of the anatomic complexities of the hand and wrist. However, with a strong understanding of the relevant anatomy and a systematic approach to patient evaluation, a logical plan of treatment can be formulated.

PATIENT EVALUATION

A systematic framework, which divides the hand and wrist into four anatomic regions, should be followed in examining a deformed hand and wrist. First, the wrist should be evaluated for localized areas of pain, tenderness, and swelling indicative of synovitis or tenosynovitis. Changes in range of motion over time are important when evaluating disease progression. Next, the thumb joints, carpometacarpal (CMC), metacarpophalangeal (MCP), and interphalangeal (IP) joints are examined. Deformity and active and passive ranges of motion are all assessed. Third, the index through small fingers are evaluated for swelling, deformity, and range of motion at the MCP joint. Lastly, the proximal IP (PIP) and distal IP (DIP) joints are assessed for articular destruction and tendon imbalance.

NONSURGICAL TREATMENT

Rest, exercise, splinting, and corticosteroid injections play a critical role during early and late stages of the disease. Inflamed painful joints will commonly respond to rest with diminished acute synovitis. However, diseased joints require use to prevent worsening contractures, as active motion is needed to maintain tendon gliding and muscle tone. In general, short frequent periods of exercise are preferable to longer periods, which have the potential to aggravate the inflammation. A hand therapist is invaluable in achieving the appropriate balance between rest and exercise and monitoring the patient's activity.

Patients are commonly treated with resting and dynamic splints. Resting splints are effective in relieving pain, yet allow many functional activities. Dynamic splints provide slow constant stretching to help alleviate deformity.

Corticosteroid injections, which can lessen synovitis and tenosynovitis, are commonly used to treat carpal tunnel syndrome, extensor tenosynovitis, and individual joints with inflammation refractory to medical treatment. Although serious complications of injections are uncommon, tendon ruptures may be caused by frequent or repeated steroid administration. Steroid injections should, therefore, be limited to two or three times annually. Any joint or tendon sheath in the hand with synovitis prompting repeat steroid injection may benefit from surgical intervention.

SURGICAL REFERRAL

Referral to a hand surgeon is indicated for failure of nonsurgical treatment of any of the disorders discussed below. In particular, when mechanical and articular changes have progressed to substantial clinical deformities (e.g., ulnar deviation at the MCP joints), the biomechanical alterations will cause the deformity to progress even if the inflammatory process is halted. As discussed previously, recurrences of symptoms following a symptom-free interval after a corticosteroid injection or two suggest an ongoing inflammatory process. Commonly, the joint or tendon sheath involved may be a candidate for a surgical procedure. Certain scenarios are more time sensitive; patients with the sudden loss of the ability to flex or extend a digit typically have ruptured a tendon from infiltrative tenosynovitis. The urgency of this process is to protect other tendons at risk as the functional results worsen with a greater number of tendons involved. Continued pain, swelling, limited function, and progressive deformities despite medical therapy constitute the most common reasons for referral. In addition, patients are also increasingly referred when deformities have progressed to the point where self-image and social interactions are impaired more than overall hand function.

RHEUMATOID ARTHRITIS OF THE WRIST

RA of the wrist causes soft tissue, articular, and osseous destruction. Management of the rheumatoid wrist includes treatment of the distal radioulnar joint (DRUJ), radiocarpal and

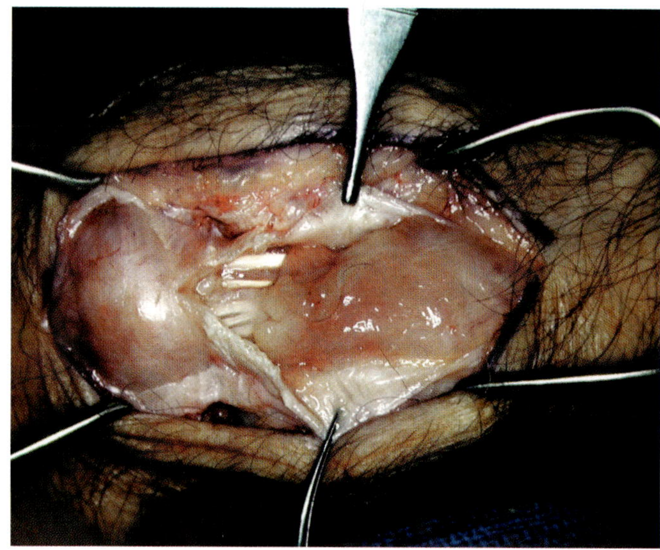

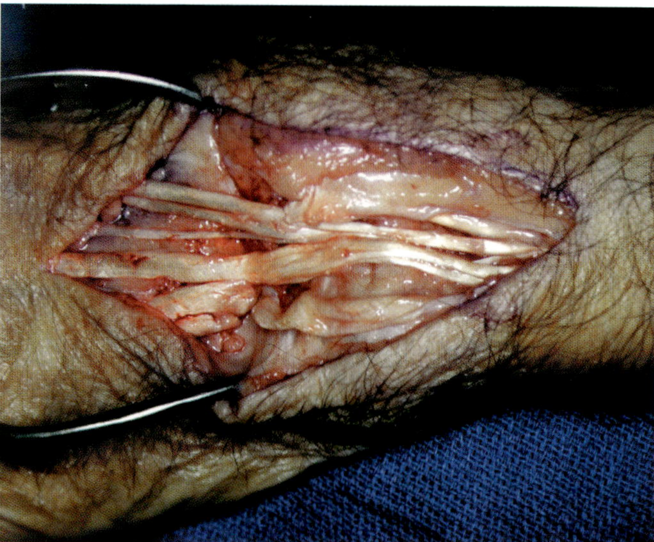

A B

Figure 42.1. A representative case of changes in chronic rheumatic extensor tenosynovitis. **A:** Note the prominent proliferative tenosynovium. **B:** After tenosynovectomy. Note the ruptured tendons.

ulnocarpal articulations, and flexor and extensor tendons for tenosynovitis, instability, and tendon rupture.

Tenosynovitis involving extensor and flexor tendons is a common finding in RA. Medical management is the primary treatment for persistent tenosynovitis. Surgical referral is appropriate for persistent tenosynovitis of more than 3 months that is refractory to medical therapy. Patients with DRUJ destruction are at particular risk for extensor tendon rupture from dorsal tenosynovitis. Surgical intervention for tenosynovitis is indicated when marked soft tissue swelling is present, indicating an active inflammatory process that has failed medical therapy over a period of 4 to 6 months (1–3). Immediate intervention is indicated when tendon rupture has occurred (3). Additional surgical indications include carpal tunnel syndrome secondary to tenosynovitis and decreased active motion with maintenance of passive motion (evidence of decreased tendon excursion secondary to tenosynovitis or invasion of the tendon). Immediate complete tenosynovectomy of the respective volar or dorsal compartments should be performed when a single flexor or extensor rupture has occurred (Fig. 42.1). The volar aspect of the wrist is the most frequent site of flexor tendon ruptures and should be aggressively treated with tenosynovectomy when diminished active motion is identified (6). Prevention of ruptures with aggressive tenosynovectomy is optimal, as functional restoration after chronic ruptures is difficult (6).

Flexor tenosynovectomy is performed with a longitudinal incision; care must be taken to avoid damage to the palmar cutaneous branch and motor branch of the median nerve. All flexor tendons are débrided of proliferative tissue, and the dorsal floor of the flexor compartment and carpal canal are débrided of remaining tenosynovium. The floor is inspected for osteophytes or capsular damage with communication of articular synovitis into the carpal canal. Osteophyte resection is performed where bone spurs could lead to tendon rupture (e.g., the Mannerfelt lesion).

Long-term results of flexor tenosynovectomy have revealed very low rates of recurrence or rupture, despite findings of tendon invasion by tenosynovium (4). Flexor tenosynovitis at the wrist must be differentiated from digital flexor tenosynovitis, which may require excision of the flexor digitorum superficialis (FDS) and recurs in up to 31% of hands at 4 years (5). Carpal tunnel release is performed with exposure of the flexor tendons at the wrist. Outcomes with surgical treatment of carpal tunnel syndrome in RA patients with more extensive volar incisions and flexor tenosynovectomy are similar to the excellent surgical outcomes in patients with primary carpal tunnel syndrome without inflammatory arthropathy (7).

Flexor tendon ruptures should be prevented but, nevertheless, can occur at the wrist level secondary to attrition, rather than overt tenosynovial invasion (6). When rupture occurs, function of an individual finger can be drastically reduced, and other tendons are at risk. Treatment depends on the number of tendons ruptured or attenuated, the extent of inflammation, and articular damage. Options include primary repair, repair with free tendon graft, two-stage repair with silicone rods, and arthrodesis of the joint affected with flexion loss, depending on associated pathologies (3). The surgical technique involves a volar approach with tenosynovectomy, identification of the level of rupture (most often at the carpal level), and reconstruction with a tendon transfer or tendon graft.

Extensor tenosynovitis is diagnosed earlier than flexor tenosynovitis because of the dorsal prominence and the obvious swelling about the tendons. Indications for extensor tenosynovectomy include rupture, failed medical management, or the need for other procedures using a dorsal wrist exposure. Sites of tendon attrition include Lister's tubercle and the DRUJ (Vaughn-Jackson lesion). Proliferative articular synovium from radiocarpal or radioulnar joints is excised with capsular closure where possible. With extensive DRUJ involvement, additional procedures may be necessary, as discussed later. Postoperative complications include skin slough and tendon adhesions, both caused by hematoma. Functional outcome after extensor tenosynovectomy is good, with very low recurrence rates (4,8).

Extensor tendon ruptures are diagnosed clinically by extensor lag at the MCP articulation. Extensor repair at the time of synovectomy is more successful than flexor repair, with the absence of marked retraction and a fibroosseous sheath and a plentiful supply of additional extensor tendons for transfer. Treatment of extensor tendon rupture is obtained with suturing of distal extensor tendons to adjacent tendons, transfer of redundant extensors (extensor indicis proprius or extensor digit quinti) when available, transfer of unused extensors (e.g., wrist extensors after wrist fusion or thumb extensors after distal thumb fusions), and FDS transfer or tendon graft (3,8,9).

Postoperative management after tenosynovectomy includes early motion when tendon repair is not performed. In cases requiring tendon repair, splinting to allow early passive excursion is used and individualized to the patient. Extensor tendon repair outcomes are good, although an increase in extension lags is observed when more tendons are involved (8,9).

Articular involvement of the wrist in RA includes proliferative synovitis at both the radiocarpal and DRUJ articulations, leading to osseous destruction, ulnar translocation of the carpus, and pain. Early radiographic evidence includes erosion at the ulnar styloid base, scalloping of the ulnar aspect of the radius at the DRUJ, ulnar head prominence as triangular fibrocartilage destruction occurs with pannus erosion, and scaphoid waist erosion (1). Natural progression includes extensor carpi ulnaris subluxation volarly with carpus supination and radial deviation, scaphoid flexion with radioscaphocapitate ligament attrition, volar ulnar carpus subluxation, dorsal distal ulna prominence (caput ulna syndrome), and eventual radial deviation of the metacarpals (1,10). Early procedures for RA address the inflammatory process in an effort to prevent joint destruction and deformity, whereas later procedures are reconstructive.

Synovectomy of the radiocarpal and ulnocarpal joints is indicated when pain persists despite medical therapy, and joint destruction is minimal. Articular synovectomy is often performed in conjunction with tenosynovectomy. The wrist is splinted for 3 weeks, followed by active range of motion exercises. The DRUJ capsule can be treated with synovectomy as well; however, complete synovectomy of the DRUJ is difficult, unless significant instability exists. The distal radioulnar ligaments must be preserved to prevent DRUJ instability and may require reconstruction. Although motion may be lost with synovectomy and subsequent capsular scarring, 95% of patients had excellent pain relief in one study, with a mean of 7 years' follow-up (11). Arthroscopic synovectomy in RA has been used with limited short-term studies showing improved grip strength, motion, and 50% reduction in pain at 6 months (12). In a study with a mean follow-up of 3.8 years after arthroscopy, pain was significantly reduced, and radiographic progression of disease was slowed in patients with no or very early radiographic changes at the time of arthroscopy. Motion was not improved, however, and no change was observed in long-term destruction of the wrist (13).

When progressive carpal subluxation or destruction occurs, simple synovectomy is no longer sufficient for pain relief or restoration of function. Arthrodesis or arthroplasty constitute the operative options for treatment of the painful degenerative wrist in RA. Surgical goals include pain relief, restoration of function, prevention of further disease, and cosmesis.

Arthrodesis eliminates pain, limits motion without further upper extremity disability, places the wrist in a durable and functional position, and allows use of ambulatory aids but diminishes dexterity. RA patients with extensive osseous destruction, young age, or high demand on their wrists are candidates for arthrodesis. Many techniques of arthrodesis have been described using various forms of internal fixation and external immobilization (15–19). Surgical technique involves a dorsal approach similar to tenosynovectomy with appropriate soft tissue procedures when indicated. Postoperative management calls for active and passive finger motion to prevent tendon adhesion and cast immobilization of the radiocarpal articulation pending radiographic evidence of fusion, which occurs between 4 and 10 weeks.

Total wrist fusion in neutral to mild extension and slight ulnar deviation provided satisfactory pain relief without sensory or motor deficits in the hand and no additional upper limb functional loss in one study, with a mean follow-up of 7 years (20). Fusion is strongly advocated for those RA patients who depend on upper extremity use for ambulating with assistive devices (21). In patients with radiocarpal changes or mild ulnar translocation of the carpus but preservation of the midcarpal articulation, an isolated radiolunate arthrodesis can be performed to prevent volar subluxation of the carpus and maintain some wrist motion (22). Five-year follow-up of radiolunate fusion revealed a high frequency of midcarpal changes and a 15% incidence of pain, with 50% reduced motion (23). Patients must be properly selected for a limited arthrodesis. This procedure cannot be used to correct a significant radiocarpal deformity (ulnar translation, volar dislocation) because of the high incidence of midcarpal changes that occur postoperatively (23).

Although arthroplasty of the wrist maintains motion, the durability of these procedures has not been established with long-term studies. Surgical technique uses a dorsal exposure of the wrist, as described for synovectomy or arthrodesis. Indications for wrist arthroplasty include extensive radiocarpal degenerative changes, diminished function, or bilateral wrist involvement in less physically active RA patients. Modern implant arthroplasty began with silastic implants, although the longevity of the implant has limited its use (27). Silicone synovitis, implant fracture, and recurrent pain occur in up to 50% of patients at 5-year follow-up (28–30). Arthrodesis has a lower complication rate and improved outcome, compared with silicone arthroplasty (21). Limited success with silastic implants has driven the design of improved wrist implants.

Several designs for total wrist arthroplasty exist and vary in the extent of constraint and technique for fixation (cemented vs. uncemented with screw fixation). Surgical technique uses a dorsal approach with differing amounts of carpal bone resection, depending on implant design. Postoperative management depends on the patient and implant but typically involves splinting for 2 to 6 weeks, depending on stability of the wrist; most patients return to full activity within 3 months. Reoperation rates range from 14% to 33%, with complication rates as high as 32% and failure of the implant as high as 44% (31–35). Total wrist arthroplasty preserves motion and leads to pain relief but has risks of early failure of the prosthesis and dislocation. Future design modifications may provide improved function and durability over current designs.

The DRUJ is an integral part of the wrist and is essential to pain-free forearm rotation. This joint is frequently involved in RA of the wrist with extensor carpi ulnaris instability, progressive volar and ulnar carpus subluxation, and dorsal ulna subluxation or dislocation (39,40). Treatment of the DRUJ in RA frequently accompanies soft tissue procedures on the dorsal aspect of the wrist. Indications for surgical intervention include failure of 3 to 6 months of medical therapy for obvious synovitis, persistent pain with forearm rotation, or clinical instability.

Many procedures are available for distal ulna resection and differ based on the amount of bone resected and the soft tissue reconstruction (39). Distal ulna resection (Darrach procedure) is performed through a dorsal exposure with elevation of the extensor retinaculum from the ulnar aspect of the wrist. The distal portion of the ulna is subperiosteally excised. Outcome studies demonstrate 77% to 86% pain relief, depending on the level of activity (43,45).

THUMB DEFORMITY

Thumb deformity is found in up to 66% of patients with RA. Despite obvious pathology, not all deformed thumbs are symptomatic (67). Most deformities of the thumb consist of a boutonnière or swan-neck deformity, resulting in a zig-zag appearance. The deformities have been categorized into six types based on the deformity of the digit at the IP, MCP, and CMC joints (68,69). Type I deformity is most common, occurring in 70% of rheumatoid thumb deformities, and is a boutonnière deformity with

MCP flexion and IP extension (70). A type II deformity is a boutonnière deformity with thumb adduction and CMC subluxation. Type III is the second most common deformity and is characterized by a swan-neck deformity, MCP hyperextension, and IP flexion with CMC subluxation. A type IV deformity is radial deviation of the thumb MCP due to ulnar collateral ligament (UCL) attenuation. A type V deformity is a swan-neck deformity without associated CMC pathology. Finally, a type VI deformity is arthritis mutilans with destruction of all three joints and loss of longitudinal support due to phalangeal and metacarpal erosions.

Synovitis, extensor pollicis brevis attrition or rupture, and extensor pollicis longus subluxation or rupture can produce the MCP flexion deformity of a boutonnière. IP pathology may be responsible for a boutonnière deformity and includes flexor pollicis longus rupture (Mannerfelt lesion) or IP hyperextension from synovitis with volar plate attrition. If the deformity can be passively corrected, soft tissue procedures can be used for treatment. Arthrodesis or arthroplasty are used for treatment of fixed deformities. The MCP is addressed initially as this joint or surrounding extensor tendon apparatus is frequently involved. Mobile MCP deformities can be treated with synovectomy followed by extensor pollicis brevis reconstruction with extensor pollicis longus rerouting. Soft tissue procedures are complicated by frequent recurrence of the deformity in 13% to 64% of patients (70,72). Soft tissue procedures for boutonnière deformity in the rheumatoid thumb can be performed when there is a mobile deformity without underlying joint destruction and good medical control of the inflammatory process.

Arthrodesis and arthroplasty are options for treating fixed deformities or mobile deformities with underlying joint destruction. With the exception of arthritis mutilans, arthrodesis of all three joints (IP, MCP, and CMC) is contraindicated. If the CMC is preserved, both the IP and MCP can be fused and provide a stable thumb post with improved pinch strength (75). Arthrodesis is indicated in patients with fixed MCP deformities or severe MCP joint destruction (75,77). IP fusion is performed in extension and stabilized with K wires or screws (70). Postoperative splinting is maintained for 6 weeks or until radiographic evidence of union has occurred. In a comparison of MCP arthrodesis with MCP synovectomy, Inglis et al. determined arthrodesis predictably relieves pain and provides thumb function, but, relative to arthrodesis, synovectomy has a 50% reduced incidence of CMC degeneration and IP hyperextension (75). However, synovectomy is only indicated in patients with a normal MCP articular surface and passively correctable deformity. Complications of arthrodesis include symptomatic hardware, CMC degeneration, and nonunion (70). Incidence of nonunion is 20% at the MCP and 15% at the IP; however, only a minority of nonunions are symptomatic (74).

Arthroplasty at the thumb MCP is indicated with CMC ankylosis or severely compromised IP and CMC articulations. Maintenance of one mobile joint optimizes function in an older, less physically active patient. Postoperative immobilization of the MCP lasts 4 weeks with progression to gradual motion under therapy guidance. Terrano et al. accepts up to 30 degrees of ulnar instability, as this improves function of the thumb with a compromised CMC (74). In this series, 23% of patients experienced IP instability, which suggests the need for IP arthrodesis simultaneously with MCP arthroplasty (74).

Type II deformity is similar to type I boutonnière deformity but includes CMC subluxation. CMC arthroplasty is commonly chosen for treating this problem (discussed below); however, the adduction contracture of type II deformity requires soft tissue release (78). MCP and IP procedures are then selected based on criteria previously described for boutonnière deformities.

Arthrodesis for type VI deformity (arthritis mutilans) requires additional considerations. Bone graft is often needed for longitudinal support at the IP and MCP because of extensive bone destruction. CMC arthrodesis is rarely needed, as ankylosis is common, and any limited motion is beneficial, provided it is pain free. Functional improvement in an opera glass hand (arthritis mutilans resulting in shortening of the rays with skin redundancy but correctable length with traction) with arthrodesis has been well documented (71,76).

Treatment of the swan-neck deformity of type III thumbs is indicated for instability or pain after failed steroid injections or 2- to 6-month course of spica splinting. CMC treatment is the first step in treating this multiple joint deformity with subsequent treatment of residual deformity at the MCP and IP. Motion is maintained at the CMC, with interposition arthroplasty as described by Burton and Pellegrini (78). Postoperative management includes spica splinting for 6 weeks progressing to motion and grip strengthening with therapy guidance. Eaton et al. and Tomaino et al. have described excellent pain relief and function using interposition arthroplasty in osteoarthritic CMC joints in separate series (79,80). Reports on patients with RA have demonstrated excellent pain relief, with lesser gains in grip strength than patients with osteoarthritis. This has been attributed to the diffuse arthropathy involving the entire hand in RA (81).

Once the CMC has been addressed in swan-neck thumbs, attention is turned to the hyperextended MCP. Many mild deformities can be treated with splinting after CMC arthroplasty (80). However, passively correctable MCP joints with substantial deformity but without extensive joint destruction can be stabilized from hyperextended positions using soft tissue procedures. In cases with extensive MCP destruction or fixed deformity, arthrodesis is performed.

Type IV deformities secondary to UCL attrition require UCL repair or reconstruction. MCP joints without fixed radial deformity, maintained articular surfaces, and no deformity of flexion or extension are treated with capsulotomy, synovectomy, and advancement of the UCL distally into the proximal phalanx, preventing radial deviation secondary to ligamentous laxity (71). Mild persistent UCL laxity may improve thumb function when other joints are ankylosed (75).

The two most common deformities of the thumb in RA are the boutonnière deformity involving MCP flexion and IP hyperextension and the swan-neck deformity with CMC dorsoradial subluxation and MCP hyperextension. Indications for surgical intervention include a painful or dysfunctional thumb that has failed conservative management with splinting or steroid injection over a 4-month period. Surgical treatment depends on the extent of articular degeneration. Arthrodesis of the MCP and IP joints is performed for rigid or in the presence of extensive degeneration. Soft tissue realignment and synovectomy are appropriate in passively correctable joints with preserved articular surfaces. In less physically active patients, an MCP arthroplasty will allow some maintained motion in the thumb ray. CMC treatment is with ligament reconstruction and interposition arthroplasty. Overall function of the thumb is predictably improved in patients treated with arthrodesis, although increasing incidence of proximal and distal joint degeneration about the arthrodesed MCP occurs. Soft tissue procedures are limited in success and must be used in carefully selected patients.

FINGER METACARPOPHALANGEAL JOINTS

The normal MCP joints are a single condylar joint allowing 90 degrees of flexion. They play an important role for positioning the fingers; loss of motion or poor position can severely compromise hand function. The extensor tendons are immediately dorsal to the MCP joints and stretching or attenuation of the supporting attachments of the tendon from chronic synovitis leads to subluxation of the tendon ulnarly. The MCP joint is the most common site in the upper extremity of involvement of RA. The capsular laxity of the MCP joints that allows radial and ulnar deviation, as well as flexion–extension motion, makes subluxation and dislocation common sequela of synovitis. When capsular laxity is combined with extensor subluxation, joint deformity progresses to a fixed volarly subluxated proximal phalanx with ulnar deviation. Attempts at finger extension lead to ulnar deviation. Additional ulnar deviation forces come from deformity of the wrist and tenosynovitis of the flexor tendons resulting in ulnar displacement of the flexors. With progressive subluxation, the radial-sided structures stretch, and the ulnar ligaments and intrinsic muscles shorten. The fixed flexion deformities interfere with opening the hand to grasp large objects and fine manipulation of objects between the index and long fingers and the thumb.

Surgical Indications

The general indications for MCP joint surgery are pain, deformity, and loss of function refractory to medical measures.

Clinical Assessment

Evaluation of a patient with RA of the MCP joints requires an assessment of the global function of the extremity and, in particular, the deformities of the adjacent joints. Progressive deformity of the wrist, in particular, may predispose MCP arthroplasty to early recurrent ulnar deviation. The long flexor and extensor tendons should be evaluated for synovitis and the potential for rupture. Changes in the PIP joints have substantial effects on global hand function and, therefore, the ultimate success of any MCP procedure. Surgical intervention for these joints is frequently performed at the same time as MCP arthroplasty. Involvement of the thumb may need to be addressed concurrently or at a separate surgery if deformity is substantial (50,60,61).

Deformity of the MCP joint has been classified in stages (50). Treatment and surgical indications vary with the stage of disease. Stage I disease shows MCP synovitis, the ability to fully extend the joint, and little ulnar deviation or articular changes. Typically, patients are managed medically for the synovitis, with splinting or corticosteroid injection for symptomatic relief. Night splints that hold the MCP joints in extension and correct ulnar deviation are frequently used.

Stage II is marked by the development of early erosions but with preservation of cartilage space. Pain is generally the chief complaint. The extensor tendons show a tendency to move toward the web spaces. An extensor lag commonly exists, but flexion is well preserved. Clinical intervention focuses on maximizing medical management. Surgical intervention is infrequently performed in this setting, but synovectomy and extensor tendon balancing in patients with well-preserved joint spaces is occasionally indicated. Synovectomy does not alter the long-term prognosis of the disease but is widely accepted for alleviating local symptoms.

Stage III disease is characterized by advancement in joint destruction and an increase in the deformity. Stage III patients frequently have substantial PIP disease. Surgery is indicated at this stage for patients with substantial pain and functional loss.

Stage IV disease is marked by fixed subluxation and destruction as seen on radiographs. MCP arthroplasty and extensor tendon realignment is the treatment of choice at this stage. However, in a young patient with a functional range of motion of the MCP joint (an active arc of motion of 60–70 degrees), the surgeon must determine whether surgical intervention is indicated, as there is unlikely to be functional improvement. Pain and deformity are reliably improved. Examination of the wrist and PIP joints must be performed, as changes in these areas are more common with advanced disease and may need to be surgically addressed before performing an MCP arthroplasty (50,60).

The silastic implants used in MCP arthroplasty function differently than those used in the more common large joint replacements. MCP silastic arthroplasties are not fixed to the skeleton, and patients have motion between the implant and the bones, as well as within the implant. Attempts at engineering MCP arthroplasties similar to larger joint replacements continue, but they are not widely accepted at this time.

The traditional postoperative therapy protocol begins within 1 week of surgery; the patient is fitted with a dynamic splint holding the MCP joints in extension and neutral to radial deviation. A static resting splint is also fabricated. The patient is encouraged to actively flex the MCP joints in a controlled fashion to protect the extensor realignment and prevent prosthetic dislocation. The patient is weaned from the dynamic splint at 6 weeks, but static splinting is continued at night for 3 to 4 months (60,62).

Patterson et al. have used an alternative therapy protocol (83). The patients are placed in a hand-based cast with the MCP joints in extension and 10 to 15 degrees of radial deviation. The wrist and distal joints are left free. The cast is removed at 5 weeks, and the patients begin a therapy program of active and passive motion with a static nighttime splint for an additional 6 weeks.

The results of MCP arthroplasty discussed in the literature include range of motion, ulnar deviation, pain relief, and patient satisfaction. Realistic expectations are important to discuss with patients, as the arthroplasties do not achieve a full range of MCP motion. The arc of motion will be in a more functional position but, commonly, is not increased. Numerous factors have been identified as affecting the ultimate result, including the strength and stability of the controlling muscles, the status of adjacent joints, and the use of postoperative therapy. Commonly reported results include realigning ulnar drift to less than 10 degrees, predictable pain relief, and a 30- to 60-degree arc of active motion (53,56–58).

The patient's subjective appraisal of outcome has been investigated for its relationship to deformity, strength, range of motion, pain relief, and other traditional parameters of success. The strongest determinant of patient satisfaction was with appearance and correction of deformity (Fig. 42.2). Pain relief was also found to be important, but the other traditionally examined parameters

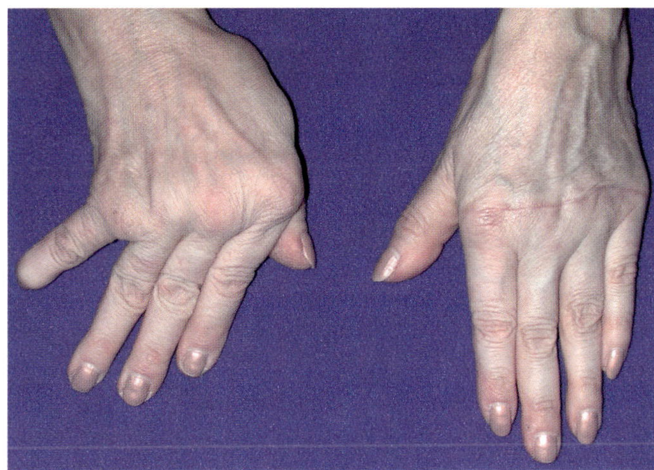

Figure 42.2. The typical appearance of rheumatoid metacarpophalangeal deformities. Both hands had similar deformities before surgery. The left is 6 months postoperative silastic metacarpophalangeal arthroplasties.

(motion, strength, etc.) were not found to have a statistical correlation (84). Correction within a few degrees of neutral is reported in most series. Recurrent ulnar drift has been reported in up to 43% of patients; however, the recurrent deformities reported are less than 20 to 25 degrees in most series (48,49,51–54,62).

Clinical experience suggests that pain relief has consistently been achieved, although this has been examined in follow-up studies infrequently. Kirschenbaum et al. reported that of 144 arthroplasties in 36 hands, none of the patients complained of pain (54). Beckenbaugh reported recurrence of pain in 2% of patients (49).

Silicone rubber MCP joint implants generally have a low rate of complications (48–54,62). Extensive changes in the bone surrounding the implant are found in 4% of silicone rubber implants (53). Implant fracture rates vary from 0% to 38% and may depend on how extensively the investigator looks for evidence of fracture (48–52). The majority of patients with fractured implants have acceptable function and do not require revision. The low morbidity of fractured prosthesis has been related to the function of the implant as a spacer, rather than as an articulated prosthesis (48–52,62).

In a metaanalysis, Foliart noted infection in 0.6% of reported implants (53). All of the infection in a series described by Millender presented within 8 weeks of implantation (57). *Staphylococcus aureus* was the most common organism isolated, and most of the infected prostheses ultimately required removal and an average of 2 weeks of intravenous antibiotic treatment (57).

Particulate synovitis and silicone-induced lymphadenopathy have received substantial attention. Foliart recorded both of these complications in less than 0.1% of reported cases (53). Synovitis in MCP implants occurred almost exclusively in fractured implants or implants with substantial signs of wear at removal. Non-Hodgkin's lymphoma has been reported in four patients with lymphadenopathy, although the relationship is unclear, given the increased incidence of lymphoma in this population.

DIGITS

Problems in the ulnar four digits in RA may originate with the flexor tendons (tenosynovitis), an imbalance between the flexor, extensor, and intrinsic tendons (boutonnière and swan-neck deformities), or the PIP and DIP joints proper. Many patients have digital pathology that is multifactorial (most boutonnières in RA present with some degree of articular destruction). They will be considered separately for clarity.

Flexor Tenosynovitis

The hypertrophied tenosynovium (synovial lining of the flexor tendons) in rheumatoid digits results in three important clinical entities. Tenosynovitis may present with painful triggering (stenosing tenosynovitis), loss of active motion with preserved passive motion (digital tenosynovitis), or flexor tendon rupture. These latter two processes can commonly be differentiated, as tenosynovitis without rupture will typically demonstrate some active function of the involved tendon, whereas rupture will not.

Palmar stenosing tenosynovitis (trigger finger) occurs when proliferation of the tenosynovium results in a mechanical block to smooth gliding of the flexor tendons within the tendon sheath. Commonly, patients can actively flex the involved digit(s), but the synovial nodule catches on the A1 pulley with extension. The digit may be locked in flexion and unable to be actively extended. Passive extension occurs with a painful snap as the nodule is brought into the sheath. Tenosynovitis along the tendon may result in crepitation throughout the arc of motion.

Treatment begins with medical management of the disease process. For patients with substantial pain or symptoms refractory to appropriate medical management, corticosteroid injection into the flexor sheath is very effective. Surgical intervention (palmar tenosynovectomy with or without division of the A1 pulley region of the flexor sheath) is indicated for failure to improve after injection or recurrence of symptoms after one or two injections (1,2). Tenosynovectomy may also be indicated to maximize functional recovery concurrently with another procedure on the same hand.

Digital flexor tenosynovitis is due to proliferation of tenosynovium within the finger. The tenosynovium within the sheath blocks full active flexion of the digits. Some active flexion is preserved, and, commonly, patients present with preserved passive flexion. Crepitation is common, as in palmar tenosynovitis, but locking is less common. A mobile fullness within the finger can be seen or felt. Stiffness of the IP joints can accompany flexor tenosynovitis. This may occur secondarily to the tenosynovitis, limiting motion of the digit, or may occur from disease intrinsic to the joints themselves.

Treatment consists of injection of corticosteroid within the flexor sheath. Surgical intervention is indicated for failure of relief or recurrence of the problem after injection (2). Associated PIP joint stiffness may need to be addressed at the same time (4). Manipulation or release of the PIP joint followed by aggressive postoperative hand therapy can restore substantial active and passive motion (5).

Flexor tendon rupture can occur within the carpal canal, palm, or digit (6). The most common site is within the carpal canal (discussed earlier). Rupture of flexor tendons in the digit is less common, as patients with substantial inflammatory changes in the digit commonly present earlier as trigger digits.

Tendon rupture is a strong indication for tenosynovectomy (1–3,6). Removal of the cause (tenosynovectomy or removal of bony protrusions) is performed to prevent damage to other tendons. In the thumb, if the IP joint is diseased, arthrodesis may be preferable. If a rupture of one tendon within a finger occurs, prompt tenosynovectomy to protect the other tendon is indicated. If both tendons are ruptured, both DIP and PIP flexion will be lost. The results of tendon grafting in this situation are often disappointing. In patients with substantial joint deformity, PIP and DIP arthrodeses in a position of function are typically recommended.

Boutonnière Deformity

A finger with flexion of the PIP joint and hyperextension of the DIP joint has a boutonnière deformity (Fig. 42.3). The cause is synovitis of the PIP joint with attenuation of the central slip of the extensor mechanism. The lateral bands of the extensor mechanism move laterally and palmarly and change from extensors of the PIP joint to flexors. The resulting traction on the terminal extensor tendon hyperextends the DIP joint. Early boutonnière deformities are passively correctable, but, with time, the palmar structures contract, and the deformity becomes fixed.

Treatment of boutonnière deformity depends on the flexibility of the deformity and the status of the articular structures. Passively correctable and small fixed boutonnière deformities and well-preserved joints are managed medically. Nighttime splinting is used to maintain passive extension. Synovectomy and mobilization of the lateral bands into a dorsal position can be considered as the deformity progresses; however, loss of flexion at both the PIP and DIP can result. A terminal tenotomy may be required if the DIP joint is fixed in hyperextension. If the deformity has progressed to more than 50 degrees of fixed PIP flexion or the joint shows substantial deterioration, arthrodesis of the PIP joint is the procedure of choice. Arthroplasty is con-

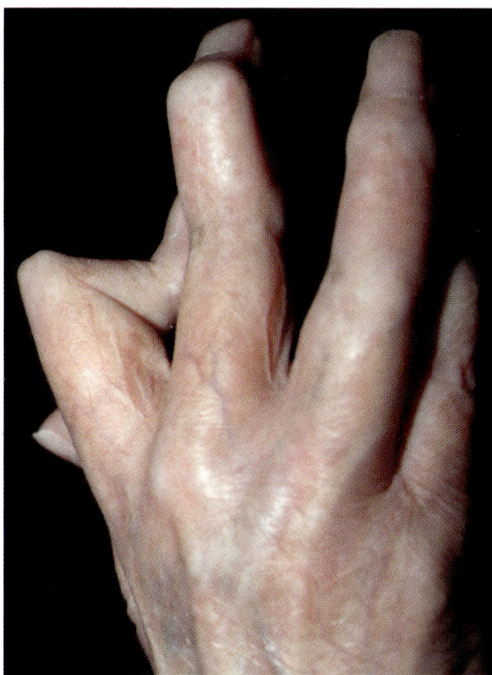

Figure 42.3. Rheumatoid arthritis finger deformities. The index finger has a severe boutonnière deformity, and the middle finger has a swan-neck deformity.

sidered when there is substantial articular destruction but the fixed flexion deformity is milder (1,85).

Swan-Neck Deformity

A swan-neck deformity is caused by synovitis leading to soft tissue attenuation; however, the primary structures involved are the restraints to hyperextension at the PIP joint. Along with PIP hyperextension, DIP flexion occurs secondary to the more proximal changes or imbalance between the flexor and extensor forces (Fig. 42.3). Fixed MCP flexion deformities contribute to the development of PIP hyperextension and swan-neck deformity. In the setting of MCP flexion and swan-neck deformity, correction of the more proximal deformity is required, typically with MCP arthroplasty, or the PIP hyperextension will recur (49,53,85).

Mild swan-neck deformity may lead to minimal functional changes and is well tolerated. As the deformity progresses, the lateral bands subluxate centrally, and patients may have a popping sensation as the tendons relocate with PIP flexion. This can be eliminated with the use of a splint that blocks hyperextension of the PIP joint. If the patient's symptoms are eliminated but the patient is unable or unwilling to consider chronic splinting, a block to PIP hyperextension can be created surgically using one slip of the FDS tendon (FDS tenodesis). If the deformity is fixed but adequate articular cartilage remains, the joint can be manipulated into flexion and held with a percutaneous K wire for 3 weeks. Joint manipulation is commonly done at the time of MCP arthroplasty and requires a relaxing incision over the dorsum of the digit that heals by secondary intention (1,85). Depending on the degree of flexion obtained with manipulation, surgical release of the lateral bands from the central extensor tendon is used if the extensor is blocking PIP flexion (85).

When a swan-neck deformity exists and the joint surfaces show substantial destruction, the options of PIP arthrodesis and arthroplasty may also be considered (86). In addition, PIP joints can also be manipulated into flexion and allowed to stiffen in that position.

The PIP joints are a hinge joint normally allowing 110 degrees of motion. Motion of the PIP joint is central to the act of the hand encompassing objects. For disease at the PIP joint, the surgical options include arthrodesis and arthroplasty. Arthroplasty of the PIP joints most commonly use silastic implants analogous to the MCP joints. In general, the results of PIP arthroplasty are better for patients with swan-neck deformity than for boutonnière deformity (86,87). Long-term follow-up studies have not shown improvement in motion, but pain relief has been predictable (86,87). Because of the limited motion achieved and problems with stability, many authors favor arthrodesis. Arthroplasties using prostheses analogous to larger joint replacements are currently under investigation but have not demonstrated conclusive advantages at this time. In the index finger, the need for stability typically steers surgical intervention to arthrodesis (1). The advantage of PIP flexion for encompassment and powerful grasp becomes more pronounced with the ulnar digits, and arthroplasty is more likely to be performed in these digits than in the index finger. The position chosen for arthrodesis of the ring and small fingers is in more flexion than the radial digits.

The DIP joints also function as hinge joints. Normal motion is 60 to 70 degrees of flexion. The collateral ligaments confer stability to lateral stress, and the volar plate and flexor digitorum profundus tendon resist hyperextension stress. The terminal extensor tendon that attaches to the bases of the distal phalanges provides extension. Joint destruction is typically treated with arthrodesis if medical management of symptoms is not adequate. Although arthroplasty can be performed, it is less durable than an arthrodesis, and the added functional gain is minimal, except in highly selected cases.

Arthrodesis is performed with the digit in slight (0 to 10 degrees) flexion. This results in a near-normal appearance with the digits extended, and the lack of flexion is rarely of functional significance. This position enhances pinch between the pulp of the finger(s) and thumb that is more functional than tip-to-tip pinch (88).

Fusion at the DIP level may also help digital deformities. Alignment in a neutral position can balance flexor and extensor forces that can be disrupted in RA, leading to digital deformities. For example, a mild swan-neck deformity (PIP hyperextension, DIP flexion) may be secondary to attenuation of the terminal extensor tendon and can be improved by DIP arthrodesis (1).

REFERENCES

1. Feldon P, Terrano AL, Nalebuff EA, et al. Rheumatoid arthritis and other connective tissue diseases. In: Green DP, Hotchkiss RN, Pederson WC, eds. *Green's operative hand surgery*, 4th ed. Philadelphia: Churchill Livingstone, 1999:1651–1737.
2. Nalebuff EA. Surgical treatment of rheumatoid tenosynovitis in the hand. *Surg Clin North Am* 1969;49:799–810.
3. Nalebuff EA. Surgical treatment of tendon rupture in the rheumatoid hand. *Surg Clin North Am* 1969;49:811–822.
4. Brown FE, Brown ML. Long-term results after tenosynovectomy to treat the rheumatoid hand. *J Hand Surg* 1988;13A:704–708.
5. Wheen DJ, Tonkin MA, Green J, et al. Long-term results following digital flexor tenosynovectomy in rheumatoid arthritis. *J Hand Surg* 1995;20A:790–794.
6. Ertel AN, Millender LH, Nalebuff E, et al. Flexor tendon ruptures in patients with rheumatoid arthritis. *J Hand Surg* 1988;13A:860–866.
7. Katz JN, Keller RB, Simmons BP, et al. Maine carpal tunnel study: outcomes of operative and nonoperative therapy for carpal tunnel syndrome in a community based cohort. *J Hand Surg* 1998;23A:697–710.
8. Millender LH, Nalebuff EA, Albin R, et al. Dorsal tenosynovectomy and tendon transfer in the rheumatoid hand. *J Bone Joint Surg* 1974;56A:601–610.
9. Bora FW, Osterman AL, Thomas VJ, et al. The treatment of ruptures of multiple extensor tendons at wrist level by a free tendon graft in the rheumatoid patient. *J Hand Surg* 1987;12A:1038–1040.
10. Backdahl M. The caput ulnae syndrome in rheumatoid arthritis. A study of the morphology, abnormal anatomy, and clinical picture. *Acta Rheumatol Scan* 1963;5:1–75.
11. Thirupathy RG, Ferlic DC, Clayton ML. Dorsal wrist synovectomy in rheumatoid arthritis: a long-term study. *J Hand Surg* 1983;8:848–856.
12. Adolfsson L, Nylander G. Arthroscopic synovectomy of the rheumatoid wrist. *J Hand Surg* 1993;18B:92–96.

13. Adolfsson L, Frisen M. Arthroscopic synovectomy of the rheumatoid wrist. A 3.8 year follow-up. *J Hand Surg* 1997;22B:711–713.
14. Reference deleted.
15. Haddad RJ, Riordan DC. Arthrodesis of the wrist. A surgical technique. *J Bone Joint Surg* 1967;49A:950–954.
16. Louis DS, Hankin FM. Arthrodesis of the wrist: past and present. *J Hand Surg* 1986;11A:787–789.
17. Clendenin MB, Green DP. Arthrodesis of the wrist—complications and their management. *J Hand Surg* 1981;6:253–257.
18. Rehak DC, Hagberg WC, Kasper P, et al. A comparison of plate and pin fixation for arthrodesis of the rheumatoid wrist. *Orthopedics* 2000;23:43–48.
19. Zachary SV, Stern PJ. Complications following AO/ASIF wrist arthrodesis. *J Hand Surg* 1995;20A:339–344.
20. Barbier O, Saels P, Rombouts JJ, et al. Long-term functional results of wrist arthrodesis in rheumatoid arthritis. *J Hand Surg* 1999;24B:27–31.
21. Vicar AJ, Burton RI. Surgical management of the rheumatoid wrist—fusion or arthroplasty. *J Hand Surg* 1986;11A:790–797.
22. Linscheid RL, Dobyns JH. Radiolunate arthrodesis. *J Hand Surg* 1985;10A:821–829.
23. Borisch N, Haussmann P. Radiolunate arthrodesis in the rheumatoid wrist: a retrospective clinical and radiological long-term follow-up. *J Hand Surg* 2002;27B:61–72.
24. Reference deleted.
25. Reference deleted.
26. Reference deleted.
27. Stanley JK, Tolat AR. Long-term results of Swanson silastic arthroplasty in the rheumatoid wrist. *J Hand Surg* 1993;18B:381–388.
28. Fatti JF, Palmer AK, Greenky S, et al. Long-term results of Swanson interpositional wrist arthroplasty: Part II. *J Hand Surg* 1991;16A:432–437.
29. Jolly SL, Ferlic DC, Clayton ML, et al. Swanson silicone arthroplasty of the wrist in rheumatoid arthritis: a long-term follow-up. *J Hand Surg* 1992;17A:142–149.
30. Brase DW, Millender LH. Failure of silicone rubber wrist arthroplasty in rheumatoid arthritis. *J Hand Surg* 1986;11A:175–183.
31. Cooney WP, Beckenbaugh RD, Linscheid RL. Total wrist arthroplasty: problems with implant failures. *Clin Orthop* 1984;187:121–128.
32. Divelbiss BJ, Sollerman C, Adams BD. Early results of the universal total wrist arthroplasty in rheumatoid arthritis. *J Hand Surg* 2002;27A:195–204.
33. Menon J. Universal total wrist implant: experience with a carpal component fixed with three screws. *J Arthroplasty* 1998;13:515–523.
34. Cobb TK, Beckenbaugh RD. Biaxial total-wrist arthroplasty. *J Hand Surg* 1996;21A:1011–1021.
35. Menon J. Total wrist replacement using the modified Volz prosthesis. *J Bone Joint Surg* 1987;69A:998–1006.
36. Reference deleted.
37. Reference deleted.
38. Reference deleted.
39. Blank JE, Cassidy C. The distal radioulnar joint in rheumatoid arthritis. *Hand Clin* 1996;12:499–513.
40. Clawson MC, Stern PJ. The distal radioulnar joint complex in rheumatoid arthritis: an overview. *Hand Clin* 1991;7:373–381.
41. Reference deleted.
42. Reference deleted.
43. Newman RJ. Excision of the distal ulna in patients with rheumatoid arthritis. *J Bone Joint Surg* 1987;69B:203–206.
44. Reference deleted.
45. DjMikic Z, Helal B. The value of the Darrach procedure in the surgical treatment of rheumatoid arthritis. *Clin Orthop* 1977;127:175–185.
46. Reference deleted.
47. Reference deleted.
48. Adams BD, Blair WF, Shurr DG. Schultz metacarpophalangeal arthroplasty: a long-term follow-up study. *J Hand Surg* 1990;15A:641–645.
49. Beckenbaugh RD, Dobyns JH, Linscheid RL, Bryan RS. Review and analysis of silicone-rubber metacarpophalangeal implants. *J Bone Joint Surg* 1976;58A:483–487.
50. Beckenbaugh RD, Linscheid RL. Arthroplasty in the hand and wrist. In: DP Green, ed. *Operative hand surgery*. New York: Churchill Livingstone, 1993:143–188.
51. Bieber EJ, Weiland AJ, Volenec-Dowling S. Silicone-rubber implant arthroplasty of the metacarpophalangeal joints for rheumatoid arthritis. *J Bone Joint Surg* 1986;68A:206–209.
52. Blair WF, Shurr DG, Buckwalter JA. metacarpophalangeal joint implant arthroplasty with a silastic spacer. *J Bone Joint Surg* 1984;66A:365–370.
53. Foliart DE. Swanson silicone finger joint implants: a review of the literature regarding long-term complications. *J Hand Surg* 1995;20A:445–449.
54. Kirschenbaum D, Schneider L, Adams DC, Cody RP. Arthroplasty of the metacarpophalangeal joints with use of silicone-rubber implants in patients who have rheumatoid arthritis. *J Bone Joint Surg* 1993;75A:3–12.
55. Reference deleted.
56. Millender L, Nalebuff E. Metacarpophalangeal joint arthroplasty utilizing the silicone rubber prosthesis. *Orthop Clin North Am* 1973;4:349–371.
57. Millender LH, Nalebuff EA, Hawkins RB, Ennis R. Infection after silicone prosthetic arthroplasty in the hand. *J Bone Joint Surg* 1975;57A:825–829.
58. Minamikawa Y, Peimer CA, Ogawa R, et al. In vivo experimental analysis of silicone implants used with titanium grommets. *J Hand Surg* 1994;19A:567–574.
59. Reference deleted.
60. Stirrat CR. Metacarpophalangeal joints in rheumatoid arthritis of the hand. *Hand Clin* 1996;12:515–529.
61. Swanson AB. A flexible implant for replacement of arthritic or destroyed joints in the hand. *New York University, Post-Graduate Medical School Inter-Clin Inform Bull* 1966;6:16–19.
62. Swanson AB. Flexible implant arthroplasty for arthritic finger joints. *J Bone Joint Surg* 1972;54A:435–455.
63. Reference deleted.
64. Reference deleted.
65. Reference deleted.
66. Reference deleted.
67. Ratliff AHC. Deformities of the thumb in rheumatoid arthritis. *Hand* 1971;3:138–143.
68. Nalebuff EA. Diagnosis, classification and management of rheumatoid thumb deformities. *Bull Hosp Joint Dis* 1968;29:119–137.
69. Stein AB, Terrono AL. The rheumatoid thumb. *Hand Clin* 1996;12:541–550.
70. Feldon P, Terrano AL, Nalebuff EA, et al. Rheumatoid arthritis and other connective tissue diseases. In: Green DP, Hotchkiss RN, Pederson WC, eds. *Green's operative hand surgery*, 4th ed. Philadelphia: Churchill Livingstone, 1999:1651–1737.
71. Brumfield RH, Conaty JP. Reconstructive surgery of the thumb in rheumatoid arthritis. *Orthopedics* 1980;3:529–533.
72. Terrono A, Millender L. Surgical treatment of the rheumatoid thumb deformity. *Hand Clin* 1989;5:239–248.
73. Reference deleted.
74. Terrano A, Millender L, Nalebuff E. Boutonnière rheumatoid thumb deformity. *J Hand Surg* 1990;15A:999–1003.
75. Inglis AE, Hamlin C, Sengelmann RP, et al. Reconstruction of the metacarpophalangeal joint of the thumb in rheumatoid arthritis. *J Bone Joint Surg* 1972;54A:704–712.
76. Nalebuff EA, Garrett J. Opera-glass hand in rheumatoid arthritis. *J Hand Surg* 1976;1:210–220.
77. Kessler I. Aetiology and management of adduction contracture of the thumb in rheumatoid arthritis. *Hand* 1973;5:170–174.
78. Burton RI, Pellegrini VD. Surgical management of basal joint arthritis of the thumb part II: ligament reconstruction with tendon interposition arthroplasty. *J Hand Surg* 1986;11A:324–332.
79. Tomaino MM, Pellegrini VD, Burton RI. Arthroplasty of the basal joint of the thumb. Long-term follow-up after ligament reconstruction with tendon interposition. *J Bone Joint Surg* 1995;77A:346–355.
80. Eaton RG, Lane LB, Littler JW, et al. Ligament reconstruction for the painful thumb carpometacarpal joint: a long-term assessment. *J Hand Surg* 1984;9A:692–699.
81. Millender LH, Nalebuff EA, Amadio P, et al. Interpositional arthroplasty for rheumatoid carpometacarpal joint disease. *J Hand Surg* 1978;3:533–541.
82. Reference deleted.
83. Patterson P, Simmons BP, Ring D, Earp B. Static versus dynamic splinting and early motion after metacarpophalangeal arthroplasty. Paper presented at: Annual Meeting of the American Society for Surgery of the Hand; September 1999; Boston, Massachusetts.
84. Mandl LA, Galvin DH, Bosch JP, et al. Metacarpophalangeal arthroplasty in rheumatoid arthritis: what determines satisfaction with surgery? *Rheumatology* 2002;12:2488–2491.
85. Boyer MI, Gelberman RH. Operative correction of swan-neck and boutonnière deformities in the rheumatoid hand. *J Am Acad Orthop Surg* 1999;7:92–100.
86. Swanson AB, Maupin BK, Gajjar NV, Swanson GD. Flexible implant arthroplasty in the proximal interphalangeal joint of the hand. *J Hand Surg* 1985; 10A;796–805.
87. Adamson GJ, Gellman H, Brumfield RH Jr, et al. Flexible implant resection arthroplasty of the proximal interphalangeal joint in patients with systemic inflammatory arthritis. *J Hand Surg* 1994;19A:1064.
88. Jones BF, Stern PJ. Interphalangeal joint arthrodesis. *Hand Clin* 1994;10:267–275.

CHAPTER 43

Foot and Ankle Surgery

Mark E. Easley and James A. Nunley

Rheumatoid arthritis (RA) commonly affects the foot and ankle (1–3). More than 90% of rheumatoid patients experience foot pain at some point in the course of their disease, and ankle involvement occurs in up to 50%. It has been estimated that at any given time, 50% or more of rheumatoid patients have active foot or ankle symptoms (2). In a cohort of 1,000 RA patients, Vainio reported that foot and ankle problems occurred in 91% of women and 85% of men (3). More recently, Michelson et al. (2) observed a prevalence of foot and ankle complaints in 94% of 99 randomly selected patients with RA. Foot pain is the presenting symptom of RA in 28% of patients and, for 8%, foot symptoms are the major source of disability. Metatarsalgia (plantar forefoot pain) is generally the earliest symptom, although, occasionally, the hindfoot or ankle may be initially involved. Given the multiple synovial joints within the foot, synovial inflammation in active rheumatoid disease often produces diffuse foot pain.

To best define rheumatoid involvement, the foot and ankle are viewed as the following components: (a) forefoot [interphalangeal and metatarsophalangeal (MTP) joints], (b) midfoot (tarsometatarsal and intercuneiform joints), (c) hindfoot (talonavicular, calcaneocuboid, and subtalar joints), and (d) ankle (tibiotalar joint). Although this classification defines the bony anatomy and articulations, soft tissue structures, including tendons, are frequently affected as well.

Synovitis and tenosynovitis are initially characterized by a chronic inflammatory response, producing pain and swelling in the foot and ankle. Chronic articular inflammation eventually promotes synovial hypertrophy and ligamentous incompetence, and chronic tenosynovitis may lead to tendon attenuation or rupture. Furthermore, the inflammatory cascade can lead to a destruction of the articular cartilage and adjacent capsular tissues. Over time, patients typically report fewer acute synovitis symptoms, as foot or ankle deformities become the dominant problem, with persistent pain. Spiegel and Spiegel (4) reported a prevalence of MTP joint synovitis in 65% of patients with disease duration of 1 to 3 years but only an 18% prevalence in patients having disease for more than 10 years. Moreover, the same authors found an 8% prevalence of hindfoot deformities in patients with RA of less than 5 years' duration, whereas 25% of patients with disease of more than 5 years' duration had abnormal hindfoot alignment.

Whether caused by acute synovitis or chronic disease, degree and frequency of foot and ankle problems in RA tend to correlate with disease duration. Spiegel and Spiegel (4) noted an increase of forefoot and hindfoot deformity during the first 10 years of the disease process. Michelson et al. (2) observed foot and ankle symptoms in 55% of patients with RA whose disease duration was less than 10 years, compared to a prevalence of these symptoms in 76% of patients with a disease duration in excess of 20 years.

When the foot is involved in RA, the forefoot is generally affected early in the disease process. It has been estimated that, with disease duration beyond 10 years, forefoot involvement approaches 100%. Furthermore, in a study of 200 patients with chronic RA, 70% had hallux valgus, 67% had lesser MTP joint subluxation, and more than 80% had hammer toe deformity (5).

Complaints of rheumatoid midfoot pain are less common than those related to the fore- or hindfoot. Although evidence for rheumatoid midfoot involvement may be frequently observed radiographically, stable bony or fibrous ankylosis typically results in relatively few symptoms and minimal midfoot deformity. In a study by Michelson et al., the midfoot was the most symptomatic part of the foot in only 5% of RA patients. However, Vidigal et al. observed radiographic evidence of midfoot disease in 65% of feet (5).

Relative to the forefoot, rheumatoid hindfoot disease generally occurs later in the disease process. Progressive joint erosion combined with destruction of the supporting ligamentous structures often leads to a valgus hindfoot deformity. Prevalence of hindfoot joint disease has been reported as follows: (a) talonavicular joint (39%), (b) calcaneo-cuboid joint (25%), and (c) subtalar joint (20%) (6). Reports have suggested that there is some disability related to the hindfoot in 42% of rheumatoid patients; in 34%, hindfoot symptoms were the predominant complaint; and in 16%, hindfoot pain was deemed most responsible for difficulty with walking.

Although the ankle has been reported to be involved in up to 50% of rheumatoid patients, the prevalence of ankle arthritis is less than that of the foot and other major weightbearing joints, such as the hip and knee. Vidigal et al. (5) noted ankle involvement in 29% of rheumatoid patients, and Vainio (3) reported tibiotalar disease in only 9% of patients with RA. Michelson et al. (2) suggested that 42% of RA patients have ankle involvement, but the relative contributions of ankle and hindfoot symptoms were not distinguished (1). Ankle deformity does not occur with the same frequency as foot deformity in RA; generally, ankle deformity is thought to develop secondarily to hindfoot valgus deformity that creates eccentric loading at the tibiotalar joint (1).

The etiology for rheumatoid hindfoot valgus deformity remains controversial. The posterior tibial tendon (PTT) is occasionally diseased in RA, but it remains unclear whether hindfoot joint destruction leads to PTT dysfunction (PTTD) (7) or if primary PTTD accelerates hindfoot valgus deformity (8,9). Regardless, PTTD has been identified in 11% of a patient cohort with RA (10).

PATHOPHYSIOLOGY

The mechanism of joint destruction in RA involves synovial invasion and erosion of bone, as well as destruction of the ligament capsule and articular cartilage. The classic deformity of RA is forefoot hallux valgus with intraarticular involvement of the MTP joints. The lesser toes drift laterally with dorsal subluxation or dislocation, and the metatarsal heads are directed toward the plantar-ward. The toes frequently show a hammer toe or claw toe deformity, and the protective plantar fat pad is drawn distal from its normal location underneath the metatarsal heads. Frequently, large bursa will be seen overlying the plantar aspects of the lesser metatarsals associated with hypertrophic keratotic callus formation. Such calluses are most common under the second and third metatarsal heads but may involve all of the metatarsals.

Symptoms of numbness, tingling, and burning in the forefoot, much like a neuroma, can be an early sign of forefoot involvement with pressure on the digital nerves from enlarged intermetatarsal bursa. Other forefoot deformities, such as hallux varus and varus drift of the lesser metatarsals, can occur, but usually this is seen only in bedridden patients and is an uncommon finding.

Midfoot synovitis and subsequent deformity are extremely uncommon and are usually seen only after long-standing disease. The destruction that does occur is erosion of the Lisfranc joints with pain, but it is uncommon to see actual deformity occur at these joints.

Hindfoot disease and ankle pathology are often subtle but can progress quite rapidly. Synovitis typically involves the talonavicular joint and the subtalar joints. Hindfoot disease commonly appears as a tenosynovitis of the tendons surrounding the hindfoot and ankle, most frequently, the tibialis posterior and the peroneals. Visualization of this involvement is quite easy, as the tendons are subcutaneous and the synovitis can easily be seen or palpated. If the tenosynovitis of the tibialis posterior is not recognized and treated early, it can lead to severe hindfoot deformities. The tibialis posterior is the major dynamic stabilizer of the medial longitudinal arch of the foot, and, when elongation occurs from tenosynovitis, the tendon becomes dysfunctional and may actually rupture, resulting in a severe planovalgus deformity of the hindfoot.

A planovalgus deformity is the most common deformity seen in the rheumatoid hindfoot and has been seen in 87.4% of rheumatoid patients by Vahvanen (11,12). Varus deformity of the hindfoot is much less common, seen between 4% and 10% of the time (12).

CLINICAL EVALUATION

History

The patient's chief complaint(s) should be assessed to define the site or source of pain and extent of deformity. Given the variability of the clinical course of RA, an attempt should be made to identify the status of the patient's disease progression. Despite variability from patient to patient, it is typically possible to determine if acute inflammation, long-standing disease, or a combination is responsible for the symptoms. Acute inflammation rarely necessitates surgical intervention; long-standing disease may be best managed operatively.

Current and past medications of the patient need to be reviewed. Several newer antirheumatic therapies have been introduced recently and are the focus of other chapters in this book. However, for the rheumatoid patient being considered for surgery, long-term use of corticosteroids, aspirin, and nonsteroidal antiinflammatory agents may pose an increased surgical risk. Generally, for patients on long-term steroids, a perioperative corticosteroid bolus should be administered to diminish the risk of acute adrenal insufficiency. Aspirin should be discontinued 7 to 10 days preoperatively to minimize bleeding complications. The antiplatelet effects of nonsteroidal antiinflammatory agents are generally reversible more quickly than aspirin; cyclooxygenase-2 inhibitors do not prolong bleeding. Wound complications for patients who continue methotrexate perioperatively are no greater than for patients who discontinue methotrexate perioperatively (13,14). Therefore, it is generally considered unnecessary to alter the prescribed administration of methotrexate if a rheumatoid patient is to undergo foot and ankle surgery. The effects of the newer rheumatoid medications on wound healing need to be defined.

RA is a systemic disease, often involving multiple joints, including the cervical spine. The surgeon contemplating foot and ankle surgery on the RA patient should identify cervical spine disease. Although most rheumatoid foot and ankle procedures can be performed under regional anesthesia, in the event that there are anesthetic complications, the surgeon should be familiar with the patient's cervical spine status if general anesthesia should become necessary intraoperatively. Furthermore, if multiple joints are involved, the surgeon must identify other joints that may be limiting mobility. Often, the RA patient requires several months of protective weightbearing postoperatively and, if other joints are diseased, safe mobilization or use of assistive devices may not be possible. Proper postoperative arrangements will be needed to help the RA patient maintain independence or receive adequate assistance.

Physical Examination

Even if the primary complaint of the patient is foot or ankle pain, the physical examination should be comprehensive. A brief examination of the cervical spine and upper extremities is important. If surgery is contemplated, potential cervical spine pathology that may complicate intubation must be identified. Upper extremity rheumatoid involvement may limit use of assistive devices and should also be documented.

The examination of the foot and ankle should include the entire limb, with the patient standing and walking. Problems related to the hip, knee, or possible limb malalignment need to be identified, particularly if foot or ankle arthrodesis (fusion) is being considered. In general, proximal orthopedic procedures should precede distal procedures to optimize proper limb alignment. The physical examination should include evaluation of the patient's shoes. Symptoms and foot–ankle malalignment often correlate with wear patterns on the shoe soles.

With the patient standing and barefoot, ankle and foot alignment is assessed. Occasionally, the rheumatoid patient will develop a pes planus (flatfoot) alignment, which may be poorly appreciated on a nonweightbearing examination. The patient is best observed from behind to appreciate hindfoot and ankle malalignment. With pes planus, the heel is in valgus, the physiologic longitudinal arch is lost, and the forefoot is abducted (producing a "too many toes sign") (15). The patient is asked to perform a heel rise. With a functioning PTT, the hindfoot should invert into a varus position. This test should be performed not only with a double limb stance, but particularly with a single limb stance to demonstrate PTT insufficiency.

Next, the remainder of the examination is performed with the patient seated on the examining table and the physician seated in front of the patient. Inspection of the skin may reveal callus formation, skin lesions, or edema. Callosities suggest areas of increased pressure due to foot malalignment or insufficient padding. Other manifestations of RA include rheumatoid nodules, vasculitis, and neurologic involvement (16). Rheumatoid nodules generally occur on extensor surfaces of joints and adjacent long bones (16). In the foot and ankle, symptomatic nodules typically occur on the plantar surface of the heel, metatarsal heads, and toes (16). It is important to identify the location of these nodules because surgical correction of the bones in the rheumatoid foot may not completely relieve symptoms; excision of rheumatoid nodules may be necessary. Vasculitis may be manifest in the rheumatoid foot and ankle as digital infarcts, diffuse rashes, or cutaneous ulcers, and typically occur late in the disease process of seropositive patients (17,18). The presence of cutaneous manifestations of rheumatoid vasculitis should prompt investigation of pulmonary, pericardiac, and gastrointestinal involvement (19,20).

Neurologic deficits in the rheumatoid foot and ankle may be manifest as decreased sensation and loss of motor function. The majority of neurologic deficits are secondary to compression on the nerves by foot deformity, rheumatoid nodules, and proliferative tenosynovitis and synovitis in an enclosed space (tarsal canal) (16). The tibial nerve courses through the tarsal canal posterior to the medial malleolus under the flexor retinaculum. With increasing valgus deformity of the hindfoot, tension may be created on the tibial nerve, producing intrinsic muscle dysfunction (claw toes) and decreased sensation on the plantar foot. Proliferative posterior tibial tenosynovitis within the tarsal canal may create pressure on the adjacent tibial nerve, and adjacent rheumatoid nodules may directly compress the tibial nerve as well.

Physical examination includes palpation, percussion, and compression of the tibial nerve along the tarsal canal to identify potential compression of the tibial nerve. Decreased sensation or forefoot tenderness, similar to that of Morton's neuralgia, is a frequent finding on clinical examination. MTP joint synovitis and rheumatoid nodules may create direct pressure on digital nerves, whereas forefoot deformity, such as claw toes, may place tension on the digital nerves. Occasionally, the medial plantar nerve or peroneal nerve branches may be compressed by inflamed flexor or extensor tendons, respectively. Finally, neurologic deficits may be due to spinal cord compression (atlanto-occipital instability) or steroid-induced diabetes mellitus with secondary peripheral neuropathy and should be investigated if suspected based on clinical examination.

As previously noted, the forefoot is commonly involved in RA (1,21). Typically, the MTP joints subluxate or dislocate, creating claw toe deformities (Fig. 43.1). With this deformity, the plantar fat pad is displaced distally. With severe deformity, hallux valgus (bunion) develops. On clinical examination, tenderness is noted on the plantar aspect of the forefoot, generally directly on the prominent metatarsal heads. Occasionally, plantar synovial cysts and nodules are palpable. Clawing of the toes also leads to tenderness and callus formation on the dorsal aspects of the proximal interphalangeal joints.

Motor function and muscle strength are assessed with active resisted dorsiflexion, plantarflexion, inversion, and eversion while the respective tendons are palpated. Particularly important is evaluation of the PTT. If PTT insufficiency is suspected based on the single limb heel rise, manual testing of the PTT should be performed. With the ankle plantar-flexed and the hindfoot everted, the patient is asked to invert against resistance while the PTT is palpated.

Range of motion of the ankle, subtalar, transverse tarsal, and MTP joints is assessed, while noting restriction of motion, instability, and crepitance. Physiologic ankle range of motion is generally in a single sagittal axis of 15 degrees of dorsiflexion and 50 degrees of plantarflexion. With a hindfoot valgus deformity, the subtalar joint should be reduced (if possible) to a neutral position to assess accurately dorsiflexion. Often, with hindfoot valgus, dorsiflexion of the ankle beyond neutral is possible, but with the hindfoot held in an anatomic position, a contracted Achilles tendon becomes obvious, highlighting an equinus contracture. Subtalar joint motion is evaluated while cupping the heel with one hand and supporting the mid- and forefoot with the other; physiologic inversion is 20 degrees and eversion is 10 degrees. In simple terms, inversion should generally be twice as much as eversion. Transverse tarsal joint (talonavicular and calcaneocuboid) motion is assessed in two planes: dorsiflexion (15 degrees), plantarflexion (15 degrees), abduction (10 degrees), and adduction (20 degrees). Generally, adduction is twice that of abduction. Plantarflexion and dorsiflexion of the transverse tarsal joint must be distinguished from ankle motion. To assess the transverse tarsal joint, one hand is used to cup the heel and talus (the talar head can be palpated and stabilized) while the other is used to move the midfoot. The MTP joints are assessed with the ankle in neutral position; typical motion is dorsiflexion of 50 degrees and plantarflexion of 15 degrees.

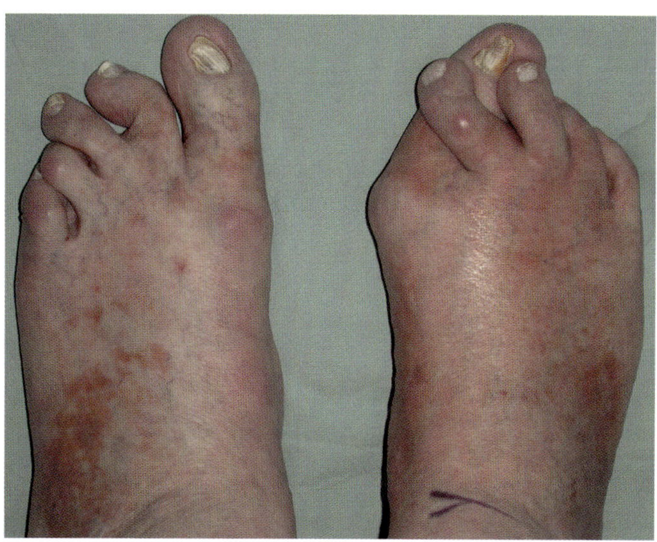

Figure 43.1. Typical appearance of a patient with rheumatoid arthritis, showing two separate types of deformity. On the right, the more classic deformity, with severe hallux valgus, which completely underlaps the second and third toes. Note the dorsal corn on the second toe. On the left foot, notice the tendency toward valgus. The big toe is straight. There is no bunion deformity, but there are marked angular deformities at the proximal interphalangeal joints and nail irregularities.

Recommendations for orthotics, bracing, or surgery are often in part determined by range of motion. With fixed deformity, arthrodeses (fusions) may be required, rather than joint-sparing procedures. One important assessment is the relationship of the hindfoot to the forefoot. With the hindfoot in neutral position, the forefoot should also maintain a neutral position; however, with a fixed hindfoot valgus deformity, forefoot varus becomes evident with the first metatarsal positioned dorsally relative to the fifth metatarsal.

Imaging Studies

Although the focus may be the foot and ankle, imaging studies should include cervical spine radiographs, if surgery is considered to identify any advanced disease that may put the patient at risk

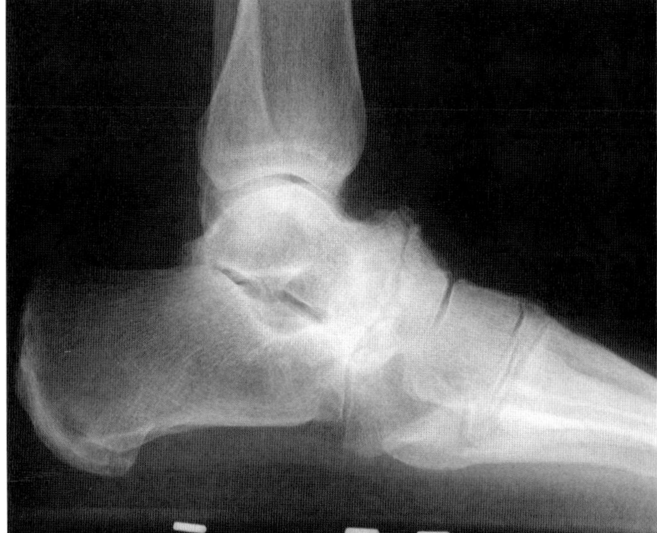

Figure 43.2. A lateral radiograph of a patient with advanced rheumatoid arthritis of the talonavicular joint. Notice hypertrophic spurring on the dorsal surface of the talonavicular joint, but with preservation of the subtalar joint.

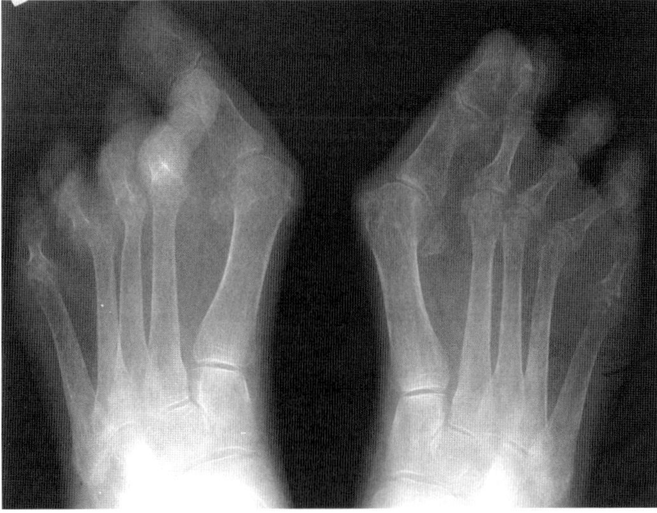

Figure 43.3. Anteroposterior radiograph of a patient with rheumatoid arthritis. On the right foot, notice the osteopenia, hallux valgus, and deviation of the fourth and fifth metatarsophalangeal (MTP) joints and cystic erosion at the fifth MTP joint. On the left foot, severe hallux valgus with near complete dislocation of the MTP joint and total dislocation of the MTP joint of the second, third, fourth, and fifth toes.

for spinal cord damage during intubation. The foot and ankle cannot be viewed in isolation; the entire extremity needs to be evaluated. If hip or knee pathology is suspected based on clinical examination, particularly with limb malalignment, radiographs should include a hip and knee series. Furthermore, mechanical axis views may be helpful in defining the apex of limb malalignment.

Routine plain radiographic views of the foot and ankle include standing (a) anteroposterior (AP), (b) oblique, and (c) lateral. Radiographs serve to confirm the diagnosis of an inflammatory arthropathy, monitor disease progression, and assess deformity for operative planning. It is imperative to obtain weightbearing radiographs of the foot and ankle to determine accurately malalignment and joint congruence with physiologic stance. Nonweightbearing x-rays generally lead to underestimation of deformity.

Typically, RA manifests as symmetric joint space narrowing of involved articulations due to articular cartilage erosion. Commonly, the MTP, cuneiform, and talonavicular joints are involved (Fig. 43.2). Metatarsal head erosions occur at the articular cartilage margins, in the synovial reflection; periarticular osteopenia is also commonly seen (Fig. 43.3). Osteopenia is seen in the periarticular region in 68% of patients, most commonly in the calcaneocuboid joint area, where the changes are moderate to severe 91% of the time. Spontaneous ankylosis, especially of the tarsal joints, has been reported in up to 25% of rheumatoid patients followed for 19 years. Frequently, rheumatoid patients develop planovalgus deformity; radiographs are useful in defining the exact location and extent of the deformity. On the AP radiograph, forefoot abduction can be appreciated with talar head uncovering (the navicular subluxates dorsally and laterally on the talar head). On the lateral x-ray, the midfoot subluxates plantarward relative to the hindfoot, usually at the transverse tarsal joints (Fig. 43.4). A simple evaluation is to assess talo–first metatarsal axis on both the AP and lateral views. On the AP and lateral view, the physiologic congruent alignment of the first metatarsal with the talus is lost. Planovalgus deformity of the foot may lead to ankle valgus alignment, evident on the AP and oblique ankle radiographs (21,22). Serial ankle radiographs are important to identify progression of ankle arthrosis.

For surgical planning, deformity needs to be measured. Planovalgus is objectively determined by measuring the talo–first metatarsal angle. On the AP radiograph, this angle is documented as the degree of talar head uncovering; on the lateral radiograph, the talar declination angle can be measured. In the forefoot, the hallux valgus and first through second intermetatarsal angles should be measured (22).

Other imaging studies that may have application in the evaluation of the rheumatoid foot and ankle include the three-phase bone scan and magnetic resonance imaging (MRI). Bone scans may demonstrate areas of subtle synovitis early in the disease process, before radiographic changes are evident. MRI is useful in defining tenosynovitis, rheumatoid nodules, and bursal expansions. Although PTT insufficiency is generally a diagnosis made based on clinical examination alone, MRI may be used to confirm suspected PTT disease in RA.

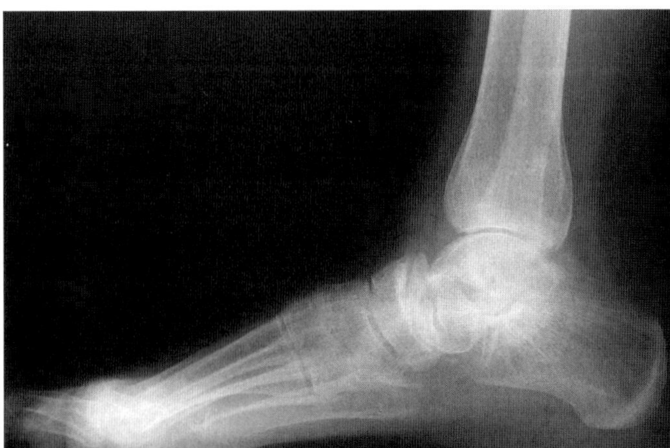

Figure 43.4. Lateral radiograph of a patient with rheumatoid arthritis involving the hindfoot. Notice the plantar flexed position of the talus and subluxation of the talonavicular joint. This can occur from rupture of the spring ligament or from attenuation of the posterior tibial tendon and results in a flat foot.

TREATMENT

Overview

Treatment of the rheumatoid forefoot deformity requires a team approach with input from primary care practitioners, rheumatologists, orthopedic surgeons, and pedorthists. The approach typically begins with medical therapy under the care of rheumatologists. Although medical management relieves symptoms related to the foot and ankle, rheumatoid patients frequently need to be considered for a graduated sequence of further treatments, progressing from injection to orthoses, synovectomy, selected joint arthrodesis, and total joint replacement (1).

Nonoperative Management

Assisted skin and nail care is routinely required, especially because rheumatoid patients frequently have concomitant upper-extremity disease leading to difficulty trimming nails and paring painful corns. Aspiration and injection of swollen intermetatarsal bursae may provide temporary relief of neuritic symptoms resulting from digital nerve compression. Furthermore, judicious intraarticular MTP joint injections often reduce symptomatic synovitis. Proper footwear is essential. With advancing synovitis, the forefoot swells, often causing the dorsal corns on the toes in standard footwear. Using an accommodative shoe with a deeper and wider toe box can obviate this problem. With progressive disease, clawing of the toes may result in plantar metatarsal pain and increase dorsal toe pressure. To alleviate plantar metatarsal pain, orthotic management should be considered. The use of simple metatarsal pads proximal to the area of increased pressure generally provides relief. With added padding in the shoe, the clawed toes will be subject to further dorsal shoe impingement, and, therefore, a larger toe box shoe is recommended.

If the metatarsal pain is more diffuse, custom orthotics can be used within the shoe. Custom orthotics include inserts fabricated on the basis of gait studies to determine accurately areas of increased pressure. Alternatively, a low-profile metatarsal bar can be attached to the (external) sole of the shoe; this device is placed proximal to the area of the pain to concentrate the weight on the metatarsal bar as the patient steps, rather than the painful metatarsal area.

When the midfoot or tarsometatarsal joints are involved, semirigid orthotics can provide midfoot support. Shoe modifications consist of inserting either a steel shank or carbon graphite to stiffen the sole in the area of the painful synovitis. A discrete rocker-bottom modification should be added to the sole of the shoe to permit a smooth transition from the stance phase to the push-off phase of gait, thereby unloading the metatarsal heads to diminish midfoot pressure.

Orthotic management for hindfoot disease presents a greater challenge than for the forefoot. With acute posterior tibial tenosynovitis, cast immobilization will frequently reduce the pain and swelling; if the tendon remains competent, no further management beyond the acute phase is needed. However, in a majority of patients, the PTT weakens, necessitating orthotic management to prevent progressive valgus hindfoot collapse. For mild disease, a medial longitudinal arch support generally suffices in reducing medial arch stress. A University of California at Berkeley Laboratory orthotic can be considered for moderate disease to control hindfoot alignment, but these rigid orthotics can be painful for the rheumatoid patient. For longer-term management of the patient with moderate to severe valgus deformity, the relatively practical and functional Arizona brace (Fig. 43.5) can replace the more traditional ankle–foot orthosis (AFO). This custom lace-up brace extends from the midfoot to the ankle and has proven effective in reducing hindfoot pain and limiting progressive deformity.

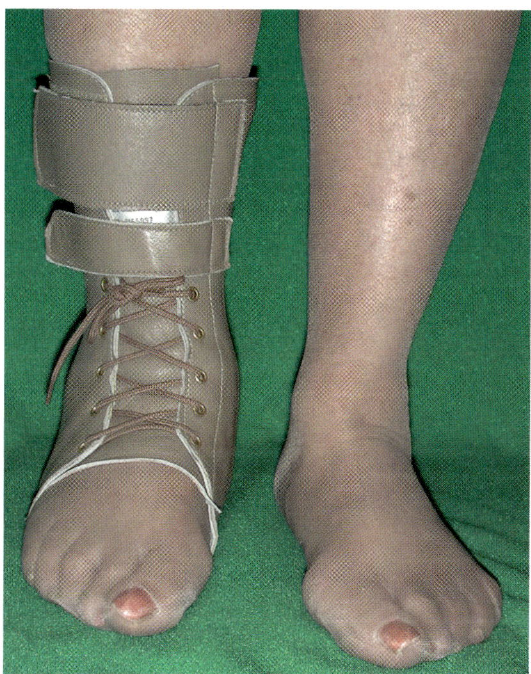

Figure 43.5. Arizona brace for nonoperative treatment of the rheumatoid hindfoot.

For significant ankle pain and deformity, the in-shoe AFO remains the standard of nonoperative care. However, an extended Arizona brace may prove equally effective. Because both the AFO and extended Arizona brace immobilize the ankle and hindfoot, the addition of a rocker-bottom shoe modification can improve the efficiency of gait. In patients with severe disease and avascular changes of the talus, a clamshell patellar tendon–bearing orthotic is needed not only to immobilize the ankle–hindfoot complex but also to unload the talus when surgery is contraindicated. The patellar tendon–bearing orthotic should be used cautiously in the rheumatoid patient, because it transfers approximately 20% of the weight to the knee.

SURGICAL PROCEDURES

General Principles

Most surgical procedures for rheumatoid foot and ankle disorders can be performed under regional anesthesia. However, should the lower-extremity anesthetic prove inadequate intraoperatively, the anesthesiologist may be forced to convert to general anesthesia. For this reason, the rheumatoid patient's cervical spine status should be defined preoperatively so as to minimize any complications related to intubation. Also, upper-extremity disease needs to be identified, because it may limit the patient's ability to unload the operated lower extremity in the postoperative period. Finally, surgical correction of multiple joints in the lower extremity should proceed from proximal to distal to ensure that anatomic limb alignment is maintained. If, for instance, the ankle is fused before correction of a valgus knee, total knee replacement after ankle fusion may lead to the ankle and hindfoot being positioned in varus. Therefore, in this example, if possible, the knee should be replaced (and realigned) first, followed by ankle or foot reconstruction. The same holds true for concomitant hindfoot and forefoot deformity. This principle is violated, however, if ankle replacement

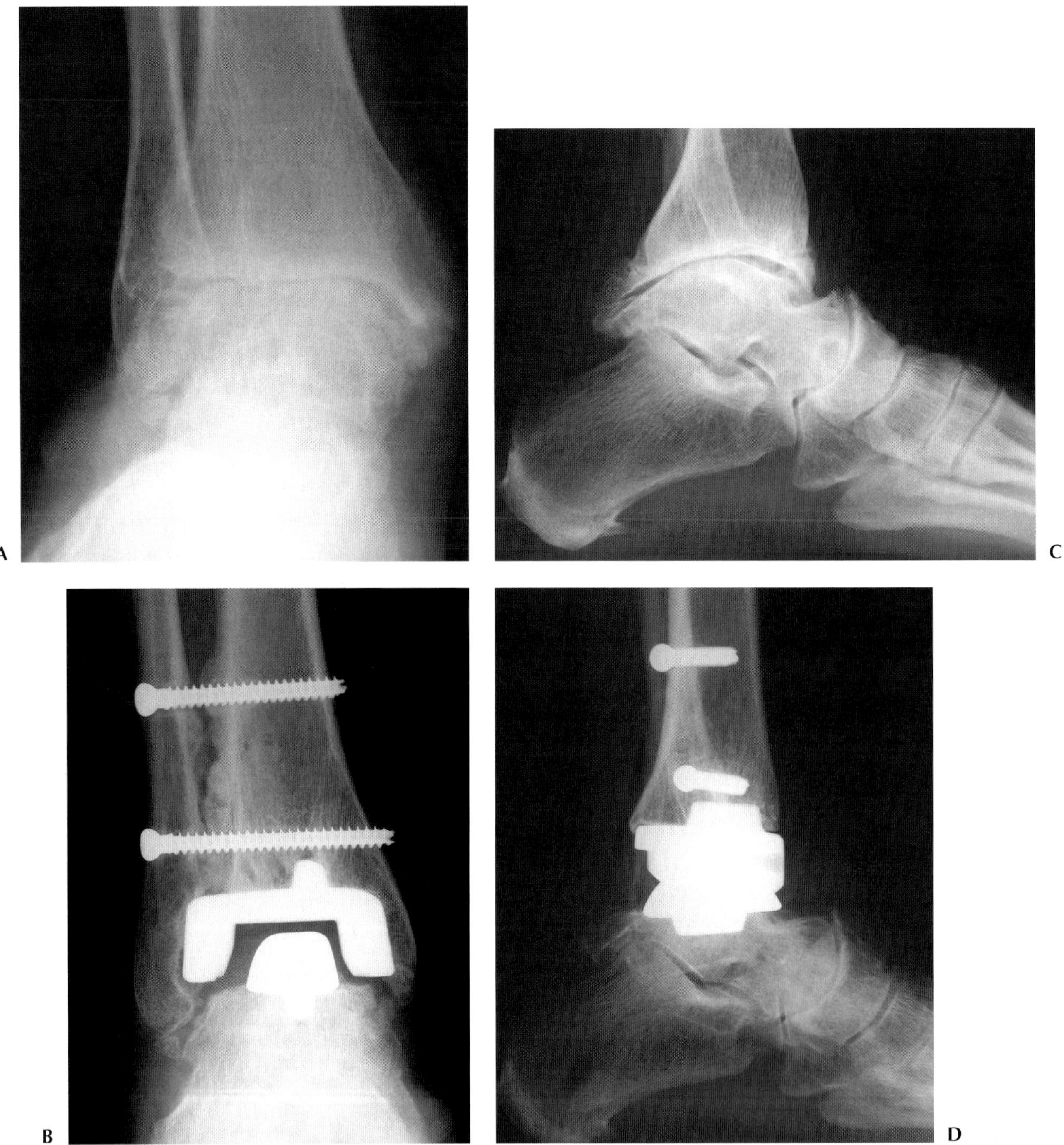

Figure 43.6. A: Preoperative anteroposterior x-ray. **B:** Postoperative anteroposterior x-ray. **C:** Preoperative lateral x-ray. **D:** Postoperative lateral x-ray. Total ankle arthroplasty in rheumatoid ankle arthritis. Note the associated hindfoot (talonavicular) involvement. Ankle arthrodesis would accelerate hindfoot erosion and degeneration. Total ankle arthroplasty reduces stress on the hindfoot articulations.

is contemplated; in this instance, the hindfoot may need to be properly positioned before ankle replacement to ensure that the ankle prosthesis has a well-balanced platform for support (23).

Ankle

Currently, two surgical options exist for the management of ankle arthritis in the rheumatoid patient, failing nonoperative measures: (a) ankle arthrodesis and (b) total ankle arthroplasty (23). In general, the gold standard for surgical management of ankle arthritis is ankle arthrodesis; however, in the rheumatoid patient, arthrodesis may have debilitating effects (24). Long-term studies of ankle arthrodesis demonstrate that, within 20 years, an ankylosed ankle leads to hindfoot arthritis; these outcomes are also found in patients with ankle arthritis of other causes. In patients with RA who have hindfoot inflammatory arthritis, ankle arthrodesis can lead to accelerated hindfoot joint degeneration (25). In addition, ankle arthrodesis may restrict a patient's ability to arise from a seated position in the setting of an associated severe knee deformity. Thus, some rheumatoid patients are candidates for total ankle replacement (26). Historically, first-generation total ankle implants were unsuccessful; the optimism of the 1970s and 1980s was diminished by the finding of poor outcomes in long-term follow-up studies. Since the early 1990s, newer-generation prostheses and improved surgical technique have rekindled enthusiasm for total ankle arthroplasty. Intermediate-term follow-up of these modern prostheses and refined methods of implantation demonstrate acceptable results in rheumatoid patients (Fig. 43.6) (27).

Hindfoot

Surgical treatment ideally begins with synovectomy in early stages of the disease. In patients with tibialis posterior tenosynovitis that persists, simple tenosynovectomy generally yields excellent long-term results. The tendon is approached through a long medial incision, and a complete tenosynovectomy is performed, from proximal to the medial malleolus to the navicular.

Rheumatoid patients can develop isolated talonavicular joint erosion and degeneration. Isolated talonavicular joint arthrodesis is typically a successful procedure in this situation (Fig. 43.7) (28,29). A medial incision will allow excellent exposure of the joint. Taking care to protect the PTT, the articular surfaces are initially prepared and the foot anatomically repositioned to reduce the joint. The joint is then stabilized with internal fixation. If there is concern that the talonavicular joint lacks inadequate stability or that the foot position cannot be restored to its anatomic alignment with talonavicular joint repositioning alone, consideration is given to double (talonavicular, calcaneocuboid) or triple (talonavicular, calcaneocuboid, subtalar) arthrodesis (23).

Triple arthrodesis is the standard procedure for all rigid hindfoot deformities (Fig. 43.8). This procedure produces reliable and predictable benefits that can be expected to last for approximately 30 years. Good to excellent long-term results have been reported for more than 85% of patients, including rheumatoid patients undergoing triple arthrodesis (12,28,30). These excellent results are also observed in patients with RA (23,31). Triple arthrodesis is accomplished through medial and lateral incisions or through a single curvilinear laterodorsal incision. The articular surfaces of the talonavicular, calcaneocuboid, and subtalar joints are denuded of any remaining cartilage. The subtalar joint is positioned in a neutral to slight valgus position and stabilized with a screw, followed by pronation and abduction through the talonavicular joint. The transverse tarsal (talonavicular and calcaneocuboid) joints are transfixed with three screws or staples (Fig. 43.9).

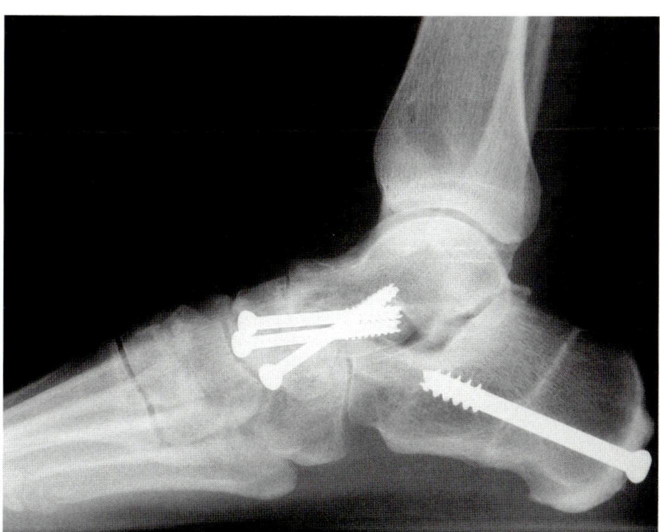

Figure 43.7. Lateral radiograph of a patient who underwent isolated talonavicular fusion in combination with joint-sparing calcaneal osteotomy. Three screws traverse the talonavicular joint, which stabilizes the hindfoot complex and can be used to correct rotational forefoot deformities. A single screw in the calcaneus across the osteotomy is used to correct hindfoot valgus. Note the preservation of the posterior facet of the subtalar joint and the ankle joint.

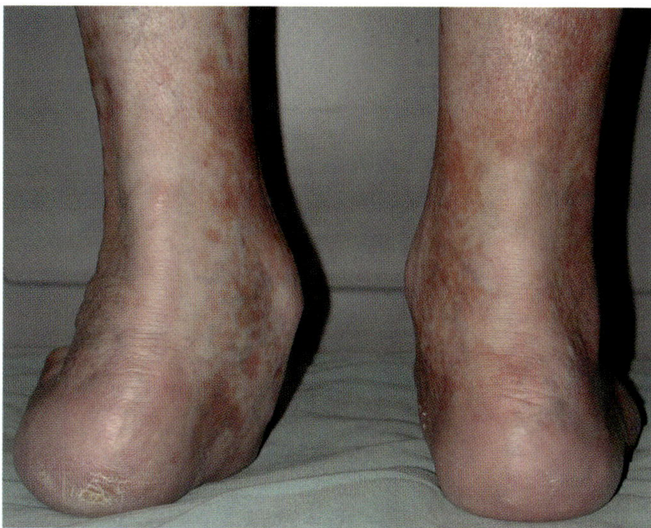

Figure 43.8. Rheumatoid patient with uncorrected left hindfoot and corrected right hindfoot, after triple arthrodesis.

Midfoot

Occasionally, rheumatoid patients present with midfoot disease. Persistent erosive and degenerative changes of the naviculocuneiform, intercuneiform, or tarsometatarsal articulations cause midfoot pain and may eventually lead to loss of the longitudinal arch and produce fixed forefoot abduction, making footwear more uncomfortable. Early in the course of midfoot involvement, orthotics with midfoot support are effective; eventually, however, surgical intervention may be required for adequate pain relief and restoration of acceptable alignment (Fig. 43.10). Because the midfoot articulations exhibit minimal physiologic motion, arthrodesis rarely changes the biomechanics of the foot during gait. Midfoot arthrodesis is typically performed through one or two longitudinal medial or dorsal incisions. To ensure the forefoot remains adaptive during stance phase, the fourth and fifth metatarsal articulation with the cuboid is not included in the fusion (23).

Forefoot

The favored forefoot corrective procedure for RA involving the MTP joints remains first MTP joint arthrodesis combined with second through fifth metatarsal head excisions (Fig. 43.11) (32). The first MTP joint procedure addresses both the erosive and degenerative changes and hallux valgus deformity. The great toe can be corrected either through arthrodesis or arthroplasty. If there is no involvement of the great toe MTP joint, a standard bunion procedure can be attempted, but, in a majority of the cases, there is significant disease in the great toe. Although attempts can be made to realign the lesser toe MTP joints, advanced erosive and degenerative changes, combined with severe claw toe or hammer toe deformity, generally warrant metatarsal head excisions. Often the lesser toe MTP joints are dislocated, and attempted realignment with joint preservation may compromise the toes' vasculature (1).

The arthrodesis-excision combination procedure uses three dorsal incisions; one along the dorsal medial aspect of the big

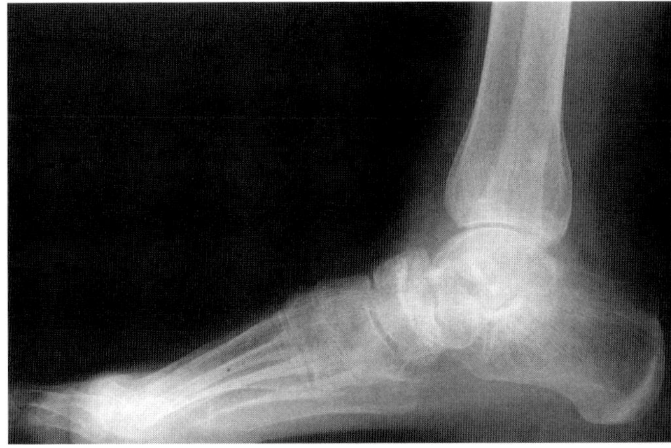

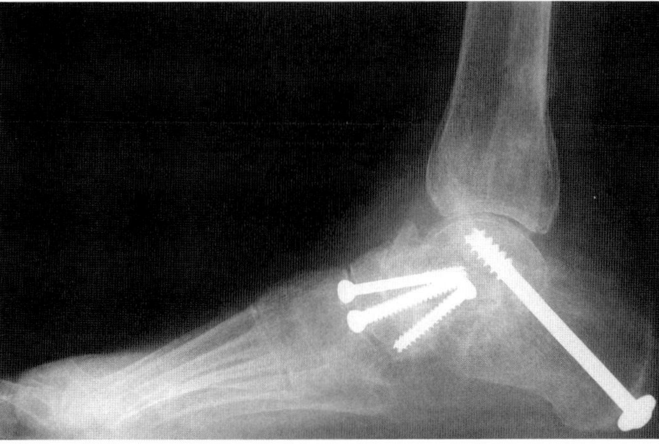

Figure 43.9. **A:** Preoperative lateral radiograph of a patient with rheumatoid arthritis seen in Figure 43.8 with pronounced hindfoot valgus and collapse. **B:** Note repositioning of the foot by arthrodesis of the talonavicular, calcaneocuboid, and subtalar joints. Two screws are used across the talonavicular, one across the calcaneocuboid, and one screw with a washer used across the subtalar joint. Note the normal relationship now of the talus to the long axis of the first metatarsal.

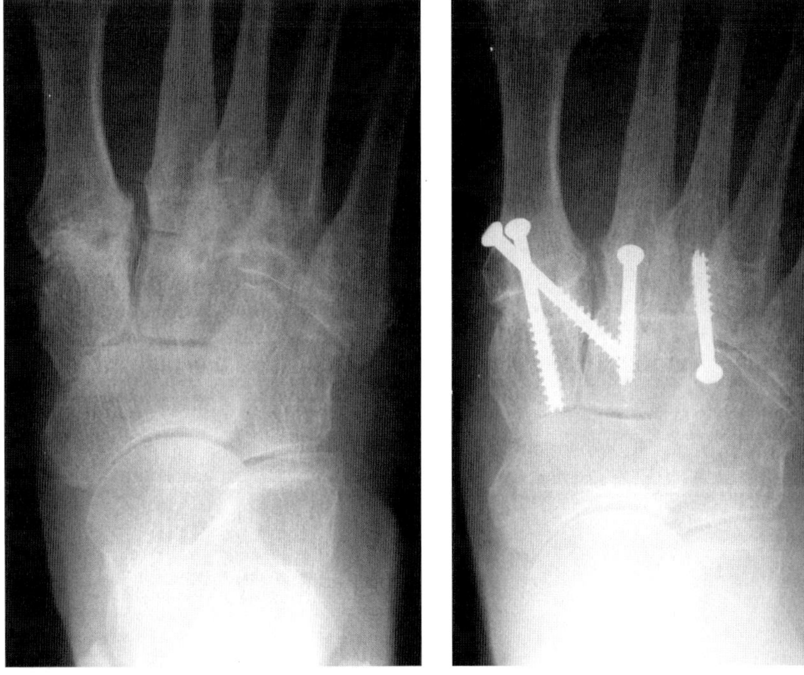

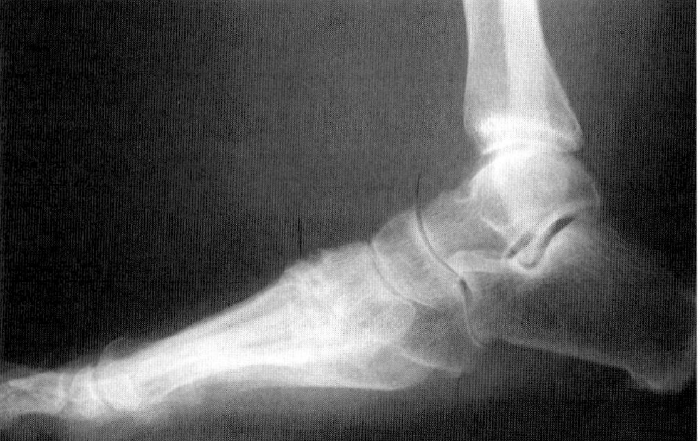

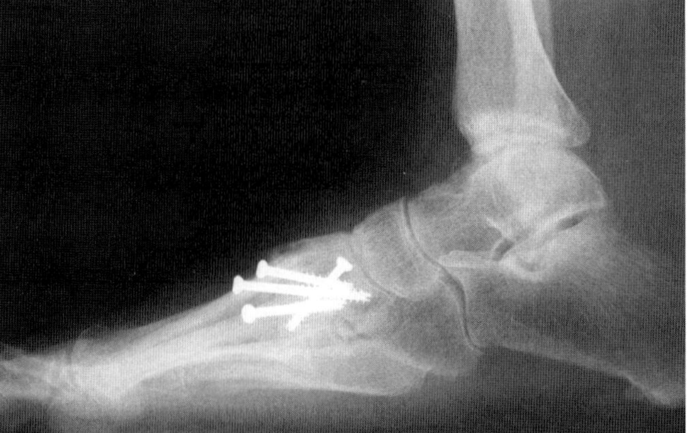

Figure 43.10. Anteroposterior **(A,B)** and lateral **(C,D)** radiographs of midfoot (tarsometatarsal) rheumatoid arthritis. **A,C:** Preoperative. **B,D:** Postoperative.

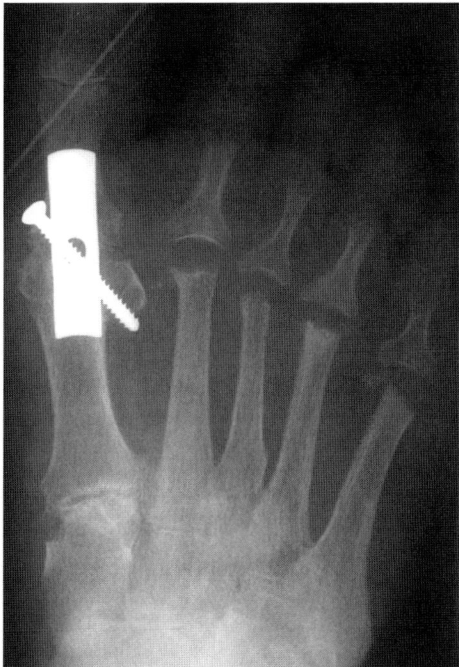

Figure 43.11. Anteroposterior radiograph of a patient seen in Figure 43.1. Forefoot is corrected with arthrodesis of the great toe metatarsophalangeal (MTP) joint. Note the improvement in valgus position and arthrodesis accomplished by single screw and dorsal plate. Dislocation of the lesser MTP joints is reduced by excising the metatarsal heads.

toe, for a correction of the great toe; a second incision in the web space between the second and third toes; and a third incision in the web space between the fourth and fifth toes. The lesser toe extensor tendons and the lesser MTP joints are released, and the metatarsal heads are excised. The lesser toes are realigned with the use of temporary longitudinal Kirschner wires; the wires are left in place for approximately 4 to 5 weeks to allow for adequate scarring to form at the MTP joints to maintain alignment. Long-term studies have shown the effectiveness of first MTP joint arthrodesis to reestablish the weightbearing axis of the first ray and to prevent recurrence of lesser toe valgus malalignment (32,33).

Excision of all five metatarsal heads has been described as another treatment option; however, without the stabilizing effect of the first metatarsal arthrodesis, recurrence of deformity is common (34).

Currently, the use of implant arthroplasty for the great toe is discouraged, especially in rheumatoid patients. With severe MTP joint dislocations, the lesser toe metatarsal heads can also be excised through a plantar approach (35). This approach may facilitate access to the metatarsal heads in severe disease and allows for repositioning of the fat pad and simultaneous removal of any coexisting rheumatoid nodules. Although plantar incisions on weightbearing areas of the foot are generally contraindicated, with resection of the metatarsal heads, pressure relief is adequate to avoid wound complications.

Rheumatoid Nodules

Rheumatoid nodules occur in approximately 25% of patients with RA (16,18,36). They probably arise due to a vasculitis mediated by immune complexes; possibly, rheumatoid factor and immunoglobulin G initiate the vasculitic response that, in turn, stimulates nodule formation (16). The diameter of the nodules can vary from as small as a few millimeters to as large as 5 cm. In the foot and ankle, rheumatoid nodules may occur in the following locations: (a) the malleoli of the ankle; (b) the prominences of the first and fifth metatarsals; and (c) plantar surfaces of the heel, metatarsal heads, and toes. The rheumatoid nodule comprises three zones: (a) superficial layer of chronic inflammatory cells; (b) intermediate layer of histocytic cells; and (c) central fibrinoid necrosis (16,36).

Shoe modifications and orthotics with pressure relief are occasionally effective in relieving symptoms created by rheumatoid nodules. However, surgical excision is occasionally warranted to eliminate symptoms related to the nodule. Often, the nodules are closely associated with adjacent structures (including neurovascular bundles), making complete excision difficult; for this reason, recurrence or persistence of the nodule is rather common. With carefully planned incisions, rheumatoid nodule excision can often be combined with the rheumatoid reconstructive procedures previously described.

Surgical Complications

Rheumatoid patients are probably at a higher risk for postsurgical complications because of their underlying systemic disease, immunosuppressive medications, often severe deformities, and potential need for multiple operations to adequately correct foot and ankle deformities. In general, patients undergoing foot and ankle surgery may have a slightly increased risk of wound problems, compared to surgery on other parts of the body, because of the thin subcutaneous tissues about the foot and ankle. In RA, this risk is probably increased, given the risk factors cited. The potential for superficial and deep infections is probably also increased for the same reasons (37).

Nonunion occasionally occurs. In rheumatoid patients, the prevalence of nonunion or delayed union has been reported to be 0% to 40% in the ankle, 0% to 10% in the hindfoot, and 0% to 6% in the forefoot (37). Nonunion does not necessarily indicate failure of the surgical procedure; a fibrous nonunion may be relatively asymptomatic for the lower demand rheumatoid patient, leading to a significant improvement over the preoperative status. Symptomatic nonunions require revision arthrodesis. Improved operative techniques developed since the mid-1980s will most likely reduce the prevalence of nonunion in rheumatoid foot and ankle surgery. However, with systemic disease and immunosuppressive medications, the nonunion rate will probably always exceed that of the general population (1,37).

Recurrence of hammer toe or claw toe deformity is the most common complication after rheumatoid forefoot surgery. Rheumatoid patients often have severe forefoot deformity that warrants correction at multiple foot and/or toe articulations. Simultaneous correction at multiple levels may compromise the vascular status of the toe and, therefore, rheumatoid forefoot correction is typically limited to the MTP joint at the time of the index procedure. If recurrence or persistence of deformity is symptomatic, secondary procedures may be added at a second stage. Occasionally, ectopic bone may form at the residual lesser metatarsal heads, leading to recurrent plantar callus formation, despite metatarsal head resection. Revision metatarsal resection is typically successful in solving this problem (1).

CONCLUSION

RA is commonly seen in the foot and ankle. Generally, the deformity follows one of several patterns. In the hindfoot, the normal pattern is to spare the ankle until late in the disease but to have significant hindfoot valgus in forefoot abduction, occurring either because of attritional disease in the PTT or because of joint involvement in the subtalar as well as the talonavicular joints.

The midfoot is generally spared until quite late in RA, but involvement of the tarsal metatarsal (Lisfranc joint) can be seen.

Most commonly, RA involves the forefoot much as it does the fingers in the upper extremity. The classic deformity is severe hallux valgus of the great toe, with synovitis eventually leading to dorsal dislocation of the second, third, fourth, and fifth MTP joints. As the synovitis produces stretching and subluxation of the MTP joint, the plantar fat pad is pulled distally, resulting in secondary hammer toe deformities.

Management of deformities is virtually impossible without surgical correction, although accommodative footwear can relieve some discomfort. Preservation of a plantar grade foot with reestablishment of a normal gait pattern should be the goal of treatment.

REFERENCES

1. Mann RA, Horton GA. Management of the foot and ankle in rheumatoid arthritis. *Rheum Dis Clin North Am* 1996;22:457–476.
2. Michelson J, Easley M, Wigley FM, Hellmann D. Foot and ankle problems in rheumatoid arthritis. *Foot Ankle Int* 1994;15:608–613.
3. Vainio K. Rheumatoid foot: clinical study with pathological and roentgenographic comments. *Ann Chir Gynaecol* 1956;45[Suppl]:1–107.
4. Spiegel TM, Spiegel JS. Rheumatoid arthritis in the foot and ankle—diagnosis, pathology, and treatment. The relationship between foot and ankle deformity and disease duration in 50 patients. *Foot Ankle* 1982;2:318–324.
5. Vidigal E, Jacoby R, Dixon A, et al. The foot in chronic rheumatoid arthritis. *Ann Rheum Dis* 1975;34:292.
6. Seltzer SE, Weissman BN, Braunstein EM, et al. Computed tomography of the hindfoot with rheumatoid arthritis. *Arthritis Rheum* 1985;28:1234–1242.
7. Kirkham BW, Gibson T. Comment on the article by Downey et al. *Arthritis Rheum* 1989;32:359.
8. Downey DJ, Simkin PA, Mack LA, et al. Tibialis posterior tendon rupture: a cause of rheumatoid flat foot. *Arthritis Rheum* 1988;31:441–446.
9. Simkin PA, Downey DJ, Richardson ML. More on the posterior tibial tendon in rheumatoid arthritis. *Arthritis Rheum* 1989;32:1050.
10. Michelson J, Easley M, Wigley FM, Hellmann D. Posterior tibial tendon dysfunction in rheumatoid arthritis. *Foot Ankle Int* 1995;16:156–161.
11. Vahvanen V. Arthrodesis of the TC or pantalar joints in rheumatoid arthritis. *Acta Orthop Scand* 1969;40:642–652.
12. Vahvanen VA. Rheumatoid arthritis in the pantalar joints. A follow-up study of triple arthrodesis on 292 adult feet. *Acta Orthop Scand* 1967;[Suppl].
13. Perhala RS, Wilke WS. Methotrexate in the treatment of inflammatory arthritis. *Compr Ther* 1991;17:51–60.
14. Sany J, Anaya JM, Canovas F, et al. Influence of methotrexate on the frequency of postoperative infectious complications in patients with rheumatoid arthritis. *J Rheumatol* 1993;20:1129–1132.
15. Funk DA, Cass JR, Johnson KA. Acquired adult flat foot secondary to posterior tibial-tendon pathology. *J Bone Joint Surg Am* 1986;68:95–102.
16. O'Brien TS, Hart TS, Gould JS. Extraosseous manifestations of rheumatoid arthritis in the foot and ankle. *Clin Orthop* 1997;340:26–33.
17. Westedt ML, Herbrink P, Molenaar JL. Clinical background of rheumatoid vascular disease. *Rheumatol Int* 1985;5:209–214.
18. Wilkinson M, Torrance WN. Clinical background of rheumatoid vascular disease. *Ann Rheum Dis* 1967;26:475–480.
19. Callen JP, Ahrens EM. Granulomatous cutaneous rheumatoid vasculitis. *J Rheumatol* 1988;15:1005–1008.
20. Geirsson AJ, Sturfelt G, Truedsson L. Clinical and serological features of severe vasculitis in rheumatoid arthritis: prognostic implication. *Ann Rheum Dis* 1987;46:727–733.
21. Cimino WG, O'Malley MJ. Rheumatoid arthritis of the ankle and hindfoot. *Rheum Dis Clin North Am* 1998;24:157–172.
22. Resnick D. Roentgen features of the rheumatoid mid- and hindfoot. *J Can Assoc Radiol* 1976;27:99–107.
23. Toolan BC, Hansen ST Jr. Surgery of the rheumatoid foot and ankle. *Curr Opin Rheumatol* 1998;10:116–119.
24. Cracchiolo A III, Cimino WR, Lian G. Arthrodesis of the ankle in patients who have rheumatoid arthritis. *J Bone Joint Surg Am* 1992;74:903–909.
25. Coester LM, Saltzman CL, Leupold J, Pontarelli W. Long-term results following ankle arthrodesis for post-traumatic arthritis. *J Bone Joint Surg Am* 2001;3A:219–228.
26. Kofoed H, Sorensen TS. Ankle arthroplasty for rheumatoid arthritis and osteoarthritis: prospective long-term study of cemented replacements. *J Bone Joint Surg Br* 1998;80:328–332.
27. Easley ME, Vertullo CJ, Urban WC, Nunley JA. Total ankle arthroplasty. *J Am Acad Orthop Surg* 2002;10:157–167.
28. Cracchiolo A. Rheumatoid arthritis: hindfoot disease. *Clin Orthop* 1997; 340:58–68.
29. Kindsfater K, Wilson MG, Thomas WH. Management of the rheumatoid hindfoot with special reference to talonavicular arthrodesis. *Clin Orthop* 1997;340:69–74.
30. Adam W, Ranawat C. Arthrodesis of the hindfoot in rheumatoid arthritis. *Orthop Clin North Am* 1976;7:827.
31. Pell RF, Myerson MS, Schon LC. Clinical outcome after primary triple arthrodesis. *J Bone Joint Surg Am* 2000;82:47–57.
32. Coughlin MJ. Rheumatoid forefoot reconstruction: a long-term follow-up study. *J Bone Joint Surg Am* 2000;82:322–341.
33. Thordarson DB, Aval S, Krieger L. Failure of hallux MP preservation surgery for rheumatoid arthritis. *Foot Ankle Int* 2002;23:486–490.
34. Hamalainen M, Raunio P. Long-term followup of rheumatoid forefoot surgery. *Clin Orthop* 1997;340:34–38.
35. Tillman K. Surgery of the rheumatoid forefoot with special reference to the plantar approach. *Clin Orthop* 2003;340:39–47.
36. Moore CP. The subcutaneous nodule: its significance in the diagnosis of rheumatic disease. *Semin Arthritis Rheum* 1977;7:63–79.
37. Nassar J, Cracchiolo A III. Complications in surgery of the foot and ankle in patients with rheumatoid arthritis. *Clin Orthop* 2001;391:140–152.

CHAPTER 44

Cervical Spine Surgery

William James Richardson, Wayne K. Cheng, and Robert E. Lins

Rheumatoid arthritis (RA) affects approximately 1% of the adult populations of both the United States and Europe (1). Cervical spine involvement is second only to metatarsophalangeal joint as the most common skeletal manifestation (2) and affects 15% to 86% of the patient population. Twenty-five percent of hospitalized rheumatoid patients have cervical involvement (3–5), and up to 26% of patients with RA require surgical intervention (1,6–8). The three abnormalities most commonly seen in rheumatoid cervical spine disease are atlanto-axial subluxation (AAS), atlanto-axial impaction (AAI), and subaxial subluxation (SAS).

AAS is the most common of the abnormalities in the cervical spine in RA, occurring in 43% to 86% of patients. The subluxation can be anterior (19–71%), lateral (21%), or posterior (6.7%) (9–12). Anterior AAS is a result of transverse ligament insufficiency and allows excessive anterior translation of atlas, primarily in flexion. Lateral AAS is defined as 2 mm or more of subluxation of the lateral masses of the atlas on the axis and is often accompanied by rotational deformity, which may be irreducible (9). Posterior AAS most commonly results from erosion of the odontoid process but may be caused by incompetence of the anterior arch of the atlas or superior and posterior migration of the atlas. Although considered more benign than anterior AAS, posterior AAS may cause cervical myelopathy due to posterior kinking of the spinal cord without demonstrable compression on tomography (13).

AAI, evident in 5% to 34% of rheumatoid patients, is the most concerning sequelae of cervical RA. It is also referred to as *cranial settling*, upward migration of the odontoid, basilar invagination, and vertical subluxation (13,14). AAI results from bone and cartilage loss in the occipito-atlantal and atlanto-axial joints that allows the odontoid to migrate superiorly and potentially impinge on the brain stem.

SAS represents instability of the subaxial cervical spine from rheumatoid involvement of the facets, interspinous ligaments, and intervertebral discs and affects 10% to 25% of patients (11,15,16). The most frequent levels involved are C2-C3 and C3-C4. The forward translation of one vertebra in relation to an adjacent vertebra at multiple levels causes a staircase appearance on radiographs. Subaxial end plate erosive changes are found in 12% to 15% of this patient population (11).

CLINICAL PRESENTATION

Pain (40–88%), neurologic deficit (7–34%), and sudden death from brain stem compression (10%) are common clinical manifestations of cervical involvement (9,17). The earliest symptoms are usually pain and neck stiffness. Pain frequently results from irritation of the second cervical nerve root at the craniocervical junction and may be aggravated by sudden or jarring movements (5). Occipital headaches are common, and neurologic symptoms are multiple and often vague. They may range from paresthesias in the hands to Lhermitte's phenomenon, with an electric shock sensation traveling through the body with head flexion (4). A high index of suspicion of craniovertebral involvement is paramount during the examination. Change in ambulatory status and urinary dysfunction always warrants a complete evaluation (18).

Careful physical examination looking for long-tract signs, such as a hyperactive reflex, positive Babinski sign, pathologic clonus, and loss of proprioception, is essential to distinguish myelopathy from more distal involvement. Peripheral rheumatoid disease may mask cord or brain stem compression until it is too late for a reasonable recovery of function. Vertebrobasilar insufficiency, especially with AAI, may cause a loss of equilibrium, tinnitus, vertigo, diplopia, and visual disturbances (9). An unexpected high rate of sudden death in RA patients with atlanto-axial dislocation was reported by Mikulowski et al. (17) based on systematic postmortem examinations of 104 patients. Out of 11 patients with severe cord compression, atlanto-axial dislocation was the sole or main cause of death for eight patients and contributory in two others. Neurologic symptoms were not helpful in identifying those at risk of developing sudden fatal cord compression.

A classification system based on neural deficits was proposed by Ranawat and colleagues (8). This system divides neural deficits into three categories: I, II, and IIIA and IIIB. Class I implies no neural deficit. Class II represents subjective weakness with hyperreflexia and dysesthesia, whereas class III involvement represents objective findings of weakness and long-tract signs. IIIA patients are ambulatory, and IIIB patients are quadriparetic and not ambulatory.

RADIOLOGIC EVALUATION

Plain radiographs, magnetic resonance imaging (MRI), and computerized tomography (CT) with and without intrathecal contrast are the three most commonly used diagnostic modalities to delineate rheumatoid involvement. Plain roentgenograms are the best preliminary screening tool and include lateral flexion–extension dynamic views, an open-mouth odontoid view, and an anteroposterior view. MRI allows visualization of soft tissues,

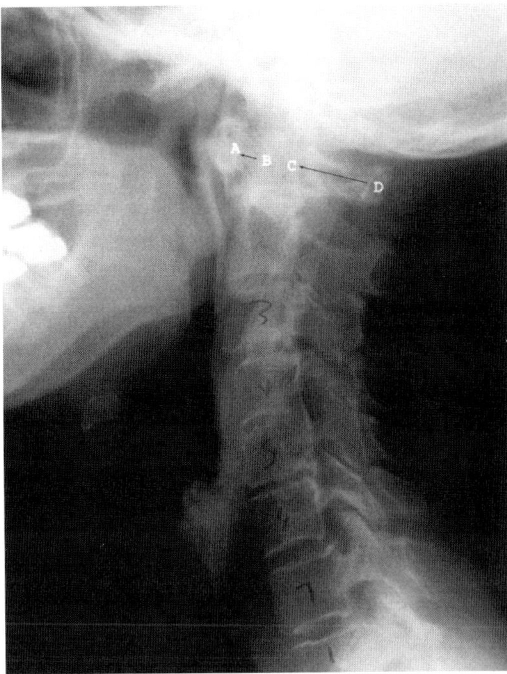

Figure 44.1. Lateral x-ray of cervical spine. Line *A–B* is anterior atlanto-dens interval. Line *C–D* is posterior atlanto-dens interval.

TABLE 44.1. Radiographic Criteria for Atlanto-Axial Impaction

Name	Definition	Abnormal Criteria
McRae & Barnum	Line across foramen magnum (basion to opisthion)	Any protrusion of dens above the line
Chamberlain	Line from hard palate to opisthion	Dens >3 mm above the line
McGregor	Line from hard palate to most caudal point on the midline occipital curve	Dens >4.5 mm above the line
Wackenheim	Line along the superior surface of the clivus	Tip of dens posterior to the line
Fischgold & Metzger	Line between digastric grooves (where mastoid process connects to the skull) on anteroposterior open-mouth view	Tip of dens <10 mm from the line
Clark station	Dividing C2 into thirds (station I, II, III) on sagittal plane	Middle or lower third of C2 at the level of arch of C1
Ranawat	Distance between transverse axis of C1 and middle of pedicle of C2	Male <15 mm; female <13 mm
Redlund-Johnell & Pettersson	Distance between McGregor line and inferior end plate of C2	Male <34 mm; female <29 mm
Kauppi & Sakaguchi	Line along the lowest part of arch of C1 (lower atlas arch line)	Tip of superior facet of C2 above the line

including pannus formation, spinal cord, as well as the cervicomedullary junction. CT provides the best bony details for preoperative planning. CT with intrathecal contrast can be useful in demonstrating spinal cord compression (19).

AAS has been traditionally defined as an atlanto-dens interval (ADI) of more than 3 mm with translation noted on lateral flexion–extension radiographs. ADI (Fig. 44.1) is the distance between the posterior edge of the anterior ring of atlas and the anterior surface of the odontoid process and measured along the transverse axis of the atlas ring (20). Biomechanical data have shown that an ADI greater than 10 to 12 mm indicates complete disruption of the atlanto-axial ligaments (21). It is important to realize that the ADI can falsely appear to be improving with an increasing degree of vertical translocation of the dens (7,12,13,22). As the odontoid moves superiorly, its wider base and the body of the second cervical vertebra approach the level of anterior arch of C1, filling the space and falsely appearing to decrease the arch-odontoid distance (7). Multiple authors have pointed out that the ADI does not reliably correlate with neurologic outcome (12,13,15,19,22).

The posterior atlanto-dental interval (PADI), or space available for the cord (SAC), is measured from the posterior aspect of the dens to the anterior aspect of the atlas lamina (Fig. 44.1). Boden has advocated using the PADI as a reliable screening tool for identifying high-risk patients who require further evaluation with MRI or CT/myelography (19). A PADI measurement of 14 mm or less has a sensitivity (the ability to detect those with paralysis) of 97% and negative predictive value of 94%. This means that if a patient has PADI more than 14 mm, then there is 94% chance that this patient will not have paralysis.

MRI allows the clinician to visualize inflammatory tissue around the odontoid and is the gold standard for cord evaluation (3,18,23–25). Hamilton et al. (3) suggested that, if cord compromise is evident on MRI, deterioration is likely, regardless of initial clinical and plain x-ray features. The use of flexed versus neutral position during MRI examination has been controversial. There is a significant difference between the diameter of the spinal cord in the neutral and flexed position (23). However, placement of the patient with cord compromise in a flexed position during MRI examination has the possibility of potential neurologic complications and requires an alert, cooperative patient.

Numerous radiographic criteria have been described for AAI (8,26–32), as indicated in Table 44.1. Plain radiographs are often difficult to interpret, due to erosion of the apex of the dens and projection of the mastoid over the osteoporotic dens. Riew et al. (33) studied the cervical radiographs of 131 patients with RA, with 67 patients further evaluated by CT and MRI. Radiographic parameters to diagnose AAI were compared. The most sensitive criteria were the Wackenheim line (88%) (Fig. 44.2) and the Clark station (83%). The specificity was highest with the Redlund-Johnell measurement (76%). The Clark station was the most consistently measured criterion measured on the same radiographs by the same observer. Because no single test had a sensitivity and specificity of greater than 90%, the study recommended using a combination of the Clark station, the Redlund-Johnell criterion, and the Ranawat criterion (Fig. 44.3) as screening test for basilar invagination. If any of these three are positive, then the patient is considered to have basilar invagination. The sensitivity of the combined measurements was 94%, with a negative predictive value of 91%. The authors also suggest that, if plain radiographs leave any doubt about the diagnosis, MRI or CT should be used to confirm the diagnosis, because plain radiographic criteria will miss 6% of patients.

Lateral cervical spine radiographs with flexion and extension views are used as a screening tool for SAS. Anterior translation of greater than 3.5 mm is considered abnormal (4). Cervical height index is measured by the distance from the center of the C2 pedicle to the inferior end plate of C7 divided by the distance from the center of the C2 pedicle to tip of C2 spinous process. A cervical height index of less than 2 is a significant independent predictor of neurologic compromise (34). Boden recommends MRI scanning if the posterior subaxial canal diameter is less than 14 mm on plain radiographs. The SAC in the subaxial region is best assessed by MRI (15,25,35).

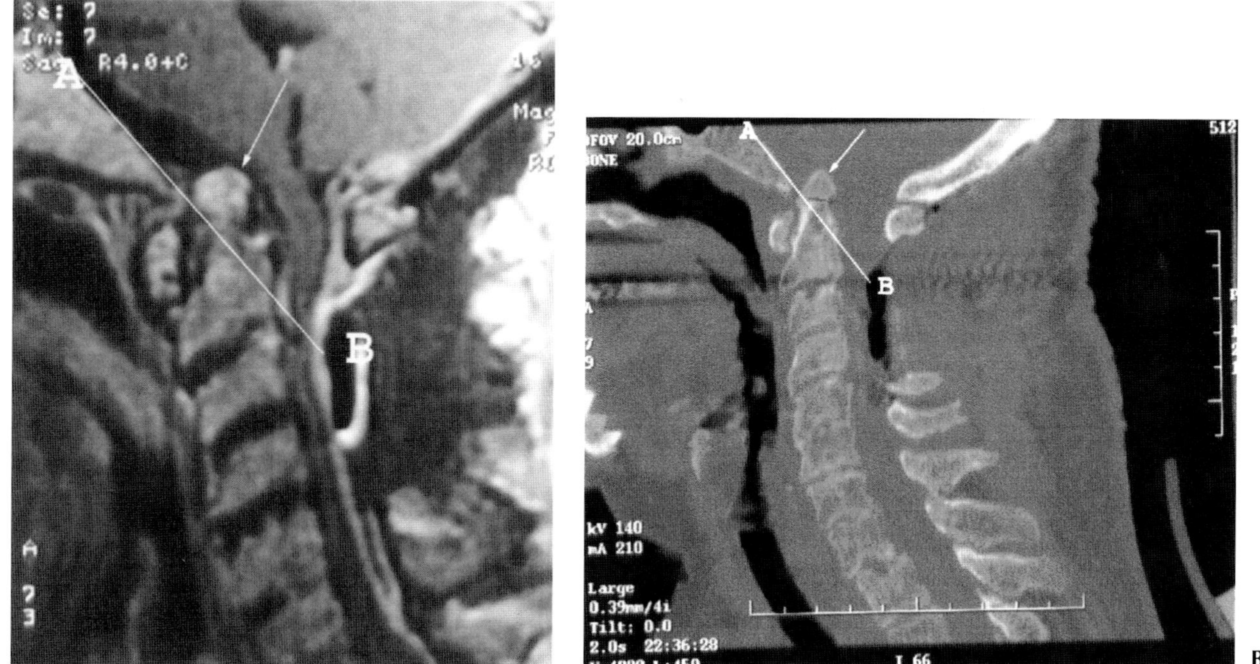

Figure 44.2. Magnetic resonance image of cervical spine mid-sagittal T2 view **(A)** and computed tomography scan sagittal reconstruction **(B)**. Line *A–B* along clivus marks the Wackenheim line. Arrows point to the tip of odontoid, which extends abnormally above the Wackenheim line.

NATURAL HISTORY

RA of the cervical spine is a progressive disease. Radiographic progression occurs to a greater degree than neural involvement, and the majority of patients can be treated medically without surgical intervention. A prospective study of the progression of the rheumatoid cervical spine was done by following 106 patients starting in 1974 over 5 years (7). At the start of the study, 46 patients already had radiographic evidence of rheumatoid involvement of the cervical spine. Cervical disease was evaluated based on pain levels, neural involvement, and radiographic abnormalities. Eighty percent of the patients had radiographic progression, but only 36% had neurologic deterioration. Pain was the only feature of the disease that showed any tendency to improve. The authors concluded that only 10% of patients with radiographic involvement deteriorate to a level requiring sur-

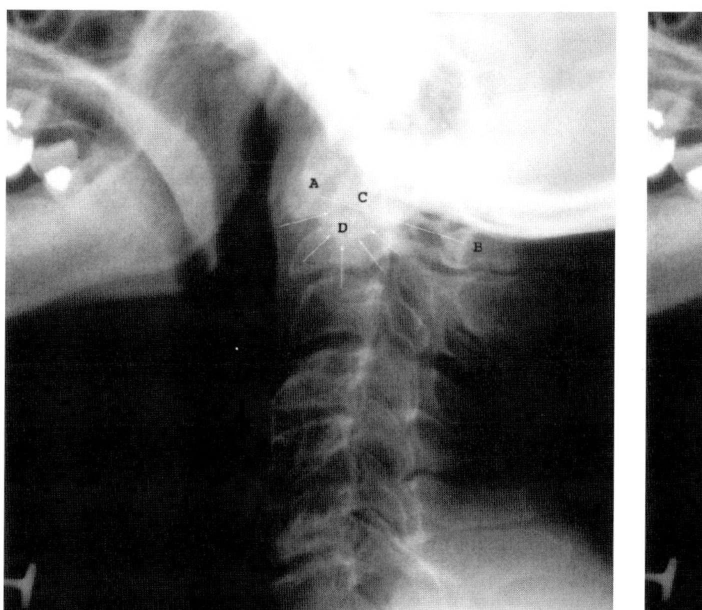

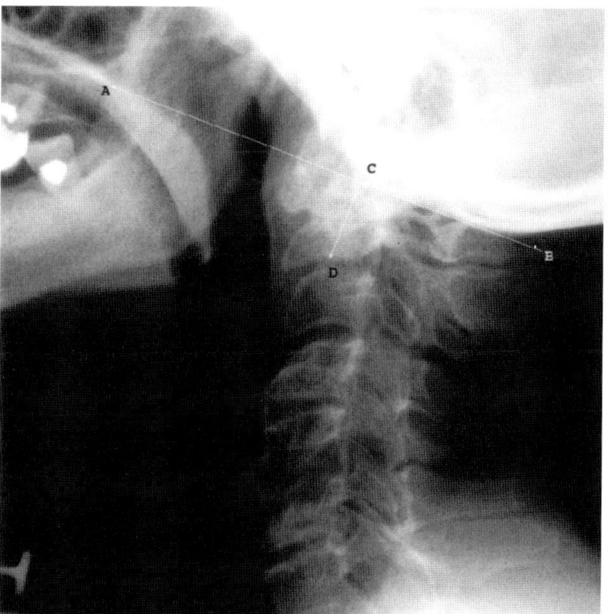

Figure 44.3. Lateral x-ray of cervical spine. **A:** Ranawat measurement. Measuring the length of the line *C–D* in millimeters from the sclerotic ring of C2 (outlined by arrows) to the line *A–B*, marking the ring of C1. **B:** Redlund-Johnell measurement. It is the perpendicular line *C–D* from the McGregor line (*A–B*) to the end plate of C2 at midbody in millimeters.

gery. Another prospective study assessed 41 cases of AAS over a 10-year period (36). Roentgenographically, 61% were unchanged and 27% showed progressive subluxation. Twelve patients had died, but only two had evidence of neurologic damage.

In contrast, rheumatoid patients with cervical myelopathy who do not undergo surgical intervention have an extremely poor prognosis. Sunahara et al. reported on 21 rheumatoid patients with myelopathy secondary to AAS who declined surgery (37). Neural deterioration was found in 76% of cases at 3 to 7 years' follow-up. All patients became bedridden within 3 years of the onset of myelopathy, and seven of the patients died suddenly from unknown reasons. The cumulative probability of survival was 0% in the first 7 years after the onset of myelopathy. In another study, Meijers et al. reported on nine myelopathic patients who were not operated on secondary to patient refusal and poor health. All nine patients died within a year, and four out of the nine patients died secondary to cord compression (38). Postmortem analysis of 11 patients with paralysis secondary to RA of the cervical spine revealed abnormal histology of the spinal cord, due to ongoing mechanical and vascular impairment in nine cases (39).

PREDICTOR OF PROGRESSION, PARALYSIS, AND RECOVERY

Factors associated with the progression of subluxation are a history of medical treatment with corticosteroids, seropositivity, the presence of rheumatoid nodules, and the presence of erosive and deforming articular disease (11). Omura et al. in 2002 demonstrated that seropositivity and deforming joint involvement are the two most important factors associated with cervical spine deterioration (40). The study further compared 11 patients who underwent surgical treatment to six patients who refused surgery. All 17 patients were seropositive with deforming type joint involvement. Four of the six patients who refused surgery ended up completely bedridden, whereas the two remaining patients died after minor trauma. In contrast, all of the 11 operated-on patients either improved or maintained their activities of daily living score.

Boden et al. (15) assessed radiographic predictors of paralysis in a series of 73 patients with an average follow-up of 7 years. PADI and subaxial sagittal canal measurement on plain radiographs correlated with the presence and severity of paralysis (15,41). All the patients with weakness and long tract signs (Ranawat class III) in this study had a measurement of less than 14 mm. In an MRI study of 15 rheumatoid patients, all patients with a cervicomedullary angle less than 135 degrees had evidence of brain stem compression, cervical myelopathy, or C2 root pain. The cervicomedullary angle is defined by the angle subtended by lines drawn parallel to the ventral surfaces of the medulla and upper cervical cord. Cervicomedullary angle criterion is a specific but not sensitive test, as three out of seven patients with neurologic dysfunction had normal angles (42). Dvorak et al. reported that six out of seven patients with clinical and neurophysiologic signs of cervical myelopathy had a spinal cord diameter of less than 6 mm either in the neutral or flexed position on MRI (23). Kawaida et al. found evidence of compression of the cord when the true SAC is less than 13 mm (43). Weissman reported that the male sex, AAS greater than 9 mm, the presence of AAI, and lateral subluxation were all factors associated with upper spinal cord compression (12).

Boden et al., in their study, suggested that the most important predictor of recovery is the preoperative PADI. No recovery occurred if the PADI was less than 10 mm in patients with AAS. In contrast, patients with PADI greater than 10 mm had recovery of at least one neurologic class. For patients with both AAS and AAI, clinically important neurologic recovery occurred only when PADI was at least 13 mm. For patients with SAS, complete motor recovery occurred only if the subaxial canal diameter was greater than 14 mm (15). Other authors suggest that other factors, such as preoperative neurologic function, spinal cord area, and the degree of vertical translocation, are more important factors influencing the final neurologic outcome (13). Klein et al. also stated that the duration of neurologic signs and symptoms referable to cervical spine was the most significant predictor of neurologic outcome (34).

INDICATIONS FOR CERVICAL SPINE SURGERY

Intractable pain, progressive neurologic impairment, and the presence of myelopathy are the three most well-accepted indications for cervical spine surgery in rheumatoid patients (5,11,19). Controversy surrounds patients with severe radiographic evidence of instability and with minimal or absent clinical symptoms. Some authors refer to this group of patients as having an *impending neurologic deficit* (19,20). The argument for prophylactic surgery in this patient population is supported by a large volume of data showing that early surgical intervention leads to a better outcome and fewer complications (6,20,44–47). The prognosis for rheumatoid patients with myelopathy is so poor that intervention before a severe neurologic deficit is warranted (11,19,20,41). The argument against prophylactic surgery is based on the previously mentioned prospective study on progression of RA of the cervical spine. Radiographic findings do not necessarily correlate with clinical symptoms. One-half of patients with radiographic evidence of instability are asymptomatic (7,36).

Boden et al. have proposed an algorithm for the treatment of rheumatoid patients with minimal pain and without a neurologic deficit. For the group of patients with AAS, they were observed clinically, unless the PADI measured less than 14 mm. MRI was then used to evaluate the cord anatomy in these patients. Surgery was considered if the cord diameter in flexion was less than 6 mm, the cervicomedullary angle was less than 135 degrees, or the canal diameter was less than 13 mm. Asymptomatic patients with AAI on plain films required an MRI. Surgery was considered if there was any evidence of cord compression. Patients with SAS without neurologic deficits were followed by the posterior subaxial canal diameter on plain radiographs. MRI was performed if the subaxial canal diameter was less than 14 mm on plain films, and surgery was suggested if the SAC was less than 13 mm on MRI (15,19,41).

SURGICAL CONSIDERATIONS

Surgical treatment is individualized for each patient. A significant number of rheumatoid patients have been treated chronically with corticosteroids and may be frail, malnourished, osteoporotic, and immunosuppressed (48,49). All medical problems, including nutrition, should be optimized preoperatively to provide patients with the best chance for recovery. Careful preoperative planning with liberal use of imaging studies may be necessary to delineate the distorted anatomy. Patients need to be informed and understand that rheumatoid cervical spine surgery is associated with a high morbidity and mortality (22,44,45,50,51).

Preoperative Cervical Traction

Preoperative cervical traction is used most often for patients with AAI and severe subluxation. The goals of traction are to reduce the subluxation and relieve compression of the brain stem or spinal cord (5,11,20). If relief of pain and neurologic symptoms is achieved with traction, stabilization with fusion alone without decompression may be all that is required (14,52). Constant skeletal traction is applied using either Gardner-Wells tongs or the Halo ring apparatus. Traction begins with 7 lb in patients with AAI and may be increased to 15 lb. In severe subluxation, traction is started at 8 lb and may be increased to 25 lb. Frequent neurologic checks and radiographic examination are required. Plain radiographs, tomograms, or CT may be used to evaluate reduction. Length of time in traction has been variably reported from overnight to several weeks (8,11,14,38). Halo-wheelchair can be used during daytime to decrease morbidity associated with prolonged immobilization. Cove and Lipson reported the result of using halo traction in bed and halo-wheelchair traction for 44 patients (53). Thirty-six out of 44 patients had neurologic improvement of at least one Ranawat grade, and pain improved in 27 patients. Radiographic changes in traction failed to show a reduction in subluxation in ten patients.

Airway Management

Awake fiber-optic–assisted intubation is preferred over non–fiber-optic intubation. Wattenmaker et al. reviewed the records of 128 posterior cervical cases for problems related to RA (54). Upper-airway obstruction after extubation occurred in 14% of patients who had non–fiber-optic intubation and in 1% of patients who had fiber-optic–assisted intubation. This finding suggests that the development of upper-airway obstruction is mainly attributed to edema caused by trauma during the non–fiber-optic intubation process. It is recommended that all patients, especially those who have non–fiber-optic intubation, should be monitored carefully for evidence of stridor for at least 12 hours after extubation. The study did not demonstrate an advantage of keeping these patients intubated overnight to protect against upper-airway obstruction.

Decompression

Decompression is considered for patients with a persistent neurologic deficit despite a trial of continuous cervical skeletal traction. The level of decompression depends on the location of cord impingement. Large inflammatory pannus anterior to the odontoid may require a transoral, retropharyngeal, or transmaxillary approach (55–57). Impingement at the posterior aspect of the cord may require decompression involving the posterior elements or posterior foramen magnum.

Despite advances in methods of retraction and microsurgical techniques, wound infection, cerebrospinal fluid fistulas, and meningitis are still major concerns of transoral decompression. The overall complication rate has decreased from approximately 32% to 15% in patients who do not undergo splitting of soft palate (58). Moreover, Zygmunt et al. have questioned the need for transoral decompression (59). In a study to visualize periodontoid pannus after posterior occipitocervical fusion, the postoperative MRI revealed resorption of pannus in all nine cases after stabilization. Casey et al. conducted a prospective study in 116 patients with RA and AAI who underwent cervical spine surgery for symptomatic myelopathy (13). The authors reported a very low complication rate as a direct result of transoral odontoidectomy. However, the degree of neurologic recovery was the same for patients who underwent posterior fusion alone and those who underwent both anterior decompression and posterior fusion. Forty-four percent to 46% of both groups improved by at least one Ranawat class.

The role of decompressive laminectomy without simultaneous fusion in rheumatoid patients with cervical myelopathy and without evidence of instability on flexion and extension radiographs was addressed by Christensson et al. in a prospective study of 15 patients (60). The study found that 14 out of 15 patients had no evidence of increased motion at the operated levels postoperatively. However, one patient developed severe vertical translocation 28 months after undergoing an isolated C1 laminectomy without fusion, which led to sudden quadriplegia. The author concluded that laminectomy with preservation of facets could be performed on rheumatoid patients without preoperative evidence of instability. C1 laminectomy should always be followed by an occipitocervical arthrodesis if there is any evidence of vertical translocation.

Bone Graft versus No Bone Graft

Autologous iliac crest bone grafting has been routinely used for posterior cervical arthrodesis. However, there is a definite morbidity associated with graft harvesting and graft site problems. Moskovich et al. reported on instrumented occipitocervical fusion with and without bone grafting (1). There was no significant difference with respect to radiographic craniovertebral motion, neck-pain rating, and presence of subaxial abnormalities or vertical subluxation. The author concluded that avoiding the harvesting of autogenous bone reduced the morbidity of occipitocervical fusion without compromising the outcome.

SURGICAL PROCEDURES

The goals of surgery are stabilization of the cervical spine, recovery from neurologic compression, and pain relief (5,61). The general rule is to include all unstable levels in the arthrodesis (20) and to include any unstable subaxial levels. A posterior C1-C2 arthrodesis is recommended for isolated, reducible AAS. If the AAS is not reducible, the fusion may need to be extended to the occiput with a concomitant decompressive laminectomy of C1. With any pathology involving AAI, an occipitocervical arthrodesis will be necessary (8).

C1-C2 Fusion

The most common methods of C1-C2 fusion are Gallie (62) or modified Gallie fusion (63), Brooks and Jenkins fusion (35), Magerl transarticular screw fixation (64), and Halifax interlaminar clamp techniques (65). Grob et al. performed a biomechanical evaluation of all four fixation techniques and concluded that the Magerl technique tended to allow the least rotation (66). The Gallie technique allowed significantly more rotation than the other three fixation techniques. The anteroposterior translation was equal for all fixation techniques.

A modified Gallie fusion is a frequently used method. A central H-shaped iliac crest bone graft is secured between the posterior arch of both the atlas and axis with an 18- or 20-gauge wire. The wire is passed cephalad under the arch of C1, then looped back and down over the spinous process of C2. The end of the wire is tightened around the graft between C1 and C2. Halo immobilization is required postoperatively. A Brooks fusion involves two pieces of beveled rectangular iliac crest bone grafts placed between C1 and C2 arches in a paracentral fashion. Sublaminar wires are passed under both C1 and C2 and tightened over the graft. Because of the osteoporotic nature of bone in chronic RA, the original authors do not ordinarily recommend its use in this patient population (35). Magerl screws are inserted from base of C2, through the C1-C2 facet, and into the lateral mass of C1 (Fig. 44.4).

Careful evaluation of the patient's vertebral artery anatomy on a preoperative CT scan is required before C1-C2 screw fixa-

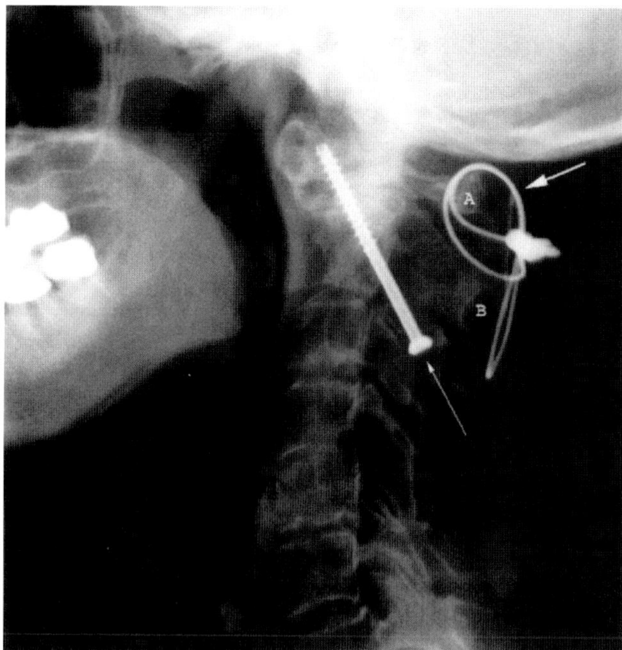

Figure 44.4. Lateral cervical spine x-ray demonstrating a posterior C1-C2 fusion using the Magerl screw technique (*small arrow*). Also, Gallie posterior wire technique using wire cable (*large arrow*) around C1 lamina (*A*) and C2 spinous process (*B*).

tion. Up to 20% of patients have vertebral artery anatomy that precludes safe use of screws.

Posterior Occipitocervical Fusion

Multiple fixation techniques have been reported for occipitocervical fusion and include the Bohlman triple wiring technique (67), Hartshill rectangle with wire (68), Ransford loop with wire (1,13), threaded Steinmann pin loop with wire (69), Y plate and lateral mass screws (45), T plate with lateral mass screws (52), wiring with methylmethacrylate stabilization (6,70), and a loop and cable construct with split thickness calvarial bone graft (71). Rigid internal fixation with a rod-plate and screw construct with iliac crest bone graft provides the most rigid fixation (72). A cross-link between the two rods at the upper cervical spine is added to provide a posterior fixation point for a sublaminar wire if the posterior arch of C1 is preserved. Autologous iliac crest bone graft is used on all patients to bridge the occipitocervical junction and cervical facets. Methylmethacrylate stabilization is not used because of its associated increased rate of infection (70,73). Post-surgical immobilization with a Miami-J collar for 6 to 12 weeks is used in the majority of patients. The authors do not hesitate to place patients in halo-vest immobilization if stable fixation could not be achieved during surgery.

Lower Cervical Spine Arthrodesis

Multiple fixation methods have been described for lower cervical fusion and include the triple wire technique, Wisconsin button wires with the Hartshill rectangle, a Halifax clamp, and lateral mass plates and screws. Lateral mass screws are directed 25 to 30 degrees lateral to avoid the vertebral artery and 15 degrees cephalad to safeguard the nerve root and facet joints (74). Local bone graft is packed within the facet joints after decortication to help the joints to fuse. If there is instability at the cervicothoracic junction, extension of the fusion to the upper thoracic levels using pedicle screw techniques is undertaken.

TABLE 44.2. Surgical Outcomes of Cervical Spine Surgery in Rheumatoid Arthritis

Year	Author	Number of Patients	Pain Relief (%)	Neurologic Improvement (%)
2001	Van Asselt	31	62	67
1999	Grob	39	96	77
1998	Eyres	26	92	89
1998	Mori	25	96	67
1989	Clark	41	91	27
1987	Sakou	16	100	100
1985	Menezes	45	100	100

Adapted from references 8, 13, 14, 20, 45, 50, 61, 68, 75, and 76.

SURGICAL OUTCOMES

Because the indications for cervical spine surgery are intractable pain and neurologic deficit, surgical outcomes are best determined by assessing the operative success in these two categories (Table 44.2).

Pain Relief

The relief of upper cervical neck pain, occipital neuralgia, headache, and facial pain is the most encouraging outcome of rheumatoid cervical spine surgery. At least partial pain relief is achieved between 62% and 100% of patients (8,14,20,45,50,61,67,68,75,76). Eight out of the ten studies reported at least partial relief of pain in at least 90% of the patients who had surgery. It was noted by Clark that many patients, although they had not complained of severe pain preoperatively, stated the neck felt much better postoperatively (20).

Neurologic Recovery

The extent of neurologic improvement alternates greatly between studies (Table 44.2) (8,13,14,20,45,50,61,68,75,76). Peppelman et al. conducted a study of 90 rheumatoid patients looking specifically for improvement of the neurologic deficit after cervical spine fusion (47). Approximately 85% of patients improved at least one Ranawat class. This increased to 94% of patients with isolated AAS or isolated SAS and dropped to 71% of patients with AAI involvement. The author concluded that the most important factor affecting neurologic recovery is the presence of superior migration of the odontoid. McRorie et al. reported that 69% of patients had subjective neurologic improvement but only 27% of patients had objective improvement based on Ranawat classification. The author attributed this difference mainly to the relative insensitivity of the Ranawat classification in detecting change in neurologic status (46). It is also important to note that surgery arrested progression of neurologic deficit in 87% of patients who had neurologic compromise before operation.

COMPLICATIONS

Mortality

The leading cause of postoperation fatality is of cardiopulmonary origin, including myocardial infarction, heart failure, and bronchopneumonia (44,46,76). Santavirta et al. reported that patients who had cardiac disease at the time of the operation and those who had more than 3 mm of cranial subluxation of the odontoid had the highest risk. The age of the patient and the magnitude of

AAS did not correlate with mortality (51). Immediate postoperative mortality was 0% to 13% (5,6,8,38,44,46,61,76). Approximately 25% of myelopathic patients with AAI were dead by 15 months after surgery (13). The accumulated survival in patients with myelopathy was only 27.5% at 10 years after surgery (50). The long-term survival of Ranawat class IIIB patients was extremely poor—58% were dead within 3 years postoperatively (44).

Pseudarthrosis

The pseudarthrosis rate is highest in isolated C1-2 fusions (20), with a nonunion rate as high as 50% for Gallie fusions. The fusion rate is fairly high for occipitocervical and lower cervical fusion and ranges between 74% and 100% (1,4,5,8,13,14,20,45,67,68,75). The pseudarthrosis rate has been noted to be higher in patients treated with corticosteroid for more than 4 years. Santavirta et al. also stated that there was no correlation between clinical outcome and postoperative radiologic findings (51).

Progressive Instability after Arthrodesis

The incidence of SAS below a rigid arthrodesis varies between 5.5% and 50% (4,16,20,50,51) and depends on the type of arthrodesis performed on the patients. Although the rate of subluxation below an occipitocervical fusion was noted to be 36% in 2.6 years, this rate is significantly higher than the reported rate of 5.5% at 9 years for a C1-2 fusion. The high incidence of early SAS in those patients who underwent an occipitocervical fusion is secondary to the biomechanical stresses from a longer lever arm (4). Matsunaga et al. noted that motion segments that manifest abnormal buckling before surgery are predisposed to develop subluxation after occipitocervical fusion (16). Cervical arthrodesis should, thus, include all unstable levels.

CONCLUSION

The majority of patients with RA can be treated conservatively. However, patients with intractable pain, progressive neurologic impairment, and myelopathy require surgical intervention. A high index of suspicion of craniovertebral involvement during examination is important. Identifying patients with impending neurologic deficit on radiographs is invaluable to the surgical decision-making process. Surgical intervention for patients with RA is technically demanding and fraught with complications. Clear understanding of the anatomy, careful preoperative planning, and implementation of the most suitable procedure for each individual patient are the keys to success.

REFERENCES

1. Moskovich R, Crockard A, Shott S, Ransford A. Occipitocervical stabilization for myelopathy in patients with rheumatoid arthritis: implications of not bone-grafting. *J Bone Joint Surg Am* 2000;82A:349–365.
2. Bland JH. Rheumatoid arthritis of the cervical spine. *J Rheumatol* 1974;1:319–342.
3. Hamilton JD, Johnston RA, Madhok R, Capell A. Factors predictive of subsequent deterioration in rheumatoid cervical myelopathy. *Rheumatology* 2001;40:811–815.
4. Kraus DR, Peppelman WC, Agarwal AK. Incidence of subaxial subluxation in patients with generalized rheumatoid arthritis who have had previous occipitocervical fusions. *Spine* 1991;16[Suppl 10]:S486–S489.
5. Zoma A, Sturrock RD, Fisher WD, et al. Surgical stabilization of the rheumatoid cervical spine: a review of indications and results. *J Bone Joint Surg Am* 1987;69B:8–12.
6. Hamilton JD, Gordon MM, McInnes IB, et al. Improved medical and surgical management of cervical spine disease in patients with rheumatoid arthritis over 10 years. *Ann Rheum Dis* 2000;59:434–438.
7. Pellicci PM, Ranawat CS, Tsairis P, Bryan WJ. A prospective study of the progression of rheumatoid arthritis of the cervical spine. *J Bone Joint Surg Am* 1981;63A:342–350.
8. Ranawat CS, O'Leary P, Pellicci P, et al. Cervical spine fusion in rheumatoid arthritis. *J Bone Joint Surg Am* 1979;61A:1003–1010.
9. Lipson SJ. Rheumatoid arthritis of the cervical spine. *Clin Orthop* 1984;182:143–149.
10. Lipson SJ. Cervical myelopathy and posterior atlanto-axial subluxation in patients with rheumatoid arthritis. *J Bone Joint Surg Am* 1985;67A:593–597.
11. Lipson SJ. Rheumatoid arthritis in the cervical spine. *Clin Orthop* 1989; 239:121–127.
12. Weissman BN, Aliabadi P, Weinfeld M, et al. Prognostic features of atlantoaxial subluxation in rheumatoid arthritis patients. *Radiology* 1982;14:745–751.
13. Casey AT, Crockard HA, Stevens J. Vertical translocation. Part II. Outcomes after surgical treatment of rheumatoid cervical myelopathy. *J Neurosurg* 1997;87:863–869.
14. Menezes AH, Van Gilder JC, Clark CR, El-Khoury G. Odontoid upward migration in rheumatoid arthritis: an analysis of 45 patients with "cranial settling." *J Neurosurg* 1985;63:500–509.
15. Boden SD, Dodge LD, Bohlman HH, Rechtine G. Rheumatoid arthritis of the cervical spine: a long-term analysis with predictors of paralysis and recovery. *J Bone Joint Surg Am* 1993;75A:1282–1297.
16. Matsunaga S, Sakou T, Sunahara N, et al. Biomechanical analysis of buckling alignment of the cervical spine: predictive value for subaxial subluxation after occipitocervical fusion. *Spine* 1997;22:765–771.
17. Mikulowski P, Wollheim FA, Rotmil P, Olsen I. Sudden death in rheumatoid arthritis with atlanto-axial dislocation. *Acta Med Scand* 1975;198:445–451.
18. Hey LA. Rheumatoid arthritis of the cervical spine. In: *Neurosurgery*. New York: McGraw-Hill, 1995:3789–3793.
19. Boden SD. Rheumatoid arthritis of the cervical spine: surgical decision making based on predictors of paralysis and recovery. *Spine* 1994;19:2275–2280.
20. Clark CR, Goetz DD, Menezes AH. Arthrodesis of the cervical spine in rheumatoid arthritis. *J Bone Joint Surg Am* 1989;71A:381–392.
21. Fielding W, Cochran GB, Lawsing JF, Hohl M. Tears of the transverse ligament of the atlas: a clinical and biomechanical study. *J Bone Joint Surg Am* 1974;56A:1683–1691.
22. Casey AT, Crockard HA, Bland JM, et al. Predictors of outcome in the quadriparetic nonambulatory myelopathic patient with rheumatoid arthritis: a prospective study of 55 surgically treated Ranawat class IIIB patients. *J Neurosurg* 1996;85:574–581.
23. Dvorak J, Grob D, Baumgartner H, et al. Functional evaluation of the spinal cord by magnetic resonance imaging in patients with rheumatoid arthritis and instability of upper cervical spine. *Spine* 1989;14:1057–1064.
24. Glew D, Watt I, Dieppe PA, Goddard PR. MRI of the cervical spine: rheumatoid arthritis compared with cervical spondylosis. *Clin Radiol* 1991;44:71–76.
25. Kawaida H, Sakou T, Morizono Y. Vertical settling in rheumatoid arthritis: diagnostic value of the Ranawat and Redlund-Johnell methods. *Clin Orthop* 1989;239:128–135.
26. Chamberlain WE. Basilar impression (platybasia): a bizarre developmental anomaly of the occipital bone and upper cervical spine with striking and misleading neurologic manifestations. *Yale J Biol Med* 1939;11:487–496.
27. Hinck VC, Hopkins CE, Savara BS. Diagnostic criteria of basilar impression. *Radiology* 1961;76:572–585.
28. Kauppi M, Sakaguchi M, Konttinen YT, Hamalainen M. A new method of screening for vertical atlantoaxial dislocation. *J Rheumatol* 1990;17:167–172.
29. McGregor M. The significance of certain measurements of the skull in the diagnosis of basilar impression. *Br J Radiol* 1948;21:171–181.
30. McRae DL, Barnum AS. Occipitalization of the atlas. *AJR Am J Roentgenol* 1953;70:23–45.
31. Redlund-Johnell I, Pattersson H. Radiographic measurements of the craniovertebral region: designed for evaluation of abnormalities in rheumatoid arthritis. *Acta Radiol Diagn (Stockh)* 1984;25:23–28.
32. Roentgen WA. *Diagnosis of the craniovertebral region*. New York: Springer, 1974.
33. Riew DK, Hilibrand AS, Palumbo MA, et al. Diagnosing basilar invagination in the rheumatoid patients: the reliability of radiographic criteria. *J Bone Joint Surg Am* 2001;83A:194–200.
34. Klein JD, Hey LA, Lipson SJ. Predictors of the preoperative neurologic deficit and postoperative outcome in patients with rheumatoid arthritis of the subaxial cervical spine. *Orthop Transaction* 1994;18:716.
35. Brooks AL, Jenkins EB. Atlanto-axial arthrodesis by the wedge compression method. *J Bone Joint Surg Am* 1978;60A:279–284.
36. Rana NA. Natural history of atlanto-axial subluxation in rheumatoid arthritis. *Spine* 1989;14:1054–1056.
37. Sunahara N, Matsunaga S, Mori T, et al. Clinical course of conservatively managed rheumatoid arthritis patients with myelopathy. *Spine* 1997;22: 2603–2608.
38. Meijers KAE, Cats A, Kremer HPH, et al. Cervical myelopathy in rheumatoid arthritis. *Clin Exp Rheumatol* 1984;2:239–245.
39. Delamarter RB, Dodge L, Bohlman HH, Bambetti PL. Postmortem neuropathologic analysis of eleven patients with paralysis secondary to rheumatoid arthritis of the cervical spine. *Orthop Transaction* 1988;12:54–55.
40. Omura K, Huikuda S, Katsuura A, et al. Evaluation of posterior long fusion versus conservative treatment for the progressive rheumatoid cervical spine. *Spine* 2002;27:1336–1345.
41. Dreyer SJ, Boden SD. Natural history of rheumatoid arthritis of the cervical spine. *Clin Orthop* 1999;366:98–106.

42. Bundschuh C, Modic MT, Kearney F, et al. Rheumatoid arthritis of the cervical spine: surface-coil MR imaging. *AJR Am J Roentgenol* 1988;151:181–187.
43. Kawaida H, Sakou T, Morizono Y, Yashikuni N. Magnetic resonance imaging of upper cervical disorder in rheumatoid arthritis. *Spine* 1989;14:1144–1148.
44. Casey AT, Crockard HA, Bland JM, et al. Surgery on the rheumatoid cervical spine for the non-ambulant myelopathic patient—too much, too late? *Lancet* 1996;347:1004–1007.
45. Grob D, Schutz U, Plotz G. Occipitocervical fusion in patients with rheumatoid arthritis. *Clin Orthop* 1999;366:46–53.
46. McRorie ER, McLoughline P, Russell T, et al. Cervical spine surgery in patients with rheumatoid arthritis: an appraisal. *Ann Rheum Dis.* 1996;55:99–104.
47. Peppelman WC, Kraus DR, Donaldson WF, Agarwal A. Cervical spine surgery in rheumatoid arthritis: improvement of neurologic deficit after cervical spine fusion. *Spine* 1993;18:2375–2379.
48. Sandeline J, Santavirta S, Laasonen E, Slatis P. Spontaneous fracture of atlas of cervical spine affected by rheumatoid arthritis. *Scand J Rheumatol* 1985;14:167–170.
49. McGrath H, McCormick C, Carey ME. Pyogenic cervical osteomyelitis presenting as a massive prevertebral abscess in a patient with rheumatoid arthritis. *Am J Med* 1988;84:363–365.
50. Mori T, Matsunaga S, Sunahara N, Sakou T. 3- to 11-year followup of occipitocervical fusion for rheumatoid arthritis. *Clin Orthop* 1998;351:169–179.
51. Santavirta S, Knottinen YT, Laasonen E, et al. Ten-year results of operations for rheumatoid cervical spine disorders. *J Bone Joint Surg Br* 1991;73B:116–120.
52. Vale FL, Oliver M, Cahill W. Rigid occipitocervical fusion. *J Neurosurg* 1999; 91:144–150.
53. Cove J, Lipson SJ. The role of preoperative management by halo-wheelchair traction in patients with rheumatoid arthritic subluxations of the cervical spine. *Orthop Transaction* 1996–1997;20:436.
54. Wattenmaker I, Concepcion M, Hibberd P, Lipson S. Upper-airway obstruction and perioperative management of the airway in patients managed with posterior operations on the cervical spine for rheumatoid arthritis. *J Bone Joint Surg Am* 1994;76A:360–365.
55. Cocke EW, Roberson JH, Roberson JT, Crook JP. The extended maxillotomy and subtotal maxillectomy for excision of skull base tumors. *Arch Otolaryngol Head Neck Surg* 1990;116:92–104.
56. Crockard HA, Calder I, Ransford AO. One-stage transoral decompression and posterior fixation in rheumatoid atlanto-axial subluxation. *J Bone Joint Surg Br* 1990;72B:682–685.
57. Hadley MN, Spetzler RF, Sonntag VKH. The transoral approach to the superior cervical spine: a review of 53 cases of extradural cervicomedullary compression. *J Neurosurg* 1989;72:16–23.
58. Jones DC, Vanghan ED, Findlay GF. Oropharyngeal morbidity following transoral approaches to the upper cervical spine. *Int J Oral Maxillofac Surg* 1998;27:295–298.
59. Zygmunt S, Saveland H, Brattstrom H, et al. Reduction of rheumatoid periodontoid pannus following posterior occipita-cervical fusion visualized by magnetic resonance imaging. *Br J Neurosurg* 1988;2:315–320.
60. Christensson D, Saveland H, Zygmunt S, et al. Cervical laminectomy without fusion in patients with rheumatoid arthritis. *J Neurosurg* 1999;90:186–190.
61. Santavirta S, Slatis P, Kankaanpaa U, et al. Treatment of the cervical spine in rheumatoid arthritis. *J Bone Joint Surg Am* 1988;70A:658–667.
62. Gallie W. Fracture and dislocation of C spine. *Am J Surg* 1939;46:495–499.
63. Fielding W, Hawkins R, Ratzan SA. Spine fusion for atlanto-axial instability. *J Bone Joint Surg Am* 1976;58A:400–407.
64. Magerl F, Seemann P. Stable posterior fusion of the atlas and axis by transarticular screw fixation. In: Kehr P, Weidner A, eds. *Cervical spine.* Strassbourg: Springer Verlag, 1987:322–327.
65. Statham P, O'Sullivan M, Russell T. The Halifax interlaminar clamp for posterior cervical fusion: initial experience in the United Kingdom. *Neurosurgery* 1993;32:396–399.
66. Grob D, Crisco J, Panjabi M, et al. Biomechanical evaluation of four different posterior atlantoaxial fixation techniques. *Spine* 1992;17:430–490.
67. Wertheim SB, Bhlman HH. Occipitocervical fusion: indications, technique, and long-term results in thirteen patients. *J Bone Joint Surg Am* 1987;69A:833–836.
68. Sakou T, Kawaida H, Morizono Y, et al. Occipitoatlantoaxial fusion utilizing a rectangular rod. *Clin Orthop* 1989;239:136–144.
69. Apostolides PJ, Dickman CA, Golfinos JG, et al. Threaded Steinmann pin fusion of the craniovertebral junction. *Spine* 1996;21:1630–1637.
70. Clark CR, Keggi KJ, Panjabi MM. Methylmethacrylate stabilization of the cervical spine. *J Bone Joint Surg Am* 1984;66A:40–46.
71. Roberson SC, Menezes AH. Occipital calvarial bone graft in posterior occipitocervical fusion. *Spine* 1998;23:249–253.
72. Huckell CB, Buchowski JM, Richardson WJ, et al. Functional outcome of plate fusions for disorders of the occipitocervical junction. *Clin Orthop* 1999;359:136–145.
73. Bryan WJ, Inglis AE, Sculco TP, Ranawat CS. Methylmethacrylate stabilization for enhancement of posterior cervical arthrodesis in rheumatoid arthritis. *J Bone Joint Surg Am* 1982;64A:1045–1050.
74. Anderson PA, Henley MB, Grady MD, et al. Posterior cervical arthrodesis with AO Reconstruction plates and bone graft. *Spine* 1991;16[Suppl 3]:S72–S79.
75. Eyres KS, Gray DH, Roberson P. Posterior surgical treatment for the rheumatoid cervical spine. *Br J Rheumatol* 1998;37:756–759.
76. Van Asselt KM, Lems WF, Bongartz EB, et al. Outcome of cervical spine surgery in patients with rheumatoid arthritis. *Ann Rheum Dis* 2001;60:448–452.

CHAPTER 45

Extraarticular Disease

John S. Sundy, Glenn J. Jaffe, and Rex M. McCallum

Extraarticular manifestations occur in 40% of patients with rheumatoid arthritis (RA). The high prevalence of extraarticular manifestations has led some authors to suggest that RA should be considered a systemic disease with primarily articular manifestations. Extraarticular disease causes severe morbidity and may account for a significant percentage of the excess mortality related to RA. Effective management of extraarticular RA requires broad knowledge of the spectrum of possible manifestations. The physician should incorporate this knowledge into an approach for anticipating potential extraarticular disease in RA patients. This task is made challenging by the fact that some extraarticular manifestations have clinical features similar to other complications associated with RA, such as drug toxicity, secondary infection, or comorbid diseases. Some authors have speculated that extraarticular disease has become less prevalent, perhaps because of more aggressive treatment of RA. Long-term observational studies are needed to characterize the impact that therapy with biologic agents has on the expression and course of extraarticular disease.

The purpose of this chapter is to describe the management of extraarticular manifestations of RA. We have taken an organ system approach to describe the typical clinical presentation of extraarticular disease. The focus is on conditions that are directly related to the inflammatory process of RA. Organ system damage related to drug toxicity and other comorbid illness is discussed elsewhere. Recommendations for the diagnosis and treatment of extraarticular disease are incorporated into each section.

OCULAR MANIFESTATIONS

Ocular manifestations, particularly keratoconjunctivitis sicca (KCS), are common in RA and occur in as many as 25% of patients (1,2). Other common ocular manifestations are episcleritis and scleritis, followed less frequently by peripheral ulcerative keratitis and central or paracentric ulcerative keratitis (1) (Table 45.1, Fig. 45.1).

Keratoconjunctivitis Sicca

KCS (aqueous tear deficiency, or dry eyes) is common in patients with RA, often in association with xerostomia, a combination referred to as *secondary Sjögren's syndrome* (SS) (1,3). Patients report foreign body sensation and dry, painful eyes that are worse in the evening or with reading. Additional symptoms may include burning, redness, photophobia, itching, excessive tearing, inability to tear, and intermittent blurring of vision (3). Ocular signs include absence or diminution of the inferior tear meniscus, a viscous corneal tear film with mucous strands and particulate matter, abnormal Schirmer's test, abnormal rose bengal or fluorescein staining of the cornea (typically in the interpalpebral area), loss of corneal sensitivity, and punctate epithelial erosions (3,4). Breaks in the corneal epithelium are associated with increased risk of infectious keratitis and, less frequently, paracentral corneal ulceration that can perforate the globe (4). SS is associated with lymphocytic infiltration of the lacrimal glands, epithelial tissue atrophy, and replacement of epithelial tissue with connective tissue, leading to secretory dysfunction of the glands with KCS and xerostomia (3,5).

The treatment of KCS is symptomatic, with the goals of relieving symptoms, promoting healing of the ocular surface, and preventing complications, such as corneal epithelial breaks, erosions, and ulcers (3,6). Treatment strategies focus on lubricating the ocular surface and conserving endogenously produced tears. Topically applied lubricating drops and ointments are the major treatments for KCS and provide at least temporary relief in almost all patients. Many artificial tear options are available for consideration, varying in pH, viscosity, and the presence or absence of preservatives, but there are no true biologically active tear replacements available (3). One therapeutic approach is to begin tear supplementation every 2 hours while awake. With symptomatic improvement, the frequency of the artificial tears should be tapered to the lowest frequency that provides improvement similar to that of every 2-hour therapy (1). Major questions from the patient are often: (a) How often is the topical therapy administered? (b) Does it burn immediately after instillation into the eyes? (c) How long does the relief last? If a topical therapy is useful but does not last long enough, a product with greater viscosity to increase the retention time should be chosen. A particular artificial tear preparation may burn, often secondary to the preservative used; therefore, all artificial tear preparations are not the same or interchangeable. A new choice with a different preservative may serve the patient.

The development of preservative-free artificial tears is a significant advance and may be necessary in patients who do not tolerate several different varieties of preservative-containing preparations or in those who use these topical therapies more than four times per day (3). Ointment lubricants can be used before going to bed and coat the cornea during sleep (3). In severe disease, ointments may be used during the day, although blurry vision and sticky sensation of the eyes complicate their

TABLE 45.1. Major Ocular Manifestations of Rheumatoid Arthritis and Major Treatments

Manifestations	Most Frequent Treatments
Keratoconjunctivitis sicca	Artificial tears, avoid dry environments, punctal occlusion
Episcleritis and scleritis	
Anterior	
Diffuse	Topical NSAIDs, topical corticosteroids, oral NSAIDs
Nodular	Systemic corticosteroids, oral NSAIDs
Necrotizing with inflammation	Systemic corticosteroids, oral NSAIDs, cyclophosphamide
Necrotizing without inflammation (scleromalacia perforans)	Treatment of underlying rheumatoid arthritis joint disease
Posterior	Systemic corticosteroids, oral NSAIDs, cyclophosphamide
Corneal ulceration	
Peripheral ulcerative keratitis	Systemic corticosteroids, artificial tears, punctal occlusion, cyclophosphamide
Central/paracentral corneal ulcers	Tissue adhesive, bandage contact lenses, topical cyclosporine 2%

NSAIDs, nonsteroidal antiinflammatory drugs.

use. Sustained-release lubricant preparations exist and work best for patients with mild to moderate disease. Often, patients with severe disease who lack the tear volume to dissolve the polymer delivery device do not tolerate them (3). Artificial tears made from autologous sera may have symptomatic efficacy in patients who do not respond to other approaches (7). Autologous serum-derived tears can also be effective in the healing of persistent corneal epithelial defects associated with KCS (7). Topical cyclosporine 2% improved tear film break-up time and rose bengal staining over a 2-month period in 30 patients who participated in a randomized double-blind placebo-controlled trial of 30 patients with secondary SS, 22 of whom had RA (8). Topical cyclosporine 1% was associated with symptomatic improvement in a small randomized double-blind crossover pilot trial (9). Topical steroids and nonsteroidal antiinflammatory drugs (NSAIDs) have both been efficacious in the treatment of KCS in the short term (10).

Systemic therapies have also been used in the treatment of KCS and secondary SS (6). Oral cyclosporine may have efficacy (6). Alternate-day therapy with 40 mg of prednisone for 6 months was effective in a small prospective study of seven patients with primary SS. Although this approach is not recommended, improved Schirmer's test and reduced punctate staining, rose bengal staining, corneal filaments, tear lysozyme levels, and lymphocytic infiltration of labial salivary gland biopsy were observed (11). No systemic treatment has been widely used because of concerns about side effects in a disease that is not fatal and can often be adequately treated with topical therapy. In addition, ophthalmologists do not believe that the aggressive medical treatment of RA in patients with secondary SS improves the patient's KCS (4).

Lid massage, to express meibomian gland secretion, and applying warm compresses can benefit patients (6). Patients symptomatic on maximal lubricant therapy may benefit from approaches to conserve naturally produced tears. Room humidification is particularly useful in dry climates and at high altitudes (3). Air conditioning, as well as windy and smoky environments, should be avoided (4). Side-shields on glasses and covering the eyes at night (e.g., swim goggles) may help reduce dry eye symptoms. Punctal occlusion is frequently used to conserve naturally produced tears. The occlusion should initially be performed on a temporary basis to assess response and potential excess tearing. Some patients may worsen symptomatically with punctal occlusion, perhaps related to prolonged contact with inflammatory agents in the tears exacerbating epithelial disease (4). Collagen plugs, plastic plugs, and chromic suture are used to create temporary punctal occlusion. Permanent punctal occlusion is typically performed with a disposable thermocautery under topical anesthesia in the clinic. Tarsorrhaphy, the closing of the lateral 20% to 30% of the lid margin surgically, can also be performed to conserve naturally produced tears (3,11).

Episcleritis and Scleritis

Episcleritis refers to inflammation of the episclera, the loose, highly vascular connective tissue that is under Tenon's capsule and is superficial to the sclera (3,12). Episcleritis can be mild, transient, recurrent, bilateral, and diffuse or localized. Pain is uncommon and, when present, is localized to the eye. If therapy is necessary, topical antiinflammatory treatment with NSAIDs is generally effective. Topical corticosteroids can be effective but are not generally necessary. Patients who do not respond to topical therapy usually respond to oral NSAIDs (3,12).

Scleritis is a severe chronic destructive inflammation of the sclera (3,12). Scleritis is noted in 0.15% to 6.3% of patients with RA, and approximately 10% to 33% of patients with scleritis will have RA (13). Anterior scleritis is further subdivided into diffuse nodular necrotizing with inflammation and necrotizing without inflammation (scleromalacia perforans) (3,12). Anterior scleritis occurs ten times more frequently than posterior scleritis, although the latter is likely underdiagnosed (13–15). Up to 50% of patients with scleritis and RA develop bilateral disease (14). If scleral inflammation extends to the ciliary body, uveitis may result (<50% of patients) and is called *sclerouveitis* (14). In posterior scleritis, the inflammation may extend to adjacent structures and result in choroiditis, choroidal effusion, nonrhegmatogenous (without a retinal hole) retinal detachment, retinal vasculitis, cystoid macular edema, and optic disc swelling (3,14). Scleritis in association with RA may be an immune complex–mediated vasculitis (15). Pain in scleritis is typically boring, constant, with facial radiation, and is worse in the morning. Scleritis pain involves the eye and periorbital region. In necrotizing disease, the pain can become disabling (3,16). Other symptoms may include ocular redness, photophobia, lacrimation, and overflowing tears (epiphora) (3). Scleromalacia perforans is largely asymptomatic and occurs in patients with advanced RA (3,13,14). Tenderness of the globe is common, and sclera edema is evident on slit lamp examination (SLE) (3,12).

Diffuse anterior scleritis involves large areas of sclera; when widespread, severe, and diffuse, it can cause intense injection, redness, and chemosis (2,3,12,14). Nodular scleritis is the second most common form of anterior uveitis. Multiple attacks are frequent and occur in approximately 50% of patients. Nodular scleritis is characterized by the presence of single or multiple localized nonmobile elevations of firm tender scleral edema associated with intense dilatation of the deep episcleral vessels of the sclera, typically found posterior to the limbus (2,3,12,14). Necrotizing anterior scleritis is the most severe form of anterior scleritis. It is bilateral in 25% of patients, and approximately 25% develop multiple attacks. Two forms of necrotizing anterior scleritis exist: with and without inflammation. With inflammation, pain is severe and excruciating, with worsening in the early morning. Examination reveals scleral edema, intense vasodilatation of deep vessels with less injection centrally, and foci of capillary closure evident on SLE. In advanced disease,

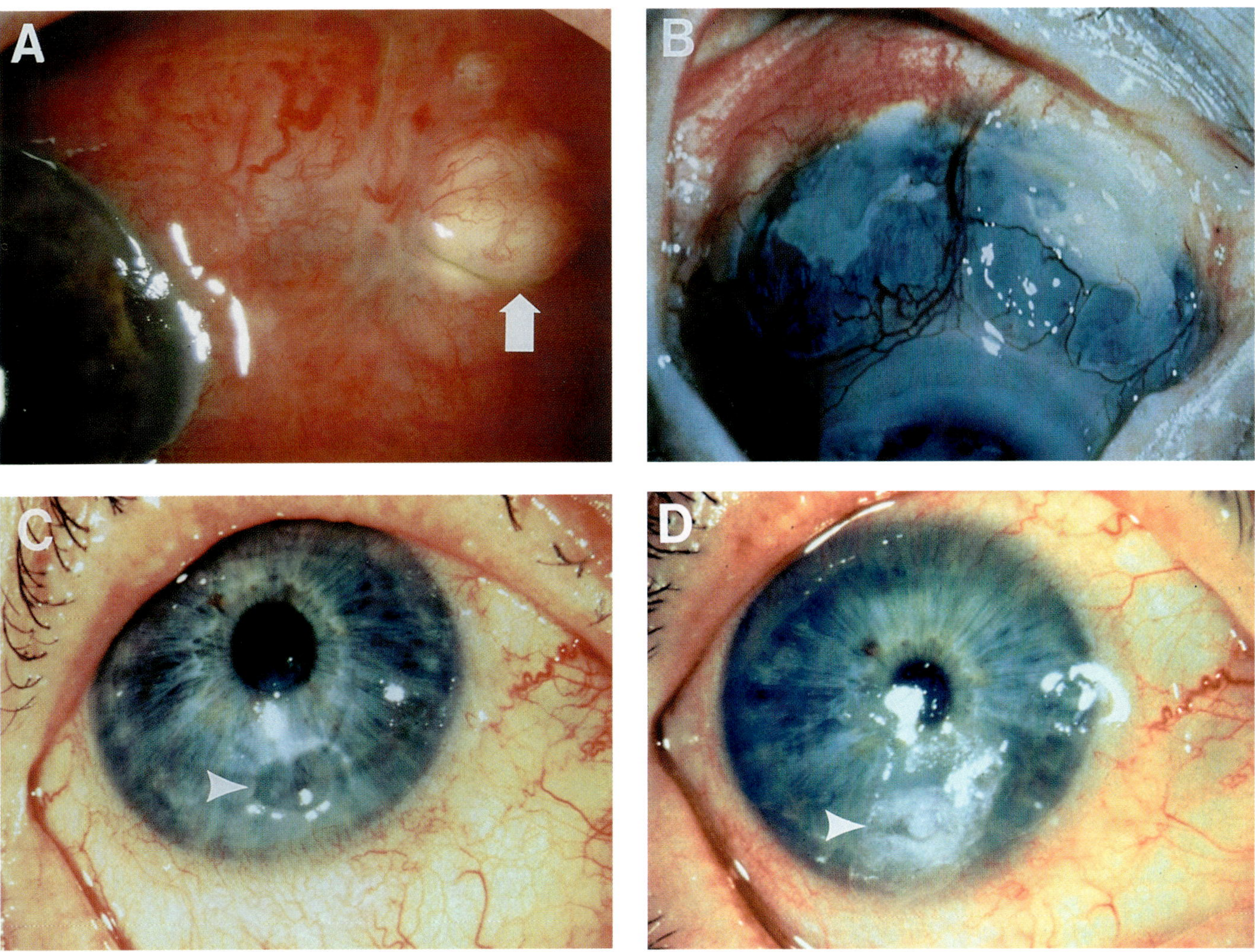

Figure 45.1. Ocular manifestations of rheumatoid arthritis. **A:** Nodular scleritis (*white arrow*) in an eye with diffuse scleritis. **B:** Severe scleromalacia perforans. **C:** Paracentral corneal ulceration (*white arrowhead*). **D:** Paracentral corneal ulceration, postapplication of tissue adhesive (*white arrowhead*). (Courtesy of Dr. Terry Kim, Duke Department of Ophthalmology, and Wills Eye Hospital Corneal Collection.)

the eye may be exquisitely tender and examination may show thinning and color change of the sclera, parchment-white avascular areas of sclera, and blue, thinned areas of sclera revealing the underlying choroid. Progression of inflammatory scleritis is expected without therapy. Scleral thinning is the inevitable result. In the face of intraocular pressure elevation, staphyloma (bulging of the sclera due to inflammatory softening) may form in areas of thinned sclera, but spontaneous perforation is unusual (2,3,12,14,17). Necrotizing scleritis without inflammation, also called *scleromalacia perforans*, is rare and seen almost exclusively in patients with RA. Scleromalacia perforans is characterized by an almost complete lack of symptoms. Patients may notice a change in eye color from scleral thinning or reduced visual acuity from induced astigmatism. SLE reveals loss of normal episcleral vasculature, localized lesions of yellow-white infarcted tissue without vascular dilatation, tenderness, and other signs of inflammation (2,3,12,14).

Posterior scleritis involves the sclera posterior to the ora serrata, occurring in isolation or in association with anterior uveitis. Posterior scleritis has protean manifestations and can be difficult to diagnose. This condition is bilateral; in one-third of patients, its symptoms are ocular pain, reduced vision, ocular redness, diplopia, and pain on eye movement. Common signs of posterior scleritis include exudative retinal detachment, annular choroidal detachment, optic disc edema, retinal folds, choroidal folds, subretinal mass, maculopathy, uveitis, retinal vasculitis, and elevated intraocular pressure. Inflammation associated with posterior scleritis can also affect Tenon's capsule and the surrounding orbital tissue, producing the following manifestations: proptosis, severe pain, pain on eye movement, limitation of eye movement, ptosis, and chemosis (3,14,15). Visual loss is common, occurring in 10% of patients with diffuse anterior scleritis, 25% of those with nodular anterior scleritis, and 75% to 80% of those with necrotizing or posterior scleritis (3).

The treatment of scleritis demands systemic therapy with NSAID, corticosteroids, or other immunosuppressive agents (3,18). Therapy is individualized based on severity of disease, side effects, and concomitant illnesses. Therapeutic goals include the preservation of vision, relief of symptoms, prevention of scleritis complications, and prevention of treatment complications (3). Diffuse scleritis and mild nodular scleritis can be treated with an NSAID at high doses to obtain maximum antiinflammatory effect. Indomethacin at a dose of 75 mg orally twice a day is often chosen, although any NSAID will likely be efficacious. If one NSAID lacks efficacy, another should be used (18). Topical NSAID, topical corticosteroid therapy, and retroorbital injections of corticosteroids can supplement oral NSAIDs (17,18). Initial evidence of response is resolution of pain, which can be rapid and dramatic. Scleral tenderness and injection are the next features to improve. Scleral nodules and uveitis respond over a more prolonged time, from weeks to months (17,18).

Patients who do not respond to an oral NSAID and supplemental local treatment with topical NSAID or corticosteroid or those with moderate to severe symptoms initially require systemic corticosteroid therapy. Systemic corticosteroid therapy is the initial treatment for patients with severe nodular or necrotizing scleritis. Corticosteroids can be administered orally or intravenously, starting at 1 mg per kg per day in a single dose for those with moderately severe nodular disease and at 1 to 2 mg per kg per day in a divided dose for patients with severe nodular or necrotizing disease (18). After control of the eye inflammation, corticosteroids should be tapered slowly to avoid recurrence.

Nodular or necrotizing scleritis and posterior scleritis not adequately controlled with oral corticosteroids require immunosuppressive therapy. The decision to use immunosuppressives requires input from the patient's ophthalmologist and rheumatologist, with consideration given to the risk of permanent visual loss balanced against the risks of immunosuppressive therapy. The threshold for the use of additional immunosuppressive therapy in necrotizing and posterior scleritis is extremely low; most patients with these problems require intensive immunosuppressive therapy (3,17,18). In addition, local corticosteroid therapy, given as a posterior subtenon's injection, can be used to supplement systemic therapy. Triamcinolone acetonide, 40 mg, is frequently used for this purpose.

A number of immunosuppressive agents have been used in the treatment of severe nodular, necrotizing, and posterior scleritis. No double-blind controlled trials of therapy exist for these conditions. Experience is derived from anecdotal reports and retrospective and prospective case series from tertiary referral centers. Drugs used include cyclophosphamide, cyclosporine, methotrexate (MTX), azathioprine, and chlorambucil.

Cyclophosphamide is one of the most effective agents for the treatment of severe nodular, necrotizing, and posterior scleritis. Whereas cyclophosphamide can be given intravenously as pulses or daily oral, scleritis is usually treated with daily oral therapy. Pretreatment laboratory evaluation includes complete blood count (CBC), chemistry panel (electrolytes, renal parameters, liver function tests, and proteins), and urinalysis. Cyclophosphamide is started at 2 mg per kg per day in a single oral dose in the a.m. if the white blood cell (WBC) count is greater than or equal to 4,000 per mm^3, platelets are greater than 100,000 per mm^3, and hematocrit is greater than 30%. Starting with a lower dose (1 mg per kg per day) is advisable if the creatinine is greater than 2.5 or liver tests are more than moderately abnormal. The patient should be instructed to drink 2 to 3 liters of fluid early in the day to minimize the potential bladder toxicity of cyclophosphamide. The dose is subsequently adjusted to keep the WBC count greater than 3,500 per mm^3, platelets greater than 100,000 per mm^3, and hematocrit at least 30%. CBCs are monitored every 1 to 2 weeks initially and may be obtained every month after reaching a stable dose of cyclophosphamide. In tapering corticosteroid therapy, it is important to recognize that, as the dose of corticosteroid is reduced, the patient's WBC will also drop and require a decrease in cyclophosphamide dose. The dose can be adjusted upward, depending on clinical response and the results of laboratory monitoring. The dose of cyclophosphamide given will have a maximal effect on the WBC 10 to 12 days later. Trends should be noted and changes in dose anticipated before the extreme hematologic parameters above are reached. The dose of cyclophosphamide can be increased 25 to 50 mg every 2 weeks if the scleritis does not respond adequately to treatment. Every-2-week CBCs are recommended as the dose is increased. Limiting cyclophosphamide therapy to less than 1 year may minimize cyclophosphamide risks of bladder cancer and cystitis and may require substituting another immunosuppressive drug for cyclophosphamide.

MTX and cyclosporine are the most frequently used alternatives to cyclophosphamide. MTX is an appropriate choice for patients responding to corticosteroid therapy who require steroid-sparing treatment, such as moderate nodular anterior scleritis (3,18). The initial dose is 15 to 20 mg weekly. See Chapter 25 for the details of MTX, as its use in inflammatory eye disease is similar to that in RA joint disease. MTX can be used as long as needed to control ocular inflammation. Cyclosporine is a possible option for patients who do not respond to cyclophosphamide therapy because of lack of efficacy or toxicity. The initial dose is 4 to 5 mg per kg per day given in two equal daily doses. Renal dysfunction and hypertension are the major side effects of cyclosporine therapy. See Chapter 29 for the details on cyclosporine therapy (17,18).

Surgical procedures are rarely required for the treatment of scleritis, but they may be necessary to repair scleral defects, repair globe perforations, and manage complications of scleritis (3,16,17). Surgery should be performed only in the context of established medical therapy; otherwise, the surgery will be complicated by unchecked inflammation in the eye (16,17). Rarely, episclera biopsy may be necessary to rule out tumor masquerading as inflammatory disease.

Corneal Ulceration

Corneal ulceration in patients with RA is categorized as peripheral ulcerative keratitis and central or paracentral corneal ulceration (2,19,20). KCS is associated with both of these RA ocular complications (2,19,20). Peripheral ulcerative keratitis is a crescent-shaped peripheral corneal stromal ulceration with an epithelial defect and an active intrastromal white blood cell infiltrate adjacent to the limbus. Peripheral ulcerative keratitis may be associated with adjacent scleritis (2). Central or paracentral corneal ulceration is distinguished by location that is central or paracentral and the almost complete lack of intrastromal white blood cell infiltration at initial presentation (20).

Peripheral ulcerative keratitis is treated similarly to nodular or necrotizing scleritis (2,20). KCS must be aggressively managed. Systemic corticosteroid therapy is instituted as soon as infection is ruled out. Most patients require additional immunosuppressive drugs, as discussed earlier (2,20). MTX is considered before cyclophosphamide in a patient whose disease seems mild or has a slower tempo (2). Surgical procedures are risky and may be required in patients with peripheral ulcerative keratitis to repair corneal or scleral defects and to repair globe perforations. Globe perforations may be temporarily repaired with tissue adhesive, but lamellar grafts (thin piece of conjunctiva and sclera from distant location) or corneal transplantation are often required to maintain anatomic integrity (2,16,21,22). The success rate for these procedures is best when the patient is treated aggressively with immunosuppressive therapy, but even with immunosuppressive therapy, the visual outcome can be limited (2,16,21,22).

Central or paracentral corneal ulceration can be treated with tissue adhesive, bandage contact lenses, and topical cyclosporine 2% (20). Tissue adhesive is particularly useful when the cornea has perforated. Eyes that perforate and do not heal with the above approach will require a penetrating keratoplasty (21,22). Topical cyclosporine may be sufficient in some patients, but systemic immunosuppression with cyclophosphamide or systemic cyclosporine, used in a manner similar to that described for scleritis above, should be undertaken for recurrent central or paracentral ulceration or for patients requiring large penetrating keratoplasties (21,22).

RHEUMATOID VASCULITIS

Whereas vascular inflammation is inherent in RA, *rheumatoid vasculitis* (RV) refers to widespread manifestations secondary to vascular inflammation. In the absence of an accepted definition of RV, many authors define RV as a syndrome characterized by deep cutaneous ulcer, cutaneous gangrene, purpura, petechiae, mononeuritis multiplex, or a positive tissue biopsy revealing vasculitis (23,24). RV occurs more often in male than female patients and has been associated with erosions, deformities, nodules, high-titer rheumatoid factor, hypocomplementemia, cryoglobulinemia, use of three or more disease-modifying antirheumatic drugs, and treatment (ever) with D-penicillamine or azathioprine (23–25). RV can involve the heart, lungs, eyes, peripheral nervous system, liver, spleen, and kidneys. RV presents with mononeuritis multiplex in 15% to 40% of patients (23,24,26), and clinical findings of mononeuritis multiplex in the face of long-standing RA without other evident etiology should be considered RV until proven otherwise. Biopsy or angiographic documentation of RV is desirable but not always possible (23–26). Patients with RV have increased mortality, compared to similar RA patients not manifesting RV (23,24,26,27).

Cutaneous RV may be treated with aggressive topical therapy, oral corticosteroids, and second-line drugs, such as MTX (23,24,27). Nail fold infarcts in isolation require no specific therapy. RV manifesting as mononeuritis multiplex or other visceral organ disease should be treated with oral corticosteroids and cyclophosphamide (23,24,27). Corticosteroids are started at 1 mg per kg per day. With clinical response, corticosteroids can be tapered over several months to 10 mg per day or less, monitoring carefully for evidence of recurrent disease activity. Whereas cyclophosphamide can be given as intravenous pulses and by a daily oral route, RV is usually treated orally because of the severity of its clinical consequences (23,28). Cyclophosphamide is started at 2 mg per kg per day (see Episcleritis and Scleritis) and is continued as the corticosteroid dose is tapered to a dose of 7.5 mg per day or less. If the RV achieves remission for 9 to 12 months at a prednisone dose of 7.5 mg per day or less, then cyclophosphamide can be withdrawn over 2 to 3 months.

CUTANEOUS MANIFESTATIONS

Cutaneous manifestations of RA are common (Table 45.2). As many as 9% of patients with RA have had a leg ulcer (29). The causes of cutaneous ulcers in RA are varied and include the following: venous insufficiency, ineffective venous pump secondary to ankle joint disease, arterial disease, vasculitis, skin fragility secondary to corticosteroids or poor nutrition, trauma, foot deformity, peripheral neuropathy, pyoderma gangrenosum, and factitious illness (30,31). Treatment is directed at the underlying cause(s), which may be multiple (30–34). Cutaneous leg ulcers occur more commonly in patients with Felty's syndrome than in patients who have RA without Felty's syndrome (31,33). Vasculitis may be a factor in 10% to 38% of patients with RA and cutaneous ulceration (31–33). Vasculitic ulcers are typically painful, deep, and punched-out in appearance (31–33). Cutaneous ulcers in patients with RA are most often lower extremity in location (31–33).

TABLE 45.2. Major Cutaneous Manifestations of Rheumatoid Arthritis

Manifestations	Most Frequent Treatments
Rheumatoid nodules	None, surgical removal
Steroid-related bruisability	Taper corticosteroid dose
Lower-extremity ulceration	
Venous	Occlusive dressings, compressive dressings, elevation
Arterial	Occlusive dressings, angioplasty or surgical revascularization
Vasculitis-related	Occlusive dressings, oral corticosteroids, cyclophosphamide
Steroid-related	Occlusive dressings, taper corticosteroid dose
Malnutrition-related	Occlusive dressings, improve caloric intake and nutrition
Pyoderma gangrenosum	Occlusive dressings
Vasculitis-related	
Petechiae	None (in isolation)
Palpable purpura	None (in isolation)
Nail fold infarcts	None
Erythema elevatum diutinum	Dapsone

The mainstay of treatment is occlusive dressings to create a physiologic moist environment for healing, to reduce eschar formation, and encourage epidermal migration. Dressings are supplemented with leg elevation and sustained lower-extremity compression (una boots), unless contraindicated secondary to significant arterial disease (30,31). Clinically evident infection (cellulitis, pain, lymphangitis, etc.) is treated with antibiotics. Colonization of the ulcer is expected, and antibiotic therapy is not needed, unless there is clinical evidence of infection (30,31). Topical growth factors, such as transforming growth factor β, may also be of benefit (31). Leg elevation when sitting is indicated for patients with a component of venous insufficiency to decrease the likelihood of recurrence (31,32,34).

Patients with evidence of arterial disease by ankle-brachial pressure index should be studied with angiography. Where treatable lesions are found, arterial reconstructive surgery or percutaneous transluminal angioplasty should be undertaken (31,32,34). Skin grafting should be considered on failure of other conservative measures, particularly with large ulcers (31,32,34). Skin grafting is associated with a reduction in pain related to cutaneous ulcers (32).

A trial of corticosteroids and cyclophosphamide, given as described for RV, should be considered in patients with biopsy-proven vascular inflammation, evidence of RV in other locations, and no other clear explanation for a cutaneous ulcer. Corticosteroids and cyclophosphamide should also be considered in patients with biopsy-proven vascular inflammation and lack of cutaneous ulcer improvement, despite optimal topical and other therapies. Immunosuppressive therapy may be needed to heal cutaneous ulcers in certain patients. MTX, dapsone, intravenous prostacyclin, topical tacrolimus, and other agents have also been reportedly successful in treating vasculitic skin ulcers (30–36).

Rheumatoid nodules are one of the most common extraarticular manifestations of RA, occurring in 15% to 20% of patients. Rheumatoid nodules infrequently require treatment. The major indications for therapy are pain, interference with function, and persistent growth (37). MTX promotes the development of multiple rheumatoid nodules, particularly on the hands, in some patients (38,39). Rheumatoid nodules are most commonly treated with surgical removal (37).

A rare type of cutaneous vasculitis, erythema elevatum diutinum, causes erythematous patches, plaques, and skin nodules; it has been associated with RA. The clinical picture and histologic findings on biopsy allow for the diagnosis and distinction from rheumatoid nodules. Treatment is dapsone given at 50 to 100 mg per day (40).

MUSCULAR MANIFESTATIONS

Muscle wasting and atrophy have been associated with inflammatory arthritis since the early descriptions of RA. Muscle weakness and atrophy are felt secondary to disuse, inflammation-related processes in the muscle and periarticular tissues, and inflammation-related processes in the joints. Weakness and atrophy can be demonstrated early in the course of patients with RA (38,39). Prospective studies show that strength training can reverse much of the weakness and atrophy associated with RA, without deterioration in the patient's control of joint inflammation (38,39).

Myositis fulfilling the American College of Rheumatology criteria for the diagnosis of polymyositis can occur in RA (41,42). Biopsy can reveal diffuse inflammation or (rarely) muscle vasculitis (42). Muscle pathology on biopsies obtained at the time of joint surgery reveals nodular myositis and lymphocytic accumulations in 61% of cases. This percentage is higher than the frequency of clinically evident muscle disease (42). Muscle disease with clinically evident vasculitis can be treated with MTX, azathioprine, or cyclophosphamide, depending on the severity of disease and involvement of other organ systems. Classic-appearing polymyositis in a patient with RA could be called an *overlap syndrome* and should be treated with corticosteroids at 1 mg per kg per day. MTX or azathioprine should be added if the response is inadequate or additional therapy is needed to control the patient's polyarthritis. Myositis has also been described in association with D-penicillamine therapy for RA. This drug is rarely used in the treatment of RA because of the widespread use of MTX and other disease-modifying antirheumatic agents. Discontinuation of the D-penicillamine may require supplementation with corticosteroid therapy, depending on disease severity and the time course of improvement (43).

LIVER MANIFESTATIONS

Nodular regenerative hyperplasia has been associated with RA and Felty's syndrome. This unusual condition is characterized by transformation of the hepatic parenchyma into nodules of hyperplastic hepatocytes without significant fibrosis. The etiology is unclear, but intrahepatic microvascular occlusive mechanisms, increased portal flow, and perisinusoidal fibrosis have all been implicated (44,45). Nodular regenerative hyperplasia is more common in Felty's syndrome than in RA (44–46). Associated clinical findings include altered liver function tests, chronic abdominal pain, portal hypertension, hepatosplenomegaly, bleeding esophageal varices, and ascites. Hepatic failure is not seen (44,45). Specific therapy does not exist. Portosystemic shunts have led to excellent results in the face of recurrent gastrointestinal bleeding (44,45).

Hepatitis C virus (HCV)–associated arthritis occurs in 2% to 20% of infected patients, can fulfill the American College of Rheumatology criteria for the diagnosis of RA, may be associated with normal liver function tests, and may occur with or without associated cryoglobulinemia. Distinguishing HCV-infected patients with polyarthritis from patients who are not HCV infected is important because therapies used to treat RA are hepatotoxic and may allow proliferation of HCV. Patients with HCV-associated arthritis may respond to treatment with interferon α (47).

RESPIRATORY MANIFESTATIONS

Up to 70% of patients with RA have evidence of respiratory tract involvement, but most do not have clinically significant manifestations requiring treatment (48). The estimated prevalence of respiratory tract involvement in RA varies widely based on differences in the patient populations studied. Asymptomatic respiratory tract disease in RA is commonly an incidental finding in patients undergoing chest radiography. Conversely, clinically significant pulmonary disease in RA may not be apparent because articular disease limits the physical activity of patients and masks symptoms. For purposes of classification, respiratory tract manifestations may be divided into those involving the upper and lower airway (Table 45.3). Interstitial lung disease (ILD) and pleural disease are the most prevalent respiratory tract manifestations of RA. With the exception of rheumatoid nodules in the lung, the respiratory manifestations of RA are not unique to this disease.

Upper Respiratory Tract

CRICOARYTENOID AND VOCAL CORD INVOLVEMENT

Laryngeal involvement in RA results from inflammatory arthritis of the cricoarytenoid joints or rheumatoid nodule formation on the vocal cords (49,50). Up to 75% of RA patients have evidence of laryngeal involvement when assessed using a combination of history, spirometry, radiography, and fiber-optic laryngoscopy, although fewer than 30% of RA patients have symptoms (51). Common symptoms include hoarseness, sore throat, and difficulty with inspiration related to edema and altered mobility of the vocal cords. In one series, 75% of patients with vocal cord involvement reported occasional difficulty breathing (51).

The greatest risk related to vocal cord involvement in RA is progressive edema and immobility of the cords, leading to obstruction of the airway (52–54). Partial airway obstruction may be exacerbated by instrumentation, such as endotracheal intubation, resulting in respiratory collapse. Occasionally, RA patients may experience spontaneous airway obstruction and present to the emergency department with stridor or respiratory distress (52). Intubation may be required to ensure adequate ventilation.

Appropriate management of laryngeal involvement in RA is focused on preventing acute complications of airway compromise and reducing symptoms of breathing difficulty, sore throat, and hoarseness. Symptoms of laryngeal involvement should be elicited at the time of diagnosis and during regular follow-up of RA patients. When symptoms are present, referral for direct laryngoscopy is appropriate to define the severity of disease. Routine spirometry may be normal in patients with hoarseness. Characteristic changes in the flow-volume loop are seen during episodes of acute airway obstruction. An elevated ratio of forced expiratory flow in 1 second per peak expiratory flow rate to values greater than 10 may indicate upper airway obstruction (52). Manifesta-

TABLE 45.3. Major Respiratory Tract Manifestations of Rheumatoid Arthritis

Upper respiratory tract
Cricoarytenoid arthritis
Rheumatoid nodules of vocal cords
Lower respiratory tract
Interstitial lung disease
Bronchiolitis obliterans with organizing pneumonia
Obliterative bronchiolitis
Pleural effusions/pleurisy
Rheumatoid nodules of the lung
Caplan's syndrome
Bronchiectasis

tions of airway compromise and dyspnea should be treated aggressively, whereas sore throat and hoarseness may be treated according to their impact on the patient's quality of life. Therapeutic intervention includes increasing the intensity of antirheumatic therapy. An oral corticosteroid taper can provide relatively rapid relief of symptoms. Intraarticular injection of the cricoarytenoid joints by the otolaryngologist can lead to symptomatic relief (55).

Patients with RA, especially those with known laryngeal involvement, should be closely monitored after procedures that may exacerbate vocal cord inflammation. A period of risk follows endotracheal extubation (56,57). Personnel experienced in managing emergent airway collapse should be immediately available during this vulnerable period.

Lower Respiratory Tract

INTERSITIAL LUNG DISEASE

The prevalence of ILD in RA appears to be highly variable based on the case definition used and characteristics of the patient study population (58,59). Pulmonary fibrosis has been detected by open lung biopsy in 60% of RA patients with abnormal pulmonary function studies or imaging studies (60). Impaired pulmonary diffusion capacity has been reported in 40% of an unselected cohort of RA patients (61). Radiologic evidence of pulmonary fibrosis is detected in only 1% to 5% of RA patients (62,63). The onset of ILD is gradual in most cases and follows the diagnosis of RA by several years. There is a male predominance (48). Smoking appears to be a risk factor for both advanced disease (pulmonary fibrosis) and asymptomatic disease (59,62). Commonly associated RA manifestations include nodules and high titers of rheumatoid factor (62–64). Further complicating the clinical evaluation of RA patients with possible ILD is lung disease related to medication, infection, or other environmental exposures. As a result, the clinician must consider a broad differential in the RA patient with pulmonary symptoms (Fig. 45.2).

The symptom typically associated with ILD is dyspnea, particularly during exertion (65). Wheezing and chest pain are uncommon. Often, patients will report fatigue and may experience weight loss with more advanced disease. Physical examination reveals bibasilar end-expiratory crackles (65). Cyanosis,

A

	Ref	Best	%Ref
FVC	2.71	1.83	67
FEV1	2.13	1.54	72
FEV1/FVC	78	84	
FEF25-75	2.11	2.13	101
PEF	5.35	5.07	95

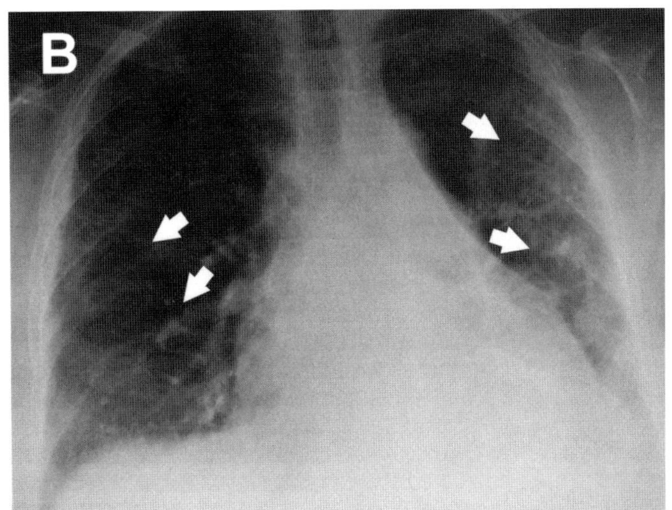

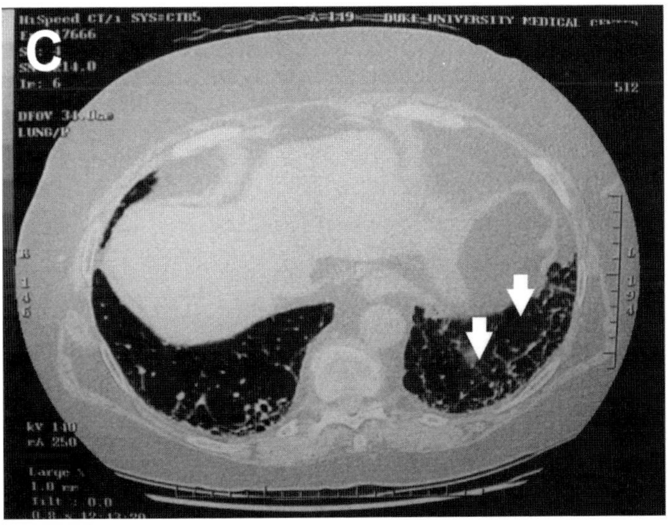

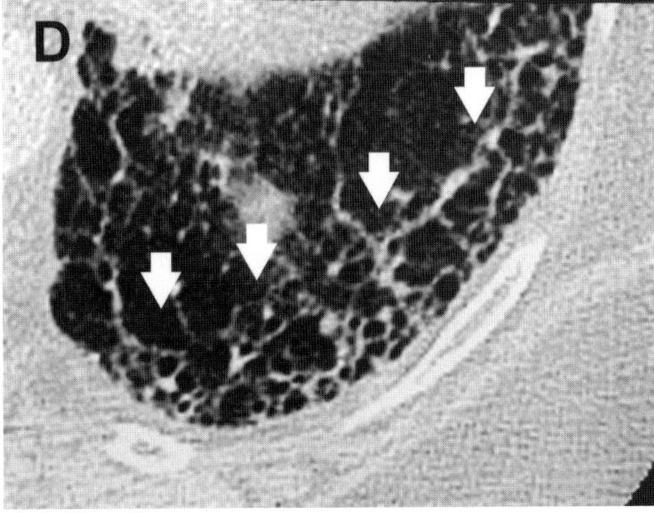

Figure 45.2. Pulmonary function studies and imaging studies of the lung in a patient with rheumatoid arthritis and interstitial lung disease (ILD). **A:** Pulmonary function studies demonstrate a restrictive pattern. **B:** Chest x-ray showing regions of diffuse hazy opacities (*arrows*). **C:** Computed tomography scan of the chest with basilar pulmonary opacities consistent with advanced ILD. **D:** Magnified view of basilar region showing honeycomb changes. FEF25-75, mid-expiratory flow volume; FEV1, forced expiratory volume in first second; FVC, forced vital capacity; PEF, peak expiratory flow.

evidence of right heart failure, and digital clubbing may be seen in advanced disease. The arterial blood gas will usually be normal but may show hypoxemia in the setting of more advanced disease. It is important to note that patients with normal oxygen saturation at rest may have hypoxemia occurring with exercise or sleep (65).

Pulmonary function studies commonly demonstrate a restrictive pattern with decreased total lung capacity, functional residual capacity, and residual volume (65). As a result, the forced expiratory volume in the first second of expiration and the forced vital capacity may be reduced, but the ratio of the forced expiratory volume in the first second of expiration to the forced vital capacity is usually normal or increased. The diffusion capacity is typically reduced, but this finding is nonspecific and does not necessarily correlate with the severity of ILD.

Imaging studies play an important role in the evaluation of RA patients with possible ILD. Characteristic findings on chest radiographs are bibasilar reticular opacities. However, the sensitivity of chest radiograph for ILD is approximately 2% to 6% (48). The chest radiograph can be normal, even with significant crackles on physical examination. High-resolution computed tomography (CT) of the chest is more sensitive than chest radiography and is better able to define the location and extent of ILD (58,66,67). Radionuclide scans to measure pulmonary uptake of technetium-99m–diethylenetriamine pentaacetate is considered a reliable, but not widely available, noninvasive method to assess disease activity and response to therapy (65).

Cardiopulmonary exercise testing with assessment of arterial blood gas parameters (or pulse oximetry) and pulmonary function is useful in assessing patients with ILD (65). A common finding includes oxygen desaturation during exercise. Physiologic abnormalities include failure to reduce dead space and excessive increases in respiratory rate with inadequate recruitment of tidal volume. Serial measurement of rest and exercise gas exchange may be used to assess disease activity over time.

Definitive diagnosis of ILD requires a lung biopsy, which should be performed before initiating specific therapy. Controversy remains as to the ideal sequence of procedures used to obtain tissue for diagnosis. Bronchoscopy with transbronchial biopsy is less invasive than an open or thoracoscopic biopsy but is also less sensitive. However, bronchoscopy also allows for microbiologic studies to be obtained when infectious causes of lung disease are in the differential diagnosis. Video-assisted thoracoscopic biopsy or open lung biopsy carry greater morbidity but often provide the most useful specimens for tissue diagnosis.

In general, ILD should be viewed as a progressive process that may lead to irreversible fibrosis. Therefore, the goals of treatment are similar to those in managing articular disease: reduce inflammation and prevent irreversible damage. Although no randomized controlled trials of drug therapy of ILD in RA have been performed, many of the agents used to treat articular disease appear effective in managing ILD (68–74). The efficacy of the biologic agents, such as etanercept, infliximab, anakinra, and adalimumab, for ILD has not been established. Early case reports suggest that these drugs may be effective (74).

Given that ILD is common in RA but may not be clinically significant, the challenge to the clinician is distinguishing those patients who require intervention from those who do not. The approach to the RA patient with ILD will continue to evolve as RA therapy evolves. ILD may not appear to be clinically important in the daily activities of RA patients. However, ILD can progress in such an insidious manner that pulmonary symptoms may become a greater impediment to adequate aerobic exercise than musculoskeletal symptoms in RA patients. For instance, the RA patient who reports difficulty climbing stairs should be questioned about the relative roles that joint pain and respiratory symptoms play in this impairment. Further studies are needed to determine if more aggressive therapy of ILD in RA patients leads to improved outcomes.

PLEURAL DISEASE

Pleural involvement has been described in up to 73% of RA patients in autopsy series (75,76). However, only approximately 20% to 30% of RA patients report symptoms of pleural disease (77). Men are more commonly affected than women. Clinically apparent pleural disease usually presents with pleuritic chest pain, fever, or dyspnea. Physical examination may reveal a pleural rub or evidence of a pleural effusion. Chest radiograph reveals pleural effusions in fewer than 25% of RA patients with pleuritic symptoms (64,77). Effusions may be unilateral or bilateral.

Management of pleural disease in RA starts with a broad differential diagnosis. The patient with new onset of pleuritic chest pain should be evaluated for clinical evidence of pulmonary embolism, infection, and malignancy. A radiograph of the chest should be performed to rule out evidence of pulmonary infiltrates or masses and to determine if a pleural effusion is present. If the clinical and radiographic examination is consistent with pleurisy related to RA and pleural effusion is not present, then intensifying the patient's antiinflammatory therapy is appropriate to provide symptomatic relief and hasten recovery. NSAIDs are the initial drugs of choice if not contraindicated. If NSAIDs are not effective or the patient is already using an NSAID, intermediate doses of a corticosteroid (10–20 mg prednisone per day) may be beneficial. Therapy may be tapered gradually over several weeks to prevent relapse of symptoms. Spontaneous resolution of pleuritis and pleural effusions may take several months.

The presence of a new pleural effusion generally requires further investigation. RA patients may be at increased risk of *Mycobacterium* tuberculosis (78). Thoracentesis should be performed to determine if the effusion is exudative or transudative (Table 45.4) and to rule out infection or malignancy (79). If the effusion is exudative, additional studies on the pleural fluid should include glucose, amylase, differential cell count, microbiologic studies, and cytology. No single study is diagnostic of a pleural effusion related to RA. However, usual findings include exudative effusion, low glucose levels, and cell counts of approximately 5,000 to 10,000 cells per mm^3 (48). Occasionally, therapeutic thoracentesis is necessary to relieve symptoms from large pleural effusions (80). On rare occasions, large effusions may recur and require pleurodesis for long-lasting resolution.

BRONCHIOLITIS OBLITERANS WITH ORGANIZING PNEUMONIA

Bronchiolitis obliterans with organizing pneumonia (BOOP; also known as *cryptogenic organizing pneumonia*) is a proliferative bronchiolitis characterized by patchy infiltration of respiratory bronchioles with fibroblast tissue (48,81). It is differentiated from

TABLE 45.4. Criteria for Exudative versus Transudative Pleural Effusions

Pleural effusion exudative if one of the following present:
- Pleural fluid protein/serum protein >0.5
- Pleural fluid LDH/serum LDH >0.6
- Pleural fluid LDH more than two-thirds normal upper limit for serum

LDH, lactate dehydrogenase.
Adapted from Light RW. Disorders of the pleura, mediastinum, and diaphragm. In: Braunwald E, Fauci AS, Isselbacher KJ, et al., eds. *Harrison's textbook of medicine.* New York: McGraw-Hill, 2002:1.

TABLE 45.5. Bronchiolitis Obliterans with Organizing Pneumonia versus Obliterative Bronchiolitis

Feature	Bronchiolitis Obliterans with Organizing Pneumonia	Obliterative Bronchiolitis
Sex predominance	Male	Female
Symptoms	Dyspnea, cough, fever, malaise, weight loss	Dyspnea, cough
Physical examination	Crackles	Diffuse wheezing, crackles less prominent
Chest radiograph	Patchy infiltrates	Normal or hyperinflation
Spirometry	Restrictive	Obstruction
Microscopic pathology	Exudative, lymphocyte infiltration, well-preserved bronchiole wall and interstitium	Bronchial wall destruction, obliteration of airway lumen, nonexudative
Response to therapy/prognosis	Good	Poor

Adapted from Tanoue LT. Pulmonary manifestations of rheumatoid arthritis. *Clin Chest Med* 1998;19:667–685, viii, and Pritikin JD, Jensen WA, Yenokida GG, et al. Respiratory failure due to a massive rheumatoid pleural effusion. *J Rheumatol* 1990;17:673–675.

obliterative bronchiolitis (OB) on both clinical and histologic grounds (Table 45.5). The clinical presentation of BOOP is usually associated with cough, dyspnea, weight loss, and fever. Typically, the onset of symptoms will be more rapid than that of ILD. Physical examination demonstrates crackles. Restrictive physiology and decreased diffusing capacity of the lung for carbon monoxide is present on pulmonary function studies. Bilateral lung opacities are noted on chest radiograph. Findings on high-resolution chest CT include a patchy consolidation, usually in distal lung segments. Ordinarily, the diagnosis of BOOP is established by thoracoscopic or open lung biopsy, although adequate tissue for diagnosis may be obtained by transbronchial lung biopsy.

Treatment of BOOP is initiated with oral corticosteroids at a dose of 1 to 1.5 mg per kg daily for 4 to 6 weeks, which is then tapered over the next 2 to 4 months, depending on clinical response (81). Rapid responses to corticosteroids, after as little as 1 to 2 days of treatment, will be seen in many patients. Symptoms can recur quickly if treatment is tapered too rapidly. Serial chest radiographs and pulmonary function studies should be performed at least every 2 months to detect relapse. Rapidly progressing BOOP may require initial therapy with divided parenteral doses of corticosteroids (0.5–10 g per day of methylprednisolone). Cyclophosphamide or other immunosuppressive therapy may also be effective in controlling severe disease or disease that does not respond to corticosteroids. No randomized, controlled trials of BOOP in RA or any disease have been performed. Although most patients with BOOP respond readily to corticosteroids, rapidly progressive disease occurs in a small minority. Early diagnosis is imperative to achieve favorable outcomes and to prevent permanent lung damage.

OBLITERATIVE BRONCHIOLITIS

OB, also known as *bronchiolitis obliterans*, is a severe manifestation of rheumatoid lung disease (48,81). Constrictive and proliferative variants of OB are recognized histologically. Each variant destroys respiratory bronchioles, leading to distal airway obstruction. Several clinical features distinguish OB from BOOP (Table 45.5). In RA, OB develops rapidly with onset and progression of dyspnea in the absence of significant fever or other systemic symptoms. Patients affected are usually women with long-standing RA in the fifth or sixth decade of life. Secondary SS and use of penicillamine have been associated with OB (82,83). Physical examination is notable for diffuse wheezing, although crackles are less prominent than in BOOP. The chest radiograph is often normal but may also demonstrate a miliary or diffuse nodular pattern with postobstructive hyperlucency. High-resolution chest CT scan may reveal evidence of air trapping (84). Spirometry reveals an obstructive pattern (83). Initial therapy with high-dose corticosteroids is appropriate, but the prognosis is generally poor. There is some evidence that early diagnosis and treatment may improve outcomes, but no definitive studies have been performed in this regard. In addition to corticosteroid therapy, treatment with β-agonists may relieve symptoms of dyspnea and wheezing associated with airway obstruction.

RHEUMATOID NODULES OF THE LUNG

Rheumatoid nodules of the lung occur in less than 1% of patients with RA as assessed by chest radiograph (76). However, nodules have been reported in up to one-third of patients undergoing high-resolution CT scan or lung biopsy for suspected lung involvement in RA (85,86). Histologically, rheumatoid lung nodules are identical to those found in the extremities (48). Usually, they are located in subpleural and interlobular septal areas. Multiple nodules are more common than solitary nodules.

Rheumatoid lung nodules are usually asymptomatic and often raise concern about underlying malignancy when seen on chest radiographs. Solitary nodules may require serial imaging studies or fine needle aspiration to rule out malignancy. Rheumatoid nodules may become symptomatic if they expand or undergo spontaneous necrosis leading to pneumothorax, pleural effusion, bronchopleural fistula, or hemoptysis (48,64,87). As a result, no specific therapy is required for asymptomatic rheumatoid nodules of the lung.

CAPLAN'S SYNDROME

Caplan's syndrome refers to nodular lung disease in patients with RA and a pneumoconiosis from exposure to coal dust other silica dusts (48,88). Patients develop dyspnea in association with airflow obstruction. Chest radiograph demonstrates multiple basilar lung nodules. Treatment does not alter the course of disease, which usually does not progress rapidly. Maximizing therapy for RA and removing the patient from the precipitating exposure are the most important interventions in Caplan's syndrome.

BRONCHIECTASIS

Thirty percent of patients with RA had bronchiectasis by high-resolution CT scan, despite a normal chest radiograph (67,85). Symptoms of bronchiectasis are less severe and the course seemingly more benign than in the non-RA population. Most patients with bronchiectasis in the setting of RA have subclinical disease, and treatment is not necessary, unless patients are symptomatic.

CARDIAC MANIFESTATIONS

Pericarditis

Pericarditis is the most common cardiovascular abnormality in RA. Autopsy series and echocardiographic studies have demonstrated that approximately one-half of RA patients have pericardial involvement (89–91). However, symptomatic pericarditis may be present only in 1% to 10% of those with RA. The typical patient with this manifestation is older and has had long-standing disease. The manifestations are similar to those of classic pericarditis: chest pain, dyspnea, palpitations, and pericardial rub. The electrocardiogram may show typical signs of pericarditis. It is usually normal, owing to the typical chronic nature of pericardial disease in RA. Many patients will have coexisting pleural effusions. Pericardial calcification or constrictive pericarditis may occur after long-standing disease (89). Pericardial fluid findings mimic those of pleural effusions. Leukocyte counts are elevated in the range of 5,000 to 30,000 cells per mm^3, predominantly neutrophils. Glucose levels may be quite low.

Pericarditis in RA is usually treated with NSAIDs or by increasing the intensity of antirheumatic therapy with corticosteroids or other disease-modifying drugs. A pericardial window may be used to treat moderate to large effusions that fail to resolve with medical therapy or effusions causing hemodynamic compromise. Constrictive pericarditis may require surgical intervention.

Myocarditis

Granulomatous myocarditis is a very rare complication of RA that can result in mitral insufficiency or conduction system disturbances (92–94). Diagnosis is more commonly made at autopsy than on the basis of clinical manifestations. Few data are available on the treatment of myocarditis in RA.

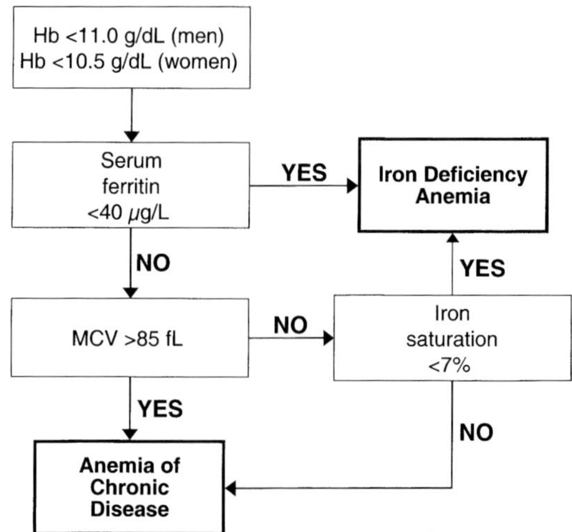

Figure 45.3. Algorithm for diagnosis of iron deficiency anemia in active rheumatoid arthritis. Hb, hemoglobin; MCV, mean corpuscular volume. (Adapted from Mulherin D, Skelly M, Saunders A, et al. The diagnosis of iron deficiency in patients with rheumatoid arthritis and anemia: an algorithm using simple laboratory measures. *J Rheumatol* 1996;23:237–240.)

HEMATOLOGIC MANIFESTATIONS

Anemia of Chronic Disease

Anemia of chronic disease (ACD) is the most common hematologic manifestation of RA (95). However, evaluation of the RA patient with anemia should also include consideration of iron deficiency, the second most common cause of anemia in RA (95). The distinction between ACD and iron deficiency anemia in RA is often complicated by the coexistence of these two conditions, and by the observation that serum markers of iron stores may not be accurate in the setting of systemic inflammation (96–98). Therefore, iron deficiency should be considered in all RA patients with anemia. A serum ferritin level less than 50 μg per L in RA indicates iron deficiency, and patients should be evaluated and treated accordingly (99). Iron deficiency is more difficult to diagnose when serum ferritin levels are greater than 50 μg per L. A simple algorithm based on measurement of mean corpuscular volume, serum ferritin, and iron saturation has been shown to reliably diagnose iron deficiency in 94% of anemic patients with RA (100) (Fig. 45.3). Finally, bone marrow biopsy may be performed to assess the adequacy of iron stores in RA patients.

Once a diagnosis of ACD has been confirmed, the most appropriate strategy is to institute appropriate antirheumatic therapy and monitor the patient's anemia. It is common for anemia to resolve as RA disease activity improves. The rare patients with symptomatic anemia (fatigue, lethargy, impaired exercise tolerance), despite therapy of RA, may benefit by a trial of recombinant erythropoietin (101–104). Treatment of ACD in RA should be targeted to patients with hematocrit less than 30%, despite appropriate therapy of arthritis (105). Iron deficiency anemia should be ruled out before initiating therapy (106). The treatment goal is to increase the hematocrit by 16% over 6 to 8 weeks or to alleviate the symptoms of anemia (105). ACD often requires a higher dose of erythropoietin than that used in patients without inflammatory disease (105,106).

Felty's Syndrome

Felty's syndrome is a rare disorder characterized by neutropenia, splenomegaly, and RA (107). Fewer than 1% of patients with RA develop Felty's syndrome (107). Usually, Felty's syndrome occurs in patients with a long-standing history of seropositive deforming nodular RA (107,108). It is not necessary for arthritis manifestations to be active at the time of diagnosis (108). Felty's syndrome is more common in women (109,110). Splenomegaly is present in 90% of patients (111). Other clinical manifestations include recurring infections, lymphadenopathy, rheumatoid nodules, and, rarely, leg ulcers (107). Laboratory evaluation usually demonstrates a markedly elevated erythrocyte sedimentation rate (112). Positive titers of antinuclear antibody and antineutrophil cytoplasmic antibodies are common in Felty's syndrome (107,113,114).

No randomized controlled studies of drug therapy for Felty's syndrome have been performed. Favorable treatment responses have been reported for corticosteroids, MTX, gold salts, cyclosporine, and cytotoxic agents (115–124). Granulocyte colony-stimulating factor or granulocyte-monocyte colony-stimulating factor will resolve neutropenia in a majority of patients. However, adverse events, such as increased arthritis symptoms, skin rash, and vasculitis, have been reported (125–127). The role of splenectomy in the treatment of Felty's syndrome remains unresolved. Up to 50% of patients resolve their neutropenia, but recurrence rates may be as high as 20% (128).

Current therapy involves initial treatment with MTX. Colony-stimulating factors may be added initially to increase WBC (129). Splenectomy should be reserved for patients who do not respond appropriately to medical therapy (130). Patients with Felty's syndrome have a poor prognosis because of the risk of fatal infection.

Large Granular Lymphocyte Syndrome

The large granular lymphocyte (LGL) syndrome is similar to Felty's syndrome in the occurrence of neutropenia, splenomegaly, and recurring infections. However, patients have a significant elevation in circulating LGLs, which are thought to be natural killer cells or cytotoxic T cells. In contrast to Felty's syndrome, up to 14% of patients may progress to leukemia. Diagnosis is confirmed by immunophenotyping of peripheral blood cells. Infection is the most common cause of death in patients with LGL syndrome. Treatment is similar to that of Felty's syndrome (131–133).

Pure Red Cell Aplasia

Pure red cell aplasia is a rare complication associated with RA. Patients usually present with moderate or severe anemia and low reticulocyte counts. Bone marrow biopsy reveals selective hypoplasia of the red cell lines. Drug-induced disease is a major concern in this setting, and all medications should be stopped. Spontaneous remission has been reported in 10% to 15% of patients (105). Failure of anemia to improve within 3 to 4 weeks of drug withdrawal should prompt medical therapy. Treatment options include corticosteroids, cyclosporine, danazol, cytotoxic drugs, plasmapheresis, and intravenous immunoglobulin (105,134,135). Medical therapy resolves red cell aplasia in up to two-thirds of patients (105).

Thrombocytosis

Elevated platelet counts are present in many patients with RA. Generally, the degree of thrombocytosis correlates with RA clinical activity and responds to treatment of the underlying disease. Platelet counts usually range between 400,000 to 700,000 per mm^3 and generally do not exceed 1,000,000 per mm^3. Thrombocytosis is not clinically significant and does not require specific therapy.

CONCLUSION

Extraarticular manifestations are common in patients with RA. Appropriate care of RA patients requires an appreciation for the varied extraarticular manifestations of this disease. Accurate diagnosis is made difficult by the overlapping manifestations of extraarticular disease with other RA complications, such as infection and drug toxicity. Once recognized, extraarticular disease is usually effectively managed by increasing the intensity of therapy with usual RA medications. Situations characterized by severe organ system damage may require aggressive immunosuppressive therapy or surgery to achieve the best possible outcome.

REFERENCES

1. Weinberg RS. The eye and rheumatic diseases. In: Kelly WN, Harris ED, Russy S, Sledge CB, eds. *Textbook of rheumatology*, 5th ed. Philadelphia: W.B. Saunders, 1997:488–495.
2. Messmer EM, Foster CS. Destructive corneal and scleral disease associated with rheumatoid arthritis. Medical and surgical management. *Cornea* 1995;14:408–417.
3. Pflugfelder SC, Whitcher JP, Daniels TE. Sjögren syndrome. In: Pepose JS, Holland GN, Wilhelmus DI, eds. *Ocular infection and immunity*. St. Louis: Mosby, 1996:313–333.
4. Rolando M. Sjögren's syndrome as seen by an ophthalmologist. *Scand J Rheumatol* 2001[Suppl]:27–31, discussion 31–33.
5. Fox RE. Sjögren's syndrome. In: Kelly WN, Harris ED, Russy S, Sledge CB, eds. *Textbook of rheumatology*, 5th ed. Philadelphia: W.B. Saunders, 1997:955–968.
6. Tabbara KF, Vera-Cristo CL. Sjögren syndrome. *Curr Opin Ophthalmol* 2000;11:449–454.
7. Poon AC, Geerling G, Dart JK, et al. Autologous serum eyedrops for dry eyes and epithelial defects: clinical and in vitro toxicity studies. *Br J Ophthalmol* 2001;85:1188–1197.
8. Gunduz K, Ozdemir O. Topical cyclosporin treatment of keratoconjunctivitis sicca in secondary Sjögren's syndrome. *Acta Ophthalmol (Copenh)* 1994;72:438–442.
9. Laibovitz RA, Solch S, Andriano K, et al. Pilot trial of cyclosporine 1% ophthalmic ointment in the treatment of keratoconjunctivitis sicca. *Cornea* 1993;12:315–323.
10. Tseng SC, Tsubota K. Important concepts for treating ocular surface and tear disorders. *Am J Ophthalmol* 1997;124:825–835.
11. Tabbara KF, Frayha RA. Alternate-day steroid therapy for patients with primary Sjögren's syndrome. *Ann Ophthalmol* 1983;15:358–361.
12. Watson PG. The diagnosis and management of scleritis. *Ophthalmology* 1980;87:716–720.
13. Pavesio CE, Meier FM. Systemic disorders associated with episcleritis and scleritis. *Curr Opin Ophthalmol* 2001;12:471–478.
14. Sainz de la Maza M, Foster CS, Jabbur NS. Scleritis associated with rheumatoid arthritis and with other systemic immune-mediated diseases. *Ophthalmology* 1994;101:1281–1286, discussion 1287–1288.
15. Riono WP, Hidayat AA, Rao NA. Scleritis: a clinicopathologic study of 55 cases. *Ophthalmology* 1999;106:1328–1333.
16. Nguyen QD, Foster CS. Scleral patch graft in the management of necrotizing scleritis. *Int Ophthalmol Clin* 1999;39:109–131.
17. Legmann A, Foster CS. Noninfectious necrotizing scleritis. *Int Ophthalmol Clin* 1996;36:73–80.
18. Sainz de la Maza M. Scleritis immunopathology and therapy. *Dev Ophthalmol* 1999;30:84–90.
19. Kervick GN, Pflugfelder SC, Haimovici R, et al. Paracentral rheumatoid corneal ulceration. Clinical features and cyclosporine therapy. *Ophthalmology* 1992;99:80–88.
20. Squirrell DM, Winfield J, Amos RS. Peripheral ulcerative keratitis "corneal melt" and rheumatoid arthritis: a case series. *Rheumatology (Oxford)* 1999;38:1245–1248.
21. Bernauer W, Ficker LA, Watson PG, Dart JK. The management of corneal perforations associated with rheumatoid arthritis. An analysis of 32 eyes. *Ophthalmology* 1995;102:1325–1337.
22. Palay DA, Stulting RD, Waring GO III, Wilson LA. Penetrating keratoplasty in patients with rheumatoid arthritis. *Ophthalmology* 1992;99:622–627.
23. Vollertsen RS, Conn DL, Ballard DJ, et al. Rheumatoid vasculitis: survival and associated risk factors. *Medicine (Baltimore)* 1986;65:365–375.
24. Scott DG, Bacon PA, Tribe CR. Systemic rheumatoid vasculitis: a clinical and laboratory study of 50 cases. *Medicine (Baltimore)* 1981;60:288–297.
25. Voskuyl AE, Zwinderman AH, Westedt ML, et al. Factors associated with the development of vasculitis in rheumatoid arthritis: results of a case-control study. *Ann Rheum Dis* 1996;55:190–192.
26. Puechal X, Said G, Hilliquin P, et al. Peripheral neuropathy with necrotizing vasculitis in rheumatoid arthritis. A clinicopathologic and prognostic study of thirty-two patients. *Arthritis Rheum* 1995;38:1618–1629.
27. Voskuyl AE, Zwinderman AH, Westedt ML, et al. The mortality of rheumatoid vasculitis compared with rheumatoid arthritis. *Arthritis Rheum* 1996;39:266–271.
28. Abel T, Andrews BS, Cunningham PH, et al. Rheumatoid vasculitis: effect of cyclophosphamide on the clinical course and levels of circulating immune complexes. *Ann Intern Med* 1980;93:407–413.
29. Thurtle OA, Cawley MI. The frequency of leg ulceration in rheumatoid arthritis: a survey. *J Rheumatol* 1983;10:507–509.
30. Hafner J, Ramelet AA, Schmeller W, Brunner UV. Management of leg ulcers. *Curr Probl Dermatol* 1999;27:4–7.
31. McRorie ER, Jobanputra P, Ruckley CV, Nuki G. Leg ulceration in rheumatoid arthritis. *Br J Rheumatol* 1994;33:1078–1084.
32. Oien RF, Hakansson A, Hansen BU. Leg ulcers in patients with rheumatoid arthritis—a prospective study of aetiology, wound healing and pain reduction after pinch grafting. *Rheumatology (Oxford)* 2001;40:816–820.
33. Hafner J, Trueb RM. Management of leg ulcers in rheumatoid arthritis and in systemic sclerosis. *Curr Probl Dermatol* 1999;27:271–276.
34. Hafner J, Schneider E, Burg G, Cassina PC. Management of leg ulcers in patients with rheumatoid arthritis or systemic sclerosis: the importance of concomitant arterial and venous disease. *J Vasc Surg* 2000;32:322–329.
35. Schuppe H, Richter-Hintz D, Stierle HE, et al. Topical tacrolimus for recalcitrant leg ulcer in rheumatoid arthritis. *Rheumatology (Oxford)* 2000;39:105–106.
36. Dash S, Seibold JR, Tiku ML. Successful treatment of methotrexate induced nodulosis with D-penicillamine. *J Rheumatol* 1999;26:1396–1399.
37. Abraham Z, Rozenbaum M, Rosner I. Colchicine therapy for low-dose-methotrexate-induced accelerated nodulosis in a rheumatoid arthritis patient. *J Dermatol* 1999;26:691–694.
38. van den Ende CH, Breedveld FC, le Cessie S, et al. Effect of intensive exercise on patients with active rheumatoid arthritis: a randomized clinical trial. *Ann Rheum Dis* 2000;59:615–621.
39. Hakkinen A, Hannonen P, Hakkinen K. Muscle strength in healthy people and in patients suffering from recent-onset inflammatory arthritis. *Br J Rheumatol* 1995;34:355–360.
40. Balbir-Gurman A, Schapira D, Bergman R, Nahir AM. Erythema elevation diutinum—a rare cause of nodulosis in a patient with rheumatoid arthritis. *J Rheumatol* 2000;27:2291–2293.
41. Van den Ende CH, Vliet Vlieland TP, Munneke M, Hazes JM. Dynamic exercise therapy in rheumatoid arthritis: a systematic review. *Br J Rheumatol* 1998;37:677–687.
42. Magyar E, Talerman A, Mohacsy J, et al. Muscle changes in rheumatoid arthritis. A review of the literature with a study of 100 cases. *Virchows Arch A Pathol Anat Histol* 1977;373:267–278.
43. Halla JT, Fallahi S, Koopman WJ. Penicillamine-induced myositis. Observations and unique features in two patients and review of the literature. *Am J Med* 1984;77:719–722.
44. Perez Ruiz F, Orte Martinez FJ, Zea Mendoza AC, et al. Nodular regenerative hyperplasia of the liver in rheumatic diseases: report of seven cases and review of the literature. *Semin Arthritis Rheum* 1991;21:47–54.
45. Thorne C, Urowitz MB, Wanless I, et al. Liver disease in Felty's syndrome. *Am J Med* 1982;73:35–40.
46. Rosenstein ED, Kramer N. Felty's and pseudo-Felty's syndromes. *Semin Arthritis Rheum* 1991;21:129–142.
47. Zuckerman E, Keren D, Rozenbaum M, et al. Hepatitis C virus-related arthritis: characteristics and response to therapy with interferon alpha. *Clin Exp Rheumatol* 2000;18:579–584.
48. Tanoue LT. Pulmonary manifestations of rheumatoid arthritis. *Clin Chest Med* 1998;19:667–685, viii.
49. Lofgren RH, Montgomery WW. Incidence of laryngeal involvement in rheumatoid arthritis. *N Engl J Med* 1962;267:193–195.
50. Darke CS, Wolman L, Young A. Laryngeal stridor in rheumatoid arthritis. *BMJ* 1958;ii:1279–1284.

51. Lawry GV, Finerman ML, Hanafee WN, et al. Laryngeal involvement in rheumatoid arthritis. A clinical, laryngoscopic, and computerized tomographic study. *Arthritis Rheum* 1984;27:873–882.
52. Bossingham DH, Simpson FG. Acute laryngeal obstruction in rheumatoid arthritis. *BMJ* 1996;312:295–296.
53. Pinels RS. Rheumatoid arthritis presenting with laryngeal obstruction. *BMJ* 1966;i:842.
54. Ten Holter JB, Van Buchem FL, Van Beusekom HJ. Cricoarytenoid arthritis may be a case of emergency. *Clin Rheumatol* 1988;7:288–290.
55. Habib MA. Intra-articular steroid injection in acute rheumatoid arthritis of the larynx. *J Laryngol Otol* 1977;91:909–910.
56. Lehmann T, Nef W, Stalder B, et al. Fatal postoperative airway obstruction in a patient with rheumatoid arthritis. *Ann Rheum Dis* 1997;56:512–513.
57. Bamshad M, Rosa U, Padda G, Luce M. Acute upper airway obstruction in rheumatoid arthritis of the cricoarytenoid joints. *South Med J* 1989;82:507–511.
58. Gabbay E, Tarala R, Will R, et al. Interstitial lung disease in recent onset rheumatoid arthritis. *Am J Respir Crit Care Med* 1997;156:528–535.
59. Saag KG, Kolluri S, Koehnke RK, et al. Rheumatoid arthritis lung disease. Determinants of radiographic and physiologic abnormalities. *Arthritis Rheum* 1996;39:1711–1719.
60. Cervantes-Perez P, Toro-Perez AH, Rodriguez-Jurado P. Pulmonary involvement in rheumatoid arthritis. *JAMA* 1980;243:1715–1719.
61. Roschmann RA, Rothenberg RJ. Pulmonary fibrosis in rheumatoid arthritis: a review of clinical features and therapy. *Semin Arthritis Rheum* 1987;16:174–185.
62. Hyland RH, Gordon DA, Broder I, et al. A systematic controlled study of pulmonary abnormalities in rheumatoid arthritis. *J Rheumatol* 1983;10:395–405.
63. Jurik AG, Davidsen D, Graudal H. Prevalence of pulmonary involvement in rheumatoid arthritis and its relationship to some characteristics of the patients. A radiological and clinical study. *Scand J Rheumatol* 1982;11:217–224.
64. Shannon TM, Gale ME. Noncardiac manifestations of rheumatoid arthritis in the thorax. *J Thorac Imaging* 1992;7:19–29.
65. King TE. The interstitial lung diseases. In: Braunwald E, Fauci AS, Isselbacher KJ, et al., eds. *Harrison's manual of medicine*. New York: McGraw-Hill, 2002:7–11.
66. Fujii M, Adachi S, Shimizu T, et al. Interstitial lung disease in rheumatoid arthritis: assessment with high-resolution computed tomography. *J Thorac Imaging* 1993;8:54–62.
67. Remy-Jardin M, Remy J, Cortet B, et al. Lung changes in rheumatoid arthritis: CT findings. *Radiology* 1994;193:375–382.
68. Alegre J, Teran J, Alvarez B, Viejo JL. Successful use of cyclosporine for the treatment of aggressive pulmonary fibrosis in a patient with rheumatoid arthritis. *Arthritis Rheum* 1990;33:1594–1596.
69. Brown CH, Turner-Warwick M. The treatment of cryptogenic fibrosing alveolitis with immunosuppressant drugs. *Q J Med* 1971;40:289–302.
70. Cohen JM, Miller A, Spiera H. Interstitial pneumonitis complicating rheumatoid arthritis. Sustained remission with azathioprine therapy. *Chest* 1977;72:521–524.
71. A controlled trial of cyclophosphamide in rheumatoid arthritis. *N Engl J Med* 1970;283:883–889.
72. Puttick MP, Klinkhoff AV, Chalmers A, Ostrow DN. Treatment of progressive rheumatoid interstitial lung disease with cyclosporine. *J Rheumatol* 1995;22:2163–2165.
73. Scott DG, Bacon PA. Response to methotrexate in fibrosing alveolitis associated with connective tissue disease. *Thorax* 1980;35:725–732.
74. Vassallo R, Matteson E, Thomas CF Jr. Clinical response of rheumatoid arthritis-associated pulmonary fibrosis to tumor necrosis factor-alpha inhibition. *Chest* 2002;122:1093–1096.
75. Kelly CA. Rheumatoid arthritis: classical rheumatoid lung disease. *Baillieres Clin Rheumatol* 1993;7:1–16.
76. Walker WC, Wright V. Pulmonary lesions and rheumatoid arthritis. *Medicine (Baltimore)* 1968;47:501–520.
77. Walker WC, Wright V. Rheumatoid pleuritis. *Ann Rheum Dis* 1967;26:467–474.
78. Jones FL Jr, Blodgett RC Jr. Empyema in rheumatoid pleuropulmonary disease. *Ann Intern Med* 1971;74:665–671.
79. Light RW. Disorders of the pleura, mediastinum, and diaphragm. In: Braunwald E, Fauci AS, Isselbacher KJ, et al., eds. *Harrison's manual of medicine*. New York: McGraw-Hill, 2002:1.
80. Pritikin JD, Jensen WA, Yenokida GG, et al. Respiratory failure due to a massive rheumatoid pleural effusion. *J Rheumatol* 1990;17:673–675.
81. DuBois RM, Wells AU. The lungs and connective tissue diseases. In: Murray JF, Nadel JA, Mason RJ, Boushey HA, eds. *Murray and Nadel: textbook of respiratory medicine*, 3rd ed. Philadelphia: W.B. Saunders Company, 2000:1691–1715.
82. Begin R, Masse S, Cantin A, et al. Airway disease in a subset of nonsmoking rheumatoid patients. Characterization of the disease and evidence for an autoimmune pathogenesis. *Am J Med* 1982;72:743–750.
83. Geddes DM, Corrin B, Brewerton DA, et al. Progressive airway obliteration in adults and its association with rheumatoid disease. *QJM* 1977;46:427–444.
84. Aquino SL, Webb WR, Golden J. Bronchiolitis obliterans associated with rheumatoid arthritis: findings on HRCT and dynamic expiratory CT. *J Comput Assist Tomogr* 1994;18:555–558.
85. Cortet B, Flipo RM, Remy-Jardin M, et al. Use of high resolution computed tomography of the lungs in patients with rheumatoid arthritis. *Ann Rheum Dis* 1995;54:815–819.
86. Yousem SA, Colby TV, Carrington CB. Lung biopsy in rheumatoid arthritis. *Am Rev Respir Dis* 1985;131:770–777.
87. Dieppe PA. Empyema in rheumatoid arthritis. *Ann Rheum Dis* 1975;34:181–185.
88. Caplan A. Certain unusual radiologic appearances in the chest of coal miners suffering from rheumatoid arthritis. *Thorax* 1953;8:29–36.
89. McRorie ER, Wright RA, Errington ML, Luqmani RA. Rheumatoid constrictive pericarditis. *Br J Rheumatol* 1997;36:100–103.
90. Hara KS, Ballard DJ, Ilstrup DM, et al. Rheumatoid pericarditis: clinical features and survival. *Medicine (Baltimore)* 1990;69:81–91.
91. Kelly CA, Bourke JP, Malcolm A, Griffiths ID. Chronic pericardial disease in patients with rheumatoid arthritis: a longitudinal study. *QJM* 1990;75:461–470.
92. Nomeir AM, Turner RA, Watts LE. Cardiac involvement in rheumatoid arthritis. Followup study. *Arthritis Rheum* 1979;22:561–564.
93. Gravallese EM, Corson JM, Coblyn JS, et al. Rheumatoid aortitis: a rarely recognized but clinically significant entity. *Medicine (Baltimore)* 1989;68:95–106.
94. Levine AJ, Dimitri WR, Bonser RS. Aortic regurgitation in rheumatoid arthritis necessitating aortic valve replacement. *Eur J Cardiothorac Surg* 1999;15:213–214.
95. Baer AN, Dessypris EN, Krantz SB. The pathogenesis of anemia in rheumatoid arthritis: a clinical and laboratory analysis. *Semin Arthritis Rheum* 1990;19:209–223.
96. Vreugdenhil G, Wognum AW, van Eijk HG, Swaak AJ. Anaemia in rheumatoid arthritis: the role of iron, vitamin B_{12}, and folic acid deficiency, and erythropoietin responsiveness. *Ann Rheum Dis* 1990;49:93–98.
97. Vreugdenhil G, Swaak AJ. Anaemia in rheumatoid arthritis: pathogenesis, diagnosis and treatment. *Rheumatol Int* 1990;9:243–257.
98. Cartwright GE, Lee GR. The anaemia of chronic disorders. *Br J Haematol* 1971;21:147–152.
99. Bentley DP, Williams P. Serum ferritin concentration as an index of storage iron in rheumatoid arthritis. *J Clin Pathol* 1974;27:786–788.
100. Mulherin D, Skelly M, Saunders A, et al. The diagnosis of iron deficiency in patients with rheumatoid arthritis and anemia: an algorithm using simple laboratory measures. *J Rheumatol* 1996;23:237–240.
101. Kaltwasser JP, Kessler U, Gottschalk R, et al. Effect of recombinant human erythropoietin and intravenous iron on anemia and disease activity in rheumatoid arthritis. *J Rheumatol* 2001;28:2430–2436.
102. Peeters HR, Jongen-Lavrencic M, et al. Recombinant human erythropoietin improves health-related quality of life in patients with rheumatoid arthritis and anaemia of chronic disease; utility measures correlate strongly with disease activity measures. *Rheumatol Int* 1999;18:201–206.
103. Peeters HR, Jongen-Lavrencic M, Vreugdenhil G, Swaak AJ. Effect of recombinant human erythropoietin on anaemia and disease activity in patients with rheumatoid arthritis and anaemia of chronic disease: a randomised placebo controlled double blind 52 weeks clinical trial. *Ann Rheum Dis* 1996;55:739–744.
104. Pincus T, Olsen NJ, Russell IJ, et al. Multicenter study of recombinant human erythropoietin in correction of anemia in rheumatoid arthritis. *Am J Med* 1990;89:161–168.
105. Weinstein IM, Rosenbloom BE. Hematologic problems in patients with cancer and chronic inflammatory disorders. In: Hoffman R, Benz EJ, Shattil SJ, et al., eds. *Hematology: basic principles and practice*, 3rd ed. Philadelphia: Churchill Livingstone, 2000:2411–2420.
106. Nordstrom D, Lindroth Y, Marsal L, et al. Availability of iron and degree of inflammation modifies the response to recombinant human erythropoietin when treating anemia of chronic disease in patients with rheumatoid arthritis. *Rheumatol Int* 1997;17:67–73.
107. Goldberg J, Pinals RS. Felty syndrome. *Semin Arthritis Rheum* 1980;10:52–65.
108. Ruderman M, Miller LM, Pinals RS. Clinical and serologic observations on 27 patients with Felty's syndrome. *Arthritis Rheum* 1968;11:377–384.
109. Campion G, Maddison PJ, Goulding N, et al. The Felty syndrome: a case-matched study of clinical manifestations and outcome, serologic features, and immunogenetic associations. *Medicine (Baltimore)* 1990;69:69–80.
110. Sibley JT, Haga M, Visram DA, Mitchell DM. The clinical course of Felty's syndrome compared to matched controls. *J Rheumatol* 1991;18:1163–1167.
111. Laszlo J, Jones R, Silberman HR, Banks PM. Splenectomy for Felty's syndrome. Clinicopathological study of 27 patients. *Arch Intern Med* 1978;138:597–602.
112. Sienknecht CW, Urowitz MB, Pruzanski W, Stein HB. Felty's syndrome. Clinical and serological analysis of 34 cases. *Ann Rheum Dis* 1977;36:500–507.
113. Coremans IE, Hagen EC, van der Voort EA, et al. Autoantibodies to neutrophil cytoplasmic enzymes in Felty's syndrome. *Clin Exp Rheumatol* 1993;11:255–262.
114. Juby A, Johnston C, Davis P, Russell AS. Antinuclear and antineutrophil cytoplasmic antibodies (ANCA) in the sera of patients with Felty's syndrome. *Br J Rheumatol* 1992;31:185–188.
115. Isasi C, Lopez-Martin JA, Angeles Trujillo M, et al. Felty's syndrome: response to low dose oral methotrexate. *J Rheumatol* 1989;16:983–985.
116. Allen LS, Groff G. Treatment of Felty's syndrome with low-dose oral methotrexate. *Arthritis Rheum* 1986;29:902–905.
117. Dillon AM, Luthra HS, Conn DL, Ferguson RH. Parenteral gold therapy in the Felty syndrome. Experience with 20 patients. *Medicine (Baltimore)* 1986;65:107–112.

118. Gowans JD, Salami M. Response of rheumatoid arthritis with leukopenia to gold salts. *N Engl J Med* 1973;288:1007–1008.
119. Canvin JM, Dalal BI, Baragar F, Johnston JB. Cyclosporine for the treatment of granulocytopenia in Felty's syndrome. *Am J Hematol* 1991;36:219–220.
120. Kaprove RE. Felty's syndrome: case report and rationale for disease-suppressant immunosuppressive therapy. *J Rheumatol* 1981;8:791–796.
121. Talip F, Walker N, Khan W, Zimmermann B. Treatment of Felty's syndrome with leflunomide. *J Rheumatol* 2001;28:868–870.
122. Pixley JS, Yoneda KY, Manalo PB. Sequential administration of cyclophosphamide and granulocyte-colony stimulating factor relieves impaired myeloid maturation in Felty's syndrome. *Am J Hematol* 1993;43:304–306.
123. Mant MJ, Akabutu JJ, Herbert FA. Lithium carbonate therapy in severe Felty's syndrome. Benefits, toxicity, and granulocyte function. *Arch Intern Med* 1986;146:277–280.
124. Schapira DV, Gordon PA, Herbert FA. Reduction of infections in Felty's syndrome through use of lithium. *Arthritis Rheum* 1977;20:1556–1557.
125. Stanworth SJ, Bhavnani M, Chattopadhya C, et al. Treatment of Felty's syndrome with the haemopoietic growth factor granulocyte colony-stimulating factor (G-CSF). *QJM* 1998;91:49–56.
126. Hellmich B, Schnabel A, Gross WL. Treatment of severe neutropenia due to Felty's syndrome or systemic lupus erythematosus with granulocyte colony-stimulating factor. *Semin Arthritis Rheum* 1999;29:82–99.
127. Moore DF Jr, Vadhan-Raj S. Sustained response in Felty's syndrome to prolonged administration of recombinant human granulocyte-macrophage colony-stimulating factor (rhGM-CSF). *Am J Med* 1995;98:591–594.
128. Blumfelder TM, Logue GL, Shimm DS. Felty's syndrome: effects of splenectomy upon granulocyte count and granulocyte-associated IgG. *Ann Intern Med* 1981;94:623–628.
129. Pinels RS. Drug therapy in Felty's syndrome. In: Rose BD, ed. *UpToDate*. Wellesley, MA: UpToDate, 2002.
130. Pinels RS. Indications for splenectomy in Felty's syndrome. In: Rose BD, ed. *UpToDate*. Wellesley, MA: UpToDate, 2002.
131. Hamidou MA, Sadr FB, Lamy T, et al. Low-dose methotrexate for the treatment of patients with large granular lymphocyte leukemia associated with rheumatoid arthritis. *Am J Med* 2000;108:730–732.
132. Loughran TP Jr, Kidd PG, Starkebaum G. Treatment of large granular lymphocyte leukemia with oral low-dose methotrexate. *Blood* 1994;84:2164–2170.
133. Loughran TP Jr, Starkebaum G, Clark E, et al. Evaluation of splenectomy in large granular lymphocyte leukaemia. *Br J Haematol* 1987;67:135–140.
134. Rodrigues JF, Harth M, Barr RM. Pure red cell aplasia in rheumatoid arthritis. *J Rheumatol* 1988;15:1159–1161.
135. Dessypris EN, Baer MR, Sergent JS, Krantz SB. Rheumatoid arthritis and pure red cell aplasia. *Ann Intern Med* 1984;100:202–206.

CHAPTER 46

Pregnancy

Monika E. Østensen and J. Lee Nelson

The interface of pregnancy and rheumatoid arthritis (RA) generates questions about interactions between these two conditions for patients and their families and for practicing clinicians. Because pregnancy is known to affect the activity of RA, it is also a subject of considerable research. The primary focus of this chapter is the clinical management of RA during pregnancy. However, the chapter is structured to also provide a background in understanding the biology of pregnancy and RA, which is discussed initially. Thereafter, common issues in clinical management are discussed and illustrated in a series of case histories. Information on antirheumatic drugs that can affect male reproduction is also provided.

EFFECT OF PREGNANCY ON DISEASE ACTIVITY IN WOMEN WITH RHEUMATOID ARTHRITIS

The amelioration of symptoms and signs of RA during pregnancy was initially described more than 60 years ago by Philip Showalter Hench (1). Numerous subsequent studies, both retrospective and prospective, confirmed this observation, citing improvement rates ranging from 54% to 86% of pregnancies (2–9). Improvement was less marked in a recent report (10) that used the Health Assessment Questionnaire administered during the third trimester as a major assessment for disease activity. However, the Health Assessment Questionnaire includes questions such as "Are you able to bend down to pick up clothing from the floor? Dress yourself including tying shoelaces. . . etc." and is not a validated measure of RA activity during pregnancy (11). An overall review of studies indicates that improvement of RA occurs in approximately three-fourths of pregnancies. Whether pregnancy affects extraarticular manifestations of RA is not known. Improvement of RA occurs early in gestation, with most patients experiencing initial abating of arthritis during the first trimester (1,3,4,6,8). Patients who experience amelioration during the first trimester are very likely to sustain this effect or improve further as gestation progresses. Most studies indicate that a woman whose RA improves during one pregnancy is likely to show improvement in subsequent pregnancies. Variables such as rheumatoid factor, age, functional class, or disease duration have not been found to predict whether a woman will experience pregnancy-induced disease amelioration (5,8,12).

PREGNANCY COMPLICATIONS, DELIVERY, AND POSTPARTUM DISEASE ACTIVITY

Pregnancy complications, such as preeclampsia and premature labor, are not increased in women with RA (2). Women who have advanced hip disease or who have undergone prior total hip replacement can potentially experience difficulty in vaginal delivery (13), but neither preclude normal vaginal delivery. In patients with cervical spine involvement, caution is indicated in anesthesia and intubation. In the postpartum period, RA is active for the large majority of women regardless of whether disease has improved during pregnancy. For those who have experienced pregnancy-induced disease amelioration, more than one-third have recurrent disease by 1 month and two-thirds by 2 months postpartum (3–6,8,14). Almost all women have recurrent disease within 3 to 4 months of delivery. It is not clear whether the timing of a flare is related to lactation. Although a study suggested a correlation between lactation and increased disease activity postpartum, among women in the study who had RA, it was described only when the woman was breast-feeding for the first time (15), and earlier studies indicated no correlation (6,8).

PROGNOSIS FOR THE FETUS AND NEWBORN

The prognosis for the fetus and newborn of women with RA is excellent. Despite occasional case reports about adverse outcomes (2,16), case series have indicated no increase of any adverse pregnancy outcome (6,8). Further, women with RA do not have an overall increase in spontaneous abortions or prematurity (2,6,8). A few studies have also examined pregnancy outcome before disease onset. Although an increase of spontaneous abortions before disease onset was suggested in one study (17), it was not confirmed in subsequent studies (18–20). Similarly, the suggestion of an increase in stillbirths before disease onset (18) was not confirmed in subsequent reports (19,20).

EFFECT OF PREGNANCY ON THE PROGNOSIS OF RHEUMATOID ARTHRITIS

Women with RA sometimes ask how one or multiple pregnancies or childbirths will affect the long-term prognosis for their disease. Theoretically, the long-term effect could be either beneficial or adverse, as improvement usually occurs during pregnancy, but active disease almost invariably occurs postpartum. One older retrospective study described no difference in long-term disease outcome between women who had pregnancies after RA onset and those who did not, but conclusions were confounded by differences in the comparison groups and an inability to distinguish term from nonterm pregnancies (21). In a more recent report, having more than three children increased the risk of severe RA, but the comparison was made to women with fewer children without a group who were childless or had never been pregnant (22). In contrast, a prospective study evaluated women with a 12-year follow-up and found no significant influence of pregnancy on long-term RA outcome but did find a trend for patients with multiple pregnancies to have less radiographic joint damage and a better functional level (23). Thus, additional studies will be necessary to fully determine the effects—whether beneficial, neutral, or adverse—of pregnancy, multiple pregnancies, and type of pregnancy on the long-term prognosis of RA in the mother.

FECUNDITY AND FERTILITY

Fertility is usually measured as the ability to conceive a child and *fecundity* as the time it takes to achieve pregnancy. A number of studies have suggested that fertility or fecundity may be decreased among women with RA (24,25). If fertility or fecundity are evaluated after disease onset, confounding may occur due to a decrease in the frequency of intercourse due to pain from RA (26). In a study of fertility and fecundity before disease onset, no decrease of fertility was observed, but a significant decrease in fecundity was found (27). In other words, women who subsequently developed RA were able to achieve pregnancy at a rate similar to controls but experienced a prolonged time to conception. Similar results were described in another study (28). The reason(s) for this observation are not known, but potential factors that could result in decreased fecundity without infertility include ovulatory dysfunction, abnormalities of tubal transport or implantation, antibodies to spermatozoa, or insufficient progesterone secretion by the corpus luteum (luteal phase defect).

PREGNANCY AND SUSCEPTIBILITY TO NEW ONSET OF RHEUMATOID ARTHRITIS

A number of studies support an immunomodulatory role of pregnancy in affecting susceptibility to RA and suggest that the risk of developing RA is modestly reduced for women who have given birth (29–31). Case control studies indicate that, overall, there is also a reduced likelihood that a woman will first develop RA during pregnancy (32,33). However, risk is transiently increased in the initial 3 to 12 months postpartum (4,16,32,33). In a large study of healthy pregnant subjects, rheumatoid factor predicated the new onset of RA in the postpartum period (34). In women who breast-feed, magnification of RA risk in the year after a first pregnancy has been described and postulated to be due to a proinflammatory role for increased levels of prolactin (35).

PREGNANCY-INDUCED AMELIORATION AND POSTPARTUM RELAPSE OF RHEUMATOID ARTHRITIS

The biologic basis for the pregnancy-induced amelioration of RA has been the subject of a number of clinical research studies. Hench's initial investigation into this intriguing biologic phenomenon contributed to the eventual discovery of cortisol, for which he shared a Nobel Prize. Although a very important discovery, subsequent studies showed that increased serum cortisol concentrations did not explain the improvement of RA during pregnancy (7,36). Other early studies failed to support the idea that elevated levels of sex hormones (notably estrogens) might be responsible (37,38). Interest in a role for a serum protein termed *pregnancy-associated* α_2 *globulin* (15), dwindled also after variable results in subsequent studies (9,39–41). Patients with RA often have abnormalities in the percentage of immunoglobulin G lacking the terminal galactose units in the oligosaccharide chains attached to CH_2 regions, and a reversion to normal has been described in association with amelioration of RA during pregnancy (42,43). Neuroendocrine changes represent another potential factor that could contribute to fluctuations in disease activity during pregnancy (44–47). Prolactin has been proposed to play a role in the postpartum relapse and in the increased risk of new-onset RA in the postpartum period (35), a possibility that is also supported by the observation that collagen-induced arthritis can be suppressed by treatment with bromocriptine, an inhibitor of prolactin (48).

A unique immunologic aspect of pregnancy is exposure of the mother to HLA molecules that are foreign to her because the child inherits one set of HLA genes from the father. HLA molecules play an essential role in the self versus nonself discrimination and regulate the generation of immune responses. Particular HLA class II molecules are associated with an increased susceptibility to RA (see Chapter 10). In studies of mother–child pairs in which the mother experienced RA improvement during pregnancy, compared to those who did not, fetal–maternal disparity in the HLA class II molecules HLA-DR and -DQ was observed significantly more often in the former than in the latter (13). A subsequent study confirmed this observation (49). The conclusions of another report differed from these two studies (50), but the study was not comparable, in that women who were in remission before becoming pregnant were included, and one-third of patients did not meet criteria for RA.

The mechanism(s) by which fetal paternally inherited HLA molecules could contribute to amelioration of RA during pregnancy is unknown. Recent studies in other diseases indicate that fetal cells enter the maternal circulation and also persist for many years thereafter (51). A potential role for maternal antibody response to paternal HLA antigens is suggested by experimental studies in which antibodies to HLA class II molecules modulate autoimmune diseases, including collagen-induced arthritis (52), and early studies suggesting placenta-eluted γ-globulins have a beneficial effect when administered to RA patients (53–55). Another possibility for amelioration of RA during pregnancy is that regulatory T cells are induced that suppress maternal autoimmune responses. Alternatively, the beneficial effect of fetal (paternal) HLA disparity could be mediated by soluble HLA molecules or peptides. A shift in cytokine production from a T helper 1 to a T helper 2 profile during pregnancy could also be important (56,57). These possibilities are not exclusive, and it is likely that the explanation for disease amelioration is multifactorial.

ISSUES IN THE MANAGEMENT OF RHEUMATOID ARTHRITIS DURING PREGNANCY AND POSTPARTUM

Although pregnancy has a beneficial effect on the majority of women with RA, approximately 25% of pregnant RA patients still have active disease or even experience a flare. Although less common, some women do not experience improvement until later in pregnancy. These observations indicate that approximately one-third of pregnant RA patients will have active disease and need medication at some time during pregnancy. Additionally, patients with active disease need therapy until pregnancy occurs and probably for some time thereafter. In the patient who is planning pregnancy, consideration must be given to the type of drug therapy that is compatible with

TABLE 46.1. Immunosuppressive Drugs and Biologic Agents in Pregnancy

Source	Drugs	Developmental Toxicity Reported	Comment
Animal and human data	Hydroxychloroquine, sulfasalazine, aurothiomalate, azathioprine, and cyclosporine	Sporadic; cause–effect relationship not conclusive	Compatible with pregnancy
Animal and human data	Prednisone and chloroquine	Sporadic; related to high doses or combination therapies	Compatible when adequate measures are taken (limiting dose)
Animal and human data	Methotrexate, cyclophosphamide, chlorambucil, and penicillamine	Evidence of developmental toxicity	Avoid
Animal data; insufficient data on human pregnancy	Infliximab and etanercept	No toxicity in animals	See text
Animal data	Leflunomide	Toxicity shown in animals	Avoid

pregnancy. In the postpartum period, treatment needs to be adjusted if the patient nurses her child.

Therapeutic problems arising in pregnant women with RA are presented by three typical cases from a pregnancy clinic for women with rheumatic diseases (headed by M. Østensen). Among the 358 consultations during the years 2000 and 2001, 52% dealt with questions related to drug treatment during pregnancy, with possible teratogenicity or other adverse effects on the fetus and neonate as the main issues. Counseling of patients has been based on published reports on gestational use of antirheumatic, immunosuppressive, and cytostatic drugs. Unfortunately, the number of controlled studies performed in pregnant women is small, and experience with therapy often derives from other diseases. With lack of sufficient data, decisions about therapy during pregnancy are in many instances based on animal studies and the known pharmacologic properties of a drug. Clearly, prescribing during pregnancy has legal aspects, and these must also be taken into account (Table 46.1).

Case 1: Nonsteroidal Antiinflammatory Drugs in Pregnancy

A 30-year-old patient with a history of RA of 2 years' duration has active disease during her second pregnancy. Because of synovitis in some metacarpophalangeal joints and wrist and knee joints, she is treated with 50 mg of diclofenac three times a day throughout the first and second trimester. She contacts her physician at week 32 and asks if she can continue this medication or should change to a selective cyclooxygenase 2 (COX-2) inhibitor because her disease is still active.

Nonsteroidal antiinflammatory drugs (NSAIDs) can be used in the first half of gestation, as there is no indication for teratogenic effects of salicylates, indomethacin, fenoprofen, ibuprofen, ketoprofen, naproxen, diclofenac, mefenamic acid, and piroxicam (58). However, both selective and nonselective inhibitors of COX can interfere with pregnancy. Inhibition of prostaglandin synthesis in the fetus can alter circulation and lead to possible side effects of NSAIDs. A reduction of fetal renal output and a decrease in the volume of amniotic fluid have been shown for indomethacin, ketoprofen, and ibuprofen and may also occur with other inhibitors of prostaglandin synthesis (59–61). Development of oligohydramnios has been shown to be dose dependent. Impairment of renal function has been demonstrated as early as in gestational week 27. There is evidence that renal function in the fetus recovers quickly after drug withdrawal (60). In cases of premature delivery and exposure to NSAIDs within 72 hours before delivery, neonatal renal function may be impaired, sometimes severely (61).

Effects on the fetal ductus arteriosus have been shown for most nonselective NSAIDs (62). Due to its frequent use for inhibition of premature labor, indomethacin has been the most thoroughly studied NSAID during human pregnancy (63). Fetal echocardiography has shown constriction of the ductus independent of the fetal serum concentration of indomethacin but related to gestational age, being rare before week 27 and increasing to affect approximately 10% to 50% of the fetuses after week 31 (64). However, NSAID-induced constriction of the ductus has been shown to resolve within 24 hours or a few days after discontinuation of the drug (64,65). Premature closure of the ductus arteriosus can result in pulmonary hypertension in the newborn and has been reported in neonates exposed to NSAIDs prenatally (66). There is no agreement on whether NSAIDs such as indomethacin increase the risk for necrotizing enterocolitis and intracranial hemorrhage in the neonate after exposure shortly before delivery (65). Many of the side effects observed in neonates after indomethacin exposure have occurred in very premature infants of low birth weight, a risk factor for perinatal morbidity.

Because both COX-1 and COX-2 are involved in the regulation of reproductive events, similar side effects should be expected from selective and nonselective NSAIDs. In lambs and baboons, COX-2 regulates the tone of the fetal ductus arteriosus and is present in the fetal kidney. Consequently, fetal cardiovascular and renal side effects may also occur in pregnancies exposed to selective COX-2 inhibitors.

In a study by Østensen et al. of pregnant patients with rheumatologic disorders, including 12 women with RA, use of standard doses of different nonselective NSAIDs for an average of 15.3 weeks during gestation did not cause adverse maternal or neonatal effects in the 49 users, compared to the 45 nonusers of NSAIDs (67). Of note, NSAIDs were always discontinued 6 weeks before term in this study. If treatment with NSAIDs is necessary after gestational week 32, effects on fetal renal function and on the ductus arteriosus can be monitored by ultrasonography. Weekly fetal monitoring may be useful in cases in which NSAIDs have to be continued up to term.

Control of joint symptoms in pregnancy can also be attempted by analgesics such as acetaminophen or low-dose (<10 mg of prednisone per day) corticosteroids. Joint swelling and effusion in one or a limited number of joints can be effectively treated with intraarticular administration of corticosteroids. No untoward fetal effects of intraarticular injections during pregnancy have been reported.

Case 2: How to Treat the Prepregnant Patient with Active Rheumatoid Arthritis

A 32-year-old patient has newly diagnosed severe RA that is not responsive to NSAIDs, antimalarials, and low-dose prednisone. Her physician wants to start treatment with a combination therapy. His suggestions are leflunomide and methotrexate (MTX) or a tumor necrosis factor α (TNF-α) inhibitor in combination with MTX. The patient wishes for a second child and does not want to postpone pregnancy because of drug therapy.

This case illustrates the problems of treating women with RA who desire children but need potent drug treatment for control of progressive erosive joint disease. The issues concern which suitable monotherapies or combination therapies are compatible with first-trimester exposure and which must be prophylactically withdrawn. The drugs suggested for the patient are discussed below.

METHOTREXATE

MTX is a folic acid antagonist that impairs dihydrofolate reductase and interferes with the production of purines. Absolute or functional folic acid deficiency during early pregnancy will typically lead to neural tube defects in the offspring. Other anomalies can also be induced. The congenital anomalies observed in animals and humans exposed to MTX in the first trimester most often involve the central nervous system, cranial ossification, and the palate (68).

Review of the literature on first-trimester exposure to MTX (once-weekly doses of 20 mg of MTX or less) disclosed 22 pregnancies (69,70). In the pregnancies not terminated electively, four (22%) ended in miscarriage. Among the terminated pregnancies, one fetus had a complete ventricular septum defect and an extensive diaphragmatic hernia (70). Of the 14 pregnancies that proceeded to delivery, one child (8%) was born with the aminopterin syndrome. Typical features of the syndrome are bony malformations of the skull, micrognathia, and hypertelorism. Birth weights of the full-term infants were within normal range. A follow-up ranging from 0.1 to 16.7 years of seven of the children revealed no developmental or other serious health problems.

Comment. Low-dose weekly MTX either as monotherapy or in combination with other immunosuppressive or biologic drugs is widely used for RA treatment but is not compatible with pregnancy. In any patient on MTX, attempts to conceive must be postponed until 3 months after withdrawal of the drug, as active metabolites can remain in cells or tissues for approximately 3 months after cessation of therapy. Safe contraception is therefore necessary throughout treatment. Folate supplementation should be continued antenatally and throughout pregnancy.

LEFLUNOMIDE

Among the new disease-modifying antirheumatic drugs (DMARDs), leflunomide is contraindicated because of skeletal and central nervous system malformations observed in animals. Data on human pregnancy are lacking. One abstract has reported the occurrence of pregnancy during treatment with leflunomide. Of the 60 pregnancies with leflunomide exposure, 22 were interrupted, details of 35 pregnancies are lacking, and three pregnancies went to delivery, but the status of the neonates are not known (71).

Comment. Leflunomide is contraindicated during pregnancy, and women of childbearing potential should be started on the drug only under safe contraception. Due to its long half-life and protracted elimination from plasma, leflunomide must be withdrawn before a planned pregnancy. Elimination of the drug should be enhanced by administering cholestyramine, 8 g three times daily for 11 days. When plasma levels of less than 0.02 μg per mL after two subsequent measurements with an interval of 28 days are achieved, pregnancy can be attempted.

ETANERCEPT AND INFLIXIMAB

The TNF-α antagonists etanercept (soluble TNF-α receptor) and monoclonal antibodies (infliximab) have not been found to be teratogenic or fetotoxic in animal studies (72). Experience from human pregnancy comprises postmarketing data and a few abstracts. A postmarketing report on 27 pregnancies exposed to etanercept and an abstract on pregnancy exposure to infliximab in 59 cases did not disclose an increase in birth defects or adverse pregnancy outcomes (73).

Comment. No clear statement on the gestational use of TNF-α antagonists can be made. Infliximab has an elimination half-life of 2 to several weeks. The manufacturer recommends waiting 6 months after drug discontinuation before conception is attempted. Etanercept has an elimination half-life of 1 to 2 weeks. In view of the lack of animal toxicity, it may be reasonable to assume that withdrawal of etanercept at the first missed period is without harmful effects.

Case 3: Prophylactic Withdrawal of Disease-Modifying Drugs

A 31-year-old patient with active RA of 3 years' duration wants to have a child. Because of the patient's desire to have a child, her rheumatologist has treated her with an NSAID and aurothiomalate, in the belief that gold is safe in pregnancy. Due to continuous disease activity, MTX was added during the last year. The patient wants to stop MTX but asks for an effective disease-modifying therapy that is compatible with pregnancy and can be continued also during lactation.

This case shows several of the therapeutic problems arising when the desire for children occurs in the setting of active disease. In that case, effective therapy must sometimes be withdrawn, leaving the patient with uncertainty if a new drug will work. Regarding DMARD therapy, no existing data support the prophylactic withdrawal of gold salts, antimalarials, or sulfasalazine. Cessation of DMARD therapy before conception can result in exacerbation of disease, particularly if conception is delayed.

Because several of the most effective new therapies for RA are not compatible with pregnancy either because they are fetotoxic or due to lack of experience with human pregnancy, other DMARDs must be applied. Treatment options for the prepregnancy RA patient include antimalarials, sulfasalazine, gold compounds, azathioprine, and cyclosporine, either as monotherapy or in combination with low-dose prednisone (Table 46.2). These agents are described below. Penicillamine should not be used because it can inhibit collagen cross-linking in the fetus and act as a human teratogen (74).

TABLE 46.2. Antirheumatic Drugs and Breast-Feeding: Recommendations of the American Academy of Pediatrics

Compatible	Not Compatible	Insufficient Data
Diclofenac	Aspirin (high dose or long-term)	Celecoxib
Ibuprofen	Cyclosporine	Rofecoxib
Indomethacin	Methotrexate	Etanercept
Ketoprofen	Cyclophosphamide	Infliximab
Mefenamic acid	Chlorambucil	Penicillamine
Naproxen		Leflunomide
Piroxicam		Azathioprine
Corticosteroids		
Chloroquine		
Hydroxychloroquine		
Gold salts		
Sulfasalazine (with caution)		
Paracetamol		

SULFASALAZINE

Reports comprising more than 2,000 pregnancies exposed to sulfasalazine have been published but only exclusively for the treatment of inflammatory bowel disease. Concerns that sulfasalazine and its metabolites could displace bilirubin and cause neonatal jaundice have not been substantiated. When patients were treated with either sulfasalazine alone or sulfasalazine in combination with corticosteroids at some time during pregnancy, no increase in birth defects, pathologic jaundice, or small-for-gestational-age babies was detected (75,76). There have been isolated reports of children born with congenital malformations to mothers treated with sulfasalazine during pregnancy (77). However, a causal relationship to the drug treatment was not established.

Comment. Sulfasalazine is a dihydrofolate reductase inhibitor associated with a risk for congenital cardiovascular defects and oral clefts for first-trimester exposure (78). Folate supplementation before and throughout pregnancy decreases this risk substantially and should, therefore, be given to fertile women on sulfasalazine. Because a case report has described neutropenia in a newborn exposed antenatally to sulfasalazine, maternal doses of this drug should not exceed 2 g daily (79).

GOLD COMPOUNDS

Although once widely used to treat RA, sodium aurothiomalate, aurothioglucose, and auranofin (oral gold) have played only a limited role as DMARDs since the development of more effective and faster-acting agents. Uneventful pregnancies concluding in the delivery of healthy children have been reported in women receiving gold therapy (80). One case of multiple fetal malformations in a mother who received 20 mg of aurothiomalate weekly during the first 20 weeks of pregnancy has been reported, but a relation to gold therapy has been disputed (81). To date, little is known about the effect of oral gold (auranofin) on the human fetus (82).

Comment. Rheumatologists differ in their view on the gestational use of gold compounds (83). Patients on long-term treatment with parenteral gold should receive their monthly injection on the first day of the menses. Such a regimen assures that gold can be withdrawn as soon as pregnancy is recognized. However, due to the long elimination half-life of gold, the fetus will still be exposed to this drug, albeit not to high doses.

ANTIMALARIAL DRUGS

Most rheumatologists continue antimalarials during pregnancy in systemic lupus erythematosus patients, particularly in patients with antiphospholipid antibodies or discoid lupus. Discontinuation in early pregnancy does not prevent fetal exposure because of the long elimination half-life. Published studies on more than 200 pregnancies exposed to standard doses of chloroquine or hydroxychloroquine during the first trimester did not show an increase of congenital malformations (84–88). Chloroquine and hydroxychloroquine cross the placenta (88,89). Chloroquine accumulates preferentially in melanin-containing structures in the fetal uveal tract and inner ear (89). Malformations of the inner ear were reported in the offspring of a woman treated with higher than the recommended doses of chloroquine (500 mg per day) throughout pregnancy (90). A recent retrospective study of children exposed to chloroquine or hydroxychloroquine antenatally showed no malformations or ocular toxicity at follow-up (91).

Comment. Chloroquine and hydroxychloroquine show little risk for birth defects and visual abnormalities in exposed children. The continuation of these drugs during pregnancy seems justified.

CYCLOSPORINE

More than 600 pregnancies exposed to cyclosporine for several weeks or throughout gestation have been reported. The majority of mothers were transplant recipients treated with cyclosporine, prednisone, and azathioprine (92–95). Daily doses of cyclosporine ranged from 1.4 to 14 mg per kg, with a mean dose of 5 mg per kg. The observed rate of congenital malformations of 3% has not exceeded the rate reported in the general population nor has any particular pattern of abnormalities emerged. Likewise, a recent metaanalysis of 400 exposed pregnancies did not show a significant increase in congenital abnormalities (94). Renal and liver function were normal in 166 neonates exposed to cyclosporine *in utero* (96). Major problems of cyclosporine-treated pregnancies were prematurity (<37 weeks) in 40% to 46% and low birth weight (<2,500 g) in 44% to 65% of cases (92,94). It has been difficult to ascribe a causative role to drug treatment or the underlying maternal disorder.

Cyclosporine can induce autoimmunity in rodents after exposure *in utero*, but several studies on children of transplant recipients have found normal immune function during a follow-up ranging from 0.5 to 9 years of age (97).

Comment. Cyclosporine is a treatment option for the RA patient in whom tolerance or efficacy of other eligible DMARDs is insufficient. Renal side effects can be minimized by close monitoring and, eventually, dose reduction.

AZATHIOPRINE

Accumulated data from renal transplant centers in North America and Europe on pregnancies in renal allograft recipients treated with corticosteroids and azathioprine found no predominant or frequent birth defects (98,99). Although case reports have described congenital malformations and immunosuppression in several infants of mothers on azathioprine, a causal relationship to this agent has not been proven (99). Fetal growth restriction has sometimes been related to the gestational use of azathioprine and corticosteroids. The possible contribution of the underlying maternal disease is unclear. Studies of pregnancies in SLE showed that azathioprine-controlled disease activity reduced the rate of pregnancy losses and did not cause congenital malformations (100,101).

Comment. Intrauterine exposure to azathioprine may occasionally cause slight suppression of the bone marrow, as shown by decreased leucocyte counts and thrombocytopenia at birth (102). Doses should be kept at 1.5 to 2 mg per kg per day to avoid neonatal depression of hemopoiesis.

CORTICOSTEROIDS

Prednisone is often prescribed in combination with a DMARD. Data in experimental animals clearly demonstrate an association of corticosteroids with neonatal malformations, particularly cleft palate (103). Most cohort studies have not been able to demonstrate an increased rate of congenital malformations in humans induced by corticosteroids (104,105). A recent metaanalysis of epidemiologic studies found a slight, although significant, increase in oral clefts after first-trimester exposure to corticosteroids (105). The results of the metaanalysis have been disputed, as there is lack of information on dose and exclusion of the largest epidemiologic study from the analysis.

Other reported side effects of corticosteroids during pregnancy are growth retardation, neonatal cataracts, and adrenal suppression in neonates (106–108). The latter two are rare, as is an increased risk for infection.

Comment. High doses of corticosteroids, such as 1 to 2 mg per kg per day, should be avoided in the first trimester. At a prednisone maintenance therapy at or below 15 mg per day, only 5% to 10% of free prednisone will be present in maternal plasma. Furthermore, prednisone and prednisolone are inactivated by 11β-hydroxylases of the placenta. For women who take corticosteroids during pregnancy, stress doses are to be given for labor and delivery.

RARE PROBLEMS

After the introduction of the TNF-α antagonists, the indication for cytotoxic drugs, such as cyclophosphamide and chlorambucil, is rare in RA and probably reserved for patients with vasculitis or amyloidosis. As alkylating agents, cyclophosphamide and chlorambucil are teratogenic and must be avoided in the first trimester (109,110). Safe contraception is necessary when fertile women are treated with cytotoxic drugs. Attempts of conception should be delayed until 3 months after cessation of therapy. Cytotoxic agents given during the second half of gestation can induce intrauterine growth restriction, bone marrow suppression, and increased risk of infection in the newborn. Previous treatment with cytotoxic drugs does not increase the risk for congenital malformations (109).

OTHER TREATMENT DURING PREGNANCY

Some patients refuse all types of drug treatment during pregnancy, despite the need for therapy. Alternative treatment includes physiotherapy, acupuncture, and modification of nutrition. Pain relief during pregnancy can be accomplished by transcutaneous nerve stimulation and by the use of orthotics and splints. Supplementation with omega-3 fatty acids has been shown to improve the symptoms of active RA and to reduce the need for NSAIDs (111).

POSTPARTUM PERIOD AND LACTATION

No study has dealt with the prevention of the postpartum flare, which occurs in approximately 90% of RA women. It is impossible to say whether lactation should be avoided or shortened to a few months. In principle, it seems reasonable to start effective drug therapy as soon as disease symptoms return after delivery. Treatment with low-dose corticosteroids for several months after parturition may be beneficial for the transient corticoid deficiency after pregnancy, although this has not been proven. Therapy raises the question of the excretion of drugs into breast milk, an issue that is insufficiently studied. A survey of the use of antirheumatic drugs during lactation is given in Table 46.2.

ANTIRHEUMATIC DRUGS WITH AN EFFECT ON MALE REPRODUCTION

Some drugs used to treat RA carry a risk for male reproduction. Adverse effects include disturbances of male fertility and chromosomal defects (Table 46.3). Cytotoxic drugs infer a risk of genotoxicity either by inducing chromosomal aberrations or through single-gene mutations. It is at present unknown whether chromosomal changes in sperm cells represent a risk for the offspring. Chromosomally altered sperm cells may be less likely to fertilize an egg, or, if so, the abnormal zygote may fail to develop. In case of single-gene mutations, adverse effects on the offspring might be greater. At present, there are no data to confirm or refute the risk for congenital abnormalities or second-generation effects (such as the development of cancer) of presumable mutagenic drugs given to men.

TABLE 46.3. Antirheumatic Drugs and Male Reproduction

Drug	Impairment of Fertility	Chromosomal Abnormalities Reported
Sulfasalazine	Yes (transient)	No
Cyclosporine	No	No
Leflunomide	No	No
Azathioprine	No	Yes
Methotrexate	Anecdotal oligospermia	Yes
Cyclophosphamide	Yes	Yes

Oligo- or azoospermia can be induced by sulfasalazine and cyclophosphamide (112). It occurs only rarely during therapy with MTX (113). Azathioprine and cyclosporine do not impair male fertility. Reproductive risks for men taking leflunomide are related to its possible effect on DNA synthesis. Tests for genotoxicity have not shown adverse effects. However, the manufacturer of the drug has recommended safe contraception during use and a washout (see Chapter 30) after discontinuation before a man tries to impregnate his sexual partner (71).

Several studies have shown that the sulfapyridine moiety of salazopyrine acts on the late stages of sperm maturation (114). This leads to abnormalities in sperm morphology and function with oligospermia, reduced sperm motility, and abnormal forms but no chromosomal aberrations. Hormonal profiles of men on salazopyrine are generally normal. The sperm alterations are reversible at an average of 2.5 months after discontinuation of the drug (114).

Cyclophosphamide is toxic to all generations of germ cells and causes oligospermia or azoospermia and reduced Leydig cell function at a total dose exceeding 10 g (112). Recovery of spermatogenesis and Leydig cell function has been observed, even 10 years after treatment (115). Chromosomal abnormalities of spermatozoa have been detected in some male patients receiving anticancer therapy, including cyclophosphamide (116). Chromosomal abnormalities have also been found in some, but not all, studies investigating cells derived from patients treated with MTX and azathioprine (117,118). Anecdotal reports are of healthy children fathered by men on ongoing therapy with MTX.

Previous completed therapy with cytoxic drugs in survivors of childhood cancer (119) or testicular cancer found no excess of malformations in children fathered by these men nor was there an increase in childhood cancer (120).

Because of the uncertainty regarding genotoxicity of several of the antirheumatic drugs, it seems prudent to wait for 3 months (one cycle of spermatogenesis takes 74 days) after discontinuation of leflunomide, MTX, and cyclophosphamide until an attempt of pregnancy is made. Sperm storage before start of treatment can be recommended. In case pregnancy occurs during cytotoxic treatment, search for structural fetal anomalies by ultrasonography or chromosome analysis of fetal cells is possible.

CONCLUSION

It is prudent to consider pregnancy a possibility in every fertile patient and to clarify a desire for children before prescribing antirheumatic drugs. Clinical assessment before a planned pregnancy and regular follow-up during gestation should guide drug therapy. Knowledge of the disease course of the individual patient assists in finding the smallest effective dose of a given drug and limiting the duration of treatment during pregnancy. If potential fetotoxic or genotoxic treatment is necessary, effective contraception must be discussed both with female and male patients. Comprehensive information on benefits and possible side effects of therapy help to reduce anxiety.

REFERENCES

1. Hench PS. The ameliorating effect of pregnancy on chronic atrophic (infectious rheumatoid) arthritis, fibrositis, and intermittent hydrarthrosis. *Proc Staff Meet Mayo Clinic* 1938;13:161–167.
2. Morris WI. Pregnancy in rheumatoid arthritis and systemic lupus erythematosus. *Aust N Z J Obstet Gynaecol* 1969;9:136–144.
3. Betson JR, Dorn RV. Forty cases of arthritis and pregnancy. *J Intl College Surg* 1964;42:521–526.
4. Oka M. Effect of pregnancy on the onset and course of rheumatoid arthritis. *Ann Rheum Dis* 1953;12:227–229.
5. Neely NT, Persellin RH. Activity of rheumatoid arthritis during pregnancy. *Tex Med* 1977;73:59–63.
6. Østensen M, Aune B, Husby G. Effect of pregnancy and hormonal changes on the activity of rheumatoid arthritis. *Scand J Rheumatol* 1983;12:69–72.
7. Smith WD, West HF. Pregnancy and rheumatoid arthritis. *Acta Rheum Scand* 1960;6:189–201.
8. Østensen M, Husby G. A prospective clinical study of the effect of pregnancy on rheumatoid arthritis and ankylosing spondylitis. *Arthritis Rheum* 1983;26:1155–1159.
9. Unger A, Kay A, Griffin AJ, et al. Disease activity and pregnancy associated A_2-glycoprotein in rheumatoid arthritis during pregnancy. *BMJ* 1983;286: 750–752.
10. Barrett JH, Brennan P, Fiddler M, et al. Does rheumatoid arthritis remit during pregnancy and relapse postpartum? Results from a nationwide study in the United Kingdom performed prospectively from late pregnancy. *Arthritis Rheum* 1999;42:1219–1227.
11. Nelson JL. Rheumatoid arthritis remission/relapse and the Health Assessment Questionnaire comment on the article by Barret et al. *Arthritis Rheum* 2000;43:234–238.
12. Nelson JL, Hughes KA, Smith AG, et al. Maternal-fetal disparity in HLA class II alloantigens and the pregnancy-induced amelioration of rheumatoid arthritis. *N Engl J Med* 1993;329:466–471.
13. Østensen M. Pregnancy in patients with a history of juvenile rheumatoid arthritis. *Arthritis Rheum* 1991;34:881–887.
14. Persellin RH. The effect of pregnancy on rheumatoid arthritis. *Bull Rheum Dis* 1977;27:922–928.
15. Barrett JH, Brennan P, Fiddler M, Silman A. Breast-feeding and postpartum relapse in women with rheumatoid and inflammatory arthritis. *Arthritis Rheum* 2000;43:1010–1015.
16. Duhring JL. Pregnancy, rheumatoid arthritis, and intrauterine growth retardation. *Am J Obstet Gynecol* 1970;108:325–326.
17. Kaplan J. Fetal wastage in patients with rheumatoid arthritis. *J Rheumatol* 1986;13:875–877.
18. Silman AJ, Roman E, Veral V, Brown A. Adverse reproductive outcomes in women who subsequently develop rheumatoid arthritis. *Ann Rheum Dis* 1988;47:979–981.
19. Spector TD, Silman AJ. Is poor pregnancy outcome a risk factor in rheumatoid arthritis? *Ann Rheum Dis* 1990;49:12–14.
20. Nelson JL, Voigt LF, Koepsell TD, et al. Pregnancy outcome in women with rheumatoid arthritis before disease onset. *J Rheumatol* 1992;19:18–21.
21. Oka M, Vainio U. Effect of pregnancy on the prognosis and serology of rheumatoid arthritis. *Acta Rheum Scand* 1966;12:47–52.
22. Jorgensen C, Picot MC, Bologna C, et al. Oral contraception, parity, breast feeding, and severity of rheumatoid arthritis. *Ann Rheum Dis* 1966;55:94–98.
23. Drossaers-Bakker KW, Zwinderman AH, van Zeen D, et al. Pregnancy and oral contraceptive use do not significantly influence outcome in long term rheumatoid arthritis. *Ann Rheum Dis* 2002;61:405–408.
24. Hargreaves ER. A survey of rheumatoid arthritis in West Cornwall. A report to the empire rheumatism council. *Ann Rheum Dis* 1957;16:61–75.
25. Kay A, Bach F. Subfertility before and after the development of rheumatoid arthritis in women. *Ann Rheum Dis* 1965;24:169–173.
26. Yoshino S, Uchida S. Sexual problems of women with rheumatoid arthritis. *Arch Phys Med Rehabil* 1981;62:122–123.
27. Nelson JL, Koepsell TD, Dugowson CE, et al. Fecundity before disease onset in women with rheumatoid arthritis. *Arthritis Rheum* 1993;36:7–14.
28. del Junco DJ. The relationship between rheumatoid arthritis and reproductive function (thesis). Houston: University of Texas, 1988.
29. Hazes JMW, Dijkmans BAC, Vandenbroucke JP, et al. Pregnancy and the risk of developing rheumatoid arthritis. *Arthritis Rheum* 1990;33:1770–1775.
30. Spector TD, Roman E, Silman AJ. The pill, parity, and rheumatoid arthritis. *Arthritis Rheum* 1990;33:782–789.
31. Dugowson CE, Nelson JL, Koepsell TD, et al. Nulliparity as a risk factor for rheumatoid arthritis. *Arthritis Rheum* 1991;34:S48(abst).
32. Silman A, Kay A, Brennan P. Timing of pregnancy in relation to the onset of rheumatoid arthritis. *Arthritis Rheum* 1992;35:152–155.
33. Lansink M, de Boer A, Dijkmans B, et al. The onset of rheumatoid arthritis in relation to pregnancy and childbirth. *Clin Exp Rheumatol* 1993;11:171–174.
34. Iijima T, Tada H, Hidaka Y, et al. Prediction of postpartum onset of rheumatoid arthritis. *Ann Rheum Dis* 1998;57:460–463.
35. Brennan P, Silman A. Breast-feeding and the onset of rheumatoid arthritis. *Arthritis Rheum* 1994;37:808–813.
36. Wolfson WQ, Robinson WD, Duff IF. The probability that increased secretion of oxysteroids does not fully explain improvement in certain systemic diseases during pregnancy. *J Mich State Med Soc* 1951;50:1019–1022.
37. Gilbert M, Rotstein J, Cunningham C, et al. Norethynodrel with mestranol in treatment of rheumatoid arthritis. *JAMA* 1964:190:235.
38. van den Brink H, van Everdingen A, van Wijk M, et al. Adjuvant oestrogen therapy does not improve disease activity in postmenopausal patients with rheumatoid arthritis. *Ann Rheum Dis* 1993;52:862–865.
39. Persellin RH, Wiginton D, Rutstein J, et al. Pregnancy alpha-glycoprotein (PAG) and rheumatoid arthritis (RA) activity: a prospective analysis during gestation. *Arthritis Rheum* 1982;25(S):S6–S21.
40. Østensen M, von Schoultz B, Husby G. Comparison between serum α_2-pregnancy-associated globulin and activity of rheumatoid arthritis and ankylosing spondylitis during pregnancy. *Scand J Rheumatol* 1983;12:315–318.
41. Quinn C, Mulpeter K, Casey E, et al. Changes in levels of IgM RF and α-2 PAG correlate with increased disease activity in rheumatoid arthritis during the puerperium. *Scand J Rheumatol* 1993;22:273–279.
42. Rahman A, Isenberg D. Does it take sugar? *Ann Rheum Dis* 1995;54:689–691.
43. Rook G, Steele J, Brealey R, et al. Changes in IgG glycoform levels may be relevant to remission of arthritis during pregnancy. *J Autoimmun* 1991;4:779–794.
44. Chowdrey H, Lightman H. Interaction between the neuroendocrine system and arthritis. *Br J Rheumatol* 1993;32:441–444.
45. Berczi I. Prolactin, pregnancy and autoimmune disease. *J Rheumatol* 1993;20: 1095–1100.
46. Chikanza IC, Petrou P, Chrousos G, et al. Excessive and dysregulated secretion of prolactin in rheumatoid arthritis: immunopathogenetic and therapeutic implications. *Br J Rheumatol* 1993;32:445–448.
47. Chikanza IC, Petrou P, Kingsley G, et al. Defective hypothalamic response to immune and inflammatory stimuli in patients with rheumatoid arthritis. *Arthritis Rheum* 1992;35:1281–1288.
48. Whyte A, Williams RO. Bromocriptine suppresses postpartum exacerbation of collagen-induced arthritis. *Arthritis Rheum* 1988;31:927–928.
49. Van der Horst-Bruinsma IE, de Vries RRP, de Buck PDM, et al. Influence of HLA-class II incompatibility between mother and fetus on the development and course of rheumatoid arthritis of the mother. *Ann Rheum Dis* 1998;57:286–290.
50. Brennan P, Barrett J, Fiddler M, et al. Maternal-fetal HLA incompatibility and the course of inflammatory arthritis during pregnancy. *J Rheumatol* 2000; 27:2843–2848.
51. Nelson JL. Microchimerism: incidental byproduct of pregnancy or active participant in human health? *Trends Mol Med* 2002;8:109–113.
52. Wooley PH, Luthra HS, Lafuse WP, et al. Type II collagen-induced arthritis in mice. III. Suppression of arthritis by using monoclonal and polyclonal anti-Ia antisera. *J Immunol* 1985;134:2366–2374.
53. Sany J, Clot J, Bonneau M, et al. Immunomodulating effect of human placenta-eluted gamma globulins in rheumatoid arthritis. *Arthritis Rheum* 1982;25:17–24.
54. Combe B, Cosso B, Clot J, et al. Human placenta-eluted gamma globulins in immunomodulating treatment of rheumatoid arthritis. *Am J Med* 1985;78: 920–928.
55. Moynier M, Cosso B, Brochier J, et al. Identification of class II HLA alloantibodies in placenta-eluted gamma globulins used for treating rheumatoid arthritis. *Arthritis Rheum* 1987;30:375–381.
56. Wegmann TG, Lin H, Gilbert L, et al. Bi-directional cytokine interactions in the maternal-fetal relationship: is successful pregnancy a TH_2 phenomenon? *Immunol Today* 1993;14:353–356.
57. Mosmann TR. Properties and functions of interleukin-10. *Adv Immunol* 1994;56:1–11.
58. Østensen M. Safety of non-steroidal anti-inflammatory drugs during pregnancy and lactation. *Inflammopharmacology* 1996;4:31–41.
59. Hickok DE, Hollenbach KA, Reilley SF, et al. The association between decreased amniotic fluid volume and treatment with nonsteroidal anti-inflammatory agents for preterm labor. *Am J Obstet Gynecol* 1989;160:1525–1531.
60. Wiggins DA, Elliott JP. Oligohydramnios in each sac of a triplet gestation caused by Motrin—fulfilling Kock's postulates. *Am J Obstet Gynecol* 1990;162: 460–461.
61. Llanas B, Cavert MH, Apere H, et al. Les effets secondaires du ketoprofène après exposition intra-utérine. Intérêt du dosage plasmatique. *Arch Pediatr* 1996;3:248–253.
62. Momma K, Takeuchi H. Constriction of the ductus arteriosus by non-steroidal anti-inflammatory drugs. *Prostaglandins* 1983;26:631–643.
63. Norton ME, Merril J, Cooper BAB, et al. Neonatal complications after the administration of indomethacin for preterm labor. *N Engl J Med* 1993;329: 1602–1607.
64. Vermillion ST, Scardo JA, Lashus AG, et al. The effect of indomethacin tocolysis on fetal ductus arteriosus constriction with advancing gestational age. *Am J Obstet Gynecol* 1997;177:256–261.
65. Macones GA, Marder SJ, Clothier B, et al. The controversy surrounding indomethacin for tocolysis. *Am J Obstet Gynecol* 2001;184:264–272.
66. Alano MA, Ngougmna E, Ostrea EM, et al. Analysis of nonsteroidal antiinflammatory drugs in meconium and its relation to persistent pulmonary hypertension of the newborn. *Pediatrics* 2001;107:519–523.

67. Østensen M, Østensen H. Safety of nonsteroidal antiinflammatory drugs in pregnant patients with rheumatic disease. *J Rheumatol* 1996;23:1045–1049.
68. Lloyd ME, Carr M, McElhatton P, et al. The effects of methotrexate on pregnancy, fertility and lactation. *QJM* 1999;92:551–563.
69. Østensen M, Hartmann H, Salvesen K. Low dose weekly methotrexate in early pregnancy. A case series and review of the literature. *J Rheumatol* 2000; 27:1872–1875.
70. Krähenmann F, Østensen M, Stallmach T, et al. In utero first trimester exposure to low-dose methotrexate with increased fetal nuchal translucency and associated malformations. *Prenat Diagn* 2002;22:489–490.
71. Brent RL. Teratogen update: reproductive risks of leflunomide (Arava), a pyrimidine synthesis inhibitor: counseling women taking leflunomide before or during pregnancy and men taking leflunomide who are contemplating fathering a child. *Teratology* 2001;63:106–112.
72. Goroir BP, Peppel K, Silva M, et al. The biosynthesis of tumor necrosis factor during pregnancy: studies with a CAT reporter transgene and TNF inhibitors. *Eur Cytokine Netw* 1992;3:533–537.
73. Antoni CE, Furst D, Manger B, et al. Outcome of pregnancy in women receiving Remicade (Infliximab) for the treatment of Crohn's disease or rheumatoid arthritis. *Arthritis Rheum* 2001;44:S84.
74. Rosa FW. Teratogen update: penicillamine. *Teratology* 1986;33:127–131.
75. Willoughby CP, Truelove SC. Ulcerative colitis and pregnancy. *Gut* 1980; 21:469–474.
76. Mogadam M, Dobbins WO, Korelitz BI, et al. Pregnancy in inflammatory bowel disease: effect of sulfasalazine and corticosteroids on fetal outcome. *Gastroenterology* 1981;80:72–76.
77. Hoo JJ, Hadro TA, von Behrens P. Possible teratogenicity of sulfasalazine. *N Engl J Med* 1988;318:1128.
78. Hernandez-Diaz S, Werler MM, Walker AM, et al. Folic acid antagonists during pregnancy and the risk of birth defects. *N Engl J Med* 2000;343:1608–1614.
79. Levi AJ, Liberman M, Levi AJ. Reversible congenital neutropenia associated with maternal sulfasalazine therapy [Letter]. *Eur J Pediatr* 1988;148:174–175.
80. Miyamoto T, Miyaji S, Horiuchi Y, et al. Gold therapy in bronchial asthma with special emphasis upon blood levels of gold and its teratogenicity. *Nippon Naika Gakkai Zasshi* 1974;63:1190–1197.
81. Rogers JG, Anderson R, Chow CW, et al. Possible teratogenic effects of gold. *Aust Paediatr J* 1980;16:194–195.
82. Tozman ECS, Gottlieb NL. Adverse reactions with oral and parenteral gold preparations. *Med Toxicol* 1987;2:177–189.
83. Gibbons RB. Complications of chrysotherapy. *Arch Intern Med* 1979;139:343–346.
84. Buchanan NMM, Toubi E, Khamashta KE, et al. Hydroxychloroquine and lupus pregnancy: review of a series of 36 cases. *Ann Rheum Dis* 1996;55:486–488.
85. Parke AL. Antimalarial drugs, systemic lupus erythematosus and pregnancy. *J Rheumatol* 1988;15:607–610.
86. Parke AL, West B. Hydroxychloroquine in pregnant patients with systemic lupus erythematosus. *J Rheumatol* 1996;23:1715–1718.
87. Levy M, Buskila D, Gladman DD, et al. Pregnancy outcome following first trimester exposure to chloroquine. *Am J Perinatol* 1991;8:174–178.
88. Phillips-Howard PA, Wood D. The safety of antimalarial drugs in pregnancy. *Drug Saf* 1996;14:131–145.
89. Costedoat-Chalumeau N, Amoura Z, Aymard G, et al. Evidence of transplacental passage of hydroxychloroquine in humans. *Arthritis Rheum* 2002; 46:1124–1125.
90. Hart CN, Naunton RF. The ototoxicity of chloroquine phosphate. *Arch Otolaryngol Head Neck Surg* 1964;80:407–412.
91. Klinger G, Morad Y, Westall CA, et al. Ocular toxicity and antenatal exposure to chloroquine or hydroxychloroquine for rheumatic diseases. *Lancet* 2001;358:813–814.
92. Cockburn I, Krupp P, Monka C. Present experience of Sandimmune in pregnancy. *Transplant Proc* 1989;21:3730–3732.
93. Gaughan WJ, Moritz MJ, Radomski JS, et al. National Transplantation Pregnancy Registry: report on outcomes in cyclosporine-treated female kidney transplant recipients with an interval from transplant to pregnancy of greater than five years. *Am J Kidney Dis* 1996;28:266–269.
94. Bar Oz, Hackman R, Einarson T, et al. Pregnancy outcome after cyclosporine therapy during pregnancy: a meta-analysis. *Transplantation* 2001;71:1051–1055.
95. Lamarque V, Leleu MF, Monka C, et al. Analysis of 629 pregnancy outcomes in transplant recipients treated with Sandimmune. *Transplant Proc* 1997;29: 2480.
96. Shaheen FAM, Al-Sulaiman MH, Al-Khader AA. Long-term nephrotoxicity after exposure to cyclosporine in utero. *Transplantation* 1993;56:224–225.
97. Di Paolo S, Schena A, Morrone LF, et al. Immunologic evaluation during the first year of life of infants born to cyclosporine-treated female kidney transplant recipients. *Transplantation* 2000;69:2049–2054.
98. Registration Committee of the European Dialysis and Transplant Association. Successful pregnancies in women treated by dialysis and kidney transplantation. *Br J Obstet Gynaecol* 1980;87:839–845.
99. Williamson RA, Karp LE. Azathioprine teratogenicity: review of the literature and case report. *Obstet Gynecol* 1981;58:247–250.
100. Meehan RT, Dorsey JK. Pregnancy among patients with systemic lupus erythematosus receiving immunosuppressive therapy. *J Rheumatol* 1987;14: 252–258.
101. Ramsey-Goldman R, Mientus JM, Kutzer JE, et al. Pregnancy outcome in women with systemic lupus erythematosus treated with immunosuppressive drugs. *J Rheumatol* 1993;20:1152–1157.
102. Davison JM, Dellagrammatikos H, Parkin JM. Maternal azathioprine therapy and depressed haemopoiesis in the babies of renal allograft patients. *Br J Obstet Gynaecol* 1985;92:233–239.
103. Pinsky L, DiGeorge AM. Cleft palate in the mouse: a teratogenic index of glucocorticoid potency. *Science* 1965;147:402–403.
104. Fraser FC, Sajoo A. Teratogenic potential of corticosteroids in humans. *Teratology* 1985;51:45–46.
105. Park-Wyllie L, Mazzotta P, Pastuszak A, et al. Birth defects after maternal exposure to corticosteroids: prospective cohort study and meta-analysis of epidemiological studies. *Teratology* 2000;62:385–392.
106. Reinisch JM, Simon NG. Prenatal exposure to prednisone in humans and animals retards intrauterine growth. *Science* 1978;202:436–438.
107. Kraus AM. Congenital cataract and maternal steroid injection. *J Pediatr Ophthalmol Strabismus* 1975;12:107–108.
108. Kozlowska-Boszko B, Soluch L, Rybus J, et al. Does chronic glucosteroid therapy in pregnant renal allograft recipients affect cortisol levels in neonates? *Transplant Proc* 1996;28:3490–3491.
109. Doll CD, Ringenberg QS, Yarbro JW. Antineoplastic agents and pregnancy. *Semin Oncol* 1989;16:337–346.
110. Mirkes PE. Cyclophosphamide teratogenesis: a review. *Teratog Carcinog Mutagen* 1985;5:75–88.
111. Panush RS, Chuzchin Y, Cintron M, et al. Nutritional therapy for active arthritis in pregnant or breast feeding women. Preliminary observations. *J Rheumatol* 1994;21:967.
112. Morris LF, Harrod MJ, Menter MA, Silverman AK. Methotrexate and reproduction in men: case report and recommendations. *J Am Acad Dermatol* 1993;29:913–916.
113. Waxman J. Chemotherapy and the adult gonad: a review. *J R Soc Med* 1983; 76:144–148.
114. O'Moràin C, Smethurst P, Doré CJ, Levi A. Reversible male infertility due to sulfasalazine: studies in man and rat. *Gut* 1984;25:1078–1084.
115. Watson AR, Rance CP, Bain J. Long term effects of cyclophosphamide on testicular function. *Br Med J* 1985;291:1457–1460.
116. Vinson RK, Hales BF. Expression of base excision, mismatch, and recombination repair genes in the organogenesis-stage rat conceptus and effects of exposure to a genotoxic teratogen, 4-hydroxyperoxycyclophosphamide. *Teratology* 2001;64:283–291.
117. Genescà A, Caballin MR, Miro R, et al. Human sperm chromosomes. Long-term effect of cancer treatment. *Cancer Genet Cytogenet* 1990;46:251–260.
118. Krogh Jensen M, Nyfors A. Cytogenetic effect of methotrexate on human cells in vivo. *Mutat Res* 1979;64:339–343.
119. Li FP, Jaffe N. Progeny of childhood-cancer survivors. *Lancet* 1974;2:707–709.
120. Senturia YD, Peckham CS. Children fathered by men treated with chemotherapy for testicular cancer. *Eur J Cancer* 1990;26:429–432.

CHAPTER 47

Osteoporosis

Qaiser Rehman and Nancy E. Lane

Osteoporosis is commonly associated with rheumatoid arthritis (RA). In fact, it is the principal bone abnormality of this disease. Bone loss in the juxtaarticular region is an important radiographic diagnostic criterion and occurs early in the disease. However, bone loss in RA is not limited to the joints. It occurs in the axial and the appendicular skeleton and involves both the cortical and cancellous bone. The rapid bone remodeling in RA results in loss of bone volume and strength, leading to an increased risk of fragility fractures. RA has been shown to be an independent risk factor for bone loss and increased fracture risk. As RA and osteoporosis are both common diseases with significant association with each other, there is a significant burden in terms of morbidity, premature mortality, economic cost, and quality of life. Unfortunately, this important aspect of rheumatoid disease is underappreciated and undertreated (Fig. 47.1) (1).

EPIDEMIOLOGY

RA is the most common inflammatory arthritis, with a prevalence range from 0.5% to 1.0% and a mean of 0.8% (2). The sex ratio is two- to threefold higher in favor of women, with peak incidence occurring in the fifth and sixth decades of life. Osteoporosis is the most common metabolic bone disease in the western hemisphere, with demographic features similar to RA, being more common in women and with a peak incidence in midlife. It is not uncommon, therefore, for the two to coexist.

It is difficult to assess the true prevalence or incidence of osteoporosis in RA, as most of the risk factors (e.g., age, sex, postmenopausal status, and decreased physical activity) are common to both diseases, and treatment of RA can also add significantly to the bone morbidity. However, the association appears to be more than just chance, as demonstrated in several epidemiologic studies. In a cross-sectional study of 925 consecutive women with RA attending rheumatology clinics in Europe, 29% were found to have osteoporosis (*t* score <–2.5) at the lumbar spine (LS) and 36.2% at the femoral neck (FN) (3). In addition, 74 of the 925 (8%) women were found to have at least one vertebral fracture in this cohort. Increased prevalence of osteoporosis in the RA population was associated with advanced age; increased disease activity, characterized by high scores on Health Assessment Questionnaires (HAQ); elevated sedimentation rate; and the use of glucocorticoids (GCs). The prevalence of osteoporosis increases linearly with worsening stages of rheumatoid disease ($p = .0001$) (Table 47.1) (3).

Patients diagnosed with juvenile RA (JRA) have a high incidence of significant bone loss, although it is difficult to diagnose osteoporosis in this younger population, due to lack of data regarding a young normal reference population. In a follow-up study (average, 27 years) of patients diagnosed with JRA at less than 16 years old, 41% (13 of 57) of the subjects tested using dual energy x-ray absorptiometry (DEXA) scan had significant osteopenia (*t* score ≤–1.0) at the LS or FN (28% and 32%, respectively) (4). A controlled trial of postpubertal women with JRA showed a lower bone mineral content (BMC) in the study population, compared to age- and race-matched controls (4.5% lower than controls), with 30% having significant osteopenia (BMC *z* score <–1, compared to controls) in the absence of prior corticosteroid therapy (5).

The risk of fractures is significantly increased in the rheumatoid population (6). A threefold increased risk of hip fractures has been observed in the rheumatoid population, after adjusting for age and sex (7). The increased hip fracture risk is independently associated with rheumatoid disease and previous corticosteroid use (8). These fractures are associated with significantly increased mortality (9) and complication rate (10). In addition, stress fractures are also common, albeit frequently missed, in rheumatoid patients. Lower extremities, including distal tibia, fibula, and metatarsals, are a common site and add to the rheumatoid foot deformities and dysfunction. Insufficiency fractures have also been reported at the FN, pubic rami, and the sternum (11,12). Most of the rheumatoid patients with fractures are postmenopausal women with low bone mass. The diagnosis of fracture is commonly delayed by several weeks, as it can be difficult to differentiate fracture pain from chronic rheumatoid foot pain.

BONE LOSS OCCURS EARLY IN RHEUMATOID ARTHRITIS

Bone loss is the earliest radiographic feature of RA (13,14). Within weeks of onset of symptoms, and much before any joint damage occurs, periarticular osteopenia is a common finding. The etiology may be multifactorial, including the release of various proinflammatory cytokines, matrix degrading enzymes, and decreased physical activity due to pain. The result is an accentuated bone turnover and significant bone loss. As much as 30% of bone mineral loss occurs before it can be detected on plain radiography. In a study, patients with inflammatory polyarthropathy of recent onset (median, 4 months) who were later classified as having RA showed a significant reduction in hand BMD measured by DEXA scan at 6-month and 12-month intervals after the onset of the disease (15). Another randomized

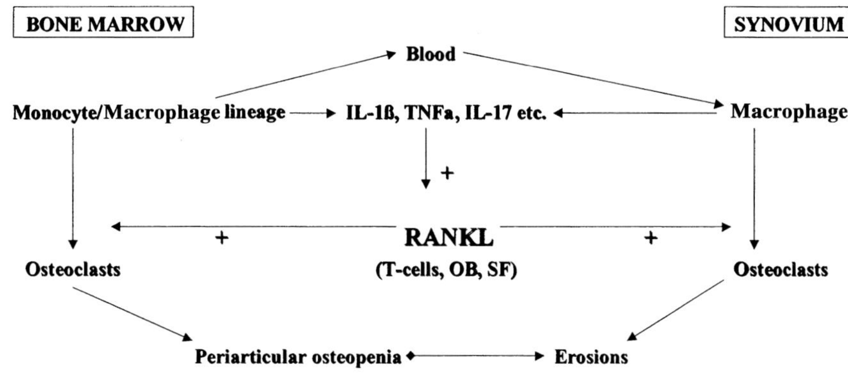

Figure 47.1. Mechanisms of bone loss in rheumatoid arthritis. OB, osteoblast; RANKL, receptor activator of nuclear factor–κB ligand; SF, synovial fibroblast.

controlled prospective study using serial DEXA scan of the hand to measure BMC in RA patients demonstrated significant bone loss within 2 years of disease onset (16).

Other studies have demonstrated significant generalized bone loss in patients with early RA (17,18). The rate of bone loss is also highest among early RA patients. In a randomized controlled trial, DEXA scan of the axial skeleton demonstrated a bone loss of 2.5% at the vertebrae and 5% at the proximal femur within the first year of RA diagnosis. After 2 years of uncontrolled RA associated with a high level of inflammatory disease activity, the bone loss increased from 5.5% to 10% at the sites (19). In general, bone loss tends to be worst in postmenopausal elderly women with more severe joint involvement who have been treated with GCs. RA patients have a significantly increased risk of fractures involving pelvis, proximal femur, proximal humerus, spine, and distal forearm (6,20–23).

MECHANISM OF BONE LOSS IN RHEUMATOID ARTHRITIS

It is well established that bone loss in RA tends to be both localized and generalized (24). Localized bone loss can be attributed to increased inflammation, local cytokine and metalloproteinase release (autocrine and paracrine), increased perfusion, and decreased use. Generalized bone loss can be explained by systemic inflammatory cytokines associated with active disease, hormonal perturbations, lack of activity, and side effects of RA therapies.

Role of Inflammatory Cytokines

Proinflammatory cytokines, such as tumor necrosis factor α (TNF-α), interleukin-1 (IL-1), and IL-6, are significantly elevated in the joints and sera of patients with active RA. These cytokines stimulate osteoclast differentiation, proliferation, and function, thus leading to increased bone resorption and resultant bone loss. They play a pivotal role in inflammatory arthritis and bone loss (25). In postmenopausal women with RA and high disease activity, IL-6 is a critical determinant of increased bone resorption (22,26). Significantly higher concentrations of these inflammatory cytokines occur both locally and systemically in active RA and contribute to both local and generalized bone loss. In addition, prostaglandins contribute to rheumatoid inflammation and bone loss, as prostaglandin E_2 produced in the rheumatoid synovium has been shown to stimulate bone resorption (27–29). Studies using markers of bone turnover have consistently demonstrated uncoupling in active RA with an increase in bone resorption without significant or consistent increase in bone formation rate (22).

Recently, a new member of the TNF family has been discovered that induces differentiation and maturation of osteoclast precursor cells into active bone-resorbing osteoclasts and plays a significant role in bone loss associated with inflammatory arthritis (30). This factor has been variably named as *osteoclast differentiation factor, TNF-related activation-induced cytokine (TRANCE), receptor activator of nuclear factor–κB ligand* (RANKL), and *osteoprotegerin ligand.* According to the American Society of Bone and Mineral Research nomenclature, this molecule will be referred to as *RANKL.* It is probably the most significant osteoclast activator protein in osteoclastogenesis, as its absence in TRANCE-deficient mice is associated with profound osteoclastopenia and severe osteopetrosis (31).

Osteoclasts play a pivotal role in bone loss associated with RA. Osteoclast numbers are increased in patients with RA (32,33). RANKL, the key osteoclast-stimulating factor responsible for this bone loss in RA, is derived from activated T cells and synovial fibroblasts (34,35), although osteoblasts and bone marrow stromal cells may also contribute (36,37). Patients with active RA have deficient expression of osteoprotegerin on the endothelium and synovial lining cells, and the expression of RANKL is demonstrated in the synovial tissue (38). Various cytokines responsible for active rheumatoid inflammation converge on T cells and synovial fibroblasts, stimulating the production of RANKL. Macrophages obtained from the synovium of RA patients have the capability to differentiate into mature bone-resorbing osteoclasts (39) and are probably responsible for quite a substantial part of the localized bone loss in RA patients. The juxtaarticular bone loss and erosions in RA most likely

TABLE 47.1. National Osteoporosis Foundation Guidelines for the Diagnosis and Treatment of Osteoporosis

Who should be tested?
- Postmenopausal women <65 yr with ≥ one additional risk factors for osteoporotic fracture (e.g., family or personal history of fractures, white or Asian, body weight <127 lb, early menopause, excessive alcohol abuse, smoking, low calcium intake, and chronic use of medications such as glucocorticoid or thyroid hormone)
- Women ≥65 yr, regardless of additional risk factors
- Postmenopausal women with fractures (to confirm diagnosis and determine disease severity)
- Women who are considering therapy for osteoporosis, if bone mineral density (BMD) testing would facilitate the decision
- Women on hormone replacement therapy for prolonged periods

Who should be treated?
- Women with BMD testing scores below –2.0 in the absence of risk factors and in women with BMD testing scores below –1.5 if other risk factors are present
- Women >70 yr with multiple risk factors (especially those with previous nonhip, nonspine fractures)

Adapted from National Osteoporosis Foundation. Osteoporosis Physician's Guide to Prevention and Treatment of Osteoporosis. Available at www.NOF.org. Accessed November 20, 2002.

occur from inflammatory-mediated osteoclast action, both within the bone, moving through and perforating the subchondral plate, and osteoclast-induced erosion of the bone surface.

Role of Hormonal Abnormalities

Many studies have suggested an abnormal androgen metabolism in patients with RA (40,41). Decreased levels of testosterone, dehydrotestosterone (DHEA), and DHEA-sulfate have been found in blood, synovial, and salivary fluids of both male and female patients with RA (42). Given their immunosuppressive potential, androgens may have a pathogenic role in rheumatoid disease. More important, androgens have a protective effect on bone and muscle mass, and their deficiency may contribute to the loss of bone and muscle mass so commonly seen in active RA. The androgen deficiency in RA may result from decreased testicular steroid synthesis or reduced gonadotropin stimulation (43,44). Chronic GC therapy may also contribute to reduced androgen levels in male RA patients by either directly suppressing testicular steroidogenesis in the hypothalamic-pituitary-adrenal axis, or inhibiting hypothalamic gonadotropin-releasing hormone secretion (45,46). Similar GC-induced reduction in estrogen production has also been demonstrated in female patients.

Role of Reduced Functional Activity

Active rheumatoid disease is associated with reduced physical activity and weightbearing. Physical activity and weightbearing exercises are positively correlated with increased bone mass. Physical incapacitation leads to less outdoor activities among rheumatoid patients, less exposure to sunlight, and, therefore, increased risk of vitamin D deficiency. Active rheumatoid disease is characterized by high scores on physical disability index, as assessed by HAQ, and correlates strongly with low bone mass at the spine and proximal femur (47–49). In a cross-sectional study of 30 ambulatory female patients with RA (average duration, 4.9 years), BMD at the LS was normal, with only slight reduction at the FN, compared to age-matched healthy controls (50). BMD was independent of disease activity or previous disease-modifying drug use. Physical impairments, reduced stability, muscle atrophy, and anemia also predispose to an increased risk of falls and resultant fractures in RA patients, as well as in the general population.

Role of Drug Therapy

In addition to the risk of osteoporosis associated with rheumatoid disease activity and associated morbidity, bone loss in RA can also occur as a side effect of RA drug therapy.

GLUCOCORTICOIDS

Although it has been argued that, by gaining a better control of inflammatory rheumatoid disease and the resultant increase in physical activity, GCs can have a positive effect on the attainment of bone mass (51), the evidence overwhelmingly implicates GC therapy with increased risk of osteoporosis in RA patients. In addition to their negative influence on gonadal hormones, as previously discussed, these agents can directly suppress bone formation and increase bone resorption. GCs act by inhibiting collagen synthesis and osteoclastogenesis and can induce early osteoblast apoptosis (52). The result is a decrease in collagen synthesis. GCs also activate osteoclasts via the RANKL pathway, with consequent increased bone resorption, at least in the short term. Histomorphometric studies have demonstrated a reduced mineral apposition rate, decreased osteoid seam, and reduced trabecular mean wall thickness in the iliac crest biopsies from GC-treated patients (Table 47.2) (53).

TABLE 47.2. Recommendations for the Prevention and Treatment of Glucocorticoid-Induced Osteoporosis

Prevention
- For patients initiating glucocorticoid (GC) therapy at a dose equivalent to ≥5 mg prednisone/day for ≥3 mo:
  - Risk factor modification (smoking cessation, decrease excessive alcohol consumption, etc.)
  - Regular weightbearing physical exercise
  - Calcium (total 1,500 mg/day) and vitamin D (400–800 IU/day) intake
  - Consider bone mineral density (BMD) testing to predict risk of fracture and bone loss
  - Bisphosphonate therapy (alendronate, 5 mg/day or 35 mg/wk, or risedronate, 5 mg/day or 35 mg/wk for prevention of glucocorticoid-induced osteoporosis)

Treatment
- Patients on long-term GC therapy should be tested for osteoporosis using BMD measurement and if BMD testing score is <–1, consider the following in addition to preventive measures as above:
  - Replace gonadal steroids, if deficient
  - Bisphosphonate therapy (alendronate, 10 mg/day or 70 mg/wk, or risedronate, 5 mg/day or 35 mg/wk)
  - If bisphosphonates are contraindicated or not tolerated, consider calcitonin as second-line agent or intravenous bisphosphonate (pamidronate or zoledronate) or parathyroid hormone (1-34)
  - Repeat BMD measurement annually or biannually

Adapted from Recommendations for the prevention and treatment of glucocorticoid-induced osteoporosis 2001 update. *Arthritis Rheum* 2001;44:1496–1503.

Another proposed mechanism for GC-induced bone loss is secondary hyperparathyroidism, induced by decreased intestinal calcium absorption and hypercalciuria associated with GC therapy (54). However, other studies have failed to confirm these findings (55,56). Rheumatoid patients taking GCs have approximately twice the risk of hip fractures, compared to non–GC-treated patients (57). In a study comparing 52 GC-treated RA patients with age- and sex-matched controls, vertebral deformities were much more common in the former group [relative risk (RR), 2.31; 95% confidence interval (CI): 1.36–3.90]. GC-treated RA patients had nearly five times higher incidence of vertebral deformities, compared to the control RA group (58). The fracture risk is highest among rheumatoid patients with preexisting low bone mass, high-dose GC therapy (>5 mg per day of prednisone), increased disability, and risk of falls.

METHOTREXATE

Methotrexate (MTX) forms the cornerstone of RA therapy. It is the anchor drug against which the new RA therapies, including the biologics, are compared. It is also the most common disease-modifying drug used to treat RA in the United States.

A syndrome known as *MTX osteopathy*, associated with the use of this drug, has been described in the literature. This syndrome is characterized by bone pain, fractures of the lower extremities, osteoporosis, and radiologic signs resembling scurvy. It was first described in childhood leukemia survivors who received low-dose long-term MTX therapy over 6 months to 3 years. These patients developed multiple fractures involving fibula and feet, severe osteoporosis, and radiologic findings suggestive of scurvy, such as ring epiphysis, corner sign, and multiple growth arrest lines (59).

The pathogenesis remains unclear and is probably related to the antiproliferative effects of MTX, including suppression of osteoblastic activity. Short-term treatment with MTX in rats is associated with 60% reduction in bone formation rate and reduced osteoid volume and thickness (60). Two patients, one with psoriasis and the other with RA, are described in the literature who developed features consistent with MTX osteopathy after long-term low-dose treatment with MTX (25 mg per week and 10 mg per week, respectively). In both patients, the symptoms of bone pain and radiologic findings of osteoporosis resolved when MTX was stopped, and the syndrome recurred in the rheumatoid patient on rechallenge with MTX (61). However, in a rat model of adjuvant-induced arthritis, daily MTX administration prevented the expected decrease in mineral apposition and bone formation rate and preserved BMD at the LS and FN, compared to the control arthritic animals (62).

Human studies conducted among RA patients comparing MTX users against MTX nonusers do not show any significant difference in BMD at the LS or FN (63,64). Conflicting data exist regarding the effects of concomitant use of MTX and GC and their effect on bone mass. In a prospective randomized placebo-controlled trial of RA patients using various disease-modifying antirheumatic drugs, BMD at the LS and FN was measured at baseline and every year for 3 years. At the end of the study, patients taking MTX and prednisone (≥5 mg per day) had a significantly greater bone loss at the LS (8.08%), compared to the prednisone-only group ($p = .004$) (64). The significant bone loss with combination therapy could be because of the augmented inhibitory action of prednisone and MTX therapy on osteoblasts. However, the same combination, when compared against prednisone only, was found to be protective against vertebral bone loss, measured by DEXA in a cohort of patients with polymyalgia rheumatica followed for 1 year (65). In conclusion, low-dose MTX appears safe in regards to bone mass in patients with active RA, because of its ability to suppress inflammation and, thus, increase physical activity. As the number of patients on chronic MTX therapy increases, our understanding of the relation between MTX and bone mass will improve. Chronically low intake of folic acid, particularly if it coexists with other nutritional deficiencies, may also predispose to osteoporosis (66). Therefore, folic acid supplementation with MTX therapy can be beneficial.

CYCLOSPORINE A

It is quite difficult to study the effects of cyclosporine A (CsA) alone on bone metabolism in a clinical setting, as it is almost always used in combination with other drugs known to perturb bone turnover. Although, theoretically, CsA therapy can lead to bone loss, given its ability to decrease osteoprotegerin messenger RNA production (67), and cause negative effects on renal function, sex hormone production, and calcium absorption, most clinical studies in rheumatic patients have failed to show any deleterious effects. In fact, at the low doses used to treat RA (<5 mg per kg per day), CsA has been shown to reduce the rate of erosions and joint damage without any increase in local or systemic osteoporosis (68,69). In a prospective cohort of 10 rheumatoid factor–positive patients with early, aggressive, erosive disease and poor response to 6 months of MTX therapy, CsA, 3 mg per kg per day, was added, and patients were followed for another 6 months. The addition of CsA resulted in a significant increase in BMD (3.9 ± 0.97%) and anabolic variables, including serum insulin-like growth factor–1 (+42.4%), serum osteocalcin (+34.3%), and serum DHEA (+34.2%) levels (70). Higher doses of CsA have been associated with increased bone turnover and uncoupling in favor of bone resorption.

BIOLOGICS

Although certain drugs can, at least theoretically, increase the risk of bone loss in RA patients, other therapies may be beneficial. Given the pivotal role of TNF-α and IL-1β in inflammatory bone loss, their inhibition using TNF-α blockers and an IL-1 receptor antagonist may have a direct bone-protective effect in RA patients. TNF-α and IL-17 can directly stimulate osteoclasts by interaction with these bone-resorbing cells (71). Moreover, TNF-α and IL-1β can also enhance osteoclast-mediated bone loss indirectly by stimulating RANKL production from osteoblast cells (72). However, change in bone mass or reduction in fracture risk were not prespecified end points in the published studies evaluating the use of biologics in RA. Therefore, further studies are needed to specifically address this issue.

TREATMENT

Although a major clinical problem, bone loss in RA has not received adequate attention in evaluating long-term outcomes. Most prospective long-term clinical outcome studies of RA have focused on disease activity markers (erythrocyte sedimentation rate, C-reactive protein, etc.), loss of function and disability (HAQ score), and development of erosions. In fact, the various measures of rheumatoid activity and responder indices, such as American College of Rheumatology core set of criteria 20, 50, and 70, as well as criteria for disease remission in RA, have not included any measure of bone loss. Recent publications have highlighted this blind spot regarding the prevention and treatment of osteoporosis in RA (1).

Most of the existing data regarding the efficacy of currently available antiosteoporosis therapies is derived from the trials of postmenopausal and GC-induced osteoporosis (GIOP). A significant number of patients in the GIOP trials have RA, but subgroup analysis is mostly unavailable for this cohort. A specific mention will be made regarding the efficacy of antiosteoporotic drugs in the treatment of bone loss in RA subgroup, if these data are reported in the trial. Moreover, any treatment that will control rheumatoid disease activity, improve function, and reduce disability is likely to improve bone mass because the pathophysiologies of inflammatory rheumatoid disease and osteoporosis are intertwined and related at the level of cytokines (TNF-α, IL-1β, IL-6, IL-17, RANKL, etc.). Suppression of inflammatory cytokines is expected to have beneficial effect in both diseases. Following is an overview of additional therapies designed more specifically to address bone loss (Table 47.3).

Exercise and Physical Activity

Physical activity is a powerful and independent factor that influences bone mass acquisition and maintenance. Bone is a dynamic tissue and accommodates the loads imposed on it by altering its mass and the distribution of this mass. Immobility is associated with substantial bone loss, and up to 40% of the original bone mass can be lost within 1 year of complete immobilization. Athletes tend to have greater bone mass than nonathletes, particularly the ones involved in power sports requiring high muscle

TABLE 47.3. Approved Therapies for the Prevention and Treatment of Osteoporosis

Calcium
Vitamin D (plain or activated form)
Estrogens (prevention only)
Raloxifene (prevention and treatment)
Alendronate (prevention and treatment)
Risedronate (prevention and treatment)
Calcitonin (treatment only, ≥5 yr postmenopausal)
Recombinant human parathyroid hormone 1-34

forces (73). However, the improvement in BMD with exercise in healthy sedentary individuals is modest, in the order of 1% to 5%.

In RA patients with osteoporosis, there are many benefits of exercise. The improvement in bone mass may be greater than healthy individuals, as RA patients have a bone deficit, compared to healthy age-matched adults, due to disease activity and reduced mobility. Lack of physical activity adds to rheumatoid cachexia and predisposes to increases in fat mass (74). In addition, regular exercise training improves muscle mass, balance, and coordination that can reduce the risk of falls and subsequent fractures. Moreover, regular outdoor activity means more sun exposure and conversion of 7-dehydrocholesterol to vitamin D_3, with its positive effects on calcium metabolism. Vitamin D deficiency is common in RA patients and serum 25(OH)D_3 levels are inversely related to functional class (75,76).

In women with RA, calcaneal bone quality and FN BMD correlates significantly with quadriceps strength (77). Women with subnormal BMD at the FN (t score <–1) had a 20% lower quadriceps strength, compared to those with normal BMD (p <.0001). A combination of skeletal muscle strength training and aerobic exercise is recommended for RA patients, in accordance with their disease status, overall health, and safety (74). However, every RA patient should have some form of daily exercise routine.

Calcium

RA patients are often in a negative calcium balance. Increased disease activity associated with elevated inflammatory cytokines and reduced physical activity leads to increased bone resorption and calcium release. Treatment with GCs can reduce intestinal calcium absorption and worsen hypercalciuria. In addition, patients with RA may not be taking adequate dietary calcium (78). Adequate calcium supplementation is helpful in counteracting all of these processes.

The beneficial effects of calcium supplementation depend on the age group of patients treated. The maximum beneficial association between calcium intake and BMD occurs before the attainment of peak bone mass (79). In a randomized study of premenopausal women aged 30 to 42 years, dietary calcium increase by 610 mg per day over a 3-year period prevented against vertebral bone loss of approximately 1% per year, compared to age-, weight-, and sex-matched controls (80). However, calcium supplementation itself is not sufficiently adequate to prevent or replenish bone loss during the early years of menopause. Hormone replacement therapy (HRT), which improves both the gastrointestinal absorption of calcium and reduces osteoclast activity, is better than calcium supplementation alone (81–83).

In late-postmenopausal and elderly women, calcium supplementation is beneficial in preventing bone loss, probably by suppressing secondary hyperparathyroidism and preventing the activation of new bone remodeling units (84). It also protects against seasonal femoral bone loss and incident vertebral fractures in calcium-deficient women with existing vertebral fractures (85,86). In a randomized prospective placebo-controlled trial of 3,270 healthy ambulatory white women aged 84 ± 6 years (age ± SD), the effect of calcium (1.2 g per day) and vitamin D_3 (800 IU per day) supplementation on hip and other nonvertebral fractures was studied. After 18 months of therapy, a 43% reduction in the risk of hip fracture (p = .043) and 32% decrease in nonvertebral fractures (p = .015) were noticed in the active treatment group (87). This study underscores the critical role both calcium and vitamin D supplementation play in the aging skeleton.

Very little information is available regarding the use of calcium supplementation in RA. Rheumatoid patients may differ considerably in their rate of bone turnover, intestinal calcium absorption, and rate of calcium excretion depending on disease activity, physical activity, and the use of GCs. Hence, it is difficult to assess the effects of calcium supplementation alone. Calcium supplementation at 1,000 mg a day has been shown to suppress increased bone turnover induced by average prednisone dose of 15 mg per day (88). However, in most randomized prospective trials of GIOP, calcium alone has been ineffective in improving bone mass; rather, the placebo group receiving calcium at only 500 mg per day supplement showed significant bone loss at the spine and hip (89–92).

Therefore, it appears that calcium supplementation at a dose of 500 to 1,000 mg a day is ineffective against preventing bone loss during GC therapy equivalent to more than 7.5 mg per day of prednisone. In such cases, calcium supplementation can be used in addition to other antiresorptives, as discussed later.

Vitamin D

Vitamin D is essential for the maintenance of normal serum calcium, intestinal calcium absorption, and, with the help of osteoprotegerin, the commitment of stem cells to the osteoblast lineage. Vitamin D occurs in various forms, including the plant sterol ergocalciferol (vitamin D_2) and the human form cholecalciferol (vitamin D_3), produced in the body from conversion of 7-dehydrocholesterol after exposure to ultraviolet B light (93). Cholecalciferol (vitamin D_3) makes up approximately 90% of the physiologic vitamin D supply (94). Vitamin D_3 is converted to the biologically inert 25(OH) vitamin D_3 in the liver. After a second hydroxylation in the kidneys by 1α-hydroxylase, the rate-limiting enzyme, it is converted to the active form, $1{,}25(OH)_2D_3$. It is essential for normal bone mineralization, and its deficiency adversely affects peak bone mass.

Low vitamin D levels are probably responsible for the loss of BMD during winter season, and decreased $1{,}25(OH)_2D_3$ levels are associated with an increased risk of hip fracture in elderly white women (RR, 2.1; 95% CI: 1.2–2.5) (95). Postmenopausal women with acute hip fractures tend to have low serum $25(OH)_D$ and elevated parathyroid hormone (PTH) levels (96). The adequate intake value for cholecalciferol increases steadily from 5 μg per day in premenopausal women to 10 μg per day in the 51 to 70 years age group and to 15 μg per day for those older than 70 years (97).

The use of vitamin D supplements in RA patients at risk of bone loss can be beneficial in many ways. First, active vitamin D metabolites are potent antiresorptives that can suppress the high bone turnover and associated bone loss seen in active RA. Secondly, GC therapy in active RA is associated with increased osteoblast apoptosis and decreased bone formation, as previously mentioned. Vitamin D analogues have a trophic effect on osteoblast function and act in synergy with osteoprotegerin to promote the commitment of stem cells to osteoblastic lineage (98,99). Finally, $1{,}25(OH)_2D_3$ may have antiinflammatory and immunomodulating properties that may be helpful in preventing RA-associated bone loss. It has been shown to affect the differentiation and proliferation of T lymphocytes and the regulation of immunoglobulin production by B lymphocytes and may affect chondrocyte function, including proteoglycan and collagen synthesis (100–103).

In a large cohort of 92 RA patients starting long-term GC therapy, calcitriol (0.6 μg per day) plus calcium (1 g per day) was more effective than calcium alone in preventing bone loss at the LS at 1 year (–0.2% vs. –4.3%; p = .0035) (88). Various other prospective randomized placebo-controlled studies have confirmed the effectiveness of vitamin D plus calcium versus calcium alone in preventing vertebral bone loss in GC-treated patients (104,105).

The use of calcium and vitamin D supplementation is required for GC-treated patients, according to the American College of Rheumatology guidelines for the prevention and treatment of GIOP (106).

Hormone Replacement Therapy

The peak incidence of RA occurs in postmenopausal years, and alterations of estrogen levels may be related to the pathophysiology of RA. A population study of 564 patients suggests that an average woman develops the first symptom of RA at the time of her menopause (107). Similarly, the radiographic joint destruction, Disease Activity Score, and physical disability tend to be worse in postmenopausal, compared to premenopausal, women with early RA (108). A role for estrogen receptor polymorphism has been suggested in the development of RA (109), and estrogen therapy has been shown to suppress disease activity in collagen-induced arthritis, an animal model for studying RA (110).

Estrogen replacement therapy (ERT) is approved for the prevention of postmenopausal osteoporosis (PMO). However, recently, it is used only for the treatment of vasomotor instability, rather than for protection of bone mass. It has also been used for the treatment of this disease. PMO- and RA-associated bone loss is characterized by increased bone turnover, increased osteoclast-mediated bone resorption, and similar inflammatory cytokine profiles, with elevated systemic levels of IL-1 and IL-6, and so forth (111,112). Estrogen treatment is associated with the suppression of IL-6 production and inhibition of the proliferation and differentiation of osteoclast precursor (113). Serum estrogen also correlates positively with circulating osteoprotegerin levels and absolute bone density at total body, total hip, and FN (114).

Conjugated equine estrogen is the best-studied oral estrogen preparation in postmenopausal women and, in the Postmenopausal Estrogen Progestin Intervention trial (115), was shown to increase spine BMD by 5% and hip BMD by 2.5%. A few small prospective trials evaluating the effect of ERT in prevention of GIOP in postmenopausal women demonstrated a modest increase in vertebral BMD, with an inconsistent effect on hip BMD (116–120). Subanalyses of RA patients in two of these studies revealed a BMD gain of 0.7% to 3.5% at the LS and 1.6% at the hip after 2 to 4 years of treatment with ERT (117,120). No randomized placebo-controlled prospective studies are available regarding the effect of ERT on incident hip and vertebral fractures. Findings from the Women's Health Initiative study have been published that also raise concern regarding long-term use of estrogen and progesterone combination (121). The clinical arm of the study evaluating the effects of estrogen (0.625 mg per day) and progesterone (medroxyprogesterone acetate, 2.5 mg per day) on the incidence of heart disease and breast cancer included more than 16,000 healthy postmenopausal women. The study was intended to last approximately 8.5 years but was prematurely terminated at approximately 5.2 years because of a high incidence of breast cancer in the active treatment group. There was a substantial increase in the risk of invasive breast cancer (26%), coronary heart disease (CHD) (29%), stroke (41%), and venous thromboembolism (twofold) in the HRT treatment group. The beneficial effects were a 37% reduction in colorectal cancer and a one-third reduction in the incidence of hip and clinical vertebral fractures, compared to placebo (p <.05). There was a statistically significant reduction in other osteoporotic fractures (23%) and total fractures (24%). These findings corroborated the earlier observations of the Heart and Estrogen/Progestin Replacement Study (HERS) (122). HERS was a randomized controlled trial of postmenopausal women with preestablished CHD and confirmed that HRT was associated with early harm and did not confer benefit from preventing CHD. An extension of this study, HERS II, followed 93% of the patients on HRT from the initial study for an additional 2.8 years and failed to notice any cardiovascular benefits (123).

Hormone therapy in men taking GCs is effective in preventing bone loss and improving bone mass when followed for 1 to 2 years (+17% vertebral BMD using quantitative computed tomography and +5% using DEXA) (124,125). Testosterone replacement therapy may be considered in men with RA with low testosterone levels (<300 ng per mL) and taking chronic GCs, provided there is no contraindication to their use. Periodic monitoring of serum testosterone and regular prostate evaluation is essential.

Selective Estrogen Receptor Modulators

Selective estrogen receptor modulators are a group of nonhormonal agents that can act as an estrogen agonist or antagonist, depending on the target tissue. These agents have an estrogen-like effect on the bone and lipid metabolism (with the exception of high-density lipoprotein) but act as estrogen antagonists in the breast and uterine tissues. Thus, they are not associated with the undesirable side effects seen with ERT, such as mastalgia, uterine bleeding, and an increased risk of breast carcinoma. Currently, tamoxifen and raloxifene are the only selective estrogen receptor modulators approved for human use, with only raloxifene having an indication for the prevention and treatment of PMO.

Raloxifene has been demonstrated in a clinical trial to suppress urinary calcium excretion and bone resorption (126). The approved dose is 60 mg per day. In randomized double-blind clinical trial for the prevention of PMO, raloxifene treatment for 24 months significantly increased vertebral and total hip BMD, compared to the calcium-supplemented placebo group (127). Raloxifene significantly reduces the risk of vertebral fractures in postmenopausal women with osteoporosis. In the Multiple Outcomes of Raloxifene Evaluation trial, 7,705 postmenopausal women with osteoporosis (t score <–2.5 or prevalent vertebral fracture) were randomized to receive raloxifene, 60 mg per day, 120 mg per day, or placebo. In addition, all women received elemental calcium, 500 mg per day, and vitamin D, 400 to 600 IU per day. After 3 years, the RR of incident vertebral fractures in women treated with raloxifene, 60 mg per day, was 0.45 (95% CI: 0.29–0.71) and 0.7 (95% CI: 0.56–0.86), compared to placebo in low BMD and prevalent fracture groups, respectively (128). No significant reduction in nonvertebral fractures was found that could be due to lack of adequate statistical power to detect such a change in this study.

Recently, 4-year data from the Multiple Outcomes of Raloxifene Evaluation trial has been published (129). The cumulative risk of at least one new vertebral fracture at 4 years was 0.64 (95% CI: 0.53–0.76). The reduction in new vertebral fracture risk in the fourth year alone was 36% (RR, 0.61; 95% CI: 0.43–0.88), not significantly different from the RR observed during the first 3 years. The nonvertebral risk was not significantly reduced (RR, 0.93; 95% CI: 0.81–1.06). Raloxifene use has been recommended for the prevention and treatment of osteoporosis in RA patients who may be at a high risk of gastrointestinal complications from oral bisphosphonate therapy (130). Their use is associated with increased risk of thromboembolism, hot flashes, and leg cramps. Therefore, patients treated with raloxifene should be counseled about these side effects.

Bisphosphonates

Bisphosphonates are nonhydrolyzable analogues of pyrophosphates and act as powerful antiresorptives in the prevention and treatment of PMO and GIOP. They act primarily by inhibiting osteoclastogenesis and osteoclast function, and the nitrogen-containing bisphosphonates (alendronate and risedronate) appear to induce osteoclast apoptosis (131–133). The specific mechanism of action and potency varies according to the structural composition of various bisphosphonates. The non–nitrogen-containing bisphosphonates (e.g., etidronate and clodronate) are the oldest known agents of the bisphosphonate family and are less potent compared to the newer, nitrogen-containing bisphosphonates, such as alendronate and risedronate. The former acts by forming toxic analogues of adenosine triphosphate inside the osteoclasts, leading to reduced bone resorption and cell death (134). The latter class of bisphosphonates acts by interfering with protein prenylation through the 3-hydroxy-3-methylglutaryl coenzyme A-mevalonate pathway. Protein prenylation is an essential step, characterized by the addition of 15 to 20 carbon side chains to specific intracellular messenger guanosine triphosphates, and is essential for normal cell function and survival. Inhibition of this critical step results in a decrease in osteoclast number and function and increased apoptosis (133,135,136).

Oral bisphosphonates have poor intestinal absorption (<5%), no significant hepatic metabolism, and predominantly renal excretion. Of the various bisphosphonates, only alendronate and risedronate are approved by the U.S. Food and Drug Administration (FDA) for the prevention and treatment of osteoporosis and GIOP.

ETIDRONATE

Etidronate is administered intermittently at a dose of 400 mg per day orally for 14 days, followed by 76 days of calcium supplementation. This cycle is repeated every 3 months. Prospective studies have demonstrated a beneficial effect of cyclical etidronate therapy in GC-treated patients. Increases of 5% to 7% at the LS and 2.5% to 6.0% at the hip have occurred in placebo-controlled trials, including patients with RA (90,91,137).

A metaanalysis of the prevention and treatment studies in GIOP using cyclical etidronate showed a significant increase in BMD at the LS and FN (3.7% and 1.7%, respectively) in the prevention trials and in the spine only (4.8%) in the treatment group after 1 year of therapy with the active drug. A benefit in vertebral fracture rate was observed in the postmenopausal women group only (138). In addition, GIOP studies of 2 to 3 years' duration using cyclic etidronate found loss of BMD at the hip. If this agent is used alone in GIOP, BMD monitoring at the hip is required.

ALENDRONATE

Alendronate therapy increases BMD at the spine and hip and reduces incident vertebral fractures in postmenopausal women with low bone mass. In a 3-year randomized placebo-controlled prospective study enrolling 994 postmenopausal women with osteoporosis, the effect of oral alendronate (average, 10 mg per day) plus calcium, 500 mg per day, on BMD was evaluated using DEXA scan (139). Alendronate therapy was associated with a BMD increase of 8.8% ± 0.4 (± SE), 5.9% ± 0.5 (± SE), and 2.5% ± 0.3 (± SE) in the spine, FN, and total body, respectively, compared to the placebo (p <.001 for all comparisons).

The largest study evaluating the benefit of alendronate therapy in fracture risk reduction in postmenopausal women with significant bone loss is the Fracture Intervention Trial. This study recruited almost 7,000 postmenopausal women in a randomized placebo-controlled study, subsequently divided into those with prevalent vertebral fracture(s) (fracture arm, N = 2,027) and those with low bone mass with t score greater than or equal to –2 and no prevalent vertebral fracture(s) (clinical arm, N = 4,432). The fracture arm of the study was prematurely terminated at 3 years because of a significant difference in the incident fracture risk between the treatment groups. Patients taking alendronate had a 47%, 51%, and 48% reduction in the risk of incident vertebral, hip, and forearm fractures, compared to placebo (p <.001, p <.05, and p <.05, respectively) (140).

In the clinical arm of the study (patients without prevalent vertebral fractures), 31% of the patients recruited were found not to meet the entry criteria of t score of –2 or more because of revision of the normative values for the FN BMD by the manufacturer. However, at the end of 4 years, there was a statistically significant difference only in the incident vertebral fractures between the alendronate and the placebo groups (2.5 vs. 4.8 fractures, 48%) (141). In a 2-year double-blind placebo-controlled study of men with significant bone loss (t score <–2 at FN or baseline osteoporotic fracture plus t score <–1 at FN), alendronate, 10 mg per day, significantly increased BMD at LS, FN, and total body (5.3%, 2.6%, and 1.6%, respectively; p <.001) (142).

Alendronate in doses of 5 and 10 mg per day was tested in the prevention of GIOP in two separate, but similar, studies of 1-year duration each. Together, 560 men and women with different chronic inflammatory diseases, including RA, taking at least 7.5 mg per day of prednisone or equivalent, were recruited. In the placebo group, taking only supplemental calcium and vitamin D, bone loss occurred at the spine, FN, and the trochanter at 1 year. However, increase in BMD of similar magnitude was seen at the spine, FN, and trochanter between the 5 and 10 mg per day alendronate groups, except in the postmenopausal group not receiving ERT. In these women, a greater increase in BMD at the spine and trochanter was seen with the higher 10 mg per day dose of alendronate compared to 5 mg per day (4.1% vs. 1.6% and 2.8% vs. 1.7%) (143).

In the year 2000, 70 mg per week dose of alendronate was found to have similar efficacy in terms of increase in BMD at the spine and hip but better gastrointestinal tolerance and compliance, compared to the 10 mg per day dose (144). The FDA has approved the 10 mg per day or 70 mg per week dose for the treatment of PMO. The recommended dose is 10 mg per day for the treatment of GIOP in postmenopausal women not taking ERT. For PMO prevention or treatment of GIOP in men and estrogen-replete women, the recommended dose of oral alendronate is 5 mg per day or 35 mg per week.

RISEDRONATE

Risedronate treatment improves BMD at the spine and hip and reduces the risk of fractures at these sites. This beneficial activity was established in a large cohort of 2,485 postmenopausal women with established osteoporosis [i.e., low bone mass plus fragility fracture(s)] treated with risedronate (2.5 or 5 mg per day) or placebo (145). Both groups received supplemental calcium, 1,000 mg per day. Vitamin D, 500 IU per day, was added, if baseline levels were low (≤40 nmol per L). The 2.5 mg per day arm was discontinued after 1 year, and final analysis involved 5 mg per day versus placebo at 3 years. The increase in BMD in risedronate versus placebo group was 5.4% versus 1.1% at the LS, 1.6% versus –1.2% at the FN, and 0.2% versus –1.4% at the midshaft of radius. The cumulative incidence of new vertebral fracture(s) was 11.3% versus 16.3% (p = .003), respectively, a 41% decrease with active drug treatment (95% CI: 18–58%). The cumulative incidence of nonvertebral fracture(s) in the risedronate versus placebo group was 5.2% versus 8.4% (p = .02), a 39% reduction (95% CI: 6–61%).

A similar study conducted in Europe and Australia involved 1,226 postmenopausal women with similar inclusion criteria, treatment groups, and duration (146). The 2.5 mg per day risedronate group was discontinued after 2 years. Risedronate,

5 mg per day, reduced the risk of incident vertebral fractures by 49%, compared with the control group (p <.001). The reduction in the risk of nonvertebral fractures was 33%, compared to the placebo (p <.06). Risedronate was shown to significantly reduce the risk of incident hip fracture(s) in women age 70 to 79 years with low BMD (t score <–4 or <–3 plus a nonskeletal risk factor for fracture) (147). After 3 years of therapy with 5 mg per day of active drug, compared to placebo, the incidence was 1.9% versus 3.2%, respectively (RR, 0.6; 95% CI: 0.4–0.9; p = .009). However, in women older than 80 years with unknown BMD and only nonskeletal risk factors, there was no significant difference in the two treatment groups at 3 years (fracture incidence, 4.2% vs. 5.1% in risedronate vs. placebo groups; p = .35).

Risedronate at 2.5 mg per day was shown to prevent bone loss at the spine and trochanter in a cohort of 120 postmenopausal women with RA taking chronic prednisone therapy greater than 2.5 mg per day, compared to placebo at 2 years (p = .009 and p = .02, respectively) (148). It is effective in preventing and treating GIOP in men and women who are either initiating or continuing GC therapy, when given as 5 mg per day (149–152). Risedronate, 35 mg per week, was approved in the year 2002 for the prevention and treatment of PMO. Additional studies are now in progress with GIOP and risedronate at 35 mg per week.

PAMIDRONATE

Pamidronate, a second-generation aminobisphosphonate, is approved in the United States for the treatment of tumor-induced hypercalcemia, Paget's disease, and for patients with osteolytic bone disease from multiple myeloma or other cancer metastases to the bone. Although not specifically approved for the prevention or treatment of osteoporosis, it is used off label for patients who cannot tolerate oral bisphosphonates or have trouble with enteral absorption of bisphosphonates. Cyclical pamidronate has been shown to suppress bone turnover markers and increase LS BMD by almost 3% in a year (153). Continuous daily pamidronate (150 mg per day) can significantly increase BMD at the LS, femoral trochanter, and total body, compared to placebo after 2 years of treatment for PMO (154). Lesser vertebral fractures were reported in the pamidronate group (13% vs. 24% patient-years; p = .07). Typically, pamidronate is given intravenously as a loading dose of 90 mg, followed by 30-mg infusions every 3 months.

ZOLEDRONATE

Recently, zoledronic acid has been approved for the treatment of hypercalcemia of malignancy. A phase 2, dose-ranging clinical study was performed to evaluate intravenous zoledronic acid for the prevention of PMO in 351 women. Interestingly, the bone mass in the LS increased nearly 5% in all dose groups, including one group that was given zoledronate, 4 mg, only at the beginning of the study. The markers of bone resorption also decreased within a few months of the initial treatment and remained suppressed for the 12-month study period. There was no dose response observed, and the duration of the effect of the one dose of zoledronate is not known. However, if these results are reproduced and fracture efficacy is determined, an intravenous bisphosphonate therapy that can be given only once a year would provide a convenient alternative to our patients with osteoporosis (155). Zoledronic acid is not FDA approved for the prevention or treatment of osteoporosis.

Combination of Bisphosphonate and Hormone Replacement Therapy

Despite the use of effective antiosteoporosis drugs, some patients will either continue to lose bone mass or may fracture while taking an antiresorptive. Theoretically, these patients could benefit from combination therapy, usually the addition of another antiosteoporosis drug. Ideally, drugs with different mechanisms of action and different toxicity profiles may be used (e.g., combination of anabolic and antiresorptive agents), and this may be possible in the near future. However, all the currently available and approved therapies are antiresorptives and act by suppressing bone resorption.

Although calcium and vitamin D have been commonly used with the more potent antiresorptives with modest benefit, significant additive effect on bone mass has been observed without much added toxicity by combining bisphosphonates and HRT. However, long-term safety concerns about profound suppression of bone turnover and fracture healing remains, and close follow-up of these patients is needed. In addition, any added benefit on fracture risk reduction, although likely, is yet unproven.

A 2-year double-blind placebo-controlled study of women with PMO (N = 425) evaluated the effects of conjugated equine estrogen (0.625 mg per day), alendronate (10 mg per day), and the combination on LS BMD (156). After 2 years, a significantly greater increase (8.3%) was seen in the combination group, compared to either drug alone (approximately 6%). The changes in total hip BMD were +4.0%, +3.4%, +4.7%, and 0.3% for the alendronate, estrogen, alendronate plus estrogen, and placebo groups, respectively. In another study, alendronate, 10 mg per day, was added to existing regimen of estrogen plus progesterone in postmenopausal women with osteoporosis. Combination therapy was associated with a 3.7% and 2.7% increase in 1 year at the LS and the trochanter, compared to 1% and 0.5% gain at the same sites in the estrogen and placebo group (p <.001) (157). The suppression of bone turnover is more profound, as confirmed by a greater reduction in biochemical bone turnover markers and confirmed by bone histomorphometry.

Similar additive benefit has been seen with the combination of risedronate (5 mg per day) and estrogen (0.625 mg per day) plus or minus progesterone in a 1-year double-blind placebo-controlled study of 524 postmenopausal women with osteoporosis (158). Increase in LS and FN BMD in the combination versus HRT-only groups was 5.2% versus 4.6% and 2.7% versus 1.8%, respectively. The difference between the groups was significant at the FN and midshaft radius only. Yet, another study evaluated the beneficial effects of combining raloxifene and alendronate, compared to either agent alone, in postmenopausal women with osteoporosis (FN t score <–2) over 1 year (159). The improvement in LS BMD in the alendronate, raloxifene, and alendronate plus raloxifene groups was 4.3%, 2.1%, and 5.3% (p <.05 between raloxifene and raloxifene plus alendronate groups). The increase in FN BMD for the same groups was 2.7%, 1.7%, and 3.7%, respectively (p <.001 raloxifene plus alendronate vs. raloxifene alone). Overall, the combination therapies were well tolerated, with no significant added toxicity in these short-term trials. A review of other possible combination therapies has been published (160).

Parathyroid Hormone Therapy

Human PTH (hPTH) is a promising new treatment that was approved at the end of 2002 for the treatment of severe bone loss and fragility fractures. Unlike the existing antiosteoporosis drugs, intermittent hPTH acts as an anabolic agent, promotes osteoblast survival and function, and prevents GC-induced osteoblast apoptosis (161). Both 1-34 and 1-84 amino terminal fragments have been studied and proven effective in improving and preserving bone mass. hPTH by itself has been shown to increase BMD within 1 year in the trabecular-rich LS by at least 8% in randomized placebo-controlled trials in both men and women with idiopathic osteoporosis and PMO, respectively (162,163).

Although hPTH (1-34) and other PTH fragments activate osteoblast activity, continued daily treatment also stimulates osteoblast production of RANKL. Continued treatment with daily injections of hPTH (1-34) also increases osteoclast activity and bone resorption. Therefore, daily treatment with hPTH (1-34) leads to a dramatic increase in bone turnover or remodeling. However, with the initiation of hPTH (1-34) therapy, there is a more rapid increase in the markers of bone formation, compared to bone resorption markers. Most studies of hPTH (1-34) find that, by 6 months of daily injections of hPTH (1-34), bone resorption markers are similar in elevation over baseline levels to bone formation markers. Measurement of bone turnover markers at baseline and 3-month follow-up was the best predictor of skeletal response to hPTH (1-34).

Combination therapy using hPTH plus ERT, compared to ERT alone, is associated with a significant increase in vertebral, femoral, and total-body BMD and a reduction in incident vertebral fractures (164,165). The increase in BMD after 3 years of combination therapy was 13% ($p < .001$), 2.7% ($p < .05$), and 8%, respectively, from the baseline, whereas the ERT group had no significant change in BMD at any of the measured sites (164). These studies confirm the synergistic effect of hPTH plus ERT in improving bone mass at the spine without any loss of bone at the distal radius.

The effect of hPTH (1-34) therapy in fracture reduction was studied in 1,637 postmenopausal women with prior vertebral fracture(s). Patients were randomly assigned to 20 μg per day, 40 μg per day, or placebo subcutaneous injections daily for median observation duration of 21 months. The incidence of new vertebral fracture(s) was 5% (RR, 0.35; 95% CI: 0.22–0.55), 4% (RR, 0.31; 95% CI: 0.19–0.50), and 14% in the 20 μg, 40 μg, and placebo daily groups. New nonvertebral fracture incidence was 6% in the placebo and 3% in both the active treatment groups. As expected, the reduction in fracture risk was associated with significant increase in LS, FN, and total-body BMD in the hPTH (1-34) groups. Hypercalcemia and injection site reactions, the most common side effects, were more common in the higher dose group, which was also associated with a 2% reduction in the BMD at the radial shaft.

The combination of hPTH and ERT can not only prevent bone loss, but also significantly increase BMD in women with PMO taking chronic GC therapy. In a randomized placebo-controlled trial, 51 osteopenic estrogen-replete postmenopausal women with chronic inflammatory conditions (including RA) requiring chronic GC therapy were randomized to either continue ERT (N = 28) or add hPTH (1-34), 400 IU per day (N = 23) (166). After 1 year, the hPTH plus ERT group had 11% and 35% increase in LS BMD by DEXA and quantitative computed tomography, respectively, compared to 1.7% increase in LS BMD by DEXA in the ERT-only group ($p < .001$ for LS BMD difference between two groups). Interestingly, when the combination group was followed for another year while off of hPTH therapy, BMD at the total hip and FN continued to increase and was significantly elevated at 24 months, compared to baseline [4.7 ± 0.9% (mean ± SEM) ($p < .01$) and 5.2 ± 1.3%, respectively] (167). Therefore, hPTH therapy appears to be promising. The combination of hPTH with other antiresorptives has a lot of potential for patients with severe bone loss or nonresponders to traditional antiresorptive therapy.

Calcitonin

Calcitonin is a 32–amino acid polypeptide hormone approved by the FDA for the treatment of late PMO. Initially, injectable calcitonin was approved by the FDA in 1984 based on its positive effects on calcium balance in postmenopausal women with osteoporosis (168–170). Subsequently, an increase in LS BMD was demonstrated with calcitonin injection therapy in postmenopausal women with osteoporosis (171–173). In a retrospective cohort study, the injectable calcitonin group had a greater decrease in the risk of hip fracture, compared to the calcium-only group (RR, 0.69 vs. 0.75) (174). A significant reduction in vertebral fracture risk in PMO has also been demonstrated (173).

Nasal calcitonin became available in the United States in 1995. However, it is not very effective in preventing early postmenopausal bone loss. In late PMO, nasal calcitonin therapy significantly decreases the risk of incident vertebral fractures, compared to calcium alone (RR, 0.23; 95% CI: 0.07–0.77; $p = .04$) (175). The largest study of calcitonin in the treatment of PMO is the Prevent Recurrence of Osteoporotic Fracture trial (176), in which 1,255 women with an average age of 68 years and established osteoporosis [prevalent vertebral fracture(s) plus t score <–2.0] were randomized to receive placebo or nasal calcitonin spray at doses of 100 IU, 200 IU, and 400 IU for 5 years. Calcium and vitamin D supplements (1,000 mg plus 400 IU, respectively) were provided to all patients.

Despite a high dropout rate (approximately 60%), an intent-to-treat analysis showed a 36% reduction in incident vertebral fractures in the 200 IU calcitonin group, compared to placebo (RR, 0.64; $p = .03$). This fracture risk reduction was associated with a 1.2% increase in LS BMD in the first year of therapy and significant reduction in markers of bone resorption. No dose-response association was seen in the active treatment group. The reduction in the rate of nonvertebral fractures was nonsignificant (46% for hip fractures and 28% for wrist fractures in the 200 IU group). Nasal calcitonin appears to be effective in preventing LS BMD loss in GC-treated patients (177–180). No data are available on hip BMD prevention or fracture risk reduction in GIOP. In comparison to other antiresorptives, calcitonin has the advantage of better tolerability, ease of administration, and having an analgesic effect on bone pain (179,181,182). However, it is considered to be a second-line agent for the treatment of osteoporosis, especially in patients who have contraindications to or cannot tolerate bisphosphonates.

How to Monitor Therapy

Currently, there is no consensus on how to monitor patients with osteoporosis therapy. In general, if a bone mineral density is obtained, it should only be done after approximately 2 years of treatment to be able to determine if the change is significant. The least significant change should be determined for the DEXA machine being used for monitoring osteoporosis therapy. The least significant change is 2.77 × coefficient of variation for the machine being used. Usually, for the LS, it is approximately 1%, and for the hip it is approximately 2%. A change of 3% in BMD at LS and 6% at the hip is considered significant. Therefore, repeat BMD testing to monitor response to antiresorptive therapy should be performed at approximately 2-year intervals. Table 47.4 outlines a suggested protocol for monitoring response to antiosteoporosis therapy. It should be noted that increase in BMD only accounts for a fraction of the overall fracture risk reduction, and currently available densitometers only measure the mineral quantity. A significant beneficial effect of the approved antiosteoporosis agents is an improvement in bone quality and connectivity, which cannot be measured with the currently available noninvasive instruments. Therefore, even if the BMD numbers do not improve much and if the patient has not had any incident fragility fracture(s) during

TABLE 47.4. Monitoring Response to Osteoporosis Therapy

Periodic evaluation with
- A modified medical history.
- Physical examination targeted to older women's health, including breast and pelvic examination, mammography, and Papanicolaou smear, if indicated.
- Inquire regarding adherence to osteoporosis regimen, including calcium, vitamin D, exercise, and any pharmacologic therapy.
- Assessment of stature and skeletal integrity, including a reliable measurement of height and a radiographic assessment if new deformities are present.
- Reinforcement of the therapeutic program and evaluation of the patient's level of understanding and concern.

Periodic assessment of bone mineral density (BMD)
- For patients with normal baseline BMD (testing score >–1.0), follow-up measurement every 3–5 yr.
- For patients in an osteoporosis prevention program, follow-up measurement at least 2 yr after antiresorptive agent was started when least significant change (LSC) in bone mass can be detected.
- For patients on a therapeutic program, perform a follow-up measurement after 2 yr when LSC can be detected.

Adapted from Hodgson SF, Watts NB, Bilezikian JP, et al. American Association of Clinical Endocrinologists 2001 medical guidelines for clinical practice for the prevention and management of postmenopausal osteoporosis. *Endocr Pract* 2001;7:293–311.

treatment, he or she should be encouraged to continue therapy. As discussed in detail above, the concordance between BMD improvement and fracture risk reduction is good for bisphosphonates, poor for raloxifene and calcitonin, and nonexistent for fluoride treatment.

CONCLUSION

RA is commonly associated with significant bone loss, both localized and generalized. The etiology is multifactorial with disease activity, poor physical conditioning, and activity, age, disability, and side effects of drug therapy as major contributors. Fortunately, effective treatment options are available for both the prevention and treatment of bone loss in these patients, and many new potent antiosteoporosis drugs are on the horizon. It is important to recognize and screen at-risk patients and, preferably with early intervention, prevent significant bone loss and fractures in this high-risk patient population.

REFERENCES

1. Jolles BM, Bogoch ER. Current consensus recommendations for rheumatoid arthritis therapy: a blind spot for osteoporosis prevention and treatment. *J Rheumatol* 2002;29:1814–1817.
2. Silman AJ, Hockberg MC. *Epidemiology of the rheumatoid disease.* Oxford: Oxford University Press, 1993.
3. Sinigaglia L, Nervetti A, Mela Q, et al. A multicenter cross sectional study on bone mineral density in rheumatoid arthritis. Italian study group on bone mass in rheumatoid arthritis. *J Rheumatol* 2000;27:2582–2589.
4. French AR, Mason T, Nelson AM, et al. Osteopenia in adults with a history of juvenile rheumatoid arthritis. A population based study. *J Rheumatol* 2002; 29:1065–1070.
5. Henderson CJ, Specker BL, Sierra RI, et al. Total-body bone mineral content in non-corticosteroid-treated postpubertal females with juvenile rheumatoid arthritis: frequency of osteopenia and contributing factors. *Arthritis Rheum* 2000;43:531–540.
6. Hooyman JR, Melton LJ III, Nelson AM, et al. Fractures after rheumatoid arthritis. A population-based study. *Arthritis Rheum* 1984;27:1353–1361.
7. Huusko TM, Korpela M, Karppi P, et al. Threefold increased risk of hip fractures with rheumatoid arthritis in Central Finland. *Ann Rheum Dis* 2001;60:521–522.
8. Cooper C, Coupland C, Mitchell M. Rheumatoid arthritis, corticosteroid therapy and hip fracture. *Ann Rheum Dis* 1995;54:49–52.
9. Davidson CW, Merrilees MJ, Wilkinson TJ, et al. Hip fracture mortality and morbidity—can we do better? *N Z Med J* 2001;114:329–332.
10. Stromqvist B. Hip fracture in rheumatoid arthritis. *Acta Orthop Scand* 1984;55:624–628.
11. Thienpont E, Simon JP, Spaepen D, Fabry G. Bifocal pubic stress fracture after ipsilateral total knee arthroplasty in rheumatoid arthritis. A case report. *Acta Orthop Belg* 2000;66:197–200.
12. Elkayam O, Paran D, Flusser G, et al. Insufficiency fractures in rheumatic patients: misdiagnosis and underlying characteristics. *Clin Exp Rheumatol* 2000;18:369–374.
13. Shenstone BD, Mahmoud A, Woodward R, et al. Longitudinal bone mineral density changes in early rheumatoid arthritis. *Br J Rheumatol* 1994;33:541–545.
14. Kroot EJ, Nieuwenhuizen MG, de Waal Malefijt MC, et al. Change in bone mineral density in patients with rheumatoid arthritis during the first decade of the disease. *Arthritis Rheum* 2001;44:1254–1260.
15. Daragon A, Krzanowska K, Vittecoq O, et al. Prospective x-ray densitometry and ultrasonography study of the hand bones of patients with rheumatoid arthritis of recent onset. *Joint Bone Spine* 2001;68:34–42.
16. Deodhar AA, Brabyn J, Jones PW, et al. Longitudinal study of hand bone densitometry in rheumatoid arthritis. *Arthritis Rheum* 1995;38:1204–1210.
17. Shenstone BD, Mahmoud A, Woodward R, et al. Longitudinal bone mineral density changes in early rheumatoid arthritis. *Br J Rheumatol* 1994;33:541–545.
18. Kroot EJ, Nieuwenhuizen MG, de Waal Malefijt MC, et al. Change in bone mineral density in patients with rheumatoid arthritis during the first decade of the disease. *Arthritis Rheum* 2001;44:1254–1260.
19. Gough AK, Lilley J, Eyre S, et al. Generalized bone loss in patients with early rheumatoid arthritis. *Lancet* 1994;344:23–27.
20. Cooper C, Coupland C, Mitchell M. Rheumatoid arthritis, corticosteroid therapy and hip fracture. *Ann Rheum Dis* 1995;54:49–52.
21. Peel NF, Moore DJ, Barrington NA, et al. Risk of vertebral fracture and relationship to bone mineral density in steroid treated rheumatoid arthritis. *Ann Rheum Dis* 1995;54:801–806.
22. Deodhar AA, Woolf AD. Bone mass measurement and bone metabolism in rheumatoid arthritis: a review. *Br J Rheumatol* 1996;35:309–322.
23. Alonso-Bartolome P, Martinez-Taboada VM, Blanco R, Rodriguez-Valverde V. Insufficiency fractures of the tibia and fibula. *Semin Arthritis Rheum* 1999;28:413–420.
24. Kennedy AC, Smith DA, Anton HC, Buchanan WW. Generalized and localized bone loss in patients with rheumatoid arthritis. *Scand J Rheumatol* 1975;4:209–215.
25. Rehman Q, Lane NE. Bone loss. Therapeutic approaches for preventing bone loss in inflammatory arthritis. *Arthritis Res* 2001;3:221–227.
26. Oelzner P, Franke S, Muller A, et al. Relationship between soluble markers of immune activation and bone turnover in post-menopausal women with rheumatoid arthritis. *Rheumatology (Oxford)* 1999;38:841–847.
27. Joffe I, Epstein S. Osteoporosis associated with rheumatoid arthritis: pathogenesis and management. *Semin Arthritis Rheum* 1991;20:256–272.
28. Bijlsma JW. Bone metabolism in patients with rheumatoid arthritis. *Clin Rheumatol* 1988;7:16–23.
29. Robinson DR, Tashjian AH Jr, Levine L. Prostaglandin-stimulated bone resorption by rheumatoid synovia. A possible mechanism for bone destruction in rheumatoid arthritis. *J Clin Invest* 1975;56:1181–1188.
30. Goldring SR, Gravallese EM. Mechanisms of bone loss in inflammatory arthritis: diagnosis and therapeutic implications. *Arthritis Res* 2000;2:33–37.
31. Kim N, Odgren PR, Kim DK, et al. Diverse roles of the tumor necrosis factor family member TRANCE in skeletal physiology revealed by TRANCE deficiency and partial rescue by a lymphocyte-expressed TRANCE transgene. *Proc Natl Acad Sci U S A* 2000;97:10905–10910.
32. Gravallese EM, Harada Y, Wang JT, et al. Identification of cell types responsible for bone resorption in rheumatoid arthritis and juvenile rheumatoid arthritis. *Am J Pathol* 1998;152:943–951.
33. Shimizu S, Shiozawa S, Shiozawa K, et al. Quantitative histologic studies on the pathogenesis of periarticular osteoporosis in rheumatoid arthritis. *Arthritis Rheum* 1985;28:25–31.
34. Kong YY, Feige U, Sarosi I, et al. Activated T cells regulate bone loss and joint destruction in adjuvant arthritis through osteoprotegerin ligand. *Nature* 1999;402:304–309.
35. Takayanagi H, Iizuka H, Juji T, et al. Involvement of receptor activator of nuclear factor κB ligand/osteoclast differentiation factor in osteoclastogenesis from synoviocytes in rheumatoid arthritis. *Arthritis Rheum* 2000;43:259–269.
36. Yasuda H, Shima N, Nakagawa N, et al. Osteoclast differentiation factor is a ligand for osteoprotegerin/osteoclastogenesis-inhibitory factor and is identical to TRANCE/RANKL. *Proc Natl Acad Sci U S A* 1998;95:3597–3602.
37. Tsurukai T, Udagawa N, Matsuzaki K, et al. Roles of macrophage-colony stimulating factor and osteoclast differentiation factor in osteoclastogenesis. *J Bone Miner Res* 2000;18:177–184.
38. Haynes DR, Barg E, Crotti TN, et al. Osteoprotegerin expression in synovial tissue from patients with rheumatoid arthritis, spondyloarthropathies and osteoarthritis and normal controls. *Rheumatology (Oxford)* 2003;42:123–134.
39. Fujikawa Y, Sabokbar A, Neale S, Athanasou NA. Human osteoclast formation and bone resorption by monocytes and synovial macrophages in rheumatoid arthritis. *Ann Rheum Dis* 1996;55:816–822.
40. Bijlsma JW, Cutolo M, Masi AT, Chikanza IC. The neuroendocrine immune basis of rheumatic diseases. *Immunol Today* 1999;20:298–301.

41. Masi AT, Bijlsma JW, Chikanza IC, et al. Neuroendocrine, immunologic, and microvascular systems interactions in rheumatoid arthritis: physiopathogenetic and therapeutic perspectives. *Semin Arthritis Rheum* 1999;29:65–81.
42. Cutolo M, Sulli A, Villaggio B, et al. Relations between steroid hormones and cytokines in rheumatoid arthritis and systemic lupus erythematosus. *Ann Rheum Dis* 1998;57:573–577.
43. Gordon D, Beastall GH, Thomson JA, Sturrock RD. Prolonged hypogonadism in male patients with rheumatoid arthritis during flares in disease activity. *Br J Rheumatol* 1988;27:440–444.
44. Spector TD, Perry LA, Tubb G, et al. Low free testosterone levels in rheumatoid arthritis. *Ann Rheum Dis* 1988;47:65–68.
45. Martens HF, Sheets PK, Tenover JS, et al. Decreased testosterone levels in men with rheumatoid arthritis: effect of low dose prednisone therapy. *J Rheumatol* 1994;21:1427–1431.
46. MacAdams MR, White RH, Chipps BE. Reduction of serum testosterone levels during chronic glucocorticoid therapy. *Ann Intern Med* 1986;104:648–651.
47. Celiker R, Gokce-Kutsal Y, Cindas A, et al. Osteoporosis in rheumatoid arthritis: effect of disease activity. *Clin Rheumatol* 1995;14:429–433.
48. Sambrook PN, Eisman JA, Champion GD, et al. Determinants of axial bone loss in rheumatoid arthritis. *Arthritis Rheum* 1987;30:721–728.
49. Laan RF, Buijs WC, Verbeek AL, et al. Bone mineral density in patients with recent onset rheumatoid arthritis: influence of disease activity and functional capacity. *Ann Rheum Dis* 1993;52:21–26.
50. Eggelmeijer F, Camps JA, Valkema R, et al. Bone mineral density in ambulant, non-steroid treated female patients with rheumatoid arthritis. *Clin Exp Rheumatol* 1993;11:381–385.
51. Lane NE, Goldring SR. Bone loss in rheumatoid arthritis: what role does inflammation play? *J Rheumatol* 1998;25:1251–1253.
52. Weinstein RS. The pathogenesis of glucocorticoid-induced osteoporosis. *Clin Exp Rheumatol* 2000;18:S35–S40.
53. Dempster DW. Bone histomorphometry in glucocorticoid-induced osteoporosis. *J Bone Miner Res* 1989;4:137–141.
54. Suzuki Y, Ichikawa Y, Saito E, Homma M. Importance of increased urinary calcium excretion in the development of secondary hyperparathyroidism of patients under glucocorticoid therapy. *Metabolism* 1983;32:151–156.
55. Hahn TJ, Halstead LR, Baran DT. Effects of short term glucocorticoid administration on intestinal calcium absorption and circulating vitamin D metabolite concentrations in man. *J Clin Endocrinol Metab* 1981;52:111–115.
56. Paz-Pacheco E, Fuleihan GE, LeBoff MS. Intact parathyroid hormone levels are not elevated in glucocorticoid-treated subjects. *J Bone Miner Res* 1995;10:1713–1718.
57. Bijlsma JWJ. Long-term glucocorticoid treatment of rheumatoid arthritis: risk or benefit? *Rheumatol Eur* 1998;27:67.
58. Lems WF, Jahangier ZN, Raymakers JA, et al. Methods to score vertebral deformities in patients with rheumatoid arthritis. *Br J Rheumatol* 1997;36:220–224.
59. Ragab AH, Frech RS, Vietti TJ. Osteoporotic fractures secondary to methotrexate therapy of acute leukemia in remission. *Cancer* 1970;25:580–585.
60. Friedlaender GE, Tross RB, Doganis AC, et al. Effects of chemotherapeutic agents on bone. I. Short-term methotrexate and doxorubicin (adriamycin) treatment in a rat model. *J Bone Joint Surg Am* 1984;66:602–607.
61. Preston SJ, Diamond T, Scott A, Laurent MR. Methotrexate osteopathy in rheumatic disease. *Ann Rheum Dis* 1993;52:582–585.
62. Segawa Y, Yamaura M, Aota S, et al. Methotrexate maintains bone mass by preventing both a decrease in bone formation and an increase in bone resorption in adjuvant-induced arthritic rats. *Bone* 1997;20:457–464.
63. Carbone LD, Kaeley G, McKown KM, et al. Effects of long-term administration of methotrexate on bone mineral density in rheumatoid arthritis. *Calcif Tissue Int* 1999;64:100–101.
64. Buckley LM, Leib ES, Cartularo KS, et al. Effects of low dose methotrexate on the bone mineral density of patients with rheumatoid arthritis. *J Rheumatol* 1997;24:1489–1494.
65. Ferraccioli G, Salaffi F, De Vita S, et al. Methotrexate in polymyalgia rheumatica: preliminary results of an open, randomized study. *J Rheumatol* 1996;23:624–628.
66. Bunker VW. The role of nutrition in osteoporosis. *Br J Biomed Sci* 1994;51:228–240.
67. Hofbauer LC, Shui C, Riggs BL, et al. Effects of immunosuppressants on receptor activator of NF-kappaB ligand and osteoprotegerin production by human osteoblastic and coronary artery smooth muscle cells. *Biochem Biophys Res Commun* 2001;280:334–339.
68. Forre O. Radiologic evidence of disease modification in rheumatoid arthritis patients treated with cyclosporine. Results of a 48-week multicenter study comparing low-dose cyclosporine with placebo. Norwegian Arthritis Study Group. *Arthritis Rheum* 1994;37:1506–1512.
69. Pasero G, Priolo F, Marubini E, et al. Slow progression of joint damage in early rheumatoid arthritis treated with cyclosporin A. *Arthritis Rheum* 1996;39:1006–1015.
70. Ferraccioli G, Casatta L, Bartoli E. Increase of bone mineral density and anabolic variables in patients with rheumatoid arthritis resistant to methotrexate after cyclosporin A therapy. *J Rheumatol* 1996;23:1539–1542.
71. Kotake S, Udagawa N, Takahashi N, et al. IL-17 in synovial fluids from patients with rheumatoid arthritis is a potent stimulator of osteoclastogenesis. *J Clin Invest* 1999;103:1345–1352.
72. Hofbauer LC, Lacey DL, Dunstan CR, et al. Interleukin-1β and tumor necrosis factor-α, but not interleukin-6, stimulate osteoprotegerin ligand gene expression in human osteoblastic cells. *Bone* 1999;25:255–259.
73. Snow-Harter C, Marcus R. Exercise, bone mineral density, and osteoporosis. *Exerc Sport Sci Rev* 1991;19:351–388.
74. Walsmith J, Roubenoff R. Cachexia in rheumatoid arthritis. *Int J Cardiol* 2002;85:89.
75. Kroger H, Penttila IM, Alhava EM. Low serum vitamin D metabolites in women with rheumatoid arthritis. *Scand J Rheumatol* 1993;22:172–177.
76. Als OS, Riis B, Christiansen C. Serum concentration of vitamin D metabolites in rheumatoid arthritis. *Clin Rheumatol* 1987;6:238–243.
77. Madsen OR, Sorensen OH, Egsmose C. Bone quality and bone mass as assessed by quantitative ultrasound and dual energy x-ray absorptiometry in women with rheumatoid arthritis: relationship with quadriceps strength. *Ann Rheum Dis* 2002;61:325–329.
78. Stone J, Doube A, Dudson D, Wallace J. Inadequate calcium, folic acid, vitamin E, zinc, and selenium intake in rheumatoid arthritis patients: results of a dietary survey. *Semin Arthritis Rheum* 1997;27:180–185.
79. Nieves JW, Golden AL, Siris E, et al. Teenage and current calcium intake are related to bone mineral density of the hip and forearm in women aged 30–39 years. *Am J Epidemiol* 1995;141:342–351.
80. Baran D, Sorensen A, Grimes J, et al. Dietary modification with dairy products for preventing vertebral bone loss in premenopausal women: a three-year prospective study. *J Clin Endocrinol Metab* 1990;70:264–270.
81. Aloia JF, Vaswani A, Yeh JK, et al. Calcium supplementation with and without hormone replacement therapy to prevent postmenopausal bone loss. *Ann Intern Med* 1994;120:97–103.
82. Riis B, Thomsen K, Christiansen C. Does calcium supplementation prevent postmenopausal bone loss? A double-blind, controlled clinical study. *N Engl J Med* 1987;316:173–177.
83. Elders PJ, Netelenbos JC, Lips P, et al. Calcium supplementation reduces vertebral bone loss in perimenopausal women: a controlled trial in 248 women between 46 and 55 years of age. *J Clin Endocrinol Metab* 1991;73:533–540.
84. McKane WR, Khosla S, Egan KS, et al. Role of calcium intake in modulating age-related increases in parathyroid function and bone resorption. *J Clin Endocrinol Metab* 1996;81:1699–1703.
85. Storm D, Eslin R, Porter ES, et al. Calcium supplementation prevents seasonal bone loss and changes in biochemical markers of bone turnover in elderly New England women: a randomized placebo-controlled trial. *J Clin Endocrinol Metab* 1998;83:3817–3825.
86. Recker RR, Hinders S, Davies KM, et al. Correcting calcium nutritional deficiency prevents spine fractures in elderly women. *J Bone Miner Res* 1996;11:1961–1966.
87. Chapuy MC, Arlot ME, Duboeuf F, et al. Vitamin D_3 and calcium to prevent hip fractures in the elderly women. *N Engl J Med* 1992;327:1637–1642.
88. Reid IR, Ibbertson HK. Calcium supplements in the prevention of steroid-induced osteoporosis. *Am J Clin Nutr* 1986;44:287–290.
89. Sambrook P, Birmingham J, Kelly P, et al. Prevention of corticosteroid osteoporosis. A comparison of calcium, calcitriol, and calcitonin. *N Engl J Med* 1993;328:1747–1752.
90. Roux C, Oriente P, Laan R, et al. Randomized trial of effect of cyclical etidronate in the prevention of corticosteroid-induced bone loss. Ciblos Study Group. *J Clin Endocrinol Metab* 1998;83:1128–1133.
91. Adachi JD, Bensen WG, Brown J, et al. Intermittent etidronate therapy to prevent corticosteroid-induced osteoporosis. *N Engl J Med* 1997;337:382–387.
92. Cohen S, Levy RM, Keller M, et al. Risedronate therapy prevents corticosteroid-induced bone loss: a twelve-month, multicenter, randomized, double-blind, placebo-controlled, parallel-group study. *Arthritis Rheum* 1999;42:2309–2318.
93. Favus MJ. *Primer on the metabolic bone diseases and disorders of mineral metabolism*. Philadelphia: Lippincott–Raven, 1996.
94. McKenna MJ. Osteoporosis prevention: from vitamin D to HRT. *Ir J Med Sci* 1997;166:143–148.
95. Cummings SR, Browner WS, Bauer D, et al. Endogenous hormones and the risk of hip and vertebral fractures among older women. Study of Osteoporotic Fractures Research Group. *N Engl J Med* 1998;339:733–738.
96. LeBoff MS, Kohlmeier L, Hurwitz S, et al. Occult vitamin D deficiency in postmenopausal US women with acute hip fracture. *JAMA* 1999;281:1505–1511.
97. Institute of Medicine. *Dietary reference intakes: the role of calcium and vitamin D in the prevention and treatment of osteoporosis*. Washington, DC: National Academy Press, 1997.
98. Tsurukami H, Nakamura T, Suzuki K, et al. A novel synthetic vitamin D analogue, 2 beta-(3-hydroxy propoxy)1 alpha, 25-dihydroxyvitamin D_3 (ED-71), increases bone mass by stimulating the bone formation in normal and ovariectomized rats. *Calcif Tissue Int* 1994;54:142–149.
99. Shiraishi A, Takeda S, Masaki T, et al. Alfacalcidol inhibits bone resorption and stimulates formation in an ovariectomized rat model of osteoporosis: distinct actions from estrogen. *J Bone Miner Res* 2000;15:770–779.
100. Tetlow LC, Woolley DE. The effects of 1 alpha, 25-dihydroxyvitamin D(3) on matrix metalloproteinase and prostaglandin E(2) production by cells of the rheumatoid lesion. *Arthritis Res* 1999;1:63–70.
101. Suda T. The role of 1 alpha, 25-dihydroxyvitamin D_3 in the myeloid cell differentiation. *Proc Soc Exp Biol Med* 1989;191:214–220.
102. Lemire JM. Immunomodulatory role of 1,25 dihydroxyvitamin D_3. *J Cell Biochem* 1992;49:26–31.
103. Gerstenfeld LC, Kelly CM, von Deck M, Lian JB. Effect of 1,25 dihydroxyvitamin D_3 on induction of chondrocyte maturation in culture: extracellular matrix gene expression and morphology. *Endocrinology* 1990;126:1599–1609.

104. Lakatos P, Nagy Z, Kiss L, et al. Prevention of corticosteroid-induced osteoporosis by alfacalcidol. *Z Rheumatol* 2000;59[Suppl 1]:48–52.
105. Reginster JY, Kuntz D, Verdickt W, et al. Prophylactic use of alfacalcidol in corticosteroid-induced osteoporosis. *Osteoporos Int* 1999;9:75–81.
106. Recommendations for the prevention and treatment of glucocorticoid-induced osteoporosis: 2001 update. American College of Rheumatology Ad Hoc Committee on Glucocorticoid-Induced Osteoporosis. *Arthritis Rheum* 2001;44:1496–1503.
107. Goemaere S, Ackerman C, Goethals K, et al. Onset of symptoms of rheumatoid arthritis in relation to age, sex and menopausal transition. *J Rheumatol* 1990;17:1620–1622.
108. Kuiper S, van Gestel AM, Swinkels HL, et al. Influence of sex, age, and menopausal state on the course of early rheumatoid arthritis. *J Rheumatol* 2001;28:1809–1816.
109. Wluka AE, Cicuttini FM, Spector TD. Menopause, estrogens and arthritis. *Maturitas* 2000;35:183–199.
110. Holmdahl R, Jansson L, Meyerson B, Klareskog L. Oestrogen induced suppression of collagen arthritis: I. Long term oestradiol treatment of DBA/1 mice reduces severity and incidence of arthritis and decreases the anti type II collagen immune response. *Clin Exp Immunol* 1987;70:372–378.
111. Ershler WB, Harman SM, Keller ET. Immunologic aspects of osteoporosis. *Dev Comp Immunol* 1997;21:487–499.
112. Manolagas SC. Role of cytokines in bone resorption. *Bone* 1995;17[Suppl 2]:63S–67S.
113. Papanicolaou DA, Wilder RL, Manolagas SC, Chrousos GP. The pathophysiologic roles of interleukin-6 in human disease. *Ann Intern Med* 1998;128:127–137.
114. Rogers A, Saleh G, Hannon RA, et al. Circulating estradiol and osteoprotegerin as determinants of bone turnover and bone density in postmenopausal women. *J Clin Endocrinol Metab* 2002;87:4470–4475.
115. Effects of hormone therapy on bone mineral density: results from the postmenopausal estrogen/progestin interventions (PEPI) trial. The Writing Group for the PEPI. *JAMA* 1996;276:1389–1396.
116. Lukert BP, Johnson BE, Robinson RG. Estrogen and progesterone replacement therapy reduces glucocorticoid-induced bone loss. *J Bone Miner Res* 1992;7:1063–1069.
117. Sambrook P, Birmingham J, Champion D, et al. Postmenopausal bone loss in rheumatoid arthritis: effect of estrogens and androgens. *J Rheumatol* 1992;19:357–361.
118. Studd JW, Savvas M, Johnson M. Correction of corticosteroid-induced osteoporosis by percutaneous hormone implants. *Lancet* 1989;1:339.
119. Hall GM, Spector TD, Delmas PD. Markers of bone metabolism in postmenopausal women with rheumatoid arthritis. Effects of glucocorticoids and hormone replacement therapy. *Arthritis Rheum* 1995;38:902–906.
120. Hall GM, Daniels M, Doyle DV, Spector TD. Effect of hormone replacement therapy on bone mass in rheumatoid arthritis patients treated with and without steroids. *Arthritis Rheum* 1994;37:1499–1505.
121. Writing Group for the Women's Health Initiative Investigators. Risks and benefits of estrogen plus progestin in healthy postmenopausal women: principal results from the Women's Health Initiative randomized controlled trial. *JAMA* 2002;288:321–333.
122. Grady D, Herrington D, Bittner V, et al. HERS Research Group. Cardiovascular disease outcomes during 6.8 years of hormone therapy: Heart and Estrogen/Progestin Replacement Study follow-up (HERS II). *JAMA* 2002;288:49–57.
123. Hulley S, Furberg C, Barrett-Connor E, et al. HERS Research Group. Noncardiovascular disease outcomes during 6.8 years of hormone therapy: Heart and Estrogen/Progestin Replacement Study follow-up (HERS II). *JAMA* 2002;288:58–66.
124. Grecu EO, Weinshelbaum A, Simmons R. Effective therapy of glucocorticoid-induced osteoporosis with medroxyprogesterone acetate. *Calcif Tissue Int* 1990;46:294–299.
125. Reid IR, Wattie DJ, Evans MC, Stapleton JP. Testosterone therapy in glucocorticoid-treated men. *Arch Intern Med* 1996;156:1173–1177.
126. Heaney RP, Draper MW. Raloxifene and estrogen: comparative bone-remodeling kinetics. *J Clin Endocrinol Metab* 1997;82:3425–3429.
127. Delmas PD, Bjarnason NH, Mitlak BH, et al. Effects of raloxifene on bone mineral density, serum cholesterol concentrations, and uterine endometrium in postmenopausal women. *N Engl J Med* 1997;337:1641–1647.
128. Ettinger B, Black DM, Mitlak BH, et al. Reduction of vertebral fracture risk in postmenopausal women with osteoporosis treated with raloxifene: results from a 3-year randomized clinical trial. Multiple Outcomes of Raloxifene Evaluation (MORE) Investigators. *JAMA* 1999;282:637–645.
129. Delmas PD, Ensrud KE, Adachi JD, et al. Multiple Outcomes of Raloxifene Evaluation Investigators. Efficacy of raloxifene on vertebral fracture risk reduction in postmenopausal women with osteoporosis: four-year results from a randomized clinical trial. *J Clin Endocrinol Metab* 2002;87:3609–3617.
130. Sewell K, Schein JR. Osteoporosis therapies for rheumatoid arthritis patients: minimizing gastrointestinal side effects. *Semin Arthritis Rheum* 2001;30:288–297.
131. van Rooijen N. Extracellular and intracellular action of clodronate in osteolytic bone diseases? A hypothesis. *Calcif Tissue Int* 1993;52:407–410.
132. Boonekamp PM, van der Wee-Pals LJ, van Wijk-van Lennep MM, et al. Two modes of action of bisphosphonates on osteoclastic resorption of mineralized matrix. *Bone Miner* 1986;1:27–39.
133. Luckman SP, Hughes DE, Coxon FP, et al. Nitrogen-containing bisphosphonates inhibit the mevalonate pathway and prevent post-translational prenylation of GTP-binding proteins, including Ras. *J Bone Miner Res* 1998;13:581–589.
134. Frith JC, Monkkonen J, Blackburn GM, et al. Clodronate and liposome-encapsulated clodronate are metabolized to a toxic ATP analog, adenosine 5'-(beta, gamma-dichloromethylene) triphosphate, by mammalian cells in vitro. *J Bone Miner Res* 1997;12:1358–1367.
135. Fisher JE, Rogers MJ, Halasy JM, et al. Alendronate mechanism of action: geranylgeranyl, an intermediate in the mevalonate pathway, prevents inhibition of osteoclast formation, bone resorption, and kinase activation in vitro. *Proc Natl Acad Sci U S A* 1999;96:133–138.
136. Russell RG, Rogers MJ, Frith JC, et al. The pharmacology of bisphosphonates and new insights into their mechanisms of action. *J Bone Miner Res* 1999;14[Suppl 2]:53–65.
137. Jenkins EA, Walker-Bone KE, Wood A, et al. The prevention of corticosteroid-induced bone loss with intermittent cyclical etidronate. *Scand J Rheumatol* 1999;28:152–156.
138. Adachi JD, Roux C, Pitt PI, et al. A pooled data analysis on the use of intermittent cyclical etidronate therapy for the prevention and treatment of corticosteroid induced bone loss. *J Rheumatol* 2000;27:2424–2431.
139. Liberman UA, Weiss SR, Broll J, et al. Effect of oral alendronate on bone mineral density and the incidence of fractures in postmenopausal osteoporosis. The Alendronate Phase III Osteoporosis Treatment Study Group. *N Engl J Med* 1995;333:1437–1443.
140. Black DM, Cummings SR, Karpf DB, et al. Randomized trial of effect of alendronate on risk of fracture in women with existing vertebral fractures. Fracture Intervention Trial Research Group. *Lancet* 1996;348:1535–1541.
141. Cummings SR, Black DM, Thompson DE, et al. Effect of alendronate on risk of fracture in women with low bone density but without vertebral fractures: results from the Fracture Intervention Trial. *JAMA* 1998;280:2077–2082.
142. Orwoll E, Ettinger M, Weiss S, et al. Alendronate for the treatment of osteoporosis in men. *N Engl J Med* 2000;343:604–610.
143. Saag KG, Emkey R, Schnitzer TJ, et al. Alendronate for the prevention and treatment of glucocorticoid-induced osteoporosis. Glucocorticoid-Induced Osteoporosis Intervention Study Group. *N Engl J Med* 1998;339:292–299.
144. Schnitzer T, Bone HG, Crepaldi G, et al. Therapeutic equivalence of alendronate 70 mg once-weekly and alendronate 10 mg daily in the treatment of osteoporosis. Alendronate Once-Weekly Study Group. *Aging (Milano)* 2000;12:1–12.
145. Reginster J, Minne HW, Sorensen OH, et al. Randomized trial of the effects of risedronate on vertebral fractures in women with established postmenopausal osteoporosis. Vertebral Efficacy with Risedronate Therapy (VERT) Study Group. *Osteoporos Int* 2000;11:83–91.
146. Reginster J, Minne HW, Sorensen OH, et al. Randomized trial of the effects of risedronate on vertebral fractures in women with established postmenopausal osteoporosis. Vertebral Efficacy with Risedronate Therapy (VERT) Study Group. *Osteoporos Int* 2000;11:83–91.
147. McClung MR, Geusens P, Miller PD, et al. Hip Intervention Program Study Group. Effect of risedronate on the risk of hip fracture in elderly women. Hip Intervention Program Study Group. *N Engl J Med* 2001;344:333–340.
148. Eastell R, Devogelaer JP, Peel NF, et al. Prevention of bone loss with risedronate in glucocorticoid-treated rheumatoid arthritis patients. *Osteoporos Int* 2000;11:331–337.
149. Cohen S, Levy RM, Keller M, et al. Risedronate therapy prevents corticosteroid-induced bone loss: a twelve-month, multicenter, randomized, double-blind, placebo-controlled, parallel-group study. *Arthritis Rheum* 1999;42:2309–2318.
150. Reid DM, Hughes RA, Laan RF, et al. Efficacy and safety of daily risedronate in the treatment of corticosteroid-induced osteoporosis in men and women: a randomized trial. European Corticosteroid-Induced Osteoporosis Treatment Study. *J Bone Miner Res* 2000;15:1006–1013.
151. Wallach S, Cohen S, Reid DM, et al. Effects of risedronate treatment on bone density and vertebral fracture in patients on corticosteroid therapy. *Calcif Tissue Int* 2000;67:277–285.
152. Reid DM, Adami S, Devogelaer JP, Chines AA. Risedronate increases bone density and reduces vertebral fracture risk within one year in men on corticosteroid therapy. *Calcif Tissue Int* 2001;69:242–247.
153. Peretz A, Body JJ, Dumon JC, et al. Cyclical pamidronate infusions in postmenopausal osteoporosis. *Maturitas* 1996;25:69–75.
154. Reid IR, Wattie DJ, Evans MC, et al. Continuous therapy with pamidronate, a potent bisphosphonate, in postmenopausal osteoporosis. *J Clin Endocrinol Metab* 1994;79:1595–1599.
155. Reid I, Reid IR, Brown JP, et al. Intravenous zoledronic acid in postmenopausal women with low bone mineral density. *N Engl J Med* 2002;346:653–661.
156. Bone HG, Greenspan SL, McKeever C, et al. Alendronate and estrogen effects in postmenopausal women with low bone mineral density. Alendronate/Estrogen Study Group. *J Clin Endocrinol Metab* 2000;85:720–726.
157. Lindsay R, Cosman F, Lobo RA, et al. Addition of alendronate to ongoing hormone replacement therapy in the treatment of osteoporosis: a randomized, controlled clinical trial. *J Clin Endocrinol Metab* 1999;84:3076–3081.
158. Harris ST, Eriksen EF, Davidson M, et al. Effect of combined risedronate and hormone replacement therapies on bone mineral density in postmenopausal women. *J Clin Endocrinol Metab* 2001;86:1890–1897.
159. Johnell O, Scheele WH, Lu Y, et al. Additive effects of raloxifene and alendronate on bone density and biochemical markers of bone remodeling in postmenopausal women with osteoporosis. *J Clin Endocrinol Metab* 2002;87:985–992.
160. Wimalawansa SJ. Prevention and treatment of osteoporosis: efficacy of combination of hormone replacement therapy with other antiresorptive agents. *J Clin Densitom* 2000;3:187–201.
161. Jilka RL, Weinstein RS, Bellido T, et al. Increased bone formation by prevention of osteoblast apoptosis with parathyroid hormone. *J Clin Invest* 1999;104:439–446.

162. Kurland ES, Cosman F, McMahon DJ, et al. Parathyroid hormone as a therapy for idiopathic osteoporosis in men: effects on bone mineral density and bone markers. *J Clin Endocrinol Metab* 2000;85:3069–3076.
163. Rittmaster RS, Bolognese M, Ettinger MP, et al. Enhancement of bone mass in osteoporotic women with parathyroid hormone followed by alendronate. *J Clin Endocrinol Metab* 2000;85:2129–2134.
164. Lindsay R, Nieves J, Formica C, et al. Randomized controlled study of effect of parathyroid hormone on vertebral-bone mass and fracture incidence among postmenopausal women on oestrogen with osteoporosis. *Lancet* 1997;350:550–555.
165. Neer RM, Arnaud CD, Zanchetta JR, et al. Effect of parathyroid hormone (1-34) on fractures and bone mineral density in postmenopausal women with osteoporosis. *N Engl J Med* 2001;344:1434–1441.
166. Lane NE, Sanchez S, Modin GW, et al. Parathyroid hormone treatment can reverse corticosteroid-induced osteoporosis. Results of a randomized controlled clinical trial. *J Clin Invest* 1998;102:1627–1633.
167. Lane NE, Sanchez S, Modin GW, et al. Bone mass continues to increase at the hip after parathyroid hormone treatment is discontinued in glucocorticoid-induced osteoporosis: results of a randomized controlled clinical trial. *J Bone Miner Res* 2000;15:944–951.
168. Caniggia A, Gennari C, Bencini M, et al. Calcium metabolism and 47-calcium kinetics before and after long-term thyrocalcitonin treatment in senile osteoporosis. *Clin Sci* 1970;38:397–407.
169. Gruber HE, Ivey JL, Baylink DJ, et al. Long-term calcitonin therapy in postmenopausal osteoporosis. *Metabolism* 1984;33:295–303.
170. Milhaud G, Talbot JN, Coutris G. Calcitonin treatment of post-menopausal osteoporosis. Evaluation of efficacy by principal components analysis. *Biomedicine* 1975;22:223–232.
171. Mazzuoli GF, Passeri M, Gennari C, et al. Effects of salmon calcitonin in postmenopausal osteoporosis: a controlled double-blind clinical study. *Calcif Tissue Int* 1986;38:3–8.
172. Mazzuoli GF, Tabolli S, Bigi F, et al. Effects of salmon calcitonin on the bone loss induced by ovariectomy. *Calcif Tissue Int* 1990;47:209–214.
173. Rico H, Revilla M, Hernandez ER, et al. Total and regional bone mineral content and fracture rate in postmenopausal osteoporosis treated with salmon calcitonin: a prospective study. *Calcif Tissue Int* 1995;56:181–185.
174. Kanis JA, Johnell O, Gullberg B, et al. Evidence for efficacy of drugs affecting bone metabolism in preventing hip fracture. *BMJ* 1992;305:1124–1128.
175. Overgaard K, Hansen MA, Jensen SB, Christiansen C. Effect of salcatonin given intranasally on bone mass and fracture rates in established osteoporosis: a dose-response study. *BMJ* 1992;305:556–561.
176. Chesnut CH III, Silverman S, Andriano K, et al. A randomized trial of nasal spray salmon calcitonin in postmenopausal women with established osteoporosis: the prevent recurrence of osteoporotic fractures study. PROOF Study Group. *Am J Med* 2000;109:267–276.
177. Montemurro L, Schiraldi G, Fraioli P, et al. Prevention of corticosteroid-induced osteoporosis with salmon calcitonin in sarcoid patients. *Calcif Tissue Int* 1991;49:71–76.
178. Luengo M, Pons F, Martinez de Osaba MJ, Picado C. Prevention of further bone mass loss by nasal calcitonin in patients on long term glucocorticoid therapy for asthma: a two-year follow-up study. *Thorax* 1994;49:1099–1102.
179. Sambrook P, Birmingham J, Kelly P, et al. Prevention of corticosteroid osteoporosis. A comparison of calcium, calcitriol, and calcitonin. *N Engl J Med* 1993;328:1747–1752.
180. Ringe JD, Welzel D. Salmon calcitonin in the therapy of corticoid-induced osteoporosis. *Eur J Clin Pharmacol* 1987;33:35–39.
181. Pun KK, Chan LW. Analgesic effect of intranasal salmon calcitonin in the treatment of osteoporotic vertebral fractures. *Clin Ther* 1989;11:205–209.
182. Lyritis GP, Paspati I, Karachalios T, et al. Pain relief from nasal salmon calcitonin in osteoporotic vertebral crush fractures. A double blind, placebo-controlled clinical study. *Acta Orthop Scand Suppl* 1997;275:112–114.

CHAPTER 48

Depression

Jerry C. Parker and James R. Slaughter

Depression is a common worldwide health care problem. In the United States, the point prevalence of major depression for men ranges from 2% to 3%; the lifetime prevalence ranges from 7% to 12% (1). The point prevalence of major depression for women ranges from 5% to 9%; the lifetime prevalence ranges from 20% to 25% (1). The reason for the difference in the prevalence of major depression between men and women is not entirely clear, although gender-related variations in hormonal patterns, social roles, and socioeconomic burdens all have been suggested as potential explanations.

The same general prevalence patterns for major depression appear to hold for persons with rheumatoid arthritis (RA) as for the broader population, but the prevalence patterns in RA tend to be exacerbated. Subpopulations of persons with RA vary widely in terms of sociodemographic variables (e.g., education and income), so generalizations about the prevalence of major depression in RA must be made with caution. Indeed, studies have yielded highly discrepant findings. On the low side, Fifield et al. (2), on the basis of a national cohort study, reported that the point prevalence of major depression for persons with RA was only 3%. Conversely, Rimón and Laakso (3) reported that as many as 80% of persons with RA showed symptoms of depression. Clearly, sampling methods, diagnostic criteria, and measurement strategies vary widely across studies, which contributes to the diverse findings. Based on a review of studies that used structured diagnostic interviews, Creed and Ash (4) estimated the point prevalence of major depression in RA to be between 17% and 27%. A metaanalysis by Dickens et al. (5) examined the association between depression and the diagnosis of RA; these authors found small to moderate effect sizes, indicating that depression is more common in persons with RA than in healthy comparison groups. Not surprisingly, a high pain level was consistently found to be associated with higher depression in RA.

RISK FACTORS

A key risk factor for major depression is a history of previous episodes (6). With a history of one previous episode of major depression, the probability of a second episode increases to approximately 50%. With a history of two previous episodes of major depression, the probability of a third episode increases to approximately 70%. With three previous episodes of major depression, the probability of recurrence is approximately 90%. Similarly, a history of past suicide attempts greatly increases the risk of subsequent episodes of major depression (1).

Family history is another risk factor for major depression. If a person has a first-degree biologic relative with a history of major depression, the probability of a diagnosis of major depression is 1.5 to 3.0 times higher than for the general population (7). Nevertheless, the evidence for a genetic linkage is not definitive; child-rearing practices, nutritional circumstances, and socioeconomic conditions, among others, are all environmental factors that might account for the higher prevalence of major depression among first-degree relatives. Female gender is another key risk factor for major depression; women also are three to four times more likely than men to have RA. Hence, one of the strongest risk factors for major depression (female gender) is heavily overrepresented within the RA population.

Medical comorbidity is an additional risk factor for major depression (8). Many persons with RA (because of the typical age of onset) encounter other concomitant health problems and must cope with chronic pain, loss of mobility, and gradually increasing disability. Specifically, Katz and Yelin (9) have shown that loss of valued activities is a significant predictor of depression in persons with RA. Similarly, Newman et al. (10) found that physical disability, longer disease duration, greater social isolation, and greater economic distress were all significantly related to depressed mood in persons with RA. Interestingly, Wright et al. (11) found that younger persons with RA were more likely to report depression than were persons of advancing age. Specifically, persons with RA who were age 45 or younger reported significantly more depression than those who were older, even after controlling for gender, marital status, antidepressant medication, arthritis medication, functional class, and disease duration. Younger persons are more likely to be raising children and coping with the stresses of the workforce, and Turner and Beiser (12) have shown that stressful life events themselves are risk factors for major depression. Lastly, Revenson et al. (13) have shown that lack of social support is related to reports of depression in persons with arthritis; numerous factors (e.g., decreased mobility, low income, and reduced self-esteem) can limit social contact for persons with RA.

DEPRESSION AND DISABILITY

RA is a potentially disabling condition in its own right (14), but depression as a comorbidity can make the situation even worse (15). Wells et al. (16) found that persons who were depressed exhibited higher levels of disability than did persons with eight other chronic medical conditions, including arthritis. Von Korff et al. (17) found a significant association between level of depression and level of functional disability; this association also appears to hold for persons with RA. For example, McFarlane and Brooks (18) found that psychological factors were better predictors of disability in persons with RA than were conventional disease activity measures. Katz and Yelin (19) found that functional status was significantly more impaired for persons with RA who reported depression than for persons with RA who did not report depression. In addition, several studies have shown that environmental factors, such as loss of employment or economic distress, can exacerbate depressed mood (10,20). Overall, the evidence is strong for a significant association between depression and higher levels of disability in RA.

DEPRESSION AND HEALTH CARE COSTS

The available data reveal that depression is an extremely costly condition in the United States. Even in 1980, a population-based study revealed an estimated 4.8 million cases of major depression over a 6-month interval, including 16,000 suicides (21); these researchers also reported 7.4 million hospital days and 13 million annual outpatient visits. Abraham et al. (22) estimated the annual cost of depression in the United States to be approximately $29 billion.

The efficient delivery of self-management and educational programs has been shown to be associated with lower health care costs. For example, Lorig and Fries (23) developed an Arthritis Self-Management Program for persons with arthritis that included information about the nature of arthritis, medications, exercises, relaxation techniques, joint protection, and interactions of patients with physicians, among other topics. Participants in the Arthritis Self-Management Program had a 40% reduction in outpatient visits, which translated into $648 in savings per patient over a 4-year interval (24). This finding by Lorig et al. (24) is consistent with the Hawaii Medicaid Study, which demonstrated that patients with chronic diseases, including RA, revealed lower health care costs after brief psychoeducational interventions (25). Therefore, the evidence suggests that appropriate treatment of depression and other related psychological conditions has the potential to reduce health care costs for persons with RA.

SCARRING HYPOTHESIS

One key reason that early recognition and treatment of depression is so important involves what has been described as the *scarring phenomenon*. Lewinsohn et al. (26) described a phenomenon in which the long-term consequences of an episode of major depression may exist for a substantial period of time after the original depressive episode has resolved. Specifically, Fifield et al. (27) demonstrated that persons with RA with a past history of depression reported higher levels of pain than persons without a past history of depression, even after the original depression was resolved. This interesting finding illustrates the importance of depression management for long-term clinical outcomes in RA.

NEUROBIOLOGY

The neurobiology of depressive disorders is an area of rapidly emerging scientific discovery. In the 1960s, investigators were able to measure catecholamine metabolites in body fluids and indoleamine metabolites in cerebrospinal fluid, which opened up interesting lines of investigation. Indeed, the central role of norepinephrine (NE) and serotonin [5-hydroxytryptamine (5-HT)] in the pathophysiology of depressive disorders remains unquestioned, although there is increasing evidence that dopamine (DA) also may play an important role in the development of some forms of depression (28). Current research and theory on the neurobiology of depression, however, do not tend to focus exclusively on the role of single neurotransmitters. Instead, there is increasing emphasis on neurobehavioral systems, neural circuits, and more intricate regulatory mechanisms (28). New lines of research on the etiology of depression involve postsynaptic receptors, presynaptic autoreceptors or heteroreceptors, second messengers, and gene transcription factors (28). Studies of depressed persons also have revealed alterations in sleep neurophysiology, disruption of circadian rhythms, structural changes in the brain (as revealed by computed tomography and magnetic resonance imaging scans), and alterations in cerebral metabolism (as revealed by positron emission tomography scans) (28). The role of stress mechanisms, learned helplessness, and abusive conditions in early life (and their neurobiologic sequelae) are additional areas of active research in the context of depressive disorders. Three broad research domains involving the neurobiology of depression are biogenic amine dysfunction, alterations of hormonal regulation, and immune system dysregulation.

Biogenic Amine Dysfunction

The evidence is clear that some persons with depression manifest one or more abnormalities of monoamine neurotransmission (28). Central nervous system 5-HT and the catecholamines (NE and DA) are important to both mood regulation and pain modulation. Specifically, low 5-HT and low NE-DA have been found to be associated with depression (28); 5-HT also has been found to be low in the brains of patients who have committed suicide (29). Brain stem centers that produce 5-HT, NE, and DA down-regulate nociception, which has relevance for persons who experience chronic pain (such as those with RA). Specifically, patients with chronic pain are known to have higher rates of depression (30).

Alterations of Hormonal Regulation

Hypothalamic-pituitary-adrenal (HPA) mechanisms are centrally related to the mammalian response to stress. Not surprisingly, severe depression in some patients has been shown to be associated with cortisol dysregulation, although cortisol has not been found to be universally suppressed in depressed persons who have been administered dexamethasone (28). Increased cortisol secretion is more likely in elderly patients and those who manifest psychotic features; hypercortisolism is a common feature in melancholic depression (28). Evidence also exists suggesting that some depressed patients show thyroid dysfunction, blunted growth hormone response to clonidine (an α_2-receptor agonist), low somatostatin levels in cerebrospinal fluid, and blunted prolactin response to 5-HT agonists (28); these findings further support the apparent involvement of hormonal dysregulation in some depressed patients.

Immune System Dysregulation

Research has shown that some persons with depressive disorders present with immunologic abnormalities, such as decreased lymphocyte proliferation, in response to mitogens and other forms of cellular immunity (28). A few studies also have examined cytokine regulation in major depression. Maes et al. (31) observed elevated plasma concentrations and increased *in vitro*

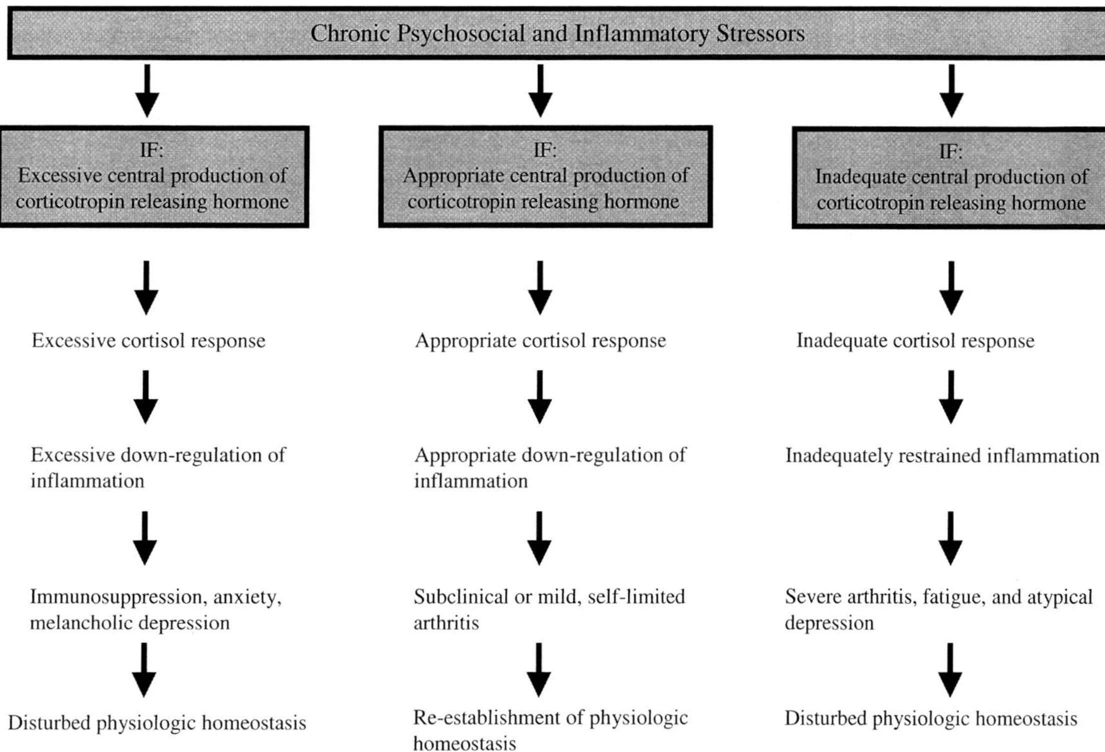

Figure 48.1. Model of possible relationships among stress response, depression, and arthritis susceptibility. (Adapted from Cash JM, Wilder RL. Stress, depression, and rheumatoid arthritis. *Contemp Intern Med* 1991;3:13–16.)

production of interleukin-1 (IL-1) in patients with major depression. Similar elevations have been reported for IL-6 (32). Clearly, symptoms that are common in depression (e.g., decreased appetite, decreased libido, and increased sleep) are similar to the known effects of IL-1 (33); tumor necrosis factor α also is known to induce depressive-like symptoms of anorexia and fatigue (34). Although anti–tumor necrosis factor antibodies have been used in the treatment of RA, the effects on mood and other psychiatric symptoms have not yet been determined (34). Dantzer et al. (35) have reviewed an extensive literature on the possible association between various cytokines and depression; these authors concluded that the evidence for causative linkage was insufficient. Hence, the role of immune system dysregulation in the pathophysiology of depressive disorders remains speculative (34).

Stress Response, Depression, and Arthritis

Cash and Wilder (36) have provided an interesting framework for conceptualizing the manifestation of depression in RA. These authors point out that the HPA axis is highly relevant for both RA disease characteristics and the manifestation of depressive symptoms. Specifically, the HPA axis is activated by a wide range of stressors, including biologic, psychological, sociologic, and environmental factors. The hypothalamus produces corticotropin-releasing hormone (CRH), which, in turn, activates the sympathetic-adrenal-medullary axis and induces the anterior pituitary to release adrenocorticotropic hormone (ACTH) into the bloodstream; ACTH stimulates the adrenal cortex to produce cortisol. As cortisol levels increase, feedback mechanisms operate to down-regulate the production of both CRH and ACTH.

Cash and Wilder (36) suggested that dysregulation of the HPA axis may contribute to both disease manifestations and depressive patterns in RA (Fig. 48.1). If stressors result in excessive central production of CRH, there may be the occurrence of excessive cortisol, excessive down-regulation of inflammation, and the appearance of depressive symptoms, characterized by hyperarousal, insomnia, and agitation. If stressors result in inadequate central production of CRH, there may be the occurrence of inadequate cortisol, inadequately restrained inflammation, and the appearance of depressive symptoms, characterized by hypoarousal, excessive sleep, and passivity. The implication is that RA may represent a multisystem syndrome in which disease activity and depressive mood are linked via neurohormonal pathways.

DIAGNOSTIC CONSIDERATIONS

Depression is a distinctly underdiagnosed condition, especially in general medical settings (8). Possibly, as many as 50% of cases of depression are not diagnosed by general medical practitioners working in primary care environments (37), and there is no evidence that rheumatologists are any more effective in the diagnosis of depression than are their primary care colleagues. In the context of RA, the symptoms of depression may be dismissed by some practitioners as simply secondary to the disease process itself. Once present, however, depression does not necessarily subside, even after the remission of RA; direct treatment for depression is frequently required.

Several diagnostic challenges exist for practitioners who care for persons with RA. For example, some practitioners may simply use a depressed versus nondepressed categorization, which is not adequate for the formulation of effective treatment strategies. In addition, the potential overlap of symptoms between depression and RA can be confusing. Symptoms such as fatigue and loss of energy may be attributable to either depression or RA. Regardless, a correct diagnosis is required for the effective management of depression.

DEPRESSION SUBTYPES

The fourth edition of the *Diagnostic and Statistical Manual of Mental Disorders* (7) provides the necessary framework for the diagnosis of specific forms of depression; several subtypes must be distinguished. An overview of the characteristic symptoms of selected depressive disorders is provided in Table 48.1.

Uncomplicated Bereavement

A depressive syndrome sometimes emerges after the death of a loved one or some other profound personal loss. In such situations, depression can be a normal, but temporary, reaction to the loss. The symptoms of bereavement are sometimes severe and may include feelings of guilt about things left undone or unsaid during a loved one's life. Sometimes spouses experience a general feeling that they no longer wish to live. Prolonged functional impairment, however, is uncommon, and the depressive symptoms must be clearly associated with a major personal loss. Although there may be a slight delay in the emergence of depressive symptoms after a personal loss, the delay is rarely longer than 3 months.

Adjustment Reaction with Depressed Mood

Depressive symptoms also can occur as a reaction to other identifiable life stressors. The adjustment reaction must occur within 3 months of the onset of the stressor and must last no longer than 6 months. The depressive reaction must be sufficiently severe to impair occupational or social functioning or must be distinctly overreactive in relation to the stressor itself. Symptoms of an adjustment reaction typically include depressed mood, tearfulness, and feelings of hopelessness. However, the reaction must not be the person's characteristic mode of responding to a stressful event (i.e., long-standing personality trait).

Dysthymic Disorder

Dysthymic disorder is characterized by chronic depressive symptoms on a near-daily basis. Indeed, to meet criteria for dysthymia, a person cannot be free of depressive symptoms for more than 2 months during the previous 2 years. In addition, at least two of the following symptoms must be present: (a) poor appetite or overeating, (b) insomnia or hypersomnia, (c) fatigue, (d) low self-esteem, (e) poor concentration or indecisiveness, or (f) feeling of hopelessness. Persons with dysthymic disorder typically do not experience severe impairment of social or occupational functioning; hospitalization is rare. In dysthymia, depressive symptoms becomes chronic, to the point of appearing to be the person's usual manner of responding to the stresses of everyday life.

Major Depression

The diagnosis of major depression is based on a constellation of nine symptoms: (a) depressed mood, (b) diminished pleasure, (c) significant weight loss or gain, (d) insomnia or hypersomnia, (e) psychomotor agitation or retardation, (f) fatigue or loss of energy, (g) feelings of worthlessness or excessive guilt, (h) diminished ability to think or concentrate, and (i) recurrent thoughts of death. To meet criteria for major depression, there must be a total of five symptoms present out of the constellation of nine, but either depressed mood or diminished pleasure (or both) must always be present. A severe depressive reaction must endure for at least 2 weeks, and there must be evidence of substantial occupational or social dysfunction. Alternative depressive diagnoses must be ruled out.

There are two subtypes of major depression (38). The melancholic subtype is characterized by symptoms of hyperarousal, including ruminative thoughts, anorexia, insomnia, and diurnal mood variation; depressive symptoms are frequently worse in the early morning. The atypical subtype is characterized by a state of hypoarousal, including hyperphagia, hypersomnia, anhedonia, and a worsening of symptoms at night. Consistent with the Cash and Wilder (36) model, the melancholic and atypical subtypes appear to differ in terms of their underlying neurobiologic mechanisms, so they also may differ with regard to their possible associations with RA disease activity.

Depression Due to a General Medical Condition

The symptoms of depression may sometimes be directly attributable to a general medical condition. For example, the depressive affect associated with a high dose of corticosteroid is an example

TABLE 48.1. Characteristic Symptoms of Selected Depressive Disorders

Symptoms	Adjustment Disorder with Depressed Mood[a]	Uncomplicated Bereavement[b]	Dysthymia[c]	Major Depression[d]
Depressed mood	+	+	+	+
Diminished pleasure	+	+		+
Weight or appetite change	+	+	+	+
Sleep disturbance	+	+	+	+
Psychomotor changes				+
Loss of energy	+	+	+	+
Feelings of worthlessness or guilt	+			+
Concentration problems		+	+	+
Thoughts of death				+
Low self-esteem	+		+	+
Hopelessness	+		+	+
Functional impairment	+			+
Identifiable stressor	+	+		+

Note: Refer to the fourth edition of the *Diagnostic and Statistical Manual of Mental Disorders* of the American Psychiatric Association for more complete diagnostic criteria. Listed symptoms are characteristic but not necessarily required or sufficient for the diagnoses.

[a]Either depressed mood *or* diminished pleasure is required for the diagnosis of major depression. Duration must be for a minimum of 2 weeks.

[b]A maladaptive reaction must occur within 3 months after the onset of an identifiable psychosocial stressor and persist for no longer than 6 months.

[c]A full depressive syndrome may occur secondary to the loss of a loved one; duration varies among different cultural groups.

[d]Symptoms must be present for a minimum of 2 years and never absent for more than 2 months.

Adapted form Morrow K, Parker J, Russell J. Clinical implications of depression in rheumatoid arthritis. *Arthritis Care Res* 1994;7:58–63.

of depression due to a general medical condition, although many other examples exist. Purely secondary depressive reactions to the stresses of a medical condition, however, do not meet criteria. There must be a direct biologic link between a disease state or medication side effect and the depressed affect to make a diagnosis of depression due to a general medical condition. A comprehensive list of disease conditions and medications that have been linked to depressed mood is provided by Stoudemire (39).

Bipolar Disorder

In some cases, a depressive manifestation is one phase of a bipolar disorder, which involves a cycling between depressive and manic (or hypomanic) mood states. In the manic-hypomanic phase, patients may present with elevated mood; expansive, grandiose ideation; or extreme irritability. The behavioral manifestations of a manic episode may include an extremely high energy level, decreased need for sleep, and marked impulsivity. In bipolar disorder, severe impairment of occupational, social, and interpersonal functioning is typical, and hospitalization may be needed to prevent harm to self or others. Hence, careful questioning about a history of mania or hypomania is an extremely important component of the diagnostic interview; treatment for bipolar disorder is distinctly different from treatments for other forms of depression. If a history of bipolar disorder is identified, early psychiatric consultation is typically indicated.

TREATMENT

After a diagnosis of depression, a key element in the formulation of a treatment plan is the identification of possible comorbidities or medication side effects that may play an etiologic role. For example, substance use disorders can affect mood. So, if present, substance use disorders should be directly treated. The possibility of various medication side effects also should be carefully considered, as medication changes may be indicated. In addition, optimal management of comorbidities (e.g., RA) should always occur, because improved functional status or decreased pain level can sometimes (but not always) alleviate the symptoms of depression. For example, approximately 20% of persons with RA also meet criteria for fibromyalgia (40), which is a comorbidity that typically requires comprehensive biopsychosocial management in its own right. Interestingly, Ahles et al. (41) have reported that the lifetime occurrence of major depression in primary fibromyalgia syndrome is 34%, which is not substantially different from that found in RA (39%).

Patients who are diagnosed with depression are at heightened risk for suicide (42). Therefore, assessment of suicide potential is a critical obligation for any practitioner who is treating a depressed patient. Risk factors for suicide include hopelessness, medical comorbidity, substance abuse, family history of substance abuse, male gender, white race, psychotic symptoms, living alone, and prior suicide attempts (6). Direct questioning about suicidal ideation, intent, and plans must occur. If suicide risk is found to be high, immediate psychiatric consultation or emergency hospitalization may be indicated.

The treatment of major depression typically proceeds in three phases: the acute phase, the continuation phase, and the maintenance phase. The objective in the acute phase, which typically lasts for 6 to 12 weeks, is to effect a remission of the depressive symptoms. The objective of the continuation phase, which typically lasts for 4 to 9 months, is to avoid relapse and to sustain recovery. The objective of the maintenance phase, which typically lasts for 1 year or longer, is to sustain recovery and to prevent recurrence. For less severe forms of depression, the duration of treatment may be shorter, but the successful management of depression is generally a long-term process.

The four major options for the treatment of major depression are psychological interventions, antidepressant medications, combined psychological and medication approaches, and electroconvulsive therapy (ECT).

Psychological Interventions

The psychological interventions most commonly used for the treatment of depression include cognitive therapy, behavioral therapy, interpersonal therapy, brief dynamic therapy, and marital therapy (6). In general, psychological intervention as the sole treatment for major depression should be used only in relatively mild cases or when antidepressant medications are contraindicated. A metaanalysis by Dobson (43) revealed that 50% of cases of major depression responded effectively to psychotherapy alone, although a skilled practitioner must be available for psychological intervention to be a viable option.

Antidepressant Medication

The key antidepressant medication categories are tricyclic antidepressants (TCAs), selective serotonin reuptake inhibitors (SSRIs), newer non-SSRIs, and monoamine oxidase inhibitors (MAOIs).

TRICYCLIC ANTIDEPRESSANTS

TCAs block the transporter sites for 5-HT and NE and, thereby, inhibit their reuptake. The major TCAs include amitriptyline, desipramine, doxepin, imipramine, nortriptyline, protriptyline, and trimipramine. Hundreds of randomized controlled trials have conclusively demonstrated the efficacy of TCAs for the treatment of major depressive disorder. In adult intent-to-treat studies, TCAs have been shown to induce a clinical response in approximately 50% of cases (6). In TCA versus placebo comparisons, TCAs have been shown to induce a clinical response in approximately 21% to 25% more cases than placebo (6). TCA side effects can include tachycardia, orthostatic hypotension, anticholinergic effects, sedation, weight gain, and mild myoclonus. Amitriptyline and imipramine are tertiary amines metabolized by hepatic cytochrome P450 (CYP) enzymes 1A2, 2C, and 3A4 (44). TCA levels and, therefore, potential side effects, will be increased by inhibitors of these enzymes (Table 48.2). In addition, smoking increases the clearance of TCAs, so doses may need to be higher in smokers to achieve saporific effects and analgesia (44). A discussion of drug metabolism and drug interactions for antidepressants (and other common medications) has been provided by DeVane and Nemeroff (44).

In the context of RA, Frank et al. (45) reported that amitriptyline was equivalent to desipramine and trazodone for the treatment of depression in RA, but amitriptyline was found to be superior to desipramine, trazodone, and placebo in the amelioration of pain. Imipramine (46) and trimipramine (47) have been evaluated in a small series of RA patients, with equivocal results.

SELECTIVE SEROTONIN REUPTAKE INHIBITORS

The major SSRIs include citalopram, escitalopram, fluoxetine, fluvoxamine, paroxetine, and sertraline. SSRIs are the most widely prescribed class of antidepressant medication, due to their efficacy in the treatment of depression in combination with a relatively low side effect profile. In adult intent-to-treat studies, SSRIs induce a clinical response in approximately 50% of cases (6). In SSRI versus placebo trials, SSRIs have been shown to induce a clinical response in approximately 20% to 26% more cases than placebo (6). SSRI side effects can include nausea, vomiting, diarrhea, activation or insomnia, sexual side effects (e.g.,

TABLE 48.2. Overview of Antidepressant Medications

Antidepressant	Cytochrome P450 Inhibition	Initial Dose (Older Adult)	Adult Range (mg/d)	Older Adult Range (mg/d)
TCAs				
Amitriptyline (Elavil)[a]	1A2, 2C, 3A4 (?+)	25 (10)	100–300	25–100
Imipramine (Tofranil)[a]	1A2, 2C, 3A4 (?+)	25 (10)	100–300	25–100
Desipramine (Norpramin)[b]	2D6 (?+)			
Nortriptyline (Pamelor)[b]	2D6 (?+)			
SSRIs[c]				
Citalopram (Celexa)	2D6 (1+)	20 (10)	20–60	10–40
Escitalopram (Lexapro)	2D6 (1+)	10 (5)	10–20	5–10
Fluoxetine (Prozac)	2C (2+), 2D6 (4+), 3A4 (2+)	20 (5)	20–60	5–30
Fluvoxamine (Luvox)	1A2 (4+), 2C (2+), 3A4 (3+)	50 (25)	50–300	50–150
Paroxetine (Paxil)	2D6 (4+)	20 (10)	20–60	20–50
Sertraline (Zoloft)	2C (1+), 2D6 (1+), 3A4 (1+)	25 (25)	50–200	25–150
Newer non-SSRIs[d]				
Bupropion SR (Wellbutrin SR)	2D6 (3+)	150 (100)	300–400	100–300
Venlafaxine XR (Effexor XR)	2D6 (1+)	37.5 (37.5)	75–375	37.5–225
Mirtazapine (Remeron)	0	15 (7.5)	15–45	7.5–30
Nefazodone (Serzone)	3A (4+)	50 (50)	150–600	50–300
Trazodone (Desyrel)	3A (4+)	50 (50)	75–300	75–200
MAOIs[e]				
Phenelzine (Nardil)	NA	15 (7.5)	15–90	7.5–45
Tranylcypromine (Parnate)	NA	10 (5)	30–60	5–30
Moclobemide (Manerix)	NA	150 (75)	300–600	75–300

?+, suggestive positive influence, but not definitive; 0, unknown or insignificant; 1+, mild and usually insignificant; 2+, moderate and possibly significant; 3+, moderate and usually significant; 4+, potent; MAOIs, monoamine oxidase inhibitors; NA, not available to authors; SR, sustained-release; SSRIs, selective serotonin reuptake inhibitors; TCAs, tricyclic antidepressants; XR, extended-release.

[a]Tertiary amine. Side effects include anticholinergic effects, hypotension (α-adrenergic blockade), sedation, analgesia, weight gain, and sexual dysfunction.

[b]Secondary amines. Side effects involve less anticholinergic effects, less hypotension, less sedation, less weight gain, and less sexual dysfunction.

[c]Side effects include sexual dysfunction, weight gain, agitation, sedation, and gastrointestinal disturbance.

[d]Side effects include agitation, anxiety, insomnia, and weight loss.

[e]Side effects include hypotension, hypertensive crisis, serotonin syndrome, stroke fatalities, and anticholinergic effect.

Adapted from Cozza KL, Armstrong SC. *Concise guide to the cytochrome p450 system: drug interaction principles for medical practice.* Washington, DC: American Psychiatric Publishing, Inc, 2001; DeVane CL, Nemeroff C. 2002 Guide to psychotropic drug interactions. *Primary Psychiatry* 2002;9(3):28–57; American Psychiatric Association. Practice guideline for the treatment of patients with major depressive disorder (revision). *Am J Psychiatry* 2000;157(4S):1–45; Lam RW, Wan DDC, Cohen NL, et al. Combining antidepressants for treatment-resistant depression: a review. *J Clin Psychiatry* 2002;63(8):685–693; and Preskorn SH. *Outpatient management of depression: a guide for the practitioner.* Caddo, OK: Professional Communications, Inc, 1999.

erectile or ejaculatory dysfunction in men and loss of libido and anorgasmia in both genders), headaches, extrapyramidal reactions, weight changes, and excessive serotonergic activity (serotonin syndrome). Although rare, serotonin syndrome deserves further discussion; it can involve confusion, myoclonus, nausea, vomiting, diarrhea, tremor, fever, elevated blood pressure, and ataxia. Serotonin syndrome is dose dependent and, therefore, may complicate the use of markedly elevated doses of SSRIs, but reduction in dosage or discontinuation resolves the syndrome. MAOIs markedly increase the risk of serotonin syndrome and, hence, never should be used in combination with SSRIs. In addition, sexual dysfunction is a more common side effect of SSRIs than of other classes of antidepressant medication (42).

Although all of the SSRIs possess similar mechanisms of action, they vary according to half-life and CYP enzymatic metabolism inhibition (Table 48.2). Fluoxetine possesses a long half-life and significant enzyme inhibition of CYP 2C, 2D6, and 3A4. Fluvoxamine possesses a brief half-life and extensive inhibition of CYP 1A2, 2C, and 3A4. A disadvantage of long half-life SSRIs is prolongation of side effects. Conversely, a disadvantage of short half-life SSRIs is serotonin withdrawal symptoms, including flu-like manifestations, nausea, diarrhea, and emesis. Sertraline and citalopram possess moderate half-lives and limited enzyme inhibition.

Slaughter et al. (48) studied 54 RA patients who were treated with sertraline for major depression. At the 15-month follow-up, 100% of the patients who successfully completed the trial (N = 41) were no longer depressed by Hamilton Rating Scale for Depression criteria. The Slaughter et al. study demonstrated that an SSRI (sertraline) is highly effective for the treatment of major depression in the context of RA.

NEWER, NONSELECTIVE SEROTONIN REUPTAKE INHIBITORS

Several newer antidepressant medications are available that differ structurally from TCAs and SSRIs. The mechanisms of action for these newer antidepressants include NE-DA reuptake inhibition, 5-HT–NE reuptake inhibition, 5-HT–NE modulation, and 5-HT modulation. The major medications in the newer non-SSRI category include bupropion, venlafaxine, mirtazapine, nefazodone, and trazodone.

Bupropion increases synaptic NE by inhibiting its reuptake, but bupropion also has a secondary effect of elevating DA in the synapse, which may also contribute to its antidepressant effect. By increasing NE and DA, bupropion exerts its antidepressant effect without causing the sexual dysfunction that sometimes accompanies SSRI treatment. In fact, bupropion has been used to potentially reverse the sexual side effects of SSRIs (49) and may actually enhance baseline sexual functioning and libido (49). Bupropion also has been used to reverse SSRI-induced side effects and to enhance SSRI antidepressant effects, particularly by increasing energy level and improving concentration. Increased seizure risk, however, has been reported with the use of immediate-release bupropion when initiated at high dosage (450 mg per day), but bupropion is now available in a sustained-release (SR) formulation that may not convey an increased risk of seizures; the manufacturer recommends waiting at least 4 days after initiating bupropion at 150-mg SR in the morning before adding a second 150-mg SR dose (most often administered in the afternoon or early evening to minimize sleep disruption). Bupropion possesses significant CYP 2D6 inhibition (Table 48.2).

Venlafaxine inhibits both NE and 5-HT reuptake and, therefore, provides a potent antidepressant effect (50). Venlafaxine also has been found to cause an appreciable elevation of blood pressure in 2% of treated patients, although blood pressure elevation is more evident with higher doses in the range of 300 to 375 mg per day. Venlafaxine is available in both immediate-release and extended-release forms. A relatively unique side effect of venlafaxine, which is encountered with some frequency, is sweating, but this symptom is often time limited (4–6 weeks); the need to discontinue venlafaxine secondary to sweating is infrequent. Venlafaxine conveys only modest CYP 2D6 inhibition and is not tightly protein bound. Venlafaxine is partially excreted renally, which minimizes its drug interaction profile (Table 48.2).

Mirtazapine, which has mixed effects on serotonin, acts as a 5-HT_2 and 5-HT_3 blocker, as well as a presynaptic α_2-receptor antagonist (44). Mirtazapine provides potential soporific effects, in addition to antidepressant activity. The sedative effects of mirtazapine, in combination with its tendency to increase appetite, are paradoxical; more sedation and greater weight gain occur at lower doses. As doses of mirtazapine increase, patients may observe an improvement in their mood but increasing difficulty sleeping. Mirtazapine has no appreciable CYP system interaction and, therefore, should not typically interfere with RA medications (Table 48.2).

Trazodone is a weak inhibitor of serotonin reuptake but a potent antagonist at 5-HT_{2a} and 5-HT_{2c} receptors. Substantial data exist regarding the efficacy of trazodone, although the findings have been somewhat inconsistent (42). Some studies have suggested comparable efficacy to TCAs (51); other studies have suggested inferior efficacy (52). One of the most common side effects of trazodone is sedation, which can be an asset when insomnia is a clinical problem. Trazodone possesses significant CYP 3A inhibition (Table 48.2).

Nefazodone is similar in structure to trazodone but differs in its pharmacologic properties and, hence, in its side effect profile (42). Nefazodone is a 5-HT_2 antagonist and a serotonin reuptake inhibitor (44); the efficacy of nefazodone has been shown to be comparable to that of TCAs (53). The sedating effect of nefazodone is not as pronounced as that of trazodone, but dry mouth, nausea, constipation, and blurred vision have been observed. Nefazodone is a potent CYP 3A4 inhibitor (44) and has the potential to raise levels of antihistamines, benzodiazepines, and digoxin (42) (Table 48.2).

MONOAMINE OXIDASE INHIBITORS

The major MAOIs include moclobemide, phenelzine, and tranylcypromine. In adult intent-to-treat studies, MAOIs have been shown to induce a clinical response in approximately 55% of cases (6). In MAOI versus placebo trials, MAOIs have been shown to induce a clinical response in approximately 18% to 31% more cases than placebo (6). MAOIs may be particularly useful for treating patients in the atypical subgroup of major depressive disorder (54,55); they also have been found to be effective in the treatment of patients who have not responded to other categories of antidepressants (56). MAOI side effects can include hypertensive crisis, serotonin syndrome, orthostatic hypotension, weight gain, sexual effects, and neurologic effects (e.g., headaches, insomnia, sedation, myoclonic jerks, paresthesia, and peripheral neuropathy). Hypertensive crises, when they occur, are typically related to the combination of a MAOI with large quantities of tyramine or other pressor amines, so dietary restrictions and avoidance of sympathomimetic and stimulant drugs is necessary. Given these potentially serious side effects, MAOIs are not recommended as first-line antidepressants and must be prescribed with great caution.

Failure to Respond to First-Line Antidepressants

Responsiveness to first-line antidepressants has been reported to be in the 50% to 75% range (42), although a 4- to 8-week trial is required before clinical responsiveness can be ascertained. Nevertheless, there is a substantial percentage of patients with major depressive disorder (≥25%) who do not respond to the initial antidepressant. In the case of nonresponders, the first step is to reevaluate the accuracy of the diagnosis, the patient's adherence to the medication regimen, the potential contribution of coexisting medical conditions, and the impact of complicating psychosocial stressors. If such factors appear to be involved, direct remediation of the circumstances contributing to the nonresponse should be pursued. Otherwise, partial responders may benefit from a brief extension of the first-line trial or a higher dose of the original medication. In addition, switching to an alternative non–MAOI agent has been shown to induce a clinical response in up to 50% of patients who do not respond to the initial medication (57). When treatment with an SSRI is complicated by side effects specific to one medication (e.g., insomnia with fluoxetine, gastrointestinal distress with sertraline, somnolence or weight gain with paroxetine), switching to an alternative SSRI is indicated. Alternatively, a switch from an SSRI to venlafaxine can be considered, due to the combined 5-HT–NE reuptake inhibition mechanism of action of venlafaxine. If the side effect is characteristic of a medication class (e.g., sexual dysfunction for SSRIs), the addition of bupropion or sildenafil should be considered. Alternatively, monotherapy with bupropion can be considered, when sexual dysfunction is a concern.

Based on practice guidelines (6,42), augmentation strategies involving multiple non-MAOI medications can be considered, if monotherapy proves ineffective. However, Lam et al. (58) have clarified that the evidence for the efficacy of antidepressant combinations is rather sparse. Bupropion can be used to augment the antidepressant effect of SSRIs because of its NE-DA effect. In addition, because the use of a saporific agent is frequently indicated in RA, there is no contraindication to the use of an SSRI in the morning, in combination with amitriptyline, trazodone, or mirtazapine at bedtime. However, the metabolism of amitriptyline may be decreased by SSRI medications, so the level of available amitriptyline may increase. Other augmentation agents include lithium, liothyronine (T_3), and methylphenidate.

Combined Psychological and Medication Approaches

Interestingly, the evidence for clinical benefits from combined treatments involving both medication and psychological approaches is equivocal (59). At best, there appears to be only a modest advantage in the addition of psychotherapy to an existing antidepressant medication regimen. In a randomized clinical trial, Parker et al. (60) found that persons with concomitant RA and major depression obtained an excellent clinical response from sertraline, but that the inclusion of cognitive-behavioral therapy to the treatment regimen did not confer an additional benefit. The combination of antidepressant medication and cognitive-behavioral approaches possibly should be used sequentially, rather than simultaneously, because the literature shows that cognitive-behavioral interventions are distinctly beneficial for the broad population of nondepressed persons with RA (61). Hence, by inference, cognitive-behavioral interventions may be most appropriately introduced after the acute phase treatment with antidepressant medication has been completed.

Electroconvulsive Therapy

ECT is indicated for only a small, select subgroup of patients, but efficacy data are generally positive (6). Specifically, ECT can be considered an option in cases of major depression that have proven highly resistant to antidepressant medication, especially when melancholic features are present. ECT may be particularly beneficial for medication-resistant patients who present with psychotic features, catatonic stupor, severe suicidality, or nutritional compromise due to refusal of food (62). Weiner (63) reported that 80% to 90% of cases of major depressive disorder improve after treatment with ECT. In addition, approximately 50% of cases of major depressive disorder that have failed antidepressant medications respond favorably to ECT (64). Overall, ECT has been shown to be a generally safe treatment, but there are inherent risks associated with anesthesia, especially in the context of certain medical comorbidities. Specifically, caution should be exercised in the use of ECT in cases involving severe cervical RA or osteoarthritis with wasting and osteopenia. However, with anesthesia and muscle blockade, the risk of injury from convulsion is generally minimal.

The major side effect associated with ECT is cognitive impairment (42), although brief-pulse stimulators and electrode placement within the nondominant hemisphere reduces the chances for adverse cognitive outcomes (65). Nevertheless, a transient postictal confusional state can occur, and there also can be both anterograde and retrograde memory interference. Although the anterograde impairment typically resolves within a few weeks posttreatment, some degree of retrograde amnesia may persist for longer periods (42). Squire et al. (66) reported that, in rare cases, more pervasive cognitive impairment can occur after ECT. The potential side effects of ECT must be weighed against the necessity for treatment in cases of severe, medication-resistant depression (e.g., psychosis, catatonia, suicidality, and nutritional compromise).

PRACTICE GUIDELINES

Excellent resources exist for the evidence-based management of major depression. The Agency for Health Care Policy and Research (AHCPR) has published practice guidelines for the detection, diagnosis, and treatment of depression in primary care settings (1,6). The AHCPR guidelines are particularly useful for nonpsychiatrists when confronted with depressive disorders in primary care or general medical settings. For rheumatologists, the AHCPR practice guidelines provide a useful, evidence-based framework for detecting, diagnosing, and treating uncomplicated depressive conditions as they inevitably present in rheumatologic practice.

The American Psychiatric Association (APA) also has published evidence-based practice guidelines for the treatment of patients with major depressive disorder (42). The APA guidelines are aimed primarily at psychiatrists, so they address management issues that are more complicated than most rheumatologists should undertake. Yet, general familiarity with the APA practice guidelines can facilitate collaboration between rheumatologists and psychiatrists, especially in complex cases of depression that do not respond to first-line treatments.

CLINICAL IMPLICATIONS

The literature on depression in the context of medical conditions (such as RA) elucidates several considerations for rheumatologic practice. First, numerous biopsychosocial issues operate for persons with RA (67), and depression is a particularly prevalent comorbidity (17–27%). Management of depression, when it exists, is a powerful source of potential therapeutic gain in the context of RA, because depression can be a major contributor to overall disability and a key amplifier of perceived pain.

A second implication is that rheumatologists should be proactive regarding the detection of cases of depression, because the literature shows that unrecognized depression (up to 50%) is a major issue in primary care environments. Although many patients will not independently discuss depressive symptoms in the context of a rheumatologic visit, they are much more likely to do so if asked relevant questions or are given an opportunity to respond to a depression screening questionnaire. Failure to detect cases of depression in a rheumatologic practice constitutes a missed opportunity to improve functional status and to enhance quality of life for persons with RA.

A third implication is that rheumatologists should possess the ability to make general distinctions among the various depression subtypes to identify those cases of major depression that need immediate antidepressive management. Specifically, a general awareness of the *Diagnostic and Statistical Manual of Mental Disorders*, fourth edition, diagnostic framework for depression should be core knowledge for rheumatologists, especially given that one in four to five patients seen in rheumatology clinics is likely to meet criteria for major depression.

A fourth implication is that rheumatologists should be proactive regarding the treatment of major depression when it occurs in the context of RA. Practice guidelines are available to inform the management of uncomplicated depression by nonpsychiatrists. Clearly, the familiarity of rheumatologists with first-line treatments for major depression is highly advantageous for persons with RA, so that comprehensive, biopsychosocial care can be provided.

A fifth implication is that an effective working alliance between rheumatologists and psychiatrists is beneficial in the management of complex cases of major depression. Some depressed patients will not respond to first-line interventions and will require more complex antidepressive strategies, including combination therapies. Psychiatry referral is specifically indicated when the symptoms of depression include psychosis, catatonia, suicidality, nutritional compromise, or bipolar features.

Lastly, there should be a keen awareness among rheumatologists that depression is a highly treatable condition; truly treatment-resistant depression is relatively rare. A wide variety of antidepressant interventions with proven efficacy are available, and these evidence-based treatments for major depression can be highly beneficial to a sizable subgroup of persons with RA.

REFERENCES

1. Depression Guideline Panel. Depression in primary care: Volume 1. Detection and diagnosis. *Clinical practice guideline, number 5*. Rockville, MD: U.S. Department of Health and Human Services, Public Health Service, 1993:73.
2. Fifield J, Reisine S, Tennen H, et al. Depressive symptom reports and depression diagnoses among patients with RA. *Arthritis Care Res* 1995;8:S15.
3. Rimón R, Laakso RL. Overt psychopathology in rheumatoid arthritis: a fifteen-year follow-up study. *Scand J Rheumatol* 1984;13:324–328.
4. Creed F, Ash G. Depression in rheumatoid arthritis: aetiology and treatment. *Int Rev Psychiatry* 1992;4:23–34.
5. Dickens C, McGowan L, Clark-Carter D, et al. Depression in rheumatoid arthritis: a systematic review of the literature with meta-analysis. *Psychosom Med* 2002;64:52–60.
6. Depression Guideline Panel. Depression in primary care: Volume 2. Treatment of major depression. *Clinical practice guideline, number 5*. Rockville, MD: U.S. Department of Health and Human Services, Public Health Service, 1993.
7. American Psychiatric Association. *Diagnostic and statistical manual of mental disorders*, 4th ed. Washington, DC: American Psychiatric Association, 1994.
8. Rodin G, Craven J, Littlefield C. *Depression in the medically ill: an integrated approach*. New York: Brunner-Mazel, 1991.
9. Katz PP, Yelin EH. The development of depressive symptoms among women with rheumatoid arthritis: the role of function. *Arthritis Rheum* 1995;38:49–56.
10. Newman SP, Fitzpatrick R, Lamb R, et al. The origins of depressed mood in rheumatoid arthritis. *J Rheumatol* 1989;16:740–744.
11. Wright GE, Parker JC, Smarr KL, et al. Age, depressive symptoms, and rheumatoid arthritis. *Arthritis Rheum* 1998;41:298–305.
12. Turner RJ, Beiser M. Major depression and depressive symptomatology among the physically disabled: assessing the role of chronic stress. *J Nerv Ment Dis* 1990;178:343–350.

13. Revenson TA, Schiaffino KM, Majerovitz SD, et al. Social support as a double-edged sword: the relation of positive and problematic support to depression among rheumatoid arthritis patients. *Soc Sci Med* 1991;33:807–813.
14. Yelin EH, Feshbach DM, Meenan RF, et al. Social problems, services and policy for persons with chronic disease: the case of rheumatoid arthritis. *Soc Sci Med* 1979;13:13–20.
15. Ormel J, Kempen GIJM, Deeg DJH, et al. Functioning, well being and health perception in late middle-aged and older people: comparing the effects of depressive symptoms and chronic medical conditions. *J Am Geriatr Soc* 1998;46:39–48.
16. Wells KB, Stewart A, Hays RD, et al. The functioning and well-being of depressed patients: results from the medical outcomes study. *JAMA* 1989; 262:914–919.
17. Von Korff MC, Ormel J, Katon W, et al. Disability and depression among high utilizers of health care: a longitudinal analysis. *Arch Gen Psychiatry* 1992;49:91–100.
18. McFarlane AC, Brooks PM. Determinants of disability in rheumatoid arthritis. *Br J Rheumatol* 1988;27:7–14.
19. Katz PP, Yelin EH. Prevalence and correlates of depressive symptoms among persons with rheumatoid arthritis. *J Rheumatol* 1993;20:790–796.
20. Fifield J, Reisine ST, Grady K. Work disability and the experience of pain and depression in rheumatoid arthritis. *Soc Sci Med* 1992;33:579–585.
21. Stoudemire A, Frank R, Hedemark N, et al. The economic burden of depression. *Gen Hosp Psychiatry* 1986;8:387–394.
22. Abraham IL, Neese JB, Westerman PS. Depression: nursing implications of a clinical and social problem. *Nurs Clin North Am* 1991;26:527–536.
23. Lorig K, Fries J. *The arthritis helpbook*, 1st ed. Reading: Addison-Wesley, 1980.
24. Lorig KR, Mazonson PD, Holman HR. Evidence suggesting that health education for self-management in patients with chronic arthritis has sustained health benefits while reducing health care costs. *Arthritis Rheum* 1993;36:439–446.
25. Pallak MS, Cummings NA, Dörken H, et al. Medical costs, Medicaid, and managed mental health treatment: the Hawaii study. *Managed Care Q* 1994;2:64–70.
26. Lewinsohn PM, Zeiss AM, Duncan EM. Probability of relapse after recovery from an episode of depression. *J Abnorm Psychol* 1989;98:107–116.
27. Fifield J, Tennen H, Reisine S, et al. Depression and the long-term risk of pain, fatigue, and disability in patients with rheumatoid arthritis. *Arthritis Rheum* 1998;41:1851–1857.
28. Thase ME. Mood disorders: neurobiology. In: Sadock BJ, Sadock VA, eds. *Kaplan & Sadock's comprehensive textbook of psychiatry*. vol 1. New York: Lippincott Williams & Wilkins, 2000:1318–1327.
29. Mann JJ, Arango V, Underwood MD. Serotonin and suicidal behavior. *Ann N Y Acad Sci* 1990;600:476–484.
30. Ward NG. Pain and depression. In: Bonica JJ, ed. *The management of pain*. vol 1. Philadelphia: Lea & Febiger, 1990:310–319.
31. Maes M, Bosmans E, Meltzer HY, et al. Interleukin-1β: a putative mediator of HPA axis hyperactivity in major depression? *Am J Psychiatry* 1993;150:1189–1193.
32. Maes M, Meltzer HY, Bosmans E, et al. Increased plasma concentrations of interleukin-6, soluble interleukin-6, soluble interleukin-2 and transferrin receptor in major depression. *J Affective Disord* 1995;34:301–309.
33. Krueger JM, Majde JA. Microbial products and cytokines in sleep and fever regulation. *Crit Rev Immunol* 1994;14:355–379.
34. Kronfol Z, Remick DG. Cytokines and the brain: implications for clinical psychiatry. *Am J Psychiatry* 2000;157:683–694.
35. Dantzer R, Wollman E, Vitkovic L, et al. Cytokines and depression: fortuitous or causative association? *Mol Psychiatry* 1999;4:328–332.
36. Cash JM, Wilder RL. Stress, depression, and rheumatoid arthritis. *Contemp Intern Med* 1991;3:13–16.
37. Kessler LG, Cleary PD, Burke JD. Psychiatric disorders in primary care. *Arch Gen Psychiatry* 1985;42:583–587.
38. Gold PW, Goodwin FK, Chrousos GP. Clinical and biochemical manifestations of depression: relation to the neurobiology of stress (first of two parts). *N Engl J Med* 1988;319:348–353.
39. Stoudemire GA. Selected organic mental disorders. In: Hales RE, Yudofsky SC, eds. *Textbook of neuropsychiatry*. Washington, DC: American Psychiatric Press, Inc., 1987:125–139.
40. Clauw DJ, Paul P. The overlap between fibromyalgia and inflammatory rheumatoid diseases: when and why does it occur? *J Clin Rheumatol* 1995; 1:335–341.
41. Ahles TA, Khan SA, Yunus MB, et al. Psychiatric status of patients with primary fibromyalgia, patients with rheumatoid arthritis, and subjects without pain: a blind comparison of DSM-III diagnoses. *Am J Psychiatry* 1991;148:1721–1726.
42. American Psychiatric Association. Practice guideline for the treatment of patients with major depressive disorder (revision). *Am J Psychiatry* 2000; 157:1–45.
43. Dobson KS. A meta-analysis of the efficacy of cognitive therapy for depression. *J Consult Clin Psychol* 1989;57:414–419.
44. DeVane CL, Nemeroff C. 2002 Guide to psychotropic drug interactions. *Primary Psychiatry* 2002;9:28–57.
45. Frank RG, Kashani JH, Parker JC, et al. Antidepressant analgesia in rheumatoid arthritis. *J Rheumatol* 1988;15:1632–1638.
46. Fowler PD, MacNeill A, Spencer D, et al. Imipramine, rheumatoid arthritis and rheumatoid factor. *Curr Med Res Opin* 1977;5:241–246.
47. Grant-Macfarlane J, Jalali S, Grace EM. Trimipramine in rheumatoid arthritis: a randomized double-blind trial in relieving pain and joint tenderness. *Curr Med Res Opin* 1986;10:89–93.
48. Slaughter JR, Parker JC, Martens MP, et al. Clinical outcomes following a trial of sertraline in rheumatoid arthritis. *Psychosomatics* 2002;43:36–41.
49. Phillips RL Jr., Slaughter JR. Depression and sexual desire. *Am Fam Physician* 2000;62:782–786.
50. Thase ME, Entsuah AR, Rudolph RL. Remission rates during treatment with venlafaxine or selective serotonin reuptake inhibitors. *Br J Psychiatry* 2001;178:234–241.
51. Schatzberg AF. Trazodone: a 5-year review of antidepressant efficacy. *Psychopathology* 1987;20[Suppl 1]:48–56.
52. Cunningham LA, Borison RL, Carman JS, et al. A comparison of venlafaxine, trazodone, and placebo in major depression. *J Clin Psychopharmacol* 1994; 14:99–106.
53. Feighner JP, Pambakian R, Fowler RC, et al. A comparison of nefazodone, imipramine, and placebo in patients with moderate to severe depression. *Psychopharmacol Bull* 1989;25:219–221.
54. Quitkin FM, McGrath PJ, Stewart JW, et al. Atypical depression, panic attacks, and response to imipramine and phenelzine. *Arch Gen Psychiatry* 1990;47:935–941.
55. Zisook S, Braff DL, Click MA. Monoamine oxidase inhibitors in the treatment of atypical depression. *J Clin Psychopharmacol* 1985;5:131–137.
56. Thase ME, Mallinger AG, McKnight D, et al. Treatment of imipramine-resistant recurrent depression, IV: a double-blind crossover study of tranylcypromine for anergic bipolar depression. *Am J Psychiatry* 1992;149: 195–198.
57. Thase ME, Rush AJ. Treatment-resistant depression. In: Bloom F, Kupfer DJ, eds. *Psychopharmacology: the fourth generation of progress*. New York: Raven Press, 1995:1081–1097.
58. Lam RW, Wan DDC, Cohen NL, et al. Combining antidepressants for treatment-resistant depression: a review. *J Clin Psychiatry* 2002;63:685–693.
59. Manning DW, Frances AJ. Combined therapy for depression: critical review of the literature. In: Manning DW, Frances AJ, eds. *Combined pharmacotherapy and psychotherapy for depression*. Washington, DC: American Psychiatric Press, Inc., 1990:3–33.
60. Parker JC, Smarr KL, Slaughter JR, et al. Management of depression in rheumatoid arthritis: a combined pharmacologic and cognitive-behavioral approach. *Arthritis Care Res* 2003;49:766–777.
61. Parker JC, Iverson GL, Smarr KL, et al. Cognitive-behavioral approaches to pain management in rheumatoid arthritis. *Arthritis Care Res* 1993;6:207–212.
62. The American Psychiatric Association Task Force on Electroconvulsive Therapy. *The practice of electroconvulsive therapy: recommendations for treatment, training, and privileging*. 1990:1–177.
63. Weiner RD. Electroconvulsive therapy. In: Gabbard GO, ed. *Treatments of psychiatric disorders*. vol 1. Washington, DC: American Psychiatric Press, 1995: 1237–1262.
64. Devanand DP, Sackeim HA, Prudic J. Electroconvulsive therapy in the treatment-resistant patient. *Psychiatr Clin North Am* 1991;14:905–923.
65. Isenberg KE, Zorumski CF. Electroconvulsive therapy. In: Sadock BJ, Sadock VA, eds. *Kaplan & Sadock's comprehensive textbook of psychiatry*. vol II. New York: Lippincott Williams & Wilkins, 2000:2503–2515.
66. Squire LR, Slater PC. Electroconvulsive therapy and complaints of memory dysfunction: a prospective three-year follow-up study. *Br J Psychiatry* 1983;142:1–8.
67. Parker JC, Bradley LA, DeVellis RM, et al. Biopsychosocial contributions to the management of arthritis disability: blueprints from an NIDRR-sponsored conference. *Arthritis Rheum* 1993;36:885–889.

APPENDIX A

1987 Revised Criteria for the Classification of Rheumatoid Arthritis (Traditional Format)*

For classification purposes, a patient shall be said to have rheumatoid arthritis if he or she has satisfied at least four of the seven criteria listed below. Criteria 1 through 4 must have been present for at least 6 weeks. Patients with two clinical diagnoses are not excluded.

1. Morning stiffness: Morning stiffness in and around the joints, lasting at least 1 hour before maximal improvement.
2. Arthritis of three or more joint areas: At least three joint areas simultaneously have had soft tissue swelling or fluid (not bony overgrowth alone) observed by a physician. The 14 possible areas are right or left proximal interphalangeal joint, metacarpophalangeal joint, wrist, elbow, knee, ankle, and metatarsophalangeal joints.
3. Arthritis of hand joints: At least one area swollen (as defined above) in a wrist, metacarpophalangeal joint, or proximal interphalangeal joint.
4. Symmetric arthritis: Simultaneous involvement of the same joint areas (as defined in Criterion 2) on both sides of the body (bilateral involvement of proximal interphalangeal joints, metacarpophalangeal joints, or metatarsophalangeal joints is acceptable without absolute symmetry).
5. Rheumatoid nodules: Subcutaneous nodules over bony prominences or extensor surfaces, or in juxtaarticular regions, observed by a physician.
6. Serum rheumatoid factor: Demonstration of abnormal amounts of serum rheumatoid factor by any method for which the result has been positive in greater than 5% of healthy control subjects.
7. Radiographic changes: Radiographic changes typical of rheumatoid arthritis on posteroanterior hand and wrist radiographs, which must include erosions or unequivocal bony decalcification localized in or most marked adjacent to the involved joints (osteoarthritis changes alone do not qualify).

*From Arnett FC, Edworthy SM, Bloch DA, et al. The American Rheumatism Association 1987 revised criteria for the classification of rheumatoid arthritis. *Arthritis Rheum* 1988;31:315–324.

APPENDIX B

American College of Rheumatology Preliminary Definition of Improvement in Rheumatoid Arthritis*

American College of Rheumatology (ACR) preliminary definition of improvement in rheumatoid arthritis (RA):

At least 20% improvement in tender joint count
At least 20% improvement in swollen joint count
plus
At least 20% improvement in three of the following five items:

- Patient's assessment of pain
- Patient's global assessment of disease activity
- Physician's global assessment of disease activity
- Patient's assessment of physical function
- Acute phase reactant (erythrocyte sedimentation rate or C-reactive protein)

DISEASE ACTIVITY MEASURES AND METHODS OF ASSESSMENT

1. Tender joint count: ACR tender joint count, an assessment of 28 or more joints. The joint count should be done by scoring several different aspects of tenderness, as assessed by pressure and joint manipulation on physical examination. The information on various types of tenderness should then be collapsed into a single tender-versus-nontender dichotomy.
2. Swollen joint count: ACR swollen joint count, an assessment of 28 or more joints. Joints are classified as either *swollen* or *not swollen*.
3. Patient's assessment of pain: A horizontal visual analog scale (usually 10 cm) or Likert scale assessment of the patient's current level of pain.
4. Patient's global assessment of disease activity: The patient's overall assessment of how the arthritis is doing. One acceptable method for determining this is the question from the Arthritis Impact Measurement Scales instrument: "Considering all the ways your arthritis affects you, mark 'X' on the scale for how well you are doing." An anchored, horizontal, visual analog scale (usually 10 cm) should be provided. A Likert scale response is also acceptable.
5. Physician's global assessment of disease activity: A horizontal visual analog scale (usually 10 cm) or Likert scale measure of the physician's assessment of the patient's current disease activity.
6. Patient's assessment of physical function: Any patient self-assessment instrument that has been validated, has reliability, has been proven in RA trials to be sensitive to change, and measures physical function in RA patients is acceptable. Instruments that have been demonstrated to be sensitive in RA trials include the Arthritis Impact Measurement Scales, the Health Assessment Questionnaire, the Quality (or Index) of Well Being, the McMaster Health Index Questionnaire, and the McMaster Toronto Arthritis Patient Preference Disability Questionnaire.
7. Acute phase reactant value: A Westergren erythrocyte sedimentation rate or a C-reactive protein level.

*From Felson DT, Anderson JJ, Boers M, et al. American College of Rheumatology preliminary definition of improvement in rheumatoid arthritis. *Arthritis Rheum* 1995;38:727–735.

APPENDIX C

Paulus Criteria for Improvement of Patients with Rheumatoid Arthritis*

The Paulus criteria for improvement of patients with rheumatoid arthritis are listed below. *Improvement* is defined as at least 20% improvement (or on a 1 to 5 scale, reduction by at least two grades or improvement to grade 1) in at least four of the six variables.

- Duration of morning stiffness (minutes)
- Joint tenderness score
- Joint swelling score
- Patient's overall assessment of current disease activity (1 to 5 scale)
- Physician's overall assessment of current disease activity (1 to 5 scale)
- Westergren erythrocyte sedimentation rate

*From Paulus HE, Egger MJ, Ward JR, et al. Analysis of improvement in individual rheumatoid arthritis patients treated with disease-modifying antirheumatic drugs, based on the findings in patients treated with placebo. *Arthritis Rheum* 1990;33:477–484.

APPENDIX D

Disease Activity Score, Disease Activity Score 28, and European League Against Rheumatism Response Criteria*

The Disease Activity Score (DAS) is a combined index designed to measure disease activity in patients with rheumatoid arthritis. It has been extensively validated in clinical trials in concert with the European League Against Rheumatism (EULAR) response criteria (Table 1). The original DAS included the Ritchie articular index, the 44 swollen joint count, the erythrocyte sedimentation rate, and a general health assessment on a visual analog scale. Later, a 28-joint count for tenderness and swelling was used to develop the DAS28 (Table 2). The DAS and the DAS28 do not produce the same results, as the DAS has a range of one to nine and the DAS28 has a range of two to ten. A transformation formula has been developed to calculate the DAS28 from the DAS:

$$DAS28 = (1.072 \times DAS) + 0.938$$

Using the DAS, response criteria were developed called the *EULAR response criteria*. The EULAR response criteria include a change in disease activity, as well as current disease activity. Three categories are defined: good, moderate, and nonresponders. A DAS less than or equal to 1.6 or a DAS28 less than or equal to 2.6 is considered to be remission.

TABLE 1. European League Against Rheumatism Response Criteria

Current DAS28	DAS28 Improvement >1.2	0.6–1.2	<0.6
<3.2	Good response	Moderate response	No response
3.2–5.1	Moderate response	Moderate response	No response
>5.1	Moderate response	No response	No response

DAS28, Disease Activity Score 28.

TABLE 2. Disease Activity Score 28 (DAS28) Form

		Left		Right	
		Swollen	Tender	Swollen	Tender
Shoulder					
Elbow					
Wrist					
MCP	1				
	2				
	3				
	4				
	5				
PIP	1				
	2				
	3				
	4				
	5				
Knee					
Subtotal					
Total		Swollen		Tender	

No disease activity — High disease activity

Swollen (0–28)	
Tender (0–28)	
Erythrocyte sedimentation rate	
Visual analog scale observer's disease activity (0–100 mm)	
DAS28 = 0.56 * ÷(t28) + 0.28 * ÷(sw28) + 0.70 * Ln(erythrocyte sedimentation rate) + 0.014 * GH	

GH, general health or global disease measure; Ln, natural logarithm; MCP, metacarpophalangeal joint; PIP, proximal interphalangeal joint; sw, swollen joint count; t, tender joint count.

*From the following sources: Home of the DAS. Department of Rheumatology, University Medical Centre, Nijmegen, The Netherlands. http://www.das-score.nl/www.das-score.nl/index.html.

Prevoo ML, van Gestel AM, van't Hof MA, et al. Remission in a prospective study of patients with rheumatoid arthritis. American Rheumatism Association preliminary remission criteria in relation to the disease activity score. *Br J Rheumatol* 1996;35:1101–1105.

van der Heijde DM, van't Hof MA, van Riel PLCM, et al. Judging disease activity in clinical practice in rheumatoid arthritis. First step in the development of a "disease activity score." *Ann Rheum Dis* 1990;49:916–920.

van der Heijde DM, van't Hof MA, van Riel PLCM, et al. Validity of single variables and composite indices for measuring disease activity in rheumatoid arthritis. *Ann Rheum Dis* 1992;51:177–181.

van der Heijde DM, van't Hof M, van Riel PL, van de Putte LB. Development of a disease activity score based on judgment in clinical practice by rheumatologists. *J Rheumatol* 1993;20:579–581.

van der Heijde DM, van't Hof M, van Riel PL, van de Putte LB. Validity of single variables and indices to measure disease activity in rheumatoid arthritis. *J Rheumatol* 1993;20:538–541.

van Gestel AM, Prevoo ML, van't Hof MA, et al. Development and validation of the European League Against Rheumatism response criteria for rheumatoid arthritis. Comparison with the preliminary American College of Rheumatology and the World Health Organization/International League Against Rheumatism Criteria. *Arthritis Rheum* 1996;39:34–40.

APPENDIX E

Clinical Health Assessment Questionnaire

Instructions

1. You will need a blue or black pen that won't bleed through the paper. Please do not use pencil or red ink.

2. You will see a lot of small squares like this: ☐ Yes ☐ No

   These squares should be marked with an X like this: ☒ Yes ☐ No

   Be sure to make your X inside the box, and fairly heavy, so the computer can read it.

3. You will also see some boxes that look like this:

   For optimum accuracy, please print carefully and avoid contact with the edges of the box. The following will serve as an example:

   0 1 2 3 4 5 6 7 8 9

   Please--no fractions or decimals!!

4. You will also see some scales like the one below. You will need to make a mark in the box that best corresponds to your answer. These scales are usually 0-100. Read carefully to determine what the question is asking. In this example, the box marked with an X represents a person having a great deal of pain.

   0 100

   NO PAIN ☐ ☐ ☐ ☐ ☐ ☐ ☐ ☐ ☐ ☐ ☐ ☐ ☐ ☐ ☐ ☐ ☐ ☐ ☒ ☐ ☐ SEVERE PAIN

First Name MI Last Name

Street Address

City State Zip Area Code and Telephone Number

Best time to call you?

Alternate Area Code and Telephone Number

How many years of school have you completed? Please X the box to the left of the number of years

☐ 1 ☐ 2 ☐ 3 ☐ 4 ☐ 5 ☐ 6 ☐ 7 ☐ 8 ☐ 9 ☐ 10 ☐ 11 ☐ 12 ☐ 13 ☐ 14 ☐ 15 ☐ 16 ☐ 17+

------------Grade School------- ----High School-- -------College------- Post college or Other

Please tell us your date of birth: mm / dd / yyyy 1 9 And are you: ☐ Male ☐ Female

Please tell us your ethnic background: ☐ White ☐ Asian ☐ American Indian/Alaska Native ☐ Black ☐ Hispanic ☐ Puerto Rican ☐ Other

Do you have: Rheumatoid Arthritis? ☐ Osteoarthritis? ☐ Fibromyalgia? ☐ Other? ☐

Clinical Health Assessment Questionnaire (CLINHAQ)

Date of birth: ☐☐ / ☐☐ / ☐☐☐☐   Last 4 digits of your social security number: ☐☐☐☐

Your Initials: ☐☐☐   Name: (Optional) ____________________

We are interested in learning how your illness affects your ability to function in daily life. Place an X in the box which best describes your usual abilities OVER THE PAST WEEK:

Visit Date: ☐☐ (mm) / ☐☐ (dd) / ☐☐☐☐ (yyyy)

Are you able to:	**Without Any Difficulty (0)**	**With Some Difficulty (1)**	**With Much Difficulty (2)**	**Unable To Do (3)**	
Dress yourself, including shoelaces and buttons?	☐	☐	☐	☐	
Shampoo your hair?	☐	☐	☐	☐	___ (D)
Get in and out of bed?	☐	☐	☐	☐	
Stand up from a straight chair?	☐	☐	☐	☐	___ (A)
Lift a full cup or glass to your mouth?	☐	☐	☐	☐	
Cut your meat?	☐	☐	☐	☐	
Open a new milk carton?	☐	☐	☐	☐	___ (E)
Walk outdoors on flat ground?	☐	☐	☐	☐	
Climb up five steps?	☐	☐	☐	☐	___ (W)

Please place an X in the box beside any aids or devices that you usually use for any of the above activities:

☐ Cane (W)   ☐ Crutches (W)   ☐ Walker (W)   ☐ Wheelchair (W)   ☐ Built up or special utensils (E)

☐ Devices used for dressing (button hook, zipper pull, long handled shoe horn) (D)   ☐ Special or built up chair (A)

Place an X in the box beside any categories for which you usually need HELP FROM ANOTHER PERSON:

☐ Dressing and Grooming (D)   ☐ Arising (A)   ☐ Eating (E)   ☐ Walking (W)

We are also interested in learning whether or not you are affected by pain because of your illness.

How much pain have you had because of your illness in the past week? Place an X in the box that best describes the severity of your pain on a scale of 0-10.

NO PAIN 0 ○ ☐ ☐ ☐ ○ ☐ ☐ ☐ ○ ☐ ☐ ☐ ○ ☐ ☐ ☐ ○ ☐ ☐ ☐ ○ 10 SEVERE PAIN

How much of a problem has sleep (i.e., resting at night) been for you IN THE PAST WEEK? Place an X in the box below that best describes how much of a problem sleep has been for you on a scale of 0-10.

SLEEP IS NO PROBLEM 0 ○ ☐ ☐ ☐ ○ ☐ ☐ ☐ ○ ☐ ☐ ☐ ○ ☐ ☐ ☐ ○ ☐ ☐ ☐ ○ 10 SLEEP IS A MAJOR PROBLEM

Place an X in the box which best describes your usual abilities OVER THE PAST WEEK:

ARE YOU ABLE TO:	Without Any Difficulty (0)	With Some Difficulty (1)	With Much Difficulty (2)	Unable To Do (3)	
Wash and dry your body?	☐	☐	☐	☐	
Take a tub bath?	☐	☐	☐	☐	
Get on and off the toilet?	☐	☐	☐	☐	___ (H)
Bend down to pick up clothing from the floor?	☐	☐	☐	☐	
Reach and get down a 5 pound object (such as a bag of sugar) from just above your head?	☐	☐	☐	☐	___ (R)
Turn faucets on and off?	☐	☐	☐	☐	
Open jars which have been previously opened?	☐	☐	☐	☐	
Open car doors?	☐	☐	☐	☐	___ (G)
Get in and out of a car?	☐	☐	☐	☐	
Run errands and shop?	☐	☐	☐	☐	
Do chores such as vacuuming or yardwork?	☐	☐	☐	☐	___ (E/C)
Go up two or more flights of stairs?	☐	☐	☐	☐	
Do yard work (outside work or activities)?	☐	☐	☐	☐	
Move heavy objects?	☐	☐	☐	☐	
Lift heavy objects?	☐	☐	☐	☐	
Wait in a line for 15 minutes?	☐	☐	☐	☐	

Please place an X in the box beside any AIDS or DEVICES that you usually use for any of these activities:

☐ Bathtub bar (H) ☐ Raised toilet seat (H) ☐ Jar opener for jars previously opened (G)

☐ Long-handled appliances in bathroom (H) ☐ Long-handled appliances for reach (R)

☐ Other (please specify) ______________________ (H,G,R, E/C)

Please place an X in the box beside any categories for which you usually need HELP FROM ANOTHER PERSON:

☐ Hygiene (H) ☐ Reach (R) ☐ Gripping and opening things (G) ☐ Errands and Chores (E/C)

We are interested in knowing about any problems that you may have been having with fatigue. How much of a problem has fatigue or tiredness been for you IN THE PAST WEEK? Place an X in the box below that best describes the severity of your fatigue on a scale of 0-10.

FATIGUE IS NO PROBLEM **0** ○ ☐ ☐ ☐ ○ ☐ ☐ ☐ ○ ☐ ☐ ☐ ○ ☐ ☐ ☐ ○ ☐ ☐ ☐ ○ **10** FATIGUE IS A MAJOR PROBLEM

Please place an X in the box under the most appropriate answer for each question. Try to answer every question.

DURING THE PAST MONTH:	Always	Very Often	Fairly Often	Some-times	Almost Never	Never
1. How much of the time have you enjoyed the things you do?	☐	☐	☐	☐	☐	☐
2. How much of the time have you felt tense or "high strung"?	☐	☐	☐	☐	☐	☐
3. How much have you been bothered by nervousness, or your "nerves"?	☐	☐	☐	☐	☐	☐
4. How often did you find yourself having difficulty trying to calm down?	☐	☐	☐	☐	☐	☐
5. How much of the time have you been in low or very low spirits?	☐	☐	☐	☐	☐	☐
6. How much of the time did you feel relaxed and free of tension?	☐	☐	☐	☐	☐	☐
7. How much of the time have you felt downhearted and blue?	☐	☐	☐	☐	☐	☐
8. How often did you feel that nothing turned out for you the way you wanted it to?	☐	☐	☐	☐	☐	☐
9. How much of the time have you felt calm and peaceful?	☐	☐	☐	☐	☐	☐
10. How often did you feel that others would be better off if you were dead?	☐	☐	☐	☐	☐	☐
11. How much of the time were you able to relax without difficulty?	☐	☐	☐	☐	☐	☐
12. How often have you felt so down in the dumps that nothing could cheer you up?	☐	☐	☐	☐	☐	☐

Considering ALL THE WAYS THAT YOUR ILLNESS AFFECTS YOU, RATE HOW YOU ARE DOING on the following scale. Place an X in the box below that best describes how you are doing on a scale of 0-10.

VERY WELL **0** ○ ☐ ☐ ☐ ○ ☐ ☐ ☐ ○ ☐ ☐ ☐ ○ ☐ ☐ ☐ ○ ☐ ☐ ☐ ○ **10** VERY POORLY

APPENDIX F

Clinical Health Assessment Questionnaire II

Instructions

1. You will need a blue or black pen that won't bleed through the paper. Please do not use pencil or red ink.

2 . You will see a lot of small squares like this: ☐ Yes ☐ No

These squares should be marked with an X like this: ☒ Yes ☐ No

Be sure to make your X inside the box, and fairly heavy, so the computer can read it.

3. You will also see some boxes that look like this:

For optimum accuracy, please print carefully and avoid contact with the edges of the box. The following will serve as an example:

0	1	2	3	4	5	6	7	8	9

Please--no fractions or decimals!!

4. You will also see some scales like the one below. You will need to make a mark in the box that best corresponds to your answer. These scales are usually 0-100. Read carefully to determine what the question is asking. In this example, the box marked with an X represents a person having a great deal of pain.

0 — 100

NO PAIN ☐ ☐ ☐ ☐ ☐ ☐ ☐ ☐ ☐ ☐ ☐ ☐ ☐ ☐ ☐ ☐ ☐ ☐ ☒ ☐ ☐ SEVERE PAIN

First Name   MI   Last Name

Street Address

City   State   Zip   Area Code and Telephone Number ___ - ___ - ___

Best time to call you?

Alternate Area Code and Telephone Number ___ - ___ - ___

☐ 1 ☐ 2 ☐ 3 ☐ 4 ☐ 5 ☐ 6 ☐ 7 ☐ 8 ☐ 9 ☐ 10 ☐ 11 ☐ 12 ☐ 13 ☐ 14 ☐ 15 ☐ 16 ☐ 17+

------------Grade School------- ----High School-- -------College------ Post college or Other

Please tell us your date of birth: mm / dd / yyyy 1 9

And are you: ☐ Male ☐ Female

Please tell us your ethnic background: ☐ White, not of hispanic origin ☐ Asian or Pacific Islander ☐ American Indian or Alaska Native ☐ Black, not of hispanic origin ☐ Hispanic ☐ Other

What is your primary rheumatic disease diagnosis (e.g., rheumatoid arthritis, osteoarthritis, other rheumatic disease,etc.) Rheumatoid Arthritis? ☐ Osteoarthritis? ☐ Fibromyalgia? ☐ Other? (e.g., lupus, psoriatic arthritis, back pain, tendonitis, etc.) ☐

If you selected "other" for your diagnosis above, please give us the name of your diagnosis (for example: lupus, psoriatic arthritis, back pain, tendonitis, etc.): ______________________

Clinical Health Assessment Questionnaire (CLINHAQ II)

Date of birth: ☐☐ / ☐☐ / ☐☐☐☐ Last 4 digits of social security number: ☐☐☐☐

Patient Initials: ☐☐☐ Patient Name: ____________

Visit Date: ☐☐ (mm) / ☐☐ (dd) / ☐☐☐☐ (yyyy)

How much of a problem has sleep (i.e., resting at night) been for you IN THE PAST WEEK? Place an X in the box below that best describes how much of a problem sleep has been for you on a scale of 0-10.

SLEEP IS NO PROBLEM 0 ○ ☐ ☐ ☐ ○ ☐ ☐ ☐ ○ ☐ ☐ ☐ ○ ☐ ☐ ☐ ○ ☐ ☐ ☐ ○ 10 SLEEP IS A MAJOR PROBLEM

We are also interested in learning whether or not you are affected by pain because of your illness.
How much pain have you had because of your illness in the past week? Place an X in the box that best describes the severity of your pain on a scale of 0-10.

NO PAIN 0 ○ ☐ ☐ ☐ ○ ☐ ☐ ☐ ○ ☐ ☐ ☐ ○ ☐ ☐ ☐ ○ ☐ ☐ ☐ ○ 10 SEVERE PAIN

We are interested in learning how your illness affects your ability to function in daily life. Place an X in the box which best describes your usual abilities OVER THE PAST WEEK:

Are you able to:	Without Any Difficulty (0)	With Some Difficulty (1)	With Much Difficulty (2)	Unable To Do (3)
Stand up from a straight chair?	☐	☐	☐	☐
Walk outdoors on flat ground?	☐	☐	☐	☐
Get on/off toilet?	☐	☐	☐	☐
Reach and get down a 5 pound object (such as a bag of sugar) from just above your head?	☐	☐	☐	☐
Open car doors?	☐	☐	☐	☐
Do outside work (such as yard work)?	☐	☐	☐	☐
Wait in a line for 15 minutes?	☐	☐	☐	☐
Lift heavy objects?	☐	☐	☐	☐
Move heavy objects?	☐	☐	☐	☐
Go up two or more flights of stairs?	☐	☐	☐	☐

How much trouble have you had with your stomach (i.e., nausea, heartburn, bloating, pain, etc.) in the past week? Place an X in the box that best describes the severity of your stomach problems on a scale of 0-10.

NO STOMACH PROBLEMS 0 ○ ☐ ☐ ☐ ○ ☐ ☐ ☐ ○ ☐ ☐ ☐ ○ ☐ ☐ ☐ ○ ☐ ☐ ☐ ○ 10 SEVERE STOMACH PROBLEMS

Considering ALL THE WAYS THAT YOUR ILLNESS AFFECTS YOU, RATE HOW YOU ARE DOING on the following scale. Place an X in the box below that best describes how you are doing on a scale of 0-10.

VERY WELL **0** ○ □ □ □ ○ □ □ □ ○ □ □ □ ○ □ □ □ ○ □ □ □ ○ **10** VERY POORLY

These questions are about how you feel and how things have been with you during the past month. For each question, please give the one answer that comes closest to the way you have been feeling. How much of the time during the 4 weeks:	All of the time	Most of the time	A good bit of the time	Some of the time	A little of the time	None of the time
Have you been a very nervous person?	□	□	□	□	□	□
Have you felt so down in the dumps that nothing could cheer you up?	□	□	□	□	□	□
Have you felt calm and peaceful?	□	□	□	□	□	□
Have you felt downhearted and blue?	□	□	□	□	□	□
Have you been a happy person?	□	□	□	□	□	□

We are interested in knowing about any problems that you may have been having with fatigue. How much of a problem has fatigue or tiredness been for you IN THE PAST WEEK? Place an X in the box below that best describes the severity of your fatigue on a scale of 0-10.

FATIGUE IS NO PROBLEM **0** ○ □ □ □ ○ □ □ □ ○ □ □ □ ○ □ □ □ ○ □ □ □ ○ **10** FATIGUE IS A MAJOR PROBLEM

How satisfied are you with your HEALTH NOW?

□ Very satisfied □ Somewhat satisfied □ Neither satisfied nor dissatisfied □ Somewhat dissatisfied □ Very dissatisfied

FOR PHYSICIAN'S USE ONLY

ESR: ________ *mm/hr* **CRP:** ________ □ *mg/dl* □ *mg/L*

Number of joints: Swollen ________ **Tender** ________ **Which joint count used?** □ 28 □ 32-34 □ 68 □ Other ________

Date of first symptom: (i.e., date of onset)
If month is not known, just enter year. □□ / □□ / □□□□

Diagnoses: Please indicate all rheumatic disease diagnoses by checking the appropriate boxes below.

□ Rheumatoid Arthritis □ Fibromyalgia □ Osteoarthritis of the hands

□ Osteoarthritis of the knee □ Osteoarthritis of the hip

□ Other arthritis-type diagnosis (e.g., lupus, psoriatic arthritis, etc.) ________

Index

Note: Page numbers followed by *t* indicate tables; those followed by *f* indicate figures.

D

U

V

W

X

Y

Z